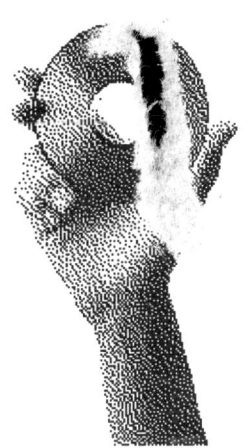

Customer Support Information

Plunkett's Health Care Industry Almanac 2005

Please register your book immediately...

if you did not purchase it directly from Plunkett Research, Ltd. This will enable us to fulfill your replacement request if you have a damaged product, or your requests for assistance. Also it will enable us to notify you of future editions, so that you may purchase them from the source of your choice.

If you are an actual, original purchaser but did not receive a FREE CD-ROM version with your book...*

you may request it by returning this form.

____ YES, please register me as a purchaser of the book.
I did not buy it directly from Plunkett Research, Ltd.

____ YES, please send me a free CD-ROM version of the book.
I am an actual purchaser, but I did not receive one with my book. (Proof of purchase may be required.)

Customer Name _____

Title _____

Organization _____

Address _____

City_____State_____Zip_____

Country (if other than USA) _____

Phone_____Fax _____

E-mail _____

Mail or Fax to: Plunkett Research, Ltd.
Attn: FREE CD-ROM and/or Registration
P.O. Drawer 541737, Houston, TX 77254-1737 USA
713.932.0000 · Fax 713.932.7080 · www.plunkettresearch.com

* Purchasers of used books are not eligible to register. Use of CD-ROMs is subject to the terms of their end user license agreements.

PLUNKETT'S HEALTH CARE INDUSTRY ALMANAC 2005

The Only Comprehensive
Guide to the Health Care Industry

Jack W. Plunkett

Published by:
Plunkett Research, Ltd., Houston, Texas
www.plunkettresearch.com

INSTALLATION
KEY CODE: 11064

SOUTH UNIVERSITY LIBRARY

PLUNKETT'S HEALTH CARE INDUSTRY ALMANAC 2005

Editor and Publisher:
Jack W. Plunkett

Executive Editor and Database Manager:
Martha Burgher Plunkett

Senior Editors and Researchers:
Tish Bastian
Elisa Gabbert
Ryan Muir
McAllister Yeomans

Editors, Researchers and Assistants:
Jessica Frey
Christie Manck
Benjamin Reike
Russell Simon
Emily Skaftun
Suzanne Zarosky
Tatiana Lindsay Zecher

Director of Corporate Accounts
Austin N. Goings

Information Technology Director:
Alex Preskovsky

E-Commerce Managers:
Jason Carmichael
Ian Markham
Sara Solbach

Cover Design:
Kim Paxson, Just Graphics
Junction, TX

Special Thanks to:
U.S. Department of Commerce,
*International Trade Administration
National Technical Information Service*
U.S. Department of Health
and Human Services
*National Institutes of Health,
Centers for Disease Control,
National Center for Health Statistics,
Centers for Medicare and Medicaid Services*

Plunkett Research, Ltd.
P. O. Drawer 541737, Houston, Texas 77254 USA
Phone: 713.932.0000   Fax: 713.932.7080
www.plunkettresearch.com

INSTALLATION
KEY CODE: 11064

Copyright © 2004 by Plunkett Research, Ltd.   3 1257 01645 5981

All rights reserved. No part of this book may be reproduced or transmitted in any form by any means, electronic or mechanical, including by photocopying or by any information storage or retrieval system, without the written permission of the publisher.

Published by:
Plunkett Research, Ltd.
P. O. Drawer 541737
Houston, Texas 77254-1737

Phone: 713.932.0000
Fax: 713.932.7080
Internet: www.plunkettresearch.com

ISBN # 1-59392-018-0

**Disclaimer of liability
for use and results of use:**

The editors and publishers assume no responsibility for your own success in making an investment or business decision, in seeking or keeping any job, in succeeding at any firm or in obtaining any amount or type of benefits or wages. Your own results and the job stability or financial stability of any company depend on influences outside of our control. All risks are assumed by the reader. Investigate any potential employer or business relationship carefully and carefully verify past and present finances, present business conditions and the level of compensation and benefits currently paid. Each company's details are taken from sources deemed reliable; however, their accuracy is not guaranteed. The editors and publishers assume no liability, beyond the actual payment received from a reader, for any direct, indirect, incidental or consequential, special or exemplary damages, and they do not guarantee, warrant nor make any representation regarding the use of this material. Trademarks or tradenames are used without symbols and only in a descriptive sense, and this use is not authorized by, associated with or sponsored by the trademarks' owners. Ranks and ratings are presented as an introductory and general glance at corporations, based on our research and our knowledge of businesses and the industries in which they operate. The reader should use caution.

PLUNKETT'S HEALTH CARE INDUSTRY ALMANAC 2005

CONTENTS

A Short Health Care Industry Glossary	i
Introduction	1
How to Use This Book	3
Chapter 1: Major Trends Affecting the Health Care Industry	7
1) Introduction to the Health Care Industry	8
2) Continued Rise in Health Care Costs	9
3) Employers Push Health Care Costs onto Employees	10
4) Medicare Changes Include Drug Benefits for Seniors for the First Time	10
5) Health Savings Accounts and Health Reimbursement Accounts Gain Traction	10
6) Vast Number of Uninsured and Underinsured Americans	12
7) Pharmaceutical Manufacturers Face Challenges, Massive Costs in New Drug Development	12
8) Cost of Pharmaceuticals Soars in U.S., Controvery over Drug Prices Rages On	13
9) Boom in Surgery Centers	14
10) Managed Care Becomes More Patient-Friendly	15
11) Growing Use of Managed Care by Medicare	16
12) Giant Mergers at Managed Care Providers	16
13) Critical Lack of Qualified Nurses	17
14) Malpractice Suits are Blamed for Rising Health Care Costs	17
15) Patients' Rights Evolve	18
16) Health Care Technology Introduction	19
17) Information Technology and Health Care	19
18) Stem Cells and Tissue Engineering	25
19) Personalized Medicine, New Drugs and New Drug Delivery Methods	29
20) Advances in Cancer Research	31
21) Advances in Diagnostic Imaging and Monitoring	32
22) Advances in Laboratory Testing	34
23) Advances in Surgery	36
24) Other Treatment Technologies	38
Chapter 2: Health Care Industry Statistics	43
I. U.S. Health Care Industry Overview	45
II. U.S. Health Care Expenditures & Costs	47
The Nation's Health Dollar 2004 - Where it Came From	48
The Nation's Health Dollar 2004 - Where It Went	49
National Health Expenditures and Average Annual Percent Change: 1980-2013	50
National Health Expenditures and Selected Economic Indicators: 1980-2013	51
National Health Expenditures, by Type of Expenditure: 1980-2013	52
Hospital Care Expenditures and Average Annual Percent Change, U.S.: 1980-2013	53
Hospital Care Expenditures, Percent Distribution and Per Capita Amount, U.S.: 1980-2013	54
U.S. Hospital Expenses: 1980-2003	55
Home Health Care Expenditures and Average Annual Percent Change, U.S.: 1980-2013	56
Home Health Care Expenditures, Percent Distribution and Per Capita Amount, U.S.: 1980-2013	57

Continued on next page

Continued from previous page

Nursing Home Care Expenditures and Average Annual Percent Change, U.S.: 1980-2013	58
Nursing Home Care Expenditures, Percent Distribution and Per Capita Amount, U.S.: 1980-2013	59
Prescription Drug Expenditures and Average Annual Percent Change, U.S.: 1980-2013	60
Prescription Drug Expenditures, Percent Distribution and Per Capita Amount, U.S.: 1980-2012	61
Index Levels of Medical Prices	62
Hospitals, Beds and Occupancy Rates, U.S.: Selected Years 1997-2003	63
U.S. Community Hospital Statistics: 2000-2003	64
III. Medicare & Medicaid	65
Medicare and Medicaid Spending: 2002-2005	66
Where the Medicare Dollar Went, 2004	67
Number of Medicare Beneficiaries, 1970-2030	68
Medicare Enrollment Trends, Hospital and/or Supplemental Medical Insurance: July 1970-2003	69
Medicare Enrollment Trends, Hospital Insurance: July 1970-2003	70
Medicare Enrollment Trends, Supplemental Medical Insurance: July 1970-2003	71
Medicare Deductible, Co-insurance and Premium Amounts, 2005	72
IV. U.S. Health Insurance Coverage & the Uninsured	73
People Without Health Insurance for the Entire Year, U.S.: 2001, 2002 and 2003	74
Number and Percent of Persons Without Health Insurance Coverage, by Age Group, U.S.: 1997-2004	75
Percent of Persons of All Ages Without Health Insurance Coverage, by Race/Ethnicity, U.S., 2004	76
Percent of Persons of All Ages Without Health Insurance Coverage, U.S.: 1997-2004	77
Percent of Persons Under Age 65 With Public and Private Coverage, U.S.: 1997-2004	78
Percent of Persons Under Age 65 Years Without Health Insurance Coverage, by Age Group and Sex, U.S., 2003	79
Employers' Costs for Health Insurance, U.S.: Selected Years 1991-2003	80
V. U.S. Vital Statistics & Population Indicators	81
Percent of Population in Three Age Groups, U.S.: 1950, 2000 and 2050	82
Life Expectancy at Birth, U.S.	83
Life Expectancy at Age 65, U.S.	84
Infant Mortality Rates, U.S.: Selected Years 1985-2004	85
Percentage of Children 19-35 Months Vaccinated for Select Diseases, U.S.: 2000-2003	86
AIDS Statistics: 1998-2003	87
Percentage of Binge Alcohol Use Among Students in Grades 8, 10 and 12, U.S.: 1980-2003	88
Cigarette Smoking Among Students in Grades 8, 10 and 12, U.S.: 1980-2003	89
Employment, Hours, and Earnings in Private Health Service Establishments, U.S.: 1999-2004	90
Chapter 3: Important Health Care Industry Contacts	91
(Addresses, Phone Numbers and World Wide Web Sites)	
Chapter 4: THE HEALTH CARE 500:	
Who They Are and How They Were Chosen	141
Industry List, With Codes	142
Index of Rankings Within Industry Groups	144
Alphabetical Index	157
Index of Headquarters Location by U.S. State	161
Index of Non-U.S. Headquarters Location by Country	166
Index by Regions of the U.S. Where THE HEALTH CARE 500 Have Locations	167
Index by Firms with Operations Outside the U.S.	176
Individual Data Profiles on Each of THE HEALTH CARE 500	179
Additional Indexes	
Index of Hot Spots for Advancement for Women/Minorities	696
Index by Subsidiaries, Brand Names and Selected Affiliations	697

A Short Health Care Industry Glossary

510 K: An application filed with the FDA for a new medical device to show that the apparatus is "substantially equivalent" to one that is already marketed.

Accountable Health Plan: A network of health care providers, such as hospitals and primary and specialty care physicians, that provides care and services and competes with other systems in the region for enrollees.

ADME (Absorption, Distribution, Metabolism and Excretion): In clinical trials, the bodily processes studied to determine the extent and duration of systemic exposure to a drug.

AE (Adverse Event): In clinical trials, a condition not observed at baseline or worsened if present at baseline. Sometimes called Treatment Emergent Signs and Symptoms (TESS).

Alternate Site Care: Health care that was previously provided in general hospitals, but is now offered in less costly, alternate sites. Examples of alternate care include home IV therapy, outpatient surgery centers, rehabilitation units within nursing homes and free-standing centers providing dialysis, radiation therapy and imaging.

Amino Acid: Any of a class of 20 molecules that combine to form proteins.

ANDA (Abbreviated New Drug Application): An application filed with the FDA showing that a substance is the same as an existing, previously approved drug (i.e., a generic version).

Angiogenesis: Blood vessel formation, typically in the growth of malignant tissue.

Angioplasty: The re-opening of a blood vessel by non-surgical techniques such as balloon dilation or laser, or through surgery.

Antibody: A protein produced by white blood cells in response to a foreign substance (see "Antigen"). Each antibody can bind only to one specific antigen.

Antigen: A foreign substance that causes the immune system to create an antibody (see "Antibody").

Apoptosis: A normal cellular process leading to the termination of a cell's life.

Applied Research: The application of compounds, processes, materials or other items discovered during "basic research" to practical uses. The goal is to move discoveries along to the final development phase.

Arthroscopy: The examination of the interior of a joint using a type of endoscope that is inserted into the joint through a small incision. (See: Endoscope)

Assay: A laboratory test to identify and/or measure the amount of a particular substance in a sample. Types of assays include endpoint assays, in which a single measurement is made at a fixed time; kinetic assays, in which increasing amounts of a product are formed with time and are monitored at multiple points; microbiological assays, which measure the concentration of antimicrobials in biological material; and immunological assays, in which analysis or measurement is based on antigen-antibody reactions.

Baseline: A set of data used in clinical studies for control or comparison.

Basic Research: Attempts to discover compounds, materials, processes or other items that may be largely or entirely new and/or unique. Basic research may start with a theoretical concept that has yet to be proven. The goal is to create discoveries that can be moved along to "applied research." Basic research is sometimes referred to as "blue sky" research.

Behavioral Health: The assessment and treatment of mental health and/or substance abuse disorders. Substance abuse includes alcohol and other drugs.

Bioavailability: In pharmaceuticals, the rate and extent to which a drug is absorbed or is otherwise available to the treatment site in the body.

Bioequivalence: In pharmaceuticals, the demonstration that a drug's rate and extent of absorption are not significantly different from those of an existing drug that is already approved by the FDA.

Bioinformatics: Research, development or application of computational tools and approaches for expanding the use of biological, medical, behavioral or health data, including those to acquire, store, organize, archive, analyze or visualize such data. Bioinformatics applies principles of information sciences and technologies to make vast, diverse and complex life sciences data more understandable and useful.

Biologic: Any virus, therapeutic serum, toxin, antitoxin, vaccine, blood, blood component or derivative, allergenic or analogous product, or arsphenamine or one of its derivatives (or any other trivalent organic arsenic compound) applicable to the prevention, treatment or cure of disease or injury.

Biotechnology: A set of powerful tools that employ living organisms (or parts of organisms) to make or modify products, improve plants or animals (including humans) or develop microorganisms for specific uses. Early uses of biotechnology included traditional animal and plant breeding techniques, based on improving genetic lineage in order to create a plant or animal with desirable characteristics. Early uses also included the use of yeast in making bread, beer, wine and cheese. Today, biotechnology is most commonly thought of to include the development of human medical therapies and processes using recombinant DNA, cell fusion, other genetic techniques and bioremediation. Modern biotechnology uses advanced technologies to modify the genes of cells so they will produce new substances or perform new functions. A good example is recombinant DNA technology, in which a copy of DNA containing one or more genes is transferred between organisms or recombined within an organism.

Boutique Medicine: A medical practice in which patients receive unlimited access to physicians for an annual retainer fee. Services include same-day or next-day appointments, unrestricted examination times and after-hours access to physicians via pagers or cell phone numbers.

Branding: A marketing strategy that takes a well-known brand and utilizes brand capital in order to increase the brand's market share, sales and availability, establish credibility, improve satisfaction, raise the profile of the firm and increase profits.

B-to-B, or B2B: See "Business-to-Business" below.

B-to-C, or B2C: See "Business-to-Consumer" below.

B-to-E, or B2E: See "Business-to-Employee" below.

B-to-G, or B2G: See "Business-to-Government" below.

Business-to-Business: An organization focused on selling products, services or data to commercial customers rather than individual consumers.

Business-to-Consumer: An organization focused on selling products, services or data to individual consumers rather than commercial customers.

Business-to-Employee: A corporate communications system, such as an intranet, aimed at conveying information from a company to its employees.

Business-to-Government: An organization focused on selling products, services or data to government units rather than commercial businesses or consumers.

CANDA (Computer-Assisted New Drug Application): An electronic submission of a new drug application (NDA) to the FDA.

Capitation: A fee method in which care providers offer a standard, or capped, per-member fee for services to participants in a particular HMO.

CAPLA (Computer-Assisted Product License Application): An electronic submission of a biological product license application (PLA) to the FDA.

Carcinogen: A substance capable of causing cancer. A suspected carcinogen is a substance that may cause cancer in humans or animals but for which the evidence is not conclusive.

Cardiac Catheterization Laboratory: Facilities offering special diagnostic procedures for cardiac patients, including the introduction of a catheter into the interior of the heart by way of a vein or artery or by direct needle puncture. Procedures must be performed in a laboratory or a special procedure room.

Cardiac Intensive Care Services: Services provided in a unit staffed with specially trained nursing personnel and containing monitoring and specialized support or treatment equipment for patients who (because of heart seizure, open-heart surgery or other life-threatening conditions) require intensified, comprehensive observation and care. May include myocardial infarction care, pulmonary care, and heart transplant units.

Catheter: A tubular instrument used to add or withdraw fluids. Heart or cardiac catheterization involves the passage of flexible catheters into the great vessels and chambers of the heart. IV catheters add intravenous fluids to the veins. Foley catheters withdraw fluid from the bladder. Significant recent advances in technology allow administration of powerful drug and diagnostic therapies via catheters.

CBER (Center for Biologics Evaluation and Research): The branch of the FDA responsible for the regulation of biological products, including blood, vaccines, therapeutics and related drugs and devices, to ensure purity, potency, safety, availability and effectiveness. www.fda.gov/cber

CDER (Center for Drug Evaluation and Research): The branch of the FDA responsible for the regulation of drug products. www.fda.gov/cder

CDRH (Center for Devices and Radiological Health): The branch of the FDA responsible for the regulation of medical devices. www.fda.gov/cdrh

Centers for Medicare and Medicaid Services (CMS): The federal agency responsible for administering Medicare and monitoring the states' operations of Medicaid.

CFR (Code of Federal Regulations): The CFR is a codification of the general and permanent rules published in the Federal Register by the executive departments and agencies of the Federal Government. The code is divided into 50 titles that represent broad areas subject to federal regulation. Title 21 of the CFR covers FDA regulations.

Chemotherapy: The treatment of cancer using anticancer drugs, often conducted in association with radiation therapy. (See "Radiation Therapy.")

Chromosome: A structure in the nucleus of a cell that contains genes. Chromosomes are found in pairs.

Class I Device: An FDA classification of medical devices for which general controls are sufficient to ensure safety and efficacy.

Class II Device: An FDA classification of medical devices for which performance standards and special controls are sufficient to ensure safety and efficacy.

Class III Device: An FDA classification of medical devices for which pre-market approval is required to ensure safety and efficacy, unless the device is substantially equivalent to a currently marketed device. (See "510 K.")

Clone: A group of identical genes, cells or organisms derived from one ancestor, an identical copy. "Dolly" the sheep is a famous case of a clone of an animal. Also see "Cloning (Reproductive)" and "Cloning (Therapeutic)."

Cloning (Reproductive): A method of reproducing an exact copy of an animal or, potentially, an exact copy of a human being. A scientist removes the nucleus from a donor's unfertilized egg, inserts a nucleus from the animal to be copied and then stimulates the nucleus to begin dividing to form an embryo. In the case of a mammal, such as a human, the embryo would then be implanted in the uterus of a host female. Also see "Cloning (Therapeutic)."

Cloning (Therapeutic): A method of reproducing exact copies of cells needed for research or for the development of replacement tissue or organs. A scientist removes the nucleus from a donor's unfertilized egg, inserts a nucleus from the animal whose cells are to be copied and then stimulates the nucleus to begin dividing to form an embryo. However, the embryo is never allowed to grow to any significant stage of development. Instead, it is allowed to grow for a few hours or days, and stem cells are then removed from it for use in regenerating tissue. Also see "Cloning (Reproductive)."

COBRA (Consolidated Omnibus Budget Reconciliation Act): A federal law that requires employers to offer uninterrupted health care coverage to certain employees and their beneficiaries whose group coverage has been terminated.

Concierge Care: See "Boutique Medicine."

Continuing Care Retirement Communities (CCRCs): CCRCs provide coordinated housing and health-related services to older individuals under an agreement which may last as little as one year or as long as the life of the individual.

Coordinator: In clinical trials, the person at an investigative site who handles the administrative responsibilities of the trial, acts as a liaison between the investigative site and the sponsor, and reviews data and records during a monitoring visit.

COSTART: In medical and drug product development, a dictionary of adverse events and body systems used for coding and classifying adverse events.

CPMP (Committee on Proprietary Medicinal Products): A committee, composed of two people from each EU Member State (see "EU" below), that is responsible for the scientific evaluation and assessment of marketing applications for medicinal products in the EU. The CPMP is the major body involved in the harmonization of pharmaceutical regulations within the EU and receives administrative support from the European Medicines Evaluation Agency. (See "EMEA" below.)

CRA (Clinical Research Associate): An individual responsible for monitoring clinical trial data to ensure compliance with study protocol and FDA GCP regulations.

CRF (Case Report Form): In clinical trials, a standard document used by clinicians to record and report subject data pertinent to the study protocol.

CRM (Customer Relationship Management): The automation of integrated business processes involving customers, including sales (contact management, product configuration), marketing (campaign management, telemarketing) and customer service (call center, field service).

CRO (Contract Research Organization): An independent organization that contracts with a sponsor of a clinical investigation to conduct part of the work on a clinical study. Drug makers and medical device makers frequently outsource work to CROs.

CRT (Case Report Tabulation): In clinical trials, a tabular listing of all data collected on study case report forms.

CT Scanner: A computed tomographic scanner used for head or whole body scans.

Current Procedural Terminology (CPT): The most widely accepted medical nomenclature used to report medical procedures and services under public and private health insurance programs. CPT is also used for administrative management purposes, such as claims processing and developing guidelines for medical care review.

CVMP (Committee for Veterinary Medicinal Products): A committee that is a veterinary equivalent of the CPMP (see "CPMP" above) in the EU (see "EU" below).

d.b.a: Doing Business As.

Defibrillator: In medicine, an instrument used externally (as electrodes on the chest) or implanted (as a small device similar in size to a pacemaker) that delivers an electric shock to return the heart to its normal rhythm.

Demographics: The breakdown of the population into statistical categories such as age, income, education and sex.

Development: The phase of research and development in which researchers attempt to create new products from the results of discoveries and applications created during basic and applied research.

Device: In medical product development, according to the FDA, an instrument, apparatus, implement, machine, contrivance, implant, in vitro reagent or other similar or related article, including any component, part or accessory, that 1) is recognized in the official National Formulary or United States Pharmacopoeia or any supplement to them, 2) is intended for use in the diagnosis of disease or other conditions, or in the cure, mitigation, treatment or prevention of disease, in man or animals or 3) is intended to affect the structure of the body of man or animals and does not achieve any of its principal intended purposes through chemical action within or on the body of man or animals and is not dependent upon being metabolized for the achievement of any of its principal intended purposes.

Diagnostic Radioisotope Facility: A medical facility in which radioactive isotopes (radiopharmaceuticals) are used as tracers or indicators to detect an abnormal condition or disease in the body.

Dialysis: An artificial blood-filtering process used to clean the blood of patients with malfunctioning kidneys.

Dietary Supplements Sold as Food: Legal diet aids that do not require licensing under medical regulations. Typically, dietary supplements sold as food are offered in powder, tablet, pill or capsule form.

Distributor: Distributors do not manufacture but may be involved in sales, marketing, warehousing or shipping of drugs and/or medical devices. In medicine, distributors are subject to medical device incident reporting, record keeping, tracking and registration and certification requirements under the Safe Medical Devices Act.

DMB (Data Monitoring Board): A committee that monitors the progress of a clinical trial and carefully observes the safety data.

DNA (Deoxyribonucleic Acid): The carrier of the genetic information that cells need to replicate and to produce proteins.

DNA Chip: The DNA microchip is a revolutionary tool used to identify mutations in genes like BRCA1 and BRCA2. The chip, which consists of a small glass plate encased in plastic, is manufactured using a process similar to the one used to make computer microchips. On the surface, each chip contains synthetic single-stranded DNA sequences identical to a normal gene.

Drug Utilization Review: A quantitative assessment of patient drug use and physicians' patterns of prescribing drugs in an effort to determine the usefulness of drug therapy.

DSMB (Data and Safety Monitoring Board): See "DMB."

EC (European Community): See "EU" below.

Ecology: The study of relationships between all living organisms and the environment, especially the totality or pattern of interactions; a view that includes all plant and animal species and their unique contributions to a particular habitat.

E-Commerce: The use of online, Internet-based sales methods. The phrase is used to describe both business-to-consumer and business-to-business sales.

EDI (Electronic Data Interchange): An accepted standard format for the exchange of data between various companies' networks. EDI allows for the transfer of e-mail as well as orders, invoices and other files from one company to another.

EFGCP (European Forum for Good Clinical Practices): The organization dedicated to finding common ground in Europe on the implementation of Good Clinical Practices. (See "GCP.") www.efgcp.org

ELA (Establishment License Application): An ELA is required for the approval of a biologic (see "Biologic"). It permits a specific facility to manufacture a biological product for commercial purposes. (Compare to "PLA.")

EMEA (European Medicines Evaluation Agency): The European agency responsible for supervising and coordinating applications for marketing medicinal products in the European Union (see "EU" and "CPMP"). The EMEA is headquartered in the U.K. www.eudraportal.eudra.org

Employee Assistance Program (EAP): A program designed to help employees, employers and family members find solutions to workplace and personal problems.

Endoscope: A tiny, flexible tube-shaped instrument with a fiber optic light and a video camera lens at the end. It is inserted into the body through a natural body opening or a small incision, and has both diagnostic and therapeutic capabilities. Laparascopic surgery is conducted in a minimally invasive manner using the endoscope to enable the surgeon to see the tissue being operated on. Such surgery is often conducted through an incision as small as one or two centimeters in length. Consequently, patients tend to heal very quickly after such surgery.

Endpoint: A clinical or laboratory measurement used to assess safety, efficacy or other trial objectives of a test article in a clinical trial.

Enzyme: A protein that acts as a catalyst, affecting the chemical reactions in cells.

ESWL (Extracorporeal Shock Wave Lithotripter): A medical device used for treating stones in the kidney or urethra. The device disintegrates kidney stones noninvasively through the transmission of acoustic shock waves directed at the stones.

Etiology: The study of the causes or origins of diseases.

EU (European Union): Previously known as the European Community (EC), the EU is a consolidation of European countries (member states) functioning as one body to facilitate trade. The EU expanded to include much of Eastern Europe in 2004, raising the total number of member states to 25. In 2002, the EU launched a unified currency, the Euro, currently in use in 12 of the member nations. europa.eu.int

EU Competence: The jurisdiction in which the EU can taken legal action.

Exclusive Provider Organization: Technically the same as an HMO, with the exception that the organization provides coverage only for services from contracted providers. See "Health Maintenance Organization (HMO)."

Extracorporeal Shock Wave Lithotripter (ESWL): A medical device used for treating stones in the kidney or urethra. The device disintegrates kidney stones noninvasively through the transmission of acoustic shock waves directed at the stones.

FD&C Act (Food, Drug and Cosmetic Act): The federal body of law that governs the manufacture, sale and distribution of food, drugs and cosmetics.

FDA (Food and Drug Administration): The U.S. government agency responsible for the enforcement of the FD&C Act (see above), ensuring industry compliance with laws regulating products in commerce. The FDA's mission is to protect the public from harm and encourage technological advances that hold the promise of benefiting society. www.fda.gov

Fee-For-Service Equivalency: The amount of reimbursement from capitation compared to fee-for-service reimbursement.

Fee-For-Service Reimbursement: The old system of payment under which payments to providers do not exceed the billed charge for each unit of service provided.

FFDCA (Federal Food, Drug and Cosmetic Act): The law which controls, among other things, residues in food and feed.

GCP (Good Clinical Practices): FDA regulations and guidelines that define the responsibilities of the key figures involved in a clinical trial, including the sponsor, the investigator, the monitor and the Institutional Review Board. (See "IRB.")

Gene: A working subunit of DNA; the carrier of inheritable traits.

Gene Chips: See "DNA Chip."

Gene Therapy: Treatment based on the alteration of existing genes.

Genetic Code: The sequence of nucleotides, determining the sequence of amino acids in protein synthesis.

Genetically Modified (GM): Bioengineered food that is designed to resist herbicides and pests, has higher nutritional value than non-engineered food and/or lasts longer on the shelf. An example of GM food is a soybean that has been specially modified to be impervious to the application of a specific pesticide.

Genetics: The study of the process of heredity.

Genome: The genetic material (composed of DNA) in the chromosomes of a living organism.

Genomics: The study of genes, their role in diseases and our ability to manipulate them.

Globalization: The increased mobility of goods, services, labor, technology and capital throughout the world. Although globalization is not a new development, its pace has increased with the advent of new technologies, especially in the areas of telecommunications, finance and shipping.

GLP (Good Laboratory Practices): A collection of regulations and guidelines to be used in laboratories where research is conducted on drugs, biologics or devices that are intended for submission to the FDA.

GMP (Good Manufacturing Practices): A collection of regulations and guidelines to be used in manufacturing drugs, biologics and medical devices.

Group Practice Without Walls: A "quasi" group formed when a hospital sponsors or provides capital to physicians for the establishment of a practice to share administrative expenses while remaining independent practitioners.

Health Indemnity Insurance: Provides traditional insurance coverage, after a deductible, for specified health care needs. Typically, the patient can go to any physician or any hospital, and there is no aspect of managed care involved.

Health Maintenance Organization (HMO): HMOs provide managed health care services. An HMO functions as a form of health care insurance which is sold on a group basis. The HMO contracts with doctors, hospitals, labs and other medical facilities for low rates in exchange for high volume. For the patient, only visits to professionals within the HMO network are covered in the highest possible amount by the HMO. The patient selects a primary care physician who is approved by the HMO. For care, the patient first visits the primary care physician who may refer the patient to a specialist on an as-needed basis. (Also see "Managed Care," "POS" and "PPO.")

Health Reimbursement Account (HRA): A Health Reimbursement Account (HRA) is a form of health care coverage plan provided to employees by their employer. It is quite different from Health Savings Accounts. Under an HRA, the employer places a given amount of money into a special account each year for the employee to spend on health care. The employer also provides a high-deductible health coverage plan. The employee elects when and how to spend the money in the account on health care. Because of the high deductible, the employee's share of the monthly premium tends to be much lower than under an HMO or PPO, but the employee faces the burden of paying the high deductible when necessary. Unspent funds in the account can roll over from year to year so that the account grows, but the employee loses the fund balance when leaving the employer.

Health Savings Account (HSA): A Health Savings Account (HSA) is a plan that combines a tax-free savings and investment account (somewhat similar to a 401k) with a high-deductible health coverage plan. The intent is to give the consumer more incentive to control health care costs by reducing unnecessary care while shopping for the best prices. The consumer contributes pre-tax dollars annually to a savings account--up to $2,600 for an individual or $5,150 for a family. The employer may or may not match part of that contribution. The account may be invested in stocks, bonds or mutual funds. It grows tax-free, but the money may be spent only on health care. Unspent money stays in the account at the end of each year. The consumer must purchase an insurance policy or health care plan with an annual deductible of at least $1,000 for individuals or $2,000 for families.

HIPAA: The Health Insurance Portability and Accountability Act of 1996, which demands that by 2003, all billing and patient data must be exchanged electronically between care givers and insurance payors.

Home Care Agencies: Home health agencies, home care aid organizations and hospices.

Hospital Insurance (HI) – Medicare: HI is the Medicare program that pays for inpatient hospital care, skilled nursing facility care, home health care and hospice care. Payments under the HI program are made from a trust fund, which is financed primarily by payroll taxes. Employees and employers each pay a payroll tax.

ICD9: International Classification of Diseases - Version 9. A government coding system used for classifying diseases and diagnoses.

IDE (Investigational New Device Exemption): An IDE must be filed with the FDA prior to initiating clinical trials of medical devices considered to pose a significant risk to human subjects.

Imaging: In medicine, the viewing of the body's organs through external, high-tech means. This reduces the need for broad exploratory surgery. These advances, along with new types of surgical instruments, have made minimally invasive surgery possible. Imaging includes MRI (magnetic resonance imaging), CT (computed tomography or "CAT scan"), MEG (magnetoencephalography), improved x-ray technology, mammography, ultrasound and angiography.

Immunoassay: An immunological assay. Types include agglutination, complement-fixation, precipitation, immunodiffusion and electrophoretic assays. Each type of assay utilizes either a particular type of antibody or a specific support medium (such as a gel) to determine the amount of antigen present.

In Vitro: Laboratory experiments conducted in the test tube, or otherwise, without using live animals and/or humans.

In Vivo: Laboratory experiments conducted with live animals and/or humans.

IND (Investigational New Drug Exemption): An IND must be filed with the FDA prior to initiating clinical trials of drugs or biologics.

Independent Practice Association (IPA): An IPA is a legal entity that holds managed care contracts. The IPA then contracts with physicians, usually in solo practice, to provide care either on a fee-for-services or capitated basis. The purpose of an IPA is to assist solo physicians in obtaining managed care contracts.

Informed Consent: Must be obtained in writing from people who agree to be clinical trial subjects prior to their enrollment in the study. The document must explain the risks associated with the study and treatment and describe alternative therapy available to the patient. A copy of the document must also be provided to the patient.

Infusion Therapy: The introduction of fluid other than blood into a vein. (See: Intravenous Therapy)

Intravenous Therapy: The introduction of fluid other than blood into a vein. (See: Infusion Therapy)

Investigator: In clinical trials, a clinician who agrees to supervise the use of an investigational drug, device or biologic in humans. Responsibilities of the investigator, as defined in FDA regulations, include administering the drug, observing and testing the patient, collecting data and monitoring the care and welfare of the patient.

Iontophoresis: The transfer of ions of medicine through the skin using a local electric current.

IRB (Institutional Review Board): This group of individuals is found in most medical institutions. The main function of the IRB is to review protocols for ethical consideration (to ensure the rights of the patients). Secondly, the IRB evaluates the benefit-to-risk ratio of a new drug to see that the risk is acceptable for patient exposure. Responsibilities of the IRB are defined in FDA regulations.

ISO 9000, 9001, 9002: Standards set by the International Organization for Standardization for quality procedures. ISO 9000, 9001 and 9002 are the quality certifications for manufacturing.

Just-in-Time (JIT) Delivery: Refers to a supply chain practice whereby manufacturers receive components on or just before the time that they are needed on the assembly line, rather than bearing the cost of maintaining several days' or weeks' supply in a warehouse. This adds greatly to the cost-effectiveness of a manufacturing plant and puts the burden of warehousing and timely delivery on the supplier of the components.

Laparoscope: See "Endoscope."

Laparoscopic Surgery: See "Endoscope."

Ligand: Any atom or molecule attached to a central atom in a complex compound.

Lithotripsy: See "Extracorporeal Shock Wave Lithotripter."

Low-Calorie: Refers to servings with 40 or fewer calories.

Low-Cholesterol: Refers to servings with 20 or fewer milligrams of cholesterol and two or fewer grams of saturated fat.

Low-Fat: Refers to servings with three or fewer grams of fat.

Low-Sodium: Refers to servings with 140 or fewer milligrams of sodium.

Magnetic Resonance Imaging (MRI): The use of a uniform magnetic field and radio frequencies to study tissues and structures of the body. This procedure enables the visualization of biochemical activity of the cell in vivo without the use of ionizing radiation, radioisotopic substances or high-frequency sound.

Managed Care: A system of prepaid medical plans providing comprehensive coverage to voluntarily enrolled members. Managed health care typically covers professional fees, hospital services, diagnostic services, emergency services, limited mental services, medical treatment for drug or alcohol abuse, home health services and preventive health care. The most common systems in managed care are HMOs (Health Maintenance Organizations) and PPOs (Preferred Provider Organizations), but there are other variations on these models. The word "managed" is used to describe this type of coverage because the total cost and extent of a patient's care is carefully managed and controlled by the group's administrators. Part of this management includes limiting the patient's choice to physicians, hospitals and labs that have agreed to provide reduced fees in exchange for high volume. Patients who receive care outside of this network will receive lesser reimbursement from the managed care provider. Also see "HMO," "PPO," and "Utilization Management."

Management Services Organization (MSO): A corporation, owned by a hospital or a physician/hospital joint venture, that provides management services to one or more medical group practices. The MSO purchases the tangible assets of the practices and leases them back as part of a full-service management agreement, under which the MSO employs all non-physician staff and provides all supplies and administrative systems for a fee.

Marketing: Includes all activities and expenses associated with the promotion of an item, such as selling and advertising costs, market research, public relations, royalties or commissions and souvenirs.

Medicaid: A federally supported and state-administered assistance program providing medical care for certain low-income individuals and families.

Medical Device: See "Device."

Medical Savings Account (MSA): See "Health Savings Account."

Medicare: A U.S. government program that pays hospitals, physicians and other medical providers for serving patients aged 65 years and older, certain disabled people and most people with end-stage renal disease (ESRD). Medicare enrolls approximately 39 million people, including 3.5 million disabled. An estimated 97% of Medicare enrollees are elderly. Medicare consists of two basic programs: Part A, or Hospital Insurance (HI) and Part B, or Supplementary Medical Insurance (SMI).

Minimally Invasive Surgery: The use of very small incisions and advanced instruments that may be viewed through microscopes or video. Includes laparoscopy, endoscopy, electrosurgery and cryosurgery. This practice promotes rapid healing.

Minimally-Invasive Surgery: See "Endoscope."

Nanotechnology: The science of designing, building or utilizing unique structures that are smaller than 100 nanometers (one billionth of a meter). This involves microscopic structures that are no larger than the width of some cell membranes.

NDA (New Drug Application): An application requesting FDA approval, after completion of Phase III studies, to market a new drug for human use in interstate commerce. Clinical trial results generally account for approximately 80% of the NDA.

Neonatal Intensive Care Services (NICU): A unit that must be separate from the newborn nursery. It provides intensive care to all sick infants, including those with very low birth weights (less than 1500 grams). The NICU can provide mechanical ventilation, neonatal surgery and special care for the sickest infants.

NIH (National Institutes of Health): A branch of the U.S. Public Health Service that conducts experimental research. www.nih.gov

Nonclinical Studies: In vitro (laboratory) or in vivo (animal) pharmacology, toxicology and pharmacokinetic studies that support the testing of a product in humans. Usually at least two species are evaluated prior to Phase I clinical trials. Nonclinical studies continue throughout all phases of research to evaluate long-term safety issues.

Nutraceutical: Nutrient + pharmaceutical – a food or part of a food that has been isolated and sold in a medicinal form and claims to offer benefits such as the treatment or prevention of disease.

ODM (Original Design Manufacturer): A contract manufacturer that offers complete, end-to-end design, engineering and manufacturing services. ODMs can design and build products, such as consumer electronics, that client companies can then brand and sell as their own.

Offshoring: The rapidly growing tendency among U.S. and Western European firms to send knowledge-based and manufacturing work overseas. The intent is to take advantage of lower wages and operating costs in such nations as India, Hungary and Russia.

Oncology: The diagnosis, study and treatment of cancer.

Open Access: Typically found in an IPA HMO, this arrangement allows members to consult specialists without obtaining a referral from another doctor.

Orthodontics: A specialized branch of dentistry that restores the teeth to proper alignment and function. There are several different types of appliances used in orthodontics, braces being one of the most common.

OTC (Over-the-Counter): OTC drug products are FDA-regulated products that do not require a physician's prescription. Some examples are aspirin, sunscreen, nasal spray and sunglasses.

Paramedical: A person trained to assist medical professionals and supplement physicians and nurses in their activities in order to give emergency medical treatment.

Pathogen: Any microorganism (i.e., fungus, virus, bacteria or parasite) that causes a disease.

Peer Review: The process used by the scientific community, whereby review of a paper, project or report is obtained through comments of independent colleagues in the same field.

Pharmacodynamics: The study of reactions between drugs and living systems. It can be thought of as the study of what a drug does to the body.

Pharmacoeconomics: The study of the costs and benefits associated with various treatments.

Pharmacokinetics (PK): The study of the processes of bodily absorption, distribution, metabolism and excretion of compounds and medicines. It can be thought of as the study of what the body does to a drug. (See "ADME.")

Phase I Clinical Trials: Studies in this phase include initial introduction of an investigational drug into humans. These studies are closely monitored and are usually conducted in healthy volunteers. Phase I trials are conducted after the completion of extensive nonclinical or preclinical trials not involving humans. Phase I studies include the determination of clinical pharmacology, bioavailability, drug interactions and side effects associated with increasing doses of the drug.

Phase II Clinical Trials: Phase II studies include randomized, masked, controlled clinical studies conducted to evaluate the effectiveness of a drug for a particular indication(s). During Phase II trials, the minimum effective dose and dosing intervals should be determined.

Phase III Clinical Trials: These studies consist of controlled and uncontrolled trials that are performed after preliminary evidence of effectiveness of a drug has been established. They are conducted to document the safety and efficacy of the drug, as well as to determine adequate directions (labeling) for use by the physician. A specific patient population needs to be clearly identified from the results of these studies. Trials during Phase III are conducted in a large number of patients to determine the frequency of adverse events and to obtain data regarding intolerance.

Phase IV Clinical Trials: These studies are conducted after approval of a drug has been obtained to gather data supporting new or revised labeling, marketing or advertising claims.

Physician-Hospital Organization (PHO), Closed: A PHO that restricts physician membership to those practitioners who meet criteria for cost effectiveness and/or high quality.

Physician-Hospital Organization (PHO), Open: A joint venture between the hospital and all members of the medical staff who wish to participate. The PHO can act as a unified agent in managed care contracting, own a managed care plan, own and operate ambulatory care centers or ancillary services projects, or provide administrative services to physician members.

Pivotal Studies: In clinical trials, a Phase III trial that is designed specifically to support approval of a product. These studies are well-controlled (usually by placebo) and are generally designed with input from the FDA so that they will provide data that is adequate to support approval of the product. Two pivotal studies are required for drug product approval, but usually only one study is required for biologics.

PLA (Product License Agreement): Required for the approval of a biologic, a PLA permits a manufacturer to produce a biological product for commercial purposes. (Compare to "ELA.")

PMA (Pre-Market Approval): PMA is required for the approval of a new medical device or a device that is to be used for life-sustaining or life-supporting purposes, is implanted in the human body or presents potential risk of illness or injury.

Point of Service: An option provided by some HMOs that allows covered persons to go outside the plan's provider network for care, but requires they pay higher cost-sharing than they would for network providers.

Point-of-Service Plan (POS): A managed care plan in which member patients may go outside of the network to be attended by their preferred physicians, but pay a higher deductible if they so choose. Routine care is provided by a primary care physician who also provides referrals to in-network specialists.

Positron Emission Tomography (PET) Scanner: Nuclear medicine imaging technology that uses computers and radioactive (positron emitting) isotopes, which are created in a cyclotron or generator, to produce composite pictures of the brain and heart at work. PET scanning produces sectional images depicting metabolic activity or blood flow rather than anatomy.

Post-Marketing Surveillance: The FDA's ongoing safety monitoring of marketed drugs.

Preclinical Studies: See "Nonclinical Studies."

Preferred Provider Organization (PPO): PPOs provide "managed health care" services. A PPO is a modified version of the HMO model. Generally, patients who are members of PPOs have more flexibility in the personal choice of physicians than do members of HMOs. Patients pay higher premiums than HMOs because of this flexibility. Patients are encouraged to visit physicians who are part of the PPO's system, but may also receive very good reimbursement for visiting physicians who are "out-of-network." Also see "HMO" and "Managed Care."

Primary Care Network: A group of primary care physicians who pool their resources to share the financial risk of providing care to their patients who are covered by a particular health plan.

Psychiatry: A branch of medicine concerned with the study, treatment and prevention of mental, emotional and behavioral disorders. Psychiatrists are doctors and can treat patients using drugs and other physical methods.

Psychology: The scientific study of human behavior and mental processes. Psychologists treat patients using therapeutic methods, including counseling or group work.

QOL (Quality of Life): In medicine, an endpoint of therapeutic assessment used to adjust measures of effectiveness for clinical decision-making. Typically, QOL endpoints measure the improvement of a patient's day-to-day living as a result of specific therapy.

R&D: Research and development.

Radiation Therapy: Frequently used to destroy cancerous cells, this branch of medicine is concerned with radioactive substances and the usage of various techniques of imaging, with the diagnosis and treatment of disease using any of the various sources of radiant energy. Services can include megavoltage radiation therapy, radioactive implants, stereotactic radiosurgery, therapeutic radioisotope services or x-ray radiation therapy.

Radioisotope: Radioisotopes have varying properties that allow them to penetrate objects at different rates. For example, a sheet of paper can stop an alpha particle, a beta particle can penetrate tissues in the body and a gamma ray can penetrate concrete. The varying penetration capabilities allow radioisotopes to be used in different ways. (Also called radioactive isotope or radionuclide.)

Return on Investment (ROI): A measure of a company's profitability, expressed in percentage as net profit (after taxes) divided by total dollar investment.

RNA (Ribonucleic Acid): A macromolecule found in the nucleus and cytoplasm of cells; vital in protein synthesis.

SMDA (Safe Medical Devices Act): This act became law in 1990 and amends the Food, Drug and Cosmetic Act to impose additional regulations on medical devices.

SNP: See "Single-Nucleotide Polymorphism."

SPECT: Single Photon Emission Computerized Tomography. A nuclear medicine imaging technology that combines existing technology of gamma camera imaging with computed tomographic imaging technology to provide a more precise and clear image.

Sponsor: The individual or company that assumes responsibility for the investigation of a new drug, including compliance with the FD&C Act and regulations. The sponsor may be an individual, partnership, corporation or governmental agency and may be a manufacturer, scientific institution or investigator regularly and lawfully engaged in the investigation of new drugs. The sponsor assumes most of the legal and financial responsibility of the clinical trial.

Stem Cells: Found in human bone marrow, the blood stream and the umbilical cord, stem cells can be replicated indefinitely and can turn into any type of mature blood cell, including platelets, white blood cells or red blood cells. Also referred to as pluripotent cells.

Study Coordinator: See "Coordinator."

Subsidiary, Wholly-Owned: A company that is wholly controlled by another company through stock ownership.

Summary Plan Description: A description of an employee's entire benefit package as required by self-funded plans.

Supplementary Medical Insurance (SMI) – Medicare: The SMI program pays for services from physicians, outpatient hospital services, home health agencies, independent laboratories and group practice prepayments. SMI funding comes primarily from government contributions, plus premiums paid by eligible people, those over 65 years old and disabled people under 65.

Supply Chain: The complete set of suppliers of goods and services required for a company to operate its business. For example, a manufacturer's supply chain may include providers of raw materials, components, custom-made parts and packaging materials.

Targets: The proteins involved in a specific disease. Drug compounds concentrate on specific targets in order to have the greatest positive effect and cut down on the incidence of side effects.

Taste Masking: The creation of a barrier between a drug molecule and taste receptors so the drug is easier to take. It masks bitter or unpleasant tastes.

TESS: See "AE."

Third-Party Administrator: An independent person or organization that administers the group plan's benefits and claims and administration for self-insured companies.

Trial Coordinator: See "Coordinator."

Ultrasound: The use of acoustic waves above the range of 20,000 cycles per second to visualize internal body structures. Frequently used to observe a fetus.

Utilization Management (or Utilization Review): A system where utilization case managers (frequently registered nurses with several years of hospital experience) are assigned to each patient who receives hospitalization or extended treatment. These case managers constantly review the amount of care being provided to the patient in question, frequently resulting in significant cost savings. Also see "Managed Care."

Validation of Data: The procedure carried out to ensure that the data contained in a final clinical trial report match the original observations.

Vegan: A person whose diet includes only plant products and excludes all forms of animal products, including meat, fish, poultry, eggs, dairy, gelatin and honey.

Vegetarian: A person whose diet includes only plant products and animal byproducts, such as eggs and dairy, but excludes meat.

Vendor: Any firm, such as a manufacturer or distributor, from which a retailer obtains merchandise.

Videolaseroscopy: Videolaseroscopy, using an endoscope equipped with a laser, is being used in minimally-invasive surgery to excise and or cauterize damaged tissue in the abdomen and lungs.

WHO (World Health Organization): Assists governments in strengthening health services, furnishing technical assistance and aid in emergencies, working on the prevention and control of epidemics and promoting cooperation among different countries to improve nutrition, housing, sanitation, recreation and other aspects of environmental hygiene. Any country that is a member of the United Nations may become a member of the WHO by accepting its constitution. The WHO currently has 191 member states.

Xenotransplantation: The science of transplanting organs such as kidneys, hearts or livers into humans from other mammals, such as pigs or other agricultural animals grown with specific traits for this purpose.

Zoonosis: An animal disease that can be transferred to man.

Zootechnical Feed Additives: Medicines, like growth promoters and antibiotics, which are incorporated as additives into feed.

INTRODUCTION

PLUNKETT'S HEALTH CARE INDUSTRY ALMANAC, the seventh edition of our guide to the health care field, is designed to be used as a general source for researchers of all types.

The data and areas of interest covered are intentionally broad, ranging from the costs and effectiveness of the American health care system, to emerging technology, to an in-depth look at the 500 major for-profit firms (which we call THE HEALTH CARE 500) within the many industry sectors that make up the health care system.

This reference book is designed to be a general source for researchers. It is especially intended to assist with market research, strategic planning, employment searches, contact or prospect list creation (be sure to see the export capabilities of the accompanying CD-ROM that is available to book and eBook buyers) and financial research, and as a data resource for executives and students of all types.

PLUNKETT'S HEALTH CARE INDUSTRY ALMANAC takes a rounded approach for the general reader. This book presents a complete overview of the health care field (see "How To Use This Book"). For example, Medicare and Medicaid growth and expenditures are provided in exacting detail, along with easy-to-use charts and tables on all facets of health care in general: from the average hospital stay to the outlook for manufacturers of drugs and medical products.

THE HEALTH CARE 500 is our unique grouping of the biggest, most successful corporations in all segments of the health care industry. Tens of thousands of pieces of information, gathered from a wide variety of sources, have been researched and are presented in a unique form that can be easily understood. This section includes thorough indexes to THE HEALTH CARE 500, by geography, industry, sales, brand names, subsidiary names and many other topics. (See Chapter 4.)

Especially helpful is the way in which PLUNKETT'S HEALTH CARE INDUSTRY ALMANAC enables readers who have no business background to readily compare the financial records and growth plans of health care companies and major industry groups. You'll see the mid-term financial record of each firm, along with the impact of earnings, sales and strategic plans on each company's potential to fuel growth, to serve new markets and to provide investment and employment opportunities.

No other source provides this book's easy-to-understand comparisons of growth, expenditures, technologies, corporations and many other items of great importance to people of all types who may be studying this, one of the largest and most complex industries in the world today.

By scanning the data groups and the unique indexes, you can find the best information to fit your personal research needs. The major growth companies in health care are profiled and then ranked using several different groups of specific criteria. Which firms are the biggest employers? Which companies earn the most profits? These things and much more are easy to find.

In addition to individual company profiles, an overview of health care markets and trends is provided. This book's job is to help you sort through easy-to-understand summaries of today's trends in a quick and effective manner.

Whatever your purpose for researching the health care field, you'll find this book to be a valuable guide. Nonetheless, as is true with all resources, this volume has limitations that the reader should be aware of:

- Financial data and other corporate information can change quickly. A book of this type can be no more current than the data that was available as of the time of editing. Consequently, the financial picture, management and ownership of the firm(s) you are studying may have changed since the date of this book. For example, this almanac includes the most up-to-date sales figures and profits available to the editors as of late-2004. That means that we have typically used corporate financial data as of the end of 2003.

- Corporate mergers, acquisitions and downsizing are occurring at a very rapid rate. Such events may have created significant change, subsequent to the publishing of this book, within a company you are studying.

- Some of the companies in THE HEALTH CARE 500 are so large in scope and in variety of business endeavors conducted within a parent organization, that we have been unable to completely list all subsidiaries, affiliations, divisions and activities within a firm's corporate structure.

- This volume is intended to be a general guide to a vast industry. That means that researchers should look to this book for an overview and, when conducting in-depth research, should contact the specific corporations or industry associations in question for the very latest changes and data. Where possible, we have listed contact names, toll-free telephone numbers and World Wide Web site addresses for the companies, government agencies and industry associations involved so that the reader may get further details without unnecessary delay.

- Tables of industry data and statistics used in this book include the latest numbers available at the time of printing, generally through the end of 2003. In a few cases, the only complete data available was for earlier years.

- We have used exhaustive efforts to locate and fairly present accurate and complete data. However, when using this book or any other source for business and industry information, the reader should use caution and diligence by conducting further research where it seems appropriate. We wish you success in your endeavors, and we trust that your experience with this book will be both satisfactory and productive.

Jack W. Plunkett
Houston, Texas
November 2004

HOW TO USE THIS BOOK

The two primary sections of this book are devoted first to the health care industry as a whole and then to the "Individual Data Listings" for THE HEALTH CARE 500. If time permits, you should begin your research in the front chapters of this book. Also, you will find lengthy indexes in Chapter 4 and in the back of the book.

THE HEALTH CARE INDUSTRY

Glossary: A short list of health care industry terms.

Chapter 1: Major Trends Affecting the Health Care Industry. This chapter presents an encapsulated view of the major trends that are creating rapid changes in the health care industry today.

Chapter 2: Health Care Industry Statistics. This chapter presents in-depth statistics on Medicare, Medicaid, hospitals, pharmaceuticals and more.

Chapter 3: Important Health Care Industry Contacts – Addresses, Telephone Numbers and World Wide Web Sites. This chapter covers contacts for important government agencies, health care organizations and trade groups. Included are numerous important World Wide Web sites.

THE HEALTH CARE 500

Chapter 4: THE HEALTH CARE 500: Who They Are and How They Were Chosen. The companies compared in this book (the actual count is 514) were carefully selected from the health care industry, largely in the United States. 47 of the firms are based outside the U.S. For a complete description, see THE HEALTH CARE 500 indexes in this chapter.

Individual Data Listings:
Look at one of the companies in THE HEALTH CARE 500's Individual Data Listings. You'll find the following information fields:

Company Name:
The company profiles are in alphabetical order by company name. If you don't find the company you are seeking, it may be a subsidiary or division of one of the firms covered in this book. Try looking it up in the Index by Subsidiaries, Brand Names and Selected Affiliations in the back of the book.

Ranks:
Industry Group Code: An NAIC code used to group companies within like segments. (See Chapter 4 for a list of codes.)
Ranks Within This Company's Industry Group: Ranks, within this firm's segment only, for annual

sales and annual profits, with 1 being the highest rank.

Business Activities:

A grid arranged into six major industry categories and several sub-categories. A "Y" indicates that the firm operates within the sub-category. A complete Index by Industry is included in the beginning of Chapter 4.

Types of Business:

A listing of the primary types of business specialties conducted by the firm.

Brands/Divisions/Affiliations:

Major brand names, operating divisions or subsidiaries of the firm, as well as major corporate affiliations—such as another firm that owns a significant portion of the company's stock. A complete Index by Subsidiaries, Brand Names and Selected Affiliations is in the back of the book.

Contacts:

The names and titles up to 27 top officers of the company are listed, including human resources contacts.

Address:

The firm's full headquarters address, the headquarters telephone, plus toll-free and fax numbers where available. Also provided is the World Wide Web site address.

Financials:

Annual Sales (2004 or the latest fiscal year available to the editors, plus up to four previous years): These are stated in thousands of dollars (add three zeros if you want the full number). This figure represents consolidated worldwide sales from all operations. 2004 figures may be estimates or may be for only part of the year—partial year figures are appropriately footnoted.

Annual Profits (2004 or the latest fiscal year available to the editors, plus up to four previous years): These are stated in thousands of dollars (add three zeros if you want the full number). This figure represents consolidated, after-tax net profit from all operations. 2004 figures may be estimates or may be for only part of the year—partial year figures are appropriately footnoted.

Stock Ticker: When available, the unique stock market symbol used to identify this firm's common stock for trading and tracking purposes is indicated. Where appropriate, this field may contain "private" or "subsidiary" rather than a ticker symbol.

Total Number of Employees: The approximate total number of employees, worldwide, as of the end of 2003 (or the latest data available to the editors).

Apparent Salaries/Benefits:

A "Y" in appropriate fields indicates "Yes."

Due to wide variations in the manner in which corporations report benefits to the U.S. Government's regulatory bodies, not all plans will have been uncovered or correctly evaluated during our effort to research this data. Also, the availability to employees of such plans will vary according to the qualifications that employees must meet to become eligible. For example, some benefit plans may be available only to salaried workers—others only to employees who work more than 1,000 hours yearly. Benefits that are available to employees of the main or parent company may not be available to employees of the subsidiaries. In addition, employers frequently alter the nature and terms of plans offered.

NOTE: Generally, employees covered by wealth-building benefit plans do not *fully* own ("vest in") funds contributed on their behalf by the employer until as many as five years of service with that employer have passed. All pension plans are voluntary—that is, employers are not obligated to offer pensions.

Pension Plan: The firm offers a pension plan to qualified employees. In this case, in order for a "Y" to appear, the editors believe that the employer offers a defined benefit or cash balance pension plan (see discussions below). The type and generosity of these plans vary widely from firm to firm. Caution: Some employers refer to plans as "pension" or "retirement" plans when they are actually 401(k) savings plans that require a contribution by the employee.

- Defined Benefit Pension Plans: Pension plans that do not require a contribution from the employee are infrequently offered. However, a few companies, particularly larger employers in high-profit-margin industries, offer defined benefit pension plans where the employee is guaranteed to receive a set pension benefit upon retirement. The amount of the benefit is determined by the years of service with the company and the employee's salary during the later years of employment. The longer a person works for the employer, the higher the retirement benefit. These defined benefit plans are funded entirely by the employer. The benefits, up to a reasonable limit, are guaranteed by the Federal Government's Pension Benefit Guaranty Corporation. These plans are not portable—if you leave the company, you cannot transfer your benefits into a different plan. Instead, upon retirement you will receive the benefits that vested during your service with the company. If your employer offers a pension plan, it must give you a summary plan description within 90 days of the date you join the plan. You can also request a summary annual report of the plan, and once every 12 months you may request an individual benefit statement accounting of your interest in the plan.

- Defined Contribution Plans: These are quite different. They do not guarantee a certain amount of pension benefit. Instead, they set out circumstances under which the employer will make a contribution to a plan on your behalf. The most common example is the 401(k) savings plan. Pension benefits are not guaranteed under these plans.

- Cash Balance Pension Plans: These plans were recently invented. These are hybrid plans—part defined benefit and part defined contribution. Many employers have converted their older defined benefit plans into cash balance plans. The employer makes deposits (or credits a given amount of money) on the employee's behalf, usually based on a percentage of pay. Employee accounts grow based on a predetermined interest benchmark, such as the interest rate on Treasury Bonds. There are some advantages to these plans, particularly for younger workers: a) The benefits, up to a reasonable limit, are guaranteed by the Pension Benefit Guaranty Corporation. b) Benefits are portable—they can be moved to another plan when the employee changes companies. c) Younger workers and those who spend a shorter number of years with an employer may receive higher benefits than they would under a traditional defined benefit plan.

ESOP Stock Plan (Employees' Stock Ownership Plan): This type of plan is in wide use. Typically, the plan borrows money from a bank and uses those funds to purchase a large block of the corporation's stock. The corporation makes contributions to the plan over a period of time, and the stock purchase loan is eventually paid off. The value of the plan grows significantly as long as the market price of the stock holds up. Qualified employees are allocated a share of the plan based on their length of service and their level of salary. Under federal regulations, participants in ESOPs are allowed to diversify their account holdings in set percentages that rise as the employee ages and gains years of service with the company. In this manner, not all of the employee's assets are tied up in the employer's stock.

Savings Plan, 401(k): Under this type of plan, employees make a tax-deferred deposit into an account. In the best plans, the company makes annual matching donations to the employees' accounts, typically in some proportion to deposits made by the employees themselves. A good plan will match one-half of employee deposits of up to 6% of wages. For example, an employee earning $30,000 yearly might deposit $1,800 (6%) into the plan. The company will match one-half of the employee's deposit, or $900. The plan grows on a tax-deferred basis, similar to an IRA. A very generous plan will match 100% of employee deposits. However, some plans do not call for the employer to make a matching deposit at all. Other plans call for a matching contribution to be made at the discretion of the firm's board of directors. Actual terms of these plans vary widely from firm to firm. Generally, these savings plans allow employees to deposit as much as 15% of salary into the plan on a tax-deferred basis. However, the portion that the company uses to calculate its matching deposit is generally limited to a maximum of 6%. Employees should take care to diversify the holdings in their 401(k) accounts, and most people should seek professional guidance or investment management for their accounts.

Stock Purchase Plan: Qualified employees may purchase the company's common stock at a price below its market value under a specific plan. Typically, the employee is limited to investing a small percentage of wages in this plan. The discount may range from 5 to 15%. Some of these plans allow for deposits to be made through regular monthly payroll deductions. However, new accounting rules for corporations, along with other factors, are leading many companies to curtail these plans—dropping the discount allowed, cutting the maximum yearly stock purchase or otherwise making the plans less generous or appealing.

Profit Sharing: Qualified employees are awarded an annual amount equal to some portion of a company's profits. In a very generous plan, the pool of money awarded to employees would be 15% of profits. Typically, this money is deposited into a long-term retirement account. Caution: Some employers refer to plans as "profit sharing" when they are actually 401(k) savings plans. True profit sharing plans are rarely offered.

Highest Executive Salary: The highest executive salary paid, typically a 2003 amount (or the latest year available to the editors) and typically paid to the Chief Executive Officer.

Highest Executive Bonus: The apparent bonus, if any, paid to the above person.

Second Highest Executive Salary: The next-highest executive salary paid, typically a 2003 amount (or the latest year available to the editors) and typically paid to the President or Chief Operating Officer.

Second Highest Executive Bonus: The apparent bonus, if any, paid to the above person.

Other Thoughts:

Apparent Women Officers or Directors: It is difficult to obtain this information on an exact basis, and employers generally do not disclose the data in a public way. However, we have indicated what our best efforts reveal to be the apparent number of women who either are in the posts of corporate officers or sit on the board of directors. There is a wide variance from company to company.

Hot Spot for Advancement for Women/Minorities: A "Y" in appropriate fields indicates "Yes." These are firms that appear either to have posted a substantial number of women and/or minorities to high posts or that appear to have a good record of going out of their way to recruit, train, promote and retain women or minorities. (See the Index of Hot Spots For Women and Minorities in the back of the book.) This information may change frequently and can be difficult to obtain and verify. Consequently, the reader should use caution and conduct further investigation where appropriate.

Growth Plans/ Special Features:

Listed here are observations regarding the firm's strategy, hiring plans, plans for growth and product development, along with general information regarding a company's business and prospects.

Locations:

A "Y" in the appropriate field indicates "Yes."

Primary locations outside of the headquarters, categorized by regions of the United States and by international locations. A complete index by locations is also in the front of this chapter.

Chapter 1

MAJOR TRENDS AND TECHNOLOGIES AFFECTING THE HEALTH CARE INDUSTRY

Major Trends Affecting the Health Care Industry:

1) Introduction to the Health Care Industry
2) Continued Rise in Health Care Costs
3) Employers Push Health Care Costs onto Employees
4) Medicare Changes Include Drug Benefits for Seniors for the First Time
5) Health Savings Accounts and Health Reimbursement Accounts Gain Traction
6) Vast Number of Uninsured and Underinsured Americans
7) Pharmaceutical Manufacturers Face Challenges, Massive Costs in New Drug Development
8) Cost of Pharmaceuticals Soars in U.S., Controversy over Drug Prices Rages On
9) Boom in Surgery Centers
10) Managed Care Becomes More Patient-Friendly
11) Growing Use of Managed Care by Medicare
12) Giant Mergers at Managed Care Providers
13) Critical Lack of Qualified Nurses
14) Malpractice Suits Are Blamed for Rising Health Care Costs
15) Patients' Rights Evolve

The Outlook for Health Care Technology:

16) Health Care Technology Introduction
17) Information Technology and Health Care
18) Stem Cells and Tissue Engineering
19) New Drugs and New Drug Delivery Methods
20) Advances in Cancer Research
21) Advances in Diagnostic Imaging and Monitoring
22) Advances in Laboratory Testing
23) Advances in Surgery
24) Other Treatment Technologies

Major Trends Affecting the Health Care Industry:

1) Introduction to the Health Care Industry

The American health care industry faces more challenges than ever, due to a number of significant factors:

- While the advent of managed care appeared to tame health care cost inflation during the early and mid 1990s, costs have now been rising very rapidly for years.
- The number of Americans who are underinsured or are without any type of insurance coverage remains staggering.
- The U.S. population is aging rapidly. At the same time, the life expectancy of seniors is extending. Senior citizens will place a significant strain on the health care system in coming years.
- The pharmaceuticals industry faces continued financial challenges. Annual expenditures for pharmaceuticals are skyrocketing, creating a large backlash among health consumers and payors. At the same time, the drug industry remains under intense public scrutiny and is facing continued calls for increased government legislation and regulation.
- We are now entering what will long be remembered as the beginning of the Biotech Era. Breakthroughs in diagnostics and drug therapies are occurring at a rapid pace, creating financial and ethical challenges along with opportunities. Personalized medicine is beginning to emerge, but it remains to be seen who will be the early beneficiaries and who will pay the costs.
- Due to rising health care costs, employers large and small are straining under the financial burden of health care coverage costs for current employees and retirees. The percentage of health costs paid by employees continues to rise.
- The future obligations of Medicare and Medicaid are enough to cause vast problems for the federal budget. Reforms are vital. Meanwhile, the number of seniors covered by Medicare will continue to grow at an exceedingly high rate, and new prescription coverage costs will add to the government's financial problems.
- Medical Savings Accounts, used by only a small number of Americans, will get a renewed push as a result of the reelection of President Bush.
- Physicians, other care providers, pharmaceutical manufacturers and insurers face daunting pressure from litigation and potential claims regarding malpractice and denial of care. Malpractice insurance costs are out of control. Some lawsuit reform legislation has begun, but much more reform is needed.

Escalating costs have forced employers to ask workers to pay for a larger share of health care. Political and market forces and the weakness of any stabilizing influences are eroding the ability of managed care firms to control underlying health care costs. Watch for significant increases in the price of coverage in 2005.

Today, health care costs are staggering. Total U.S. health care expenditures are projected to increase from $1.8 trillion in 2004 to $3.4 trillion in 2013, with annual increases averaging about 7%. Health spending in the U.S., at 16% of Gross Domestic Product (GDP), accounts for a larger share of GDP than in any other major industrialized country. Despite the incredible investment America continues to make in health care, an astounding 15% of Americans lack health care coverage altogether.

Continuous increases in the cost of health care, growing at rates far exceeding the rate of inflation in general, are hammering health consumers and payors of all types. Managed and Medicare/Medicaid care providers continue to struggle to contain costs. Meanwhile, employers are hit hard by vast increases in the cost of providing coverage to employees and retirees. Some employers are utilizing unique new programs in efforts to reduce employee illness, and thereby reduce costs. For example, the use of preventative care programs is growing, as is the use of employee education programs aimed at better managing the effects of diseases such as diabetes.

In 2004, employers saw health coverage cost increases of as much as 12%, with small employers taking on the brunt of the increase. This figure is projected to mediate in 2005 to an increase of 8%. The greatest portion of the blame lies with rising drug costs.

Smart employers are showing their employees how to use the Internet to obtain better information about diseases and prevention. Insurance providers are jumping on the Internet bandwagon as well. For example, Humana's web-based Emphesys benefits system puts everything from monthly payments to participating physicians to claims on the Internet, at a substantial decrease in cost. Some employers are even hiring in-house physicians and nurses to provide primary care in the workplace. (See, "Employers Push Health Care Costs onto Employees.")

Patients and insurance companies are also dealing with sticker shock as the nation's prescription drug bill soars. Prescription drug costs have increased more than 10% every year since 1995, surging 13.4% in 2003, with an expected growth of 12.9% in 2004. Other factors edging costs upward are exuberance over new medical technology and patients' demand for greater plan flexibility in choosing doctors and specialists at their will. At the same time, hospitals and health systems write off record amounts of revenues to bad debt.

In the wake of the tremendous growth of all aspects of the health care industry from the end of World War Two onward, efficiency, competition and productivity were, regretfully, largely overlooked. Much of this occurred because federal and state governments paid such a large portion of the health care bill. Total Medicare and Medicaid program outlays in 2005 will reach $476.4 billion, or 20% of the total federal budget.

Meanwhile, physicians are caught between the desire for quality care and the desire for cost control on the part of payors, including HMOs, Medicare and Medicaid. The cost versus care debate has spawned an energetic movement to improve the quality of health care in the U.S., much of it centered around patients' rights.

Another major challenge facing the health care industry is the severely tarnished image of managed care companies in general. Supporters of managed care contend that its structure offers higher-quality care at a lower cost. Critics of managed care argue that the system risks lives by allowing plan managers to question, and sometimes reverse, the decisions made by medical professionals while emphasizing cost control at the expense of quality, thus sabotaging the bond of trust that should exist between doctor and patient. There is also concern among detractors of managed care about the trend of mergers creating huge managed care companies. Some metropolitan markets are dominated by as few as two major health plans. Critics are equally concerned about the lack of autonomy of physicians who are forced to deal with the growing power of managed care giants.

While both supporters and critics make valid arguments, sweeping generalizations about the state of managed care are inherently flawed, since no two managed care plans are exactly alike. Neither society nor consumers can afford to turn back the clock to the traditional, considerably more expensive fee-for-service system in which quality preventive care was largely non-existent, and patient care was generally provided without regard to cost.

2) Continued Rise in Health Care Costs

After five consecutive years of double-digit growth in health care costs, 2005 is expected to mark a slight slowdown. American employers anticipate an 8% increase in premiums paid to health plans, still a substantial increase, but certainly preferable to previous increases. In 2004, employers saw an increase of 11% to 12% over the previous year. In comparison, increases in 2003 were 13% to 14%. The reasons for the projected 2005 slowdown include fewer hospital stays and the growing use of generic drugs. The slowing trend is expected to continue; however, projections for health care cost growth still exceed those for overall economic growth. Due to steady increases, health care costs are predicted to make up more than 18% of GDP in 2013.

The catalysts for these repeated rises include the cost of prescription drugs, medical innovation and a growing acceptance of higher-premium health plans that offer greater flexibility in choice of providers. One way in which employers are attempting to control costs is to implement monitoring and preventive care plans for conditions such as diabetes and heart disease. Blue Cross and Blue Shield of Minnesota offers such a program and has used it to post annual employer savings as high as $36 million.

The U.S. continues to spend more on health care than any other developed nation, whether measured as total spending, spending per capita or spending as a percentage of GDP. Per capita expenses were $6,167 in 2004 (an estimate based on a U.S. population of 293 million). The average per capita health care spending among 30 member nations of the Organization for Economic Cooperation and Development is less than half as much.

The U.S. is also seeing greater growth in spending from one year to the next than other developed nations. Despite the higher costs, Americans have a much higher incidence of obesity, and the average life expectancy is slightly lower than that of people in Japan, Iceland, Sweden and Canada.

Many cash-strapped Americans abandon their increasingly expensive private health care plans and choose not to be insured at all. Unfortunately, patients who are not covered by managed care organizations are typically charged much higher rates for care. For example, a hospital might charge a set price of $1,900 for a CT scan procedure when billing an individual not covered by a managed care contract, but discount the cost to $1,200 for someone who is covered. This is because managed care companies insist on negotiated rates for care.

3) Employers Push Health Care Costs onto Employees

As employers face continued growth in health care costs, they are, in most cases, shifting more of the burden onto employees. In 2004, employees contributed an average of 16% of the cost for individual health care coverage and 28% of the cost for family coverage, which remains the same as their percentages in 2003. However, retirees are paying significantly higher shares, approximately 41% for those under 65, and 44% for those over 65.

Many employers have taken measures to decrease health care benefits for retirees in order to cut costs. Be it raising retirees' share of premiums, capping the total amount paid or cutting benefits, employers have been steadily placing more of the financial burden of health care onto their retired employees. For example, in 1993 IBM capped its spending on health insurance premiums for retirees over 65 (and thereby covered by Medicare) to no more than $3,500 yearly. Caterpillar, Inc. cut costs by $75 million in 2002 by raising the premiums paid by retirees. Aetna decided to cut health benefits out of the retirement package for its workers altogether, starting for those who retire in 2004. These trends will likely continue over the mid-term, with more and more of the cost of elderly health care being pushed onto retirees and Medicare.

For those still actively in the workforce, the average annual cost of insurance premiums for family coverage has risen to about $10,000. On average, employers who provide health coverage are paying about $7,500 of this premium, leaving about $2,500 to be paid by the employee. Co-payments and deductibles are also up. The average deductible is $287 for participants in preferred provider organizations (PPOs), which are the most common type of health plan. Deductibles for small company workers are up to $420 per year for PPOs and $676 for other plans. Co-payments range from $10 for generic drug prescriptions to $224 for hospitalization.

Health coverage premium increases would be much higher except for proactive measures on the part of many employers, such as sponsoring wellness or disease management programs for employees and increasing employees' share of premiums, co-payments or deductibles.

4) Medicare Changes Include Drug Benefits for Seniors for the First Time

In November 2003, Congress passed a $395-billion bill for the reform of Medicare. In a largely bi-partisan vote, legislators approved a measure that will give large private insurers a greater role in health care for senior citizens, as well as provide a prescription drug benefit that will go into effect in 2006. Part of the bill provides $25 billion for rural hospitals and health care providers; a provision that requires wealthy seniors to pay more for Medicare Part B coverage; and substantial support ($70 billion) for corporations that might otherwise eliminate existing coverage for retirees.

The new legislation creates a government-subsidized prescription drug benefit, which may vary from plan to plan. Seniors who participate will pay a monthly premium, estimated to be $35 per month in 2006. They will be issued a drug benefit identification card. Beneficiaries will be responsible for the first $250 in yearly drug expenses, and then will pay, on average, a 25% coinsurance until they reach the benefit limit, which is $2,250 in 2006. Once they reach the benefit limit, they will face a gap in coverage in which they will pay 100% of their drug costs up to $5,100 in total drug spending. Medicare will then pay 95% of drug costs above that amount.

Premiums can vary by region, and private plan providers may vary benefits so long as they are equivalent to standard coverage described above. Low-income Medicare beneficiaries, those with incomes less than 150% of the federal poverty level, including those who receive Medicaid coverage in addition to Medicare, will be eligible for varying levels of additional assistance depending on their incomes and assets.

Certain health companies will likely profit from this new Medicare drug benefit, including drug manufacturers who may have the opportunity to sell more drugs to more seniors, and health plan firms that may administer the drug benefit cards backed by Medicare.

5) Health Savings Accounts and Health Reimbursement Accounts Gain Traction

A _Health Savings Account (HSA)_ is a plan that combines a tax-free savings and investment account, somewhat similar to a 401(k), with a high-deductible health coverage plan. The intent is to give the consumer more incentive to control health care costs by reducing unnecessary care while shopping for the best prices. The consumer contributes pre-tax dollars annually to a savings account—up to $2,600 for an individual or $5,150 for a family. The employer may or may not match part of that contribution. The account may be invested in stocks, bonds or mutual funds. It grows tax-free, but the money may be spent only on health care. Unspent money stays in the account at the end of each year. The consumer must purchase an insurance policy or health care plan with an annual deductible of at least $1,000 for individuals or $2,000 for families. Funds may be withdrawn to pay a broad variety of medical expenses, including cosmetic surgery, dental care and ophthalmologist/optometrist expenses.

A <u>Health Reimbursement Account (HRA)</u> is a form of health care coverage plan provided to employees by their employer. It is quite different from a Health Savings Account. Under an HRA, the employer places a given amount of money into a special account each year for the employee to spend on health care. The employer also provides a high-deductible health coverage plan. The employee elects when and how to spend the money in the account on health care. Because of the high deductible, the employee's share of the monthly premium tends to be much lower than under an HMO or PPO, but the employee faces the burden of paying the high deductible when necessary. Unspent funds in the account can roll over from year to year so that the account grows, but the employee loses the fund balance when leaving the employer.

Detractors claim that HSAs will provide a tax shelter for the young and wealthy and also make it possible for poor or uninformed seniors to make choices that will ultimately harm rather than help them. From the employer's point of view, HSAs give employees who carefully manage their costs and investments an opportunity to build up a significant savings account. At the same time, since most employers will pay only a specific amount into an HSA each year, the plan may shield the employer from a portion of any increases in health care costs.

From the point of view of covered workers, HSAs may be a real boon, particularly for those who are relatively healthy and generally spend little on health care. However, a participating worker will be at risk for the amount of the high deductible provided for in the coverage plan until the savings account contains a substantial cushion. Consequently, some observers speculate that HSAs will appeal mainly to more affluent employees. HSAs are required to include annual out-of-pocket expense caps of no more than $5,000 for individuals or $10,000 for families. Some workers may opt to pay higher monthly premiums in exchange for lower expense caps.

From the point of view of health planners and health economists, many feel that widespread use of HSAs could create a true turning point in the American health system. Today, under most coverage plans, health consumers give little thought to the amount of or price of care they are receiving. Few covered consumers question expensive tests and other procedures when they are ordered by their physicians. Fewer still ask the price of procedures or shop around for the best care at the best price. Many hope that, by giving them control of the purchasing process and a vested stake in the balance in the savings account, consumers will begin demanding better care at lower prices. Ideally, the result would be more cost competition, greater choices for patients and an end to the continuous upward spiral of health care costs.

For example, some health analysts estimate that 20% to 30% of health care dollars are spent on needless tests or other procedures. Others feel that Americans are over-cared for—particularly those who can receive an endless stream of care at the expense of their health plans. For example, some surgical procedures, such as a hip replacement, might be eliminated through the use of much less expensive alternate care, such as physical therapy. Eventually, people who indulge in self-destructive behavior such as smoking or excessive weight gain might be motivated to change their habits when they see the actual costs in terms of health care dollars.

How quickly will the use of HSAs spread? Plans will be offered to millions of Americans starting in 2005. For example, 10 million Federal Government employees will have an HSA option. Approximately 10% of U.S. employers offer HSAs as of the beginning of 2005, but a recent survey by Mercer Human Resource Consulting found that 73% of employers are likely or somewhat likely to sponsor HSAs by 2006. Major employers that were early in offering these programs include Intel, Pitney Bowes and Textron. Approximately 160 million Americans are currently insured by employers. If 6% of them switch to HSAs yearly, which is a reasonable goal, the number of people covered by such plans could grow by nearly 10 million per year over the mid-term.

In order to encourage participants in HSAs to keep up preventative care and regular checkups, many insurers, such as Aetna and UnitedHealthcare, are offering 100% coverage of such visits to the doctor. Other providers are offering disease management and education programs. Some employers are covering 100% of the cost of drugs that are vital for people with chronic illnesses. Such innovations will help HSAs appeal to a broader range of workers.

6) Vast Number of Uninsured and Underinsured Americans

The total number of Americans who were without health insurance in 2003 was 45 million, an increase of 1.4 million from 2002. This figure accounts for 15.6% of the population, up from 15.2% the previous year. These figures are projected to rise even further due to the continued drop in employer-sponsored health care benefits. In 2003, 60.4% of Americans had insurance from employers, down from 61.3% in 2002. Put another way, the total number of people who enjoy employer-sponsored health coverage fell in 2003 by 900,000 to 175.6 million, while the total population grew by 2.8 million.

Who are the uninsured? Many are working adults. Not surprisingly, few are elderly or disabled, groups generally covered by Medicare or Medicaid. The Census Bureau estimates that of the more than 45 million uninsured Americans, more than 8 million are children. Minorities have a high rate of uninsurance as well, with Hispanics topping the list at 32.7%.

There are several possible explanations for the large number of uninsured Americans:
- As a result of the 1996 welfare-reform act, millions of people have shifted from welfare to low-wage jobs with employers that either offer no coverage whatsoever or offer plans with co-payments that lower-income workers cannot afford.
- Increases in the cost of health care coverage have outpaced increases in household income, making coverage unaffordable for the many who are self-employed or who do not qualify for employer-provided plans.
- There has been an increasing trend toward alternate employment, such as temporary and part-time work, which seldom offers health care coverage. Likewise, a growing number of people are unemployed.

In addition to the number of people with no insurance at all, the growing number of underinsured Americans is a problem. In many cases, increased limitations on care covered by payors result in costs shifting to patients in the form of high co-payments.

7) Pharmaceutical Manufacturers Face Challenges, Massive Costs in New Drug Development

Despite exponential advances in biopharmaceutical knowledge and technology, pharmaceutical companies enduring the task of getting new drugs to market continue to face long timeframes, daunting costs and immense risks. Although the number of New Drug Applications (NDAs) submitted to the FDA has grown dramatically since 1996, the number of new drugs receiving final approval remains relatively small: Out of every 1,000 experimental drug compounds in some form of preclinical testing, only one actually makes it to clinical trials. Then, only one in five of those drugs makes it to market. The amount of time required to develop a new drug and get it to market has not lessened, and development costs continue to rise rapidly for biopharmaceutical firms. The number of NDAs approved in 2003 was down to 72, from a high of 131 in 1996. The approval of entirely new compounds that have never before been submitted to the FDA, known as New Molecular Entities (NMEs), was limited to 21 in 2003, down from a height of 53, also in 1996.

Key terms, human clinical trials stages:
Phase I—small-scale human trials for safety
Phase II—preliminary trials on a drug's efficacy/safety
Phase III—large-scale controlled trials for efficacy/safety; also the last stage before a request for approval is made to the FDA
Phase IV—follow-up trials after a drug is released to the public
NDA (New Drug Application)—states results of clinical trials and asks permission to market the drug to the public
PMA (Pre-Market Approval)—application to sell a device (rather than a drug) that is implanted, life-sustaining or life-supporting

---

According to a study released in 2001 by the Tufts Center for the Study of Drug Development, the cost of developing a new drug and getting it to market averaged $802 million, up from about $500 million in 1996. (Averaged into these figures are the costs of developing and testing drugs that never reach the market.) Expanding on the study to include post-approval research (Phase IV clinical studies), Tufts increased the number to $897 million. Even more pessimistic is research done by Bain & Co., a consulting firm, which states that the cost is more on the order of $1.7 billion, including such factors as marketing and advertising expenses.

The average time elapsed from the synthesis of a new chemical compound to its introduction to the market remains 12 to 14 years—the same timeframe that drug makers have dealt with for the past decade. Considering that the patent for a new compound only lasts 20 years, a limited amount of time is left to reclaim the considerable investment. As a result of these costs and the lengthy time-to-market, young biotech companies encounter a harsh financial reality: commercial profits take years and years to emerge from promising beginnings in the laboratory.

However, advances in systems biology (the use of a combination of state-of-the-art technologies, such as molecular diagnostics, advanced computers and extremely deep, efficient genetic databases) may eventually lead to more efficient, faster drug development at reduced costs. Much of this advance will stem from the use of technology to efficiently target the genetic causes of, and develop novel cures for, niche diseases.

For example, in May 2001 the FDA approved Novartis's new drug Gleevec (a revolutionary and highly effective treatment for patients suffering from chronic myeloid leukemia) after an astonishingly brief two and a half months in the approval process (compared to a more typical six years). This fast-track approval of the drug, which promptly began saving lives, was possible because of two factors in addition to the FDA's cooperation. One, Novartis mounted a targeted approach to this niche disease. Its research determined that a specific genetic malfunction causes the disease, and its drug specifically blocks the protein that causes the genetic malfunction. Two, thanks to its use of advanced genetic research techniques, Novartis was so convinced of the effectiveness of this drug that it invested heavily and quickly in its development.

Small to mid-size biotech firms continue to look to mature, global pharmaceutical companies for cash, marketing muscle, distribution channels and regulatory expertise. Despite the problems in the ImClone partnership with Bristol-Myers Squibb with regard to control over drug development, major partnerships and acquisitions are still being signed at a rapid clip. Good examples are the agreement between Millennium Pharmaceuticals and Abbott Laboratories to develop new diagnostics for obesity and diabetes, and the Isis Pharmaceuticals deal to conduct research into new drugs for inflammatory and metabolic diseases.

Internet Research Tip:
For extensive commentary and analysis on the true costs and difficulty of developing new drugs, see:
Tufts Center for the Study of Drug Development
csdd.tufts.edu
Bain & Co.
www.bain.com
Go to "Publications" from the home page, and then click on "Healthcare" in the "Select Industry" drop-down menu.

8) Cost of Pharmaceuticals Soars in U.S., Controversy over Drug Prices Rages On

Overall, the drug industry is one of the world's most profitable business sectors. Among the Fortune 500 companies in 2003, pharmaceutical firms ranked third in return on revenues at 14.3%. These profits come at significant cost—about 20% of pharmaceutical revenue is redirected toward discovering new medicines, well above the average of 4% reinvested in research and development in most industries. Advanced technology has allowed drug companies to saturate their development programs with smarter, more promising drugs. R&D budgets are staggering. Pfizer planned to invest $8 billion in R&D in 2004, and Merck increased its R&D budget by 19% in 2003 alone, to $3.2 billion. Total spending on research and development in the U.S. in 2003 was an estimated $33.2 billion, according to Pharmaceutical Research and Manufacturers of America (PhRMA www.phrma.org), a trade organization.

Until recently, pharmaceutical research was focused primarily on curing life-threatening or severely debilitating illnesses. But a current generation of drugs, commonly referred to as "lifestyle" drugs, is transforming the pharmaceutical industry. Lifestyle drugs target a variety of medical conditions, ranging from the painful to the inconvenient, including obesity, impotence, memory loss and depression. Drug companies also continue to develop treatments for wrinkles and hair loss in an effort to capture their share of the huge anti-aging market aimed at the baby-boomer generation. The use of lifestyle drugs dramatically increases the total annual consumer intake of pharmaceuticals and creates a great deal of controversy over which drugs should be covered by managed care and which should be paid for by the consumer alone.

As demand for new and improved treatments intensifies, the abilities of modern technology grow as well. In addition to expediting the process of drug discovery and development, advanced pharmaceutical technology promises to increase the number of diseases that are treatable with drugs, enhance the effectiveness of those drugs and increase the ability to predict disease, not just the ability to react to it.

New technology aided by very fast computers will help control the cost of drug development. For example, testing of new chemical compounds for potential drug use was previously a tiresome process that could easily require a full week of a laboratory worker's effort, at a cost of $5,000 to $10,000 per compound. Now, chemists can test thousands of drugs in one day, automatically, via sophisticated, computerized equipment.

Consumers' voracious appetites for new drugs continue to grow. Insurance companies may raise co-payments for drugs, strike discount deals with drug companies and employ pharmacy benefit management tactics in an effort to fend off rising pharmaceutical costs. Also, new drugs have very high prices when they initially hit the market, since they have no generic equivalent while covered by patent protection.

In coming years, taming pharmaceutical costs will be one of the biggest challenges facing the health care system. Managed care must be able to determine which promising new drugs can deliver meaningful clinical benefits proportionate to their costs.

Several developments are fueling the fire under the controversy over drug costs in the U.S. To begin with, it has become common knowledge that drug firms tend to price their drugs at vastly lower prices outside the U.S. market. The result is that U.S. consumers and their health care payors are bearing a disproportionate share of the costs of developing new drugs. Whereas prices in the U.S. are determined by a free market and are mostly limited only by competition, nations such as Australia and Canada put a cap on drug prices that cannot exceed a given amount. Taking advantage of this discrepancy, generally a 30% to 80% difference, border-crossing U.S. citizens have saved bundles of money on prescription drugs by importing them from Canada and Mexico. Canadian Internet-based drug retailers such as RxNorth and CanadaRx have been popping up, selling to anyone with a credit card and a faxed prescription. U.S. drug companies have of course raised a furor. Many have threatened to limit Canada's supplies so it only meets the demands of Canadians, as well as putting a corporate embargo on any pharmacy or distributor suspected of selling to Internet companies.

Factors leading to soaring drug costs in the American health care system:
- The lifespan of Americans is increasing, and chronic illnesses that require drug treatment are increasing as the population ages.
- The drug industry is making an intensified sales effort. Direct-to-consumer advertising and legions of sales professionals calling on physicians increase demand for the newest, most expensive drugs.
- Convoluted and uncoordinated lists of drug "formularies" (available drugs, their uses and their interactions) require increased administrative work to sort through, thus forcing costs upward.
- Physicians often prescribe name-brand drugs when a generic equivalent may be available at a fraction of the cost.
- Research budgets are escalating rapidly. Breakthroughs in research and development are creating significant new drug therapies, allowing a wide range of popular treatments that were not previously available. An excellent example is the rampant use of antidepressants such as Prozac and Zoloft. Meanwhile, major drug companies face the loss of patent protection on dozens of leading drugs—they are counting on expensive research, partnerships and acquisitions to replace those marquis drugs.
- "Lifestyle" drug use is increasing, as shown by the popularity of such drugs as Viagra (for the treatment of sexual dysfunction), Propecia (for the treatment of male baldness) and Botox (for the treatment of facial wrinkles).
- Drug manufacturers face soaring costs from class action lawsuits when patients press claims that drugs had harmful side affects.

Source: Plunkett Research, Ltd.

9) Boom in Surgery Centers

The number of ambulatory surgery centers (ASCs), otherwise known as outpatient surgery centers, has skyrocketed since their initial Medicare approval in 1982, rising to 3,735 Medicare-certified facilities by the beginning of 2004. These centers offer a variety of outpatient surgical procedures for a broad range of medical specialties, including ear, nose and throat, gastroenterology, general surgery, gynecology, ophthalmology, orthopedics, pain management, pediatric surgery, plastic surgery and oral surgery, among others. Centers that exclusively offer services relating to ophthalmology and gastroenterology are the most commonly covered by Medicare. The trend has grown substantially since the mid-90s with the development of laparoscopic techniques and procedures using laser technology, resulting in more outpatient surgery and therefore fewer patients requiring expensive overnight hospital stays.

Most procedures performed in such centers are covered under Medicare or by most major health plans. Medicare paid $2 billion to surgery centers in 2003, up from $610 million in 1993. Most ASCs have popped up in major metropolitan areas, where there is a high volume of particular surgeries. Because of the need for a large population base to serve, 40% of ASCs are located in only five states, each containing densely populated metro areas: California, Maryland, Florida, Texas and Washington.

The rapid growth of ASCs has not been without controversy, however, since an industry leader, HealthSouth Corp., was charged in early 2003 with over-billing Medicare and inflating earnings by the billions. There is also concern regarding conflict of interest in cases where surgeons performing procedures also have financial interests in the centers. Medicare has a tendency to pay very high rates for some types of surgery, such as heart bypass or cataract removal, while paying much less for others. The type of specialty hospitals under operation is influenced heavily by the types of surgery for which Medicare is most generous.

In the midst of the specialty hospital boom, traditional hospitals are losing surgery revenues. Some are forced to cut costs, lay off staff or discontinue money-losing programs such as psychiatric care and preventive medicine. The most lucrative procedures are being performed away from traditional hospitals, many of which face increasingly difficult financial conditions. More and more, full-service hospitals are left serving patients who require money-losing treatments.

Worries about ASCs were finally brought before Congress at the beginning of 2004. The major problem in developing a fair pay scheme at Medicare is the lack of data provided by ASCs, which are not subject to the same regulatory reporting that hospitals are. Frustrated by the lack of information, Congress froze the pay scales for all ASCs at 2002 rates, pending a new payment system to be organized by the Department of Health and Human Services. Reform may take until 2008 or 2009, meaning that surgery centers are left in the lurch until then, without pay increases. Concerns about the eventual pay rates adopted by Medicare may hamper the mid-term growth of ASCs, forcing existing centers to cut costs and discouraging potential investors.

10) Managed Care Becomes More Patient-Friendly

Under the previous fee-for-service system of health care coverage, quality care suffered due to excessive paperwork, needless surgery and tests and little or no emphasis on containing costs or preventative care. Patients who were insured could receive almost any treatment they wanted with very little concern for cost.

With the advent of managed care, however, consumers' freedom of choice has been drastically reduced. Understandably, many patients resent this. What is forgotten in this upheaval of public opinion is the fact that without the cost constraint and savings instituted by the managed care system, many more Americans would have no health care coverage at all because they or their employers couldn't afford it.

Employers, seeking control of health care expenses, quickly adopted managed care. Today, only a small percentage of Americans who are insured outside of government programs are covered by unmanaged fee-for-service plans.

Drawbacks of the managed care system are sometimes more visible than its benefits. As a result, national and state governments have passed bills aimed at micro-managing the operations of managed care companies. However, the massive backlash against the Clinton Administration's early proposals for universal, government-managed care showed that there is a limit to the public's desire for government interference in health care systems.

Although Americans want unlimited health care availability, they must realize that money and services are not unlimited. At the same time, managed care firms must be sensitive to the real concerns and needs of patients. The challenge of continued reform of health care falls largely on the private sector.

The concept of managed care has engendered a plethora of organizations within which medical professionals operate. The dominant types are HMOs, POS (Point-of-Service) and PPOs.

HMOs (Health Maintenance Organizations) were the original type of managed care offerings. Initially, HMOs restricted members to visits to physicians and clinics that were within a network—a group of providers under contract with the HMO. Patients needing to see a specialist first had to be referred by a primary care physician. The intent of this referral system was to keep patients from making costly, unnecessary visits to specialists. Attending physicians were forced to obtain HMO approval for tests, such as imaging, surgery, hospital stays and other everyday care needs. Many critics bemoaned that these organizations overly restricted patients' access to care. Today's HMOs are much more patient-friendly than they were in the past. Many now give much more leeway to physicians who need to order tests and other procedures. Also, many HMOs allow members to see the most commonly used specialists, such as gynecologists, without a referral. HMO premiums tend to be lower than those of PPOs because patients have fewer choices.

PPOs (Preferred Provider Organizations) are designed to give patients much more freedom in their choice of physicians. To begin with, members typically may visit any physician within the network, including specialists, without a referral. Visits to physicians outside of the network are often allowed, but the patient is charged a higher co-payment for such visits. Overall, monthly premiums and patient co-payments tend to be a bit higher at PPOs than HMOs, but patients who want the freedom to visit specific doctors are generally much happier with this type of coverage.

POS (Point-of-Service plans) are designed to give the patient a great deal of choice of physician. For routine checkups and office visits, the patient sees a primary care physician and pays a simple co-payment. As with an HMO, the plans are designed to keep the patient's out-of-pocket costs low. At the same time, the patient is free to go outside of the network, but will be charged a higher co-payment. Another similarity to HMOs is the fact that POS operates by requiring the patient to rely on a primary care physician for referrals to specialists when needed. If the patient is referred to a specialist, the patient's fees remain low.

11) Growing Use of Managed Care by Medicare

A few years back, a combination of unfriendly Medicare rules and the high cost of care prompted managed care firms to abruptly drop Medicare patients and exit the Medicare field altogether. Tens of thousands of seniors were left scurrying for new providers, and most of these seniors were inconvenienced, disillusioned and upset.

Today, managed care's role in Medicare is an entirely different matter. The Federal Government has decided to push managed care once again, hoping that it will provide more choices for seniors who are covered by Medicare, while introducing higher levels of competition and cost control into the marketplace. As part of this program, Medicare is paying higher reimbursement rates in some cases, making senior patients more attractive to managed care firms. From 2004 through 2006, Medicare expects the number of seniors who are members of managed care plans to triple, to nearly 15 million people. "Medicare Plus Choice" plans are being sold aggressively by firms such as Humana and WellCare. These companies are using such marketing techniques as free lunches and health seminars to attract potential members to their offices, where they also learn about the managed care plans. Generally, these plans are being offered at extremely low monthly premiums that are hard for cash-strapped seniors to resist. Among choices offered under Medicare Plus Choice plans are preferred provider networks that give seniors much greater flexibility in choosing physicians.

12) Giant Mergers at Managed Care Providers

Currently, mergers are the name of the game in managed care. In late 2003, Anthem, Inc. announced its planned acquisition of WellPoint Health Networks, Inc. for $16.4 billion, which will create one of the world's largest managed care companies. By November 2004, the merger had passed the most significant of its regulatory hurdles, including approval by health regulators in the State of California. Likewise, UnitedHealth Group completed its acquisition, early in 2004, of Mid Atlantic Medical Services, Inc. for $2.6 billion. Similar to the merger trend that the banking industry has been experiencing, managed care consolidation will likely bring about more standardization in an industry that desperately needs it, as well as the economies that come with doing business on a larger scale. Larger managed care companies will be better able to foot the bill for such projects as digitization of patient records. However, mergers mean fewer companies in the marketplace, which may reduce competition.

2003 was a good year for managed care companies, which collectively saw double-digit profit increases. Despite this growth, competition is keen—most managed care companies are seeing their client companies seeking bids from other firms for better deals. The depressed economy of 2001-2002, which caused many workers to lose their jobs and, therefore, managed care companies to lose members, was an additional catalyst for the mergers.

More big news for managed care is the settlement of a lawsuit against Aetna in mid 2003. The suit, one of the largest health care industry related class action suits, in which more than 700,000 practicing physicians went up against 10 major insurance companies, concerned billing and medical decisions. As a result of the suit, Aetna pledged to change the way in which it provides information to patients and doctors, expedite the payment system and cut red tape overall. While not a change that is sweeping the industry, it is a first step toward simplifying claims processing and building a clearer relationship among doctors, patients and benefits companies. Aetna has accepted general treatment guidelines established by the American Medical Association (AMA). In a nutshell, these guidelines stipulate that patient care is to be based on the prudent and clinical judgment of the attending physician rather than the treatments that the insurance company believes to be the most cost-effective. Furthermore, Aetna agreed to publish a list of the procedures it covers, along with their costs, on its web site.

13) Critical Lack of Qualified Nurses

A report by the Joint Commission on Accreditation of Healthcare Organizations in late 2003 stated that of 1,609 types of unexpected problems (including accidental death or serious physical harm) in U.S. hospitals reported between January 1996 and March 2002, 24% took place because of an insufficient number of nurses on duty. Low staffing levels were found to contribute to 50% of ventilator-related incidents, 42% of surgery-related incidents, 25% of transfusion incidents, 19% of medication errors and 14% of patient falls.

Sadly, the nursing shortage is nothing new. In a 2001 survey conducted by the Federation of Nurses and Health Professionals, one in five nurses stated their intention to leave the profession within the next five years due to poor working conditions. Stress, irregular hours, low morale and excessive patient loads are all cited as problems serious enough to cause nurses to quit.

The implications of the staffing shortage are serious indeed. Analysis of data on nurse staffing levels confirms that there is a direct link between the number of registered nurses on staff and the hours they spend with patients. Likewise it is a determining factor in whether patients develop a number of serious complications or die while in the hospital. Additional factors include the aging population, the growing numbers of patients who will require care in assisted living centers and all-time low enrollment in nursing school.

In response to the situation, the Nurse Reinvestment Act was passed in Congress in 2002 and was signed by President Bush in 2003. The act authorizes $30 million in federal funding for scholarships and loan repayments for nursing students who agree to work in nursing shortage areas after graduation. While this may well be a boon to potential nursing school enrollment, there may still be a problem finding enough masters- and doctorate-level nurses who are qualified to teach in nursing schools.

In addition to the shortages of qualified nurses, there are significant shortages of radiology technicians, pharmacists and other allied health professionals. Watch for further efforts by the government to boost the number of students in nursing and allied health care professions.

14) Malpractice Suits Are Blamed for Rising Health Care Costs

Health care costs have become a hot political topic, and many people have pointed at malpractice lawsuits as a primary cause of rising costs. For years, punitive lawsuits for pain and suffering have levied huge settlements from doctors, hospitals and their insurers. In reaction, premiums for malpractice insurance have burgeoned, growing far faster than the costs for any other type of insurance. Doctors and hospitals, in order to offset malpractice insurance premiums, raise rates and conduct extensive and often unnecessary tests in order to protect themselves from legal accountability. All of these factors contribute significantly to the overall cost of health care in the U.S., and a political battle has ensued, particularly between lobbyists for plantiffs' lawyers and lobbyists for the health care industry.

In addition to adding immense costs to the health care system, malpractice lawsuits have done much to erode the relationship between doctors and their patients. At the same time, fear of malpractice suits can discourage young physicians from pursuing higher-risk specialties, such as obstetrics and surgery, rather than fields where they are much less likely to be sued. Relations between doctors and lawyers have also become strained, with many doctors blaming some lawyers' willingness to take even the most frivolous cases. Meanwhile, it is common for physicians in higher-risk fields to face annual malpractice insurance premiums of $100,000 or more, while clinics and hospitals are paying astronomical insurance premiums.

Some physicians have responded in self-interest. Reports have been published of physicians refusing to treat attorneys, their families or their employees except in cases of emergency. Many would-be patients have learned how hard it can be to get a physician in high-risk fields, such as OB/GYN, to take a new client. In April 2003, the Texas Medical Association reported that during 2002, 62% of Texas physicians began denying or referring high-risk cases, and 52% had stopped providing certain services to their patients. As a result, anecdotes of inconvenient or unavailable care for patients are rife.

Many states are tackling the malpractice awards issue through referendums and legislation that limit total damage awards. Texas is a prime example of a state that has limited non-economic damage awards. By 2000, the state had reached a crisis level: One report compiled in October 2002 showed that 52% of all Texas physicians in the state were subjected to malpractice claims during 2000. Another report found that in the Lower Rio Grande River Valley it was even worse. Claims were growing at 60% a year, and there were 350 claims for every 100 doctors.

In response to situations such as this, many states have passed legislation to limit rewards given to plaintiffs for "non-economic" damages, which include pain, inconvenience, suffering and disfigurement. By early 2003, 26 states had limited non-economic damages in medical malpractice cases, generally to amounts between $250,000 and $500,000 dollars. The statutes also generally limit the amount that lawyers can make off the case via contingency fees, making sure that the plaintiff receives a substantial portion of the reward. Some see such laws as contributing to a failure of the justice system. Others feel that a $250,000 to $500,000 award cap is not fair payment for a patient who has been severely disfigured for life.

On the other hand, there may be few limits on the amount of "economic" damages awarded to a patient—that is, loss of earnings due to the inability to function fully at a job or profession. Patients who earn extremely high salaries may seek damages that are proportionately high—even multimillion-dollar amounts. However, attorneys may be discouraged from taking, on contingency, clients who work in low-paying jobs.

California limits the contingency fee that an attorney can collect under a malpractice claim as follows: 40% of the first $50,000; 33.3% of the next $50,000; 25% of the next $500,000; and 15% of any amount above $600,000. These limits apply whether the damages are collected as a settlement out of court, an award under a lawsuit or an award under arbitration.

As in any other legal matter, there are two sides to the story, and arguments for and against malpractice award limits abound. California is often named as the poster child for how effective such legislation can be in lowering insurance premiums and health care costs in general. From 1975, when California first passed malpractice reform, to 2002, the state's malpractice insurance premiums rose only 167%, compared to the national average of 505% in the same period.

Under the Clinton Administration, the Department of Health & Human Services estimated that a major limit to the malpractice liability of physicians and hospitals could reduce between $60 and $108 billion from the nation's annual expenditures on health because it would reduce the practice of defensive medicine—that is, testing and procedures that are ordered largely to cut exposure to lawsuits rather than increase the quality of care. Federal legislation limiting malpractice awards has yet to be passed. The matter has come before Congress on a number of occasions, but no bill has made it through both the House and the Senate. It may come to a head in the near future, however. It is quite possible that federal legislation limiting pain and suffering rewards could be passed in 2005 or 2006, in a form similar to the laws in California.

15) Patients' Rights Evolve

Is managed care unjustly maligned? Managed care officials have vigorously defended their contributions to the health care system, averring that they have drastically cut costs while subsequently improving the quality of health care by reducing unnecessary treatments and procedures that drove up costs under the old system. It is fair to say that the large number of patient complaints about HMOs and PPOs is in part a consequence of more people using the managed care system. Industry executives are also miffed by what they claim to be one-sided reporting by the media. Individual medical situations can be highly complex, and while some of the problem stories may be one-sided, unsubstantiated or distorted, others are very real.

State legislatures have been extremely active over recent years in protecting patients' rights. Forty-one states plus the District of Columbia have enacted laws requiring that patients are provided with some type of relief when there is a disagreement regarding the type and amount of care needed between an attending physician and a patient's health plan. Typically, these laws call for a prompt review by an independent and objective system. Such a review system was upheld five to four by the U.S. Supreme Court in June 2002.

In 11 states, including Texas, laws have been enacted giving patients the right to sue their health plans for damages incurred when a plan refuses to pay for treatments recommended by a doctor. However, the Supreme Court, in a unanimous decision in June 2004, struck down the landmark Texas law. The court determined that the federal Employee Retirement Income Securities Act of 1974 (ERISA) preempted the Texas law and made it invalid. Health care plan firms involved in the case argued that, in refusing to pay for certain treatments, the companies were making plan coverage decisions, not medical decisions. The court agreed.

A key point here is that patients cannot sue for damages in such a case. However, they may sue in federal court for reimbursement for the actual cost of the denied care. Also, patients in most types of plans still have the right to take their case to an independent review commission to seek coverage. (This right may not apply to patients covered by self-funded plans.)

The Outlook for Health Care Technology

16) Health Care Technology Introduction

In recent years, the health care industry has capitalized on many remarkable advances in medical technology, including breakthroughs in computing, communications, small-incision surgery, drug therapies, diagnostics and instruments. For example, for the first time since the epidemic began, we are seeing real remission in AIDS thanks to advanced therapies that have recently been introduced. In addition, huge advances are being made in the fields of cardiovascular care, cancer care, diagnostic imaging and testing, organ transplants and minimally invasive surgery.

In the area of drug development, new methods, including robotics, miniaturization, genome mapping and high-throughput screening, are helping to provide a clearer understanding of the efficacy of drugs before they are sent into clinical trials. In addition, the FDA has hired legions of employees in recent years to help process applications for new drugs, procedures and equipment.

Meanwhile, more emphasis is being placed on the use of computers and advanced telecommunication technology in many phases of hospital operations and patient care, often in conjunction with complex equipment to diagnose and improve patients' conditions. Moreover, investors are getting into the health care act, putting $4.8 billion in venture money into U.S. health care companies in the first nine months of 2004 alone.

The first part of the 21st Century promises to bring even greater milestones in human health as we begin to reap the benefits of new therapies created through biotechnology and genetic engineering. As our understanding of human biology at the molecular level matures, genetically engineered pharmaceuticals and gene therapies will be developed that target diseases at their molecular origins, thus lessening the need for more costly elements of treatment such as invasive surgery and intensive care. If applied during the early stages of disease development, these new biotechnologies will extend and improve the quality of life for the patient. If the disease has already caused the failure or malfunction of vital organs or tissue, it may one day be possible for the patient to receive a fully functioning, genetically engineered replacement, harvested from cells in the patient's own tissues. Gene mapping and proteomics will allow researchers to halt disease before it becomes symptomatic, and future newborn children may be screened to determine whether they are genetically predisposed to certain diseases. Knowledge obtained from biomedical research will also help to improve the general health of the public by identifying beneficial behavioral changes.

17) Information Technology and Health Care

The Internet

According to a study by The Pew Internet and American Life Project, 80% of people with access to the Internet have used it for gathering health care information at one time or another. Studies by other firms have shown that nearly one-half of people seeking online health information do so to research information on a specific disease, while many others are interested in educational services, prescription drug information, fitness and alternative medicine. About 81% of those who searched for health care information online indicated that what they found was "useful" or "very useful."

Deloitte Touche Tohmatsu reported that, among those online health data seekers, 83% use the Internet at least once daily. Their most common reason for turning to the Internet for health assistance is because a loved one has been diagnosed with a medical condition (40.1%), followed by an interest in changing personal dietary habits (26.3%) and having been diagnosed with a chronic condition (22.1%).

> *Internet Research Tip:*
> According to The Medical Library Association (www.mlanet.org), the top 10 most useful web sites for health care information are:
> National Cancer Institute, www.cancer.gov
> Centers for Disease Control and Prevention (CDC), www.cdc.gov
> FamilyDoctor.org, www.familydoctor.org
> Health Finder, www.healthfinder.gov
> HIV InSite, http://hivinsite.ucsf.edu
> KidsHealth, www.kidshealth.org
> Mayo Clinic, www.mayoclinic.com
> MEDEM Medical Library, www.medem.com/medlib/medlib_entry.cfm
> MEDLINEplus, www.medlineplus.gov
> NOAH: New York Online Access to Health, www.noah-health.org

However, patients seeking health care information on the web should be wary. The bottom line is that if you think you are ill, you should seek professional medical advice. There are virtually no quality controls governing online medical advice. Therefore, while information is easy to get, credible information is not—be sure to consider the source. Since anyone can publish a web site, the depth, quality and breadth of information can vary greatly. "Cyberquacks" pose a serious threat to the integrity of online medical information. Before pouring out personal details in a chat room, be aware that your fellow chatter may not be telling the truth when claiming, for example, to be a cancer survivor or a physician.

> *Internet Research Tip:*
> When researching health care web sites, look for the seal of approval from the Health on the Net Foundation (www.hon.ch), a nonprofit organization based in Geneva, Switzerland. Founded in 1995 at the behest of international medical experts, the foundation approves medical web sites that meet or exceed its guidelines.

The Internet is also radically transforming the relationship between doctor and patient, since patients can obtain information previously not available from traditional resources. A Deloitte Touche Tohmatsu study reported that more than 66% of patients in the U.S. did not receive any informational literature about their condition or their child's condition while at the physician's office, and only one-third received information about their medication. Consumers are now demanding the information necessary to help them make educated decisions regarding medical care. The Internet has allowed patients to walk into their doctors' offices with information in their hands that doctors didn't know about or simply wouldn't supply in the past. Patients can also obtain straightforward information from the web about their diseases. This empowering of the patient forces physicians to treat the patient more like a partner. It is a fundamental shift of knowledge from physician to patient.

In another Internet development, Blue Cross Blue Shield of Florida is offering thousands of physicians the option to be paid for consulting with patients online, via a secure website.

Useful Internet sites can aid patients in finding a specialist, checking to see how a local hospital measures up and obtaining information about prescription drugs. For example, the American Medical Association (www.ama-assn.org) offers a searchable database with information on doctors' educations and specialties. RxList (www.rxlist.com) allows visitors to search for a drug by generic or brand name, learn about its potential side effects, become familiar with warnings and read about clinical studies. One of the most promising health care sites is Medscape.com (www.medscape.com), where consumers can access information on topics ranging from AIDS to women's health.

The Internet is also becoming a useful tool for medical professionals. For example, a surgeon can obtain clinical information relevant to surgical practice, both from general professional sites and through specialty and sub-specialty sites. The surgeon can also follow links to other sites offering information on updated techniques or research and educational opportunities. Online discussion groups are growing in popularity; these forums are useful for physicians with similar interests who wish to share information. Another exciting development is live surgeries that can be viewed via webcams. Surgeons and students all over the world can watch and learn from surgical procedures from the comfort of their own homes or offices.

A promising new service will soon be unveiled thanks to the combined efforts of the American Diabetes Association and the insurance group Kaiser Permanente. Together they are designing a web site for diabetics that will suggest customized treatment plans. It will be based on a complex software program, developed at a cost of several million dollars, that models health care outcomes based on specified criteria such as medication, diet, demographics and exercise. The software accesses a massive database containing years of patient data. The web site, to be called Diabetes PHD, could prove a model for web sites for dozens of other diseases and the patients who suffer from them.

Another Internet innovation that will assist diabetes patients is the ability for physicians to monitor glucose levels online. In late 2003, Medem, Inc. launched an online service that effectively saves these patients from multiple office visits to check blood-glucose levels while giving physicians the ability to evaluate the patient's blood sugar level more frequently. The new tool links glucose meters used by patients to their computers, then transmits that information to a secure server via the Internet.

RFID Inventory Systems

RFID (radio frequency identification) will be a huge breakthrough in hospital inventory management. RFID systems are based on the placement of microchips in product packaging. These chips, continuously broadcasting product identification data, are used with special sensors in handheld devices or on shelves that alert a central inventory management system as to product usage and the need to restock inventory, communicating via wireless means. From loading docks to stockroom shelves to the hospital floor, radio frequency readers will wirelessly track the movement of each and every item, replacing bar codes. These systems will lead to reductions in out-of-stock situations and the elimination of costly manual inventory counts.

This technology was first adopted by Johns Hopkins hospital in order to track bags of intravenous fluid, one of the thousands of possible applications that could save the medical industry much of the estimated $75 billion a year currently lost due to mistakes in the prescription, storage and delivery of drugs. RFID chips and the scanners that look after them are rapidly becoming smaller and cheaper and will likely be steadily adopted for more and more items in hospitals and pharmacies. The transmitter chips could even become small enough to be injectable, making it possible to place them in pills, giving doctors the ability to track prescription compliance. Beyond the monetary savings, RFID systems could save some of the many people who die every year due to medical treatment errors.

RFID tags implanted in the wristbands worn by hospital patients will also reduce patient identification errors, thereby reducing instances of errors in treatment. Data gathered electronically from RFID systems will be integrated with enterprise-wide computer systems throughout the hospital.

The U.S. pharmaceutical industry, with the cooperation of the FDA, will begin voluntary use of RFID tags on containers of prescription drugs in 2005. The FDA is relying on a nonprofit group, EPCglobal in Lawrenceville, N.J., to set standards for the tags, which have the potential to cut down on stolen drugs, counterfeiting of drugs, drug-related fraud and the dispensing of the wrong drugs.. If early use of these tags proves satisfactory, use on all drug containers could become mandatory by 2007.

Advanced Information Technology and Medical Records Technology

> **Internet Research Tip:** The Medical Records Institute, www.medrecinst.com provides in depth discussion of electronic health records at its website. In particular, see the "Health IT Library" page.

There is a strong movement in the United States, the U.K., Canada and elsewhere to implement widespread use of electronic health records (EHRs). A major goal in this movement is to create Continuity of Care Records (CCRs), which would ensure that a patient's health history could be utilized seamlessly by hospitals, primary care physicians and specialists.

The U.S. Department of Health & Human Services estimates that a national electronic health information network could save about $140 billion yearly, or 8% of the nation's health expenditures. This is due to the fact that vast amounts of time and money are wasted on redundant paperwork, billing errors, duplicated tasks and mistreatment of patients due to a lack of complete patient health information at the point of treatment.

America's health care system generates more than 35 billion transactions each year. A primary goal of the health industry is to move as many of these transactions as possible away from phone, fax and mail into electronic systems, databases and secure email. Transferring both these transactions as well as health care records, patient information and insurance information will greatly streamline the health care industry.

The elimination of errors in patient care, in addition to financial savings and productivity improvements, is a major impetus for computerizing the entire health system. The Institute of Medicine estimates that between 44,000 and 98,000 deaths occur in hospitals each year from medical errors, ranging from simple cases of neglect to giving patients incorrect medications to extreme cases such as performing the wrong surgery. Information technology (IT) is seen as a cure for accidental in-hospital mortality rates, as well as the road to the promised land of efficiencies in costs and time. The health care industry lagged behind almost all other business sectors in 2003, spending just under 4% of its revenue on IT, in contrast to many other industries that have been averaging 5% to 8%. However, this is starting to change. Gartner (a major research firm) projects health care industry spending on IT to rise from $34 billion in 2001 to nearly $48 billion in 2006—the second-fastest area for IT growth after the Federal Government. A recent survey by the Health Information Management and Systems Society found that 60% of U.S. hospitals are utilizing, installing or planning to install systems to handle electronic patient records.

Developments in the U.K.'s public health system will likely spur the American effort to digitize medical records and patient care. In December 2003, England's National Health Service (NHS) announced plans for a $17 billion project to wire every hospital, doctor's office and clinic by 2008. The British government is supplying $3.9 billion for a three-year period beginning in 2004, to be followed by another $13 billion. When complete, information on each and every one of the 50 million patients registered in the U.K. national system will reside in a central database. Appointments and referrals will be scheduled online, and doctors' orders and prescriptions will be transmitted automatically to other caregivers and pharmacies. The system could very well serve as the model for electronic records and digitized patient care for the rest of the world.

Several U.S. technology companies, including IBM, are bidding for the lucrative contracts that split the U.K. job into several multi-million-dollar projects. One major contract concerns the national database of patient records. Five additional contracts will address regional networks, which will communicate with the central database. Another $108 million contract has already been granted to SchlumbergerSema to handle online appointment booking.

In Canada, another ambitious technical initiative is underway. The Canadian government is investing $844 million in electronic health records systems. The goal is to link 50% of the country's medical community. Experts estimate that an additional $1.07 billion will be necessary to take the project from coast to coast so that all Canadian health records will be digital.

One of the most important forces in enabling health care providers to garner the power of information technology has been *Web*MD Corporation (www.webmd.com), originally known as Healtheon/*Web*MD. This firm has invested billions of dollars in creating a seamless, Internet-based system that collects and stores patient data, while providing back-office physician practice, clinical and laboratory accounting and management functions. More importantly, it keeps track of billings, presents those bills to payors automatically and collects for the health care providers. *Web*MD, conceived in 1996 by famous technology entrepreneur Jim Clark, already connects hundreds of thousands of physicians with tens of thousands of facilities, laboratories, clinics and payors. In 2003, the company processed over 2.5 billion transactions. It has made dozens of acquisitions and mergers, including the acquisition of Envoy, the world's largest electronic claims processor.

Seven of the largest health insurers banded together in 2000 to create a major competitor to *Web*MD: MedUnite. The company was a coalition by Aetna, Anthem, Cigna, Heath Net, Oxford, PacifiCare and WellPoint Health Systems. In 2002, MedUnite was acquired by ProxyMed, Inc., another online physician service provider. Though still only a tenth the size of its competitor, processing 227 million transactions in 2003, ProxyMed is rapidly growing its services to meet the standard set by WebMD.

Growth in health care transaction processing is still far from over. These two firms still make up only a small portion of the billions of transactions that occur every year, such as billing, prescription processing, insurance claims and so on.

The computer industry is also struggling to convert physicians to the use of PCs and Internet devices. For example, there are dozens of competing platforms attempting to get doctors to use wireless Palm-type devices (PDAs) to prescribe medications. This practice reduces medical errors, since electronic orders are easily legible and can be checked for conflicts with other medications currently taken by the patient. The PDAs check and notify physicians of drugs not covered by insurance or those to which a patient is allergic. Some systems can transmit physicians' orders directly to a local server, which then generates a fax to a pharmacy or clinic. To eliminate fraud, doctors submit electronic signatures for verification, and drug store systems check for recognized fax numbers.

As more physicians and clinics digitize, the need for standardization grows. A consortium, RxHub (www.rxhub.net), has created a standard electronic prescription format, and is currently looking for acceptance from the government, pharmacies and health care providers.

Other digital health care systems include electronic medical records and web sites on which patients and physicians take a team approach to care. Today, nurses using advanced systems can keep hospital patients' charts on computer screens by the bedside. Physicians can speak to voice-recognition-driven computers that instantly create patient files during examinations and procedures.

As hospitals and other major health care service providers scramble to digitize, concerns about the quality of patient care have been voiced. As a result, caregivers and insurers have combined forces to monitor the changes brought about by the technological boom. The Leapfrog Group, a coalition of over 160 companies and private organizations that provide health care benefits, was created to improve, among other things, the flow of patient data. Leapfrog has set exacting standards for the health system to strive for in the creation and utilization of digital data. "Leapfrog compliance" is a catch phrase among hospitals, which are rated on the organization's web site (www.leapfroggroup.org) with regard to compliance issues such as computerized prescription order systems and statistics on staffing and medical procedure success rates.

Many medical innovations are becoming widespread. For example, "med carts" equipped with computers and bar code scanners allow nurses to scan patients' identifying wristbands to verify identity and medication orders, improving safety and efficiency. These carts will evolve to use RFID instead of bar codes. In addition, examination and operating rooms are now often equipped with wireless laptops that transmit on-the-spot notes and evaluations for each patient to a central information system.

IT innovations continue to flood the health care market. Siemens Medical, a manufacturer of medical equipment such as MRI and ultrasound machines, has developed a patient information system called Soarian. The Soarian system is designed to optimize information-based processes throughout the entire cycle of a patient's hospitalization, including administration, diagnosis, clinic, care, therapy and dismissal. Likewise, GE Healthcare has created an IT system, marketed under the brand name Centricity, that comprises a substantial portion of the GE subsidiary's $14 billion in annual sales.

McKesson Corporation, a major pharmaceutical supply management and health care information technology company, debuted its Horizon Physician Portal in 2002. The system is an online gateway that connects various hospital systems so that physicians can view and personalize patient information including laboratory and radiology results, transcriptions, vital statistics and orders for tests and medications. Other major software firms are also getting into the act; Microsoft has a health care industry solutions group, as do SAP, PeopleSoft and Oracle.

A leader of the pack in IT-savvy medical centers is Indiana Heart Hospital, completed in 2003, which outsources all of its technology needs to GE Medical Systems. With one-fourth of its $60 million construction budget earmarked for IT systems, the 88-bed facility is almost completely digital. Staff members have received intensive training on how to alter their practices and workflow to make use of state-of-the-art systems through 650 computer terminals (there are more computers at Indiana Heart than there are doctors). By keeping transactions largely paperless, the facility has done away with nurses' stations, chart racks and a medical records department. This amounts to savings of $500,000 that would have been spent on copiers, printers and filing cabinets, as well as building space that would have amounted to about $230 per square foot. Indiana Heart operates at full capacity with a staff of 285, compared to the 400 usually needed to run a facility of that size. Patient stays are abbreviated, thanks to more efficient information retrieval. The average hospital stay for a heart attack patient is five days, while at Indiana Heart the same patient goes home in three. There is more good news in the facility's accounting department; its average time period for collection of receivables is only 45 days, compared to 60 days in most clinics.

Consolidated Health Informatics Initiative Attracts Millions in Government Funds

Since it pays over $400 billion in yearly health care bills through Medicare and Medicaid, the Federal Government has enormous clout in shaping the health care system of the future. The Consolidated Health Informatics Initiative (CHI) is a major government-backed initiative to help the health system evolve.

In his fiscal year 2005 budget, President Bush has asked Congress for several million dollars to support the development of local health information networks and to fund the build out of several demonstration projects, which would enable a physician treating a patient to have information about all other care the patient has received. These local networks would be able to communicate with one another in a dispersed national network of local and regional systems. This action moves the nation closer to having a national, interoperable health information infrastructure that would allow quick, reliable and secure access to information needed for patient care, while protecting patient privacy. Such a system would allow a doctor or health care provider to access an always-up-to-date electronic health record of a patient who has agreed to be part of the system, regardless of when and where the patient receives care. During 2004, President Bush established a national goal of assuring that most Americans have electronic health records by 2015.

The U.S. health care sector, after lagging behind other industries in IT spending for years, will now have the highest growth rate in IT spending over the mid term, resulting in vast opportunities for profits at hardware, software and consulting firms. One major hurdle to overcome is the need for different information systems to communicate with each other. This is problematic at best, since medical systems that are currently in place have been written in a variety of languages using a host of different protocols. The Institute of Medicine, an advisory group associated with the National Academy of Sciences, is working on a standardized health record, for which there is already a functional model. In Washington, D.C. the newly created position of the National Health Information Technology Coordinator will oversee the creation of standards and the transition to digital health records.

Standards Adopted for the Consolidated Health Informatics Initiative (CHI)

As part of the CHI initiative, the Department of Health and Human Services (HHS) and the other federal departments that deliver health care services–the Departments of Defense and Veterans Affairs–are working with other federal agencies to identify appropriate, existing data standards and to endorse them for use across the federal health care sector. These include:

- Health Level 7 (HL7) vocabulary standards for demographic information, units of measure, immunizations, clinical encounters and HL7's Clinical Document Architecture standard for text-based reports.
- The College of American Pathologists Systematized Nomenclature of Medicine Clinical Terms (SNOMED CT) for laboratory result contents, non-laboratory interventions and procedures, anatomy, diagnosis and problems and nursing. HHS is making SNOMED-CT available for use in the United States at no charge to users.
- Laboratory Logical Observation Identifier Name Codes (LOINC) to standardize the electronic exchange of laboratory test orders and drug label section headers.
- The Health Insurance Portability and Accountability Act of 1996 (HIPAA) transactions and code sets for electronic exchange of health related information to perform billing or administrative functions. These are the same standards now required under HIPAA for health plans, health care clearinghouses and those health care providers who engage in certain electronic transactions.
- A set of federal terminologies related to medications, including the Food and Drug Administration's names and codes for ingredients, manufactured dosage forms, drug products and medication packages; the National Library of Medicine's RxNORM for describing clinical drugs; and the Veterans Administration's National Drug File Reference Terminology (NDF-RT) for specific drug classifications.
- The Human Gene Nomenclature (HUGN) for exchanging information regarding the role of genes in biomedical research in the federal health sector.
- The Environmental Protection Agency's Substance Registry System for non- medicinal chemicals of importance to health care.

Of major concern with regard to electronic health care records is patient privacy. HIPAA rules mandate that doctors, hospitals, pharmacies and other providers must limit patient information disclosure. Doctors must now give patients written "notice of privacy practices" and post this information prominently in their offices. Patients may receive copies of their records, including doctor's notes, lab results and data collected by their insurance companies. Violation of any of the privacy compliance rules may result in a $250,000 fine and up to 10 years in prison.

Computer Modeling

In recent times, impressive advances in computer modeling have lead to accurate mapping of very complex systems, including weather, planetary systems and molecular interaction. Health care is another natural application of these capabilities. Everything from genes to bodily systems could possibly be mapped by computers, with the benefit of learning more about the complex interactions that go on. The technology for mapping genes has now been around for quite awhile; the technology for mapping other biological entities has been sadly absent. But many scientists have now realized the benefits that could be gained from advanced mapping of the body and all the processes that go on within it. Think of all the innovations computer modeling has brought to the automobile industry, which can now design a car in a matter of months, predict how the car will perform in crashes, how it will handle, its wind resistance and how it will wear down over time. Now imagine a similar instance in health care: being able to model a complete human body, where things might go wrong, or how it will react to certain chemicals. Drug development and diagnosis are two obvious areas where health care might benefit for computer modeling.

One of the most promising uses of modeling is in analyzing patient care outcomes to project the best possible treatment for specific diseases and ailments. Patient records are kept in increasingly powerful databases, which can be analyzed to find the history of treatment outcomes. For the first time, payors such as HMOs and insurance companies have vast amounts of data available to them, including answers to questions such as:

• Which procedures and surgeries do and do not bring the desired results?
• Which physicians and hospitals have the highest and lowest rates of cure (or of untimely deaths of patients)?
• What is the average length of stay required for the treatment and recovery of patients undergoing various surgeries?
• How long should it take for the rehabilitation of a patient with a worker's compensation claim for a specific type of injury?

The knowledge available will soon be essentially unlimited, and the result will be higher efficiency and common use of the most effective treatment and rehabilitation regimens.

Scientists at Oxford in England, as well as at the University of California, San Diego and several other universities, have been developing models of the heart, liver and other organs, hoping to eventually build a complete model of the human body. The project to model the heart is made to mimic everything from chemical reactions up through cellular reactions, all coalescing to make an almost perfect model of the heart. In this way, scientists can construct a "normal" heart, and then compare it to images of irregular or diseased hearts, in order to find out what goes wrong and, possibly, what could fix them. Novartis, a leading drug manufacturer, is already using a model of the heart to predict how the heart will react to different drugs, hoping to come up with a compound that can keep hearts healthy or heal them after a heart attack.

Internet Research Tip: Body Computer Modeling

There are now several companies that are working on modeling the human body:

Artesian Therapeutics, Gaithersburg, MD
    www.artesianrx.com
Immersion Medical, Gaithersburg, MD
    www.immersion.com/medical
Insilicomed, La Jolla, CA
    www.insilicomed.com
Predix Pharmaceuticals, Woburn, MA
    www.predixpharm.com

---

18)   **Stem Cells and Tissue Engineering**

Controversy in U.S. while Research Flourishes Overseas:

During the 1980s, a biologist at Stanford University, Irving L. Weissman, was the first to isolate the stem cell that builds human blood (the mammalian hematopoietic cell). Later, Weissman isolated a stem cell in a laboratory mouse and went on to co-found SysTemix, Inc. (now part of drug giant Novartis) and StemCells, Inc. to continue this work in a commercial manner.

In November 1998, two different university-based groups of researchers announced that they had accomplished the first isolation and characterization of the human embryonic stem cell (ESC). One group was led by James A. Thomson at the University of Wisconsin at Madison. The second was led by John D. Gearhart at the Johns Hopkins University School of Medicine in Baltimore. The ESC is among the most versatile basic building blocks in the human body. Embryos, when first conceived, begin creating small numbers of ESCs, and these cells eventually differentiate and develop into the more than 200 cell types that make up the distinct tissues and organs of the human body, from bones to brains. If scientists can reproduce and then guide the development of these basic ESCs, then they could theoretically grow replacement organs and tissues in the laboratory—even such complicated tissue as brain cells or heart cells.

Ethical and regulatory difficulties have arisen from the fact that the only source for human "embryonic" stem cells is, logically enough, human embryos. A laboratory can obtain these cells in one of three ways: 1) by inserting a patient's DNA into an egg, thus producing a blastocyst that is a clone of the patient—which is then destroyed after only a few days of development; 2) by harvesting stem cells from aborted fetuses; or 3) by harvesting stem cells from embryos that are left over and unused after an in vitro fertilization of a hopeful mother. (Artificial in vitro fertilization requires the creation of a large number of test tube embryos per instance, but only one of these embryos is used in the final process.)

A rich source of similar but "non-embryonic" stem cells is bone marrow. Doctors have been performing bone marrow transplants in humans for years. This procedure essentially harnesses the healing power of stem cells, which proliferate to create healthy new blood cells in the recipient. Several other non-embryonic stem cell sources have great promise (see "Potential methods of developing 'post-embryonic' stem cells without the use of human embryos" below).

In the fall of 2001, a small biotech company called Advanced Cell Technology announced the first cloning of a human embryo. The announcement set off yet another firestorm of rhetoric and debate on the scientific and ethical questions that cloning and related stem cell technologies inspire. While medical researchers laud the seemingly infinite possibilities stem cells promise for fighting disease and the aging process, conservative theologians, policy makers and pro-life groups decry the harvest of cells from aborted fetuses and the possibility of cloning as an ethical and moral abomination.

The U.S. Congress has banned the use of federal funding for the creation of new embryonic stem cell lines. This action was taken in spite of impassioned testimony regarding the healing potential of stem cells from physicians, researchers and celebrities such as actor Michael J. Fox on behalf of research for Parkinson's disease, the late Christopher Reeve for spinal injury study and former first lady Nancy Reagan on behalf of Alzheimer's research.

Stem cell research has been underway for years at biotech companies including Stem Cells, Inc., Geron and ViaCell. One company, Osiris Therapeutics, has been at work long enough to have several clinical trial programs in progress. The potential benefits are staggering. Through stem cell therapies, neurological disorders might be aided with the growth of healthy cells in the brain. Injured cells in the spinal column might be regenerated. Damaged organs such as hearts, livers and kidneys might be infused with healthy cells.

Potential methods of developing "post-embryonic" stem cells without the use of human embryos:
- Parthenogenesis—manipulation of unfertilized eggs.
- Adult Stem Cells—harvesting of stem cells from bone marrow or brain tissue.
- Other Cells—harvesting of stem cells from human placentas or other cells.
- De-Differentiation—using the nucleus of an existing cell, such as a skin cell, that is altered by an egg that has had its own nucleus removed.
- Transdifferentiation—making a skin cell de-differentiate back to its primordial state so that it can then morph into a useable organ cell, such as heart tissue.

ESCs (typically harvested from five-day-old human embryos which are destroyed during the process) are used because of their ability to evolve into any cell or tissue in the body. Their versatility is undeniable, yet the implications of the death of the embryo are at the heart of the ethical and moral concerns.

Meanwhile, scientists have discovered that there are stem cells in existence in many diverse places in the adult human body, and they are thus succeeding in creating stem cells without embryos from "post-embryonic" cells. Such cells are already showing the ability to differentiate and function in animal and human recipients. Best of all, these types of stem cells are not plagued by problems found in the use of ESCs, such as the tendency for ESCs to form tumors when they develop into differentiated cells. However, Thomas Okarma, CEO and President of Geron, argues that stem cells derived from bone marrow and other adult sources are fundamentally limited in their application, because it is nearly impossible to get them to produce anything besides blood cells, making it very difficult to harvest organ or nerve cells.

In December 2002 Stanford University in Palo Alto, California, announced plans to develop a privately funded library of human stem cell lines, meaning that it will be able to operate outside of the restrictions placed on federally funded ESC research and development. It was the first U.S. university to take this path.

Therapeutic Cloning Techniques Advance:

For scientists, the biggest challenge at present may be to discover the exact process by which stem cells are signaled to differentiate. Another big challenge lies in the fact that broad use of therapeutic cloning may require immense numbers of human eggs in which to grow blastocysts.

The clearest path to "therapeutic" cloning may lie in "autologous transplantation." In this method, a tiny amount of a patient's muscle or other tissue would be harvested. This sample's genetic material would then be de-differentiated, that is, reduced to a simple, unprogrammed state. The patient's DNA sample would then be inserted into an egg to grow a blastocyst. The blastocyst would be manipulated so that its stem cells would differentiate into the desired type of tissue, such as heart tissue. That newly grown tissue would then be transplanted to the patient's body. Many obstacles must be overcome before such transplants can become commonplace, but there is definitely potential to completely revolutionize healing through such regenerative, stem cell-based processes.

One type of bone marrow stem cell, recently discovered by scientists at the University of Minnesota, appears to have a wide range of differentiation capability, which means that it may become the first cell type to be widely used to grow useful replacement tissue in the laboratory.

It is instructive to note that there are two distinct types of embryonic cloning: "reproductive" cloning and "therapeutic" cloning. While they have similar beginnings, the desired end results are vastly different.

"Reproductive" cloning is a method of producing an exact copy of an animal—or potentially an exact copy of a human being. A scientist would remove the nucleus from a donor's unfertilized egg, insert a nucleus from the animal or human to be copied, and then stimulate the nucleus to begin dividing to form an embryo. In the case of a mammal, the embryo would then be implanted in the uterus of a host female for gestation and birth. The successful birth of a cloned human baby does not necessarily mean that a healthy adult human will result. To date, cloned animals have tended to develop severe health problems. For example, a U.S. firm, Advanced Cell Technology, reported that it had engineered the birth of cloned cows that appeared healthy at first but developed severe health problems after a few years.

On the other hand, "therapeutic" cloning is a method of reproducing exact copies of cells needed for research or for the development of replacement tissue. Once again a scientist removes the nucleus from a donor's unfertilized egg, inserts a nucleus from the animal or human whose cells are to be copied, and then stimulates the nucleus to begin dividing to form an embryo. However, in therapeutic use, the embryo would never be allowed to grow to any significant stage of development. Instead, it would be allowed to grow for a few hours or days, at which point stem cells would be removed for use in regenerating tissue.

Because it can provide a source of stem cells, cloning has uses in regenerative medicine that can be vital in treating many types of disease. The main differences between stem cells derived from clones and those derived from aborted fetuses or fertility specimens is that they are made from only one source of genes, rather than by mixing sperm and eggs. Furthermore, they are made specifically for scientific purposes, rather than being existing specimens. Cloned stem cells have the added advantage of being 100% compatible with their donors, sharing the same genes, and so would provide the best possible source for replacement organs and tissues. Although the use of cloning for regeneration has stirred heated debate, it has not resulted in universal rejection. Most of the industrialized countries, including Canada, Russia, most of Western Europe and most of Asia, have made some government-sanctioned allowances for research into this area.

As a result of this permissiveness, some countries have already made progress in the field of regenerative cloning. At Shanghai Second Medical University, for example, Dr. Huizhen Sheng managed to produce cloned embryos by placing living human skin cells inside genetically "stripped" rabbit eggs. The embryos developed long enough for stem cells to be harvested, after which they were destroyed. Another successful experiment was carried out in South Korea by a team of researchers led by Dr. Hwang Woo Suk, a professor at Seoul National University. In this instance, human female eggs were implanted with ovarian cells. Chemicals triggered a reaction that led to embryonic development in one of the 242 eggs used. These techniques are currently inefficient and unpredictable, but human cloning has now been proven possible.

In an important development in August 2004, scientists at Newcastle University in the U.K. announced that they have been granted permission by the Human Fertilisation and Embryology Authority (HFEA), a unit of the British Government, to create human embryos as a source of stem cells for certain therapeutic purposes. Specifically, researchers will clone early-stage embryos in search of new treatments for such degenerative diseases as Parkinson's disease, Alzheimer's and diabetes. The embryos will be destroyed before they are two weeks old and will therefore not develop beyond a tiny cluster of cells.

A New Era of Regenerative Medicine Begins:

Many firms are conducting product development and research in the areas of skin replacement, vascular tissue replacement, bone grafting or regeneration and stem cells, as well as transgenic organs harvested from pigs for use in humans. At its highest and most promising level, regenerative medicine may eventually utilize human stem cells to create virtually any type of replacement organ or tissue. Since the ability of most human tissue to repair itself is a result of the activity of these cells, the potential that cultured stem cells have for transplant medicine and basic developmental biology is enormous.

In one recent exciting experiment, doctors took stem cells from bone marrow and injected them into the hearts of patients undergoing bypass surgery. The study showed that the bypass patients who received the stem cells were pumping blood 24% better than patients who had not received them.

In an experiment conducted by Dr. Mark Keating at Harvard, the first evidence was gathered showing that stem cells may be used for regenerating lost limbs and organs. The regenerative abilities of amphibians have long been known, but exactly how they do it, or how it could be applied to mammals, has been little understood. Much of the regenerative challenge lies in differentiation, or the development of stem cells into different types of adult tissue such as muscle and bone. Creatures such as amphibians have the ability to turn their complex cells back into stem cells in order to regenerate lost parts. In an experiment, Dr. Keating made a serum from the regenerating nub (stem cells) of a newt's leg and applied it to adult mouse cells in a petri dish. He observed the mouse cells to "de-differentiate," or turn into stem cells. In a later experiment, de-differentiated cells were turned back into muscle, bone and fat. These experiments could be the first steps to true human regeneration.

The potential of the relatively young science of tissue engineering appears to be unlimited. Transgenics (the use of organs and tissues grown in laboratory animals for transplantation to humans) is considered by many to have great future potential, and improvements in immune system suppression will eventually make it possible for the human body to tolerate foreign tissue instead of rejecting it. There is also increasing theoretical evidence that malfunctioning or defective vital organs such as livers, bladders and kidneys could be replaced with perfectly functioning "neo-organs" (like spare parts) grown in the laboratory from the patient's own stem cells, with minimal risk of rejection.

Diabetics who are forced to cope with daily insulin injection treatments could also benefit from engineered tissues. If they could receive a fully functioning replacement pancreas, diabetics might throw away their hypodermic needles once and for all. This could also save the health care system immense sums, since diabetics tend to suffer from many ailments that require hospitalization and intensive treatment, including blindness, organ failure, diabetic coma and circulatory diseases.

Elsewhere, the harvesting of replacement cartilage, which does not require the growth of new blood vessels, is being used to repair damaged joints and treat urological disorders. Genzyme Corp. recently won FDA approval for its replacement cartilage product Carticel. Genzyme's process involves harvesting the patient's own cartilage-forming cells and re-growing new cartilage from those cells in the laboratory. The physician then injects the new cartilage into the damaged area. Full regeneration of the replacement cartilage is expected to take up to 18 months. The Genzyme process can cost up to $30,000, compared to $10,000 for typical cartilage surgery, and many patients who want this new therapy can't get their health plans to pay for it. Other companies are exploring alternative methods that may be less expensive and therefore more attractive to payors.

> ***Internet Research Tip:***
> For an excellent primer on genetics and basic biotechnology techniques, see:
> **National Center for Biotechnology Information**
> www.ncbi.nlm.nih.gov

Gene Therapy

In a groundbreaking procedure at New York-Presbyterian Hospital, a patient received gene therapy to treat Parkinson's disease. Parkinson's is a nervous disorder associated with the death of certain brain cells, causing a drop in the production of dopamine, a vital chemical for brain function. The patient was injected with a gene-laden virus that would theoretically stimulate the creation of dopamine. Though this was a controversial procedure, the possible benefits over more traditional treatments are astounding. Previous treatments of Parkinson's have involved either dopamine injections, which patients could become resistant to, or the implantation of a device that stimulates appropriate neurons in the brain, which many patients are hesitant to accept.

> ***Internet Research Tip:*** For the latest biotech developments check out www.biospace.com and www.bio.org.

> ***Companies to Watch:*** StemCells, Inc. in Palo Alto, California (www.stemcellsinc.com) has isolated and cultured human neural stem cells and is currently working on applications in the treatment of degenerative neural disorders. ViaCell, Inc. in Boston (www.viacellinc.com) develops therapies using umbilical cord and bone marrow stems.

19) Personalized Medicine, New Drugs and New Drug Delivery Methods

Genetics and Personalized Medicine

Scientists now believe that almost all diseases have some genetic component. For example, some people have a genetic predisposition to breast cancer or heart disease. Understanding of human genetics will likely lead to breakthroughs in gene therapy for many ailments, allowing us to avoid the suffering caused by hundreds of types of genetic diseases. Organizations ranging from the Mayo Clinic to drug giant GlaxoSmithKline are experimenting with personalized drugs that are designed to provide appropriate therapies based on a patient's personal genetic makeup.

The ultimate goal of all of this activity is for physicians to be able to examine a genetic model of a patient's DNA, determine from there whether a particular drug will work effectively without daunting side effects and thus prescribe the drug that is most likely to effect the desired cure. This could be described as "predictive, preventive medicine."

For example, drugs that target the genetic origins of tumors will offer more effective, longer-lasting and far less toxic alternatives to conventional chemotherapy and radiation. An exciting drug that attacks cancer at its genetic roots is called Herceptin, which was developed by Genentech. Approved by the FDA in 1998, Herceptin, when used in conjunction with chemotherapy, shows great promise in significantly reducing breast cancer. Herceptin also shows potential in treating other types of cancer, such as ovarian, pancreatic and prostate cancer.

Extensive research is also being conducted related to the genetic defects responsible for congenital diseases such as sickle cell anemia. Researchers are experimenting with inserting healthy genetic material directly into cells to replace or repair defective or missing genes. Animal research is beginning to give way to clinical trials. In a recent rodent model, gene therapy was also used to alter a donor liver prior to surgery so that the immune system of the recipient became permanently tolerant of the new organ without the aid of immunosuppressive drugs. A one-time gene therapy treatment could be a source of cost control for the health care industry, because immunosuppressive drugs are costly and make the patient vulnerable to infections, cancer and other complications. In addition, gene therapy in animal models is giving researchers a clearer understanding of rheumatoid arthritis, which currently afflicts about 2.1 million Americans.

Other applications of gene therapy are already in use for treatment of certain conditions, such as rare immune system disorders. In addition, the FDA has approved gene therapy for use in certain cancer and other disease treatments. As a result, melanoma and cystic fibrosis may be treatable by gene therapy within a few years, which would greatly extend the life span of victims and significantly reduce their rates of hospitalization. Extensive research is underway to identify myriad other possible applications.

Genetic research is rapidly leading to breakthroughs in dozens of vital areas of medicine.

For example, a recently discovered gene appears to play a major role in the most widespread of the more than 30 different types of congenital heart defects, the most common of all human birth defects. Genes that are used by bacteria to trigger the infection process have also been identified, which could lead to powerful vaccines and antibiotics against life-threatening bacteria such as salmonella.

In the area of heart disease, about 300,000 patients per year undergo bypass surgeries in an effort to increase blood flow to and from the heart. Clogged arteries are bypassed with arteries moved from the leg or elsewhere in the patient's body. Genetic experts have now developed the biobypass. That is, they have determined which genes and human proteins create a condition known as angiogenesis, which is the growth of new blood vessels that can increase blood flow without traumatic bypass surgery. This technique may become widespread in the near future.

> ***Companies to Watch:*** Amgen, Thousand Oaks, California; Aventis, Schiltigheim, France; Centocor, Malvern, Pennsylvania; ICOS, Bothell, Washington; Schering-Plough, Kenilworth, New Jersey; Genzyme Corporation, Cambridge, Massachusetts; Valentis, Burlingame, California; Targeted Genetics, Seattle, Washington.

Lifestyle Drugs

Today's era of lifestyle drugs will continue to have major effects on the pharmaceutical industry, as new drugs are developed to treat diseases or disorders commonly associated with the aging baby-boom population. These conditions range from those that cause inconvenience to problems that severely impair quality of life. They include such conditions as baldness, partial memory loss, osteoporosis, impotence and Alzheimer's disease.

Other New Drugs

The rampant overuse of antibiotics in the U.S. has given rise to a number of bacteria impervious to nearly every class of antibiotics. Subsequently, new, more effective drugs are needed to ward off drug-resistant bacteria. To meet this need, Cubist Pharmaceuticals developed a new antibiotic called Cubicin. FDA-approved in September 2003, it is an injectable form of doptamycin used for the treatment of a variety of bacterial infections including strep throat, staph infections and skin infections.

Methods of chemical tailoring have made possible the development of targeted drugs. These methods produce commercially successful drugs for treatment of hypertension, high cholesterol, ulcers, bone loss, stress, depression, severe acne and other maladies. For example, ACE (angiotensin-converting enzyme) inhibitors and other drugs aid in recovery from heart attacks, and there is growing evidence that some may be effective in preventing the onset of congestive heart failure. Two drugs, streptokinase and urokinase, are effective clot dissolvers, serving as cheaper alternatives to TPA (tissue-type plasminogen activators) for treating heart attacks. When combined with aspirin, their efficacy approaches that of TPA. Another clot-dissolving drug, anistreplase, can be administered by intravenous injection and works in five minutes or less, as opposed to one to three hours for the other drugs. This drug may expand the use of clot-dissolving therapy to ambulance teams and small emergency rooms.

Drugs for other previously untreatable diseases are in the pipeline. Novartis released the first new drug to treat the "wet form" of age-related macular degeneration, the number-one cause of blindness in people over age 50. Visudyne, is a light-activated injected drug, used in conjunction with a low-temperature laser to eliminate the abnormal blood vessels that cause the condition.

New Drug Delivery Systems

Controlling how drugs are delivered is a huge business. Sales of drugs using new drug delivery systems is expected to balloon to $30 billion by 2007, up from $9.8 billion in 1998.

Before the biotech age, drugs were generally comprised of small chemical molecules capable of being absorbed by the stomach and passed into the blood stream—drugs that were swallowed as pills or liquids. However, many new biotech drugs require delivery directly into the bloodstream, because they are based on larger molecules that cannot be absorbed by the stomach. Many new drug delivery techniques that provide an alternative to injections are in development.

In the near future there may be an implantable microchip, controlled by a miniature computer capable of releasing variable doses of multiple potent medications over an extended period, potentially up to one year. The miniscule silicon chips will bear a series of tiny wells, sealed with membranes that dissolve and release the contents when a command is received by the computer. Chips that can receive commands beamed through the skin are also conceptually possible. This technology would help treatment of conditions such as Parkinson's disease or cancer, where doctors need to vary medications and dosages. This technology must first be tested in animals and then in humans to ensure that the chips are biocompatible. The chips will more likely be used first in external applications, which may facilitate laboratory testing and drug development.

Other potential needle-free drug delivery systems include synthetic molecules attached to a drug, making it harder for the stomach to render the medicine useless before it reaches the blood. High-tech inhalers that force medicine through the lungs and biotech drugs that can be imbibed are also in the works. For the patient, this means less pain and the promise of better outcomes. Needle-free systems may also make toxic drugs safer and give older drugs new life. For example, the painkiller Fetanyl was recently converted into a lozenge. Alkermes and Alza Corp. are developing techniques to encapsulate or rearrange drug molecules into more sturdy compounds that release steady, even doses over a prolonged period. A patch being developed by Alza Corp., a subsidiary of Johnson & Johnson, has a network of microscopic needles that penetrate painlessly into the first layer of the skin. In addition, Alza is in competition with Vyteris to develop a patch that delivers drugs via a small electric current, activated by a button on the patch itself. Another device, made by Sontra Medical Corp., uses ultrasound and gel to agitate and open temporary pores in the skin that can then receive a drug.

20) Advances in Cancer Research

Improvements in Chemotherapy

Chemotherapy continues to reduce the need for surgical excision of cancers and treat cancers that are considered inoperable. Improvements in chemotherapy continue to reduce the number and severity of side effects and the length of treatment, boosting a shift from inpatient to outpatient care. Recent developments in the treatment of leukemia, for example, show much promise. Although some cancers show resistance to chemotherapy, researchers have recently discovered a unique gene that causes resistance, so compounds may be added to chemotherapy that will block the gene's ability to resist. In many cases chemotherapy is combined with radiation and/or surgery. For example, a recent study showed that chemotherapy in combination with radiation therapy might reduce death from cervical cancer by as much as 50%.

Nuclear Medicine

Radiation therapy and nuclear medicine are currently used in the treatment of cancers and benign tumors. Treatment can involve the use of radioisotopes and x-rays at various energy levels. Because different isotopes have distinct properties and are absorbed differently in the tissues of the body, nuclear medicine also plays an important role in testing and diagnosis.

This technology has been moving toward greater precision in irradiating tumors. High-energy x-ray equipment can focus on and attack tumors while doing less damage to surrounding tissue. Some newer therapeutic isotopes can shrink tumors quite rapidly. New implantation techniques put radiation sources near or directly within tumors to accelerate the destruction of malignant cells, leaving the surrounding tissue largely unaffected. An example of this is the treatment of early-stage breast cancer without a mastectomy.

Refinements in these technologies expand the role of nuclear medicine in the hospital, creating more specialties and more technical positions. At the same time, improvements in treatment and diagnosis can reduce hospitalization and lengths of stay in hospitals.

Treating Cancer with Electricity

Another new high-tech tool for treating certain types of cancer is a short burst of electricity directed at the tumor. This process, called electroporation, involves treating the tumor with chemotherapy and then sending short electrical pulses into the tumor with a needle electrode. The electrical pulse allows the tumor to become more porous and thus more susceptible to the chemotherapeutic drugs.

Genetronics is a leading company in the new field of electroporation therapy. The company's main device for the delivery of the therapy is the MedPulser Electroporation Therapy System, first introduced in 1998. The device is currently in Phase III clinical trials. In initial tests for the treatment of head and neck cancer, 10 patients were treated with electroporation. All 10 experienced tumor shrinkage, and five experienced significant tumor reduction. Genetronics is also in collaboration with several biotech and pharmaceutical companies to develop drugs to be used in conjunction with electroporation.

Viruses

A new weapon for the war on cancer is a growing assortment of viruses that replicate in tumors and kill them, sparing the healthy tissue. Viruses are also being developed with the ability to carry a gene into the cancer, making the tumor more vulnerable to radiation and chemotherapy. This new method will also lessen the side effects associated with conventional treatments.

Onyx Pharmaceuticals and Calydon (now part of Cell Genesys) pioneered the modern application of viruses to cancer cells, using variants of the adenovirus (the cause of the common cold) to attack tumorous cells. Research continues at various biotechnology companies and institutions such as Johns Hopkins and the University of Alabama. One of the most prevalent techniques is engineering the viruses to attack cells with certain active proteins or enzymes. For example, a virus that attacks cells with excessive amounts of melanin (the protein that makes cells darken) could be used for the destruction of melanoma cancer cells. Some of these viruses are currently going through Phase I and II clinical trials and may be available to the public in just a few years.

Vaccines

Though not quite as amazing as the name suggests, cancer vaccines will certainly make an impression on the way cancer is treated. The vaccines cannot prevent cancer, but they can help fight it. The basic principal is to teach the immune system to identify tumors as an enemy and help fight them. For the most part, this is done by introducing an altered, harmless form of the cancer into the patient, much like a classic vaccine. As techniques have been refined, scientists have been able to find the specific proteins that have proven to be the most effective in educating the body to fight cancer.

Pharmaceutical companies and universities in the U.S., Canada and Europe are developing dozens of vaccines. These vaccines are targeted at the most common types of cancer including melanoma, kidney, lung and breast cancer. They have proven effective enough to send the cancers into remission or, at the very least, slow the spread of the cancer. One woman with late-stage melanoma experienced a remission of the cancer for 32 months after being treated with an early vaccine. Although not all of the vaccines have proven so effective, the prospects are certainly remarkable; many have even reached late-stage human trials. Two of these are in the midst of Phase III clinical trials, including a kidney cancer vaccine being developed by Antigenics and a prostate cancer vaccine by Dendreon.

Biopharma companies have developed vaccines to carry specific proteins that can stimulate the human immune system to have a desired response against an infectious disease. For example, biotech vaccines that fight hepatitis B have been introduced. Vaccines are under development at various firms for such conditions as herpes and tuberculosis. Additional DNA therapies that are somewhat related to vaccines are being developed to fight specific cancers and immune system diseases such as AIDS. Merck & Co. is developing a combination vaccine with Aventis, based on two independent vaccines that have shown great promise when used together. In preclinical trials, the two drugs together increased cell resistance to HIV in Macaque monkeys. First-stage clinical trials began at the end of 2003.

> **Companies to Watch:**
> Antigenics, New York, NY; CancerVax, Carlsbad, CA; Cell Genesys, South San Francisco, CA; Corixa, Seattle, WA; GlaxoSmithKline Biologicals, Rixensart, Belgium; Dendreon, Seattle, WA; Progenics Pharmaceuticals, Tarrytown, NY.

21) Advances in Diagnostic Imaging and Monitoring

> **Internet research tip:**
> For descriptions of advanced imaging procedures, see the web site of the Radiological Society of North America at www.radiologyinfo.org.

Improved diagnostic imaging, diagnostic catheterization and better monitoring procedures have made earlier detection of many diseases possible and reduced the need for exploratory surgery. While x-ray technology is effective for observing general anatomical features such as bones, organs and tissue masses, recent advances in imaging technology now provide medical professionals with a deeper understanding of the molecular structure of hard and soft tissues. These new technologies, which are now in common use throughout the U.S., include infrared imaging, ultrasound, tomography and magnetic resonance imaging.

Magnetic resonance imaging (MRI) uses a combination of radio waves and a strong magnetic field to gauge the behavior of hydrogen atoms in water molecules. Improvements in hardware and software have made MRI scans faster and more thorough. Ultra-fast MRI has many important clinical applications. Recent studies show that MRI may be the best method for determining the extent of a patient's recovery after a heart attack. Rapid-imaging MRI machines also expedite the diagnosis and treatment of heart conditions and strokes, thus reducing the time and money needed to scan the patient. However, this technology has been extremely expensive, with equipment costs alone running from $1 million to $2 million. Until recently, very heavy shielding was needed to encapsulate the imaging room, which necessitated special construction of new facilities or very costly reinforcement of older building space. Progress in shielding technology and facility design, combined with more cost-effective mid-field and low-field MRI, has dramatically lowered the cost of most new installations. Some of these lighter, less powerful devices can be used in mobile settings, which makes MRI available in rural areas that could never have justified the expense of permanent installations. Low-field MRI technology has also enabled the development of open-MRI devices, which do not require a patient to be completely surrounded by a tunnel-shaped magnet. Open MRIs reduce patient anxiety and claustrophobia. In addition, the lower intensity of the magnetic field allows technicians, physicians and even family members to be present in the room at the time of the test, if the patient prefers.

Magnetoencephalography (MEG) is a newer technology derived from both MRI and electroencephalography (EEG). Like EEG, MEG registers brain patterns, but whereas EEG measures electrical activity in the brain, MEG measures magnetic waves, primarily in the cerebral cortex of the brain. Computer enhancement of the generated data is improving EEG as a diagnostic tool. Recent refinements in EEG technology make it possible to use this device to help diagnose various forms of depression and schizophrenia. Computed tomography (CT) scanners use a circular pattern of x-rays to produce high-resolution, cross-sectional images, which can help precisely locate tumors, clots, narrowed arteries and aneurysms. CT can also produce three-dimensional images, which are beneficial in reconstructive surgery. However, CT machines cost up to $1 million and are generally available only at hospitals and large clinics. In addition, a patient's CT scan can cost $500 or more. Less expensive CT units can only scan the cranium, while larger units can be used to produce cross-sections of any part of the body.

Two other imaging machines, single photon emission computed tomography (SPECT) and positron emission tomography (PET), use forms of radioisotope imaging to detect and study conditions such as stroke, epilepsy, schizophrenia and Parkinson's and Alzheimer's diseases. PET is a major research tool for understanding the human brain, and has a substantial indirect impact on medical and surgical practices.

Other improvements in x-ray technology include digital subtractive angiography (DSA) and mammography. DSA involves the use of enhanced x-ray pictures to see blood vessels and arteries. It can clearly image aneurysms and can be used in angioplasty, a procedure that reduces the need for heart bypass surgery. Mammography is another x-ray technology that has been refined over the years. While traditional mammography with film offers sufficient x-ray images of older women's breasts, the film lacks the versatility of gray values that radiologists need to interpret mammograms from younger women. A new digital x-ray sensitive camera produces digital images on a computer screen with a higher dynamic range of gray values. Modern mammography equipment gives detailed and precise images of breast tissue, resulting in high detection levels of very small malignant tumors. The sooner a malignance is discovered, the better the prognosis is for excision and follow-up treatment success. Advanced mammography techniques reduce the chance for misdiagnoses, the amount of radiation needed to develop the image and the time spent in the exam room.

Another improved imaging technique, sonography, uses ultrasound to create images of internal body tissues and fetuses. Ultrasound is a cheaper alternative to many other imaging techniques, and results are available almost immediately. This scanning technique is recommended for pregnant women, since the sound waves apparently cause no harm to human tissue. Refinements in sonography have led to excellent prenatal images, which can be used to detect even small abnormalities in a fetus. Sonography is also being used in other imaging applications. For example, a new $250,000 ultrasound device is capable of displaying a three-dimensional image of organs such as the heart. Ultrasound in real time has even become sensitive enough to show blood flow. Ultrasound units are common in all but the very smallest hospitals.

New ultrasound diagnostic devices are now being manufactured by Sonoscope, Inc. and General Electric that are small enough to carry and provide doctors with a comprehensive picture of a patient's major organs and possible problems. These devices, which resemble the handheld scanners used on *Star Trek*, use ultrasonic waves to map out the interior features of a patient and then enhance them to provide an accurate and easy-to-read picture. Not only can doctors spot heart murmurs and breathing abnormalities with a simple inspection, but they can also spot things like kidney stones and gallstones, or whether there is an abnormal amount of fluid surrounding an organ. Though the machines currently cost more than $50,000 each, they could potentially save millions in radiology and other diagnostic bills. In addition, these devices could be carried on ambulances or even on a doctor's person, allowing diagnostics to be performed wherever they are needed.

While x-rays, ultrasound, MRI and CT are all very effective imaging techniques, they are limited in their potential because they are flat. A fast new way to compute three-dimensional images of organs and anatomical features has been developed. This new technology should make medical images more useful to doctors, resulting in quicker, better-informed treatment decisions.

Another exciting monitoring technique involves measuring the levels of the chemical creatine in the heart, which indicate the extent of muscle damage caused by a heart attack. Using a combination of MRI and MRS (magnetic resonance spectroscopy), this noninvasive method allows doctors to pinpoint injured heart tissue by measuring depleted levels of creatine in areas of the heart that were difficult to view using older imaging techniques.

Some patients even carry monitoring equipment on or in their bodies for long-term diagnostic purposes relating to biochemical balances, brain and sleep disorders, heart and vascular diseases and metabolic problems. More accurate, easy-to-use equipment has been introduced. For example, Medtronic has released an implantable heart monitoring device the size of three sticks of gum. Called the Reveal, the device can detect brief heart stoppages or other abnormalities and report them to a support network.

Light and diagnostic devices have also been showing up to diagnose certain forms of cancer. Similar to spectroscopy, which has been used to analyze chemical compositions for decades, these small diagnostic devices can detect cancer by finding abnormalities in the body's reaction to light. In one instance, doctors at the University of Texas at Austin found that cervical cancer could be detected using a small ultraviolet light shown on the cervix.

Precancerous cells are distinctly more fluorescent than normal cells. A preliminary study showed that the technique was 50% more accurate than a PAP smear and microscope examination, reducing the need to perform further diagnostic biopsies on healthy women. In another instance of light diagnostics, researchers at the University of California, Irvine found that infrared light could assist in finding breast cancer.

22) Advances in Laboratory Testing

New rapid testing techniques, improved equipment and the growing list of conditions that can be detected through blood, tissue and fluid specimen tests have expanded the role of laboratory testing in routine hospital patient care. The growth in the variety of tests has caused an increase in the use of outside laboratories by hospitals, but rapid techniques are most effectively used in-house. Therefore, on-site laboratories remain necessary. New tests for AIDS, hepatitis, cancer and genetic diseases have been developed. Recently, the FDA approved the first at-home test for hepatitis C, which silently lurks in about 3.9 million Americans who are unaware that they have the virus. Hepatitis is the leading cause of liver failure and kills up to 10,000 Americans each year.

Amazing advances in the understanding of genetics have given rise to the ability to test for a predisposition towards inherited diseases with genetic testing. Based on a simple blood test that can be performed in a doctor's office, the genetic tests look for the hallmark genes that indicate whether someone is at risk for a variety of diseases. Tests for over 1,000 diseases now exist, including both common and rare diseases and life-threatening conditions such as colon and breast cancer, Alzheimer's and diabetes. These tests have also led many hospitals and medical centers to hire genetic counselors, not only to interpret the tests, but to help patients deal with the results, giving advice on the conceivably life-altering revelations as well as means of prevention if the patient is at high risk.

Early-Stage Testing

Many diseases can now be detected in their earliest stages. Such early detection often occurs before the patient has suffered significant harm, and it tends to lead to more effective treatment. Besides early cancer detection and genetic screening, an important focus is cardiovascular disease, the leading cause of death in the U.S. High blood pressure and high cholesterol levels are conditions that require testing to detect, yet control of cholesterol levels and blood pressure can lead to significant increases in longevity and general health levels. A new laboratory test can detect levels of 15 blood cholesterol-containing particles called lipoproteins, which will more accurately measure a person's risk of heart disease than the tests currently in use. The test uses NMR (proton nuclear magnetic resonance spectroscopy) to record radio signals emitted by fats in the blood. Although the equipment itself is expensive, the test can be done in minutes rather than hours, because it does not require the physical separation of blood components. Furthermore, the test will likely be more accurate than traditional blood screening, resulting in fewer misdiagnoses and underestimates of cholesterol levels.

Another exciting testing device has been developed that could detect disease from a patient's breath. As blood circulates through the body, gases in the lungs and blood equilibrate and are carried out through the lungs. Kidney problems may be diagnosed by a fishy smell produced by compounds called amines, and diabetes could be deduced from the sweet smell of acetone. Advances in breath-collection techniques and analysis have made it feasible to test for a variety of diseases, from asthma to schizophrenia, with a simple breath test. The technology is being developed to detect symptoms of a variety of cancers as well, the most prominent being lung and breast cancer. Preliminary studies have shown that breath tests can detect upwards of 85% of breast cancers, which is equivalent to mammography. Commercial versions of this new device should be available in a few years.

A new noninvasive colonoscopy is also gaining popularity. In a virtual colonoscopy, doctors take a computed tomography (CT) scan of the patient's abdomen, which is rendered into a 3-D computer-generated model of the patient's colon. To date, the virtual colonoscopy has been able to detect polyps or abnormalities that are larger than six millimeters.

Another noninvasive test for colorectal cancer on the horizon involves DNA testing of stool samples. So far, DNA tests have outperformed the traditional fecal occult blood test and could become standard procedure within a few years.

One of the most promising new fields in diagnostic medicine is molecular imaging. Molecular imaging allows doctors to inject a patient with imaging agents that cling to trace molecules that could be indicative of health problems such as cancer and diseases of the cardiovascular and nervous systems. This new technique has the capability to spot these ailments with an accuracy that ordinary x-rays and biopsies cannot match. Two of the most successful applications are in breast and colon cancer. Imaging molecules that are injected into the patient become active when they come into contact with enzymes found in cancerous cells, causing them to "light up" and expose the cancer cells. Molecular imaging also allows doctors to witness what is called apoptosis, or the dying of cells. Viewing this process is invaluable for observing the effectiveness of cancer treatment, actually providing a way to see cells in a malignant tumor die.

While the benefits of early testing are considerable, there has been criticism of the extent and cost of testing. Due to patient expectations and malpractice concerns, physicians may practice defensive medicine, which leads to greater use of diagnostic tests. Often the latest and most expensive testing procedures are used. Fortunately, the accuracy of most tests is increasing, and newer, more rapid procedures raise laboratory worker productivity, which helps hold down costs and staffing. Artificial intelligence research has produced expert systems that are beginning to help physicians gain accurate diagnosis without excessive testing. Computerized systems are being developed and implemented by third-party payors and hospital managers for review and monitoring of testing practices.

Cancer Testing

In testing for cancer, early detection leads to increased life expectancy and cure rates. Cancer cells can often be distinguished from healthy cells by microscopic inspection and biochemical tests. For decades, suspect tissue has been routinely gathered by minor exploratory surgery. Such surgery is being augmented by fiberscopic and needle incisions. In direct cancer detection, the testing for chemical or biological markers has improved. The net impact on hospital labor is unclear, but cancer survival rates are slowly rising, in part due to early detection.

Cancer testing is often done rapidly enough to be integrated with a surgical procedure that is guided by the test results. Some procedures are very complex. An example is a new procedure that excises skin cancers layer by layer and maps the presence of cancer cells and their pattern in each layer of tissue. With this process, only 2% of patients have a recurrence of cancer at the site, as opposed to a 3% recurrence rate by simple excision, burning or freezing. In addition, there is slightly less scarring due to the removal of a smaller amount of healthy tissue. The tradeoff is the transformation of a simple procedure into a complex, costly and lengthy one.

A new PSA (prostate specific antigen) test for prostate cancer could spare up to 200,000 men each year in the U.S. the pain and anxiety associated with invasive surgical biopsies to detect cancer. The test better determines which men to biopsy for cancer by providing more accurate measurements of PSA levels. Costs of prostate screening could also be cut dramatically.

A new urine test may also allow doctors to check regularly and quickly for cancers in patients at risk for developing cancer due to genetic or environmental factors. The test temporarily slows DNA production in cancer cells, causing some elements of DNA to accumulate in the blood. When these materials are excreted in large amounts in urine, they indicate the presence of cancer. Clinical human trials have been promising, but the test still needs validation through additional research.

Rapid Laboratory Procedures
More advanced and faster computerized analyzers and other laboratory technologies are being introduced to speed testing procedures. In some hospitals analyzers are linked to a central computer, and test results are sent automatically from the laboratory to the patient's ward. A variety of new test kits allow many laboratory procedures to yield results in one to three hours. Many tests are read spectrographically, using light refraction to measure the samples. Other improved laboratory procedures include monoclonal antibody technology (the extraction of specific genetic traits for cloning) and a new rapid AIDS test, which uses microscopic latex beads. Test results from rapid procedures equal the accuracy of slower methods, but more skill and care are often required for sample preparation and testing. Automated laboratory equipment is currently found in most hospitals.

Patients receiving heart treatment now benefit from tremendous advances in the monitoring of heart conditions in the cardiac catheter lab. Using catheters that probe the recesses of the heart, combined with the latest in hardware and software made by GE Medical Systems, doctors are able to pinpoint the exact location of problem spots in the heart during outpatient procedures.

Although new equipment has improved productivity in the laboratory, specimens must still be obtained manually. The expansion of available tests boosts demand for laboratory services. The net result is a growth in demand for laboratory technicians and engineers.

23) Advances in Surgery

Increasing technical skill, improved diagnostic imaging, better equipment and laparoscopic techniques have made less invasive surgery possible. Incisions are much smaller than in the past, and recovery from surgery is often more rapid. Lasers, computers, sonography, magnetic resonance imaging, stereo optiscopes, miniature precision tools, robotics, fiber optics, imaging chemicals and isotopes and better x-ray equipment are factors in these advances. In 1998, the National Science Foundation provided $12.9 billion in a grant to establish the Engineering Research Center in Computer-Integrated Surgical Systems Technology (ERC CISST). Today it is a broad reaching organization that includes both schools and hospitals. Members include Johns Hopkins University and Institutions, Carnegie Mellon University, Massachusetts Institute of Technology, Brigham and Women's Hospital in Boston, and Shadyside Hospital in Pittsburgh. Collaborating on the project are students, professors, doctors and engineers, while their communication is facilitated by a web-based Intranet that allows the transfer of ideas and technology. The ultimate goal of the project is a completely automated operating room, in which a surgeon uses a custom-tailored, computer-generated image of the patient to help diagnose the patient's condition, select the appropriate treatment option and practice the procedure before making an incision. This operating room of the future will allow surgeons to learn more from their own work, resulting in fewer mistakes and complications.

Minimally Invasive and Laparoscopic Surgery
Small-incision and micro-incision surgery may be the most cost-effective development in new technology. Surgery has evolved from large incisions at the site of entry to smaller and smaller incisions, to procedures that are performed with needles, catheters, lasers and ultrasound. Recovery periods are cut dramatically as the severity of the procedures is reduced. Because surgical procedures involve risk to the patient, surgeons are highly motivated to develop ever more efficient and rapid techniques to reduce the period of time a patient must be under anesthesia and exposed to potential infection or shock.

One example is the laparoscope (or endoscope), a device consisting of an extremely thin tube containing a video camera lighted by fiber optics, which allows a surgeon to view and operate on abdominal or pelvic organs through an incision between one and two centimeters long.

Over time, most surgical procedures have been greatly modified and simplified. In surgery for breast cancer, for example, radical and modified radical mastectomies have given way to less extensive surgeries. In some cases, simple lumpectomies are effective. Chemotherapy and radiation therapy reduce the severity of many surgical procedures for cancer. Angioplasty, a catheter procedure in which a balloon is used to open clogged arteries, is replacing some coronary bypass surgeries, or at least delaying the need for such surgeries.

Endovascular grafts are a new procedure for operating on abdominal aortic aneurysm (AAA). Where traditional AAA surgery involved an incision from the breastbone to the pubic bone, the endovascular graft only requires a small incision in the groin area. The graft is delivered to the aorta via the patient's blood vessels, where it attaches to the heart. So far, this procedure has exceeded expectations for safety and efficacy.

Using MRI and lasers or linear accelerators, stereoscopic surgery is being used to remove deep-seated brain tumors, and an operation (percutaneous automated dissectomy) is turning some herniated disk surgery into an outpatient procedure. MRI is partly replacing diagnostic knee surgery.

Breakthroughs in surgery will touch every type of operation. In one of the most exciting developments, a growing number of surgeons are now able to do revolutionary open-heart surgery, such as complicated bypass operations, by working through much smaller incisions and using the latest in minimally invasive techniques. This means that patients will have greatly reduced recovery times and will suffer fewer traumas during the operation. A technology known as MIDCAB (minimally invasive direct coronary artery bypass system) is rapidly growing in popularity.

Laser Surgery

Lasers have been used surgically for many years to reattach detached retinas, but there are several newer applications. Advanced videolaseroscopy, using an endoscope equipped with a laser, is being used in minimally-invasive surgery to excise and or cauterize damaged tissue in the abdomen and lungs. It has proven effective in treatment for appendicitis, bowel tumors and adhesions, gallstones, fibroid tumors, endometriosis, ectopic pregnancy and lung lesions.

The FDA has granted approval for the use of new lasers for a number of gynecological and other procedures. Lasers are being used to remove vulvalar cancers, destroy genital warts and remove infected toenails. They are also being used to vaporize deposits of fat in the blood vessels of the legs. Moreover, the vaporizing of fat deposits in the arteries of the heart, lungs and neck may prove feasible, reducing the need for bypass surgery and carotid artery surgery.

New diode lasers that use quantum-well technology are expected to replace most of the current gas-based lasers. This situation is analogous to the replacement of vacuum tubes by transistors and integrated circuits. Quantum-well diode lasers' greater efficiency, speed and coolness of operation will multiply the potential medical applications of laser technology, and in the coming century an even more advanced laser technology (called quantum wire) is expected to play an important role in medical research and patient care.

Microsurgery

The reattachment of limbs and digits, the implantation of middle ear prostheses and some eye surgeries are now routine microsurgery procedures. These successes required the development of precision instruments, magnifying systems, microscopically fine sutures and other closure systems. Microsurgery is also being used in fetal and infant treatments, and some applications make nerve, organ, vascular and trauma repair possible.

Surgeons have contributed to improvements in surgical tools and the development of equipment that makes possible very small incisions and repairs. However, nerve surgery advances are still highly dependent on new equipment and on progress in the use of steroids and other medications.

Robotics

Eventually, we may see widespread use of robotics in microsurgery. Experts are now using advanced computer technology to enable surgeons to control tiny, robotic pincers that can perform surgical procedures through extremely small openings. This is laparoscopic surgery carried to its highest level. Using such systems, surgeons view the interior of the body using tiny cameras. They then work from remote consoles to manipulate the robotic arms that cut, cauterize or staple the patient as needed. The use of robotics makes surgical procedures safer and more precise.

Intuitive Surgical, Inc. (www.intuitivesurgical.com) of Mountain View, California is a leader in equipment for this field. At this time, Intuitive Surgical manufactures the only operative robotic system with FDA clearance. Its da Vinci system costs around $1 million. A surgeon sits at a control console and uses a joystick control to manipulate robotic arms that are equipped with surgical instruments. The surgeon observes the operation via a camera that projects 3-D images onto a computer screen. Fatigue may cause the surgeon's hands to shake after many hours at the operating table. The da Vinci system recognizes these minute tremors and ignores them, minimizing the chances of surgical error.

Wound and Incision Closures

Surgical staples are used as an alternative to suturing. Although several times more expensive than sutures, they require less skill to insert and speed surgical procedures. They also promote more rapid healing and recovery. This concept originated abroad many years ago but was of little interest in the U.S. until improvements were made in equipment, materials and methods. Stapling allows faster surgical procedures, which benefit both the patient and the surgical team, since the shorter the surgery is the lower the chances are of complications from anesthesia, infection, blood loss and shock. Some staples are made of surgical steel, while others are made of soluble materials that dissolve as healing takes place. One study indicated that the use of staples could reduce a hospital stay by three to five days compared to a similar operation with sutures. Using staples reduces labor requirements for surgery and postoperative care. In addition, staples increase the number of surgical procedures that can be performed safely on an outpatient basis.

Some new systems use super adhesives or plastic coverings to close incisions and cuts instead of either sutures or staples. Rigid plastic coverings can be glued to the area above the wound. The stiff plastic prevents the sides of the wound from shifting while healing takes place. When the wound or incision has healed, the skin beneath the adhesive sloughs (slowly peels away), which causes the plastic or fiberglass covering to come free. This is a new approach, but it may come into common use quickly. Furthermore, there is a growing trend toward using adhesives directly to close incisions. The adhesive is absorbed or breaks down as the wound heals.

24) Other Treatment Technologies

Shock-Wave Treatment

The lithotripter is a high-intensity sound-generating device that pulverizes kidney stones with shock waves. It is widely used, mainly in larger hospitals. In most cases, it is no longer necessary to surgically remove kidney stones that cannot be passed naturally. The original version of this device required that the patient be partially immersed in water, however a newer version does not require immersion and allows a greater number of shocks to be administered in a single session, which usually lasts less than an hour. One session is generally all that is needed in either approach.

A lithotripsy facility costs about $2 million. The treatment is supervised by an M.D., usually a urologist or radiologist. Treatment is expensive, but the potential exists for cost reduction as equipment and staff costs are lowered and facility requirements are reduced due to more compact units. Reductions in average patient costs for diagnosis, treatment and follow-up appear feasible.

Lithotripsy also allows many people to avoid gallbladder surgery. Gallbladder surgery is typically followed by weeks of recuperation, although a new procedure cuts recovery periods in half. Lithotripsy treatment can be performed on an outpatient basis or, at most, requires an overnight stay in a hospital followed by a day or less of recuperation. Furthermore, the procedure costs significantly less than the surgical operation, and, as indicated above, there are good prospects that the costs of lithotripsy facilities will gradually decline.

Because it is expensive to construct a lithotripsy unit, permanent installations are found mainly in larger hospitals. Many metropolitan areas only require a single unit to meet all local demand for this service. Mobile units can be trucked to smaller communities on a regular schedule. HealthTronics, Inc. (www.healthtronics.com) is one of the leading providers of mobile lithotripsy services, serving hundreds of hospitals nationwide.

Implantable Pumps as Testing Devices

This category includes miniature pumps that administer medicines, hormones, insulin and chemotherapy agents. Miniature pumps, about the size of a cigarette pack or smaller, are used to infuse analgesics and other drugs into the body in a controlled, time-release fashion. Research in the use of such pumps to infuse insulin has been underway for some time.

Cancer patients and other victims of severe pain are already benefiting from new infusion technology. Implantable pumps and testing devices involve high levels of automation and computerized monitoring. Miniature electrocardiogram (EKG) systems, for example, are designed to be worn by patients with heart disease and to broadcast warnings of infarctions or other crises. These devices are used for long-term diagnosis and medical studies. (Also, see "Diabetes Treatment.")

Advances in Transplantation and Immunology

Transplantation of organs and other body parts has grown very rapidly, due to improvements in immune system suppression that make it possible for the human body to tolerate foreign tissue instead of rejecting it. The most common implants are plastic lenses in the eyes of cataract patients. Over 1 million of these procedures are performed each year. Thousands of synthetic blood vessels, joints, bones, middle ears and teeth are also implanted. Transplantation of living tissues includes hearts, livers, lungs, kidneys, pancreases, corneas and skin or bone from one part of a patient to another part. Advanced transgenics methods and genetic engineering will eventually provide transplantable tissues from laboratory-grown animals.

Transplantation of organs normally requires immunological treatment to prevent organ rejection. In recent years, a powerful immunosuppressive agent, cyclosporine, has dramatically reduced organ rejection rates. Steroids, cyclosporine and immuran have led the way toward the development and use of even more effective agents. Sometimes drug combinations prevent organ rejection, even after the rejection process has begun.

> **Internet research tip:**
> For more information on organ transplantation, visit www.transweb.org.

In the future, heart patients may be among the biggest beneficiaries of transgenics, the use of organs and tissues grown in laboratory animals for transplantation to humans. Over 30,000 patients per year already receive heart valve transplants from pigs. The next challenge is to use genetic engineering to produce pig hearts that contain the human immune system proteins that reduce the chance of rejection. The same techniques may eventually grow kidneys or other organs suitable for use in humans.

Lung and kidney transplants are now commonplace. Corneal eye transplants can often be performed on an outpatient basis, but the growth in other transplants is resulting in more hospitalization and surgery. The main constraint to the growth of transplant surgery is a shortage of replacement organs. On any given day, tens of thousands of patients are waiting for organs. Only 20% of the 25,000 Americans who die each year under circumstances conducive to organ use actually donate organs. It is hoped that the supply of transplantable organs and tissue will grow due to greater awareness and technological advances.

Dialysis

Dialysis is available to virtually all patients requiring it in the U.S. This government-funded system currently provides treatment to over 220,000 people. The sheer size of the program has created the proper environment for the improvement and refinement of methods and equipment. Important advances include more and better venous shunts (now usually internal), better and more compact machinery, more rapid treatment and more complete cleansing of the patient's body. Procedural simplification makes it easier for patients to be treated at home.

There are two basic types of dialysis for treating kidney failure. The older method, peritoneal dialysis, is used mainly to treat temporary kidney failure. This treatment involves a fluid exchange between an external reservoir and a patient's abdominal cavity. When introduced, this treatment required a one- or two-week period of immobility, but ambulatory peritoneal dialysis has now become common. Patients are mobile and provide much of their own care during treatment. This has reduced labor requirements related to treatment of acute kidney failure.

The second method of dialysis, hemodialysis, involves purging a patient's blood of waste products normally removed by functioning kidneys. Until long-lasting venous shunts were introduced, this treatment was impractical for more than a short period because catheters tended to destroy the patient's accessible arteries and veins. Over time, longer-lasting internal shunting systems were developed.

The Federal Government provides hemodialysis for any person with chronic kidney failure (end-stage renal disease). The number of patients in the program will probably correspond to the growth in the population over age 55. However, the patient population may remain close to its present level, assuming the number of kidney transplants grows as expected.

Most patients receive treatment in special centers, some of which are located in hospitals. The proportion of home dialysis patients can be expected to grow to one-third of the total, due to cost considerations and simpler self-care resulting from technical improvements. Annual cost of treatment in centers exceeds $20,000; the cost of home care is lower. Dialysis has many side effects, including depression and fatigue, however home treatment tends to improve a patient's feelings of control and self-worth and allows more time for work and other activities. Regardless, only a successful kidney transplant can return a patient to a nearly normal life.

Diabetes Treatment

Type I and Type II diabetes affect over 18 million Americans. Diabetes poses one of the most serious health problems, as diabetics tend to suffer from many ailments that require hospitalization and intensive treatment. These include pregnancy complications, blindness, circulatory diseases, organ failure and diabetic coma. Under the new classification standard, a person is considered diabetic after the blood level reaches 115 milligrams of sugar per deciliter of blood. (The previous standard was 150 mg.) This reclassification will lead to an expansion in the number of patients defined as diabetic, but though diabetes can lead to complications that require hospital treatment, most diabetic treatments do not require hospitalization.

Recent changes in routine treatment could improve the health of diabetics and lead to fewer hospitalizations. These new methods require diabetics to monitor blood sugar levels several times a day and to take more frequent dosages of insulin formulations that combine fast-acting insulin with intermediate forms. The diabetic must purchase a blood-glucose meter and incur other costs for testing materials.

Exciting new regimens are currently under testing. Generex Biotechnology Corp., Aradigm Corp. and Nektar Therapeutic are developing drug delivery via inhalation techniques that may eventually be used for the delivery of insulin. Two companies, Bioject Medical Technologies and Antares Pharma, have needle-free injection systems for insulin and other drugs on the market. This is a particular asset for children with diabetes who may be afraid of needles.

The use of miniature insulin pumps, instead of insulin injection via needles, has been shown to raise the quality of life for many diabetics and increase their health levels. Traditional insulin injection methods are believed to exacerbate damage to the circulatory system and the retinas of the eyes. This can shorten the life span of diabetics and subject them to blindness, gangrene and other health problems. Medtronic MiniMed manufactures the Paradigm line of insulin pumps. However, the company's implantable pump that delivers a steady insulin dose, 24 hours a day, without syringes, may be the ultimate device. Medtronic MiniMed has received regulatory approval to sell its implantable insulin pumps in Europe, and hopes to eventually receive approval in the U.S. The device is implanted in the peritoneal cavity (the abdomen) and releases insulin in small, steady bursts into the body, actually mimicking the body's natural delivery system. With a reservoir that can last up to three months, along with a long-life battery, the device requires very little maintenance and can even be regulated externally.

Another needle-free alternative may be a recently discovered simple molecule that, when swallowed, mimics the action of insulin in diabetics. Insulin currently has no benefit when taken orally because the protein is broken down in the stomach. This new molecule has been shown to control blood glucose levels in mice bred to develop diabetes. The next step is to begin testing on humans.

Other Implantable and Replacement Devices and Therapies

New technology is rapidly creating a wealth of exciting devices that can be implanted in the body to increase health or to replace human parts or functions. For example, Cyberonics (based in Clear Lake, Texas, near Houston) received FDA approval in 1997 to market its pacemaker-sized implantable electric stimulator device, which can help deter epileptic seizures by sending carefully timed impulses to the vagus nerve. The same technology may eventually prove effective in treating many other conditions, such as Parkinson's disease, headaches and depression.

Medtronic has similarly developed the Activa Parkinson's Control Therapy. It utilizes an implanted device that sends impulses to the thalamus region of the brain to counteract the effects of Parkinson's disease tremors.

By use of implanted chips, scientists can now make significant impact on harmful neural conditions, and they have also begun to study how to interact with the brain on an electric level. One experiment implanted electrodes in monkeys' brains, and then began deciphering the impulses coming out. To do this, the monkeys were given joysticks, which could move a cursor across a computer screen, and then the movements of the cursor were cross-referenced with the impulses coming from the brain. After writing programs for these thought intentions, the monkeys were able to move the cursor purely through the implants.

Another new technology called SIM (Surface Induced Mineralization) allows metal implants to be surface-coated with a water-based calcium phosphate material, which stimulates the growth of new bone. The material bonds with the natural bone surrounding the implant, offering a more secure scaffold for new bone to grow, thus extending the life of the implant.

Rutgers University professor William Craelius has designed a prosthesis for the human hand which affords recipients independent control of each finger via a computer. Sensors detect signals from nerve pathways which go through the computer to orchestrate finger movement. The prosthesis is so effective that patients have enough control and mobility to manipulate keyboards.

Advances in Organ Replacements

An exciting piece of news in prosthetic organs is the Dobelle eye, the use of which resulted in a sightless study participant successfully driving a car through a closed test course. The Dobelle eye is a combination of two electrode arrays (called pedestals) embedded through the skull and onto the visual cortex; a miniature camera mounted on a pair of eyeglasses; and a three-pound microcomputer worn around the patient's waist. While vision is not fully restored, patients receive digital information taken from the camera and processed by the microcomputer. The data is translated into strings of electrical impulses that are fed through wires into the pedestals in the brain. Points of light similar to video pixels are formed, allowing the patient to see shapes and, in some cases, colors.

There are two other similar projects underway. In one of these projects, electrodes will be implanted inside the visual cortex instead of on the surface, allowing for much finer stimulation and requiring much lower amperage. This means that the patient will not only have a higher resolution, but will be at lower risk of experiencing seizures. The other project uses an implant placed atop the retina instead of inside the brain. The device is designed to assist functional rods and cones within an eye that is mostly non-functional. Though this approach is limited, it is a much less invasive implant.

Artificial eyes are not the only big news in artificial organs. Artificial hearts are finally showing great promise. The Jarvik heart, which confines recipients to hospitals and requires a great deal of peripheral equipment, is quickly falling behind the AbioCor artificial heart. Weighing less than three pounds and roughly the size of a human heart, the AbioCor requires no additional equipment outside the body to function. The unit is designed to both extend a patient's life and to provide a reasonable quality of life. After implantation, the device does not require any tubes or wires to pass through the skin because power to drive the heart is transmitted across intact skin. Made by ABIOMED, Inc., it has received humanitarian use device (HUD) status from the FDA for use in patients with certain end-stage heart failure. In September 2004, the firm submitted a request for FDA approval to market the device to a certain subset of no more than 4,000 irreversible end-stage heart failure patients. Meanwhile, the firm is pursuing regulatory approval in Europe.

A Houston, Texas firm developed the DeBakey VAD heart assist device, a tiny turbine that pumps blood into the left ventricle. It was co-developed by NASA and famed heart surgeon Michael DeBakey. The pump is powered by an external battery pack and is designed to keep heart patients alive and active for several months while they await a transplant. Eventually, it may be useful for long-term needs. The device has now been used in over 200 patients, including a 14-year old boy and an 11-year-old girl, who was the youngest person to ever receive such an implant.

The Streamliner is another exciting device, developed by a cardiologist at the University of Pittsburgh in Pennsylvania. Using a turbine instead of the left ventricle to pump blood, the device also features magnetic levitation and a motor that can be powered externally via induction, making it one of the most powerful ideas in heart-assist devices. The chief designer of the Streamliner, Brad Paden, has since gone on to design another device, the HeartQuest VAD (Left Ventricular Assist Device), in partnership with MedQuest, a medical device manufacturer. Utilizing the same innovations found in the Streamliner, the HeartQuest also uses a circular flow design, which maximizes efficiency. The National Institute of Health recently gave $4.2 million for the development of HeartQuest.

With regard to pulmonary advances, an implantable plastic lung has been successfully tested on sheep. The BioLung is powered by the patient's heart, requiring no additional pumps or power sources. Licensed to NovaLung GmbH in Germany for development, human trials are scheduled to begin in Europe in 2005.

Chapter 2

HEALTH CARE STATISTICS

Including Medicare and Medicaid

Tables and Charts:	
I. U.S. Health Care Industry Overview	45
II. U.S. Health Care Expenditures & Costs	47
III. Medicare & Medicaid	65
IV. U.S. Health Insurance Coverage & the Uninsured	73
V. U.S. Vital Statistics & Population Indicators	81

I. U.S. Health Care Industry Overview

U.S. Health Care Industry Overview

	Amount	Units	Year	Source
National Health Care Expenditures 2004	1,794	Bil. Dollars	2004	CMS
In 2010	2,751	Bil. Dollars	2010*	CMS
National Health Care Expenditures per Capita 2004	6,167	Dollars	2004	CMS
In 2010	8,984	Dollars	2010*	CMS
National Health Care Expenditures by Type, 2004				
Hospitals	551.7	Bil. Dollars	2004	CMS
Physician and Clinical Services	386.8	Bil. Dollars	2004	CMS
Dental	78.0	Bil. Dollars	2004	CMS
Nursing Home and Home Health	152.2	Bil. Dollars	2004	CMS
Prescription drugs	207.9	Bil. Dollars	2004	CMS
Other	417.4	Bil. Dollars		
U.S. Population Less Than 65 Years of Age, 2004	254.9	Million	2004	CMS
In 2010	266.8	Million	2010*	CMS
U.S. Population Age 65 Years and Older, 2004	36.0	Million	2004	CMS
In 2010	39.4	Million	2010*	CMS
Number of Medicare Beneficiaries, 2000	34.1	Million	2000	CMS
Number of Medicare Beneficiaries, 2010	38.6	Million	2010*	CMS
Number of Medicare Beneficiaries, 2030	68.2	Million	2030*	CMS
U.S. Fertility Rate	2.07	Children Born/Woman	2004*	WFB
U.S. Birth Rate	14.13	Births /1,000 Pop.	2004*	WFB
U.S. Infant Mortality Rate	6.63	Deaths/1,000 Live Births	2004	WFB
U.S. Life Expectancy at birth	77.43	Years	2004	WFB
U.S. Death Rate	8.34	Deaths/1,000 Pop.	2004*	WFB
U.S. HIV/AIDS Adult Rate of Prevalence	0.6	%	2003*	WFB
Number of People Living with HIV/AIDS in U.S.	950,000		2003*	WFB
U.S. HIV/AIDS Deaths	14,000		2003*	WFB
Number of All U.S. Registered[1] Hospitals	5,764		2003	AHA
Staffed Beds in All U.S. Registered[1] Hospitals	965,256		2003	AHA
Admissions in All U.S. Registered[1] Hospitals	36,610,535		2003	AHA
Number of People Without Healthcare for the Entire Year	44,961	Thousand	2003	USCB
Percent of Population	15.6	%	2003	USCB

*Estimate

[1] **Registered** hospitals are those hospitals that meet AHA's criteria for registration as a hospital facility. Registered hospitals include AHA member hospitals as well as nonmember hospitals. For a complete listing of the criteria used for registration, please see www.aha.org

AHA = American Hospital Association

WFB = CIA World Fact Book 2004

CMS = Centers for Medicare & Medicaid Services

USCB = U.S. Census Bureau

II. U.S. Health Care Expenditures and Costs

Contents:

The Nation's Health Dollar 2004 - Where it Came From	48
The Nation's Health Dollar 2004 - Where It Went	49
National Health Expenditures and Average Annual Percent Change: 1980-2013	50
National Health Expenditures and Selected Economic Indicators: 1980-2013	51
National Health Expenditures, by Type of Expenditure: 1980-2013	52
Hospital Care Expenditures and Average Annual Percent Change, U.S.: 1980-2013	53
Hospital Care Expenditures, Percent Distribution and Per Capita Amount, U.S.: 1980-2013	54
U.S. Hospital Expenses: 1980-2003	55
Home Health Care Expenditures and Average Annual Percent Change, U.S.: 1980-2013	56
Home Health Care Expenditures, Percent Distribution and Per Capita Amount, U.S.: 1980-2013	57
Nursing Home Care Expenditures and Average Annual Percent Change, U.S.: 1980-2013	58
Nursing Home Care Expenditures, Percent Distribution and Per Capita Amount, U.S.: 1980-2013	59
Prescription Drug Expenditures and Average Annual Percent Change, U.S.: 1980-2013	60
Prescription Drug Expenditures, Percent Distribution and Per Capita Amount, U.S.: 1980-2012	61
Index Levels of Medical Prices	62
Hospitals, Beds and Occupancy Rates, U.S.: Selected Years 1997-2003	63
U.S. Community Hospital Statistics: 2000-2003	64

The Nation's Health Dollar, 2004 (Estimated)
Where It Came From

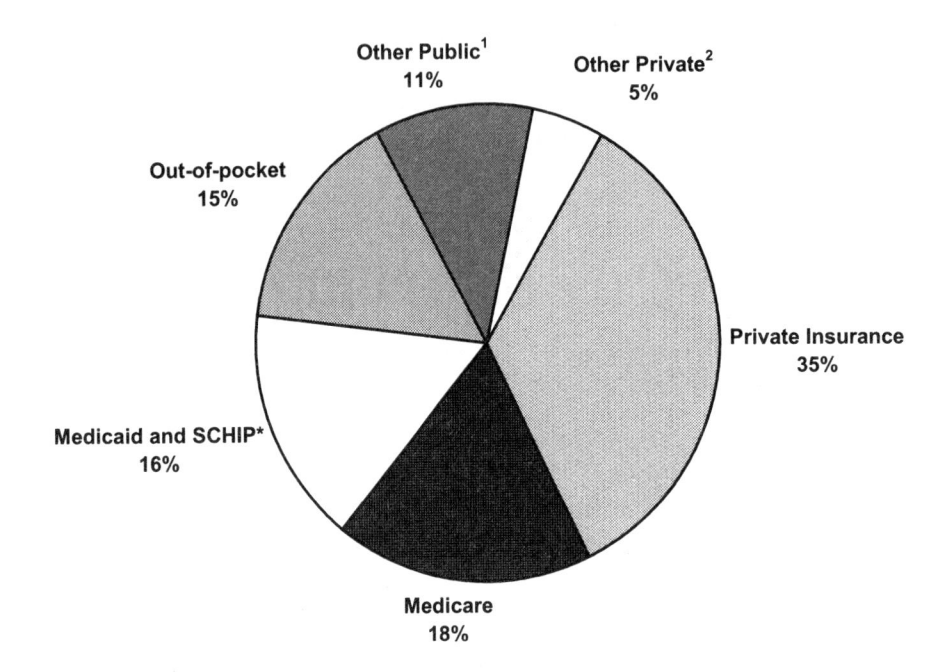

- Other Public[1]: 11%
- Other Private[2]: 5%
- Out-of-pocket: 15%
- Private Insurance: 35%
- Medicaid and SCHIP*: 16%
- Medicare: 18%

[1] "Other Public" includes programs such as workers' compensation, public health activity, Department of Defense, Department of Veterans Affairs, Indian Health Service, and State and local hospital subsidies and school health.

[2] "Other Private" includes industrial in-plant, privately funded construction, and non-patient revenues, including philanthropy.

*SCHIP=State Children's Health Insurance Program. Provides health insurance to uninsured, low-income children 18 years of age or younger, including those who are homeless.

Note: Numbers shown may not add to 100 because of rounding.

Source: Plunkett Research, Ltd.

The Nation's Health Dollar, 2004
Where It Went

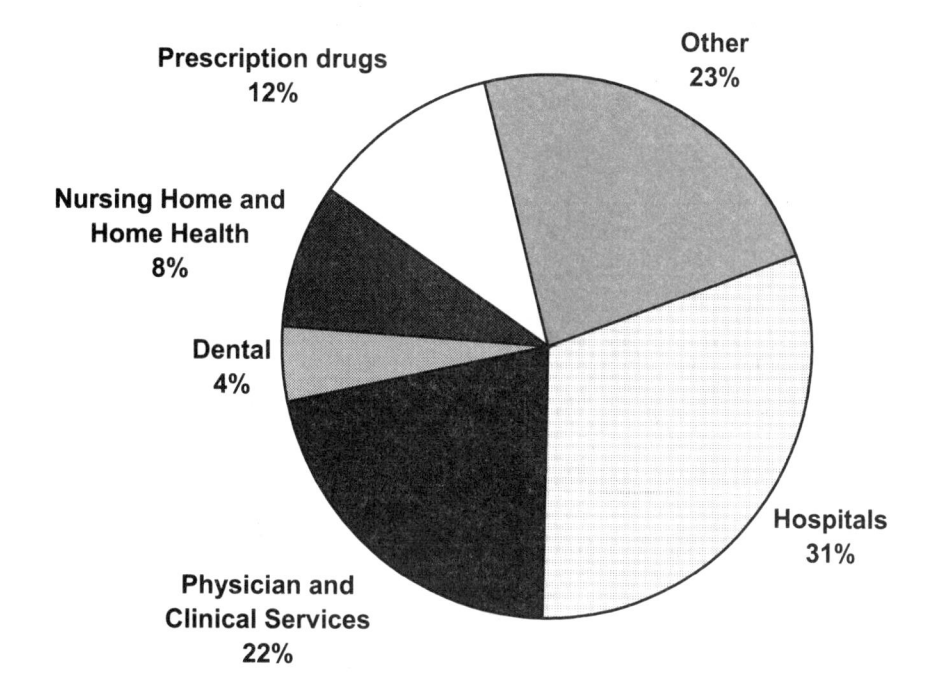

- Prescription drugs: 12%
- Nursing Home and Home Health: 8%
- Dental: 4%
- Physician and Clinical Services: 22%
- Hospitals: 31%
- Other: 23%

Source: Centers for Medicare & Medicaid Services (CMS), Plunkett Research, Ltd.

National Health Expenditures and Average Annual Percent Change: Selected Calendar Years 1980-2013[1]

By Source of Funds

Year	Total	Out-of-Pocket Payments	Third-Party Payments Total	Private Health Insurance	Other Private Funds	Public Total	Federal[2]	State and Local[2]	Medicare[3]	Medicaid[4]
Historical Estimates					Amount in Billions US$					
1980	$245.8	$58.2	$187.5	$68.2	$14.5	$104.8	$71.3	$33.5	$37.4	$26.0
1990	696.0	137.3	558.7	233.5	42.8	282.5	192.7	89.8	110.2	73.6
2000	1309.4	192.6	1116.9	449.3	72.9	594.6	416.0	178.6	225.1	203.4
2001	1420.7	200.5	1220.2	495.6	72.3	652.3	460.3	192.0	246.5	224.3
2002	1553.0	212.5	1340.5	549.6	77.5	713.4	504.7	208.7	267.1	250.4
Projected										
2003	1673.6	227.0	1446.6	606.7	80.9	759.0	535.2	223.8	280.9	269.2
2004	1793.6	243.0	1550.6	656.5	84.5	809.6	569.1	240.5	295.2	292.7
2005	1920.8	260.9	1660.0	707.0	88.7	864.2	605.0	259.3	309.3	319.2
2006	2064.0	279.7	1784.3	762.2	93.8	928.2	648.1	280.1	328.3	348.4
2007	2219.2	299.3	1919.9	821.9	99.5	998.5	695.5	303.0	349.3	380.4
2008	2387.7	319.9	2067.8	887.7	105.3	1074.8	747.1	327.7	372.9	414.9
2009	2565.0	341.7	2223.3	954.6	111.3	1157.4	803.5	354.0	399.3	452.2
2010	2751.0	364.3	2386.7	1022.2	117.6	1246.9	864.9	382.0	428.9	492.1
2011	2945.6	387.4	2558.2	1092.0	123.7	1342.5	930.6	411.9	460.8	534.8
2012	3145.8	411.3	2734.5	1160.6	129.9	1444.0	1000.3	443.6	495.1	580.2
2013	3358.1	436.2	2921.8	1233.4	136.3	1552.1	1074.8	477.3	532.1	628.5
Historical Estimates			Average Annual Percent Change from Previous Year Shown							
1990	--	--	--	--	--	--	--	--	--	--
2000	7.1	4.4	7.6	8.9	0.5	7.5	7.6	7.3	5.4	8.9
2001	8.5	4.1	9.2	10.3	-0.9	9.7	10.7	7.5	9.5	10.2
2002	9.3	6.0	9.9	10.9	7.2	9.4	9.7	8.7	8.4	11.7
Projected										
2003	7.8	6.8	7.9	10.4	4.4	6.4	6.0	7.2	5.2	7.5
2004	7.2	7.1	7.2	8.2	4.5	6.7	6.3	7.5	5.1	8.7
2005	7.1	7.3	7.1	7.7	4.9	6.8	6.3	7.8	4.8	9.0
2006	7.5	7.2	7.5	7.8	5.8	7.4	7.1	8.0	6.1	9.2
2007	7.5	7.0	7.6	7.8	6.0	7.6	7.3	8.2	6.4	9.2
2008	7.6	6.9	7.7	8.0	5.9	7.6	7.4	8.1	6.8	9.1
2009	7.4	6.8	7.5	7.5	5.7	7.7	7.5	8.0	7.1	9.0
2010	7.3	6.6	7.3	7.1	5.6	7.7	7.6	7.9	7.4	8.8
2011	7.1	6.3	7.2	6.8	5.3	7.7	7.6	7.8	7.5	8.7
2012	6.8	6.2	6.9	6.3	5.0	7.6	7.5	7.7	7.4	8.5
2013	6.7	6.1	6.9	6.3	5.0	7.5	7.4	7.6	7.5	8.3

[1] The health spending projections were based on the 2002 version of the National Health Expenditures (NHE) released in Jan. 2004.
[2] Includes Medicaid SCHIP Expansion and SCHIP.
[3] Subset of Federal funds.   [4] Subset of Federal and State and local funds. Includes Medicaid SCHIP Expansion.

Sources: Centers for Medicare & Medicaid Services (CMS), Office of the Actuary.

National Health Expenditures and Selected Economic Indicators, Levels and Average Annual Percent Change: Selected Calendar Years 1980-2013[1]

Item	1990	2000	2002	2003	2004	2010	2013
National Health Expenditures (billions)	$696.0	$1,309.4	$1,553.0	$1,673.6	$1,793.6	$2,751.0	$3,358.1
National Health Expenditures (% of GDP)	12.0	13.3	14.9	15.3	15.5	17.4	18.4
National Health Expenditures Per Capita	$2,738	$4,670	$5,440	$5,808	$6,167	$8,984	$10,709
Gross Domestic Product (billions)	$5,803.3	$9,824.7	$10,446.0	$10,947.4	$11,582.4	$15,789.4	$18,243.4
Gross Domestic Product (billions of 1996 $)	$6,707.9	$9,191.4	$9,439.9	$9,751.4	$10,170.7	$12,120.3	$12,950.6
Consumer Price Index (CPI-W) - 1982-1984 base	1.307	1.722	1.799	1.847	1.895	2.202	2.393
CMS Implicit Medical Price Deflator[2]	0.774	1.109	1.197	1.239	1.281	1.585	1.779
U.S. Population[3] (millions)	254.2	280.4	285.5	288.2	290.8	306.2	313.6
Population age less than 65 years (millions)	222.7	245.2	249.9	252.5	254.9	266.8	270.8
Population age 65 years and older (millions)	31.5	35.2	35.6	35.7	36	39.4	42.8
Private Health Insurance - NHE (billions)	$233.5	$449.3	$549.6	$606.7	$656.5	$1,022.2	$1,233.4
Private Health Insurance - PHC (billions)	$203.6	$398.7	$479.3	$522.1	$566.7	$883.7	$1,066.8
Average Annual Percent Change from Previous Year Shown (in %)							
National Health Expenditures	--	7.1	9.3	7.8	7.2	7.3	6.7
National Health Expenditures (% of GDP)	--	1.1	5.5	2.8	1.3	1.9	1.9
National Health Expenditures Per Capita	--	6.1	8.3	6.8	6.2	6.4	5.9
Gross Domestic Product (GDP)	--	5.9	3.6	4.8	5.8	5.2	4.8
GDP (1996 $)	--	3.8	2.4	3.3	4.3	2.5	2.1
Consumer Price Index (CPI-W) - 1982-1984 base	--	3.4	1.6	2.7	2.6	2.5	2.9
CMS Implicit Medical Price Deflator[2]	--	3.4	3.9	3.5	3.4	3.9	3.9
U.S. Population[3]	--	1.0	0.9	0.9	0.9	0.8	0.8
Population age less than 65 years	--	1.0	0.9	1.1	0.9	0.6	0.4
Population age 65 years and older	--	0.9	0.7	0.1	0.8	2.3	3.0
Private Health Insurance - NHE	--	8.9	10.9	10.4	8.2	7.1	6.3
Private Health Insurance - PHC	--	8.8	9.6	8.9	8.5	7.1	6.3

Note: Numbers and percents may not add to totals because of rounding. Figures for 2003-2013 are forecasts.

[1] The health spending projections were based on the 2002 version of the National Health Expenditures released in Jan. 2004.

[2] 1996 base year. Calculated as the difference between nominal personal health care spending and real personal health care spending. Real personal health care spending is produced by deflating spending on each service type by the appropriate deflator (PPI, CPI, etc.) and adding real spending by service type.

[3] July 1 Census resident based population estimates.

Sources: Centers for Medicare & Medicaid Services (CMS), Office of the Actuary.

National Health Expenditure Amounts, By Type of Expenditure: Selected Calendar Years 1980-2013[1]

(In Billions US$)

Item	1980	1990	2000	2002	2003	2004	2010	2013
National Health Expenditures	$245.8	$696.0	$1,309.4	$1,553.0	$1,673.6	$1,793.6	$2,751.0	$3,358.1
Health Services and Supplies	233.5	669.6	1,261.4	1,496.3	1,613.6	1,730.1	2,654.7	3,241.9
Personal Health Care	214.6	609.4	1,135.3	1,340.2	1,436.5	1,540.7	2,360.7	2,881.2
Hospital Care	101.5	253.9	413.2	486.5	518.1	551.7	791.5	934.3
Professional Services	67.3	216.9	426.5	501.5	535.8	572.0	876.7	1,075.8
Physician and Clinical Services	47.1	157.5	290.3	339.5	362.8	386.8	580.3	700.9
Other Professional Services	3.6	18.2	38.8	45.9	48.3	51.0	76.3	92.8
Dental Services	13.3	31.5	60.7	70.3	74.0	78.0	108.8	126.3
Other Personal Health Care	3.3	9.6	36.7	45.8	50.8	56.2	111.3	155.9
Nursing Home and Home Health	20.1	65.3	125.5	139.3	145.2	152.2	215.3	258.2
Home Health Care	2.4	12.6	31.7	36.1	38.3	40.6	60.3	73.4
Nursing Home Care	17.7	52.7	93.8	103.2	107.0	111.7	155.0	184.8
Retail Outlet Sales of Medical Products	25.7	73.3	170.1	212.9	237.4	264.8	477.2	612.9
Prescription Drugs	12.0	40.3	121.5	162.4	184.1	207.9	396.7	519.8
Other Medical Products	13.7	33.1	48.5	50.5	53.2	56.9	80.5	93.1
Durable Medical Equipment	3.9	10.6	17.7	18.8	19.6	20.6	27.8	32.6
Other Non-Durable Medical Products	9.8	22.5	30.8	31.7	33.6	36.4	52.7	60.5
Government Administration and Net Cost of Private Health Insurance	12.1	40.0	80.3	105.0	120.8	127.9	193.5	233.7
Government Public Health Activities	6.7	20.2	45.8	51.2	56.3	61.4	100.5	127.1
Investment	12.3	26.4	48.0	56.7	60.0	63.5	96.3	116.1
Research[2]	5.5	12.7	28.8	34.3	36.3	38.6	61.2	75.4
Construction	6.8	13.7	19.2	22.4	23.7	25.0	35.1	40.8

Note: Numbers and percents may not add to totals because of rounding. Figures for 2003-2013 are forecasts.

[1] The health spending projections were based on the 2002 version of the National Health Expenditures released in January 2004.

[2] Research and development expenditures of drug companies and other manufacturers and providers of medical equipment and supplies are excluded from research expenditures. These research expenditures are implicitly included in the expenditure class in which the product falls, in that they are covered by the payment received for that product.

Sources: Centers for Medicare & Medicaid Services (CMS), **Office of the Actuary.**

Hospital Care Expenditures and Average Annual Percent Change, U.S.: Selected Calendar Years 1980-2013[1]
By Source of Funds

Year	Total	Out-of-Pocket Payments	Third-Party Payments Total	Private Health Insurance	Other Private Funds	Public Total	Federal[2]	State and Local[2]	Medicare[3]	Medicaid[4]
Historical Estimates					Amount in Billions US$					
1980	**$101.5**	$5.3	$96.3	$36.1	$5.0	$55.2	$41.5	$13.7	$26.4	$10.6
1990	253.9	11.2	242.7	97.1	10.4	135.2	102.7	32.4	67.8	27.6
2000	413.2	12.7	400.5	137.5	20.2	242.8	194.2	48.6	126.9	70.2
2001	444.3	13.1	431.2	149.5	19.1	262.6	211.6	51.1	137.2	75.3
2002	486.5	14.7	471.8	165.0	20.3	286.4	229.9	56.5	149.2	83.5
Projected										
2003	518.1	15.9	502.2	181.9	21.1	299.1	240.4	58.7	156.7	86.6
2004	551.7	16.9	534.8	197.3	21.9	315.5	254.0	61.6	165.3	92.6
2005	585.8	18.1	567.7	211.0	23.0	333.7	268.9	64.8	175.1	98.8
2006	623.2	19.2	604.0	224.7	24.5	354.8	286.6	68.1	187.5	105.2
2007	661.8	20.4	641.4	238.7	26.0	376.6	304.9	71.7	200.3	111.6
2008	702.6	21.8	680.8	253.3	27.7	399.8	324.5	75.4	214.4	118.2
2009	746.1	23.3	722.8	268.7	29.4	424.7	345.7	79.0	230.1	125.0
2010	791.5	24.7	766.7	284.1	31.2	451.5	368.8	82.7	247.7	131.8
2011	838.1	26.3	811.8	299.2	33.0	479.6	393.2	86.4	266.6	138.7
2012	885.2	27.8	857.4	313.7	34.8	508.8	418.7	90.1	286.8	145.6
2013	934.3	29.4	904.9	328.4	36.8	539.7	445.9	93.8	308.8	152.4
Historical Estimates					Average Annual Percent Change from Previous Year Shown					
1990	--	--	--	--	--	--	--	--	--	--
1999	3.9	4.4	3.9	6.0	3.9	2.8	2.4	4.4	0.8	8.9
2000	5.0	1.9	5.1	7.5	-1.5	4.4	4.4	4.2	3.5	5.7
2001	7.5	3.4	7.7	8.7	-5.5	8.2	9.0	5.0	8.1	7.2
Projected										
2003	6.5	8.2	6.4	10.3	4.0	4.4	4.5	4.0	5.0	3.7
2004	6.5	6.3	6.5	8.4	3.9	5.5	5.7	4.8	5.4	6.9
2005	6.2	6.6	6.2	7.0	5.0	5.8	5.9	5.2	5.9	6.7
2006	6.4	6.5	6.4	6.5	6.4	6.3	6.6	5.2	7.1	6.4
2007	6.2	6.3	6.2	6.3	6.2	6.1	6.4	5.2	6.9	6.1
2008	6.2	6.7	6.1	6.1	6.2	6.2	6.4	5.1	7.0	5.9
2009	6.2	6.8	6.2	6.1	6.3	6.2	6.5	4.8	7.3	5.7
2010	6.1	6.2	6.1	5.7	6.1	6.3	6.7	4.6	7.6	5.5
2011	5.9	6.1	5.9	5.3	5.9	6.2	6.6	4.5	7.6	5.2
2012	5.6	5.8	5.6	4.9	5.5	6.1	6.5	4.4	7.6	4.9
2013	5.6	5.8	5.5	4.7	5.7	6.1	6.5	4.0	7.7	4.7

[1]The health spending projections were based on the 2002 version of the National Health Expenditures (NHE) released in Jan. 2004.
[2]Includes Medicaid SCHIP Expansion and SCHIP.
[3]Subset of Federal funds. [4]Subset of Federal and State and local funds. Includes Medicaid SCHIP Expansion.

Sources: Centers for Medicare & Medicaid Services (CMS), Office of the Actuary.

Hospital Care Expenditures, Percent Distribution and Per Capita Amount, U.S.: Selected Calendar Years 1980-2013[1]

By Source of Funds

Year	Total	Out-of-Pocket Payments	Third-Party Payments Total	Private Health Insurance	Other Private Funds	Public Total	Federal[2]	State and Local[2]	Medicare[3]	Medicaid[4]
Historical Estimates	\multicolumn{10}{c}{Per Capita Amount in US$}									
1980	$441	$23	$418	$157	$22	$239	$180	$59	5	5
1990	999	44	955	382	41	532	404	128	5	5
2000	1,474	45	1,428	491	72	866	692	173	5	5
2001	1,570	46	1,524	528	67	928	748	180	5	5
2002	1,704	52	1,653	578	71	1,003	805	198	5	5
Projected										
2003	1,798	55	1,743	631	73	1,038	834	204	5	5
2004	1,897	58	1,839	678	75	1,085	873	212	5	5
2005	1,996	62	1,935	719	79	1,137	916	221	5	5
2006	2,105	65	2,040	759	83	1,198	968	230	5	5
2007	2,216	68	2,148	799	87	1,261	1,021	240	5	5
2008	2,333	72	2,261	841	92	1,328	1,077	250	5	5
2009	2,457	77	2,380	885	97	1,398	1,138	260	5	5
2010	2,585	81	2,504	928	102	1,474	1,204	270	5	5
2011	2,715	85	2,630	969	107	1,554	1,274	280	5	5
2012	2,845	89	2,756	1,008	112	1,635	1,346	290	5	5
2013	2,980	94	2,886	1,047	117	1,721	1,422	299	5	5
Historical Estimates	\multicolumn{10}{c}{Percent Distribution}									
1980	100.0	5.2	94.8	35.6	4.9	54.3	40.9	13.5	26.0	10.4
1990	100	4.4	95.6	38.3	4.1	53.2	40.5	12.8	26.7	10.9
2000	100	3.1	96.9	33.3	4.9	58.8	47.0	11.8	30.7	17.0
2001	100	2.9	97.1	33.6	4.3	59.1	47.6	11.5	30.9	16.9
2002	100	3.0	97.0	33.9	4.2	58.9	47.3	11.6	30.7	17.2
Projected										
2003	100	3.1	96.9	35.1	4.1	57.7	46.4	11.3	30.3	16.7
2004	100	3.1	96.9	35.8	4.0	57.2	46.0	11.2	30.0	16.8
2005	100	3.1	96.9	36.0	3.9	57.0	45.9	11.1	29.9	16.9
2006	100	3.1	96.9	36.1	3.9	56.9	46.0	10.9	30.1	16.9
2007	100	3.1	96.9	36.1	3.9	56.9	46.1	10.8	30.3	16.9
2008	100	3.1	96.9	36.1	3.9	56.9	46.2	10.7	30.5	16.8
2009	100	3.1	96.9	36.0	3.9	56.9	46.3	10.6	30.8	16.8
2010	100	3.1	96.9	35.9	3.9	57.0	46.6	10.4	31.3	16.7
2011	100	3.1	96.9	35.7	3.9	57.2	46.9	10.3	31.8	16.6
2012	100	3.1	96.9	35.4	3.9	57.5	47.3	10.2	32.4	16.4
2013	100	3.1	96.9	35.1	3.9	57.8	47.7	10.0	33.1	16.3

[1] The health spending projections were based on the 2002 version of the National Health Expenditures (NHE) released in Jan. 2004.
[2] Includes Medicaid SCHIP Expansion and SCHIP.
[3] Subset of Federal funds. [4] Subset of Federal and State and local funds. Includes Medicaid SCHIP Expansion.
[5] Calculation of per capita estimates is inappropriate.

Notes: Per capita amounts based on July 1 Census resident based population estimates. Numbers and percents may not add to totals because of rounding.

Sources: Centers for Medicare & Medicaid Services (CMS), Office of the Actuary.

U.S. Hospital Expenses: Selected Years 1980-2003
According to Type of Ownership and Size of Hospital

Type of Ownership and Size of Hospital	1980	1990	1995	1997	1999	2001	2003
Hospitals	Amount in US$ Bil.						
All hospitals	$91.9	$234.9	$320.3	$342.3	$372.9	$426.8	$498.1
Federal	7.9	15.2	20.2	22.7	23.7	27.5	n/a
Non-Federal[1]	84.0	219.6	300.0	319.6	349.2	399.4	n/a
Community[2]	76.9	203.7	285.6	305.8	335.2	383.7	450.1
Nonprofit	55.8	150.7	209.6	225.3	251.5	287.3	n/a
For profit	5.8	18.8	26.7	31.2	31.2	37.3	n/a
State-local government	15.2	34.2	49.3	49.3	52.5	59.1	n/a
6-24 beds	0.2	0.5	1.1	1.3	1.7	1.6	n/a
25-49 beds	1.7	4.0	7.2	8.1	9.2	11.4	n/a
50-99 beds	5.4	12.6	17.8	19.5	21.0	24.0	n/a
100-199 beds	12.5	33.3	50.7	54.9	60.8	66.4	n/a
200-299 beds	13.4	38.7	55.8	57.1	61.1	68.9	n/a
300-399 beds	11.5	33.1	43.3	48.4	55.5	59.0	n/a
400-499 beds	10.5	25.3	33.7	35.0	33.9	47.3	n/a
500 beds or more	21.6	56.2	76.1	81.7	92.0	105.1	n/a
Expenses per Inpatient Day	Amount in US$						
Community[2]	$245	$687	$968	$1,033	$1,103	$1,217	n/a
Nonprofit	246	692	994	1,074	1,140	1,255	n/a
For profit	257	752	947	962	999	1,121	n/a
State-local government	239	634	878	914	1,007	1,114	n/a
6-24 beds	203	526	678	731	955	1,020	n/a
25-49 beds	197	489	696	775	846	907	n/a
50-99 beds	191	493	647	686	717	786	n/a
100-199 beds	215	585	796	853	897	974	n/a
200-299 beds	239	665	943	1,011	1,077	1,174	n/a
300-399 beds	248	731	1,070	1,129	1,215	1,338	n/a
400-499 beds	215	756	1,135	1,195	1,285	1,492	n/a
500 beds or more	239	825	1,212	1,304	1,404	1,549	n/a

[1] The category of non-Federal hospitals is comprised of psychiatric, tuberculosis and other respiratory disease hospitals and long-term and short-term hospitals. [2] Community hospitals are short-term hospitals excluding hospital units in institutions such as prison and college infirmaries, facilities for the mentally retarded and alcoholism and chemical dependency hospitals.

n/a = not available

Source: American Hospital Association (AHA).

Home Health Care Expenditures and Average Annual Percent Change, U.S.: Selected Calendar Years 1980-2013[1]

By Source of Funds

Year	Total	Out-of-Pocket Payments	Third-Party Payments Total	Private Health Insurance	Other Private Funds	Public Total	Federal[2]	State and Local[2]	Medicare[3]	Medicaid[4]
Historical Estimates	Amount in Billions US$								
1980	**$2.40**	$0.40	$2.00	$0.30	$0.40	$1.30	$0.80	$0.50	$0.60	$0.30
1990	12.6	2.3	10.3	2.9	1.0	6.5	4.4	2.0	3.3	2.1
2000	31.7	6.2	25.5	7.7	1.3	16.5	12.1	4.4	8.6	6.2
2001	33.7	6.1	27.6	6.9	1.1	19.6	14.4	5.2	10.1	7.6
2002	36.1	6.5	29.6	6.7	1.1	21.9	16.2	5.7	11.4	8.4
Projected										
2003	38.3	6.9	31.3	6.9	1.1	23.3	17.3	6.0	12.2	8.9
2004	40.6	7.3	33.2	7.1	1.2	24.9	18.5	6.4	13.1	9.6
2005	43.2	7.9	35.4	7.4	1.3	26.7	19.9	6.8	14.0	10.4
2006	46.2	8.4	37.8	7.8	1.4	28.7	21.3	7.3	15.0	11.3
2007	49.4	9.0	40.4	8.1	1.4	30.8	22.9	7.9	16.0	12.3
2008	52.7	9.6	43.1	8.6	1.5	33.1	24.6	8.4	17.1	13.3
2009	56.3	10.2	46.1	9.1	1.6	35.4	26.3	9.1	18.2	14.5
2010	60.3	11.0	49.3	9.6	1.7	37.9	28.2	9.7	19.4	15.7
2011	64.4	11.8	52.6	10.1	1.8	40.7	30.2	10.5	20.7	17.0
2012	68.7	12.6	56.1	10.7	1.9	43.5	32.3	11.2	21.9	18.5
2013	73.4	13.5	59.9	11.3	2.0	46.6	34.5	12.0	23.3	20.0
Historical Estimates	Average Annual Percent Change from Previous Year Shown								
1990	--	--	--	--	--	--	--	--	--	--
2000	-1.8	-6.5	-0.6	-5.6	-18.8	3.8	3.5	4.6	0.6	11.2
2001	6.2	-2.1	8.3	-10.5	-14.1	18.8	19.0	18.4	17.6	22.2
2002	7.2	6.4	7.4	-2.5	-6.9	11.7	12.7	9.0	13.3	10.8
Projected										
2003	5.9	6.4	5.8	3.0	8.6	6.5	6.8	5.6	7.3	5.7
2004	6.1	6.3	6.0	2.6	7.3	7.0	7.1	6.4	7.0	7.6
2005	6.6	7.0	6.5	4.2	5.4	7.2	7.2	7.0	6.8	8.3
2006	6.8	7.0	6.8	4.8	4.7	7.5	7.5	7.3	7.1	8.5
2007	6.9	7.0	6.8	4.9	5.2	7.5	7.5	7.5	7.0	8.7
2008	6.8	6.5	6.9	5.6	5.6	7.3	7.2	7.4	6.7	8.6
2009	6.8	6.8	6.8	6.0	6.2	7.1	7.0	7.4	6.3	8.6
2010	7.0	7.2	6.9	5.9	6.2	7.2	7.1	7.4	6.6	8.5
2011	6.8	7.3	6.7	5.1	6.0	7.2	7.1	7.4	6.5	8.5
2012	6.8	7.1	6.7	5.5	5.8	7.1	7.0	7.3	6.3	8.5
2013	6.8	7.3	6.7	5.5	5.9	7.0	6.9	7.3	6.2	8.4

[1]Health spending projections based on the 2002 version of the National Health Expenditures (NHE) released in January 2004.
[2]Includes Medicaid SCHIP Expansion and SCHIP.   [3]Subset of Federal funds.
[4]Subset of Federal and State and local funds. Includes Medicaid SCHIP Expansion.

Source: Centers for Medicare & Medicaid Services (CMS), Office of the Actuary.

Home Health Care Expenditures, Percent Distribution and Per Capita Amount, U.S.: Selected Calendar Years 1980-2013[1]

By Source of Funds

Year	Total	Out-of-Pocket Payments	Third-Party Payments Total	Private Health Insurance	Other Private Funds	Public Total	Federal[2]	State and Local[2]	Medicare[3]	Medicaid[4]
Historical Estimates				**Percent Distribution**						
1980	100.0	15.3	84.7	14.7	15.5	54.5	33.6	21.0	26.8	11.7
1990	100.0	18.1	81.9	22.7	7.6	51.6	35.3	16.2	26.0	17.0
2000	100.0	19.7	80.3	24.3	4.1	51.9	38.0	13.8	27.0	19.7
2001	100.0	18.1	81.9	20.5	3.4	58.0	42.6	15.4	29.9	22.6
2002	100.0	18.0	82.0	18.6	2.9	60.5	44.8	15.7	31.6	23.4
Projected										
2003	100.0	18.1	81.9	18.1	3.0	60.8	45.2	15.6	32.0	23.3
2004	100.0	18.1	81.9	17.5	3.0	61.3	45.6	15.7	32.3	23.7
2005	100.0	18.2	81.8	17.1	3.0	61.7	45.9	15.8	32.4	24.0
2006	100.0	18.2	81.8	16.8	2.9	62.0	46.2	15.8	32.5	24.4
2007	100.0	18.2	81.8	16.5	2.9	62.4	46.5	15.9	32.5	24.8
2008	100.0	18.2	81.8	16.3	2.8	62.7	46.6	16.0	32.4	25.3
2009	100.0	18.2	81.8	16.2	2.8	62.8	46.7	16.1	32.3	25.7
2010	100.0	18.2	81.8	16.0	2.8	63.0	46.8	16.2	32.2	26.1
2011	100.0	18.3	81.7	15.7	2.8	63.2	46.9	16.2	32.1	26.5
2012	100.0	18.3	81.7	15.6	2.8	63.3	47.0	16.3	31.9	26.9
2013	100.0	18.4	81.6	15.4	2.7	63.5	47.1	16.4	31.8	27.3
Historical Estimates				**Per Capita Amount in US$**						
1980	$10	$2	$9	$2	$2	$6	$3	$2	5	5
1990	49	9	41	11	4	25	17	8	5	5
2000	113	22	91	28	5	59	43	16	5	5
2001	119	22	98	24	4	69	51	18	5	5
2002	127	23	104	24	4	77	57	20	5	5
Projected										
2003	133	24	109	24	4	81	60	21	5	5
2004	140	25	114	24	4	86	64	22	5	5
2005	147	27	121	25	4	91	68	23	5	5
2006	156	28	128	26	5	97	72	25	5	5
2007	165	30	135	27	5	103	77	26	5	5
2008	175	32	143	29	5	110	82	28	5	5
2009	186	34	152	30	5	117	87	30	5	5
2010	197	36	161	32	6	124	92	32	5	5
2011	209	38	170	33	6	132	98	34	5	5
2012	221	41	180	34	6	140	104	36	5	5
2013	234	43	191	36	6	149	110	38	5	5

[1] Health spending projections based on the 2002 version of the National Health Expenditures (NHE) released in January 2004.
[2] Includes Medicaid SCHIP Expansion and SCHIP.
[3] Subset of Federal funds. [4] Subset of Federal and State and local funds. Includes Medicaid SCHIP Expansion.
[5] Calculation of per capita estimates is inappropriate.

Notes: Per capita amounts based on July 1 Census resident based population estimates. Numbers and percents may not add to totals because of rounding.

Sources: Centers for Medicare & Medicaid Services (CMS), Office of the Actuary.

Nursing Home Care Expenditures and Average Annual Percent Change, U.S.: Selected Calendar Years 1980-2013[1]

By Source of Funds

Year	Total	Out-of-Pocket Payments	Third-Party Payments Total	Private Health Insurance	Other Private Funds	Public Total	Federal[2]	State and Local[2]	Medicare[3]	Medicaid[4]
Historical Estimates				Amount in Billions US$						
1980	$17.7	$7.1	$10.6	$0.2	$0.8	$9.6	$5.7	$3.9	$0.3	$8.9
1990	52.7	19.8	32.9	3.1	3.9	25.9	15.8	10.2	1.7	23.2
2000	93.8	26.2	67.6	7.3	4.1	56.1	37.7	18.5	9.5	44.6
2001	99.1	26.7	72.4	7.6	3.7	61.1	42.2	18.9	12.0	46.9
2002	103.2	25.9	77.3	7.7	3.5	66.1	45.5	20.5	12.9	50.9
Projected										
2003	107.0	26.5	80.5	7.9	3.6	69.0	47.2	21.9	12.6	54.1
2004	111.7	27.2	84.4	8.1	3.7	72.6	49.5	23.1	13.0	57.1
2005	116.9	28.5	88.4	8.5	3.9	76.0	51.5	24.5	12.8	60.6
2006	123.3	29.8	93.5	8.8	4.1	80.6	54.5	26.1	13.4	64.4
2007	130.2	31.2	99.1	9.3	4.3	85.5	57.8	27.8	13.9	68.6
2008	137.8	32.7	105.1	9.7	4.5	90.9	61.3	29.6	14.6	73.1
2009	146.1	34.2	111.9	10.2	4.7	97.0	65.5	31.6	15.6	78.1
2010	155.0	35.8	119.2	10.6	4.9	103.7	69.9	33.7	16.7	83.4
2011	164.4	37.4	127.0	11.1	5.1	110.8	74.8	36.0	17.8	89.1
2012	174.3	39.0	135.3	11.6	5.3	118.4	79.8	38.5	19.0	95.2
2013	184.8	40.7	144.1	12.1	5.6	126.4	85.3	41.1	20.3	101.8
Historical Estimates			Average Annual Percent Change from Previous Year Shown							
1990	--	--	--	--	--	--	--	--	--	--
2000	4.7	4.2	4.9	-2.3	-8.0	7.1	9.0	3.2	9.6	6.6
2001	5.7	1.8	7.2	4.2	-10.2	8.9	12.1	2.3	26.5	5.1
2002	4.1	-2.9	6.7	0.9	-4.9	8.1	7.8	8.7	7.7	8.6
Projected										
2003	3.7	2.2	4.2	2.2	2.2	4.5	3.7	6.4	-2.7	6.3
2004	4.4	2.9	4.9	2.9	2.9	5.2	4.9	5.8	3.4	5.6
2005	4.7	4.8	4.7	4.8	4.8	4.7	4.1	6.0	-1.4	6.0
2006	5.4	4.5	5.8	4.5	4.5	6.0	5.8	6.3	4.3	6.3
2007	5.6	4.7	5.9	4.7	4.7	6.1	6.0	6.5	4.2	6.5
2008	5.8	4.8	6.1	4.8	4.8	6.3	6.2	6.6	4.8	6.6
2009	6.1	4.8	6.5	4.8	4.8	6.7	6.7	6.7	6.7	6.7
2010	6.1	4.6	6.5	4.6	4.6	6.8	6.8	6.8	7.0	6.8
2011	6.1	4.5	6.6	4.5	4.5	6.9	6.9	6.8	7.0	6.9
2012	6.0	4.2	6.5	4.2	4.2	6.8	6.8	6.9	6.6	6.9
2013	6.0	4.4	6.5	4.4	4.4	6.8	6.8	6.8	6.7	6.8

[1] Health spending projections based on the 2002 version of the National Health Expenditures (NHE) released in January 2004.
[2] Includes Medicaid SCHIP Expansion and SCHIP.
[3] Subset of Federal funds.
[4] Subset of Federal and State and local funds. Includes Medicaid SCHIP Expansion.

Sources: Centers for Medicare & Medicaid Services (CMS), Office of the Actuary.

Nursing Home Care Expenditures, Percent Distribution and Per Capita Amount, U.S.: Selected Calendar Years 1980-2013[1]

By Source of Funds

Year	Total	Out-of-Pocket Payments	Third-Party Payments Total	Private Health Insurance	Other Private Funds	Public Total	Federal[2]	State and Local[2]	Medicare[3]	Medicaid[4]
Historical Estimates					Per Capita Amount in US$					
1980	$77	$31	$46	$1	$3	$42	$25	$17	5	5
1990	207	78	130	12	16	102	62	40	5	5
2000	334	93	241	26	15	200	134	66	5	5
2001	350	94	256	27	13	216	149	67	5	5
2002	361	91	271	27	12	231	159	72	5	5
Projected										
2003	371	92	279	27	13	240	164	76	5	5
2004	384	94	290	28	13	250	170	80	5	5
2005	398	97	301	29	13	259	176	84	5	5
2006	416	101	316	30	14	272	184	88	5	5
2007	436	104	332	31	14	286	193	93	5	5
2008	458	109	349	32	15	302	204	98	5	5
2009	481	113	368	33	15	320	216	104	5	5
2010	506	117	389	35	16	339	228	110	5	5
2011	533	121	411	36	17	359	242	117	5	5
2012	560	125	435	37	17	380	257	124	5	5
2013	589	130	459	39	18	403	272	131	5	5
Historical Estimates					Percent Distribution					
1980	100.0	40.0	60.0	1.2	4.5	54.2	32.0	22.2	1.7	50.2
1990	100	37.5	62.5	5.8	7.5	49.2	30.0	19.3	3.2	43.9
2000	100	27.9	72.1	7.8	4.4	59.8	40.2	19.7	10.1	47.5
2001	100	26.9	73.1	7.7	3.8	61.7	42.6	19.1	12.1	47.3
2002	100	25.1	74.9	7.5	3.4	64.0	44.1	19.9	12.5	49.3
Projected										
2003	100	24.7	75.3	7.3	3.4	64.5	44.1	20.4	11.8	50.6
2004	100	24.4	75.6	7.2	3.3	65.1	44.3	20.7	11.6	51.2
2005	100	24.4	75.6	7.2	3.3	65.0	44.1	21.0	11.0	51.8
2006	100	24.2	75.8	7.2	3.3	65.4	44.2	21.1	10.8	52.2
2007	100	23.9	76.1	7.1	3.3	65.7	44.4	21.3	10.7	52.7
2008	100	23.7	76.3	7.0	3.2	66.0	44.5	21.5	10.6	53.1
2009	100	23.4	76.6	7.0	3.2	66.4	44.8	21.6	10.7	53.4
2010	100	23.1	76.9	6.9	3.2	66.9	45.1	21.8	10.7	53.8
2011	100	22.8	77.2	6.8	3.1	67.4	45.5	21.9	10.8	54.2
2012	100	22.4	77.6	6.6	3.1	67.9	45.8	22.1	10.9	54.7
2013	100	22.0	78.0	6.5	3.0	68.4	46.1	22.3	11.0	55.1

[1] Health spending projections based on the 2002 version of the National Health Expenditures (NHE) released in January 2004.
[2] Includes Medicaid SCHIP Expansion and SCHIP.
[3] Subset of Federal funds. [4] Subset of Federal and State and local funds. Includes Medicaid SCHIP Expansion.
[5] Calculation of per capita estimates is inappropriate.

Notes: Per capita amounts based on July 1 Census resident based population estimates. Numbers and percents may not add to totals because of rounding.

Sources: Centers for Medicare & Medicaid Services (CMS), Office of the Actuary.

Prescription Drug Expenditures and Average Annual Percent Change, U.S.: Selected Calendar Years 1980-2013[1]

By Source of Funds

Year	Total	Out-of-Pocket Payments	Third-Party Payments						Medicare[3]	Medicaid[4]
			Total	Private Health Insurance	Other Private Funds	Public Total	Federal[2]	State and Local[2]		
Historical Estimates					Amount in Billions US$					
1990	$40.30	$23.80	$16.50	$9.80	--	$6.70	$3.20	$3.40	$0.20	$5.10
1998	87.3	30.5	56.8	38.3	--	18.4	10.5	7.9	1.8	14.4
1999	104.4	34.4	70.1	47.9	--	22.2	12.8	9.4	2.1	17.3
2000	121.5	38.3	83.2	56.6	--	26.7	15.3	11.4	2.3	20.9
2001	140.8	42.5	98.3	66.8	--	31.5	18	13.5	2.5	24.8
2002	162.4	48.6	113.8	77.6	--	36.2	20.9	15.4	2.6	28.6
Projected										
2003	184.1	54.4	129.7	88.7	--	41	23.6	17.4	2.7	32.7
2004	207.9	60.8	147.1	101.2	--	45.9	26.4	19.6	2.8	37
2005	233.6	67.6	166	114.5	--	51.5	29.5	22	2.8	42
2006	261.8	74.9	186.8	129.2	--	57.7	33	24.7	2.8	47.5
2007	292.4	82.8	209.6	145	--	64.5	36.9	27.6	3	53.4
2008	325.3	91.2	234.2	162.3	--	71.9	41	30.8	3.2	59.7
2009	360.1	99.9	260.2	180.6	--	79.6	45.4	34.1	3.4	66.1
2010	396.7	109.5	287.2	199.7	--	87.6	49.9	37.6	3.7	72.8
2011	435.2	119.3	315.9	219.9	--	95.9	54.6	41.3	3.9	79.5
2012	476.2	130.3	345.9	241.4	--	104.5	59.4	45.1	4.3	86.3
2013	519.8	141.9	378	264.6	--	113.4	64.3	49.1	4.6	93.1
Historical Estimates					Average Annual Percent Change from Previous Year Shown					
1998	10.1	3.1	16.7	18.6	--	13.5	15.8	11	31.6	14
1999	19.7	12.7	23.4	24.8	--	20.4	21.4	19	20.1	20
2000	16.4	11.5	18.8	18.2	--	20.1	20	20.2	8.2	20.7
2001	15.9	10.9	18.1	18.2	--	18.1	17.9	18.5	6.9	18.8
2002	15.3	14.4	15.8	16.1	--	15.1	15.7	14.3	7	15.2
Projected										
2003	13.4	12	13.9	14.4	--	13	13	13	3.9	14.3
2004	12.9	11.7	13.4	14	--	12.1	11.8	12.6	3.4	13.3
2005	12.4	11.2	12.9	13.2	--	12.1	11.9	12.4	-0.6	13.5
2006	12.1	10.9	12.6	12.8	--	12	11.9	12.3	1.2	13.1
2007	11.7	10.5	12.2	12.3	--	11.9	11.9	12	5.2	12.5
2008	11.3	10.2	11.7	11.9	--	11.3	11.2	11.4	6.4	11.6
2009	10.7	9.6	11.1	11.3	--	10.7	10.6	10.8	7.1	10.8
2010	10.2	9.5	10.4	10.5	--	10.1	10	10.3	7.5	10
2011	9.7	9	10	10.2	--	9.5	9.4	9.7	7.7	9.3
2012	9.4	9.1	9.5	9.8	--	8.9	8.7	9.2	7.7	8.5
2013	9.2	8.9	9.3	9.6	--	8.5	8.2	8.8	7.6	7.9

[1] The health spending projections were based on the 2002 version of the National Health Expenditures (NHE) released in Jan. 2004.
[2] Includes Medicaid SCHIP Expansion and SCHIP.
[3] Subset of Federal funds.
[4] Subset of Federal and State and local funds. Includes Medicaid SCHIP Expansion.

Sources: Centers for Medicare & Medicaid Services (CMS), Office of the Actuary.

Prescription Drug Expenditures, Percent Distribution and Per Capita Amount, U.S.: Selected Calendar Years 1980-2013[1]

By Source of Funds

Year	Total	Out-of-Pocket Payments	Third-Party Payments Total	Private Health Insurance	Other Private Funds	Public Total	Federal[2]	State and Local[2]	Medicare[3]	Medicaid[4]
Historical Estimates				Per Capita Amount in US$						
1980	$52	$36	$16	$9	--	$7	$4	$4	5	5
1990	159	94	65	39	--	26	13	14	5	5
2000	433	137	297	202	--	95	55	40	5	5
2001	498	150	347	236	--	111	64	48	5	5
2002	569	170	399	272	--	127	73	54	5	5
Projected										
2003	639	189	450	308	--	142	82	60	5	5
2004	715	209	506	348	--	158	91	67	5	5
2005	796	230	566	390	--	175	100	75	5	5
2006	884	253	631	436	--	195	111	83	5	5
2007	979	277	702	486	--	216	124	93	5	5
2008	1,080	303	777	539	--	239	136	102	5	5
2009	1,186	329	857	595	--	262	150	112	5	5
2010	1,296	357	938	652	--	286	163	123	5	5
2011	1,410	387	1,023	712	--	311	177	134	5	5
2012	1,530	419	1,112	776	--	336	191	145	5	5
2013	1,658	452	1,205	844	--	362	205	157	5	5
Historical Estimates				Percent Distribution						
1980	100.0	69.4	30.6	16.7	--	13.9	7.1	6.8	--	11.7
1990	100	59.1	40.9	24.4	--	16.6	8.0	8.5	0.5	12.6
2000	100	31.5	68.5	46.5	--	21.9	12.6	9.3	1.9	17.2
2001	100	30.2	69.8	47.5	--	22.4	12.8	9.6	1.7	17.6
2002	100	29.9	70.1	47.8	--	22.3	12.8	9.5	1.6	17.6
Projected										
2003	100	29.6	70.4	48.2	--	22.2	12.8	9.4	1.5	17.8
2004	100	29.2	70.8	48.7	--	22.1	12.7	9.4	1.4	17.8
2005	100	28.9	71.1	49.0	--	22.0	12.6	9.4	1.2	18.0
2006	100	28.6	71.4	49.3	--	22.0	12.6	9.4	1.1	18.2
2007	100	28.3	71.7	49.6	--	22.1	12.6	9.5	1.0	18.3
2008	100	28.0	72.0	49.9	--	22.1	12.6	9.5	1.0	18.3
2009	100	27.8	72.2	50.2	--	22.1	12.6	9.5	0.9	18.4
2010	100	27.6	72.4	50.3	--	22.1	12.6	9.5	0.9	18.3
2011	100	27.4	72.6	50.5	--	22.0	12.6	9.5	0.9	18.3
2012	100	27.4	72.6	50.7	--	21.9	12.5	9.5	0.9	18.1
2013	100	27.3	72.7	50.9	--	21.8	12.4	9.4	0.9	17.9

[1] Health spending projections based on the 2002 version of the National Health Expenditures (NHE) released in January 2004.
[2] Includes Medicaid SCHIP Expansion and SCHIP.
[3] Subset of Federal funds. [4] Subset of Federal and State and local funds. Includes Medicaid SCHIP Expansion.
[5] Calculation of per capita estimates is inappropriate.
Notes: Per capita amounts based on July 1 Census resident based population estimates. Numbers and percents may not add to totals because of rounding.

Sources: Centers for Medicare & Medicaid Services (CMS), Office of the Actuary.

Index Levels of Medical Prices, U.S.: 2000-2004

	2000	2001	2002	2003	Q1 2004
Consumer Price Indexes, All Urban Consumers[1]					
Medical Care Services[2]	266.0	278.8	292.9	306.0	316.3
Professional Services	237.7	246.5	253.9	261.2	267.7
Physicians' Services	244.7	253.6	260.6	267.7	274.6
Dental Services	258.5	269.0	281.0	292.5	301.2
Hospital and Related Services	317.3	338.3	367.8	394.8	412.0
Hospital Services (12/96=100)	115.9	123.6	134.7	144.7	151.2
Inpatient Hospital Services (12/96=100)	113.8	121.0	131.2	140.1	146.0
Outpatient Hospital Services (12/86=100)	263.8	281.1	309.8	337.9	351.7
Nursing Home Services (12/96=100)	117.0	121.8	127.9	135.2	138.9
Medical Care Commodities	238.1	247.6	256.4	262.8	266.5
Prescription Drugs	285.4	300.9	316.5	326.3	332.2
Non-prescription Drugs & Medical Supplies (1986=100)	149.5	150.6	150.4	152.0	152.5
Internal and Respiratory Over-the-Counter Drugs	176.9	178.9	178.8	181.2	181.6
Non-prescription Medical Equipment and Supplies	178.1	178.2	177.5	178.1	179.2
Producer Price Indexes[3]					
Industry Groupings[4]					
Health Services (12/94=100)	112.8	116.4	119.4	124.2	n/a
Offices and Clinics of Doctors of Medicine (12/93=100)	115.8	119.1	119.1	120.9	123.0
Hospitals (12/92=100)	119.4	123.0	127.5	134.9	139.6
General Medical and Surgical Hospitals (12/92=100)	119.8	123.4	127.9	135.3	140.0
Medicare Patients (12/92=100)	110.3	113.0	116.1	122.1	125.1
Medicaid Patients (12/92=100)	114.3	117.3	121.0	125.5	128.2
All Other Patients (12/92=100)	124.8	129.4	136.1	147.0	154.3
Skilled and Intermediate Care Facilities (12/94=100)	131.0	139.3	144.6	149.4	153.9
Public Payers (12/94=100)	131.6	140.9	146.2	149.5	153.6
Private Payers (12/94=100)	131.5	138.3	144.1	151.2	156.3
Medical Laboratories (6/94=100)	108.0	112.1	113.9	115.7	n/a
Home Health Care Services (12/96=100)	111.1	114.0	116.6	117.0	119.5
Medicare Payers (12/96=100)	112.1	116.2	118.2	114.7	117.2
Commodity Groupings					
Drugs and Pharmaceuticals	257.4	261.8	265.8	274.7	279.6
Pharmaceutical Preparations (6/01=100)	n/a	n/a	102.7	107.3	109.6
Medical, Surgical, and Personal Aid Devices	146.0	148.3	150.9	154.7	157.7
Personal Aid Equipment	150.3	155.2	161.4	162.3	n/a
Medical Instruments and Equipment (6/82=100)	125.6	127.0	129.1	132.8	133.9
Surgical Appliances and Supplies (6/83=100)	167.1	170.4	173.9	178.2	184.7
Ophthalmic Goods (12/83=100)	118.3	118.5	119.3	120.0	120.8
Dental Equipment and Supplies (6/85=100)	164.8	170.4	172.0	179.1	182.1

Note: Q designates quarter of year. Quarterly data are not seasonally adjusted. N/a = not available
[1] Unless otherwise noted, base year is 1982-84 = 100.
[2] Includes the net cost of private health insurance.
[3] Unless otherwise noted, base year is 1982 = 100. Producer price indexes are classified by industry (price changes received for the industry's output sold outside the industry) and commodity.
[4] Further detail for Producer Price Industry groupings are available from Bureau of Labor Statistics.

Sources: U.S. Department of Labor, Bureau of Labor Statistics: *CPI Detailed Report* and *Producer Price Indexes*.

Hospitals, Beds and Occupancy Rates, U.S.: 1997-2003
According to Type of Ownership and Size of Hospital

Type of Ownership and Size of Hospital	1997	1998	1999	2000	2001	2003
Hospitals						
All hospitals	6,097	6,021	5,890	5,810	5,801	5,764
Federal	285	275	264	245	243	239
Non-Federal[1]	5,812	5,746	5,626	5,565	5,558	5,525
Community[2]	5,057	5,015	4,956	4,915	4,908	4,895
Nonprofit	3,000	3,026	3,012	3,003	2,998	2,984
For profit	797	771	747	749	754	790
State-local government	1,260	1,218	1,197	1,163	1,156	1,121
6-24 beds	281	293	299	288	281	n/a
25-49 beds	890	900	887	910	916	n/a
50-99 beds	1,111	1,085	1,082	1,055	1,070	n/a
100-199 beds	1,289	1,304	1,266	1,236	1,218	n/a
200-299 beds	679	644	642	656	635	n/a
300-399 beds	367	352	365	341	348	n/a
400-499 beds	185	183	161	182	191	n/a
500 beds or more	255	254	254	247	249	n/a
Beds						
All hospitals	1,035,390	1,012,582	993,866	983,628	987,440	965,256
Federal	61,937	56,698	55,120	53,067	51,900	n/a
Non-Federal[1]	973,453	955,884	938,746	930,561	935,540	n/a
Community[2]	853,287	839,988	829,575	823,560	825,966	813,307
Nonprofit	590,636	587,658	586,673	582,988	585,070	n/a
For profit	115,074	112,975	106,790	109,883	108,718	n/a
State-local government	147,577	139,355	136,112	130,689	132,178	n/a
6-24 beds	5,128	5,351	5,442	5,156	4,964	n/a
25-49 beds	33,138	33,510	32,816	33,333	33,263	n/a
50-99 beds	79,837	78,035	78,121	75,865	76,924	n/a
100-199 beds	182,284	186,118	181,115	175,778	174,024	n/a
200-299 beds	165,197	156,978	155,831	159,807	154,420	n/a
300-399 beds	126,307	120,512	126,259	117,220	119,753	n/a
400-499 beds	82,250	81,247	71,580	80,763	84,745	n/a
500 beds or more	179,146	178,237	178,411	175,638	177,873	n/a
Occupancy rate						
All hospitals	65.0%	65.4%	66.1%	66.1%	66.7%	n/a
Federal	79.1%	78.9%	74.4%	68.2%	69.8%	n/a
Non-Federal[1]	64.1%	64.6%	65.6%	65.9%	66.5%	n/a
Community[2]	61.8%	62.5%	63.4%	63.9%	64.5%	n/a
Nonprofit	63.6%	64.2%	64.9%	65.5%	65.8%	n/a
For profit	52.0%	53.2%	54.8%	55.9%	57.8%	n/a
State-local government	62.3%	62.7%	63.4%	63.2%	64.1%	n/a
6-24 beds	35.4%	33.2%	33.0%	31.7%	31.3%	n/a
25-49 beds	40.3%	41.2%	41.5%	41.3%	42.5%	n/a
50-99 beds	54.2%	54.7%	54.5%	54.8%	55.5%	n/a
100-199 beds	58.2%	58.4%	59.3%	60.0%	60.7%	n/a
200-299 beds	61.8%	62.9%	64.1%	65.0%	65.5%	n/a
300-399 beds	63.2%	64.7%	66.1%	65.7%	66.4%	n/a
400-499 beds	68.0%	67.3%	68.3%	69.1%	68.9%	n/a
500 beds or more	69.8%	70.9%	71.7%	72.2%	72.8%	n/a

[1] The category of non-Federal hospitals is comprised of psychiatric, tuberculosis and other respiratory disease hospitals, and long-term and short-term hospitals. [2] Community hospitals are short-term hospitals excluding hospital units in institutions such as prison and college infirmaries, facilities for the mentally retarded and alcoholism and chemical dependency hospitals.

n/a = not available

Source: American Hospital Association (AHA).

U.S. Community Hospital Statistics[1]: 2000-2003

Item	Calendar Year 2000	2001	2002	2003
Utilization				
All Ages				
Discharges in Thousands	36,328	37,141	37,348	37,441
Discharges Per 1,000 Population[2]	126	128	127	126
Inpatient Days in Thousands	188,703	190,711	191,563	192,317
Adult Length of Stay in Days	5.2	5.1	5.1	5.1
65 Years of Age or Over				
Discharges in Thousands	14,298	14,750	14,809	14,936
Discharges Per 1,000 Population[2]	404	413	412	413
Inpatient Days in Thousands	86,877	87,961	87,511	87,988
Adult Length of Stay in Days	6.1	6	5.9	5.9
Under 65 Years of Age				
Discharges in Thousands	22,029	22,391	22,539	22,505
Discharges Per 1,000 Population[2]	87	88	87	86
Inpatient Days in Thousands	101,826	102,750	104,051	104,329
Adult Length of Stay in Days	4.6	4.6	4.6	4.6
Outpatient Visits in Thousands	592,337	591,278	592,845	585,541
Adjusted Patient Days in Thousands[3]	302,674	309,295	314,047	316,207
Total Hospital Revenues in Millions[4]	$387,539	$427,804	$457,098	$488,543
Total Patient Revenues in Millions	359,688	398,857	429,041	456,592
Inpatient Revenues in Millions	224,207	245,858	261,627	277,647
Outpatient Revenues in Millions	135,481	152,998	167,414	178,945
Total Expenses				
Total Hospital Expenses in Millions	$371,580	$407,706	$434,936	$464,394
Inpatient Expense in Millions[5]	$231,595	$251,278	$265,195	$282,398
Amount per Patient Day	1,227	1,318	1,384	1,468
Amount per Discharge	6,375	6,766	7,101	7,542
Outpatient Expense in Millions[5]	$139,986	$156,427	$169,741	$181,996
Amount per Outpatient Visit	236	265	286	311

Notes: Community hospitals include all non-Federal, short-term general, and other special hospitals open to the public. They exclude hospital units of institutions; psychiatric facilities; tuberculosis, other respiratory, and chronic disease hospitals; institutions for the mentally retarded; and alcohol and chemical dependency hospitals.

[1] *National Hospital Indicators Survey* data for 1998:4-2003:4. Survey replaced *National Hospital Panel Survey*.

[2] Discharges per 1,000 population is calculated using population estimates prepared by the Social Security Administration.

[3] Adjusted patient days is an aggregate figure reflecting the number of days of inpatient care, plus an estimate of the volume of the volume of outpatient services, expressed in units equivalent to an inpatient day in terms of level of effort. It is derived by multiplying the number of outpatient visits by the ratio of outpatient revenue per outpatient visit to inpatient revenue per inpatient day, and adding the product to the number of inpatient days.

[4] Total hospital revenue is the sum of total patient revenue and all other operating revenue. Total patient revenue is the sum of inpatient revenue and outpatient revenue.

[5] Inpatient Expense and Outpatient Expense are calculated by the National Health Statistics Group. These statistics are calculated by applying the ratio of inpatient or outpatient revenue to total patient revenue multiplied by total hospital expenses.

Source: Centers for Medicare & Medicaid Services (CMS)

III. Medicare and Medicaid

Contents:

Medicare and Medicaid Spending: 2002-2005	66
Where the Medicare Dollar Went, 2004	67
Number of Medicare Beneficiaries, 1970-2030	68
Medicare Enrollment Trends, Hospital and/or Supplemental Medical Insurance: July 1970-2003	69
Medicare Enrollment Trends, Hospital Insurance: July 1970-2003	70
Medicare Enrollment Trends, Supplemental Medical Insurance: July 1970-2003	71
Medicare Deductible, Co-insurance and Premium Amounts, 2005	72

Medicare and Medicaid Spending: 2002-2005

(In Billions US$)

	2002	2003	2004	2005
Medicare (excluding premiums)	256.8	277.9	302.6	331.1
Medicare (including premiums)	230.8	249.5	270.4	294.3
Medicaid	147.5	160.7	177.3	182.1
Total*	378.3	410.2	447.7	476.4
Total Federal Spending	2,011	2,158	2,319	2,400
Medicare/Medicaid % of Federal Spending*	18.0%	19.0%	19.3%	19.9%

*Medicare/Medicaid total = Medicare with Premiums + Medicaid

Note: Figures for 2004 and 2005 are estimates.

Source: U.S. Office of Management and Budget; Plunkett Research, Ltd.

Where the Medicare Dollar Went, 2004 (Estimate)

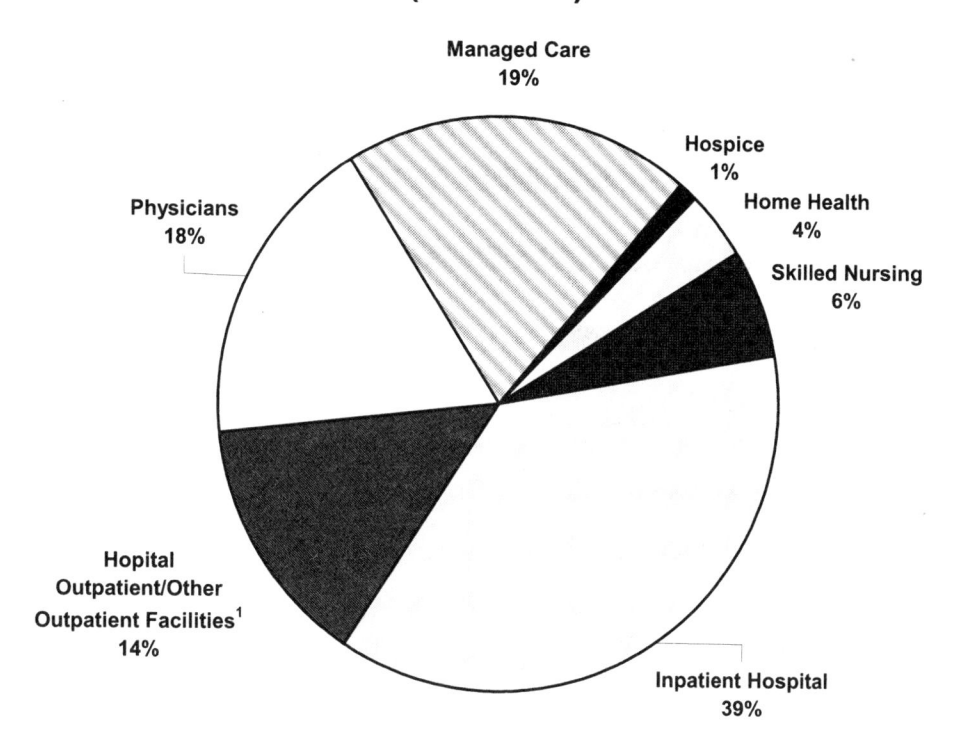

- Managed Care: 19%
- Hospice: 1%
- Home Health: 4%
- Skilled Nursing: 6%
- Inpatient Hospital: 39%
- Hopital Outpatient/Other Outpatient Facilities[1]: 14%
- Physicians: 18%

[1] Other outpatient facilities include ESRD freestanding dialysis facilities, RHCs, outpatient rehabilitation facilities, and federally qualified health centers.

Source: Plunkett Research, Ltd.

Number of Medicare Beneficiaries, 1970-2030

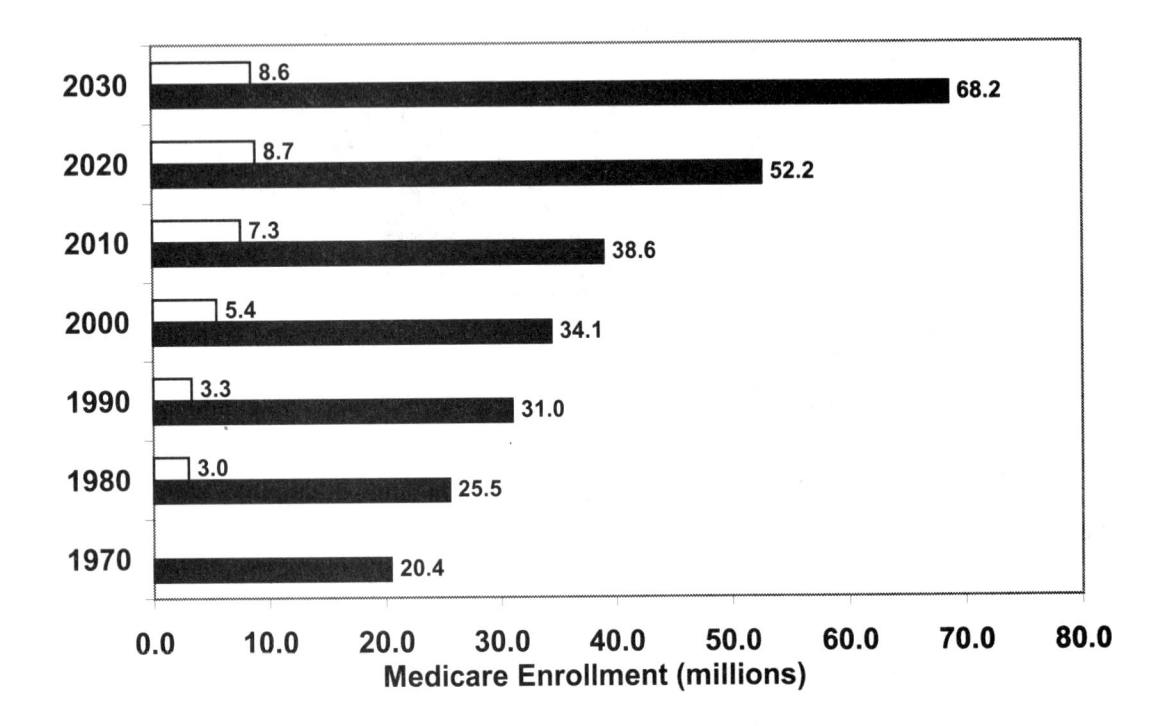

Year	Disabled & ESRD	Elderly
2030	8.6	68.2
2020	8.7	52.2
2010	7.3	38.6
2000	5.4	34.1
1990	3.3	31.0
1980	3.0	25.5
1970		20.4

Medicare Enrollment (millions)

■ ELDERLY □ DISABLED & END-STAGE RENAL DISEASE (ESRD)

Sources: Centers for Medicare & Medicaid Services (CMS), Office of the Actuary.

U.S. Medicare Enrollment Trends, Hospital And/Or Supplemental Medical Insurance (SMI)[1]: July 1970-2003

Medicare Aged and Disabled, by Type of Coverage

All Areas

Year	All Persons	Aged Persons	Disabled Persons
1970	20,490,908	20,490,908	n/a
1971	20,914,896	20,914,896	n/a
1972	21,332,120	21,332,120	n/a
1973	23,545,363	21,814,825	1,730,538
1974	24,201,042	22,272,920	1,928,122
1975	24,958,552	22,790,157	2,168,395
1976	25,662,921	23,270,739	2,392,182
1977	26,457,899	23,838,478	2,619,421
1978	27,164,222	24,370,986	2,793,236
1979	27,858,742	24,947,954	2,910,788
1980	28,478,245	25,515,070	2,963,175
1981	29,009,934	26,010,978	2,998,956
1982	29,494,219	26,539,994	2,954,225
1983	30,026,082	27,108,500	2,917,582
1984	30,455,368	27,570,950	2,884,418
1985	31,082,801	28,175,916	2,906,885
1986	31,749,708	28,791,162	2,958,546
1987	32,411,204	29,380,480	3,030,724
1988	32,980,033	29,878,528	3,101,505
1989	33,579,449	30,408,525	3,170,924
1990	34,203,383	30,948,376	3,255,007
1991	34,870,240	31,484,779	3,385,461
1992	35,579,149	32,010,515	3,568,634
1993	36,305,903	32,461,719	3,844,184
1994	36,935,366	32,800,745	4,134,621
1995	37,535,024	33,141,730	4,393,294
1996	38,064,130	33,423,945	4,640,184
1997	38,444,739	33,629,955	4,814,784
1998	38,824,855	33,802,038	5,022,817
1999	39,140,386	33,928,752	5,211,634
2000	39,619,986	34,252,835	5,367,151
2001	40,025,724	34,462,465	5,563,259
2002	40,488,878	34,679,267	5,809,611
2003	41,086,981	35,007,557	6,079,424

[1] Indicates the unduplicated count if persons are enrolled in either or both parts of the program.

Source: Centers for Medicare & Medicaid Services (CMS).

U.S. Medicare Enrollment Trends, Hospital Insurance (HI)[1]: July 1970-2003

Medicare Aged and Disabled, by Type of Coverage

All Areas

Year	All Persons	Aged Persons	Disabled Persons
1970	20,361,152	20,361,152	n/a
1971	20,742,250	20,742,250	n/a
1972	21,115,261	21,115,261	n/a
1973	23,301,082	21,570,544	1,730,538
1974	23,924,145	21,996,029	1,928,116
1975	24,640,497	22,472,104	2,168,393
1976	25,312,575	22,920,417	2,392,158
1977	26,093,919	23,474,546	2,619,373
1978	26,777,263	23,984,057	2,793,206
1979	27,459,157	24,548,391	2,910,766
1980	28,066,894	25,103,738	2,963,156
1981	28,589,504	25,590,555	2,998,949
1982	29,068,966	26,114,758	2,954,208
1983	29,587,295	26,669,745	2,917,550
1984	29,995,971	27,111,561	2,884,410
1985	30,589,468	27,682,592	2,906,876
1986	31,215,529	28,257,004	2,958,525
1987	31,852,860	28,822,152	3,030,708
1988	32,413,038	29,311,556	3,101,482
1989	33,039,977	29,869,060	3,170,917
1990	33,719,118	30,464,135	3,254,983
1991	34,428,810	31,043,371	3,385,439
1992	35,153,223	31,584,598	3,568,625
1993	35,904,436	32,060,258	3,844,178
1994	36,543,147	32,408,543	4,134,604
1995	37,134,949	32,741,662	4,393,287
1996	37,661,881	33,021,701	4,640,180
1997	38,052,242	33,237,460	4,814,782
1998	38,432,477	33,409,666	5,022,811
1999	38,432,477	33,409,666	5,022,811
2000	39,199,460	33,832,862	5,366,598
2001	39,606,975	34,044,115	5,562,860
2002	40,066,786	34,257,612	5,809,174
2003	40,656,995	34,580,961	6,076,034

[1] People enrolled in HI regardless if they are enrolled in SMI.

Source: Centers for Medicare and Medicaid Services (CMS).

U.S. Medicare Enrollment Trends, Supplemental Medical Insurance (SMI)[1]: July 1970-2003

Medicare Aged and Disabled, by Type of Coverage; All Areas

Year	All Persons	Aged Persons	Disabled Persons
1970	19,584,387	19,587,387	n/a
1971	19,974,692	19,974,692	n/a
1972	20,351,273	20,357,273	n/a
1973	22,490,534	20,920,660	1,569,874
1974	23,166,570	21,421,545	1,745,025
1975	23,904,551	21,945,301	1,959,250
1976	24,614,402	22,445,911	2,168,491
1977	25,363,468	22,990,826	2,372,642
1978	26,074,085	23,530,893	2,543,192
1979	26,757,329	24,098,491	2,658,838
1980	27,399,658	24,680,432	2,719,226
1981	27,941,227	25,181,731	2,759,496
1982	28,412,282	25,706,792	2,705,490
1983	28,974,535	26,292,124	2,682,411
1984	29,415,397	26,764,150	2,651,247
1985	29,988,763	27,310,894	2,677,869
1986	30,589,728	27,862,737	2,726,991
1987	31,169,960	28,382,203	2,787,757
1988	31,617,082	28,780,154	2,836,928
1989	32,098,770	29,216,027	2,882,743
1990	32,629,109	29,685,629	2,943,480
1991	33,237,474	30,185,162	3,052,312
1992	33,933,274	30,712,791	3,220,483
1993	34,612,360	31,146,557	3,465,803
1994	35,167,288	31,447,255	3,720,033
1995	35,684,584	31,742,132	3,942,452
1996	36,139,608	31,984,257	4,155,351
1997	36,460,143	32,164,416	4,295,727
1998	36,780,731	32,308,268	4,472,463
1999	37,039,848	32,402,760	4,637,088
2000	37,359,512	32,589,708	4,769,804
2001	37,685,281	32,748,714	4,936,567
2002	38,078,574	32,934,153	5,144,421
2003	38,589,685	32,202,715	5,386,970

[1] People enrolled in SMI regardless their enrollment in Hospital Insurance.

Source: Centers for Medicare and Medicaid Services (CMS).

Medicare Deductible, Co-insurance and Premium Amounts, 2005

Hospital Insurance (Part A)

~**Deductible** - $912 per each Benefit Period.

~**Coinsurance**

* $228 a day for the 61st through the 90th day, per Benefit Period.

* $456 a day for the 91st through the 150th day for each lifetime reserve day.

~**Skilled Nursing Facility Coinsurance** – up to $114 a day for the 21st through the 100th day per Benefit Period.

~**Hospital Insurance Monthly Premium** - $375 per month (See Note 1, below).

~**Reduced Hospital Insurance Premium** - $206 (See Note 1, below).

Medical Insurance (Part B)

~**Deductible** - $110 per year.

~**Medical Insurance Monthly Premium** - $78.20

Notes:

1. Most people age 65 or older are eligible for premium-free Hospital Insurance (Part A). However, there are some people age 65 or older who do not meet the requirements for premium-free Hospital Insurance. Also, certain disabled individuals who were entitled to premium-free Hospital Insurance lose their entitlement upon having earnings exceeding certain amounts. If you are in either of these categories, you can get Part A by paying a monthly premium. The full Part A premium in calendar year 2005 will be $375 per month. However, if you or your spouse have 30 to 39 quarters of Social Security coverage, your Part A premium, in calendar year 2005, will be $206 per month.

Source: U.S. Dept. of Health and Human Services (HHS)/Centers for Medicare and Medicaid Services (CMS).

IV. U.S. Health Insurance Coverage and the Uninsured

Contents:	
People Without Health Insurance for the Entire Year, U.S.: 2001, 2002 and 2003	**74**
Number and Percent of Persons Without Health Insurance Coverage, by Age Group, U.S.: 1997-2004	**75**
Percent of Persons of All Ages Without Health Insurance Coverage, by Race/Ethnicity, U.S., 2004	**76**
Percent of Persons of All Ages Without Health Insurance Coverage, U.S.: 1997-2004	**77**
Percent of Persons Under Age 65 With Public and Private Coverage, U.S.: 1997-2004	**78**
Percent of Persons Under Age 65 Years Without Health Insurance Coverage, by Age Group and Sex, U.S., 2003	**79**
Employers' Costs for Health Insurance, U.S.: Selected Years 1991-2003	**80**

People Without Health Insurance for the Entire Year, U.S.: 2001, 2002 and 2003

(In Thousands)

Characteristic	2001 Without Insurance	2001 Percent of Pop. (%)	2002 Without Insurance	2002 Percent of Pop. (%)	2003 Without Insurance	2003 Percent of Pop. (%)
Total	**41,207**	**14.6**	**43,574**	**15.2**	**44,961**	**15.6**
Sex						
Male	21,722	15.8	23,327	16.7	n/a	n/a
Female	19,485	13.5	20,246	13.9	n/a	n/a
Age						
Under 18 years	8,509	11.7	8,531	11.6	8,373	11.4
18 to 24 years	7,673	28.1	8,128	29.6	8,414	30.2
25 to 34	9,051	23.4	9,769	24.9	10,345	26.4
35 to 44	7,131	16.1	7,781	17.7	7,885	18.1
45 to 64	8,571	13.1	9,106	13.5	9,657	13.9
65 years and over	272	0.8	258	0.8	286	0.8
Nativity						
Native	30,364	12.2	32,388	12.8	33,146	13.0
Foreign Born	10,843	33.4	11,186	33.4	11,815	34.5
Household Income						
Less than $25,000	14,474	23.3	14,776	23.5	15,331	24.2
$25,000 to $49,999	13,516	17.7	14,638	19.3	14,823	19.9
$50,000 to $74,999	6,595	11.3	6,904	11.8	7,226	12.5
$75,000 or more	6,623	7.7	7,256	8.2	7,580	8.2
Work Experience						
Worked during year	24,230	17.0	25,679	18.0	26,581	18.6
Did not work	8,197	24.7	9,106	25.7	9,720	26.0

Source: U.S. Census Bureau, Current Population Survey, 2003 and 2004 Annual Social and Economic Supplements.

Number and Percent of Persons Without Health Insurance Coverage, by Age Group, U.S.: 1997-2004

Year	Number of Uninsured[1] in Millions				Percent Uninsured[1] (95% Confidence Interval)				
						Under 65 Years		
	All Ages	Under 65 Years	18-64 Years	Under 18 Years	All Ages	Crude	Age-Adjusted	18-64 Years	Under 18 Years
1997	41.0	40.7	30.8	9.9	15.4 (15.0-15.8)	17.4 (16.9-17.9)	17.2 (16.8-17.7)	18.9 (18.4-19.4)	13.9 (13.2-14.6)
1998	39.3	39.0	30.0	9.1	14.6 (14.1-15.1)	16.5 (16.0-17.0)	16.4 (15.9-16.9)	18.2 (17.7-18.7)	12.7 (12.0-13.4)
1999	38.7	38.3	29.8	8.5	14.2 (13.8-14.6)	16.0 (15.5-16.5)	16.0 (15.5-16.5)	17.8 (17.3-18.3)	11.8 (11.2-12.4)
2000	41.3	40.8	32.0	8.9	14.9 (14.5-15.3)	16.8 (16.3-17.2)	16.8 (16.3-17.3)	18.7 (18.1-19.2)	12.3 (11.7-12.9)
2001	40.2	39.8	31.9	7.9	14.3 (13.8-14.8)	16.2 (15.7-16.7)	16.2 (15.7-16.7)	18.3 (17.8-18.8)	11.0 (10.3-11.7)
2002	41.5	41.1	33.5	7.6	14.7 (14.3-15.1)	16.5 (16.0-16.9)	16.6 (16.1-17.1)	19.1 (18.6-19.6)	10.5 (9.9-11.1)
2003	43.6	43.2	35.9	7.3	15.2 (14.8-15.7)	17.2 (16.6-17.7)	17.3 (16.8-17.8)	20.1 (19.5-20.6)	10.1 (9.4-10.7)
2004*	42.0	41.5	35.1	6.4	14.6 (13.8-15.5)	16.4 (15.5-17.4)	16.6 (15.6-17.5)	19.5 (18.5-20.6)	8.8 (7.7-10.0)

*2004 Figures from January through March only.

[1] A person was defined as uninsured if he or she did not have any private health insurance, Medicare, Medicaid, State Children's Health Insurance Program (SCHIP), State-sponsored or other government-sponsored health plan, or military plan at the time of the interview. A person was also defined as uninsured if he or she had only Indian Health Service coverage or had only a private plan that paid for one type of service such as accidents or dental care. The analyses excluded persons with unknown health insurance status (about 1% of respondents each year). The data on health insurance status were edited using an automated system based on logic checks and keyword searches. For comparability, the estimates for all years were created using these same procedures. The resulting estimates of persons without health insurance coverage are generally 0.1-0.2 percentage points lower than those based on the editing procedures used for the final data files. The number of uninsured was calculated as the percent of uninsured multiplied by the total weighted population including persons with unknown coverage. The age-specific numbers of uninsured may not add to their respective totals due to rounding error.

Age-adjusted estimates for persons under 65 years old for this Healthy People 2010 Leading Health Indicator are adjusted to the 2000 projected U.S. standard population using three age groups: under 18 years, 18-44 years, and 45-64 years.

Notes: Beginning with the 2003 data, the National Health Interview Survey transitioned to weights derived from the 2000 census. In this Early Release, estimates for 2000-02 were recalculated using weights derived from the 2000 census.

Source: CDC; Family Core component of the 1997-2004 National Health Interview Surveys.

Percent of Persons of All Ages Without Health Insurance Coverage, by Race/Ethnicity, U.S., 2004*

	Percent (95% Confidence Interval)	
Race/Ethnicity	Age-Sex-Adjusted[1]	Age-Adjusted[2]
Hispanic or Latino	33.1 (30.8-35.4)	35.2 (32.8-37.7)
White, Single Race	10.2 (9.5-11.0)	12.0 (11.1-12.9)
Black, Single Race	16.8 (14.7-18.9)	18.7 (16.4-21.1)

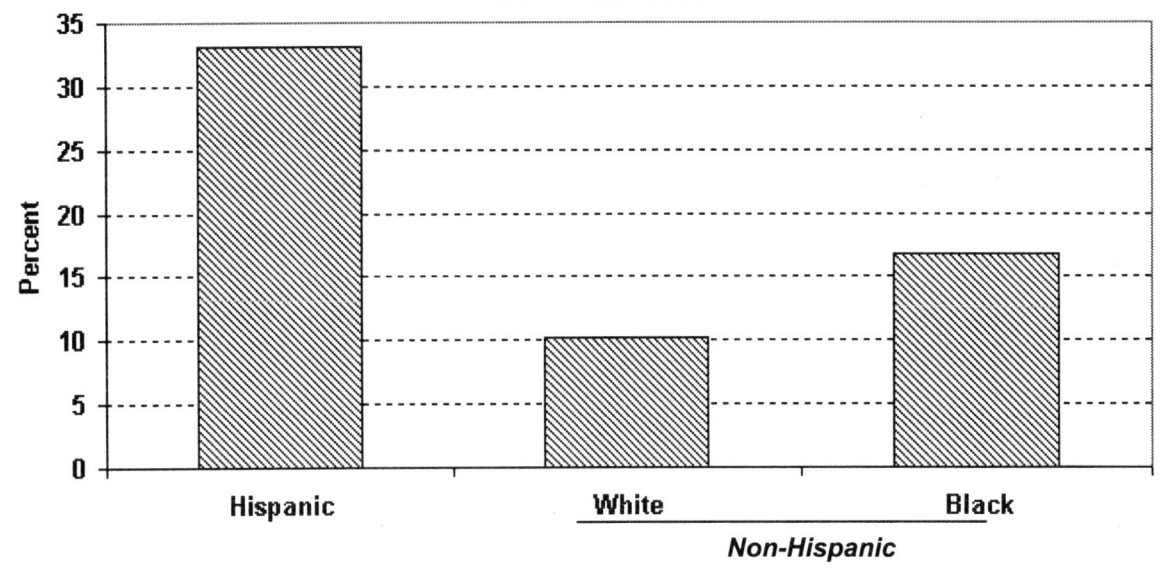

*Figures based on January-March 2004 only.
1 Age-sex-adjusted estimates are presented in the graph. Estimates are for persons of all ages and are age-sex-adjusted to the 2000 projected U.S. standard population using three age groups: under 18 years, 18-64 years, and 65 years and over.
2 Estimates for this Healthy People 2010 Leading Health Indicator are for persons under 65 years and are age-adjusted to the 2000 projected U.S. standard population using three age groups: under 18 years, 18-44 years, and 45-64 years.
Notes: A person was defined as uninsured if he or she did not have any private health insurance, Medicare, Medicaid, State Children's Health Insurance Program (SCHIP), State-sponsored or other government-sponsored health plan, or military plan at the time of the interview. A person was also defined as uninsured if he or she had only Indian Health Service coverage or had only a private plan that paid for one type of service such as accidents or dental care. The analyses excluded 1148 persons (1.3%) with unknown health insurance status. The data on health insurance status were edited using an automated system based on logic checks and keyword searches. The resulting estimates of persons not having health insurance coverage are generally 0.1-0.2 percentage points lower than those based on the editing procedures used for the final data files. Estimates are age-sex-adjusted to the 2000 projected U.S. standard population using three age groups: under 18 years, 18-64 years, and 65 years and over.

Source: CDC; Selected Estimates Based on Data From the January-March 2004 National Health Interview Survey

Percent of Persons of All Ages Without Health Insurance Coverage, U.S.: 1997-2004

Year	Percent	95% Confidence Interval
1997	15.4	15.0-15.8
1998	14.6	14.1-15.1
1999	14.2	13.8-14.6
2000	14.9	14.5-15.3
2001	14.3	13.8-14.8
2002	14.7	14.3-15.1
2003	15.2	14.8-15.7
2004*	14.6	13.8-15.5

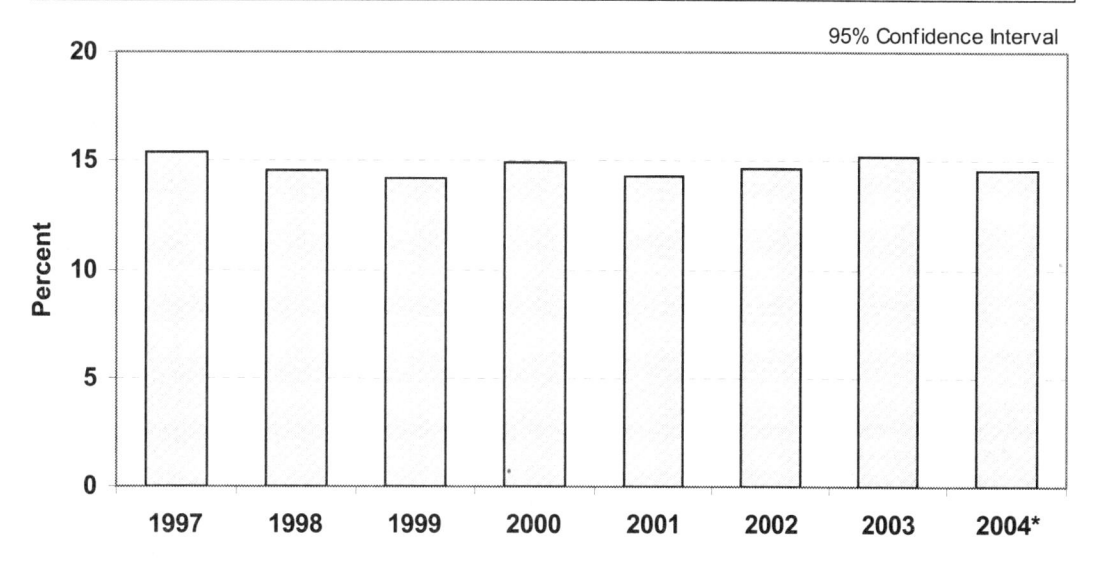

* 2004 figures for January-March only.

Notes: A person was defined as uninsured if he or she did not have any private health insurance, Medicare, Medicaid, State Children's Health Insurance Program (SCHIP), State-sponsored or other government-sponsored health plan, or military plan at the time of the interview. A person was also defined as uninsured if he or she had only Indian Health Service coverage or had only a private plan that paid for one type of service such as accidents or dental care. The analyses excluded persons with unknown health insurance status (about 1% of respondents each year). The data on health insurance status were edited using an automated system based on logic checks and keyword searches. For comparability, the estimates for all years were created using these same procedures. The resulting estimates of persons without health insurance coverage are generally 0.1-0.2 percentage points lower than those based on the editing procedures used for the final data files. CI is confidence interval. Beginning with the 2003 data, the National Health Interview Survey transitioned to weights derived from the 2000 census. In this Early Release, estimates for 2000-02 were recalculated using weights derived from the 2000 census.

Source: CDC; Family Core component of the 1997-2003 National Health Interview Surveys.

Percent of Persons Under Age 65 With Public Health Plan Coverage and Private Health Insurance Coverage, by Age Group, U.S.: 1997-2004

	Public[1]			Private[1]		
Year	Under 65 years	18-64 years	Under 18 years	Under 65 years	18-64 years	Under 18 years
	Percent (97% confidence interval)					
1997	13.6 (13.1-14.1)	10.2 (9.8-10.6)	21.5 (20.5-22.4)	70.8 (70.1-71.5)	72.8 (72.2-73.4)	66.2 (65.1-67.3)
1998	12.7 (12.2-13.2)	9.5 (9.1-9.9)	20.0 (19.0-20.9)	72.0 (71.3-72.7)	73.5 (72.9-74.1)	68.5 (67.4-69.5)
1999	12.4 (12.0-12.9)	9.0 (8.6-9.3)	20.5 (19.5-21.4)	73.1 (72.3-73.8)	74.8 (74.1-75.4)	69.1 (68.0-70.2)
2000	12.9 (12.4-13.4)	9.1 (8.7-9.4)	22.0 (21.0-23.0)	71.8 (71.1-72.5)	73.8 (73.2-74.4)	67.1 (66.1-68.2)
2001	13.6 (13.1-14.1)	9.4 (9.0-9.8)	23.6 (22.6-24.5)	71.6 (70.9-72.3)	73.7 (73.1-74.4)	66.7 (66.4-68.6)
2002	15.2 (14.6-15.8)	10.3 (9.9-10.7)	27.1 (26.0-28.2)	69.8 (69.0-70.6)	72.3 (71.6-72.9)	63.9 (62.7-65.1)
2003	16.0 (15.4-16.6)	10.9 (10.4-11.4)	28.6 (27.4-29.7)	68.2 (67.5-69.0)	70.6 (69.9-71.3)	62.6 (61.4-63.8)
2004*	16.1 (15.0-17.2)	10.9 (10.0-11.7)	28.9 (26.8-31.0)	68.7 (67.2-70.2)	70.8 (69.5-72.2)	63.4 (61.1-65.7)

*2004 Figures are for January through March only.

[1] The category "public health plan coverage" includes Medicare (disability), Medicaid, State Children's Health Insurance Program (SCHIP), State-sponsored or other government-sponsored health plan, and military plans. The category "private health insurance" excludes plans that paid for only one type of service such as accidents or dental care. A small number of persons were covered by both public and private plans and were included in both categories. The analyses excluded persons with unknown health insurance status (about 1% of respondents each year). The data on type of coverage were edited using an automated system based on logic checks and keyword searches. For comparability, the estimates for all years were created using these same procedures. The resulting estimates of persons having public or private coverage are within 0.1-0.3 percentage points of those based on the editing procedures used for the final data files.

Notes: Beginning with the 2003 data, the National Health Interview Survey transitioned to weights derived from the 2000 census. In this Early Release, estimates for 2000-02 were recalculated using weights derived from the 2000 census.

Source: CDC; Family Core component of the 1997-2004 National Health Interview Surveys.

Percent of Persons Under Age 65 Years Without Health Insurance Coverage, by Age Group and Sex: U.S., 2004*

Age and sex	Percent	95% Confidence Interval
Total: Under 18 Years	8.8	7.7-10.0
Men	8.7	7.4-10.1
Women	8.9	7.7-10.2
Total: 18-24 Years	31.5	28.7-34.3
Men	37.2	33.6-40.9
Women	25.7	22.5-29.0
Total: 25-34 Years	25.0	22.8-27.1
Men	28.6	25.9-31.4
Women	21.3	18.9-23.7
Total: 35-44 Years	17.8	16.2-19.4
Men	19.6	17.5-21.7
Women	16.0	14.2-17.9
Total: 45-64 Years	12.8	11.5-14.0
Men	12.5	11.0-13.9
Women	13.0	11.6-14.4
Total: Under 65 Years[1]	16.4	15.5-17.4
Men	17.8	16.7-18.9
Women	15.1	14.1-16.0

*Figures for January-March 2004 only.

[1] Crude estimates are presented in the graph. Estimates for this Healthy People 2010 Leading Health Indicator are for persons under 65 years and are age-adjusted to the 2000 projected U.S. standard population using three age groups: under 18 years, 18-44 years, and 45-64 years.

Notes: A person was defined as uninsured if he or she did not have any private health insurance, Medicare, Medicaid, State Children's Health Insurance Program (SCHIP), State-sponsored or other government-sponsored health plan, or military plan at the time of the interview. A person was also defined as uninsured if he or she had only Indian Health Service coverage or had only a private plan that paid for one type of service such as accidents or dental care. The analyses excluded 1065 persons (1.3%) with unknown health insurance status. The data on health insurance status were edited using an automated system based on logic checks and keyword searches. The resulting estimates of persons not having health insurance coverage are generally 0.1-0.2 percentage points lower than those based on the editing procedures used for the final data files. Early Release of Selected Estimates Based on Data From the 2003 National Health Interview Survey 6.

Source: CDC; Selected Estimates Based on Data From the January-March 2004 National Health Interview Survey.

Employers' Costs for Health Insurance, Amount and Percent of Total Compensation, U.S.: Selected Years 1991-2003

Amount per Employee-Hour Worked (in US$)

Characteristic	Health Insurance Cost per Employee-Hour Worked					Health Insurance as Percent of Total Compensation				
	1991	2000	2001	2002	2003	1991	2000	2001	2002	2003
	In US$					In Percent (%)				
State and local gov't	$1.54	$2.27	$2.56	$2.69	$2.99	6.9	7.8	8.5	8.6	9.2
Total private industry	0.92	1.09	1.28	1.29	1.41	6.0	5.5	6.2	5.9	6.3
Industry:										
Goods producing	1.28	1.62	1.85	1.84	1.98	6.9	6.9	7.6	7.2	7.5
Service producing	0.79	0.92	1.11	1.13	1.25	5.5	4.9	5.6	5.5	5.9
Manufacturing	1.37	1.69	1.93	1.92	2.08	7.5	7.2	7.9	7.6	8.0
Nonmanufacturing	0.80	0.96	1.15	1.17	1.29	5.5	5.0	5.7	5.6	5.9
Occupation:										
White collar	1.02	1.21	1.43	1.42	1.86	5.6	5.0	5.6	5.4	6.4
Blue collar	1.06	1.28	1.45	1.48	1.70	7.0	6.8	7.5	7.3	8.0
Service	0.36	0.42	0.52	0.56	0.96	4.6	4.3	5.0	5.1	7.0
Census region:										
Northeast	1.08	1.27	1.50	1.48	1.63	6.2	5.6	6.3	5.9	6.3
Midwest	0.95	1.12	1.35	1.35	1.48	6.3	5.8	6.6	6.4	6.6
South	0.76	0.96	1.16	1.14	1.24	5.5	5.4	6.2	5.8	6.2
West	0.92	1.05	1.19	1.26	1.39	5.8	5.0	5.4	5.6	6.0
Union	1.63	2.17	2.48	2.57	2.80	8.2	8.4	8.9	8.7	9.1
Nonunion	0.78	0.95	1.14	1.13	1.24	5.4	5.0	5.7	5.4	5.8
Establishment employment size:										
1–99 employees	0.68	0.82	0.94	0.96	1.05	5.1	4.8	5.3	5.2	5.5
100 or more	1.14	1.38	1.66	1.67	1.84	6.6	6.0	6.9	6.6	7.0
100–499	0.90	1.09	1.38	1.40	1.56	6.3	5.6	6.6	6.4	6.9
500 or more	1.40	1.73	2.00	1.99	2.17	6.8	6.4	7.1	6.7	7.0

Notes: Costs are calculated from March survey data each year. Total compensation includes wages and salaries, and benefits.

Sources: U.S. Department of Labor, Bureau of Labor Statistics, National Compensation Survey, Employer Costs for Employee Compensation, March release; News–292, 00–186, 01–194, 02–346, and 03–297. June 19, 1991; June 29, 2000; June 29, 2001; June 19, 2002; and June 11, 2003. Washington, DC.

V. U.S. Vital Statistics and Population Indicators

Contents:	
Percent of Population in Three Age Groups, U.S.: 1950, 2000 and 2050	82
Life Expectancy at Birth, U.S.	83
Life Expectancy at Age 65, U.S.	84
Infant Mortality Rates, U.S.: Selected Years 1985-2004	85
Percentage of Children 19-35 Months Vaccinated for Select Diseases, U.S.: 2000-2003	86
AIDS Statistics: 1998-2003	87
Percentage of Binge Alcohol Use Among Students in Grades 8, 10 and 12, U.S.: 1980-2003	88
Cigarette Smoking Among Students in Grades 8, 10 and 12, U.S.: 1980-2003	89
Employment, Hours, and Earnings in Private Health Service Establishments, U.S.: 1999-2004	90

Percent of Population in Three Age Groups, U.S.: 1950, 2000 and 2050

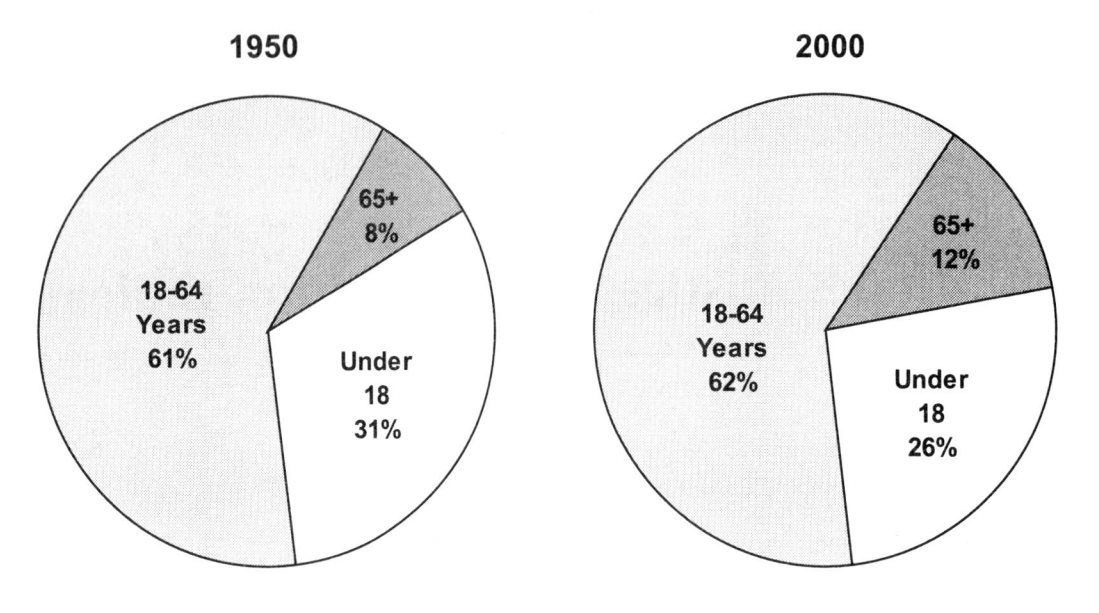

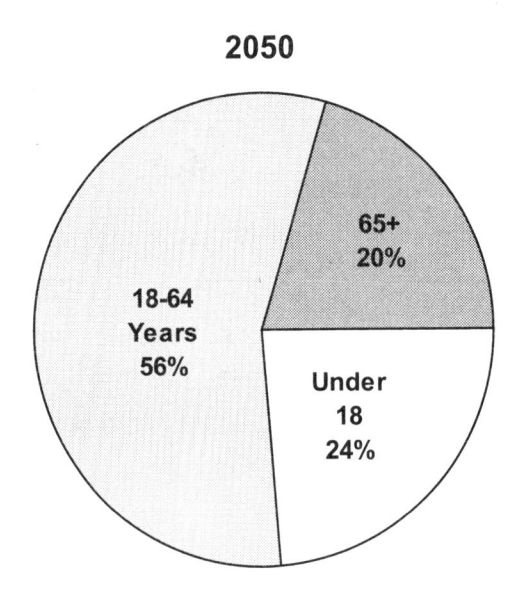

1950
- 65+: 8%
- 18-64 Years: 61%
- Under 18: 31%

2000
- 65+: 12%
- 18-64 Years: 62%
- Under 18: 26%

2050
- 65+: 20%
- 18-64 Years: 56%
- Under 18: 24%

Source: U.S. Census Bureau

Life Expectancy at Birth, U.S.

Total Lifespan in years, for those born in selected years, 1950-2003

Year	Men	Women
1950	65.6	71.1
1960	66.6	73.1
1970	67.1	74.7
1980	70.0	77.4
1990	71.8	78.8
1995	72.5	78.9
1998	73.8	79.5
1999	73.9	79.4
2000	74.3	79.7
2003	74.4	80.05

2004 expectancy average for men and women combined is 77.4

Source: Social Security Administration, Office of the Actuary, *World Factbook 2003, 2004*

Life Expectancy at Age 65, U.S.

Selected Years, 1965-2070

Year	Male	Female
1965	12.9	16.3
1980	14.0	18.4
1985	14.4	18.6
1990	15.0	19.0
1995	15.3	19.0
1998	15.6	19.0
1999	15.7	18.9
2000	15.7	19.0
2010	16.4	19.4
2020	17.0	20.0
2030	17.7	20.6
2040	18.3	21.2
2050	18.8	21.8
2060	19.4	22.4
2070	19.9	22.9

Note: Years 2000-2070 are estimated.

Sources: Social Security Administration, Office of the Actuary.

Infant Mortality Rates, U.S.: Selected Years 1985-2004

By Detailed Race of Mother

Race	1985	1990	1995 [1]	1997	1998	1999	2000	2001	2004*
Infant Deaths per 1,000 Live Births									
Total	10.4	8.9	7.6	7.2	7.2	7.0	6.9	6.8	6.6
White, non-Hispanic	8.6	7.2	6.3	6.0	6.0	5.8	5.7	5.7	n/a
Black, non-Hispanic	18.3	16.9	14.7	13.7	13.9	14.1	13.6	13.3	n/a
Hispanic[2,3]	8.8	7.5	6.3	6.0	5.8	5.7	5.6	5.4	n/a
Mexican American	8.5	7.2	6.0	5.8	5.6	5.5	5.4	5.2	n/a
Puerto Rican	11.2	9.9	8.9	7.9	7.8	8.3	8.2	8.5	n/a
Cuban	8.5	7.2	5.3	5.5	3.6	4.7	4.5	4.2	n/a
Central and South American	8.0	6.8	5.5	5.5	5.3	4.7	4.6	5.0	n/a
Other and unknown Hispanic	9.5	8.0	7.4	6.2	6.5	7.2	6.9	6.0	n/a
Asian/Pacific Islander	7.8	6.6	5.3	5.0	5.5	4.8	4.9	4.7	n/a
Chinese	5.8	4.3	3.8	3.1	4.0	2.9	3.5	3.2	n/a
Japanese	6.0	5.5	5.3	5.3	3.5	3.4	4.6	4.0	n/a
Filipino	7.7	6.0	5.6	5.8	6.2	5.8	5.7	5.5	n/a
Hawaiian and part Hawaiian	9.9	8.0	6.6	9.0	10.0	7.1	9.1	7.3	n/a
Other Asian/Pacific Islander	8.5	7.4	5.5	5.0	5.7	5.1	4.8	4.8	n/a
American Indian/Alaska Native	13.1	13.1	9.0	8.7	9.3	9.3	8.3	9.7	n/a

*Estimate. n/a = not available.

[1] Beginning with data for 1995, rates are on a period basis. Earlier rates are on a cohort basis. Race-specific data for 1995-99 are weighted to account for unmatched records.

[2] Persons of Hispanic origin may be of any race.

[3] Trend data for Hispanic women are affected by expansion of the reporting area in which an item on Hispanic origin is included on the birth certificate, as well as by immigration. These two factors affect numbers of events, composition of the Hispanic population, and maternal and infant health characteristics. The number of States in the reporting area increased from 22 in 1980 to 23 and the District of Columbia (DC) in 1983-87, 30 and DC in 1988, 47 and DC in 1989, 48 and DC in 1990, 49 and DC in 1991, and all 50 States and DC from 1993 forward.

Sources: CIA World Fact Book 2004; Centers for Disease Control and Prevention (CDC), National Center for Health Statistics, National Linked Files of Live Births and Infant Deaths; and *America's Children, 2003* at www.childstats.gov

Percentage of Children 19-35 Months Vaccinated for Select Diseases, U.S.: 2000-2003*

By Race and Poverty Level; In Percent

Characteristic	U.S. National 2000	2001	2002	2003	Below Poverty 2000	2001	2002	2003	At or Above Poverty 2000	2001	2002	2003
Total (in percent)												
Combined series (4:3:1:3)[a]	76	77	78	81	71	72	72	76	78	79	79	83
Combined series (4:3:1)[b]	78	79	79	82	72	73	73	77	79	80	80	84
DTP (4 doses or more)[c]	82	82	82	85	76	77	75	80	84	84	84	87
Polio (3 doses or more)	90	89	90	92	87	87	88	89	90	90	91	93
Measles-containing (MCV)[d]	91	91	92	93	89	89	90	92	91	92	92	93
Hib (3 doses or more)[e]	93	93	93	94	90	90	90	91	95	94	94	95
Hepatitis B (3 doses or more)[f]	90	89	90	92	87	87	88	91	91	90	90	93
Varicella[g]	68	76	81	85	64	74	79	84	69	77	81	85
White, non-Hispanic (in percent)												
Combined series (4:3:1:3)[a]	79	79	80	84	73	71	72	79	80	80	81	85
Combined series (4:3:1)[b]	80	80	81	85	74	72	73	80	81	81	82	86
DTP (4 doses or more)[c]	84	84	84	88	78	75	75	82	85	85	86	88
Polio (3 doses or more)	91	90	91	93	88	87	88	91	91	91	92	93
Measles-containing (MCV)[d]	92	92	93	93	88	87	91	90	92	92	93	94
Hib (3 doses or more)[e]	95	94	94	95	92	89	88	91	95	95	95	96
Hepatitis B (3 doses or more)[f]	91	90	91	93	88	86	86	91	92	90	92	94
Varicella[g]	66	75	79	84	58	67	75	80	68	76	80	85
Black, non-Hispanic (in percent)												
Combined series (4:3:1:3)[a]	71	71	71	75	69	69	68	70	72	74	72	79
Combined series (4:3:1)[b]	72	73	72	77	70	71	69	72	73	75	73	80
DTP (4 doses or more)[c]	76	76	76	80	75	74	74	72	78	78	77	84
Polio (3 doses or more)	87	85	87	89	85	84	87	86	87	86	87	91
Measles-containing (MCV)[d]	88	89	90	92	88	88	90	91	87	90	90	93
Hib (3 doses or more)[e]	93	90	92	92	92	87	88	90	93	91	94	95
Hepatitis B (3 doses or more)[f]	89	85	88	92	89	85	89	92	90	85	88	92
Varicella[g]	67	75	83	85	60	71	80	84	72	77	84	86
Hispanic (in percent)												
Combined series (4:3:1:3)[a]	73	77	76	79	70	73	75	78	74	79	76	81
Combined series (4:3:1)[b]	75	79	77	79	73	76	76	79	75	80	77	81
DTP (4 doses or more)[c]	79	83	79	82	76	79	78	81	80	83	80	84
Polio (3 doses or more)	88	91	90	90	88	90	89	89	87	91	91	92
Measles-containing (MCV)[d]	90	92	91	93	90	91	91	93	90	93	89	93
Hib (3 doses or more)[e]	91	93	92	93	88	91	93	92	93	94	92	95
Hepatitis B (3 doses or more)[f]	88	90	90	91	87	88	89	91	90	91	89	93
Varicella[g]	70	80	82	86	70	81	82	88	70	82	81	85

[a] The 4:3:1:3 combined series consists of 4 doses of diphtheria and tetanus toxoids and pertussis vaccine (DTP), 3 doses of polio vaccine, 1 dose of a measles-containing vaccine (MCV), and 3 doses of Haemophilus influenzae type b (Hib) vaccine. [b] The 4:3:1 combined series consists of 4 doses of diphtheria and tetanus toxoids and pertussis vaccine (DTP), 3 doses of polio vaccine and 1 dose of a measles-containing vaccine (MCV). [c] Diphtheria and tetanus toxoids and pertussis vaccine. [d] Respondents were asked about measles-containing vaccine, including MMR (measles-mumps-rubella) vaccines. [e] Haemophilus influenzae type b (Hib) vaccine. [f] The percentage of children 19 to 35 months of age who received 3 doses of hepatitis B vaccine was low in 1994, because universal infant vaccination with a 3-dose series was not recommended until November 1991. [g] Recommended in July 1996. Administered on or after the first birthday, unadjusted for history of varicella illness (chicken pox).

* 2003 figures are estimates. Children in the 2003 National Immunization Survey were born between Feb. 2000 and May 2002.

Sources: Centers for Disease Control and Prevention, National Center for Health Statistics and National Immunization Program.

AIDS Statistics

Estimated Number of AIDS Deaths Worldwide, 2003 = 2.9 Million

Estimated Numbers of Deaths of Persons With AIDS, U.S.: 1998–2002

	Year of Death					Cumulative Through 2002[a]
	1998	1999	2000	2001	2002	
Total[b]	19,005	18,454	17,347	17,402	16,371	501,669
Age At Death (yrs)						
<13	104	102	51	49	33	5,071
13--14	9	19	10	5	10	244
15--24	258	232	206	261	190	9,507
25--34	3,785	3,252	2,765	2,377	1,971	139,977
35--44	7,991	7,679	6,998	7,077	6,401	207,324
45--54	4,784	5,004	5,082	5,202	5,395	97,027
55--64	1,511	1,546	1,584	1,758	1,728	31,179
≥ 65	562	622	652	673	641	11,340
Race/Ethnicity						
White, not Hispanic	6,228	5,800	5,331	5,061	4,555	223,623
Black, not Hispanic	9,116	9,097	8,723	8,915	8,566	185,080
Hispanic	3,449	3,353	3,118	3,236	3,056	87,888
Asian/Pacific Islander	125	116	107	111	93	3,350
American Indian/Alaska Native	79	79	61	70	72	1,424
Male Adult or Adolescent	14,715	13,997	13,104	13,001	12,083	419,754
Female Adult or Adolescent	4,167	4,327	4,169	4,328	4,226	76,507
Child (<13 yrs)	122	130	75	73	62	5,407

Note: These numbers do not represent actual cases in persons who died with AIDS. Rather, these numbers are point estimates of cases in persons who died with AIDS that have been adjusted for delays in reporting of deaths and for redistribution of cases in persons initially reported without an identified risk. The estimates have not been adjusted for incomplete reporting.

[a] Includes persons who died with AIDS, from the beginning of the epidemic through 2002.

[b] Includes persons of unknown or multiple race and of unknown sex. Cumulative total includes 304 persons of unknown or multiple race and 1 person of unknown sex. Because column totals were calculated independently of the values for the subpopulations, the values in each column may not sum to the column total.

Sources: UNAIDS 2004 Report, Centers for Disease Control and Prevention (CDC).

Percentage of Binge Alcohol[1] Use Among Students in Grades 8, 10 and 12, U.S.: Selected Years 1980-2003
by Gender, Race and Hispanic Origin

Characteristic	1980	1985	1990	1995	1997	1998	1999	2000	2001	2002	2003
8th-graders (in percent)											
Total	–	–	–	14.5	14.5	13.7	15.2	14.1	13.2	12.4	11.9
Gender											
Male	–	–	–	15.1	15.3	14.4	16.4	14.4	13.7	12.5	12.2
Female	–	–	–	13.9	13.5	12.7	13.9	13.6	12.4	12.1	11.6
Race and Hispanic origin[2]											
White	–	–	–	13.9	15.1	14.1	14.3	14.9	13.8	12.7	11.8
Black	–	–	–	10.8	9.8	9.0	9.9	10.0	9.0	9.4	10.4
Hispanic[3]	–	–	–	22.0	20.7	20.4	20.9	19.1	17.6	17.8	16.6
10th-graders (in percent)											
Total	–	–	–	24.0	25.1	24.3	25.6	26.2	24.9	22.4	22.2
Gender											
Male	–	–	–	26.3	28.6	26.7	29.7	29.8	28.6	23.8	23.2
Female	–	–	–	21.5	21.7	22.2	21.8	22.5	21.4	21	21.2
Race and Hispanic origin[2]											
White	–	–	–	25.4	26.9	27.0	27.2	28.1	27.4	25.5	24.5
Black	–	–	–	13.3	12.7	12.8	12.7	12.9	12.6	12.4	12.1
Hispanic[3]	–	–	–	26.8	27.5	26.3	27.5	28.3	27.7	26.5	26.1
12th-graders (in percent)											
Total	41.2	36.7	32.2	29.8	31.3	31.5	30.8	30.0	29.7	28.6	27.9
Gender											
Male	52.1	45.3	39.1	36.9	37.9	39.2	38.1	36.7	36.0	34.2	34.2
Female	30.5	28.2	24.4	23.0	24.4	24.0	23.6	23.5	23.7	23.0	22.1
Race and Hispanic origin[2]											
White	44.3	41.5	36.6	32.3	35.1	36.4	35.7	34.6	34.5	33.7	32.4
Black	17.7	15.7	14.4	14.9	13.4	12.3	12.3	11.5	11.8	11.5	10.8
Hispanic[3]	33.1	31.7	25.6	26.6	27.6	28.1	29.3	31.0	28.4	26.4	25.9

– = not available

[1] Indicated by having five or more drinks in a row in the past two weeks.

[2] Estimates for race and Hispanic origin represent the mean of the specified year and the previous year. Data have been combined to increase subgroup sample sizes, thus providing more stable estimates.

[3] Persons of Hispanic origin may be of any race.

Source: *America's Children in Brief: Key National Indicators of Well-Being, 2004*; www.childstats.gov. Johnston, L.D., O'Malley, P.M., and Bachman, J.G. (2003). *Monitoring the Future national survey results on drug use, 1975-2002 Volume I: Secondary School Students* (NIH Publication No. 03-5375). Bethesda, MD: National Institute on Drug Abuse Tables 2-2 and 5-3. Data for 2003 are from a press release of December 19, 2003, and demographic disaggregations are from unpublished tabulations from Monitoring the Future, University of Michigan

Cigarette Smoking Among Students in Grades 8, 10 and 12, U.S.: Selected Years 1980-2003

by Gender, Race and Hispanic Origin

Characteristic	1980	1985	1990	1995	1997	1999	2000	2001	2002	2003
8th-graders (in percent)										
Total	–	–	–	9.3	9.0	8.1	7.4	5.5	5.1	4.5
Gender										
Male	–	–	–	9.2	9.0	7.4	7.0	5.9	5.4	4.4
Female	–	–	–	9.2	8.7	8.4	7.5	4.9	4.9	4.5
Race and Hispanic origin[1]										
White	–	–	–	10.5	11.4	9.7	9.0	7.5	6.0	5.3
Black	–	–	–	2.8	3.7	3.8	3.2	2.8	2.8	2.9
Hispanic[2]	–	–	–	9.2	8.1	8.5	7.1	5.0	4.4	3.7
10th-graders (in percent)										
Total	–	–	–	16.3	18.0	15.9	14.0	12.2	10.1	8.9
Gender										
Male	–	–	–	16.3	17.2	15.6	13.7	12.4	9.4	8.6
Female	–	–	–	16.1	18.5	15.9	14.1	11.9	10.8	9
Race and Hispanic origin[1]										
White	–	–	–	17.6	21.4	19.1	17.7	15.5	13.3	11.4
Black	–	–	–	4.7	5.6	5.3	5.2	5.2	5.0	4.3
Hispanic[2]	–	–	–	9.9	10.8	9.1	8.8	7.4	6.4	6.0
12th-graders (in percent)										
Total	21.3	19.5	19.1	21.6	24.6	23.1	20.6	19.0	16.9	15.8
Gender										
Male	18.5	17.8	18.6	21.7	24.8	23.6	20.9	18.4	17.2	17.0
Female	23.5	20.6	19.3	20.8	23.6	22.2	19.7	18.9	16.1	14
Race and Hispanic origin[1]										
White	23.9	20.4	21.8	23.9	27.8	26.9	25.7	23.8	21.8	19.5
Black	17.4	9.9	5.8	6.1	7.2	7.7	8.0	7.5	6.4	5.4
Hispanic[2]	12.8	11.8	10.9	11.6	14.0	14.0	15.7	12.0	9.2	8.0

– = not available

[1] Estimates for race and Hispanic origin represent the mean of the specified year and the previous year. Data have been combined to increase subgroup sample sizes, thus providing more stable estimates.

[2] Persons of Hispanic origin may be of any race.

Sources: *America's Children In Brief: Key National Indicators of Well-Being, 2004*; www.childstats.gov. Johnston, L.D., O'Malley, P.M., and Bachman, J.G. (2003). *Monitoring the Future national survey results on drug use, 1975-2002 Volume I: Secondary School Students* (NIH Publication No. 03-5375). Bethesda, MD: National Institute on Drug Abuse Tables 2-2 and 5-3. Data for 2003 are from a press release of December 19, 2003, and demographic disaggregations are from unpublished tabulations from Monitoring the Future, University of Michigan

Employment, Hours, and Earnings in Private[1] Health Service Establishments by Type of Establishment, U.S. : 1999-2004

Type of Establishment	Calendar Year 2000	2001	2002	2003	Q1 2004
Total Employment (In Thousands)					
Nonfarm Private Sector[1]	110,996	110,707	108,886	108,356	107,192
Health Care[2]	10,439	10,743	11,075	11,343	11,435
Offices of Physicians	1,840	1,911	1,968	2,004	2,034
Offices of Dentists	688	705	725	745	751
Home Health Care Services	633	639	680	727	736
Private Hospitals	3,954	4,051	4,160	4,253	4,284
Nursing and Residential Care Facilities	2,583	2,676	2,743	2,784	2,786
Nonsupervisory Employment					
Nonfarm Private Sector[1]	90,336	89,983	88,393	87,606	86,377
Health Care[2]	9,298	9,578	9,852	10,014	10,048
Offices of Physicians	1,545	1,601	1,636	1,640	1,648
Offices of Dentists	594	610	627	635	632
Home Health Care Services	583	588	626	670	675
Private Hospitals	3,649	3,746	3,841	3,904	3,926
Nursing and Residential Care Facilities	2,304	2,391	2,451	2,475	2,466
Average Weekly Hours					
Nonfarm Private Sector[1]	34.3	34.0	33.9	33.7	33.5
Health Care[2]	32.5	32.6	32.7	32.9	33.0
Offices of Physicians	32.4	32.7	33.1	33.1	33.3
Offices of Dentists	27.4	27.3	27.2	27.3	27.0
Home Health Care Services	27.4	27.7	28.4	29.0	28.7
Private Hospitals	34.1	34.3	34.3	34.8	35.0
Nursing and Residential Care Facilities	32.9	33.0	32.8	32.6	32.6
Average Hourly Earnings (in US$)					
Nonfarm Private Sector[1]	14.00	14.53	14.95	15.35	15.57
Health Care[2]	14.81	15.57	16.28	16.91	17.35
Offices of Physicians	15.65	16.25	17.04	17.91	18.23
Offices of Dentists	15.96	16.74	17.78	18.38	18.77
Home Health Care Services	12.83	13.18	13.37	13.69	14.21
Private Hospitals	16.71	17.72	18.63	19.37	19.99
Nursing and Residential Care Facilities	10.67	11.19	11.60	11.86	11.97
Hospital Employment (In Thousands)					
Total	5,141	5,253	5,375	5,480	5,528
Private	3,954	4,051	4,160	4,253	4,284
Federal	222	229	227	231	236
State	343	345	349	349	352
Local	622	628	642	652	656

[1] Excludes hospitals, clinics, and other health-related establishments run by all governments.
[2] Health care is the sum of ambulatory health services, private hospitals, nursing care facilities, residential mental health facilities, and continuing care retirement communities.
Notes: Data presented here conform to the 1987 Standard Industrial Classification.
Q designates quarter of year. Quarterly data are not seasonally adjusted.
Source: U.S. Department of Labor, Bureau of Labor Statistics: *Employment and Earnings*. Washington. U.S. Government Printing Office. Monthly reports for January 1998 - February 2003.

Chapter 3

IMPORTANT HEALTH CARE INDUSTRY CONTACTS

Contents:

I. Aging
II. AIDS/HIV
III. Alzheimer's Disease
IV. Arthritis
V. Biotech Associations
VI. Biotech Resources
VII. Blindness
VIII. Cancer
IX. Careers-Biotech
X. Careers-First Time Jobs/New Grads
XI. Careers-General Job Listings
XII. Careers-Health Care
XIII. Careers-Job Reference Tools
XIV. Child Abuse
XV. Child Development
XVI. Corporate Information
XVII. Diabetes
XVIII. Disabling Conditions
XIX. Diseases, Rare
XX. Drug & Alcohol Abuse
XXI. Economic Data & Research
XXII. Engineering Associations
XXIII. Fitness
XXIV. Headache/Head Injury
XXV. Health Associations-International
XXVI. Health Care Business & Professional Associations
XXVII. Health-General
XXVIII. Hearing & Speech
XXIX. Heart Disease
XXX. Hormonal Disorders
XXXI. Hospice Care
XXXII. Hospital Care
XXXIII. Immunization
XXXIV. Industry Research/Market Research
XXXV. Laboratories/Research
XXXVI. Learning Disorders
XXXVII. Libraries
XXXVIII. Liver Diseases
XXXIX. Managed Care Information
XL. Maternal & Infant Health
XLI. Medical & Health Indexes
XLII. Medicare Information
XLIII. Mental Health
XLIV. Neurological Disease
XLV. Nutrition
XLVI. Online Health Data
XLVII. Online Health Information, Reliability & Ethics
XLVIII. Organ Donation
XLIX. Osteoporosis
L. Patients Rights & Information
LI. Pharmaceutical Associations
LII. Privacy & Consumer Matters
LIII. Rare Disorders
LIV. Respiratory
LV. Scientific Business & Professional Associations
LVI. Sexually Transmitted Diseases
LVII. U.S. Government Agencies
LVIII. Urological Disorders

I. Aging

Administration on Aging (AOA)
One Massachusetts Ave.
Washington, DC 20201 US
Phone: 202-619-7501
Fax: 202-260-1012
E-mail Address: *aoainfo@aoa.gov*
Web Address: www.aoa.gov
The Administration on Aging (AOA) is the federal focal point and advocate agency for older persons and their concerns. In this role, AOA works to heighten awareness among other federal agencies, organizations, groups and the public.

Aging with Dignity
Toll Free: 888-594-7437
E-mail Address: *fivewishes@agingwithdignity.org*
Web Address: www.agingwithdignity.org
Aging with Dignity is a nonprofit organization that offers information, advice and legal tools needed to ensure that the wishes of the elderly concerning health and death be respected.

American Association of Home Services for the Aging (AAHSA)
2519 Connecticut Ave. NW
Washington, DC 20008 US
Phone: 202-783-2242
Fax: 202-783-2255
E-mail Address: *info@aahsa.org*
Web Address: www2.aahsa.org
The American Association of Home Services for the Aging (AAHSA) is committed to advancing the vision of healthy, affordable, ethical long-term care for America.

American Society on Aging (ASA)
833 Market St., Ste. 511
San Francisco, CA 94103 US
Phone: 415-974-9600
Fax: 415-974-0300
Toll Free: 800-537-9728
E-mail Address: *info@asaging.org*
Web Address: www.asaging.org
The American Society on Aging (ASA) is a nonprofit organization committed to enhancing the knowledge and skills of those working with older adults and their families.

National Association of Area Agencies on Aging (N4A)
1730 Rhode Island Ave. NW, Ste. 1200
Washington, DC 20005 US
Phone: 202-872-0888
Fax: 202-872-0057
Web Address: www.n4a.org
The National Association of Area Agencies on Aging (N4A) is the umbrella organization for the 655 area agencies on aging and more than 230 Title VI Native American aging programs in the U.S.

National Citizen's Coalition for Nursing Home Reform (NCCNHR)
1424 16th St. NW, Ste. 202
Washington, DC 20036 US
Phone: 202-332-2275
Fax: 202-332-2949
Web Address: www.nccnhr.org
The National Citizen's Coalition for Nursing Home Reform (NCCNHR) represents the grassroots membership of concerned advocates of quality long-term care nationwide.

National Council on the Aging (NCOA)
300 D St. SW
Washington, DC 20024 US
Phone: 202-479-1200
Fax: 202-479-0735
E-mail Address: *info@ncoa.org*
Web Address: www.ncoa.org
The National Council on the Aging (NCOA) is a group of organizations and professionals promoting the dignity, self-determination and well-being of older persons.

II. AIDS/HIV

AIDS Action
1906 Sunderland Pl. NW
Washington, DC 20036 US
Phone: 202-530-8030
Fax: 202-530-8031
E-mail Address: *aidsaction@aidsaction.org*
Web Address: www.aidsaction.org
AIDS Action is committed to advocating for people affected by HIV/AIDS.

CDC National STD and AIDS Hotline
Toll Free: 800-342-2437
Web Address: www.ashastd.org/nah/
The CDC National STD and AIDS Hotline exists to answer questions, provide referrals and send free publications through e-mail and postal mail.

HIV/AIDS Treatment Information Service
P.O. Box 6303
Rockville, MD 20849 US
Fax: 301-519-6616
Toll Free: 800-448-0440
E-mail Address: *atis@hivatis.org*
Web Address: www.aidsinfo.nih.gov
The HIV/AIDS Treatment Information Service is a central resource for federally approved treatment guidelines for HIV and AIDS.

III. Alzheimer's Disease

Alzheimer's Association
225 N. Michigan Ave., 17th Fl.
Chicago, IL 60601 US
Phone: 312-335-8700
Fax: 312-335-1110
Toll Free: 800-272-3900
E-mail Address: *info@alz.org*
Web Address: www.alz.org
The Alzheimer's Association is the largest national voluntary health organization committed to finding a cure for Alzheimer's and helping those affected by the disease.

Alzheimer's Disease Education and Referral Center (ADEAR)
P.O. Box 8250
Silver Spring, MD 20907 US
Toll Free: 800-438-4380
E-mail Address: *adear@alzheimers.org*
Web Address: www.alzheimers.org
The Alzheimer's Disease Education and Referral Center (ADEAR) provides information about Alzheimer's disease, its impact on families and health professionals and research into possible causes and cures.

IV. Arthritis

Arthritis Central
Web Address: www.arthritiscentral.com
Arthritis Central provides information and referrals, as well as articles and videos for members.

Arthritis Foundation
P.O. Box 7669
Atlanta, GA 30357-0669 US
Toll Free: 800-283-7800
Web Address: www.arthritis.org
The Arthritis Foundation supports the more than 100 types of arthritis and related conditions with advocacy, programs, services and research.

Arthritis Insight
P.O. Box 184
Smithville, IN 47458-0184 US
E-mail Address: *info@arthritisinsight.com*
Web Address: www.arthritisinsight.com
Arthritis Insight provides information and education on arthritis, as well as news and referrals.

Arthritis National Research Foundation (ANRF)
200 Oceangate, Ste. 400
Long Beach, CA 90802 US
Phone: 562-437-6808
Fax: 562-983-1410
Toll Free: 800-588-2873
E-mail Address: *anrf@ix.netcom.com*
Web Address: www.curearthritis.org
The Arthritis National Research Foundation (ANRF) provides funding for researchers associated with major research institutes, universities and hospitals throughout the country seeking to discover new knowledge for the prevention, treatment and cure of arthritis and related rheumatic diseases.

Arthritis.com
Web Address: www.arthritis.com
Arthritis.com is an online resource for arthritis information.

V. Biotech Associations

BIOCOM
4510 Executive Dr., Plz. 1
San Diego, CA 92121 US
Phone: 858-455-0300
Fax: 858-455-0022
Web Address: www.biocom.org
BIOCOM is a trade association for the life science industry in San Diego and Southern California.

Biotechnology Industry Organization (BIO)
1225 Eye St. NW, Ste. 400
Washington, DC 20005 US
Phone: 202-962-9200
Web Address: www.bio.org
The Biotechnology Industry Organization (BIO) is involved in the research and development of health care, agricultural, industrial and environmental biotechnology products.

Society for Biomaterials
17000 Commerce Pkwy.
Mt.Laurel, NJ 08054 US
Phone: 856-439-0826
Fax: 856-439-0525
E-mail Address: *info@biomaterials.org*
Web Address: www.biomaterials.org
The Society for Biomaterials is a professional society that promotes advances in all phases of materials research and development by encouragement of cooperative educational programs, clinical applications and professional standards in the biomaterials field.

VI. Biotech Resources

Bio Online
1900 Powell St., Ste. 230
Emeryville, CA 94608 US
Phone: 510-601-7194
Fax: 510-601-1862
E-mail Address: *sales@bio.com*
Web Address: www.bio.com
Bio Online is an online community of scientists, professionals, businesses and organizations supporting life science for the purpose of an exchange of information.

Biospace.com
580 Market St., 6th Fl.
San Francisco, CA 94104 US
Phone: 415-355-6500
Fax: 415-503-1070
Toll Free: 888-246-7722
Web Address: www.biospace.com
Biospace.com offers information, breaking news and profiles on biotech companies.

BioTech
Web Address: biotech.icmb.utexas.edu
This site offers a comprehensive dictionary of biotech terms, plus extensive research data regarding biotechnology.

Biotech Rumor Mill
E-mail Address: *info@biofind.com*
Web Address: www.biofind.com/rumor
Biotech Rumor Mill is an open discussion forum that attracts participants from the many biotech disciplines.

MedWeb: Biomedical Internet Resources
Web Address: www.medweb.emory.edu/medweb
MedWeb lists resources by medical field and allows users to search for articles by topic or date.

Tufts Center for the Study of Drug Development
192 South St., Ste. 550
Boston, MA 02111 US
Phone: 617-636-2170
Fax: 617-636-2425
Web Address: csdd.tufts.edu
The Tufts Center for the Study of Drug Development, an affiliate of Tuft's University, provides analyses and commentary on pharmaceutical issues. Its mission is to improve the quality and efficiency of pharmaceutical development, research and utilization.

VII. Blindness

American Council of the Blind (ACB)
1155 15th St. NW, Ste. 1004
Washington, DC 20005 US
Phone: 202-467-5081
Fax: 202-467-5085
Toll Free: 800-424-8666
Web Address: www.acb.org
The American Council of the Blind (ACB) is a leading membership organization of blind and visually impaired people.

Guide Dog Foundation for the Blind, Inc.
371 E. Jericho Tpke.
Smithtown, NY 11787-2976 US
Phone: 631-930-9000
Fax: 631-361-5192
Toll Free: 800-548-4337
Web Address: www.guidedog.org
The Guide Dog Foundation for the Blind strives to be the leading resource and provider of premier services to facilitate the independence of people who are blind or visually impaired.

Helen Keller International Organization
352 Park Ave. S., 12th Fl.
New York, NY 10010 US
Phone: 212-532-0544
Fax: 212-532-6014
Toll Free: 877-535-5374
Web Address: www.hki.org
The Helen Keller International Organization directly addresses the causes of preventable blindness, provides rehabilitation services to blind people and helps reduce micronutrient malnutrition which can cause blindness and death in children.

Lighthouse International
111 E. 59th St.
New York, NY 10022 US
Phone: 212-821-9760
Fax: 212-821-9702
Toll Free: 800-829-0500
E-mail Address: *visionrehab@lighthouse.org*
Web Address: www.lighthouse.org
Lighthouse International is a leading resource worldwide on vision impairment and vision rehabilitation.

National Association for the Visually Handicapped (NAVH)
22 W. 21st St.
New York, NY 10010 US
Phone: 212-889-3141
Fax: 212-727-2931
E-mail Address: *staff@navh.org*
Web Address: www.navh.org
The National Association for the Visually Handicapped (NAVH) works with the visually impaired so that those affected can live with as little disruption as possible.

National Eye Institute (NEI)
2020 Vision Pl.
Bethesda, MD 20892 US
Phone: 301-496-5248
Web Address: www.nei.nih.gov
The National Eye Institute (NEI) conducts and supports research that helps prevent and treat eye diseases and other disorders of vision.

National Library Service for the Blind and Physically Handicapped (NLS)
Library of Congress
1291 Taylor St. NW
Washington, DC 20542 US
Phone: 202-707-5100
Fax: 202-707-0712
Toll Free: 800-424-8567
E-mail Address: *nls@loc.gov*
Web Address: www.loc.gov/nls
National Library Service for the Blind and Physically Handicapped (NLS) administers a free library program of Braille and audio materials circulated to eligible borrowers in the United States by postage-free mail.

Prevent Blindness America (PBA)
500 E. Remington Rd.
Schaumburg, IL 60173 US
Phone: 847-843-2020
Toll Free: 800-331-2020
E-mail Address: *info@preventblindness.org*
Web Address: www.preventblindness.org
Prevent Blindness America (PBA) is a leading volunteer eye health and safety organization dedicated to fighting blindness and saving sight.

Recording for the Blind and Dyslexic (RFB&D)
20 Roszel Rd.
Princeton, NJ 08540 US
Toll Free: 866-732-3585
Web Address: www.rfbd.org
Recording for the Blind and Dyslexic (RFB&D) is an educational library serving people who cannot effectively read standard print because of visual impairment, dyslexia or other physical disability.

VISIONS
500 Greenwich St., 3rd Fl.
New York, NY 10013 US
Phone: 212-625-1616
Fax: 212-219-4078
E-mail Address: *info@visionsvcb.org*
Web Address: www.visionsvcb.org
VISIONS is a nonprofit agency that promotes the independence of people who are blind or visually impaired.

VIII. Cancer

American Cancer Society (ACS)
Toll Free: 800-227-2345
Web Address: www.cancer.org
The American Cancer Society (ACS) is a nationwide community-based voluntary health organization dedicated to eliminating cancer as a major health problem by preventing the disease, saving lives and diminishing suffering from cancer.

Association of Community Cancer Centers (ACCC)
11600 Nebel St., Ste. 201
Rockville, MD 20852 US
Phone: 301-984-9496
Fax: 301-770-1949
Web Address: www.accc-cancer.org
The Association of Community Cancer Centers (ACCC) helps oncology professionals adapt to the complex challenges of program management, cuts in reimbursement, hospital consolidation and mergers, and legislation and regulations that threaten to compromise the delivery of quality cancer care.

Lance Armstrong Foundation (LAF)
1221 S. MoPac Expy., Ste. 320
Austin, TX 78746 US
Phone: 512-236-8820
Web Address: www.laf.org
The Lance Armstrong Foundation (LAF) provides cancer patients, their families and caregivers with advocacy, education, public health and research programs relating to the treatment of and possible cures for all forms of cancer.

National Marrow Donor Program
3001 Broadway St., Ste. 500
Minneapolis, MN 55413 US
Toll Free: 800-627-7692
Web Address: www.marrow.org
The National Marrow Donor Program is an international leader in the facilitation of marrow and blood stem cell transplantation through non-family donors.

OncoLink
University of Pennsylvania Cancer Center
3400 Spruce St., 2 Donner
Philadelphia, PA 19104-4283 US
Fax: 215-349-5445
Web Address: www.oncolink.upenn.edu
OncoLink strives to help cancer patients, families, health care professionals and the general public obtain accurate cancer-related information.

Susan G. Komen Breast Cancer Foundation
5005 LBJ Fwy., Ste. 250
Dallas, TX 75244 US
Phone: 972-855-1600
Fax: 972-855-1605
Toll Free: 800-462-9273
E-mail Address: *helpline@komen.org*
Web Address: www.komen.org
This Susan G. Komen Breast Cancer Foundation strives to eradicate breast cancer as a life-threatening disease by advancing research, education, screening and treatment.

Y-Me National Breast Cancer Organization
212 W. Van Buren St., Ste. 500
Chicago, IL 60607 US
Phone: 312-986-8338
Fax: 312-294-8597
Toll Free: 800-221-2141
Web Address: www.y-me.org
The Y-Me National Breast Cancer Organization seeks to decrease the impact of breast cancer, create and increase breast cancer awareness and ensure that no one faces breast cancer alone.

IX. Careers-Biotech

Bio Online Career Center
1900 Powell St., Ste. 230
Emeryville, CA 94608 US
Phone: 510-601-7194
Fax: 510-601-1862
E-mail Address: *careers@bio.com*
Web Address:
career.bio.com/careercenter/index.jhtml
Provided by Bio Online, Bio Online Career Center enables users to search an extensive database of jobs in the life sciences field.

X. Careers-First Time Jobs/New Grads

Black Collegian Home Page
Web Address: www.black-collegian.com
Black Collegian Home Page features listings for job and internship opportunities. The site includes a list of the top 100 minority corporate employers and an assessment of job opportunities.

California Cooperative Occupational Information System
Phone: 916-262-2162
Fax: 916-262-2443
Web Address: www.calmis.ca.gov
California Cooperative Occupational Information System is a joint project of California's state and local governments to provide job information.

Collegegrad.com
P.O. Box 1703
Blue Bell, PA 19422 US
Phone: 262-675-0790
Web Address: www.collegegrad.com
Collegegrad.com offers in-depth resources for new grads seeking entry-level jobs.

Job Web
62 Highland Ave.
Bethlehem, PA 18017-9085 US
Phone: 610-868-1421
Fax: 610-868-0208
Toll Free: 800-544-5272
Web Address: www.jobweb.com
Job Web, provided by the National Association of Colleges and Employers, includes job openings and employer descriptions. The site also offers a database

of career fairs, searchable by state or keyword, with contact information.

MBAjobs.net
Fax: 413-556-8849
E-mail Address: *contact@mbajobs.net*
Web Address: www.mbajobs.net
MBAjobs.net is a unique international service for MBA students and graduates, employers and recruiters and business schools.

MonsterTrak
11845 W. Olympic Blvd., Ste. 500
Los Angeles, CA 90064 US
Fax: 310-474-2537
Toll Free: 800-999-8725
Web Address: www.monstertrak.monster.com
Features links to hundreds of university and college career centers across the U.S. with entry-level job listings categorized by industry. Major companies also utilize MonsterTrak.

National Association of Colleges and Employers
62 Highland Ave.
Bethlehem, PA 18017-9085 US
Phone: 610-868-1421
Fax: 610-868-0208
Toll Free: 800-544-5272
Web Address: www.naceweb.org
National Association of Colleges and Employers is a premier U.S. organization representing college placement offices and corporate recruiters who focus on hiring new grads. The site offers in-depth resources.

XI. Careers-General Job Listings

America's Job Bank
Toll Free: 877-872-5627
Web Address: www.jobsearch.org
Developed by the U.S. Department of Labor as part of an array of web-based job tools, America's Job Bank offers an extensive list of searchable employment vacancies as well as other job resources.

Career Exposure, Inc.
805 SW Broadway, Ste. 2250
Portland, OR 97205 US
Phone: 503-221-7779
Fax: 503-221-7780
E-mail Address: *info@careerexposure.com*
Web Address: www.careerexposure.com
Career Exposure is an online career center and job placement service, with features for employers, recruiters and job seekers.

CareerBuilder
Toll Free: 866-438-1485
Web Address: www.careerbuilder.com
CareerBuilder focuses on the needs of companies but also provides a database of job openings. Resumes are sent directly to the company, and applicants can set up a special e-mail account for job-seeking purposes.

Careers.wsj.com from the Publishers of the Wall Street Journal
Web Address: www.careers.wsj.com
The Wall Street Journal's interactive job search and career-management site posts job opportunities with employers worldwide. Provides a weekly career column and a range of articles about topics including promotion, career crisis and negotiation for higher wages.

DirectEmployers
E-Recruiting Association, Inc.
4040 Vincennes Cir., 4th Fl.
Indianapolis, IN 46268 US
Phone: 317-874-9000
Fax: 317-874-9100
Toll Free: 866-268-6206
E-mail Address: *info@directemployers.com*
Web Address: www.directemployers.com
Operated by the nonprofit E-Recruiting Association, DirectEmployers links users directly to hundreds of thousands of job opportunities posted on the sites of participating employers, thus bypassing the usual job search sites. Since employers must pay monster.com and other listing sites for each job opportunity they want to list, it can become too expensive for a growing employer to list all available jobs on third-party sites. Consequently, using directemployers.com saves the employer money and gives job seekers an opportunity to see many more jobs.

Flipdog.com
5 Clock Tower Pl., Ste. 500
Maynard, MA 01754 US
Toll Free: 877-887-3547
E-mail Address: *info@flipdog.com*
Web Address: www.flipdog.com
Flipdog.com, free to both job seekers and employers, scours the Internet to find jobs available at over 45,000 corporate sites.

HotJobs
406 W. 31st St.
New York, NY 10001 US
Web Address: hotjobs.yahoo.com
Designed for experienced professionals, HotJobs, a Yahoo-based site provides company profiles, a resume posting service and a resume workshop. The site allows posters to block resumes from being viewed by certain companies and provides a notification service of new jobs.

HRS Federal Job Search
Web Address: www.hrsjobs.com
HRS Federal Job Search features a database of federal jobs available across the U.S. The job seeker creates a profile with desired job type, salary and location to receive applicable postings by e-mail.

Monster.com
Toll Free: 800-666-7837
Web Address: www.monster.com
The Monster is an electronic career center that hosts more than 8,000 employers and serves more than 1 million job seekers each month. Job seekers can build and store a resume online and find job listings that match their profiles. Monster e-mails the results once per week.

Recruiters Online Network
E-mail Address: *info@recruitersonline.com*
Web Address: www.recruitersonline.com
Recruiters Online provides job postings from more than 7,000 recruiters, Careers Online Magazine and a resume database, as well as other resources.

TrueCareers, Inc.
11600 Sallie Mae Dr.
Reston, VA 20193 US
Toll Free: 800-441-4062
Web Address: www.truecareers.com
In addition to offering job listings, TrueCareers provides an array of career resources.

XII. Careers-Health Care

Health Care Source
Web Address: www.healthcaresource.com
Health Care Source offers career-related information for health care professionals.

HMonster
Toll Free: 800-666-7837
Web Address: healthcare.monster.com
Managed by monster.com, HMonster provides job listings, job searches and search agents for the medical field.

Medicalworkers.com
E-mail Address: *info@medicalworkers.com*
Web Address: www.medicalworkers.com
Medicalworkers.com is an employment site for medical and health care professionals.

Medjump.com
7119 E. Shea Blvd., Ste. 109-535
Scottsdale, AZ 85254 US
E-mail Address: *info@medjump.net*
Web Address: www.medjump.com
Medjump.com is dedicated to empowering health care and medical-related professionals with the necessary tools to market their abilities and skills.

Medzilla.com
Web Address: www.medzilla.com
Medzilla.com offers job searches, salary surveys, a search agent and information on health care employment.

NationJob Networks--Medical and Health Care Jobs Page
601 SW 9th St., Stes. J&K
Des Moines, IA 50309 US
Toll Free: 800-292-6083
E-mail Address: *elinebach@nationjob.com*
Web Address: www.nationjob.com/medical
This section of the NationJob web site offers information and listings for health care employment.

Nurse-Recruiter.com
2200 Defense Hwy., Ste. 101
Crofton, MD 21114 US
Phone: 410-451-7229
Fax: 410-451-7259
Web Address: www.nurse-recruiter.com
Nurse-Recruiter.com is a nurse-owned, web-centric company devoted to bringing health care employers and the nursing community together.

PracticeLink
PracticeLink & Web-CV
P.O. Box 100
Hinton, WV 25951 US
Phone: 877-847-0120
Toll Free: 800-776-8383
E-mail Address: *info@practicelink.com*
Web Address: www.practicelink.com

Established in 1994, PracticeLink is one of the largest physician employment web sites. It is a free service used by more than 15,000 practice-seeking physicians annually to quickly search and locate potential physician practice opportunities. PracticeLink is financially supported by more than 700 hospitals, medical groups, private practices and health care systems that advertise more than 4,000 opportunities.

XIII. Careers-Job Reference Tools

Newspaperlinks.com
E-mail Address: *knigj@naa.org*
Web Address: www.newspaperlinks.com
Newspaperlinks.com, a service of the Newspaper Association of America, links individuals to local, national and international newspapers. Job seekers can search through thousands of classified sections.

Society of Human Resource Management
1800 Duke St.
Alexandria, VA 22314 US
Phone: 703-548-3440
Fax: 703-535-6490
Toll Free: 800-283-7476
Web Address: www.shrm.org
The Society of Human Resource Management provides frequently updated information for hiring managers. This site also has an online library of articles by keyword and provides the latest news in employment and labor law.

Vault.com
150 W. 22nd St.
New York, NY 10011 US
Phone: 212-366-4212
Web Address: www.vault.com
Vault.com is a comprehensive career web site for employers and employees, with job postings and valuable information on the employment industry. The site focuses on helping the user understand what it's really like to work at a particular firm. Many of the features are focused on MBAs, and the site offers a wide variety of industry guides for sale.

XIV. Child Abuse

Adult Survivors of Child Abuse
The Morris Center
P.O. Box 14477
San Francisco, CA 94114 US
Phone: 415-928-4576

E-mail Address: *tmc_asca@dnai.com*
Web Address: www.ascasupport.org
Adult Survivors of Child Abuse is a support program for adult survivors of child neglect and abuse.

National Center for Missing and Exploited Children (NCMEC)
699 Prince St.
Alexandria, VA 22314 US
Phone: 703-274-3900
Fax: 703-274-2220
Toll Free: 800-843-5678
Web Address: www.ncmec.org
The National Center for Missing and Exploited Children (NCMEC) is an international resource for abducted, endangered and sexually exploited children.

National Clearinghouse on Child Abuse and Neglect Information
330 C St.
Washington, DC 20447 US
Phone: 703-385-7565
Fax: 703-385-3206
Toll Free: 800-394-3366
E-mail Address: *nccanch@calib.com*
Web Address: nccanch.acf.hhs.gov
The National Clearinghouse on Child Abuse and Neglect Information is a national resource for professionals and others seeking information on child abuse, neglect and child welfare.

XV. Child Development

Autism Society of America (ASA)
7910 Woodmont Ave., Ste. 300
Bethesda, MD 20814-3067 US
Phone: 301-657-0881
Fax: 301-657-0869
Toll Free: 800-328-8476
E-mail Address: *info@autism-society.org*
Web Address: www.autism-society.org
The Autism Society of America (ASA) seeks to promote lifelong access and opportunity for all individuals affected by autism to be fully participating members of their communities.

Human Growth Foundation
997 Glen Cove Ave., Ste. 5
Glen Head, NY 11545 US
Fax: 516-671-4055
Toll Free: 800-451-6434
E-mail Address: *hgf1@hgfound.org*

Web Address: www.hgfound.org
The Human Growth Foundation helps children and adults with disorders related to growth or growth hormone through research, education, support and advocacy.

XVI. Corporate Information

bizjournals.com
120 W. Morehead St., Ste. 200
Charlotte, NC 28202 US
Phone: 704-973-1000
Fax: 704-973-1001
E-mail Address: *info@bizjournals.com*
Web Address: www.bizjournals.com
Operated by the American Business Journals firm, the publisher of dozens of leading city business journals nationwide, bizjournals.com provides access to research into the latest news regarding companies small and large.

Business Wire
Web Address: www.businesswire.com
Business Wire strives to deliver news in an innovative manner. Smart News releases, industry-specific and company-specific news, today's headlines, conference calls, IPOs on the Internet, media services, tradeshownews.com and BW Connect On-line are all accessible through this informative and continuously updated site.

CNNfn Home Page
Web Address: money.cnn.com
CNNfn provides the same in-depth financial information online that CNN's cable television financial news unit provides to television viewers.

Edgar Online
50 Washington St., 9th Fl.
Norwalk, CT 06854 US
Phone: 203-852-5666
Fax: 203-852-5667
Toll Free: 800-416-6651
Web Address: www.edgar-online.com
Edgar Online is a gateway and search tool for viewing corporate documents, such as annual reports on form 10K, filed with the U.S. Securities and Exchange Commission.

PRNewswire
810 7th Ave., 35th Fl.
New York, NY 10019 US
Phone: 212-596-1500
Toll Free: 800-832-5522
E-mail Address: *information@prnewswire.com*
Web Address: www.prnewswire.com
PRNewswire provides comprehensive communications services for public relations and investor relations professionals ranging from information distribution and market intelligence to the creation of online multimedia content and investor relations web sites. Users can also view recent corporate press releases.

Silicon Investor
Web Address: www.siliconinvestor.com
Silicon Investor is focused on technology companies. The site serves as a financial discussion forum and offers quotes, profiles and charts.

XVII. Diabetes

American Diabetes Association
1701 N. Beauregard St.
Alexandria, VA 22311 US
Toll Free: 800-342-2383
E-mail Address: *customerservice@diabetes.org*
Web Address: www.diabetes.org
The American Diabetes Association is a nonprofit health organization providing diabetes research, information and advocacy.

Juvenile Diabetes Research Foundation (JDRF)
120 Wall St.
New York, NY 10005 US
Fax: 212-785-9595
Toll Free: 800-533-2873
E-mail Address: *info@jdrf.org*
Web Address: www.jdrf.org
The Juvenile Diabetes Research Foundation (JDRF) is the world's leading nonprofit, nongovernmental sponsor of diabetes research.

XVIII. Disabling Conditions

Americans with Disabilities Act (ADA)
950 Pennsylvania Ave.
Civil Rights Div., Disability Rights Section
Washington, DC 20530 US
Fax: 202-307-1198
Toll Free: 800-514-0301
Web Address: www.usdoj.gov/crt/ada/adahom1.htm
The Americans with Disabilities Act (ADA) web site providing information and technical assistance on the Americans with Disabilities Act.

Job Accommodation Network (JAN)
P.O. Box 6080
Morgantown, WV 26506 US
Phone: 304-293-7186
Fax: 304-293-5407
Toll Free: 800-526-7234
E-mail Address: *jan@jan.icdi.wvu.edu*
Web Address: janweb.icdi.wvu.edu
The Job Accommodation Network (JAN) is a free consulting service that provides information about job accommodations, the Americans with Disabilities Act and the employability of people with disabilities.

National Easter Seal Society
230 W. Monroe St., Ste. 1800
Chicago, IL 60606 US
Phone: 312-726-6200
Fax: 312-726-1494
Toll Free: 800-221-6827
E-mail Address: *info@easter-seals.org*
Web Address: www.easter-seals.org
The National Easter Seal Society provides services to children and adults with disabilities, as well as assistance to their families.

National Information Center for Children and Youth with Disabilities (NICHCY)
P.O. Box 1492
Washington, DC 20013 US
Phone: 202-884-8200
Fax: 202-884-8441
Toll Free: 800-695-0285
E-mail Address: *nichcy@aed.org*
Web Address: www.nichcy.org
National Information Center for Children and Youth with Disabilities (NICHCY) is a national information and referral center that provides information on disabilities and disability-related issues for families, educators and other professionals.

XIX. Diseases, Rare

American Association on Mental Retardation (AAMR)
Web Address: www.aamr.org
The American Association on Mental Retardation (AAMR) promotes progressive policies, sound research, effective practices and universal human rights for people with intellectual disabilities.

American SIDS Institute
509 Augusta Dr.
Marietta, GA 30067 US
Phone: 770-426-8746
Fax: 770-426-1369
Toll Free: 800-232-7437
Web Address: www.sids.org
The American SIDS Institute is dedicated to the prevention of sudden infant death and the promotion of infant health.

Amyotrophic Lateral Sclerosis Association (ALSA)
27001 Agoura Rd., Ste. 150
Calabasas Hills, CA 91301 US
Phone: 818-880-9007
Fax: 818-880-9006
Toll Free: 800-782-4747
Web Address: www.alsa.org
The Amyotrophic Lateral Sclerosis Association (ALSA) seeks to be the primary resource to the ALS, or Lou Gehrig's disease, community by providing information about the disease, products and services, physicians and other information.

Angelman Syndrome Foundation (ASF)
3015 E. New York St., Ste. A2265
Aurora, IL 60559 US
Phone: 630-978-4245
Fax: 630-978-7408
Toll Free: 800-432-6435
E-mail Address: *info@angelman.org*
Web Address: www.angelman.org
The mission of the Angelman Syndrome Foundation (ASF) is to advance the awareness and treatment of Angelman Syndrome through education, information exchange and research.

Cleft Palate Foundation (CPF)
1504 E. Franklin St., Ste. 102
Chapel Hill, NC 27514 US
Phone: 919-933-9044
Fax: 919-933-9604
Toll Free: 800-242-5338
E-mail Address: *help@cleft.org*
Web Address: www.cleftline.org
The Cleft Palate Foundation (CPF) is a nonprofit organization dedicated to optimizing the quality of life for individuals affected by facial birth defects.

Cystic Fibrosis Foundation (CFF)
6931 Arlington Rd.
Bethesda, MD 20814 US
Phone: 301-951-4422
Fax: 301-951-6378
Toll Free: 800-344-4823

E-mail Address: *info@cff.org*
Web Address: www.cff.org
The Cystic Fibrosis Foundation (CFF) assures the development of the means to cure and control cystic fibrosis and to improve the quality of life for those with the disease.

Dystonia Medical Research Foundation
One E. Wacker Dr., Ste. 2430
Chicago, IL 60601-1905 US
Phone: 312-755-0198
Fax: 312-803-0138
Toll Free: 800-361-8061
E-mail Address: *dystonia@dystonia-foundation.org*
Web Address: www.dystonia-foundation.org
Dystonia Medical Research Foundation seeks to advance research for more treatments and ultimately a cure for dystonia, to promote awareness and education of the disease and to support the needs and well-being of affected individuals and families.

Epilepsy Foundation of America
4351 Garden City Dr.
Landover, MD 20785 US
Phone: 301-459-3700
Toll Free: 800-332-1000
Web Address: www.epilepsyfoundation.org
The Epilepsy Foundation of America seeks to ensure that people with seizures are able to participate in all life experiences.

Hepatitis B Foundation
700 E. Butler Ave.
Doylestown, PA 18901 US
Phone: 215-489-4900
Fax: 215-489-4920
E-mail Address: *info@hepb.org*
Web Address: www.hepb.org
The Hepatitis B Foundation is a national nonprofit organization dedicated to finding a cure and improving the quality of life of those affected by hepatitis B worldwide through research, education and patient advocacy.

Huntington's Disease Society of America, Inc. (HDSA)
158 W. 29th St., 7th Fl.
New York, NY 10001 US
Phone: 212-242-1968
Fax: 212-239-3430
Toll Free: 800-345-4372
E-mail Address: *hdsainfo@hdsa.org*
Web Address: www.hdsa.org

The Huntington's Disease Society of America, Inc. (HDSA) is dedicated to finding a cure for Huntington's disease (HD) while providing support and services for those living with HD and their families.

Lupus Foundation of America
2000 L St. NW, Ste. 710
Washington, DC 20036 US
Phone: 805-339-0443
Fax: 805-339-0467
Toll Free: 800-331-1802
Web Address: www.lupus.org
The Lupus Foundation of America is the nation's leading nonprofit voluntary health organization dedicated to improving the diagnosis and treatment of lupus, supporting individuals and families affected by the disease, increasing awareness of lupus among health professionals and the public, and finding the cure.

Meniere's Network
1817 Patterson St.
Nashville, TN 37203 US
Toll Free: 800-545-4327
Web Address: www.theearfound.org
The Meniere's Network offers information and a newsletter on Meniere's disease to its members.

Muscular Dystrophy Association (MDA)
3300 E. Sunrise Dr.
Tucson, AZ 85718 US
Toll Free: 800-572-1717
E-mail Address: *mda@mdausa.org*
Web Address: www.mdausa.org
The Muscular Dystrophy Association (MDA) is a voluntary health agency aimed at conquering neuromuscular diseases that affect more than 1 million Americans.

Myasthenia Gravis Foundation of America (MGFA)
1821 University Ave. W., Ste. S256
St. Paul, MN 55104 US
Phone: 952-545-9438
Fax: 952-545-6073
Toll Free: 800-541-5454
E-mail Address: *myasthenia@myasthenia.org*
Web Address: www.myasthenia.org
The Myasthenia Gravis Foundation of America (MGFA) is the only national volunteer health agency dedicated solely to the fight against myasthenia gravis.

National Down Syndrome Congress (NDSC)
1370 Center Dr., Ste. 102
Atlanta, GA 30338 US
Phone: 770-604-9500
Toll Free: 800-232-6372
E-mail Address: *info@ndsccenter.org*
Web Address: www.ndsccenter.org
The National Down Syndrome Congress (NDSC) strives to be the national advocacy organization for Down syndrome and to provide leadership in all areas of concern related to persons with Down syndrome.

National Multiple Sclerosis Society (NMSS)
733 3rd Ave.
New York, NY 10017 US
Toll Free: 800-344-4867
E-mail Address: *info@nmss.org*
Web Address: www.nmss.org
The National Multiple Sclerosis Society (NMSS) and its network of chapters nationwide promote research, educate, advocate on critical issues and organize a wide range of programs for those living with multiple sclerosis.

National Organization for Rare Disorders (NORD)
55 Kenosia Ave.
Danbury, CT 06813 US
Phone: 203-746-0100
Fax: 203-798-2291
Toll Free: 800-999-6673
E-mail Address: *orphan@rarediseases.org*
Web Address: www.rarediseases.org
The National Organization for Rare Disorders (NORD) is a unique federation of voluntary health organizations dedicated to helping people with rare diseases and assisting the organizations that serve them.

National Peticulosis Association (NPA)
50 Kearney Rd.
Needham, MA 02494 US
Phone: 781-449-6487
Fax: 781-449-8129
E-mail Address: *npa@headlice.org*
Web Address: www.headlice.org
The National Peticulosis Association (NPA) is the only nonprofit health and education agency dedicated to protecting children from the misuse and abuse of potentially harmful lice and scabies pesticidal treatments.

National Reye's Syndrome Foundation (NRSF)
P.O. Box 829
Bryan, OH 43506 US
Phone: 419-636-2679
Fax: 419-636-9897
Toll Free: 800-233-7393
E-mail Address: *nrsf@reyessyndrome.org*
Web Address: www.reyessyndrome.org
The National Reye's Syndrome Foundation (NRSF) attempts to generate a concerted, organized lay movement to eradicate Reye's syndrome.

Paget Foundation for Paget's Disease of Bone and Related Disorders
120 Wall St., Ste. 1602
New York, NY 10005 US
Phone: 212-509-5335
Fax: 212-509-8492
Toll Free: 800-237-2438
E-mail Address: *pagetfdn@aol.com*
Web Address: www.paget.org
The Paget Foundation for Paget's Disease of Bone and Related Disorders is an informative web site dedicated to Paget's disease.

Scleroderma Foundation
12 Kent Way, Ste. 101
Byfield, MA 01922 US
Phone: 978-463-5843
Fax: 978-463-5809
Toll Free: 800-722-4673
E-mail Address: *sfinfo@scleroderma.org*
Web Address: www.scleroderma.org
The Scleroderma Foundation seeks to help patients and their families cope with scleroderma, as well as raise public awareness and stimulate research.

Sickle Cell Disease Association of America, Inc.
200 Corporate Point, Ste. 495
Culver City, CA 90230 US
Phone: 310-216-6363
Fax: 310-215-3722
Toll Free: 800-421-8453
E-mail Address: *scdaa@sicklecelldisease.org*
Web Address: www.sicklecelldisease.org
The Sickle Cell Disease Association of America is devoted to the care and cure of individuals with sickle cell disease.

Spina Bifida Association of America (SBAA)
4590 MacArthur Blvd. NW, Ste. 250
Washington, DC 20007 US
Phone: 202-944-3285

Fax: 202-944-3295
Toll Free: 800-621-3141
E-mail Address: *sbaa@sbaa.org*
Web Address: www.sbaa.org
The Spina Bifida Association of America (SBAA) seeks to promote the prevention of spina bifida and to enhance the lives of all affected.

Tourette Syndrome Association, Inc. (TSA)
42-40 Bell Blvd.
Bayside, NY 11361 US
Phone: 718-224-2999
Fax: 718-279-9596
Web Address: www.tsa-usa.org
The Tourette Syndrome Association, Inc. (TSA) seeks to identify the cause, find the cure for and control the effects of Tourette syndrome.

United Cerebral Palsy Association (UCPA)
1660 L St. NW, Ste. 700
Washington, DC 20036 US
Phone: 202-776-0406
Fax: 202-776-0414
Toll Free: 800-872-5827
E-mail Address: *webmaster@ucpa.org*
Web Address: www.ucpa.org
The United Cerebral Palsy Association (UCPA) seeks change and progress for persons with disabilities.

XX. Drug & Alcohol Abuse

Al-Anon/Alateen
1600 Corporate Landing Pkwy.
Virginia Beach, VA 23454 US
Phone: 757-563-1600
Fax: 757-563-1655
Web Address: www.al-anon.alateen.org
Al-Anon/Alateen strives to help families and friends of alcoholics recover from the effects of living with the problem drinking of a relative or friend.

Drug Information Association (DIA)
800 Enterprise Rd., Ste. 200
Horsham, PA 19044 US
Phone: 215-442-6100
Fax: 215-442-6199
E-mail Address: *dia@diahome.org*
Web Address: www.diahome.org
The Drug Information Association (DIA) provides a neutral global forum for the exchange and dissemination of information on the discovery, development, evaluation and utilization of medicines and related health care technologies.

National Clearinghouse for Alcohol and Drug Information (NCADI)
P.O. Box 2345
Rockville, MD 20847 US
Phone: 301-468-2600
Fax: 301-468-6433
Toll Free: 800-729-6686
E-mail Address: *info@health.org*
Web Address: www.health.org
The National Clearinghouse for Alcohol and Drug Information (NCADI) is the information service of the Center for Substance Abuse Prevention of the Substance Abuse and Mental Health Services Administration in the U.S. Department of Health & Human Services.

National Cocaine Hotline
Toll Free: 800-262-2463
Web Address: www.phoenixhouse.org
The National Cocaine Hotline is a drug hotline hosted by Phoenix House, a leader in drug treatment.

XXI. Economic Data & Research

STAT-USA
HCHB, Rm. 4885
U.S. Department of Commerce
Washington, DC 20230 US
Phone: 202-482-1986
Fax: 202-482-2164
Toll Free: 800-782-8872
E-mail Address: *statmail@mail.doc.gov*
Web Address: www.stat-usa.gov
STAT-USA is an agency in the Economics and Statistics Administration of the U.S. Department of Commerce. The site offers daily economic news, statistical releases, export and trade databases and information and domestic economic databases.

XXII. Engineering Associations

American Society for Healthcare Engineering (ASHE)
One N. Franklin, 28th Fl.
Chicago, IL 60606 US
Phone: 312-422-3800
Fax: 312-422-4571
E-mail Address: *ashe@aha.org*
Web Address: www.ashe.org

The American Society for Healthcare Engineering (ASHE) is the advocate and resource for continuous improvement in the health care engineering and facilities management professions.

American Society of Safety Engineers (ASSE)
1800 E. Oakton St.
Des Plaines, IL 60018 US
Phone: 847-699-2929
Fax: 847-768-3434
E-mail Address: *customerservice@asse.org*
Web Address: www.asse.org
The American Society of Safety Engineers (ASSE) is the world's oldest and largest professional safety organization. ASSE manages, supervises and consults on safety, health and environmental issues in industry, insurance, government and education.

Society of Nuclear Medicine (SNM)
1850 Samuel Morse Dr.
Reston, VA 20190 US
Phone: 703-708-9000
Fax: 703-708-9015
Web Address: www.snm.org
The Society of Nuclear Medicine (SNM) is an international scientific and professional organization founded to promote the science, technology and practical application of nuclear medicine.

XXIII. Fitness

Aerobics and Fitness Association of America (AFAA)
15250 Ventura Blvd., Ste. 200
Sherman Oaks, CA 91403 US
Toll Free: 877-968-7263
Web Address: www.afaa.com
The Aerobics and Fitness Association of America (AFAA) answers questions from the public regarding safe and effective exercise programs and practices.

American Fitness Professionals and Associates (AFPA)
P.O. Box 214
Ship Bottom, NJ 08008 US
Phone: 609-978-7583
E-mail Address: *afpa@afpafitness.com*
Web Address: www.afpafitness.com
American Fitness Professionals and Associates (AFPA) offers health and fitness professionals certification programs, continuing education courses, home correspondence courses and regional conventions.

YMCA of the USA
101 N. Wacker Dr.
Chicago, IL 60606 US
Phone: 312-977-0031
Fax: 312-977-9063
Toll Free: 800-872-9622
Web Address: www.ymca.net
The YMCA is the largest nonprofit community service organization in America, and it strives to put Christian principles into practice through programs that build healthy spirit, mind and body for all.

XXIV. Headache/Head Injury

American Council for Headache Education (ACHE)
19 Mantua Rd.
Mt. Royal, NJ 08061 US
Phone: 856-423-0258
Fax: 856-423-0082
E-mail Address: *achehq@talley.com*
Web Address: www.achenet.org
The American Council for Headache Education (ACHE) is a nonprofit patient-health professional partnership dedicated to advancing the treatment and management of headache and to raising the public awareness of headache as a valid, biologically based illness.

Brain Injury Association, Inc.
8201 Greensboro Dr., Ste. 611
McLean, VA 22102 US
Phone: 703-761-0750
Toll Free: 800-444-6443
Web Address: www.biausa.org
The mission of the Brain Injury Association is to create a better future through brain injury prevention, research, education and advocacy.

National Headache Foundation (NHF)
820 N. Orleans, Ste. 217
Chicago, IL 60610 US
Toll Free: 888-643-5552
E-mail Address: *info@headaches.org*
Web Address: www.headaches.org
The National Headache Foundation (NHF) is a nonprofit organization dedicated to educating headache sufferers and health care professionals about headache causes and treatments.

XXV. Health Associations-International

World Health Organization (WHO)
Ave. Appia 20
1211 Geneva 27
Geneva, Switzerland
Phone: 41-22-791-2111
Fax: 41-22-791-3111
Web Address: www.who.int
The World Health Organization (WHO), the United Nations' specialized agency for health, was established in April 1948. WHO's objective, as set out in its constitution, is the attainment by all people of the highest possible level of health. Health is defined in WHO's constitution as a state of complete physical, mental and social well-being and not merely the absence of disease or infirmity. WHO is governed by 191 member states through the World Health Assembly, composed of representatives from the member states.

XXVI. Health Care Business & Professional Associations

Academy of Laser Dentistry (ALD)
P.O. Box 8667
Coral Springs, FL 33075 US
Phone: 954-346-3776
Fax: 954-757-2598
Toll Free: 877-527-3776
E-mail Address: *laserexec@laserdentistry.org*
Web Address: www.laserdentistry.org
The Academy of Laser Dentistry (ALD) is an international professional membership association of dental practitioners and supporting organizations.

Academy of Medical-Surgical Nurses (AMSN)
E. Holly Ave., Box 56
Pitman, NJ 08071-0056 US
Toll Free: 866-877-2370
E-mail Address: *amsn@ajj.com*
Web Address: amsn.inurse.com
The Academy of Medical-Surgical Nurses (AMSN) is dedicated to fostering excellence in adult health and medical-surgical nursing practice.

Acute Long-Term Hospital Association (ALTHA)
1055 N. Fairfax St., Ste. 201
Alexandria, VA 22314 US
Phone: 703-299-5571
Fax: 703-299-5574
Web Address: www.altha.org
The Acute Long-Term Hospital Association (ALTHA) represents over 100 long-term care hospitals (both free-standing and "hospitals-within-hospitals") specializing in intensive care for long-stay patients.

Advanced Medical Technology Association (AdvaMed)
1200 G St. NW, Ste. 400
Washington, DC 20005-3814 US
Phone: 202-783-8700
Fax: 202-783-8750
E-mail Address: *info@advamed.org*
Web Address: www.advamed.org
The Advanced Medical Technology Association (AdvaMed) strives to be the advocate for a legal, regulatory and economic climate that advances global health care by assuring worldwide access to the benefits of medical technology.

Air and Surface Transport Nurses Association (ASTNA)
9101 E. Kenyon Ave., Ste. 3000
Denver, CO 80237 US
Fax: 303-770-1812
Toll Free: 800-897-6362
E-mail Address: *executive-director@astna.org*
Web Address: www.astna.org
The Air and Surface Transport Nurses Association (ASTNA) is a nonprofit member organization whose mission is to represent, promote and provide guidance to professional nurses who practice the unique and distinct specialty of transport nursing.

America's Health Insurance Plans (AHIP)
601 Pennsylvania Ave. NW, Ste. 500
Washington, DC 20004 US
Phone: 202-778-3200
Fax: 202-331-7487
Web Address: www.ahip.org
America's Health Insurance Plans (AHIP) is a prominent trade association representing the private health care system.

American Academy of Ambulatory Care Nursing (AAACN)
E. Holly Ave., Box 56
Pitman, NJ 08071 US
Phone: 856-256-2350
Fax: 856-589-7463
Toll Free: 800-262-6877
E-mail Address: *aaacn@ajj.com*
Web Address: www.aaacn.org

The American Academy of Ambulatory Care Nursing (AAACN) is the association of professional nurses who identify ambulatory care practice as essential to the continuum of high-quality, cost-effective health care.

American Academy of Facial Plastic and Reconstructive Surgery (AAFPRS)
310 S. Henry St.
Alexandria, VA 22314 US
Phone: 703-299-9291
Fax: 703-299-8898
Web Address: www.facial-plastic-surgery.org
The American Academy of Facial Plastic and Reconstructive Surgery (AAFPRS) is the world's largest association of facial plastic and reconstructive surgeons.

American Academy of Family Physicians (AAFP)
11400 Tomahawk Creek Pkwy.
Leawood, KS 66211 US
Phone: 913-906-6000
Toll Free: 800-274-2237
E-mail Address: *fp@aafp.org*
Web Address: www.aafp.org
The American Academy of Family Physicians (AAFP) is the national association of family doctors.

American Academy of Hospice and Palliative Medicine (AAHPM)
4700 W. Lake Ave.
Glenview, IL 60025 US
Phone: 847-375-4712
Fax: 877-734-8671
Web Address: www.aahpm.org
The American Academy of Hospice and Palliative Medicine (AAHPM) is the only organization in the United States for physicians dedicated to the advancement of hospice and palliative medicine and its practice, research and education.

American Academy of Medical Administrators (AAMA)
701 Lee St., Ste. 600
Des Plaines, IL 60016 US
Phone: 847-759-8601
Fax: 847-759-8602
E-mail Address: *info@aameda.org*
Web Address: www.aameda.org
The American Academy of Medical Administrators (AAMA) is an association for health care leaders to enhance their profession and community health.

American Academy of Nurse Practitioners (AANP)
P.O. Box 12846
Austin, TX 78711 US
Phone: 512-442-4262
Fax: 512-442-6469
E-mail Address: *admin@aanp.org*
Web Address: www.aanp.org
The American Academy of Nurse Practitioners (AANP) is the only full-service organization for nurse practitioners of all specialties.

American Academy of Nursing (AAN)
555 E. Wells St., Ste. 1100
Milwaukee, WI 53202 US
Phone: 414-287-0289
Fax: 414-276-3349
Web Address: www.aannet.org
The American Academy of Nursing (AAN) exists to help nursing leaders transform the health care system to optimize public well-being.

American Academy of Ophthalmology (AAO)
P.O. Box 7424
San Francisco, CA 94120-7424 US
Phone: 415-561-8500
Fax: 415-561-8533
Web Address: www.aao.org
The American Academy of Ophthalmology (AAO) is dedicated to advancing learning and interests of ophthalmologists to ensure the best in eye care.

American Academy of Orthotics and Prosthetics (AAOP)
526 King St.
Alexandria, VA 22314 US
Phone: 703-836-0788
Fax: 703-836-0737
E-mail Address: *academy@oandp.org*
Web Address: www.oandp.org
The American Academy of Orthotics and Prosthetics (AAOP) promotes high standards of patient care through advocacy, education, literature and research.

American Association of Blood Banks (AABB)
8101 Glenbrook Rd.
Bethesda, MD 20814-2749 US
Phone: 301-907-6977
Fax: 301-907-6895
E-mail Address: *aabb@aabb.org*
Web Address: www.aabb.org

The American Association of Blood Banks (AABB) promotes high standards of care for blood banking and transfusion medicine.

American Association of Colleges of Nursing (AACN)
One Dupont Cir. NW, Ste. 530
Washington, DC 20036 US
Phone: 202-463-6930
Fax: 202-785-8320
Web Address: www.aacn.nche.edu
The American Association of Colleges of Nursing (AACN) is the national voice for U.S. nursing education programs.

American Association of Colleges of Pharmacy (AACP)
1426 Prince St.
Alexandria, VA 22314 US
Phone: 703-739-2330
Fax: 703-836-8982
Web Address: www.aacp.org
The American Association of Colleges of Pharmacy (AACP) is the national organization representing the interests of pharmaceutical education and educators.

American Association of Critical Care Nurses (AACN)
101 Columbia
Aliso Viejo, CA 92656 US
Phone: 949-362-2000
Fax: 949-362-2020
Toll Free: 800-899-2226
E-mail Address: *info@aacn.org*
Web Address: www.aacn.org
The American Association of Critical Care Nurses (AACN) provides leadership to establish work/care environments that involve respect and healing.

American Association of Health Plans (AAHP)
601 Pennsylvania Ave. NW
South Bldg., Ste. 500
Washington, DC 20036-3421 US
Phone: 202-778-3200
Fax: 202-778-8486
Web Address: www.aahp.org
The American Association of Health Plans (AAHP) represents more than 1,000 plans that provide coverage for approximately 150 million Americans nationwide.

American Association of Healthcare Consultants (AAHC)
5938 N. Drake Ave.
Chicago, IL 60659 US
Toll Free: 888-350-2242
E-mail Address: *info@aahc.net*
Web Address: www.aahc.net
The American Association of Healthcare Consultants (AAHC) is a professional society for credentialed consultants practicing in health care organization and delivery.

American Association of Legal Nurse Consultants (AALNC)
401 N. Michigan Ave.
Chicago, IL 60611 US
Fax: 312-673-6655
Toll Free: 877-402-2562
E-mail Address: *info@aalnc.org*
Web Address: www.aalnc.org
The American Association of Legal Nurse Consultants (AALNC) is a nonprofit organization dedicated to the professional enhancement of registered nurses practicing in a consulting capacity in the legal field.

American Association of Medical Assistants (AAMA)
20 N. Wacker Dr., Ste. 1575
Chicago, IL 60606-2903 US
Phone: 312-899-1500
Web Address: www.aama-ntl.org
The American Association of Medical Assistants (AAMA) seeks to promote the professional identity and stature of its members and the medical assisting profession through education and credentialing.

American Association of Neuroscience Nurses (AANN)
4700 W. Lake Ave.
Glenview, IL 60025 US
Phone: 847-375-4733
Fax: 847-375-6333
Toll Free: 888-557-2266
E-mail Address: *info@aann.org*
Web Address: www.aann.org
The American Association of Neuroscience Nurses (AANN) is a national organization of registered nurses and other health care professionals that want to improve the care of neuroscience patients and further the interests of health professionals in the neurosciences.

American Association of Nurse Anesthetists (AANA)
222 S. Prospect Ave.
Park Ridge, IL 60068 US
Phone: 847-692-7050
Fax: 847-692-6968
E-mail Address: *info@aana.com*
Web Address: www.aana.com
The American Association of Nurse Anesthetists (AANA) is the professional association representing registered nurse anesthetists nationwide.

American Association of Occupational Health Nurses (AAOHN)
2920 Brandywine Rd., Ste. 100
Atlanta, GA 30341 US
Phone: 770-455-7757
Fax: 770-455-7271
E-mail Address: *aaohn@aaohn.org*
Web Address: www.aaohn.org
The American Association of Occupational Health Nurses (AAOHN) seeks to advance the profession of occupational and environmental health nursing as the authority on health, safety, productivity and disability management for worker populations.

American Association of Office Nurses (AAON)
109 Kinderkamack Rd.
Montvale, NJ 07645 US
Phone: 201-391-2600
Fax: 201-573-8543
Toll Free: 800-457-7504
E-mail Address: *aaonmail@aaon.org*
Web Address: www.aaon.org
The American Association of Office Nurses (AAON) is an organization for health care practitioners working in the office setting and facilitators of health care and patient education, well-being and support.

American Association of Preferred Provider Organizations (AAPPO)
P.O. Box 429
Jeffersonville, IN 47131-0429 US
Phone: 812-246-4376
Fax: 812-246-4630
Web Address: www.aappo.org
The American Association of Preferred Provider Organizations (AAPPO) is the leading national association of network-based preferred provider organizations and affiliate organizations.

American Association of Spinal Cord Injury Nurses (AASCIN)
75-20 Astoria Blvd.
Jackson Heights, NJ 11370 US
Phone: 718-803-3782
Fax: 718-803-0414
E-mail Address: *aascin@epva.org*
Web Address: www.aascin.org
The American Association of Spinal Cord Injury Nurses (AASCIN) is dedicated to promoting quality care for individuals with spinal cord impairment.

American Board of Facial Plastic and Reconstructive Surgery (ABFPRS)
115C S. St. Asaph St.
Alexandria, VA 22314 US
Phone: 703-549-3223
Fax: 703-549-3357
Web Address: www.abfprs.org
The American Board of Facial Plastic and Reconstructive Surgery (ABFPRS) is dedicated to improving the quality of facial plastic surgery available to the public by measuring the qualifications of candidate surgeons against rigorous standards.

American Board of Medical Specialties (ABMS)
1007 Church St., Ste. 404
Evanston, IL 60201 US
Phone: 847-491-9091
Fax: 847-328-3596
Toll Free: 866-275-2267
Web Address: www.abms.org
The American Board of Medical Specialties (ABMS) is an organization of 24 approved medical specialty boards.

American Burn Association (ABA)
625 N. Michigan Ave., Ste. 1530
Chicago, IL 60611 US
Phone: 312-642-9260
Fax: 312-642-9130
Toll Free: 800-548-2876
E-mail Address: *info@ameriburn.org*
Web Address: www.ameriburn.org
The American Burn Association (ABA) dedicates its efforts to the problems of burn injuries and burn victims throughout the U.S., Canada and other countries.

American Chiropractic Association (ACA)
1701 Clarendon Blvd.
Arlington, VA 22209 US

Phone: 703-276-8800
Fax: 703-243-2593
Toll Free: 800-986-4636
E-mail Address: *memberinfo@americhiro.org*
Web Address: www.amerchiro.org
The American Chiropractic Association (ACA) exists to preserve, protect, improve and promote the chiropractic profession for the benefit of the patients it serves.

American College of Emergency Physicians (ACEP)
1125 Executive Cir.
Irving, TX 75038 US
Phone: 972-550-0911
Fax: 972-580-2816
Toll Free: 800-798-1822
E-mail Address: *info@acep.org*
Web Address: www.acep.org
The American College of Emergency Physicians (ACEP) exists to support quality emergency medical care and to promote the interests of emergency physicians.

American College of Health Care Administrators (ACHCA)
300 N. Lee St., Ste. 301
Alexandria, VA 22314 US
Phone: 703-739-7900
Fax: 703-739-7901
Toll Free: 888-882-2422
Web Address: www.achca.org
The American College of Health Care Administrators (ACHCA) offers educational programming and career development for health care administrators.

American College of Healthcare Executives (ACHE)
One N. Franklin, Ste. 1700
Chicago, IL 60606-3491 US
Phone: 312-424-2800
Fax: 312-424-0023
E-mail Address: *geninfo@ache.org*
Web Address: www.ache.org
The American College of Healthcare Executives (ACHE) is an international professional society of health care executives that offers credentialing and educational programs.

American College of Legal Medicine (ACLM)
1111 N. Plaza Dr., Ste. 550
Schaumburg, IL 60173 US
Phone: 847-969-0283
Fax: 847-517-7229
E-mail Address: *info@aclm.org*
Web Address: www.aclm.org
The American College of Legal Medicine (ACLM) is the official organization for professionals who focus on the important issues where law and medicine converge.

American College of Medical Quality (ACMQ)
4334 Montgomery Ave.
Bethesda, MD 20814 US
Phone: 301-913-9149
Fax: 301-913-9142
Toll Free: 800-924-2149
E-mail Address: *acmq@acmq.org*
Web Address: www.acmq.org
The American College of Medical Quality (ACMQ) strives to provide leadership and education in health care quality management.

American College of Nurse Practitioners (ACNP)
1111 19th St., Ste. 404
Washington, DC 20036 US
Phone: 202-659-2190
Fax: 202-659-2191
E-mail Address: *acnp@acnpweb.org*
Web Address: www.nurse.org/acnp
The American College of Nurse Practitioners (ACNP) is focused on advocacy and keeping nurse practitioners current on legislative, regulatory and clinical practice issues that effect them in the rapidly changing health care arena.

American College of Physician Executives (ACPE)
4890 W. Kennedy Blvd., Ste. 200
Tampa, FL 33609 US
Phone: 813-287-2000
Fax: 813-287-8993
Toll Free: 800-562-8088
E-mail Address: *acpe@acpe.org*
Web Address: www.acpe.org
The American College of Physician Executives (ACPE) represents physicians in health care leadership.

American College of Physicians (ACP)
190 N. Independence Mall W.
Philadelphia, PA 19106 US
Phone: 215-351-2800
Toll Free: 800-523-1546
Web Address: www.acponline.org
The American College of Physicians (ACP) exists to enhance the quality and effectiveness of health care

by fostering excellence and professionalism in the practice of medicine.

American College of Prosthodontists (ACP)
211 E. Chicago Ave., Ste. 1000
Chicago, IL 60611 US
Phone: 312-573-1260
Fax: 312-573-1257
Web Address: www.prosthodontics.org
The American College of Prosthodontists (ACP) is the official sponsoring organization for the specialty of prosthodontics.

American College of Rheumatology (ACR)
1800 Century Pl., Ste. 250
Atlanta, GA 30345 US
Phone: 404-633-3777
Fax: 404-633-1870
E-mail Address: acr@rheumatology.org
Web Address: www.rheumatology.org
The American College of Rheumatology (ACR) is the professional organization of rheumatologists and associated health professionals dedicated to healing, preventing disability and curing arthritis and related disabling and sometimes fatal disorders of the joints, muscles and bones.

American College of Sports Medicine (ACSM)
401 W. Michigan St.
Indianapolis, IN 46202 US
Phone: 317-637-9200
Fax: 317-634-7817
Web Address: www.acsm.org
The American College of Sports Medicine (ACSM) promotes and integrates research, education and applications of sports medicine and exercise science to maintain and enhance quality of life.

American Correctional Health Services Association (ACHSA)
250 Gatsby Pl.
Alpharetta, GA 30022-6161 US
Fax: 770-650-5789
Toll Free: 877-918-1842
E-mail Address: achsa@mindspring.com
Web Address: www.corrections.com/achsa
The American Correctional Health Services Association (ACHSA) serves as a forum for communication addressing current issues and needs confronting correctional health care.

American Dental Association (ADA)
211 E. Chicago Ave.
Chicago, IL 60611 US
Phone: 312-440-2500
Fax: 312-440-2800
Web Address: www.ada.org
The American Dental Association (ADA) is a professional association of dentists committed to the public's oral health, ethics, science and professional advancement.

American Dental Trade Association (ADTA)
4222 King St. W.
Alexandria, VA 22302 US
Phone: 703-379-7755
Fax: 703-931-9429
E-mail Address: adta@adta.com
Web Address: www.adta.com
The American Dental Trade Association (ADTA) seeks to promote and represent the interests of its members.

American Dietetic Association (ADA)
120 S. Riverside Plaza, Ste. 2000
Chicago, IL 60606-6995 US
Toll Free: 800-877-1600
Web Address: www.eatright.org
The American Dietetic Association (ADA) is the world's largest organization of food and nutrition professionals, with nearly 70,000 members. In addition to services for its professional members, this organization's web site offers consumers a Nutrition Knowledge Center and a Healthy Lifestyle Center.

American Health Association (AHA)
One N. Franklin
Chicago, IL 60606-3491 US
Phone: 312-422-3000
Fax: 312-422-4796
Web Address: www.aha.org
The American Health Association (AHA) represents and serves all types of hospitals, health care networks and their patients and communities.

American Health Care Association (AHCA)
1201 L St. NW
Washington, DC 20005 US
Phone: 202-842-4444
Fax: 202-842-3860
Web Address: www.ahca.org
The American Health Care Association (AHCA) represents the long-term care community.

American Health Information Management Association (AHIMA)
233 N. Michigan Ave., Ste. 2150
Chicago, IL 60601 US
Phone: 312-233-1100
Fax: 312-233-1090
E-mail Address: *info@ahima.org*
Web Address: www.ahima.org
The American Health Information Management Association (AHIMA) is the professional association that represents specially educated health information management professionals who work throughout the health care industry.

American Health Lawyers Association (AHLA)
1025 Connecticut Ave. NW, Ste. 600
Washington, DC 20036 US
Phone: 202-833-1100
Fax: 202-833-1105
E-mail Address: *info@healthlawyers.org*
Web Address: www.healthlawyers.org
American Health Lawyers Association (AHLA) provides resources to address the issues facing its active members who practice in law firms, government, in-house settings and academia and who represent the entire spectrum of the health industry.

American Health Planning Association (AHPA)
7245 Arlington Blvd., Ste. 300
Falls Church, VA 22042 US
Phone: 703-573-3103
Fax: 703-573-1276
Web Address: www.ahpanet.org
The American Health Planning Association (AHPA) is a nonprofit organization committed to the creation of health policies and systems which assure access for all people to quality care at a reasonable cost.

American Health Quality Association (AHQA)
1155 21st St. NW
Washington, DC 20036 US
Phone: 202-331-5790
Fax: 202-331-9334
E-mail Address: *ahqa@ahqa.org*
Web Address: www.ahqa.org
The American Health Quality Association (AHQA) is a nonprofit national association dedicated to community-based, quality evaluation of health care.

American Holistic Nurses Association (AHNA)
P.O. Box 2130
Flagstaff, AZ 86003-2130 US
Toll Free: 800-278-2462
Web Address: www.ahna.org
The American Holistic Nurses Association (AHNA) embraces nursing as a lifestyle and a profession and provides a means to create bonds within the nursing community.

American Managed Behavioral Care Association (AMBCA)
1101 Pennsylvania Ave., 6th Fl.
Washington, DC 20004 US
Fax: 202-756-7308
Web Address: www.ambha.org
The American Managed Behavioral Care Association (AMBCA) exists to enable the leading organizations in this new industry to work together on key issues of public accountability, quality, public policy and communication.

American Medical Association (AMA)
515 N. State St.
Chicago, IL 60610 US
Phone: 312-464-5000
Web Address: www.ama-assn.org
The American Medical Association (AMA) strives to promote the science and art of medicine and the betterment of public health.

American Medical Group Association (AMGA)
1422 Duke St.
Alexandria, VA 22314-3430 US
Phone: 703-838-0033
Fax: 703-548-1890
Web Address: www.amga.org
The American Medical Group Association (AMGA) seeks to shape the health care environment by advancing high-quality, cost-effective, patient-centered and physician-directed health care.

American Medical Informatics Association (AMIA)
4915 St. Elmo Ave., Ste. 401
Bethesda, MD 20814 US
Phone: 301-657-1291
Fax: 301-657-1296
E-mail Address: *mail@mail.amia.org*
Web Address: www.amia.org
The American Medical Informatics Association (AMIA) is a nonprofit membership organization of individuals, institutions and corporations dedicated to developing and using information technologies to improve health care.

American Medical Technologists (AMT)
710 Higgins Rd.
Park Ridge, IL 60068 US
Phone: 847-823-5169
Fax: 847-823-0458
Web Address: www.amt1.com
American Medical Technologists (AMT) is a nonprofit certification agency and professional membership association representing individuals in health care.

American Medical Women's Association (AMWA)
801 N. Fairfax St., Ste. 400
Alexandria, VA 22314 US
Phone: 703-838-0500
Fax: 703-549-3864
E-mail Address: info@amwa-doc.org
Web Address: www.amwa-doc.org
The American Medical Women's Association (AMWA) is an organization of women physicians and medical students dedicated to serving as the unique voice for women's health and the advancement of women in medicine.

American National Standards Institute (ANSI)
1819 L St. NW
Washington, DC 20036 US
Phone: 202-293-8020
Fax: 202-293-9287
E-mail Address: ansionline@ansi.org
Web Address: www.ansi.org
American National Standards Institute (ANSI) is a nonprofit organization that coordinates the U.S. voluntary standardization system.

American Nephrology Nurses Association (ANNA)
E. Holly Ave., Box 56
Pitman, NJ 08071-0056 US
Phone: 856-256-2320
Fax: 856-589-7463
Toll Free: 888-600-2662
E-mail Address: anna@ajj.com
Web Address: anna.inurse.com
The American Nephrology Nurses Association (ANNA) seeks to advance nephrology nursing practice and positively influence outcomes for patients with diseases that require replacement therapies.

American Occupational Therapy Association (AOTA)
4720 Montgomery Ln., Box 31220
Bethesda, MD 20824-1220 US
Phone: 301-652-2682
Fax: 301-652-7711
Web Address: www.aota.org
The American Occupational Therapy Association (AOTA) advances the quality, availability, use and support of occupational therapy through standard-setting, advocacy, education and research on behalf of its members and the public.

American Organization of Nurse Executives (AONE)
325 7th St. NW
Washington, DC 20004 US
Phone: 202-626-2240
Fax: 202-638-5499
E-mail Address: aone@aha.org
Web Address: www.aone.org
The American Organization of Nurse Executives (AONE) is a national organization of nurses who design, facilitate and manage care.

American Osteopathic Association (AOA)
142 E. Ontario St.
Chicago, IL 60611 US
Phone: 312-202-8000
Fax: 312-202-8200
Toll Free: 800-621-1773
E-mail Address: info@aoa-net.org
Web Address: www.osteopathic.org
The American Osteopathic Association (AOA) is organized to advance the philosophy and practice of osteopathic medicine by promoting excellence in education, research and the delivery of cost-effective health care.

American Pediatric Surgical Association (APSA)
60 Revere Dr., Ste. 500
Northbrook, IL 60062 US
Phone: 847-480-9576
Fax: 847-480-9282
E-mail Address: eapsa@eapsa.org
Web Address: www.eapsa.org
The American Pediatric Surgical Association (APSA) is a surgical specialty organization composed of individuals who have dedicated themselves to the care of pediatric surgical patients.

American Psychiatric Association (APA)
1000 Wilson Blvd., Ste. 1825

Arlington, VA 22209-3901 US
Phone: 703-907-7300
Fax: 202-682-6850
Toll Free: 888-357-7924
E-mail Address: apa@psych.org
Web Address: www.psych.org
The American Psychiatric Association (APA) seeks to ensure humane care and effective treatment for all persons with mental disorders, including mental retardation and substance-related disorders.

American Public Health Association (APHA)
800 I St. NW
Washington, DC 20001 US
Phone: 202-777-2742
Fax: 202-777-2534
E-mail Address: comments@apha.org
Web Address: www.apha.org
The American Public Health Association (APHA) is an association of individuals and organizations working to improve the public's health and to achieve equity in health status for all.

American School Health Association (ASHA)
P.O. Box 708
7263 State Rte. 43
Kent, OH 44240 US
Phone: 330-678-1601
Fax: 330-678-4526
E-mail Address: asha@ashaweb.org
Web Address: www.ashaweb.org
The American School Health Association (ASHA) advocates high-quality school health instruction, health services and a healthful school environment.

American Society for Dermatologic Surgery, Inc. (ASDS)
5550 Meadowbrook Dr., Ste. 120
Rolling Meadows, IL 60008 US
Phone: 847-956-0900
Fax: 847-956-0999
E-mail Address: info@aboustskinsurgery.com
Web Address: www.asds-net.org
The American Society for Dermatologic Surgery, Inc. (ASDS) seeks to promote excellence in the subspecialty of dermatological surgery and to foster the highest standards of patient care.

American Society for Healthcare Central Service Professionals (ASHCSP)
One N. Franklin, Ste. 2800
Chicago, IL 60606 US
Phone: 312-422-3750
Fax: 312-422-4577
Web Address: www.ashcsp.org
The American Society for Healthcare Central Service Professionals (ASHCSP) exists to provide education, networking, recognition, membership advocacy and professional practices to promote innovative ideas toward the future direction of the industry.

American Society for Healthcare Environmental Services (ASHES)
One N. Franklin, Ste. 2800
Chicago, IL 60606 US
Phone: 312-422-3860
Fax: 312-422-4577
Web Address: www.ashes.org
The American Society for Healthcare Environmental Services (ASHES) is the premier health care association for environmental services, housekeeping and textile care professionals.

American Society For Healthcare Food Service Administrators (ASHFSA)
304 W. Liberty St., Ste. 201
Louisville, KY 40202 US
Phone: 312-422-3870
Fax: 312-422-4581
E-mail Address: ashfsa@aha.org
Web Address: www.ashfsa.org
The American Society For Healthcare Food Service Administrators (ASHFSA) seeks to provide members with quality education, networking and opportunities for professional growth.

American Society for Healthcare Human Resources Administrators (ASHRM)
One N. Franklin
Chicago, IL 60606 US
Phone: 312-422-3980
Fax: 312-422-4580
E-mail Address: ashrm@aha.org
Web Address: www.ashrm.org
The American Society for Healthcare Human Resources Administrators (ASHRM) is the professional society for health care risk management professionals and those responsible for decisions that will promote quality care, maintain a safe environment and preserve human and financial resources in health care organizations.

American Society of Addiction Medicine (ASAM)
4601 N. Park Ave., Arcade Ste. 101
Chevy Chase, MD 20815 US
Phone: 301-656-3920

Fax: 301-656-3815
E-mail Address: *email@asam.org*
Web Address: www.asam.org
The American Society of Addiction Medicine (ASAM) is dedicated to educating physicians and improving the treatment of individuals suffering from alcoholism and other addictions.

American Society of Directors of Volunteer Services (ASDVS)
One N. Franklin, 27th Fl.
Chicago, IL 60606 US
Phone: 312-422-3939
Fax: 312-422-4575
E-mail Address: *asdvs@aha.org*
Web Address: www.hospitalconnect.com/asdvs
The American Society of Directors of Volunteer Services (ASDVS) exists to strengthen the profession of volunteer services administration, provide opportunities for professional development and promote volunteerism as a resource in serving the health care needs of the nation.

American Society of Pain Management Nurses (ASPMN)
7794 Grow Dr.
Pensacola, FL 32514 US
Phone: 850-473-0233
Fax: 850-484-8762
Toll Free: 888-342-7766
E-mail Address: *aspmn@puetzamc.com*
Web Address: www.aspmn.org
The American Society of Pain Management Nurses (ASPMN) is an organization of professional nurses dedicated to promoting and providing optimal care of patients with pain.

American Society of Peri-Anaesthesia Nurses (ASPAN)
10 Melrose Ave., Ste. 110
Cherry Hill, NJ 08003 US
Phone: 856-616-9600
Fax: 856-616-9601
Toll Free: 877-737-9696
E-mail Address: *aspan@aspan.org*
Web Address: www.aspan.org
The American Society of Peri-Anaesthesia Nurses (ASPAN) advances nursing practice through education, research and standards.

American Society of Plastic Surgeons (ASPS)
444 E. Algonquin Rd.
Arlington Heights, IL 60005 US
Toll Free: 888-475-2784
Web Address: www.plasticsurgery.org
The American Society of Plastic Surgeons (ASPS) seeks to support its members in their efforts to provide the highest-quality patient care and maintain professional and ethical standards through education, research and advocacy of socioeconomic and other professional activities.

American Telemedicine Association (ATA)
1100 Connecticut Ave. NW, Ste. 540
Washington, DC 20006 US
Phone: 202-223-3333
Fax: 202-223-2787
E-mail Address: *info@americantelemed.org*
Web Address: www.atmeda.org
The American Telemedicine Association (ATA) is the leading resource and advocate promoting access to medical care for consumers and health professionals via telecommunications technology.

Assisted Living Federation of America (ALFA)
11200 Waples Mill Rd., Ste. 150
Fairfax, VA 22030 US
Phone: 703-691-8100
Fax: 703-691-8106
E-mail Address: *info@alfa.org*
Web Address: www.alfa.org
The Assisted Living Federation of America (ALFA) represents for-profit and not-for-profit providers of assisted living, continuing care retirement communities, independent living and other forms of housing and services.

Association of Camp Nurses (ACN)
8504 Thorsonveien NE
Bemidji, MN 56601 US
Phone: 218-586-2633
E-mail Address: *acn@campnurse.org*
Web Address: www.campnurse.org
The Association of Camp Nurses (ACN) promotes and develops the practice of camp nursing for a healthy camp community.

Association of Clinicians for the Underserved (ACU)
1420 Spring Hill Rd., Ste. 600
Tysons Corner, VA 22102 US
Phone: 703-442-5318
Fax: 707-749-5348
E-mail Address: *acu@clinicians.org*
Web Address: www.clinicians.org

The Association of Clinicians for the Underserved (ACU) is a nonprofit, interdisciplinary organization whose mission is to improve the health of underserved populations by enhancing the development and support of the health care clinicians serving these populations.

Association of Emergency Physicians (AEP)
911 Whitewater Dr.
Mars, PA 16046-4221 US
Fax: 866-422-7794
Toll Free: 866-772-1818
E-mail Address: *aep@interaccess.com*
Web Address: www.aep.org
The Association of Emergency Physicians (AEP) represents the emergency physicians who largely practice clinical emergency medicine.

Association of Nurses in AIDS Care (ANAC)
3538 Ridgewood Rd.
Akron, OH 44333-3122 US
Phone: 330-670-0101
Fax: 330-670-0109
Toll Free: 800-260-6780
E-mail Address: *anac@anacnet.org*
Web Address: www.anacnet.org
The Association of Nurses in AIDS Care (ANAC) was founded to address the specific needs of nurses working in HIV/AIDS.

Association of Operating Room Nurses (AORN)
2170 S. Parker Rd., Ste. 300
Denver, CO 80231-5711 US
Phone: 303-755-6304
Toll Free: 800-755-2676
E-mail Address: *custserv@aorn.org*
Web Address: www.aorn.org
The Association of Operating Room Nurses (AORN) supports registered nurses in achieving optimal outcomes for patients undergoing operative and other invasive procedures.

Association of Rehabilitation Nurses (ARN)
4700 W. Lake Ave.
Glenview, IL 60025 US
Phone: 847-375-4710
Fax: 847-734-9384
Toll Free: 800-229-7530
E-mail Address: *info@rehabnurse.org*
Web Address: www.rehabnurse.org
The Association of Rehabilitation Nurses (ARN) helps nurses stay on top of the skills and knowledge needed to provide quality rehabilitative and restorative care across settings, conditions and age spans.

Association of Telehealth Service Providers (ATSP)
4702 SW Scholls Ferry Rd., Ste. 400
Portland, OR 97225-2008 US
Phone: 503-222-2406
Fax: 503-223-7581
Toll Free: 800-852-3591
E-mail Address: *info@atsp.org*
Web Address: www.atsp.org
The Association of Telehealth Service Providers (ATSP) is an international membership-based organization dedicated to improving health care through growth of the telehealth industry.

Association of Women's Health, Obstetric and Neonatal Nurses (AWHONN)
2000 L St. NW, Ste. 740
Washington, DC 20036 US
Fax: 202-728-0575
Toll Free: 800-673-8499
Web Address: www.awhonn.org
The Association of Women's Health, Obstetric and Neonatal Nurses (AWHONN) serves and represents health care professionals in the U.S., Canada and abroad.

Blue Cross and Blue Shield Association
225 N. Michigan Ave.
Chicago, IL 60601-7680 US
Phone: 312-297-6000
Fax: 312-297-6609
Web Address: www.bcbs.com
Blue Cross and Blue Shield Association is a nonprofit professional association of health care insurance providers.

Chinese-American Medical Society (CAMS)
E-mail Address: *hw5@columbia.edu*
Web Address: www.camsociety.org
The Chinese-American Medical Society (CAMS) exists to promote the scientific association of medical professionals of Chinese descent, advance medical knowledge and scientific research with emphasis on aspects unique to the Chinese, and establish scholarships for medical and dental students.

Clinical Immunology Society (CIS)
555 E. Wells St., Ste. 1100
Milwaukee, WI 53202 US
Phone: 414-224-8095

Fax: 414-276-3349
E-mail Address: cis@execinc.com
Web Address: www.clinimmsoc.org
The Clinical Immunology Society (CIS) is devoted to fostering developments in the science and practice of clinical immunology.

College of Healthcare Information Management Executives (CHIME)
3300 Washtenaw Ave., Ste. 225
Ann Arbor, MI 48104 US
Phone: 734-665-0000
Fax: 734-665-4922
E-mail Address: staff@cio-chime.org
Web Address: www.cio-chime.org
College of Healthcare Information Management Executives (CHIME) was formed with the dual objective of serving the professional development needs of health care CIOs and advocating the more effective use of information management within health care.

Contact Lens Manufacturers Association (CLMA)
PO Box 29398
Lincoln, NE 68529 US
Phone: 402-465-4122
Fax: 402-465-4187
Toll Free: 800-344-9060
E-mail Address: clma@mindspring.com
Web Address: www.clma.net
The Contact Lens Manufacturers Association (CLMA) seeks to increase awareness and utilization of custom-manufactured contact lenses.

Contact Lens Society of America (CLSA)
441 Carlisle Dr.
Herndon, VA 20170 US
Phone: 703-437-5100
Fax: 703-437-7127
Web Address: www.clsa.info
The Contact Lens Society of America (CLSA) strives to educate and share knowledge among fitters of contact lenses.

Corporate Angel Network, Inc. (CAN)
Westchester County Airport
One Loop Rd.
White Plains, NY 10604 US
Phone: 914-328-1313
Fax: 914-328-3938
Toll Free: 866-328-1313
E-mail Address: info@corpangelnetwork.org
Web Address: www.corpangelnetwork.org
Corporate Angel Network (CAN) exists to ease the emotional stress, physical discomfort and financial burden of travel for cancer patients by arranging free flights to treatment centers, using the empty seats on corporate aircraft flying on routine business.

Delta Dental Plans Association
1515 W. 22nd St., Ste. 1200
Oak Brook, IL 60523 US
Phone: 630-574-6001
Fax: 630-574-6999
Web Address: www.deltadental.com
Delta Dental Plans Association is the nation's largest and most experienced dental benefits system.

Dental Trade Alliance (DTA)
4222 King St. W.
Alexandria, VA 22302 US
Phone: 215-731-9975
Fax: 215-731-9984
Web Address: www.dmanews.org
The Dental Trade Alliance (DTA) represents dental manufacturers, dental dealers and dental laboratories.

Emergency Nurses Association (ENA)
915 Lee St.
Des Plaines, IL 60016 US
Toll Free: 800-243-8362
E-mail Address: enainfo@ena.org
Web Address: www.ena.org
The Emergency Nurses Association (ENA) is the specialty nursing association serving the emergency nursing profession through research, publications, professional development and injury prevention.

Federation of American Hospitals (FAH)
801 Pennsylvania Ave. NW, Ste. 245
Washington, DC 20004 US
Phone: 202-624-1500
Fax: 202-737-6462
E-mail Address: info@fahs.com
Web Address: www.fahs.com
The Federation of American Hospitals (FAH) is the national representative of privately owned and managed community hospitals and health systems in the U.S.

Federation of Nurses and Health Professionals (FNHP)
555 New Jersey Ave. NW
Washington, DC 20001 US
Phone: 202-879-4491
Fax: 202-879-4597

E-mail Address: *fnhpaft@aft.org*
Web Address: www.aft.org/healthcare
The Federation of Nurses and Health Professionals (FNHP) represents its members in the health professions and seeks to enhance the professional norms and ethics of health care workers.

Health Industry Business Communications Council (HIBCC)
2525 E. Arizona Biltmore Cir., Ste. 127
Phoenix, AZ 85016 US
Phone: 602-381-1091
Fax: 602-381-1093
Web Address: www.hibcc.org
The Health Industry Business Communications Council (HIBCC) seeks to facilitate electronic communications by developing appropriate standards for information exchange among all health care trading partners.

Health Industry Distributors Association (HIDA)
310 Montgomery St.
Alexandria, VA 22314-1516 US
Phone: 703-549-4432
Fax: 703-549-6495
E-mail Address: *mail@hida.org*
Web Address: www.hida.org
The Health Industry Distributors Association (HIDA) is the international trade association representing medical products distributors.

Health and Science Communications Association (HeSCA)
39 Wedgewood Dr., Ste. A
Jewett City, CT 06351 US
Phone: 860-376-5915
Fax: 860-376-6621
E-mail Address: *hesca@hesca.org*
Web Address: www.hesca.org
The Health and Science Communications Association (HeSCA) is an association of communications professionals committed to sharing knowledge and resources in the health sciences arena.

Healthcare Financial Management Association (HFMA)
2 Westbrook Corporate Ctr., Ste. 700
Westchester, IL 60154-5700 US
Phone: 708-531-9600
Fax: 708-531-0032
Toll Free: 800-252-4362
Web Address: www.hfma.org
The Healthcare Financial Management Association (HFMA) is the nation's leading personal membership organization for health care financial management professionals.

Healthcare Information and Management Systems Society (HIMSS)
230 E. Ohio St., Ste. 500
Chicago, IL 60611-3269 US
Phone: 312-664-4467
Fax: 312-664-6143
E-mail Address: *himss@himss.org*
Web Address: www.himss.org
The Healthcare Information and Management Systems Society (HIMSS) provides leadership in health care for the management of technology, information and change through publications, educational opportunities and member services.

Hearing Industries Association (HIA)
515 King St., Ste. 320
Alexandria, VA 22314 US
Phone: 703-684-5744
Fax: 703-684-6048
E-mail Address: *info@hearing.org*
Web Address: www.hearing.org
The Hearing Industries Association (HIA) represents and unifies the many aspects of the hearing industry.

Home Healthcare Nurses Association (HHNA)
Web Address: www.hhna.org
The Home Healthcare Nurses Association (HHNA) is a national professional nursing organization of members involved in home health care practice, education, administration and research.

Independent Medical Distributors Association (IMDA)
414 Plaza Dr., Ste. 209
Westmont, IL 60559 US
Toll Free: 866-463-2937
Web Address: www.imda.org
The Independent Medical Distributors Association (IMDA) is an association of medical product sales and marketing organizations.

Institute for Diversity in Health Management (IDHM)
Web Address: www.diversityconnection.org
The Institute for Diversity in Health Management (IDHM) is a nonprofit organization that collaborates with educators and health services organizations to

expand leadership opportunities to ethnic minorities in health services management.

International Association of Forensic Nurses (IAFN)
E. Holly Ave., Box 56
Pitman, NJ 08071-0056 US
Phone: 856-256-2425
Fax: 856-589-7463
E-mail Address: *iafn@ajj.com*
Web Address: www.forensicnurse.org
The International Association of Forensic Nurses (IAFN) is the only international professional organization of registered nurses formed exclusively to develop, promote and disseminate information about the science of forensic nursing.

International Association of Medical Equipment Remarketers & Servicers (IAMERS)
E-mail Address: *info@iamers.org*
Web Address: www.iamers.org
The International Association of Medical Equipment Remarketers & Servicers (IAMERS) works to improve the quality of pre-owned medical equipment, both domestically and internationally.

International Council of Nurses (ICN)
3, Place Jean Marteau
1201 Geneva, Switzerland
Phone: 41-22-908-01-00
Fax: 41-22-908-01-01
E-mail Address: *icn@icn.ch*
Web Address: www.icn.ch
The International Council of Nurses (ICN) is a federation of national nurses' associations representing nurses in more than 120 countries.

International Nurses Society on Addiction (IntNSA)
P.O. Box 10752
Raleigh, NC 27605 US
Phone: 919-821-1292
Fax: 919-833-5743
Web Address: www.intnsa.org
The International Nurses Society on Addiction (IntNSA) is a global voice for nurses committed to addressing the impact of addictions on society.

International Pharmaceutical Excipients Council of the Americas (IPEC-Americas)
1655 N. Fort Myer Dr., Ste. 700
Arlington, VA 22209 US
Phone: 703-875-2127
Fax: 703-525-5157
E-mail Address: *info@ipecamericas.org*
Web Address: www.ipecamericas.org
International Pharmaceutical Excipients Council of the Americas (IPEC-Americas) is a trade organization that promotes standardized approval criteria for drug inert ingredients, or excipients, among different nations. The organization also works to promote safe and useful excipients in the U.S.

International Transplant Nurses Society (ITNS)
1739 E. Carson St., Box 351
Pittsburgh, PA 15203 US
Phone: 412-343-4867
Fax: 412-343-3959
E-mail Address: *itns@msn.com*
Web Address: www.itns.org
The International Transplant Nurses Society (ITNS) is committed to promoting excellence in transplant clinical nursing through the provision of educational and professional growth opportunities, interdisciplinary networking and collaborative activities and transplant nursing research.

Joint Commission on Accreditation of Healthcare Organizations (JCAHO)
One Renaissance Blvd.
Oakbrook Terrace, IL 60181 US
Phone: 630-792-5000
Fax: 630-792-5005
Web Address: www.jcaho.org
The Joint Commission on Accreditation of Healthcare Organizations (JCAHO) evaluates and accredits health care organizations and programs in the United States.

Medical Device Manufacturers Association (MDMA)
1900 K St. NW, Ste. 300
Washington, DC 20006 US
Phone: 202-496-7150
Web Address: www.medicaldevices.org
The Medical Device Manufacturers Association (MDMA) is a national trade association that represents independent manufacturers of medical devices, diagnostic products and health care information systems.

Medical Group Management Association (MGMA)
104 Inverness Terrace E.
Englewood, CO 80112-5306 US

Phone: 303-799-1111
Fax: 303-643-4439
Toll Free: 877-275-6462
Web Address: www.mgma.com
Medical Group Management Association (MGMA) is the nation's principal voice for medical group practice.

Michigan Medical Device Association (MMDA)
P.O. Box 170
Howell, MI 48844 US
Fax: 517-546-3356
Toll Free: 800-930-5698
E-mail Address: *info@mmda.org*
Web Address: www.mmda.org
The Michigan Medical Device Association (MMDA) sponsors educational seminars and informational programs; is active in the areas of government relations, networking and business development; and acts as a source for the dissemination of matters of interest to its members.

National Academy of Sciences (NAS)
500 5th St.
Washington, DC 20001 US
Web Address: www4.nationalacademies.org/nas/nashome.nsf
The National Academy of Sciences (NAS) is a private, nonprofit, self-perpetuating society of scholars engaged in scientific and engineering research dedicated to the furtherance of science and technology and to their use for the general welfare.

National Association for Healthcare Quality (NAHQ)
4700 W. Lake Ave.
Glenview, IL 60025 US
Toll Free: 847-375-4720
Web Address: www.nahq.org
The National Association for Healthcare Quality (NAHQ) is the nation's leading organization for health care quality professionals.

National Association for Home Care (NAHC)
228 7th St. SE
Washington, DC 20003 US
Phone: 202-547-7424
Fax: 202-547-3540
Web Address: www.nahc.org
The National Association for Home Care (NAHC) is committed to representing the interests of the home care and hospice community.

National Association for the Support of Long-Term Care (NASL)
1321 Duke St., Ste. 304
Alexandria, VA 22314 US
Phone: 703-549-8500
Fax: 703-549-8342
E-mail Address: *member@nasl.org*
Web Address: www.nasl.org
The National Association for the Support of Long-Term Care (NASL) provides a task-force-specific committee structure that focuses on payment reform, legislative policy, medical products and medical services.

National Association of Clinical Nurse Specialists (NACNS)
2090 Linglestown Rd., Ste. 107
Harrisburg, PA 17110 US
Phone: 717-234-6799
Fax: 717-234-6798
E-mail Address: *info@nacns.org*
Web Address: www.nacns.org
The National Association of Clinical Nurse Specialists (NACNS) exists to enhance and promote the contributions of clinical nurse specialists to the health of individuals, families, groups and communities.

National Association of Health Data Organizations (NAHDO)
375 Chipeta Way, Ste. A
Salt Lake City, UT 84108 US
Phone: 801-587-9104
Fax: 801-587-9125
E-mail Address: *info@nahdo.org*
Web Address: www.nahdo.org
The National Association of Health Data Organizations (NAHDO) is a not-for-profit membership organization dedicated to strengthening the nation's health information system.

National Association of Health Services Executives (NAHSE)
8630 Fenton St., Ste. 126
Silver Spring, MD 20910 US
Phone: 202-628-3953
Fax: 301-588-0011
E-mail Address: *nationalhq@nahse.org*
Web Address: www.nahse.org
The National Association of Health Services Executives (NAHSE) is a nonprofit association of black health care executives who promote the advancement and development of black health care

leaders and elevate the quality of health care services rendered to minority and underserved communities.

National Association of Hispanic Nurses (NAHN)
1501 16th St. NW
Washington, DC 20036 US
Phone: 202-387-2477
Fax: 202-483-7183
E-mail Address: *info@thehispanicnurses.org*
Web Address: www.thehispanicnurses.org
The National Association of Hispanic Nurses (NAHN) strives to serve the nursing and health care delivery needs of the Hispanic community and the professional needs of Hispanic nurses.

National Association of Neonatal Nurses (NANN)
4700 W. Lake Ave.
Glenview, IL 60025 US
Fax: 847-477-6266
Toll Free: 800-451-3795
E-mail Address: *info@nann.org*
Web Address: www.nann.org
The National Association of Neonatal Nurses (NANN) represents the community of neonatal nurses that provide evidence-based care to high-risk neonatal patients.

National Association of Orthopedic Nurses (NAON)
401 N. Michigan Ave., Ste. 2200
Chicago, IL 60611 US
Fax: 312-527-6658
Toll Free: 800-289-6266
E-mail Address: *naon@mail.ajj.com*
Web Address: www.orthonurse.org
The National Association of Orthopedic Nurses (NAON) exists to promote education and research related to nursing care of persons with orthopedic conditions.

National Association of Pediatric Nurse Practitioners (NAPNAP)
20 Brace Rd.
Cherry Hill, NJ 08034 US
Phone: 856-857-9700
Fax: 856-857-1600
E-mail Address: *info@napnap.org*
Web Address: www.napnap.org
The National Association of Pediatric Nurse Practitioners (NAPNAP) is the professional organization that advocates for children and provides leadership for pediatric nurse practitioners who deliver primary health care in a variety of settings.

National Association of Professional Geriatric Care Managers (GCM)
1604 N. Country Club Rd.
Tucson, AZ 85716 US
Phone: 520-881-8008
Fax: 520-325-7925
E-mail Address: *info@caremanager.org*
Web Address: www.caremanager.org
The National Association of Professional Geriatric Care Managers (GCM) is a nonprofit, professional organization of practitioners whose goal is the advancement of dignified care for the elderly and their families.

National Association of School Nurses (NASN)
P.O. Box 1300
Scarborough, ME 04070-1300 US
Phone: 207-883-2117
Fax: 207-883-2683
Toll Free: 877-627-6476
E-mail Address: *nasn@nasn.org*
Web Address: www.nasn.org
The National Association of School Nurses (NASN) improves the health and educational success of children and youth by developing and providing leadership to advance school nursing practice.

National Association of State Mental Health Program Directors (NASMHPD)
66 Canal Ctr. Plz., Ste. 302
Alexandria, VA 22314 US
Phone: 703-739-9333
Fax: 703-548-9517
Web Address: www.nasmhpd.org
The National Association of State Mental Health Program Directors (NASMHPD) organizes to reflect and advocate for the collective interests of state mental health authorities and their directors at the national level.

National Black Nurses Association (NBNA)
8630 Fenton St., Ste. 330
Silver Spring, MD 20910 US
Phone: 301-589-3200
Fax: 301-589-3223
E-mail Address: *nbna@erols.com*
Web Address: www.nbna.org
The National Black Nurses Association (NBNA) is a professional nursing organization representing African American nurses throughout the United States.

National Board of Medical Examiners (NBME)
3750 Market St.
Philadelphia, PA 19104-3102 US
Phone: 215-590-9500
Fax: 215-590-9555
E-mail Address: *webmail@mail.nbme.org*
Web Address: www.nbme.org
The National Board of Medical Examiners (NBME) exists to protect the health of the public through state-of-the-art assessment of health professionals.

National Family Caregivers Association (NFCA)
10400 Connecticut Ave., Ste. 500
Kensington, MD 20895-3944 US
Fax: 301-942-2302
Toll Free: 800-896-3650
E-mail Address: *info@nfcacares.org*
Web Address: www.thefamilycaregiver.org
The National Family Caregivers Association (NFCA) is a grassroots organization created to educate, support, empower and speak for the millions of Americans who care for chronically ill, aged or disabled loved ones.

National Flight Paramedics Association (NFPA)
951 E. Montana Vista
Salt Lake City, UT 84124 US
Fax: 801-534-0434
Toll Free: 800-381-6372
Web Address: www.flightparamedic.org
The National Flight Paramedics Association (NFPA) promotes the global development and growth of the paramedic profession.

National Hospice and Palliative Care Organization (NHPCO)
1700 Diagonal Rd., Ste. 625
Alexandria, VA 22314 US
Phone: 703-837-1500
Fax: 703-837-1233
E-mail Address: *info@nhpco.org*
Web Address: www.nho.org
The National Hospice and Palliative Care Organization (NHPCO) is the largest nonprofit membership organization representing hospice and palliative care programs and professionals in the United States.

National Practitioner Data Bank (NPDB)
4094 Majestic Ln., PMB 332
Fairfax, VA 22033 US
Web Address: www.npdb-hipdb.com
The National Practitioner Data Bank (NPDB) is an alert or flagging system intended to facilitate a comprehensive review of health care practitioners' professional credentials.

National Student Nurses' Association (NSNA)
45 Main St., Ste. 606
Brooklyn, NY 11201 US
Phone: 728-210-0705
Fax: 728-210-0710
E-mail Address: *nsna@nsna.org*
Web Address: www.nsna.org
The National Student Nurses' Association (NSNA) is a membership organization representing those in programs preparing students for registered nurse licensure, as well as RNs in BSN completion programs.

Nurse Practitioner Associates for Continuing Education (NPACE)
209 W. Central St., Ste. 302
Natick, MA 01760 US
Phone: 508-907-6424
Fax: 508-907-6425
E-mail Address: *npace@npace.org*
Web Address: www.npace.org
Nurse Practitioner Associates for Continuing Education (NPACE) seeks to improve health care in the U.S. by providing continuing education and professional support to nurse practitioners and other clinicians in advanced practice.

Oncology Nursing Society (ONS)
125 Enterprise Dr.
Pittsburgh, PA 15275-1214 US
Phone: 866-257-4667
Fax: 877-369-5497
Web Address: www.ons.org
The Oncology Nursing Society (ONS) is a national organization of registered nurses and other health care professionals dedicated to excellence in patient care, teaching, research, administration and education in the field of oncology.

Regulatory Affairs Professional Society (RAPS)
11300 Rockville Pike, Ste. 1000
Rockville, MD 20852 US
Phone: 301-770-2920
Fax: 301-770-2924
E-mail Address: *raps@raps.org*
Web Address: www.raps.org
The Regulatory Affairs Professional Society (RAPS) is an international professional society representing

the health care regulatory affairs profession and individual professionals worldwide.

Shriners International Headquarters
2900 Rocky Point Dr.
Tampa, FL 33607-1460 US
Phone: 813-281-0300
Web Address: www.shrinershq.org
Shriners International Headquarters is an international fraternity of approximately 500,000 members throughout the United States, Mexico, Canada and Panama.

Society for Vascular Nursing (SVN)
7794 Grow Dr.
Pensacola, FL 32514 US
Phone: 850-474-6963
Fax: 850-484-8762
Toll Free: 888-536-4786
Web Address: www.svnnet.org
The Society for Vascular Nursing (SVN) is the nursing organization dedicated to the compassionate and comprehensive care of persons with vascular disease.

Society of Critical Care Medicine (SCCM)
701 Lee St., Ste. 200
Des Plaines, IL 60016 US
Phone: 847-827-6869
Fax: 847-827-6886
Toll Free: 877-291-7226
E-mail Address: *info@sccm.org*
Web Address: www.sccm.org
The Society of Critical Care Medicine (SCCM) is the largest multidisciplinary, multiprofessional organization dedicated to ensuring excellence and consistency in the practice of critical care medicine.

Society of Gastroenterology Nurses and Associates (SGNA)
401 N. Michigan Ave.
Chicago, IL 60611-4267 US
Phone: 312-321-5165
Fax: 312-527-6658
Toll Free: 800-245-7462
Web Address: www.sgna.org
The Society of Gastroenterology Nurses and Associates (SGNA) is a professional organization of nurses and associates dedicated to the safe and effective practice of gastroenterology and endoscopy nursing.

Society of Pediatric Nurses (SPN)
7794 Grow Dr.
Pensacola, FL 32514 US
Fax: 850-484-8762
Toll Free: 800-723-2902
Web Address: www.pedsnurses.org
The Society of Pediatric Nurses (SPN) seeks to promote excellence in nursing care of children and their families through support of its members' clinical practice, education, research and advocacy.

Society of Trauma Nurses (STN)
223 N. Guadalupe, PMB 300
Santa Fe, NM 87501 US
Phone: 505-983-4923
Fax: 505-983-5109
E-mail Address: *stnexecdir@aol.com*
Web Address: www.traumanursesoc.org
The Society of Trauma Nurses (STN) is a membership-based, nonprofit organization whose members are trauma nurses from around the world.

Society of Urologic Nurses and Associates (SUNA)
E. Holly Ave., Box 56
Pitman, NJ 08071 US
Phone: 856-256-2335
Fax: 856-589-7463
Toll Free: 888-827-7862
Web Address: www.suna.org
The Society of Urologic Nurses and Associates (SUNA) is a professional organization committed to excellence in patient care standards and a continuum of quality care, clinical practice and research through education of its members, patients, families and community.

Southern Nursing Research Society (SNRS)
P.O. Box 870388
Tuscaloosa, AL 35487 US
Fax: 205-348-6614
Toll Free: 877-314-7677
E-mail Address: *info@snrs.org*
Web Address: www.snrs.org
The Southern Nursing Research Society (SNRS) exists to advance nursing research, promote the utilization of research finding and facilitate the career development of nurses as researchers.

Visiting Nurse Associations of America (VNAA)
99 Summer St., Ste. 1700
Boston, MA 02110 US
Phone: 617-737-3200
Fax: 617-737-1144

E-mail Address: *vnaa@vnaa.org*
Web Address: www.vnaa.org
Visiting Nurse Associations of America (VNAA) is the official, national association of freestanding, not-for-profit, community-based visiting nurse agencies.

Wound, Ostomy and Continence Nurses Society (WOCN)
Web Address: www.wocn.org
The Wound, Ostomy and Continence Nurses Society (WOCN) is a professional, international nursing society of nurse professionals who are experts in the care of patients with wound, ostomy and continence problems.

XXVII. Health-General

MedicAlert Foundation
2323 Colorado Ave.
Turlock, CA 95382 US
Phone: 209-668-3333
Fax: 209-669-2450
Toll Free: 888-633-4298
E-mail Address: *customer_service@medicalert.org*
Web Address: www.medicalert.org
The MedicAlert Foundation is a service that protects and saves the lives of its members by providing identification and critical personal health information in an emergency.

Society for Social Work Leadership in Health Care (SSWLHC)
1211 Locust St.
Philadelphia, PA 19107 US
Phone: 215-599-6134
Fax: 215-545-8107
Toll Free: 866-237-9542
Web Address: www.sswlhc.org
The Society for Social Work Leadership in Health Care (SSWLHC) is dedicated to promoting the universal availability, accessibility, coordination and effectiveness of health care that addresses the psychosocial components of health and illness.

XXVIII. Hearing & Speech

Alexander Graham Bell Association for the Deaf and Hard of Hearing (AGBELL)
3417 Volta Pl. NW
Washington, DC 20007 US
Phone: 202-337-5220, TTY 202-337-5220
Fax: 202-337-8314
Web Address: www.agbell.org

The Alexander Graham Bell Association for the Deaf and Hard of Hearing (AGBELL) is an international membership organization and resource center on hearing loss and spoken language approaches and related issues.

American Speech-Language-Hearing Association (ASHA)
10801 Rockville Pike
Rockville, MD 20852 US
Toll Free: 800-638-8255
E-mail Address: *actioncenter@asha.org*
Web Address: www.asha.org
The American Speech-Language-Hearing Association (ASHA) is the professional, scientific and credentialing association for audiologists, speech-language pathologists and speech, language and hearing scientists.

National Family Association for Deaf-Blind (NFADB)
141 Middle Neck Rd.
Sands Point, NY 11050 US
Phone: 202-337-5220
Fax: 516-883-9060
Toll Free: 800-255-0411
E-mail Address: *nfadb@aol.com*
Web Address: www.nfadb.org
The National Family Association for Deaf-Blind (NFADB) is the largest national network of families focusing on issues surrounding deaf blindness.

National Institute on Deafness and Other Communication Disorders (NIDCD)
31 Center Dr., MSC 2320
Bethesda, MD 20892-2320 US
Phone: 301-496-7243
Fax: 301-402-0018
Toll Free: 800-241-1044
E-mail Address: *nidcdinfo@nidcd.nih.gov*
Web Address: www.nidcd.nih.gov
The National Institute on Deafness and Other Communication Disorders (NIDCD) conducts and supports biomedical and behavioral research and research training in the normal and disordered processes of hearing, balance, smell, taste, voice, speech and language.

XXIX. Heart Disease

American Heart Association (AHA)
7272 Greenville Ave.
Dallas, TX 75231 US

Toll Free: 800-242-8721
Web Address: www.americanheart.org
The American Heart Association (AHA) seeks to reduce disability and death from cardiovascular diseases and stroke.

XXX. Hormonal Disorders

Thyroid Foundation of America, Inc. (TFA)
410 Stuart St.
Boston, MA 02114 US
Fax: 617-534-1515
Toll Free: 800-832-8321
E-mail Address: *info@allthyroid.org*
Web Address: www.allthyroid.org
The Thyroid Foundation of America, Inc. (TFA) seeks to ensure timely, accurate diagnosis, appropriate treatment and ongoing support for all individuals with thyroid disease.

XXXI. Hospice Care

Children's Hospice International (CHI)
901 N. Pitt St., Ste. 230
Alexandria, VA 22314 US
Phone: 703-684-0330
Toll Free: 800-242-4453
E-mail Address: *info@chionline.org*
Web Address: www.chionline.org
Children's Hospice International (CHI) is a nonprofit organization founded to promote hospice support through pediatric care facilities, to encourage the inclusion of children in existing and developing hospice and home-care programs and to include the hospice perspectives in all areas of pediatric care, education and the public arena.

Hospice Education Institute
3 Unity Sq., P.O. Box 98
Machiasport, ME 04655-0098 US
Phone: 207-255-8800
Fax: 207-255-8008
Toll Free: 800-331-1620
E-mail Address: *hospiceall@aol.com*
Web Address: www.hospiceworld.org
The Hospice Education Institute is an independent, not-for-profit organization serving members of the public and health care professions with information and education about the many facets of caring for the dying and the bereaved.

XXXII. Hospital Care

American Hospital Association (AHA)
One N. Franklin
Chicago, IL 60606-3421 US
Phone: 312-422-3000
Fax: 312-422-4796
Web Address: www.aha.org/aha/index.jsp
The American Hospital Association (AHA) is the national organization that represents and serves all types of hospitals, health care networks, their patients and communities.

Council of Teaching Hospitals and Health Systems (COTH)
Association of American Medical Colleges
2450 N St. NW
Washington, DC 20037-1126 US
Phone: 202-828-0400
Fax: 202-828-1125
E-mail Address: *kgserrin@aamc.org*
Web Address: www.aamc.org/teachinghospitals.htm
The Council of Teaching Hospitals and Health Systems (COTH) provides representation and services related to the special needs, concerns and opportunities facing major teaching hospitals in the United States and Canada. Its site offers a listing of member hospitals.

XXXIII. Immunization

CDC National Immunization Information Hotline (NIIH)
Toll Free: 800-232-2522
Web Address: www.vaccines.ashastd.org
The CDC National Immunization Information Hotline (NIIH) offers up-to-date immunization information, including vaccine schedules, side effects, contraindications, recommendations and more.

XXXIV. Industry Research/Market Research

Forrester Research
400 Technology Sq.
Cambridge, MA 02139 US
Phone: 617-613-6000
Fax: 617-613-5000
Web Address: www.forrester.com
Forrester Research identifies and analyzes emerging trends in technology and their impact on business. Among the firm's specialties are the financial

services, retail, health care, entertainment, automotive and information technology industries.

Marketresearch.com
641 Ave. of the Americas, 4th Fl.
New York, NY 10011 US
Fax: 212-807-2676
Toll Free: 800-298-5699
Web Address: www.marketresearch.com
Marketresearch.com is a leading broker for market research and industry analysis written by professionals. Users are able to search the company's database of more than 40,000 research publications including data on global industries, companies, products and trends.

Mindbranch
160 Water St.
Williamstown, MA 01267 US
Phone: 413-458-7600
Fax: 413-458-1706
Toll Free: 800-774-4410
E-mail Address: *jbua@mindbranch.com*
Web Address: www.mindbranch.com
Mindbranch is a broker for industry research prepared by market research professionals. The user-friendly site is organized by a broad range of industries and business topics. Customers can also receive superb telephone support and suggestions about research reports.

Plunkett Research, Ltd.
P.O. Drawer 541737
Houston, TX 77254-1737 US
Phone: 713-932-0000
Fax: 713-932-7080
E-mail Address: *info@plunkettresearch.com*
Web Address: www.plunkettresearch.com
Plunkett Research, Ltd. is a leading provider of market research, industry trends analysis and business statistics. Since 1985, it has served clients worldwide, including corporations, universities, libraries, consultants and government agencies. At the firm's web site, visitors can view product information and pricing and access a great deal of basic market information on industries such as financial services, InfoTech, e-commerce, health care and biotech.

Reuters Investor
Web Address: www.investor.reuters.com
Reuters Investor (formerly Multex) is an excellent source for industry and company reports written by professional stock and business analysts. It also offers news and advice on stocks, funds and personal finance, and it has a superb tool that allows users to screen a database of major corporations and view pertinent financial and business data on the selected firms.

XXXV. Laboratories/Research

Battelle Memorial Institute
505 King Ave.
Columbus, OH 43201 US
Phone: 614-424-6424
Toll Free: 800-201-2011
Web Address: www.battelle.org
Battelle Memorial Institute serves industry and government in developing new technologies and products. The institute adds technology to systems and processes for manufacturers; pharmaceutical and agrochemical industries; trade associations; and government agencies supporting energy, the environment, health, national security and transportation.

Commonwealth Scientific and Industrial Research Organization (CSRIO)
Bag 10
Clayton South, VIC 3169 Australia
Phone: 61-3-9545-2176
Fax: 61-3-9545-2175
E-mail Address: *enquiries@csiro.au*
Web Address: www.csiro.au
The Commonwealth Scientific and Industrial Research Organization (CSRIO) performs research and development over a broad range of areas including agriculture, minerals and energy, manufacturing, communications, construction, health and the environment.

SRI International
333 Ravenswood Ave.
Menlo Park, CA 94025-3493 US
Phone: 650-859-2000
Fax: 650-326-5512
Toll Free: 866-451-5998
E-mail Address: *inquiry.line@sri.com*
Web Address: www.sri.com
SRI International is a nonprofit organization offering a wide range of services, including engineering services, information technology, pure and applied physical sciences, product development, pharmaceutical discovery, biopharmaceutical discovery and policy issues.

XXXVI. Learning Disorders

Children and Adults with Attention Deficit Disorder (CHADD)
8181 Professional Pl., Ste. 150
Landover, MD 20785 US
Phone: 301-306-7070
Fax: 301-306-7090
Toll Free: 800-233-4050
Web Address: www.chadd.org
Children and Adults with Attention Deficit Disorder (CHADD) is the nation's leading nonprofit organization serving individuals with AD/HD.

XXXVII. Libraries

Library and Info Systems
Web Address: www.cellbio.wustl.edu/library.htm
Library and Info Systems provides information on libraries at various higher institutions of learning in the United States.

Medical Library Association (MLA)
65 E. Wacker Pl., Ste. 1900
Chicago, IL 60601-7298 US
Phone: 312-419-9094
Fax: 312-419-8950
E-mail Address: *info@mlahq.org*
Web Address: www.mlanet.org
The Medical Library Association (MLA) is dedicated to improving the quality and leadership of health information professionals in order to foster the art and science of health information services.

Multimedia Medical Reference Library (MMRL)
Web Address: www.medical-library.org
The Multimedia Medical Reference Library (MMRL) provides a free resource of medical information for both health care consumers and medical professionals.

National Library of Medicine (NLM)
8600 Rockville Pike
Bethesda, MD 20894 US
Web Address: www.nlm.nih.gov
The National Library of Medicine (NLM) site offers links to several databases of medical research, as well as a variety of online health information.

Weill Cornell Medical Library
Joan & Sanford I. Weill Medical College, Cornell University
1300 York Ave.
New York, NY 10021-4896 US
Phone: 212-746-6068
E-mail Address: *infodesk@med.cornell.edu*
Web Address: lib2.med.cornell.edu
The Weill Cornell Medical Library houses information on the biomedical sciences, as well as performing data retrieval, management and evaluation.

WWW Virtual Library: Bioscience – Medicine
Oregon Health & Science University, School of Medicine
3181 SW Sam Jackson Pk. Rd.
Portland, OR 97239-8311 US
Phone: 503-494-8220
Web Address: londonbridge.ohsu.edu/wwwvl/
Oregon State Health & Science University provides this list of companies and organizations involved in biomedical research.

XXXVIII. Liver Diseases

American Liver Foundation (ALF)
75 Maiden Ln., Ste. 603
New York, NY 10038 US
Phone: 212-668-1000
Fax: 212-483-8179
Toll Free: 800-465-4837
E-mail Address: *info@liverfoundation.org*
Web Address: www.liverfoundation.org
The American Liver Foundation (ALF) is a national, nonprofit organization dedicated to the prevention, treatment and cure of hepatitis and other liver diseases.

XXXIX. Managed Care Information

Managed Care Information Center (MCIC)
1913 Atlantic Ave., Ste. F4
Manasquan, NJ 08736 US
Phone: 888-843-6242
Fax: 888-329-6242
Web Address: www.themcic.com
The Managed Care Information Center (MCIC) is a clearinghouse for health care executives' managed care information needs. MCIC publishes newsletters, advisories, guides, manuals, special reports and books.

Managed Care On-Line (MCOL)
1101 Stanford Ave., Ste. C-3
Modesto, CA 95350 US
Phone: 209-577-4888

Fax: 209-577-3557
E-mail Address: *mcare@mcol.com*
Web Address: www.mcol.com
Managed Care On-Line (MCOL) is an Internet-based health care company delivering business-to-business managed care resources. The web site includes a knowledge center and resources. E-mail newsletters and updates are available.

XL. Maternal & Infant Health

Association of Maternal and Child Health Programs (AMCHP)
1220 19th St. NW, Ste. 801
Washington, DC 20036 US
Phone: 202-775-0436
Fax: 202-775-0061
E-mail Address: *info@amchp.org*
Web Address: www.amchp.org
The Association of Maternal and Child Health Programs (AMCHP) is the national organization representing public health leaders and others working to improve the health and well-being of women, children and youth.

La Leche League International
1400 N. Meacham Rd.
Schaumburg, IL 60173-4808 US
Phone: 847-519-7730
Fax: 847-519-0035
Web Address: www.lalecheleague.org
The La Leche League International seeks to help mothers worldwide to breastfeed through mother-to-mother support, encouragement, information and education and to promote a better understanding of breastfeeding.

National Center for Education in Maternal and Child Health (NCEMCH)
2115 Wisconsin Ave. NW
Washington, DC 20007-2292 US
Phone: 202-784-9770
Fax: 202-784-977
E-mail Address: *mchlibrary@ncemch*
Web Address: www.ncemch.org
The National Center for Education in Maternal and Child Health (NCEMCH) provides national leadership to the maternal and child health community to improve the health and well-being of the nation's children and families.

XLI. Medical & Health Indexes

MEDIC: What's New This Month
Web Address: medic.med.uth.tmc.edu/index.html
MEDIC offers annotated links to various medical sites.

Medical World Search
Phone: 914-248-6770
Web Address: www.mwsearch.com
Medical World Search is a search engine especially developed for the medical field.

XLII. Medicare Information

Medicare Rights Center (MRC)
1460 Broadway, 17th Fl.
New York, NY 10036 US
Phone: 212-869-3850
Fax: 212-869-3532
E-mail Address: *info@medicarerights.org*
Web Address: www.medicarerights.org
The Medicare Rights Center (MRC) is a not-for-profit organization that is acts as a source for Medicare consumers and professionals. Its web site is a helpful, independent source of Medicare information.

Medicare.gov
Web Address: www.medicare.gov
Medicare.gov is the official U.S. Government site for people with questions or problems relating to Medicare.

XLIII. Mental Health

American Academy of Child and Adolescent Psychiatry (AACAP)
3615 Wisconsin Ave. NW
Washington, DC 20016-3007 US
Phone: 202-966-7300
Fax: 202-966-2891
Web Address: www.aacap.org
The American Academy of Child and Adolescent Psychiatry (AACAP) is the leading national professional medical association dedicated to treating and improving the quality of life for children, adolescents and families affected by these disorders.

Depression Awareness, Recognition and Treatment (D/ART)
NIMH Office of Communications

6001 Executive Blvd., Rm. 8184, MSC 9663
Bethesda, MD 20892 US
Phone: 301-443-4513
Fax: 301-443-4279
Toll Free: 866-615-6464
E-mail Address: *nimhinfo@nih.gov*
Web Address:
www.nimh.nih.gov/healthinformation/depressionmenu.cfm
Depression Awareness, Recognition and Treatment (D/ART), a site supported by the National Institute of Mental Health, offers a wealth of information on depression.

International Society for Mental Health Online (ISMHO)
Web Address: www.ismho.org
The International Society for Mental Health Online (ISMHO) strives to promote online communication, information and technology for the mental health community.

National Foundation for Depressive Illness
P.O. Box 2257
New York, NY 10116 US
Toll Free: 800-239-1265
Web Address: www.depression.org
The National Foundation for Depressive Illness provides information on depression.

National Mental Health Association (NMHA)
2001 N. Beauregard St., 12th Fl.
Alexandria, VA 22314 US
Phone: 703-684-7722
Fax: 703-684-5968
Toll Free: 800-969-6642
Web Address: www.nmha.org
The National Mental Health Association (NMHA) is the country's oldest and largest nonprofit organization addressing all aspects of mental health and mental illness.

XLIV.	Neurological Disease

American Neurological Association (ANA)
5841 Cedar Lake Rd., Ste. 204
Minniapolis, MN 55416 US
Phone: 952-545-6284
Fax: 952-545-6073
Web Address: www.aneuroa.org
The American Neurological Association (ANA) is a professional society of academic neurologists and neuroscientists devoted to advancing the goals and science of neurology.

American Parkinson's Disease Association (APDA)
1250 Hylan Blvd., Ste. 4B
Staten Island, NY 10305 US
Fax: 718-981-4399
Toll Free: 800-223-2732
E-mail Address: *apda@apdaparkinson.org*
Web Address: www.apdaparkinson.com
The American Parkinson's Disease Association (APDA) seeks to promote a better quality of life for the Parkinson's community.

Christopher Reeve Paralysis Foundation (CRPF)
500 Morris Ave.
Springfield, NJ 07081 US
Fax: 973-912-9433
Toll Free: 800-225-0292
Web Address: www.apacure.org
The Christopher Reeve Paralysis Foundation (CRPF) is committed to funding research that develops treatments and cures for paralysis caused by spinal cord injury and other central nervous system disorders.

National Rehabilitation Information Center (NARIC)
4200 Forbes Blvd., Ste. 202
Lanham, MD 20706 US
Phone: 301-459-5900
Toll Free: 800-346-2742
E-mail Address: *naricinfo@heitechservices.com*
Web Address: www.naric.com
The National Rehabilitation Information Center (NARIC) collects and disseminates the results of federally funded research projects.

XLV.	Nutrition

Center for Science in the Public Interest (CSPI)
1875 Connecticut Ave., Ste. 300
Washington, DC 20009 US
Phone: 202-332-9110
Fax: 202-265-4954
E-mail Address: *cspi@cspinet.org*
Web Address: www.cspinet.org
The Center for Science in the Public Interest (CSPI) is a nonprofit education and advocacy organization that focuses on improving the safety and nutritional quality of our food supply and on reducing the incidence of alcohol-related injuries.

XLVI. Online Health Data

Centers for Disease Control and Prevention (CDC)
1600 Clifton Rd.
Atlanta, GA 30333 US
Phone: 404-639-3311
Toll Free: 800-311-3435
Web Address: www.cdc.gov
The Centers for Disease Control and Prevention (CDC) is recognized as the lead federal agency for protecting the health and safety of people at home and abroad, providing credible information to enhance health decisions and promoting health through strong partnerships.

Family Health Radio
Web Address: www.fhradio.org
Family Health Radio offers audio files that provide practical answers to frequently asked questions about health.

Healthfinder
P.O. Box 1133
Washington, DC 20013-113 US
E-mail Address: *healthfinder@nhic.org*.
Web Address: www.healthfinder.gov
Healthfinder is a resource for finding government and nonprofit health and human services information on the Internet.

HealthLinks
Web Address: healthlinks.washington.edu
HealthLinks, based at the University of Washington Health Sciences Center, offers health-related information and articles from the center's HealthBeat publication.

HealthWeb
Web Address: www.healthweb.org
HealthWeb is a collaborative project of the health sciences libraries of the Greater Midwest Region of the National Network of Libraries of Medicine and those of the Committee for Institutional Cooperation.

HIV InSite
Web Address: hivinsite.ucsf.edu
HIV InSite offers comprehensive, up-to-date information on HIV/AIDS treatment, prevention and policy.

Mayo Clinic
200 1st St.
Rochester, MN 55905 US
Web Address: www.mayoclinic.com
The Mayo Clinic's web site seeks to empower people to manage their health using information and tools from the clinic's experts.

MEDEM
Fax: 415-644-3950
Toll Free: 877-926-3336
Web Address: medem.com
MEDEM provides tools and secure technologies for physicians to provide patients access to trusted health information via the doctor's own web site.

MEDLINEplus
E-mail Address: *custserv@nlm.nih.gov*.
Web Address: medlineplus.gov
MEDLINEplus offers information from the National Library of Medicine, the world's largest medical library.

MEDMarket
710 Tubbs Hill Dr.
Coeur d'Alene, ID 83814 US
Phone: 866-666-4069
Fax: 208-445-8966
Web Address: www.medmarket.com
MEDMarket serves as an online guide to the health care manufacturers industry, featuring employment listings, an industry index and more.

Medscape
WebMD Medscape Health Network
224 W. 30th St.
New York, NY 10001-5399 US
Toll Free: 888-506-6098
Web Address: www.medscape.com
Medscape, an online resource for better patient care, provides links to journal articles, health care-related sites and health care information.

National Women's Health Information Center (NWHIC)
Phone: 888-220-5446
Toll Free: 800-994-9662
Web Address: www.4women.gov
The National Women's Health Information Center (NWHIC) provides a gateway to the vast array of federal and other women's health information resources.

New York Online Access to Health (NOAH)
Web Address: www.noah-health.org

New York Online Access to Health (NOAH) provides access to high-quality, full-text consumer health information in English and Spanish that is accurate, timely, relevant and unbiased.

PubMed
Web Address: www.ncbi.nlm.nih.gov/entrez/query
PubMed provides access to over 14 million MEDLINE citations dating back to the mid-1960s and additional life science journals.

RxList
16092 San Dieguito Rd.
Rancho Sante Fe, CA 92067 US
Phone: 609-882-8887
Fax: 425-671-7796
E-mail Address: *info@rxlist.com*
Web Address: www.rxlist.com
RxList provides health and medical information to consumers and medical professionals.

Virtual Hospital
Web Address: www.vh.org
The Virtual Hospital digital library exists to make the Internet a useful medical reference and health promotion tool for health care providers and patients.

WebMD
669 River Dr., Ctr. 2
Elmwood Park, NJ 07407 US
Phone: 201-703-3400
Fax: 201-703-3401
Web Address: www.webmd.com
WebMD features a broad selection of interrelated health topics, current medical news and its own search engine.

XLVII. Online Health Information, Reliability & Ethics

eHealth Ethics
Internet Healthcare Coalition
P.O. Box 286
Newtown, PA 18940 US
Phone: 215-504-4164
Fax: 215-504-5739
Web Address: www.ihealthcoalition.org/ethics/ethics.html
eHealth Ethics is a forum for the development of a universal set of ethics principles for health-related web sites.

Health Internet Ethics
E-mail Address: *cheryl@drgreene.com*
Web Address: www.hiethics.org
Hi-Ethics, Inc. unites the most widely used health Internet sites supporting high ethical standards.

Health on the Net Foundation Code of Conduct
Medical Informatics Division, University Hospital of Geneva
24, rue Micheli-du-Crest
Geneva 14, 1211 Switzerland
Phone: 41-22-372-62-50
Fax: 41-22-372-88-85
E-mail Address: *Info@hon.ch*
Web Address: www.hon.ch/HONcode
The Health on the Net Foundation Code of Conduct defines a set of rules to help standardize the reliability of medical and health information on the Internet.

XLVIII. Organ Donation

Living Bank (The)
P.O. Box 6725
Houston, TX 77265 US
Toll Free: 800-528-2971
E-mail Address: *info@livingbank.org*
Web Address: www.livingbank.org
The Living Bank is the oldest and largest donor education organization in the country and the only national organization that keeps computerized records of donor data for future retrieval in an emergency.

XLIX. Osteoporosis

National Osteoporosis Foundation (NOF)
1232 22nd St. NW
Washington, DC 20037-1292 US
Phone: 202-223-2226
Web Address: www.nof.org
The National Osteoporosis Foundation (NOF) works to fight osteoporosis and promote bone health.

L. Patients Rights & Information

FamiliesUSA
1334 G St. NW
Washington, DC 20005 US
Phone: 202-628-3030
Fax: 202-347-2417
E-mail Address: *info@familiesusa.org*

Web Address: www.familiesusa.org
FamiliesUSA is a national nonprofit, non-partisan organization dedicated to the achievement of high-quality, affordable health and long-term care for all Americans.

Medical Record Privacy
Web Address: www.epic.org/privacy/medical
Medical Record Privacy tracks recent developments in medical privacy legislation.

National Committee for Quality Assurance (NCQA)
Toll Free: 888-275-7585
Web Address: www.ncqa.org
The National Committee for Quality Assurance (NCQA) seeks to improve health care quality for everyone.

Society for Healthcare Consumer Advocacy (SHCA)
One N. Franklin
Chicago, IL 60606 US
Phone: 312-422-3907
Fax: 312-422-4575
E-mail Address: *shca@aha.org*
Web Address: www.shca-aha.org
The Society for Healthcare Consumer Advocacy (SHCA) includes patient representatives, guest relations professionals, physicians, nurses, social workers and others employed in hospitals, health maintenance organizations, home health agencies, long-term care facilities and other health-related organizations.

LI. Pharmaceutical Associations

Accreditation Council for Pharmacy Education (ACPE)
20 N. Clark St., Ste. 2500
Chicago, IL 60602-5109 US
Phone: 312-664-3575
Fax: 312-664-4652
Web Address: www.acpe-accredit.org
The Accreditation Council for Pharmacy Education (ACPE) provides accreditation for pharmaceutical programs.

American Academy of Pharmaceutical Physicians (AAPP)
1031 Pemberton Hill Rd., Ste. 101
Apex, NC 27502 US
Phone: 919-355-1000
Fax: 919-355-1010
Web Address: aapp.org
The American Academy of Pharmaceutical Physicians (AAPP) is a nonprofit organization for the professional improvement of pharmaceutical physicians.

American Pharmaceutical Association (APhA)
2215 Constitution Ave. NW
Washington, DC 20037 US
Phone: 202-628-4410
Fax: 202-783-2351
Web Address: www.aphanet.org
American Pharmaceutical Association (APhA) is the national professional society that provides news and information to pharmacists.

Association of the British Pharmaceutical Industry (ABPI)
12 Whitehall
London, SW1A 2DY UK
Phone: 44-20-7930-3477
Fax: 44-20-7747-1411
Web Address: www.abpi.org.uk
The Association of the British Pharmaceutical Industry (ABPI) is a trade association that provides research and information for the British biotech industry.

Institute for Clinical Research in the Pharmaceutical Industry (ICRPI)
P.O. Box 2962
Marlow, SL7 1XH UK
Phone: 44-0-1628-899755
Fax: 44-0-1628-899766
Web Address: www.instituteofclinicalresearch.org
The Institute for Clinical Research in the Pharmaceutical Industry (ICRPI) is a professional organization for clinical researchers in the pharmaceutical industry.

International Federation of Pharmaceutical Manufacturers Associations (IFPMA)
30 rue de St.-Jean, P.O. Box 758
1211
Geneva, 13 Switzerland
Phone: 41-22-338-32-00
Fax: 41-22-338-32-99
Web Address: www.ifpma.org
The International Federation of Pharmaceutical Manufacturers Associations (IFPMA) is a nonprofit organization that represents the world's research-based pharmaceutical companies.

Pharmaceutical Research and Manufacturers of America (PhRMA)
1100 15th St. NW
Washington, DC 20005 US
Phone: 202-835-3400
Fax: 202-835-34114
Web Address: www.phrma.org
Pharmaceutical Research and Manufacturers of America (PhRMA) represents the nation's leading research-based pharmaceutical and biotechnology companies.

LII. Privacy & Consumer Matters

Federal Trade Commission-Privacy
Web Address: www.ftc.gov/privacy
Federal Trade Commission-Privacy is responsible for many aspects of business-to-consumer and business-to-business trade and regulation.

Privacy International
Lancaster House, 2nd Fl., 33 Islington High St.
London, N1 9LH UK
Web Address: www.privacyinternational.org
Privacy International is a government and business watchdog, alerting individuals to wiretapping and national security activities, medical privacy infringement, police information systems and the use of ID cards, video surveillance and data matching.

TRUSTe
685 Market St., Ste. 560
San Francisco, CA 94105 US
Phone: 415-618-3400
Fax: 415-618-3420
Web Address: www.truste.org
TRUSTe, a nonprofit agency, formed an alliance with all major portal sites to launch the Privacy Partnership campaign, a consumer education program designed to raise the awareness of Internet privacy issues. The organization works to meet the needs of business web sites while protecting user privacy.

LIII. Rare Disorders

International Myeloma Foundation (IMF)
12650 Riverside Dr., Ste. 206
North Hollywood, CA 91607 US
Phone: 818-487-7455
Fax: 818-487-7454
Toll Free: 800-452-2873
E-mail Address: *theimf@myeloma.org*
Web Address: www.myeloma.org
The International Myeloma Foundation (IMF) is a group dedicated to the treatment of myeloma.

LIV. Respiratory

American Academy of Allergy, Asthma & Immunology (AAAAI)
555 E. Wells St., Ste. 1100
Milwaukee, WI 53202 US
Phone: 414-272-6071
Toll Free: 800-822-2762
E-mail Address: *info@aaaai.org*
Web Address: www.aaaai.org
The American Academy of Allergy, Asthma & Immunology (AAAAI) offers information and services to allergy and asthma sufferers and their families and friends.

American Lung Association (ALA)
61 Broadway, 6th Fl.
New York, NY 10006 US
Phone: 212-315-8700
Web Address: www.lungusa.org
The American Lung Association (ALA) fights lung disease in all its forms, with special emphasis on asthma, tobacco control and environmental health.

Asthma and Allergy Foundation of America (AAFA)
1233 20th St. NW, Ste. 402
Washington, DC 20036 US
Phone: 202-466-7643
Fax: 202-466-8940
E-mail Address: *info@aafa.org*
Web Address: www.aafa.org
The Asthma and Allergy Foundation of America (AAFA) is dedicated to improving the quality of life for people with asthma and allergies through education, advocacy and research.

Asthma in America Survey Project
1901 L St. NW, Ste. 300
Washington, DC 20036 US
Phone: 202-452-9429
Fax: 202-296-3727
Web Address: www.asthmainamerica.com
The Asthma in America Survey Project was conducted by Schulman, Ronca & Bucuvalas, a national research firm specializing in health issues.

LV. Scientific Business & Professional Associations

American Association for the Advancement of Science (AAAS)
1200 New York Ave. NW
Washington, DC 20005 US
Phone: 202-326-6400
E-mail Address: *webmaster@aaas.org*
Web Address: www.aaas.org
The American Association for the Advancement of Science (AAAS) is the world's largest scientific society and the publisher of Science magazine.

LVI. Sexually Transmitted Diseases

Centers for Disease Control and Prevention National STD Hotline
Toll Free: 800-227-8922
Web Address: www.ashastd.org/search/index.html
The Centers for Disease Control and Prevention National STD Hotline provides toll-free information on sexually transmitted diseases to the general public.

National Herpes Resource Center (HRC)
P.O. Box 13827
Research Triangle Park, NC 27709 US
Phone: 919-361-8400
Fax: 919-361-8425
Web Address: www.ashastd.org/hrc
The National Herpes Resource Center (HRC) focuses on increasing education, public awareness and support to anyone concerned about herpes.

LVII. U.S. Government Agencies

Agency for Health Care Research and Quality (AHCRQ)
540 Gaither Rd.
Rockville, MD 20850 US
Phone: 301-427-1364
E-mail Address: *info@ahrq.gov*
Web Address: www.ahcpr.gov
The Agency for Health Care Research and Quality (AHCRQ) provides evidence-based information on health care outcomes, quality, cost, use and access. Its research helps people make more informed decisions and improve the quality of health care services.

Bureau of Economic Analysis (BEA)
1441 L St.
Washington, DC 20230 US
Phone: 202-606-9900
Web Address: www.bea.doc.gov
The Bureau of Economic Analysis (BEA), an agency of the U.S. Department of Commerce, is the nation's economic accountant, preparing estimates that illuminate key national, international and regional aspects of the United States economy.

Bureau of Labor Statistics (BLS)
2 Massachusetts Ave. NE
Washington, DC 20212-0001 US
Phone: 202-691-5200
Fax: 202-691-6325
E-mail Address: *blsdata_staff@bls.gov*
Web Address: stats.bls.gov
The Bureau of Labor Statistics (BLS) is the principal fact-finding agency for the Federal Government in the field of labor economics and statistics. It is an independent national statistical agency that collects, processes, analyzes and disseminates statistical data to the American public, U.S. Congress, other federal agencies, state and local governments, business and labor. The BLS also serves as a statistical resource to the Department of Labor.

Cancer Information Service (CIS)
31 Center Dr., MSC 2580
Bldg. 31, Rm. 10AO3
Bethesda, MD 20892 US
Fax: 301-402-5874
Toll Free: 800-422-6237
E-mail Address: *cancermail@icicc.nci.nih.gov*
Web Address: cis.nci.nih.gov
The Cancer Information Service (CIS) is a national information and education network provided by the National Cancer Institute.

CDC National Prevention Information Network (CDCNPIN)
P.O. Box 6003
Rockville, MD 20849-6003 US
Phone: 301-562-1098
Fax: 888-282-7681
Toll Free: 800-458-5231
E-mail Address: *info@cdcnpin.org*
Web Address: www.cdcnpin.org
The CDC National Prevention Information Network (CDCNPIN) is the U.S. reference, referral and distribution service for information on HIV/AIDS, sexually transmitted diseases and tuberculosis. It is operated by the Centers for Disease Control, a Federal Government agency.

Centers for Medicare and Medicaid Services (CMMS)
7500 Security Blvd.
Baltimore, MD 21244-1850 US
Phone: 410-786-3000
Toll Free: 877-267-2323
Web Address: cms.hhs.gov
The Centers for Medicare and Medicaid Services (CMMS) runs the Medicare and Medicaid programs in the U.S., as well as State Children's Health Insurance Program.

Clinical Trials
U.S. National Library of Medicine
8600 Rockville Pike
Bethesda, MD 20894 US
Phone: 301-594-5983
Fax: 301-402-1384
Toll Free: 888-346-3656
Web Address: www.clinicaltrials.gov
Clinical Trials offers up-to-date information for locating federally and privately supported clinical trials for a wide range of diseases and conditions. It is a service of the National Institutes of Health (NIH).

Department of Health and Human Services (HHS)
200 Independence Ave. SW
Washington, DC 20201 US
Phone: 202-619-0257
Toll Free: 877-696-6775
Web Address: www.hhs.gov
The Department of Health and Human Services (HHS) seeks to protect health and give a helping hand to those who need assistance.

Food and Drug Administration (FDA)
5600 Fishers Ln.
Rockville, MD 20857-0001 US
Toll Free: 888-463-6332
Web Address: www.fda.gov
The Food and Drug Administration (FDA) strives to promote and protect public health by helping safe and effective products reach the market in a timely way and by monitoring products for continued safety after they are approved for use.

Government Printing Office (GPO)
732 N. Capitol St. NW
Washington, DC 20401 US
Phone: 202-512-0000
Fax: 202-512-1262
Toll Free: 888-293-6498
E-mail Address: *gpoinfo@gpo.gov*
Web Address: www.gpo.gov
The U.S. Government Printing Office (GPO) is the source for many government books and documents.

Health.gov
Web Address: www.health.gov
Health.gov is a portal to the web sites of a number of multi-agency health initiatives and activities of the U.S. Department of Health and Human Services (HHS) and other federal departments and agencies.

National Cancer Institute (NCI)
6116 Executive Blvd., Ste. 3036A, MSC 8322
Bethesda, MD 20892 US
Toll Free: 800-422-6237
Web Address: www.cancer.gov
The National Cancer Institute (NCI) is the Federal Government's principal agency for cancer research and training.

National Center for Chronic Disease Prevention and Health Promotion (NCCDPHP)
Web Address: www.cdc.gov/nccdphp
The National Center for Chronic Disease Prevention and Health Promotion (NCCDPHP) strives to see all people in an increasingly diverse society leading long, healthy and satisfying lives.

National Center for Complementary and Alternative Medicine (NCCAM)
P.O. Box 7923
Gaithersburg, MD 20898 US
Phone: 301-519-3153
Fax: 866-464-3616
Toll Free: 888-644-6226
Web Address: nccam.nih.gov
The National Center for Complementary and Alternative Medicine (NCCAM) supports rigorous research on complementary and alternative medicine. It disseminates information to the public and professionals about which of these modalities work, which do not and why.

National Center for Health Statistics (NCHS)
6525 Belcrest Rd.
Hyattsville, MD 20782 US
Phone: 301-458-4636
Web Address: www.cdc.gov/nchs/Default.htm
The National Center for Health Statistics (NCHS) is the federal government's principal vital and health statistics agency.

National Center for Research Resources (NCRR)
One Democracy Plaza, 9th Fl.
6701 Democracy Blvd., MSC 4874
Bethesda, MD 20892-4874 US
Phone: 301-435-0888
Fax: 301-480-3558
E-mail Address: *info@ncrr.nih.gov*
Web Address: www.ncrr.nih.gov
The National Center for Research Resources (NCRR) supports primary research to create and develop critical resources, models and technologies.

National Heart, Lung, and Blood Institute (NHLBI)
31 Center Dr., Bldg. 31, Rm. 5A52, MSC 2486
Bethesda, MD 20824-0105 US
Phone: 301-496-4236
Fax: 301-592-8563
E-mail Address: *nhlbiinfo@rover.nhlbi.nih.gov*
Web Address: www.nhlbi.nih.gov
The National Heart, Lung, and Blood Institute (NHLBI) provides leadership for a national program in diseases of the heart, blood vessels, lung and blood; blood resources; and sleep disorders.

National Institute of Allergy and Infectious Diseases (NIAID)
6610 Rockledge Dr., MSC 6612
Bethesda, MD 20892 US
Web Address: www.niaid.nih.gov
The National Institute of Allergy and Infectious Diseases (NIAID) conducts and supports research that strives for understanding, treatment and prevention of the many infectious, immunologic and allergic diseases that threaten people worldwide.

National Institute of Child Health and Human Development (NICHD)
P.O. Box 3006
Rockville, MD 20847 US
Fax: 301-496-7101
Toll Free: 800-370-2943
Web Address: www.nichd.nih.gov
The National Institute of Child Health and Human Development (NICHD) conducts and supports laboratory, clinical and epidemiological research on the reproductive, neurobiological, developmental and behavioral processes that determine and maintain the health of children, adults, families and populations.

National Institute of Diabetes and Digestive and Kidney Disorders (NIDDK)
31 Center Dr.
Bldg. 31, Rm. 9A04, MSC 2560
Bethesda, MD 20892 US
Web Address: www.niddk.nih.gov
The National Institute of Diabetes and Digestive and Kidney Disorders (NIDDK) conducts and supports basic and clinical research on many of the most serious diseases affecting public health.

National Institute of Environmental Health Services (NIEHS)
P.O. Box 12233
Research Triangle Park, NC 27709 US
Phone: 919-541-3345
Web Address: www.niehs.nih.gov
The National Institute of Environmental Health Services (NIEHS) is the segment of the National Institutes of Health that deals with environmental effects on human health.

National Institute of General Medical Services (NIGMS)
45 Center Dr., MSC 6200
Bethesda, MD 20892 US
Phone: 301-496-7301
E-mail Address: *pub_info@nigms.nih.gov*
Web Address: www.nigms.nih.gov
The National Institute of General Medical Services (NIGMS) supports basic biomedical research that is not targeted to specific diseases or disorders.

National Institute of Mental Health (NIMH)
6001 Executive Blvd.
Rm. 8184, MSC 9663
Bethesda, MD 20892 US
Phone: 301-443-4513, TTY 301-443-8431
Fax: 301-443-4279
Toll Free: 866-615-6464
E-mail Address: *nimhinfo@nih.gov*
Web Address: www.nimh.nih.gov
The National Institute of Mental Health (NIMH) strives to better understand and respond to mental health disorders.

National Institute of Neurological Disorders and Stroke (NINDS)
P.O. Box 5801
Bethesda, MD 20824 US
Phone: 301-496-5751
Toll Free: 800-352-9424
Web Address: www.ninds.nih.gov
The National Institute of Neurological Disorders and Stroke (NINDS) strives to lead the neuroscience

community in shaping the future of research and its relationship to brain diseases.

National Institute of Nursing Research (NINR)
Phone: 301-496-0207
Web Address: www.nih.gov/ninr
The National Institute of Nursing Research (NINR) supports clinical and basic research to establish a scientific basis for the care of individuals across the life span.

National Institute on Aging (NIA)
31 Center Dr., MSC 2292
Bldg. 31, Rm. 5C27
Bethesda, MD 20892 US
Phone: 301-496-1752
Toll Free: 800-222-2225
Web Address: www.nia.nih.gov
The National Institute on Aging (NIA) is one of the 25 institutes and centers of the National Institutes of Health and leads a broad scientific effort to understand the nature of aging and to extend the healthy, active years of life.

National Institute on Alcohol Abuse and Alcoholism (NIAAA)
5635 Fishers Ln., MSC 9304
Bethesda, MD 20892-9304 US
Phone: 301-443-3885
Web Address: www.niaaa.nih.gov
The National Institute on Alcohol Abuse and Alcoholism (NIAAA) provides information on alcohol abuse.

National Institute on Arthritis and Musculoskeletal and Skin Diseases (NIAMSD)
One AMS Cir.
Bethesda, MD 20892 US
Phone: 301-495-4484
Fax: 301-718-6366
Toll Free: 877-226-4267
E-mail Address: *niamsinfo@mail.nih.gov*
Web Address: www.nih.gov/niams
The National Institute on Arthritis and Musculoskeletal and Skin Diseases (NIAMSD) serves the public, patients and health professionals by providing information, creating health information materials and participating in a national database on health information.

National Institute on Drug Abuse (NIDA)
6001 Executive Blvd., Rm. 5213
Bethesda, MD 20892-9561 US
Phone: 301-443-1124
E-mail Address: *Information@lists.nida.nih.gov*
Web Address: www.nida.nih.gov
The National Institute on Drug Abuse (NIDA) seeks to lead the nation in bringing the power of science to bear on drug abuse and addiction.

National Institutes of Health (NIH)
9000 Rockville Pike
Bethesda, MD 20892 US
Phone: 301-496-4000
E-mail Address: *nihinfo@od.nih.gov*
Web Address: www.nih.gov
The National Institutes of Health (NIH) is the steward of medical and behavioral research for the nation.

National Science Foundation (NSF)
4201 Wilson Blvd.
Arlington, VA 22230 US
Phone: 703-292-5111
Toll Free: 800-877-8339
E-mail Address: *info@nsf.gov*
Web Address: www.nsf.gov
The National Science Foundation (NSF) is an independent government agency responsible for promoting science and engineering. The foundation provides grants and funding for research.

President's Council on Physical Fitness and Sports
Web Address: www.fitness.gov
The President's Council on Physical Fitness and Sports offers information about exercise for people of all ages.

Social Security Administration (SSA)
Windsor Park Bldg.
6401 Security Blvd.
Baltimore, MD 21235 US
Phone: 800-325-0778
Toll Free: 800-772-1213
Web Address: www.ssa.gov
The Social Security Administration (SSA) site offers information on social security and retirement.

U.S. Business Advisor
Web Address: www.business.gov
U.S. Business Advisor offers a searchable directory of business-specific government information. Topics include taxes, regulations, international trade, financial assistance and business development. U.S.

Business Advisor was created by the Small Business Administration and an interagency task force.

U.S. Census Bureau
4700 Silver Hill Rd.
Washington, DC 20233 US
Web Address: www.census.gov
The U.S. Census Bureau is the official collector of data about the people and economy of the U.S. It provides official social, demographic and economic information.

U.S. Department of Labor (DOL)
Francis Perkins Bldg.
200 Constitution Ave. NW
Washington, DC 20210 US
Toll Free: 866-487-2365
Web Address: www.dol.gov
The U.S. Department of Labor (DOL) is the government agency responsible for labor regulations. This site provides tools to help citizens find out whether companies are complying with family and medical-leave requirements.

U.S. Environmental Protection Agency (EPA)
Ariel Rios Bldg.
1200 Pennsylvania Ave. NW
Washington, DC 20460 US
Phone: 202-272-0167
Web Address: www.epa.gov
The U.S. Environmental Protection Agency (EPA) seeks to protect human health and to safeguard the natural environment.

U.S. Patent and Trademark Office (PTO)
General Information Services Division
Crystal Plaza 3, Rm. 2C02
Washington, DC 20231 US
Phone: 703-308-4357
Toll Free: 800-786-9199
Web Address: www.uspto.gov
The U.S. Patent and Trademark Office (PTO) administers patent and trademark laws for the U.S. and enables registration of patents and trademarks.

U.S. Securities and Exchange Commission (SEC)
450 5th St. NW
Washington, DC 20549 US
Phone: 202-942-8088
Toll Free: 800-732-0330
Web Address: www.sec.gov
The U.S. Securities and Exchange Commission (SEC) is a nonpartisan, quasi-judicial regulatory agency responsible for administering federal securities laws. These laws are to protect investors in securities markets and ensure that they have access to disclosure of all material information concerning publicly traded securities. Visitors to the web site can access the EDGAR database of corporate financial and business information.

U.S. Technology Administration
U.S. Department of Commerce
1401 Constitution Ave. NW
Washington, DC 20230 US
Phone: 202-482-1575
E-mail Address: *info@ta.doc.gov*
Web Address: www.technology.gov
The U.S. Technology Administration seeks to maximize technology's contribution to economic growth, high-wage job creation and the social well-being of the United States. Its web site offers publications as well as information about events and services. Departments of this agency include the Office of Technology Policy and the National Technical Information Service.

White House (The)
1600 Pennsylvania Ave.
Washington, DC 20500 US
Phone: 202-456-1414
Web Address: www.whitehouse.gov
The White House site was designed for communication between the Federal Government and the American people. It provides access to all government information and services that are available on the Internet.

LVIII.	Urological Disorders

American Foundation for Urologic Disease (AFUD)
1000 Corporate Blvd., Ste. 410
Linthicum, MD 21090 US
Phone: 410-689-3990
Fax: 410-689-3998
Toll Free: 800-828-7866
E-mail Address: *admin@afud.org*
Web Address: www.afud.org
The American Foundation for Urologic Disease (AFUD) seeks the prevention and cure of urologic disease through the expansion of patient education, public awareness, research and advocacy.

National Association for Continence (NAFC)
P.O. Box 1019

Charleston, SC 29402 -1019 US
Phone: 843-377-0900
Fax: 843-377-0905
Toll Free: 800-252-3337
Web Address: www.nafc.org
National Association for Continence (NAFC) is a national, private, nonprofit organization dedicated to improving the quality of life of people with incontinence.

National Kidney Foundation
30 E. 33rd St., Ste. 1100
New York, NY 10016 US
Phone: 212-889-2210
Fax: 212-689-9261
Toll Free: 800-622-9010
E-mail Address: *info@kidney.org*
Web Address: www.kidney.org
The National Kidney Foundation seeks to prevent kidney and urinary tract diseases, improve the health and well-being of individuals and families affected by these diseases and increase the availability of all organs for transplantation.

Chapter 4

THE HEALTH CARE 500: WHO THEY ARE AND HOW THEY WERE CHOSEN

Includes Indexes by Company Name, Industry & Location, And a Complete Table of Sales, Profits and Ranks

The companies chosen to be listed in PLUNKETT'S HEALTH CARE INDUSTRY ALMANAC comprise a unique list. THE HEALTH CARE 500 (the actual count is 514 companies) were chosen specifically for their dominance in the many facets of the health care industry in which they operate. Complete information about each firm can be found in the "Individual Profiles," beginning at the end of this chapter. These profiles are in alphabetical order by company name.

THE HEALTH CARE 500 includes leading companies from all parts of the United States as well as many other nations, and from all health care and related industry segments: insurance and reinsurance companies; manufacturers and distributors of health care supplies and products; pharmaceuticals manufacturers; health care providers of all types, including major firms owning clinics, physical rehabilitation centers, hospitals, outpatient surgery centers, nursing homes, home health care offices and other types of health care specialists; specialized service companies that are vital to the health care field, such as medical information management companies and equipment leasing companies; health maintenance organizations and many others.

Simply stated, the list contains 514 of the largest, most successful, fastest growing firms in the health care and related industries in the world. To be included in our list, the firms had to meet the following criteria:

1) Generally, these are corporations based in the U.S., however, the headquarters of 47 firms are located in other nations.
2) Prominence, or a significant presence, in health care and supporting fields. (See the following Industry Codes section for a complete list of types of businesses that are covered).
3) The companies in THE HEALTH CARE 500 do not have to be exclusively in the health care field.
4) Financial data and vital statistics must have been available to the editors of this book, either directly from the company being written about or from outside sources deemed reliable and accurate by the editors. A small number of

companies that we would like to have included are not listed because of a lack of sufficient, objective data.

INDEXES TO THE HEALTH CARE 500, AS FOUND IN THIS CHAPTER AND IN THE BACK OF THE BOOK:	
Industry List, With Codes	p. 142
Index of Rankings Within Industry Groups	p. 144
Alphabetical Index	p. 157
Geographic Indexes	
Index of Headquarters Location by U.S. State	p. 161
Index of Non-U.S. Headquarters Location by Country	p. 166
Index by Regions of the U.S. Where THE HEALTH CARE 500 Have Locations	p. 167
Index by Firms with Operations Outside the U.S.	p. 176
Index of Firms Noted as "Hot Spots for Advancement" for Women/Minorities	p. 696
Index by Subsidiaries, Brand Names and Selected Affiliations	p. 697

INDUSTRY LIST, WITH CODES

This book refers to the following list of unique industry codes, based on the 1997 NAIC code system (NAIC is used by many analysts as a replacement for older SIC codes because NAIC is more specific to today's industry sectors). Companies profiled in this book are given a primary NAIC code, reflecting the main line of business of each firm.

Energy

Manufacturing, Electrical
335929 Superconducting Materials and Other Wire

Financial Services

Banking, Credit & Finance
522220A Financing--Business
522320 Payment and Transaction Processing Services
522320A Payment and Transaction Processing-- Benefits Management

Insurance
524113 Insurance-Life
524114 Insurance-Medical & Health, HMO's and PPO's
524114A Insurance-Supplemental and Specialty Health
524210 Insurance Brokerage and Management

Entertainment & Hospitality

Gambling & Recreation
713940 Fitness Centers/Health Clubs
Food Service
722310 Food Service Contractors

Health Care

Health Products, Manufacturing
325412 Drugs, Manufacturing
325413 In Vitro Diagnostic Substances, Manufacturing
325414 Biological Products, Manufacturing
325416 Drugs, Generic Manufacturing
339113 Medical/Dental/Surgical Equipment and Supplies, Manufacturing

Health Products, Wholesale Distribution
421450 Medical/Dental/Surgical Equipment and Supplies, Distribution
422210 Drugs, Distribution

Equipment Rental
532400 Equipment Rental

Veterinary Care
541940 Veterinary Clinics

Plunkett's Health Care Industry Almanac 2005

	Health Care-Clinics, Labs and Organizations
621111	Physician Practice Management
621340	Clinics--Physical Rehab Ctr.
621490	Clinics--Outpatient Clinics and Surgery
621511	Laboratories and Diagnostics--Medical
621610	Home Health Care
621991	Blood and Organ Banks
621999	Utilization Management, Health Care
	Hospitals
622110	Hospitals/Clinics--General & Specialty Hospitals
622210	Hospitals/Clinics--Psychiatric Clinics
	Nursing
623110	Long-Term Health Care and Assisted Living

InfoTech

	Computers & Electronics Manufacturing
334500	Instrument Manufacturing, including Measurement, Control, Test and Navigational
	Software
511200	Computer Software
	Information & Data Processing Services
514199	Online Publishing, Services and Niche Portals
514199A	Online Business-to-Business or to-Consumer Intermediary
514210	Data Processing Services
	Information Services-Professional
541512	Consulting--Computer and Internet

Manufacturing

	Paper Products/Forest Products
322000	Forest Products/Paper, Manufacturing
	Chemicals
325000	Chemicals, Manufacturing
	Machinery and Manufacturing Equipment
333314	Optical Instrument and Lens, Manufacturing

Retailing

	Drug Stores, Beauty Supply & Health Items Stores
446110	Pharmacies and Drug Stores
446110A	Pharmacies-Specialty
446130	Optical Goods Stores
446191	Health Supplement Stores
	Personal Services & Salons
446190	Other Health and Personal Care Stores/Weight Management

Services

	Consulting & Professional Services
541613	Consulting--Marketing
541690	Consulting--Scientific and Technical
541710	Research and Development--Physical, Engineering and Life Sciences
	Personnel, Administrative & Support Services
561400	Business Support Services
	Educational
611410	Business Schools and Computer or Management Training

Telecommunications

	Telecommunications Equipment
334200	Communications Equipment, Manufacturing
	Telecommunications
513390D	Specialty and Internet Telecommunications Services

INDEX OF RANKINGS WITHIN INDUSTRY GROUPS

Company	Industry Code	2003 Sales (U.S. $ thousands)	Sales Rank	2003 Profits (U.S. $ thousands)	Profits Rank
Biological Products, Manufacturing					
GTC BIOTHERAPEUTICS INC	325414	9,764	4	-29,537	3
HOSPIRA INC	325414	2,500,000	1		
INTERPORE CROSS INTERNATIONAL	325414	70,718	2	14,934	2
LIFECELL CORPORATION	325414	40,249	3	18,672	1
NANOBIO CORPORATION	325414				
ORGANOGENESIS INC	325414				
Blood and Organ Banks					
HEMACARE CORPORATION	621991	27,488	2	-4,679	2
SEROLOGICALS CORP	621991	146,915	1	1,506	1
Business Schools and Computer or Management Training					
HEALTHSTREAM INC	611410	18,195	1	-3,412	1
Business Support Services					
NOVATION LLC	561400				
PREMIER INC	561400				
Chemicals, Manufacturing					
BAYER AG	325000	35,914,000	1	-1,585,000	2
SIGMA ALDRICH CORP	325000	1,298,146	2	193,102	1
Clinics--Outpatient Clinics and Surgery					
AMERICA SERVICE GROUP INC	621490	549,257	5	11,875	9
AMERICAN HEALTHWAYS INC	621490	165,500	10	18,500	7
AMERICAN SHARED HOSPITAL SERVICES	621490	16,178	19	1,382	15
AMSURG CORP	621490	301,408	6	30,126	5
CURATIVE HEALTH SERVICES	621490	214,741	7	13,075	8
DAVITA INC	621490	2,016,418	3	175,791	2
DYNACQ HEALTHCARE INC	621490	90,000	14	21,000	6
FRESENIUS AG	621490	8,866,700	1	144,300	3
GAMBRO AB	621490	3,606,400	2	196,200	1
HEALTHSOUTH CORP	621490				
HEALTHTRONICS INC	621490	160,393	11	6,223	13
HEARUSA INC	621490	70,545	16	-1,109	17
HORIZON HEALTH CORP	621490	166,300	9	9,600	10
LCA VISION INC	621490	81,423	15	7,269	12
NOVAMED INC	621490	55,506	17	3,491	14
OPTICARE HEALTH SYSTEMS	621490	125,702	12	-12,353	19
PHC INC	621490	23,833	18	977	16
RENAL CARE GROUP INC	621490	1,105,319	4	102,056	4
TLC VISION CORPORATION	621490	195,680	8	-9,399	18
US PHYSICAL THERAPY INC	621490	105,568	13	7,331	11
Clinics--Physical Rehab Ctr.					
HANGER ORTHOPEDIC GROUP	621340	547,903	1	16,239	1
OCCUPATIONAL HEALTH + REHABILITATION INC	621340	53,538	3	-231	2
REHABCARE GROUP INC	621340	539,322	2	-13,699	3

Company	Industry Code	2003 Sales (U.S. $ thousands)	Sales Rank	2003 Profits (U.S. $ thousands)	Profits Rank
Communications Equipment, Manufacturing					
TELEX COMMUNICATIONS INC	334200				
Computer Hardware, Manufacturing					
TOSHIBA CORPORATION	334111	47,191,800	1	154,400	1
Computer Software					
CEDARA SOFTWARE CORP	511200	22,992	12	-10,152	10
CERNER CORP	511200	839,587	2	42,791	3
ECLIPSYS CORPORATION	511200	254,679	5	-55,964	12
EPIC SYSTEMS CORP	511200	15,300	14		
ERESEARCH TECHNOLOGY	511200	66,842	8	14,463	4
HEALTHAXIS INC	511200	20,851	13	-4,264	9
IDX SYSTEMS CORP	511200	400,000	3	58,400	2
IMS HEALTH INC	511200	1,381,800	1	639,000	1
PER SE TECHNOLOGIES INC	511200	335,200	4	12,000	5
QUALITY SYSTEMS INC	511200	54,769	9	7,035	7
QUOVADX INC	511200	71,595	7	-14,694	11
SOLUCIENT LLC	511200	50,000	11		
TRIPOS INC	511200	54,148	10	2,100	8
VITALWORKS INC	511200	111,519	6	7,963	6
Consulting--Computer and Internet					
FIRST CONSULTING GROUP	541512	287,739	1	-16,953	2
SUPERIOR CONSULTANT HOLDINGS CORP	541512	99,540	2	-1,755	1
Consulting--Marketing					
PDI INC	541613	317,448	1	12,258	1
VENTIV HEALTH INC	541613	224,453	2	5,776	2
Consulting--Scientific and Technical					
IMPATH INC	541690				
Data Processing Services					
MEDQUIST INC	514210				
TRANSCEND SERVICES INC	514210	14,663	1	1,020	1
Drugs, Distribution					
AMERISOURCEBERGEN CORP	422210	49,657,300	3	441,200	3
CARDINAL HEALTH INC	422210	56,737,000	2	1,405,800	1
D & K HEALTHCARE RESOURCES INC	422210	2,223,400	4	9,686	4
DRUGMAX INC	422210	291,800	5	-13,200	6
MCKESSON CORPORATION	422210	57,120,800	1	555,400	2
PETMED EXPRESS INC	422210	54,975	6	3,258	5
Drugs, Generic Manufacturing					
ALPHARMA INC	325416	1,297,285	2	16,936	4
ANDRX CORP	325416	1,046,300	4	48,200	3
MYLAN LABORATORIES INC	325416	1,269,200	3	272,400	2
TEVA PHARMACEUTICAL INDUSTRIES	325416	3,276,400	1	691,000	1
Drugs, Manufacturing					
ABBOTT LABORATORIES	325412	19,680,600	8	2,753,200	6
AETERNA ZENTARIS INC	325412	128,587	43	-32,426	32
ALCON INC	325412	3,406,900	18	595,400	16

Company	Industry Code	2003 Sales (U.S. $ thousands)	Sales Rank	2003 Profits (U.S. $ thousands)	Profits Rank
ALLERGAN INC	325412	1,171,400	27	-52,500	33
AMERICAN PHARMACEUTICAL PARTNERS INC	325412	351,315	40	71,693	28
AMGEN INC	325412	8,356,000	14	2,259,500	11
AVENTIS SA	325412	22,397,000	6	2,390,000	10
BARR LABORATORIES INC	325412	902,900	28	167,600	24
BAYER CORP	325412	10,999,300	12		
BIOGEN IDEC INC	325412	679,183	33	-875,097	42
BIOVAIL CORPORATION	325412	823,700	29	-27,300	31
BRISTOL MYERS SQUIBB CO	325412	20,671,000	7	2,952,000	5
CAMBREX CORP	325412	405,600	39	-54,100	34
CELLTECH GROUP PLC	325412	630,100	35	-96,100	38
CEPHALON INC	325412	714,800	31	83,900	27
CHIRON CORP	325412	1,776,361	23	227,313	22
ELAN CORP PLC	325412	746,000	30	-529,400	41
ELI LILLY & CO	325412	12,582,500	11	2,560,800	8
ENDO PHARMACEUTICALS HOLDINGS INC	325412	595,608	36	69,790	30
EON LABS INC	325412	329,538	42	70,135	29
FOREST LABORATORIES INC	325412	2,206,700	21	622,000	15
FUJISAWA PHARMACEUTICALS COMPANY LTD	325412	3,188,300	19	238,900	21
GENENTECH INC	325412	2,799,400	20	562,527	17
GENZYME CORP	325412	1,713,900	24	-67,600	36
GLAXOSMITHKLINE PLC	325412	17,251,000	9	1,949,000	13
JOHNSON & JOHNSON	325412	41,862,000	2	7,197,000	1
MERCK & CO INC	325412	22,485,900	5	6,830,900	2
MILLENNIUM PHARMACEUTICALS INC	325412	433,687	37	-483,687	40
NOVARTIS AG	325412	24,864,000	4	5,016,000	3
NOVO-NORDISK AS	325412	4,501,000	17	824,000	14
PAR PHARMACEUTICAL COMPANIES INC	325412	646,023	34	122,533	25
PFIZER INC	325412	45,188,000	1	3,910,000	4
ROCHE GROUP	325412	25,132,100	3	2,470,500	9
SANOFI-SYNTHELABO	325412	10,118,000	13	2,610,000	7
SCHERING AG	325412	6,070,000	16	557,000	18
SCHERING-PLOUGH CORP	325412	8,334,000	15	-92,000	37
SEPRACOR INC	325412	344,040	41	-135,936	39
SERONO SA	325412	1,858,000	22	390,000	19
SHIRE PHARMACEUTICALS PLC	325412	1,237,101	26	276,051	20
VALEANT PHARMACEUTICALS INTERNATIONAL	325412	685,953	32	-55,640	35
WARNER CHILCOTT PLC	325412	432,300	38	96,200	26
WATSON PHARMACEUTICALS	325412	1,457,722	25	202,864	23
WYETH	325412	15,850,600	10	2,051,600	12
Equipment Rental					
UNIVERSAL HOSPITAL SERVICES INC	532400	171,000	1	-19,500	1
Financing--Business					
GE COMMERCIAL FINANCE	522220A	18,869,000	1		
Fitness Centers/Health Clubs					
HEALTH FITNESS CORP	713940	31,478	1	632	1

Company	Industry Code	2003 Sales (U.S. $ thousands)	Sales Rank	2003 Profits (U.S. $ thousands)	Profits Rank
Food Service Contractors					
MORRISON MANAGEMENT SPECIALISTS INC	722310				
Forest Products/Paper, Manufacturing					
KIMBERLY CLARK CORP	322000	14,348,000	1	1,694,200	1
Health Supplement Stores					
GENERAL NUTRITION COMPANIES INC	446191	1,429,500	1		
Home Health Care					
ALLIED HEALTHCARE INTERNATIONAL INC	621610	294,400	6	8,000	7
AMEDISYS INC	621610	142,500	10	84,800	2
AMERICAN HOMEPATIENT INC	621610	336,181	3	14,025	5
APRIA HEALTHCARE GROUP	621610	1,380,900	1	116,000	1
ATC HEALTHCARE INC	621610	148,700	9	-2,800	12
CONTINUCARE CORP	621610	101,400	11	100	11
GENTIVA HEALTH SERVICES	621610	814,029	2	56,766	3
MATRIA HEALTHCARE INC	621610	326,847	5	7,306	8
NATIONAL HOME HEALTH CARE	621610	97,200	12	5,800	9
NEW YORK HEALTH CARE INC	621610	45,060	13	-22,052	13
ODYSSEY HEALTHCARE INC	621610	274,309	7	31,207	4
OPTION CARE INC	621610	335,440	4	8,718	6
PATIENT CARE INC	621610				
PEDIATRIC SERVICES OF AMERICA INC	621610	215,592	8	5,126	10
Hospitals/Clinics--General & Specialty Hospitals					
ADVENTIST HEALTH SYSTEM	622110	10,123,100	4		
ADVOCATE HEALTH CARE	622110	2,715,900	22	123,600	11
ALLINA HOSPITALS AND CLINICS	622110	1,940,000	32		
ASCENSION HEALTH	622110	9,054,300	5		
AVERA HEALTH	622110				
BANNER HEALTH	622110				
BJC HEALTHCARE	622110	2,500,000	27		
BON SECOURS HEALTH SYSTEM INC	622110	2,523,400	25		
CATHOLIC HEALTH INITIATIVES	622110	6,071,600	7	202,900	7
CATHOLIC HEALTHCARE PARTNERS	622110	2,874,300	18		
CATHOLIC HEALTHCARE WEST	622110	4,989,100	9	50,700	15
CHRISTUS HEALTH	622110	2,302,400	29	20,000	17
CLARIAN HEALTH PARTNERS	622110	2,102,200	31	89,000	13
COMMUNITY HEALTH SYSTEMS	622110	2,834,624	19	131,472	10
DETROIT MEDICAL CENTER	622110	1,600,000	35		
FAIRVIEW HEALTH SERVICES	622110				
HCA INC	622110	21,808,000	2	1,332,000	1
HEALTH MANAGEMENT ASSOCIATES INC	622110	2,560,600	24	283,400	6
HENRY FORD HEALTH SYSTEMS	622110	2,600,000	23		
INTERMOUNTAIN HEALTH CARE	622110	3,266,700	17	893,200	3
JEFFERSON HEALTH SYSTEM	622110	2,499,900	28		
JOHNS HOPKINS MEDICINE	622110	1,600,000	36		
KAISER PERMANENTE	622110	25,300,000	1	996,000	2
MARIAN HEALTH SYSTEMS	622110	2,804,800	20		

Company	Industry Code	2003 Sales (U.S. $ thousands)	Sales Rank	2003 Profits (U.S. $ thousands)	Profits Rank
MAYO FOUNDATION FOR MEDICAL EDUCATION AND RESEARCH	622110	4,822,200	11	348,900	5
MEDCATH CORPORATION	622110	542,986	42	-60,306	19
MEDSTAR HEALTH	622110	2,250,000	30		
MEMORIAL HERMANN HEALTHCARE SYSTEM	622110	2,500,000	26		
MEMORIAL SLOAN KETTERING CANCER CENTER	622110	1,317,700	39	422,700	4
NEW YORK CITY HEALTH AND HOSPITALS CORPORATION	622110	4,200,000	13		
NEW YORK-PRESBYTERIAN HEALTHCARE SYSTEM	622110	7,060,000	6		
OHIOHEALTH CORPORATION	622110	1,036,000	40		
PARTNERS HEALTHCARE SYSTEM	622110	4,561,200	12	85,600	14
PROVIDENCE HEALTH SYSTEM	622110	3,780,200	15	176,600	9
PROVINCE HEALTHCARE CO	622110	761,978	41	31,619	16
SENTARA HEALTHCARE	622110	1,530,000	38		
SISTERS OF MERCY HEALTH SYSTEMS	622110	2,721,900	21		
SPECTRUM HEALTH	622110	1,537,600	37		
SSM HEALTH CARE SYSTEM	622110	1,900,000	33		
ST JUDE CHILDRENS RESEARCH HOSPITAL	622110	450,800	43	17,900	18
SUTTER HEALTH	622110	5,672,000	8		
TENET HEALTHCARE CORP	622110	13,212,000	3	-1,477,000	21
TEXAS HEALTH RESOURCES	622110	1,900,000	34		
TRIAD HOSPITALS INC	622110	3,865,900	14	95,200	12
TRINITY HEALTH COMPANY	622110	4,956,700	10	-235,900	20
UNIVERSAL HEALTH SERVICES	622110	3,643,566	16	199,269	8
Hospitals/Clinics--Psychiatric Clinics					
MAGELLAN HEALTH SERVICES	622210	1,510,746	1	451,770	1
PSYCHIATRIC SOLUTIONS INC	622210	293,665	3	5,216	3
RES CARE INC	622210	961,333	2	13,387	2
In Vitro Diagnostic Substances, Manufacturing					
E-Z-EM INC	325413	133,200	1	2,700	2
MERIDIAN BIOSCIENCE INC	325413	65,864	2	7,018	1
Instrument Manufacturing, including Measurement, Control, Test and Navigational					
ART ADVANCED RESEARCH TECHNOLOGIES	334500	1,003,100	4	148,100	2
METTLER-TOLEDO INTERNATIONAL	334500	1,304,400	3	95,800	3
PERKINELMER INC	334500	1,535,200	2	52,900	4
THERMO ELECTRON CORP	334500	2,097,135	1	200,009	1
Insurance Brokerage and Management					
AON CORPORATION	524210	9,810,000	2	628,000	2
MARSH & MCLENNAN COMPANIES INC	524210	11,588,000	1	1,540,000	1
Insurance-Life					
ASSURANT EMPLOYEE BENEFITS	524113	1,450,000	1		
Insurance-Medical & Health, HMO's and PPO's					
AETNA INC	524114	17,976,400	5	933,800	3
AMERICAN MEDICAL SECURITY GROUP INC	524114	743,716	50	29,310	38
AMERICHOICE CORPORATION	524114				
AMERIGROUP CORPORATION	524114	1,622,234	38	67,324	28
ANTHEM INC	524114	16,771,400	6	774,300	4

Plunkett's Health Care Industry Almanac 2005

Company	Industry Code	2003 Sales (U.S. $ thousands)	Sales Rank	2003 Profits (U.S. $ thousands)	Profits Rank
ARKANSAS BLUE CROSS AND BLUE SHIELD	524114	907,100	47	52,400	33
ASSURANT HEALTH	524114	2,091,000	33		
ASSURANT INC	524114	7,066,213	15	185,652	19
AVMED HEALTH PLAN	524114				
AXA PPP HEALTHCARE	524114	1,200,100	42		
BLUE CARE NETWORK OF MICHIGAN	524114	1,400,000	41	53,100	32
BLUE CROSS AND BLUE SHIELD ASSOCIATION	524114	182,700,000	1		
BLUE CROSS AND BLUE SHIELD OF FLORIDA	524114	5,991,000	18	281,000	10
BLUE CROSS AND BLUE SHIELD OF GEORGIA INC	524114				
BLUE CROSS AND BLUE SHIELD OF KANSAS	524114	1,125,400	43	100,600	26
BLUE CROSS AND BLUE SHIELD OF LOUISIANA	524114				
BLUE CROSS AND BLUE SHIELD OF MASSACHUSETTS	524114	4,300,000	24	232,300	15
BLUE CROSS AND BLUE SHIELD OF MICHIGAN	524114	13,716,000	7	367,700	7
BLUE CROSS AND BLUE SHIELD OF MINNESOTA	524114	5,983,900	19	149,500	24
BLUE CROSS AND BLUE SHIELD OF MONTANA	524114	478,300	53	17,800	40
BLUE CROSS AND BLUE SHIELD OF NEBRASKA	524114	705,600	51	45,800	34
BLUE CROSS AND BLUE SHIELD OF NORTH CAROLINA	524114	3,153,900	26	196,300	18
BLUE CROSS AND BLUE SHIELD OF OKLAHOMA	524114	1,063,900	44		
BLUE CROSS AND BLUE SHIELD OF TENNESSEE INC	524114	1,965,300	35	101,000	25
BLUE CROSS AND BLUE SHIELD OF TEXAS	524114	2,549,000	29		
BLUE CROSS AND BLUE SHIELD OF VERMONT	524114				
BLUE CROSS AND BLUE SHIELD OF WYOMING	524114				
BLUE CROSS OF CALIFORNIA	524114	11,808,600	9		
BLUE CROSS OF IDAHO	524114	660,300	52		
BLUE SHIELD OF CALIFORNIA	524114	6,000,000	17	314,300	9
BRITISH UNION PROVIDENT ASSOCIATION (BUPA)	524114				
CAPITAL BLUECROSS	524114	1,675,000	37		
CAREFIRST INC	524114	7,292,300	14	171,300	20
CENTENE CORPORATION	524114	769,730	49	33,270	37
CIGNA CORP	524114	18,808,000	4	668,000	5
CONCENTRA INC	524114	1,050,700	45	43,300	36
COVENTRY HEALTH CARE INC	524114	4,535,143	23	250,145	12
FIRST CHOICE HEALTH NETWORK INC	524114				
FIRST HEALTH GROUP CORP	524114	890,926	48	152,734	23
GROUP HEALTH COOPERATIVE OF PUGET SOUND	524114	1,966,100	34	155,700	22
GROUP HEALTH INC	524114	2,157,500	31	5,600	41
HARVARD PILGRIM HEALTH CARE INC	524114	2,100,000	32	44,200	35
HEALTH CARE SERVICE CORP	524114	8,190,400	12	624,600	6
HEALTH INSURANCE PLAN OF GREATER NEW YORK	524114	3,369,900	25	274,800	11
HEALTH NET INC	524114	10,959,000	11	234,000	14
HEALTHNOW NEW YORK	524114	1,775,600	36	55,200	31
HIGHMARK INC	524114	8,104,800	13	75,700	27
HORIZON BLUE CROSS BLUE SHIELD OF NEW JERSEY	524114	5,082,400	22	171,100	21
HUMANA INC	524114	12,226,311	8	228,934	16

Company	Industry Code	2003 Sales (U.S. $ thousands)	Sales Rank	2003 Profits (U.S. $ thousands)	Profits Rank
MEDICAL MUTUAL OF OHIO	524114	1,600,000	39		
METROPOLITAN HEALTH NETWORKS	524114	143,874	54	4,402	42
MID ATLANTIC MEDICAL SERVICES INC	524114				
OXFORD HEALTH PLANS INC	524114	5,452,444	20	351,853	8
PACIFICARE HEALTH SYSTEMS	524114	11,008,511	10	242,748	13
PREMERA BLUE CROSS	524114	2,800,000	28	3,300	43
REGENCE GROUP (THE)	524114	6,700,000	16		
SIERRA HEALTH SERVICES	524114	1,485,079	40	62,326	29
TUFTS ASSOCIATED HEALTH PLANS	524114	2,300,000	30	56,900	30
UNIPRISE INCORPORATED	524114	3,107,000	27		
UNITEDHEALTH GROUP INC	524114	28,823,000	2	1,825,000	1
WELLCARE GROUP OF COMPANIES	524114	1,046,000	46	23,500	39
WELLCHOICE INC	524114	5,382,555	21	201,126	17
WELLPOINT HEALTH NETWORKS INC	524114	20,101,500	3	935,200	2
Insurance-Supplemental and Specialty Health					
AFLAC INC	524114A	11,447,000	1	795,000	1
DELTA DENTAL PLANS ASSOCIATION	524114A				
DENTAL BENEFITS PROVIDERS	524114A				
SAFEGUARD HEALTH ENTERPRISES INC	524114A	104,891	3	7,813	2
VISION SERVICE PLAN	524114A	1,970,000	2		
Laboratories and Diagnostics--Medical					
ALLIANCE IMAGING INC	621511	415,283	3	-31,610	9
BIO REFERENCE LABORATORIES INC	621511	109,033	9	6,539	5
CRYOLIFE INC	621511	59,532	10	-32,294	10
HOOPER HOLMES INC	621511	300,182	5	15,847	4
LABONE INC	621511	346,020	4	20,732	3
LABORATORY CORP OF AMERICA HOLDINGS	621511	2,939,400	2	321,000	2
PRIMEDEX HEALTH SYSTEMS	621511	140,259	7	-2,267	6
QUEST DIAGNOSTICS INC	621511	4,737,958	1	436,717	1
RADIOLOGIX INC	621511	257,014	6	-7,963	8
SPECIALTY LABORATORIES INC	621511	119,653	8	-6,361	7
Long-Term Health Care and Assisted Living					
ADVOCAT INC	623110	195,750	11	-11,221	10
ALTERRA HEALTHCARE CORP	623110				
AMERICAN RETIREMENT CORP	623110	368,096	9	-17,314	12
ASSISTED LIVING CONCEPTS	623110	168,012	12	157	8
ATRIA SENIOR LIVING GROUP	623110				
BEVERLY ENTERPRISES INC	623110	1,996,981	3	80,468	2
CAPITAL SENIOR LIVING CORP	623110	66,325	13	4,990	6
EMERITUS CORP	623110	206,657	10	-3,825	9
EXTENDICARE INC	623110	1,338,800	5	47,100	4
HARBORSIDE HEALTHCARE	623110				
KINDRED HEALTHCARE INC	623110	3,284,019	1	-75,336	13
LIFE CARE CENTERS OF AMERICAN	623110				
MANOR CARE INC	623110	3,029,441	2	119,007	1
MARINER HEALTH CARE INC	623110	1,715,400	4	-12,800	11

Company	Industry Code	2003 Sales (U.S. $ thousands)	Sales Rank	2003 Profits (U.S. $ thousands)	Profits Rank
NATIONAL HEALTHCARE CORP	623110	472,864	8	19,952	5
OUTLOOK POINTE CORP	623110				
REGENT ASSISTED LIVING INC	623110	19,100	14		
SUN HEALTHCARE GROUP	623110	834,043	7	354	7
SUNRISE SENIOR LIVING	623110	1,188,300	6	62,200	3
Medical/Dental/Surgical Equipment and Supplies, Distribution					
CARDINAL MEDICAL PRODUCTS AND SERVICES	421450				
CHINDEX INTERNATIONAL INC	421450				
FISHER SCIENTIFIC INTERNATIONAL INC	421450	3,564,400	2	78,400	3
HENRY SCHEIN INC	421450	3,353,805	3	137,501	1
MOORE MEDICAL CORP	421450	141,700	6	-1,500	6
NYER MEDICAL GROUP INC	421450	59,900	7	500	5
OWENS & MINOR INC	421450	4,244,067	1	53,641	4
PATTERSON COMPANIES INC	421450	1,657,000	4	119,700	2
PSS WORLD MEDICAL INC	421450	1,177,900	5	-54,800	7
Medical/Dental/Surgical Equipment and Supplies, Manufacturing					
3M COMPANY	339113	18,232,000	1	2,403,000	1
ABIOMED INC	339113	23,300	130	-18,200	129
ADVANCED BIONICS CORP	339113				
ADVANCED MEDICAL OPTICS	339113	601,453	35	10,357	73
ALIGN TECHNOLOGY	339113	122,725	81	-20,122	130
AMERICAN MEDICAL SYSTEMS HOLDINGS INC	339113	168,283	69	29,050	44
ANALOGIC CORP	339113	471,500	42	49,500	33
ANSELL LIMITED COMPANY	339113	862,961	30	37,291	40
APOGENT TECHNOLOGIES INC	339113	1,097,487	23	-11,746	126
APPLERA CORPORATION	339113	1,777,232	16	118,480	19
ARADIGM CORPORATION	339113	33,857	122	-25,970	131
ARROW INTERNATIONAL INC	339113	380,400	48	45,700	36
ARTHROCARE CORP	339113	118,900	84	7,500	78
ASPECT MEDICAL SYSTEMS	339113	44,091	115	-6,523	120
ATRION CORPORATION	339113	62,800	107	5,100	86
ATS MEDICAL INC	339113	18,484	132	-13,292	127
BAUSCH & LOMB INC	339113	2,019,500	13	125,500	18
BAXTER INTERNATIONAL INC	339113	8,916,000	3	881,000	3
BECKMAN COULTER INC	339113	2,192,500	10	207,200	14
BECTON DICKINSON & CO	339113	4,527,940	5	547,056	4
BESPAK PLC	339113	140,800	75	4,400	90
BIO RAD LABORATORIES INC	339113	1,003,382	27	76,171	22
BIOMET INC	339113	1,390,300	20	286,700	10
BIOPHAN TECHNOLOGIES INC	339113	0		-3,438	117
BOSTON SCIENTIFIC CORP	339113	3,476,000	8	472,000	5
CANDELA CORP	339113	80,800	99	6,800	79
CANTEL MEDICAL CORP	339113	129,300	80	7,900	76
CARDIOGENESIS CORP	339113	13,518	134	-348	105
CENTERPULSE AG	339113				
CHOLESTECH CORP	339113	48,500	112	4,900	89

Company	Industry Code	2003 Sales (U.S. $ thousands)	Sales Rank	2003 Profits (U.S. $ thousands)	Profits Rank
CIVCO MEDICAL INSTRUMENTS	339113				
CNS INC	339113	79,100	100	6,500	81
COCHLEAR LTD	339113				
COHERENT INC	339113	406,235	44	-45,891	133
COMPEX TECHNOLOGIES INC	339113	75,500	103	5,000	87
CONMED CORP	339113	497,100	39	32,100	42
CONVATEC	339113				
COOPER COMPANIES INC	339113	411,790	43	68,770	24
CORDIS CORP	339113				
CR BARD INC	339113	1,433,100	19	233,000	13
CRITICARE SYSTEMS INC	339113	28,600	127	-900	111
CTI MOLECULAR IMAGING	339113	362,289	49	20,563	57
CYBERONICS INC	339113	104,500	90	5,200	85
DADE BEHRING HOLDINGS INC	339113	1,436,400	18	48,100	34
DATASCOPE CORP	339113	328,300	54	23,300	52
DENTSPLY INTERNATIONAL INC	339113	1,570,925	17	174,183	15
DEPUY INC	339113				
DIAGNOSTIC PRODUCTS CORP	339113	381,386	47	61,795	27
DIGENE CORPORATION	339113	63,100	105	-4,300	118
DJ ORTHOPEDICS INC	339113	197,939	64	12,071	68
EDWARDS LIFESCIENCES	339113	860,500	31	79,000	21
EMERGENCY FILTRATION PRODUCTS INC	339113	764	135	-706	109
EMPI INC	339113	150,300	71	13,300	64
ENCORE MEDICAL CORP	339113	108,059	86	-2,517	115
ENVIRONMENTAL TECTONICS	339113	43,100	116	2,500	96
ESSILOR INTERNATIONAL SA	339113	2,656,500	9	251,500	12
ETHICON INC	339113				
EXACTECH INC	339113	71,255	104	6,501	80
EXCEL TECHNOLOGY INC	339113	122,681	82	11,318	70
FISCHER IMAGING CORP	339113	46,200	114	-14,400	128
GE HEALTHCARE	339113	10,200,000	2		
GISH BIOMEDICAL INC	339113				
GSI LUMONICS INC	339113	185,561	65	-2,170	113
GUIDANT CORP	339113	3,698,000	6	330,300	9
GYRUS GROUP	339113	138,900	76	10,600	72
HAEMONETICS CORPORATION	339113	337,000	51	28,400	45
HILLENBRAND INDUSTRIES	339113	2,042,000	12	138,000	16
HILL-ROM COMPANY INC	339113	1,067,000	24		
HOLOGIC INC	339113	204,035	62	2,882	93
HUNTLEIGH TECHNOLOGIES	339113	332,800	52	27,500	46
I FLOW CORPORATION	339113	47,043	113	457	100
ICU MEDICAL INC	339113	107,354	87	22,297	54
IDEXX LABORATORIES INC	339113	475,992	41	57,090	30
IMMUCOR INC	339113	98,300	93	14,400	62
INAMED CORP	339113	332,600	53	53,000	32
INSTITUT STRAUMANN AG	339113	269,400	58	62,900	26
INSTRUMENTARIUM CORP	339113				

Company	Industry Code	2003 Sales (U.S. $ thousands)	Sales Rank	2003 Profits (U.S. $ thousands)	Profits Rank
INTEGRA LIFESCIENCES HOLDINGS CORP	339113	166,695	70	26,861	48
INTUITIVE SURGICAL INC	339113	91,675	96	-9,623	124
INVACARE CORP	339113	1,247,176	22	71,409	23
INVERNESS MEDICAL INNOVATIONS INC	339113	296,712	56	12,269	67
IRIDEX CORP	339113	31,699	124	371	102
IRIS INTERNATIONAL INC	339113	31,345	125	-530	108
I-STAT CORP	339113				
KINETIC CONCEPTS INC	339113	763,800	32	60,200	28
KYPHON INC	339113	131,028	79	27,323	47
LAKELAND INDUSTRIES INC	339113	77,800	101	2,600	94
LASERSCOPE	339113	57,427	109	2,517	95
LIFECORE BIOMEDICAL INC	339113	42,400	117	-400	106
LIFESCAN INC	339113	1,004,000	26		
LUMENIS LTD	339113				
MALLINCKRODT INC	339113				
MDS INC	339113	1,364,000	21	36,000	41
MEDEX HOLDINGS CORP	339113	219,100	60	-7,400	121
MEDICAL ACTION INDUSTRIES	339113	104,800	89	8,200	75
MEDICORE INC	339113	32,110	123	273	103
MEDSOURCE TECHNOLOGIES	339113	177,300	68	-35,300	132
MEDTRONIC INC	339113	7,665,200	4	1,599,800	2
MEDTRONIC MINIMED INC	339113				
MEDTRONIC SOFAMOR DANEK	339113				
MEDTRONIC VASCULAR	339113				
MEDTRONIC XOMED SURGICAL PRODUCTS INC	339113				
MENTOR CORP	339113	382,400	46	55,900	31
MERIDIAN MEDICAL TECHNOLOGIES INC	339113				
MERIT MEDICAL SYSTEMS INC	339113	135,954	77	17,295	60
MICROTEK MEDICAL HOLDINGS	339113	98,664	92	16,023	61
MINE SAFETY APPLIANCES CO	339113	698,197	33	65,267	25
MINNTECH CORP	339113				
MISONIX INC	339113	34,900	120	1,000	98
MIV THERAPEUTICS INC	339113	0		-3,200	116
MOLECULAR DEVICES CORP	339113	115,581	85	7,742	77
NATIONAL DENTEX CORP	339113	99,274	91	5,757	84
NEKTAR THERAPEUTICS	339113	106,257	88	-65,890	134
NMT MEDICAL INC	339113	22,961	131	-1,150	112
NOVAMETRIX MEDICAL SYSTEMS INC	339113				
NOVOSTE CORPORATION	339113	62,901	106	-868	110
OCULAR SCIENCES INC	339113	310,563	55	26,554	49
ORTHOFIX INTERNATIONAL NV	339113	203,707	63	24,730	51
OSTEOTECH INC	339113	94,433	95	10,867	71
PALOMAR MEDICAL TECHNOLOGIES INC	339113	34,773	121	3,369	92
PHILIPS MEDICAL SYSTEMS	339113				
POLYMEDICA CORPORATION	339113	356,200	50	25,600	50
QUIDEL CORP	339113	95,105	94	19,651	58
RESMED INC	339113	273,600	57	45,700	37

Company	Industry Code	2003 Sales (U.S. $ thousands)	Sales Rank	2003 Profits (U.S. $ thousands)	Profits Rank
RESPIRONICS INC	339113	629,800	34	46,600	35
RITA MEDICAL SYSTEMS INC	339113	16,607	133	-11,079	125
ROTECH HEALTHCARE INC	339113	581,221	36	8,413	74
SCHICK TECHNOLOGIES INC	339113	29,817	126	11,825	69
SIEMENS MEDICAL SOLUTIONS	339113				
SMITH & NEPHEW PLC	339113	2,102,500	11	264,100	11
SOLA INTERNATIONAL INC	339113	562,700	37	3,966	91
SONIC INNOVATIONS INC	339113	87,690	97	376	101
SPAN AMERICA MEDICAL SYSTEMS INC	339113	41,575	118	1,399	97
SPECTRANETICS CORP	339113	27,869	128	929	99
SRI/SURGICAL EXPRESS INC	339113	86,474	98	-499	107
SSL INTERNATIONAL	339113	982,000	28	39,000	39
ST JUDE MEDICAL INC	339113	1,932,500	14	339,400	8
STAAR SURGICAL CO	339113	50,458	111	-8,357	122
STERIS CORP	339113	972,100	29	79,400	20
STRYKER CORP	339113	3,625,300	7	453,500	6
SUNRISE MEDICAL INC	339113				
SYBRON DENTAL SPECIALTIES	339113	526,391	38	57,452	29
SYMMETRY MEDICAL INC	339113	122,000	83	5,900	83
SYNOVIS LIFE TECHNOLOGIES	339113	58,000	108	5,000	88
TECHNE CORP	339113	145,000	73	45,400	38
THERAGENICS CORP	339113	35,600	119	-300	104
THERASENSE INC	339113	210,900	61	-4,800	119
THORATEC CORPORATION	339113	149,916	72	-2,182	114
TRIPATH IMAGING INC	339113	53,764	110	-8,538	123
TYCO HEALTHCARE GROUP	339113				
UROCOR INC	339113				
UTAH MEDICAL PRODUCTS INC	339113	27,137	129	20,761	56
UTI CORPORATION	339113				
VARIAN MEDICAL SYSTEMS INC	339113	1,041,600	25	130,900	17
VENTANA MEDICAL SYSTEMS	339113	132,380	78	5,972	82
VIASYS HEALTHCARE INC	339113	394,947	45	21,586	55
VISX INC	339113	143,905	74	23,251	53
VITAL SIGNS INC	339113	182,163	67	14,222	63
WELCH ALLYN INC	339113				
WEST PHARMACEUTICAL SERVICES INC	339113	490,700	40	31,900	43
WRIGHT MEDICAL GROUP INC	339113	248,932	59	17,397	59
YOUNG INNOVATIONS INC	339113	76,156	102	13,201	65
ZIMMER HOLDINGS INC	339113	1,901,000	15	346,300	7
ZLB BEHRING LLC	339113				
ZOLL MEDICAL CORP	339113	184,603	66	12,850	66
Online Business-to-Business or to-Consumer Intermediary					
WEBMD CORPORATION	514199A	963,980	1	-17,006	1
Online Publishing, Services and Niche Portals					
HEALTH GRADES INC	514199	8,805	1	-1,284	1

Plunkett's Health Care Industry Almanac 2005   155

Company	Industry Code	2003 Sales (U.S. $ thousands)	Sales Rank	2003 Profits (U.S. $ thousands)	Profits Rank
Optical Goods Stores					
COLE NATIONAL CORP	446130	1,148,100	1	-5,100	2
EMERGING VISION INC	446130	13,980	3	-2,967	1
US VISION INC	446130	172,100	2		
Optical Instrument and Lens, Manufacturing					
LUXOTTICA GROUP SPA	333314	3,551,100	1	336,100	1
SIGNATURE EYEWEAR INC	333314	24,420	2	3,463	2
Other Health and Personal Care Stores/Weight Management					
JENNY CRAIG INC	446190	280,000	2		
WEIGHT WATCHERS INTERNATIONAL INC	446190	943,932	1	143,941	1
Payment and Transaction Processing Services					
HEALTH MANAGEMENT SYSTEMS INC	522320	74,400	1	2,300	1
PLANVISTA CORP	522320	33,100	2		
Payment and Transaction Processing--Benefits Management					
ADVANCEPCS INC	522320A	14,110,900	2	168,400	3
EXPRESS SCRIPTS INC	522320A	13,294,517	3	249,600	2
MEDCO HEALTH SOLUTIONS	522320A	34,264,500	1	425,800	1
MIM CORP	522320A	588,770	4	9,130	4
NATIONAL MEDICAL HEALTH CARD SYSTEMS INC	522320A	573,300	5	6,400	5
Pharmacies and Drug Stores					
CVS CORPORATION	446110	26,588,000	2	847,300	2
DUANE READE INC	446110	1,383,828	5	5,074	4
LONGS DRUG STORES CORPORATION	446110	4,426,300	4	6,700	3
RITE AID CORPORATION	446110	15,800,900	3	-112,100	5
WALGREEN CO	446110	32,505,400	1	1,175,700	1
Pharmacies-Specialty					
ACCREDO HEALTH INC	446110A	1,337,400	5	29,500	5
CAREMARK RX INC	446110A	9,067,291	1	290,838	1
NEIGHBORCARE INC	446110A	2,649,000	3	32,700	4
OMNICARE INC	446110A	3,499,174	2	194,368	2
PRIORITY HEALTHCARE CORP	446110A	1,461,811	4	50,600	3
Physician Practice Management					
AMERIPATH INC	621111	485,000	4	23,400	6
CASTLE DENTAL CENTERS INC	621111	93,889	8	26,104	5
COAST DENTAL SERVICES INC	621111	56,416	10	-2,986	9
INTEGRAMED AMERICA INC	621111	93,690	9	1,044	7
LOGISTICARE INC	621111	180,000	7		
MONARCH DENTAL CORP	621111				
ORTHODONTIC CENTERS OF AMERICA INC	621111	375,380	6	49,065	3
PEDIATRIX MEDICAL GROUP INC	621111	551,197	3	84,328	1
TEAM HEALTH	621111	1,479,000	2	-2,800	8
UNITED SURGICAL PARTNERS	621111	446,269	5	29,876	4
US ONCOLOGY INC	621111	1,965,725	1	70,656	2
Research and Development--Physical, Engineering and Life Sciences					
AAIPHARMA INC	541710	282,700	5	34,300	5
APPLIED BIOSYSTEMS GROUP	541710	1,682,900	2	183,200	2

Company	Industry Code	2003 Sales (U.S. $ thousands)	Sales Rank	2003 Profits (U.S. $ thousands)	Profits Rank
ARQULE INC	541710	65,500	9	-34,800	8
CELERA GENOMICS GROUP	541710	88,300	8	-81,900	10
COVANCE INC	541710	974,210	3	76,136	3
HUMAN GENOME SCIENCES	541710	8,168	12	-185,324	12
INCYTE CORP	541710	47,092	10	-166,463	11
KENDLE INTERNATIONAL INC	541710	209,657	6	-1,690	6
MAXYGEN INC	541710	30,528	11	-44,964	9
PHARMACEUTICAL PRODUCT DEVELOPMENT INC	541710	726,983	4	46,310	4
PHARMACOPEIA INC	541710	115,064	7	-3,497	7
QUINTILES TRANSNATIONAL	541710	2,046,000	1	297,000	1
Superconducting Materials and Other Wire					
INTERMAGNETICS GENERAL	335929	147,400	1	14,900	1
Telecommunications Services-Specialty					
LIFELINE SYSTEMS INC	513390D	116,159	1	10,259	
SHL TELEMEDICINE	513390D				
Utilization Management, Health Care					
CORVEL CORP	621999	282,800	1	16,600	1
Veterinary Clinics					
VCA ANTECH INC	541940	544,665	1	43,423	1

ALPHABETICAL INDEX

3M COMPANY
AAIPHARMA INC
ABBOTT LABORATORIES
ABIOMED INC
ACCREDO HEALTH INC
ADVANCED BIONICS CORPORATION
ADVANCED MEDICAL OPTICS INC
ADVANCEPCS INC
ADVENTIST HEALTH SYSTEM
ADVOCAT INC
ADVOCATE HEALTH CARE
AETERNA ZENTARIS INC
AETNA INC
AFLAC INC
ALCON INC
ALIGN TECHNOLOGY
ALLERGAN INC
ALLIANCE IMAGING INC
ALLIED HEALTHCARE INTERNATIONAL INC
ALLINA HOSPITALS AND CLINICS
ALPHARMA INC
ALTERRA HEALTHCARE CORP
AMEDISYS INC
AMERICA SERVICE GROUP INC
AMERICAN HEALTHWAYS INC
AMERICAN HOMEPATIENT INC
AMERICAN MEDICAL SECURITY GROUP INC
AMERICAN MEDICAL SYSTEMS HOLDINGS INC
AMERICAN PHARMACEUTICAL PARTNERS INC
AMERICAN RETIREMENT CORP
AMERICAN SHARED HOSPITAL SERVICES
AMERICHOICE CORPORATION
AMERIGROUP CORPORATION
AMERIPATH INC
AMERISOURCEBERGEN CORP
AMGEN INC
AMSURG CORP
ANALOGIC CORP
ANDRX CORP
ANSELL LIMITED COMPANY
ANTHEM INC
AON CORPORATION
APOGENT TECHNOLOGIES INC
APPLERA CORPORATION
APPLIED BIOSYSTEMS GROUP
APRIA HEALTHCARE GROUP INC
ARADIGM CORPORATION
ARKANSAS BLUE CROSS AND BLUE SHIELD
ARQULE INC
ARROW INTERNATIONAL INC
ART ADVANCED RESEARCH TECHNOLOGIES
ARTHROCARE CORP
ASCENSION HEALTH
ASPECT MEDICAL SYSTEMS INC
ASSISTED LIVING CONCEPTS INC
ASSURANT EMPLOYEE BENEFITS
ASSURANT HEALTH
ASSURANT INC
ATC HEALTHCARE INC
ATRIA SENIOR LIVING GROUP
ATRION CORPORATION
ATS MEDICAL INC
AVENTIS SA
AVERA HEALTH
AVMED HEALTH PLAN
AXA PPP HEALTHCARE
BANNER HEALTH
BARR LABORATORIES INC
BAUSCH & LOMB INC
BAXTER INTERNATIONAL INC
BAYER AG
BAYER CORP
BECKMAN COULTER INC
BECTON DICKINSON & CO
BESPAK PLC
BEVERLY ENTERPRISES INC
BIO RAD LABORATORIES INC
BIO REFERENCE LABORATORIES INC
BIOGEN IDEC INC
BIOMET INC
BIOPHAN TECHNOLOGIES INC
BIOVAIL CORPORATION
BJC HEALTHCARE
BLUE CARE NETWORK OF MICHIGAN
BLUE CROSS AND BLUE SHIELD ASSOCIATION
BLUE CROSS AND BLUE SHIELD OF FLORIDA
BLUE CROSS AND BLUE SHIELD OF GEORGIA INC
BLUE CROSS AND BLUE SHIELD OF KANSAS
BLUE CROSS AND BLUE SHIELD OF LOUISIANA
BLUE CROSS AND BLUE SHIELD OF MASSACHUSETTS
BLUE CROSS AND BLUE SHIELD OF MICHIGAN
BLUE CROSS AND BLUE SHIELD OF MINNESOTA
BLUE CROSS AND BLUE SHIELD OF MONTANA
BLUE CROSS AND BLUE SHIELD OF NEBRASKA
BLUE CROSS AND BLUE SHIELD OF NORTH CAROLINA
BLUE CROSS AND BLUE SHIELD OF OKLAHOMA
BLUE CROSS AND BLUE SHIELD OF TENNESSEE INC
BLUE CROSS AND BLUE SHIELD OF TEXAS
BLUE CROSS AND BLUE SHIELD OF VERMONT
BLUE CROSS AND BLUE SHIELD OF WYOMING
BLUE CROSS OF CALIFORNIA
BLUE CROSS OF IDAHO
BLUE SHIELD OF CALIFORNIA
BON SECOURS HEALTH SYSTEM INC
BOSTON SCIENTIFIC CORP
BRISTOL MYERS SQUIBB CO
BRITISH UNION PROVIDENT ASSOCIATION (BUPA)
CAMBREX CORP
CANDELA CORP
CANTEL MEDICAL CORP
CAPITAL BLUECROSS
CAPITAL SENIOR LIVING CORP
CARDINAL HEALTH INC
CARDINAL MEDICAL PRODUCTS AND SERVICES
CARDIOGENESIS CORP
CAREFIRST INC
CAREMARK RX INC
CASTLE DENTAL CENTERS INC
CATHOLIC HEALTH INITIATIVES
CATHOLIC HEALTHCARE PARTNERS
CATHOLIC HEALTHCARE WEST
CEDARA SOFTWARE CORP
CELERA GENOMICS GROUP
CELLTECH GROUP PLC
CENTENE CORPORATION
CENTERPULSE AG
CEPHALON INC
CERNER CORP
CHINDEX INTERNATIONAL INC
CHIRON CORP
CHOLESTECH CORP
CHRISTUS HEALTH
CIGNA CORP
CIVCO MEDICAL INSTRUMENTS
CLARIAN HEALTH PARTNERS INC
CNS INC
COAST DENTAL SERVICES INC
COCHLEAR LTD
COHERENT INC
COLE NATIONAL CORPORATION
COMMUNITY HEALTH SYSTEMS INC
COMPEX TECHNOLOGIES INC
CONCENTRA INC
CONMED CORP
CONTINUCARE CORP
CONVATEC
COOPER COMPANIES INC
CORDIS CORP
CORVEL CORP
COVANCE INC
COVENTRY HEALTH CARE INC
CR BARD INC
CRITICARE SYSTEMS INC
CRYOLIFE INC
CTI MOLECULAR IMAGING
CURATIVE HEALTH SERVICES INC
CVS CORPORATION
CYBERONICS INC
D & K HEALTHCARE RESOURCES INC
DADE BEHRING HOLDINGS INC

DATASCOPE CORP
DAVITA INC
DELTA DENTAL PLANS ASSOCIATION
DENTAL BENEFITS PROVIDERS
DENTSPLY INTERNATIONAL INC
DEPUY INC
DETROIT MEDICAL CENTER
DIAGNOSTIC PRODUCTS CORPORATION
DIGENE CORPORATION
DJ ORTHOPEDICS INC
DRUGMAX INC
DUANE READE INC
DYNACQ HEALTHCARE INC
ECLIPSYS CORPORATION
EDWARDS LIFESCIENCES CORP
ELAN CORP PLC
ELI LILLY & CO
EMERGENCY FILTRATION PRODUCTS INC
EMERGING VISION INC
EMERITUS CORP
EMPI INC
ENCORE MEDICAL CORPORATION
ENDO PHARMACEUTICALS HOLDINGS INC
ENVIRONMENTAL TECTONICS CORP
EON LABS INC
EPIC SYSTEMS CORPORATION
ERESEARCH TECHNOLOGY INC
ESSILOR INTERNATIONAL SA
ETHICON INC
EXACTECH INC
EXCEL TECHNOLOGY INC
EXPRESS SCRIPTS INC
EXTENDICARE INC
E-Z-EM INC
FAIRVIEW HEALTH SERVICES
FIRST CHOICE HEALTH NETWORK INC
FIRST CONSULTING GROUP INC
FIRST HEALTH GROUP CORP
FISCHER IMAGING CORP
FISHER SCIENTIFIC INTERNATIONAL INC
FOREST LABORATORIES INC
FRESENIUS AG
FUJISAWA PHARMACEUTICALS COMPANY LTD
GAMBRO AB
GE COMMERCIAL FINANCE
GE HEALTHCARE
GENENTECH INC
GENERAL NUTRITION COMPANIES INC
GENTIVA HEALTH SERVICES INC
GENZYME CORP
GISH BIOMEDICAL INC
GLAXOSMITHKLINE PLC
GROUP HEALTH COOPERATIVE OF PUGET SOUND
GROUP HEALTH INCORPORATED
GSI LUMONICS INC

GTC BIOTHERAPEUTICS INC
GUIDANT CORP
GYRUS GROUP
HAEMONETICS CORPORATION
HANGER ORTHOPEDIC GROUP INC
HARBORSIDE HEALTHCARE CORP
HARVARD PILGRIM HEALTH CARE INC
HCA INC
HEALTH CARE SERVICE CORPORATION
HEALTH FITNESS CORP
HEALTH GRADES INC
HEALTH INSURANCE PLAN OF GREATER NEW YORK
HEALTH MANAGEMENT ASSOCIATES INC
HEALTH MANAGEMENT SYSTEMS INC
HEALTH NET INC
HEALTHAXIS INC
HEALTHNOW NEW YORK
HEALTHSOUTH CORP
HEALTHSTREAM INC
HEALTHTRONICS INC
HEARUSA INC
HEMACARE CORPORATION
HENRY FORD HEALTH SYSTEMS
HENRY SCHEIN INC
HIGHMARK INC
HILLENBRAND INDUSTRIES
HILL-ROM COMPANY INC
HOLOGIC INC
HOOPER HOLMES INC
HORIZON BLUE CROSS BLUE SHIELD OF NEW JERSEY
HORIZON HEALTH CORPORATION
HOSPIRA INC
HUMAN GENOME SCIENCES INC
HUMANA INC
HUNTLEIGH TECHNOLOGIES PLC
I FLOW CORPORATION
ICU MEDICAL INC
IDEXX LABORATORIES INC
IDX SYSTEMS CORP
IMMUCOR INC
IMPATH INC
IMS HEALTH INC
INAMED CORP
INCYTE CORP
INSTITUT STRAUMANN AG
INSTRUMENTARIUM CORPORATION
INTEGRA LIFESCIENCES HOLDINGS CORP
INTEGRAMED AMERICA INC
INTERMAGNETICS GENERAL CORP
INTERMOUNTAIN HEALTH CARE
INTERPORE CROSS INTERNATIONAL
INTUITIVE SURGICAL INC
INVACARE CORP
INVERNESS MEDICAL INNOVATIONS INC
IRIDEX CORP

IRIS INTERNATIONAL INC
I-STAT CORP
JEFFERSON HEALTH SYSTEM INC
JENNY CRAIG INC
JOHNS HOPKINS MEDICINE
JOHNSON & JOHNSON
KAISER PERMANENTE
KENDLE INTERNATIONAL INC
KIMBERLY CLARK CORP
KINDRED HEALTHCARE INC
KINETIC CONCEPTS INC
KYPHON INC
LABONE INC
LABORATORY CORP OF AMERICA HOLDINGS
LAKELAND INDUSTRIES INC
LASERSCOPE
LCA VISION INC
LIFE CARE CENTERS OF AMERICA
LIFECELL CORPORATION
LIFECORE BIOMEDICAL INC
LIFELINE SYSTEMS INC
LIFESCAN INC
LOGISTICARE INC
LONGS DRUG STORES CORPORATION
LUMENIS LTD
LUXOTTICA GROUP SPA
MAGELLAN HEALTH SERVICES INC
MALLINCKRODT INC
MANOR CARE INC
MARIAN HEALTH SYSTEMS
MARINER HEALTH CARE INC
MARSH & MCLENNAN COMPANIES INC
MATRIA HEALTHCARE INC
MAXYGEN INC
MAYO FOUNDATION FOR MEDICAL EDUCATION AND RESEARCH
MCKESSON CORPORATION
MDS INC
MEDCATH CORPORATION
MEDCO HEALTH SOLUTIONS
MEDEX HOLDINGS CORPORATION
MEDICAL ACTION INDUSTRIES INC
MEDICAL MUTUAL OF OHIO
MEDICORE INC
MEDQUIST INC
MEDSTAR HEALTH
MEDTRONIC INC
MEDTRONIC MINIMED INC
MEDTRONIC SOFAMOR DANEK
MEDTRONIC VASCULAR
MEDTRONIC XOMED SURGICAL PRODUCTS INC
MEMORIAL HERMANN HEALTHCARE SYSTEM
MEMORIAL SLOAN KETTERING CANCER CENTER
MENTOR CORP
MERCK & CO INC
MERIDIAN BIOSCIENCE INC
MERIDIAN MEDICAL TECHNOLOGIES INC
MERIT MEDICAL SYSTEMS INC

METROPOLITAN HEALTH NETWORKS
METTLER-TOLEDO INTERNATIONAL
MICROTEK MEDICAL HOLDINGS INC
MID ATLANTIC MEDICAL SERVICES INC
MILLENNIUM PHARMACEUTICALS INC
MIM CORP
MINE SAFETY APPLIANCES CO
MINNTECH CORP
MISONIX INC
MIV THERAPEUTICS INC
MOLECULAR DEVICES CORP
MONARCH DENTAL CORP
MOORE MEDICAL CORP
MORRISON MANAGEMENT SPECIALISTS INC
MYLAN LABORATORIES INC
NANOBIO CORPORATION
NATIONAL DENTEX CORP
NATIONAL HEALTHCARE CORP
NATIONAL HOME HEALTH CARE CORP
NATIONAL MEDICAL HEALTH CARD SYSTEMS INC
NEIGHBORCARE INC
NEKTAR THERAPEUTICS
NEW YORK CITY HEALTH AND HOSPITALS CORPORATION
NEW YORK HEALTH CARE INC
NEW YORK-PRESBYTERIAN HEALTHCARE SYSTEM
NMT MEDICAL INC
NOVAMED INC
NOVAMETRIX MEDICAL SYSTEMS INC
NOVARTIS AG
NOVATION LLC
NOVO-NORDISK AS
NOVOSTE CORPORATION
NYER MEDICAL GROUP INC
OCA INC
OCCUPATIONAL HEALTH + REHABILITATION INC
OCULAR SCIENCES INC
ODYSSEY HEALTHCARE INC
OHIOHEALTH CORPORATION
OMNICARE INC
OPTICARE HEALTH SYSTEMS
OPTION CARE INC
ORGANOGENESIS INC
ORTHOFIX INTERNATIONAL NV
OSTEOTECH INC
OUTLOOK POINTE CORP
OWENS & MINOR INC
OXFORD HEALTH PLANS INC
PACIFICARE HEALTH SYSTEMS INC
PALOMAR MEDICAL TECHNOLOGIES INC
PAR PHARMACEUTICAL COMPANIES INC
PARTNERS HEALTHCARE SYSTEM

PATIENT CARE INC
PATTERSON COMPANIES INC
PDI INC
PEDIATRIC SERVICES OF AMERICA INC
PEDIATRIX MEDICAL GROUP INC
PER SE TECHNOLOGIES INC
PERKINELMER INC
PETMED EXPRESS INC
PFIZER INC
PHARMACEUTICAL PRODUCT DEVELOPMENT INC
PHARMACOPEIA INC
PHC INC
PHILIPS MEDICAL SYSTEMS
PLANVISTA CORP
POLYMEDICA CORPORATION
PREMERA BLUE CROSS
PREMIER INC
PRIMEDEX HEALTH SYSTEMS INC
PRIORITY HEALTHCARE CORP
PROVIDENCE HEALTH SYSTEM
PROVINCE HEALTHCARE CO
PSS WORLD MEDICAL INC
PSYCHIATRIC SOLUTIONS INC
QUALITY SYSTEMS INC
QUEST DIAGNOSTICS INC
QUIDEL CORP
QUINTILES TRANSNATIONAL CORP
QUOVADX INC
RADIOLOGIX INC
REGENCE GROUP (THE)
REGENT ASSISTED LIVING INC
REHABCARE GROUP INC
RENAL CARE GROUP INC
RES CARE INC
RESMED INC
RESPIRONICS INC
RITA MEDICAL SYSTEMS INC
RITE AID CORPORATION
ROCHE GROUP
ROTECH HEALTHCARE INC
SAFEGUARD HEALTH ENTERPRISES INC
SANOFI-SYNTHELABO
SCHERING AG
SCHERING-PLOUGH CORP
SCHICK TECHNOLOGIES INC
SENTARA HEALTHCARE
SEPRACOR INC
SEROLOGICALS CORP
SERONO SA
SHIRE PHARMACEUTICALS PLC
SHL TELEMEDICINE
SIEMENS MEDICAL SOLUTIONS
SIERRA HEALTH SERVICES INC
SIGMA ALDRICH CORP
SIGNATURE EYEWEAR INC
SISTERS OF MERCY HEALTH SYSTEMS
SMITH & NEPHEW PLC
SOLA INTERNATIONAL INC
SOLUCIENT LLC
SONIC INNOVATIONS INC

SPAN AMERICA MEDICAL SYSTEMS INC
SPECIALTY LABORATORIES INC
SPECTRANETICS CORP
SPECTRUM HEALTH
SRI/SURGICAL EXPRESS INC
SSL INTERNATIONAL
SSM HEALTH CARE SYSTEM INC
ST JUDE CHILDRENS RESEARCH HOSPITAL
ST JUDE MEDICAL INC
STAAR SURGICAL CO
STERIS CORP
STRYKER CORP
SUN HEALTHCARE GROUP
SUNRISE MEDICAL INC
SUNRISE SENIOR LIVING
SUPERIOR CONSULTANT HOLDINGS CORP
SUTTER HEALTH
SYBRON DENTAL SPECIALTIES INC
SYMMETRY MEDICAL INC
SYNOVIS LIFE TECHNOLOGIES INC
TEAM HEALTH
TECHNE CORP
TELEX COMMUNICATIONS INC
TENET HEALTHCARE CORPORATION
TEVA PHARMACEUTICAL INDUSTRIES
TEXAS HEALTH RESOURCES
THERAGENICS CORP
THERASENSE INC
THERMO ELECTRON CORP
THORATEC CORPORATION
TLC VISION CORPORATION
TOSHIBA CORPORATION
TRANSCEND SERVICES INC
TRIAD HOSPITALS INC
TRINITY HEALTH COMPANY
TRIPATH IMAGING INC
TRIPOS INC
TUFTS ASSOCIATED HEALTH PLANS
TYCO HEALTHCARE GROUP
UNIPRISE INCORPORATED
UNITED SURGICAL PARTNERS
UNITEDHEALTH GROUP INC
UNIVERSAL HEALTH SERVICES INC
UNIVERSAL HOSPITAL SERVICES INC
UROCOR INC
US ONCOLOGY INC
US PHYSICAL THERAPY INC
US VISION INC
UTAH MEDICAL PRODUCTS INC
UTI CORPORATION
VALEANT PHARMACEUTICALS INTERNATIONAL
VARIAN MEDICAL SYSTEMS INC
VCA ANTECH INC
VENTANA MEDICAL SYSTEMS
VENTIV HEALTH INC
VIASYS HEALTHCARE INC
VISION SERVICE PLAN

VISX INC
VITAL SIGNS INC
VITALWORKS INC
WALGREEN CO
WARNER CHILCOTT PLC
WATSON PHARMACEUTICALS INC
WEBMD CORPORATION

WEIGHT WATCHERS INTERNATIONAL INC
WELCH ALLYN INC
WELLCARE GROUP OF COMPANIES
WELLCHOICE INC
WELLPOINT HEALTH NETWORKS INC

WEST PHARMACEUTICAL SERVICES INC
WRIGHT MEDICAL GROUP INC
WYETH
YOUNG INNOVATIONS INC
ZIMMER HOLDINGS INC
ZLB BEHRING LLC
ZOLL MEDICAL CORP

INDEX OF HEADQUARTERS LOCATION BY U.S. STATE

To help you locate members of THE HEALTH CARE 500 geographically, the city and state of the headquarters of each company are in the following index.

ALABAMA
HEALTHSOUTH CORP; Birmingham

ARIZONA
BANNER HEALTH; Phoenix
VENTANA MEDICAL SYSTEMS; Tucson

ARKANSAS
ARKANSAS BLUE CROSS AND BLUE SHIELD; Little Rock
BEVERLY ENTERPRISES INC; Ft. Smith

CALIFORNIA
ADVANCED BIONICS CORPORATION; Sylmar
ADVANCED MEDICAL OPTICS INC; Santa Ana
ALIGN TECHNOLOGY; Santa Clara
ALLERGAN INC; Irvine
ALLIANCE IMAGING INC; Anaheim
AMERICAN SHARED HOSPITAL SERVICES; San Francisco
AMGEN INC; Thousand Oaks
APPLIED BIOSYSTEMS GROUP; Foster City
APRIA HEALTHCARE GROUP INC; Lake Forest
ARADIGM CORPORATION; Hayward
ARTHROCARE CORP; Sunnyvale
BECKMAN COULTER INC; Fullerton
BIO RAD LABORATORIES INC; Hercules
BLUE CROSS OF CALIFORNIA; Thousand Oaks
BLUE SHIELD OF CALIFORNIA; San Francisco
CARDIOGENESIS CORP; Foothill Ranch
CATHOLIC HEALTHCARE WEST; San Francisco
CHIRON CORP; Emeryville
CHOLESTECH CORP; Hayward
COHERENT INC; Santa Clara
COOPER COMPANIES INC; Pleasanton
CORVEL CORP; Irvine
DAVITA INC; El Segundo
DIAGNOSTIC PRODUCTS CORPORATION; Los Angeles
DJ ORTHOPEDICS INC; Vista
EDWARDS LIFESCIENCES CORP; Irvine
FIRST CONSULTING GROUP INC ; Long Beach
GENENTECH INC; South San Francisco
GISH BIOMEDICAL INC; Rancho Santa Margarita
HEALTH NET INC; Woodland Hills
HEMACARE CORPORATION; Woodland Hills
I FLOW CORPORATION; Lake Forest
ICU MEDICAL INC; San Clemente
INAMED CORP; Santa Barbara
INTERPORE CROSS INTERNATIONAL; Irvine
INTUITIVE SURGICAL INC; Sunnyvale
IRIDEX CORP; Mountain View
IRIS INTERNATIONAL INC; Chatsworth
JENNY CRAIG INC; Carlsbad
KAISER PERMANENTE; Oakland
KYPHON INC; Sunnyvale
LASERSCOPE; San Jose
LIFESCAN INC; Milpitas
LONGS DRUG STORES CORPORATION; Walnut Creek
MAXYGEN INC; Redwood City
MCKESSON CORPORATION; San Francisco
MEDEX HOLDINGS CORPORATION; Carlsbad
MEDTRONIC MINIMED INC; Northridge
MEDTRONIC VASCULAR; Santa Rosa
MENTOR CORP; Santa Barbara
MOLECULAR DEVICES CORP; Sunnyvale
NEKTAR THERAPEUTICS; San Carlos
OCULAR SCIENCES INC; Concord
PACIFICARE HEALTH SYSTEMS INC; Cypress
PREMIER INC; San Diego
PRIMEDEX HEALTH SYSTEMS INC; Los Angeles
QUALITY SYSTEMS INC; Irvine
QUIDEL CORP; San Diego
RESMED INC; Poway
RITA MEDICAL SYSTEMS INC; Mountain View
SAFEGUARD HEALTH ENTERPRISES INC; Aliso Viejo
SIGNATURE EYEWEAR INC; Inglewood
SOLA INTERNATIONAL INC; San Diego
SPECIALTY LABORATORIES INC; Santa Monica
STAAR SURGICAL CO; Monrovia
SUN HEALTHCARE GROUP; Irvine
SUNRISE MEDICAL INC; Carlsbad
SUTTER HEALTH; Sacramento
SYBRON DENTAL SPECIALTIES INC; Orange
TENET HEALTHCARE CORPORATION; Santa Barbara
THERASENSE INC; Alameda
THORATEC CORPORATION; Pleasanton
VALEANT PHARMACEUTICALS INTERNATIONAL; Costa Mesa
VARIAN MEDICAL SYSTEMS INC; Palo Alto
VCA ANTECH INC; Los Angeles
VISION SERVICE PLAN; Rancho Cordova
VISX INC; Santa Clara
WATSON PHARMACEUTICALS INC; Corona
WELLPOINT HEALTH NETWORKS INC; Thousand Oaks

COLORADO
CATHOLIC HEALTH INITIATIVES; Denver
FISCHER IMAGING CORP; Denver
HEALTH GRADES INC; Lakewood
QUOVADX INC; Englewood
SPECTRANETICS CORP; Colorado Springs

CONNECTICUT
AETNA INC; Hartford
APPLERA CORPORATION; Norwalk
GE COMMERCIAL FINANCE; Stamford
IMS HEALTH INC; Fairfield
MAGELLAN HEALTH SERVICES INC; Farmington
MOORE MEDICAL CORP; New Britain
NOVAMETRIX MEDICAL SYSTEMS INC; Wallingford
OPTICARE HEALTH SYSTEMS; Waterbury
OXFORD HEALTH PLANS INC; Trumbull
UNIPRISE INCORPORATED; Hartford
VITALWORKS INC; Ridgefield

DELAWARE
INCYTE CORP; Wilmington

FLORIDA
ADVENTIST HEALTH SYSTEM; Winter Park
AMERIPATH INC; Riviera Beach
ANDRX CORP; Davie
AVMED HEALTH PLAN; Gainesville
BLUE CROSS AND BLUE SHIELD OF FLORIDA; Jacksonville
COAST DENTAL SERVICES INC; Tampa
CONTINUCARE CORP; Miami
CORDIS CORP; Miami Lakes
DRUGMAX INC; Clearwater
ECLIPSYS CORPORATION; Boca Raton
EXACTECH INC; Gainsville
HEALTH MANAGEMENT ASSOCIATES INC; Naples
HEARUSA INC; West Palm Beach
MEDICORE INC; Hialeah
MEDTRONIC XOMED SURGICAL PRODUCTS INC; Jacksonville
METROPOLITAN HEALTH NETWORKS; West Palm Beach
PEDIATRIX MEDICAL GROUP INC; Sunrise
PETMED EXPRESS INC; Pompano Beach
PLANVISTA CORP; Tampa
PRIORITY HEALTHCARE CORP; Lake Mary
PSS WORLD MEDICAL INC; Jacksonville
ROTECH HEALTHCARE INC; Orlando
SRI/SURGICAL EXPRESS INC; Tampa
WELLCARE GROUP OF COMPANIES; Tampa

GEORGIA
AFLAC INC; Columbus
BLUE CROSS AND BLUE SHIELD OF GEORGIA INC; Atlanta
CRYOLIFE INC; Kennesaw
IMMUCOR INC; Norcross
LOGISTICARE INC; Atlanta
MARINER HEALTH CARE INC; Atlanta
MATRIA HEALTHCARE INC; Marietta
MORRISON MANAGEMENT SPECIALISTS INC; Atlanta
NOVOSTE CORPORATION; Norcross
PEDIATRIC SERVICES OF AMERICA INC; Norcross
PER SE TECHNOLOGIES INC; Alpharetta
SEROLOGICALS CORP; Norcross
THERAGENICS CORP; Buford
TRANSCEND SERVICES INC; Atlanta

IDAHO
BLUE CROSS OF IDAHO; Meridian

ILLINOIS
ABBOTT LABORATORIES; Abbott Park
ADVOCATE HEALTH CARE; Oak Brook
AMERICAN PHARMACEUTICAL PARTNERS INC; Schaumburg
AON CORPORATION; Chicago
BAXTER INTERNATIONAL INC; Deerfield
BLUE CROSS AND BLUE SHIELD ASSOCIATION; Chicago
CARDINAL MEDICAL PRODUCTS AND SERVICES; McGaw Park
DADE BEHRING HOLDINGS INC; Deerfield
DELTA DENTAL PLANS ASSOCIATION; Oak Brook
FIRST HEALTH GROUP CORP; Downers Grove
HEALTH CARE SERVICE CORPORATION; Chicago
HOSPIRA INC; Lake Forest
NOVAMED INC; Chicago
OPTION CARE INC; Buffalo Grove
SOLUCIENT LLC; Evanston
WALGREEN CO; Deerfield

INDIANA
ANTHEM INC; Indianapolis
BIOMET INC; Warsaw
CLARIAN HEALTH PARTNERS INC; Indianapolis
DEPUY INC; Warsaw
ELI LILLY & CO; Indianapolis
GUIDANT CORP; Indianapolis
HILLENBRAND INDUSTRIES; Batesville
HILL-ROM COMPANY INC; Batesville
SYMMETRY MEDICAL INC; Warsaw
ZIMMER HOLDINGS INC; Warsaw

IOWA
CIVCO MEDICAL INSTRUMENTS; Kalona

KANSAS
BLUE CROSS AND BLUE SHIELD OF KANSAS; Topeka
LABONE INC; Lenexa

KENTUCKY
ATRIA SENIOR LIVING GROUP; Louisville
HUMANA INC; Louisville
KINDRED HEALTHCARE INC; Louisville
OMNICARE INC; Covington
RES CARE INC; Louisville

LOUISIANA
AMEDISYS INC; Baton Rouge
BLUE CROSS AND BLUE SHIELD OF LOUISIANA; Baton Rouge
OCA INC; Metairie

MAINE
IDEXX LABORATORIES INC; Westbrook
NYER MEDICAL GROUP INC; Bangor

MARYLAND
BON SECOURS HEALTH SYSTEM INC; Marriottsville
CAREFIRST INC; Owings Mills
CELERA GENOMICS GROUP; Rockville
CHINDEX INTERNATIONAL INC; Bethesda
COVENTRY HEALTH CARE INC; Bethesda
DENTAL BENEFITS PROVIDERS; Bethesda
DIGENE CORPORATION; Gaithersburg
HANGER ORTHOPEDIC GROUP INC; Bethesda
HUMAN GENOME SCIENCES INC; Rockville
JOHNS HOPKINS MEDICINE; Baltimore
MEDSTAR HEALTH; Columbia
MERIDIAN MEDICAL TECHNOLOGIES INC; Columbia
MID ATLANTIC MEDICAL SERVICES INC; Rockville
NEIGHBORCARE INC; Baltimore

MASSACHUSETTS
ABIOMED INC; Danvers
ANALOGIC CORP; Peabody
ARQULE INC; Woburn
ASPECT MEDICAL SYSTEMS INC; Newton
BIOGEN IDEC INC; Cambridge

BLUE CROSS AND BLUE SHIELD OF MASSACHUSETTS; Boston
BOSTON SCIENTIFIC CORP; Natick
CANDELA CORP; Wayland
GENZYME CORP; Cambridge
GSI LUMONICS INC; Billerica
GTC BIOTHERAPEUTICS INC; Framingham
HAEMONETICS CORPORATION; Braintree
HARBORSIDE HEALTHCARE CORP; Boston
HARVARD PILGRIM HEALTH CARE INC; Wellesley
HOLOGIC INC; Bedford
INVERNESS MEDICAL INNOVATIONS INC; Waltham
LIFELINE SYSTEMS INC; Framingham
MILLENNIUM PHARMACEUTICALS INC; Cambridge
NATIONAL DENTEX CORP; Wayland
NMT MEDICAL INC; Boston
OCCUPATIONAL HEALTH + REHABILITATION INC; Hingham
ORGANOGENESIS INC; Canton
PALOMAR MEDICAL TECHNOLOGIES INC; Burlington
PARTNERS HEALTHCARE SYSTEM; Boston
PERKINELMER INC; Wellesley
PHC INC; Peabody
PHILIPS MEDICAL SYSTEMS; Andover
POLYMEDICA CORPORATION; Woburn
SEPRACOR INC; Marlborough
THERMO ELECTRON CORP; Waltham
TUFTS ASSOCIATED HEALTH PLANS; Waltham
TYCO HEALTHCARE GROUP; Mansfield
ZOLL MEDICAL CORP; Chelmsford

MICHIGAN
BLUE CARE NETWORK OF MICHIGAN; Southfield
BLUE CROSS AND BLUE SHIELD OF MICHIGAN; Detroit
DETROIT MEDICAL CENTER; Detroit
HENRY FORD HEALTH SYSTEMS; Detroit
NANOBIO CORPORATION; Ann Arbor
SPECTRUM HEALTH; Grand Rapids
STRYKER CORP; Kalamazoo
SUPERIOR CONSULTANT HOLDINGS CORP; Southfield
TRINITY HEALTH COMPANY; Novi

MINNESOTA
3M COMPANY; St. Paul
ALLINA HOSPITALS AND CLINICS; Minneapolis
AMERICAN MEDICAL SYSTEMS HOLDINGS INC; Minnetonka
ATS MEDICAL INC; Minneapolis
BLUE CROSS AND BLUE SHIELD OF MINNESOTA; Eagan
CNS INC; Minneapolis
COMPEX TECHNOLOGIES INC; New Brighton
EMPI INC; St. Paul
FAIRVIEW HEALTH SERVICES; Minneapolis
HEALTH FITNESS CORP; Bloomington
LIFECORE BIOMEDICAL INC; Chaska
MAYO FOUNDATION FOR MEDICAL EDUCATION AND RESEARCH; Rochester
MEDTRONIC INC; Minneapolis
MINNTECH CORP; Minneapolis
PATTERSON COMPANIES INC; St. Paul
ST JUDE MEDICAL INC; St. Paul
SYNOVIS LIFE TECHNOLOGIES INC; St. Paul
TECHNE CORP; Minneapolis
TELEX COMMUNICATIONS INC; Burnsville
UNITEDHEALTH GROUP INC; Minnetonka
UNIVERSAL HOSPITAL SERVICES INC; Bloomington

MISSISSIPPI
MICROTEK MEDICAL HOLDINGS INC; Columbus

MISSOURI
ASCENSION HEALTH; St. Louis
ASSURANT EMPLOYEE BENEFITS; Kansas City
BJC HEALTHCARE; St. Louis
CENTENE CORPORATION; St Louis
CERNER CORP; Kansas City
D & K HEALTHCARE RESOURCES INC; St. Louis
EXPRESS SCRIPTS INC; Maryland Heights
MALLINCKRODT INC; Hazelwood
REHABCARE GROUP INC; St. Louis
SIGMA ALDRICH CORP; St. Louis
SISTERS OF MERCY HEALTH SYSTEMS; Chesterfield
SSM HEALTH CARE SYSTEM INC; St. Louis
TRIPOS INC; St. Louis
YOUNG INNOVATIONS INC; Earth City

MONTANA
BLUE CROSS AND BLUE SHIELD OF MONTANA; Helena

NEBRASKA
BLUE CROSS AND BLUE SHIELD OF NEBRASKA; Omaha

NEVADA
EMERGENCY FILTRATION PRODUCTS INC; Henderson
SIERRA HEALTH SERVICES INC; Las Vegas

NEW HAMPSHIRE
APOGENT TECHNOLOGIES INC; Portsmouth
FISHER SCIENTIFIC INTERNATIONAL INC; Hampton

NEW JERSEY
ALPHARMA INC; Fort Lee
BECTON DICKINSON & CO; Franklin Lakes
BIO REFERENCE LABORATORIES INC; Elmwood Park
CAMBREX CORP; East Rutherford
CANTEL MEDICAL CORP; Little Falls
CONVATEC; Skillman
COVANCE INC; Princeton
CR BARD INC; Murray Hill
DATASCOPE CORP; Montvale
ETHICON INC; Somerville
HOOPER HOLMES INC; Basking Ridge
HORIZON BLUE CROSS BLUE SHIELD OF NEW JERSEY; Newark
INTEGRA LIFESCIENCES HOLDINGS CORP; Plainsboro
I-STAT CORP; East Windsor
JOHNSON & JOHNSON; New Brunswick
LIFECELL CORPORATION; Branchburg
MEDCO HEALTH SOLUTIONS; Franklin Lakes
MEDQUIST INC; Mount Laurel
MERCK & CO INC; Whitehouse Station
OSTEOTECH INC; Eatontown
PATIENT CARE INC; West Orange
PDI INC; Saddle River
PHARMACOPEIA INC; Princeton
QUEST DIAGNOSTICS INC; Teterboro
SCHERING-PLOUGH CORP; Kenilworth

US VISION INC; Glendora
VENTIV HEALTH INC; Somerset
VITAL SIGNS INC; Totowa
WEBMD CORPORATION; Elmwood Park
WYETH; Madison

NEW YORK
ALLIED HEALTHCARE INTERNATIONAL INC; New York
ASSURANT INC; New York
ATC HEALTHCARE INC; Lake Success
BARR LABORATORIES INC; Pomona
BAUSCH & LOMB INC; Rochester
BIOPHAN TECHNOLOGIES INC; West Henrietta
BRISTOL MYERS SQUIBB CO; New York
CONMED CORP; Utica
CURATIVE HEALTH SERVICES INC; Hauppauge
DUANE READE INC; New York
EMERGING VISION INC; Garden City
EON LABS INC; Laurelton
EXCEL TECHNOLOGY INC; East Setauket
E-Z-EM INC; Westbury
FOREST LABORATORIES INC; New York
GENTIVA HEALTH SERVICES INC; Melville
GROUP HEALTH INCORPORATED; New York
HEALTH INSURANCE PLAN OF GREATER NEW YORK; New York
HEALTH MANAGEMENT SYSTEMS INC; New York
HEALTHNOW NEW YORK; Buffalo
HENRY SCHEIN INC; Melville
IMPATH INC; New York
INTEGRAMED AMERICA INC; Purchase
INTERMAGNETICS GENERAL CORP; Latham
LAKELAND INDUSTRIES INC; Ronkonkorna
MARSH & MCLENNAN COMPANIES INC; New York
MEDICAL ACTION INDUSTRIES INC; Hauppauge
MEMORIAL SLOAN KETTERING CANCER CENTER; New York
MIM CORP; Elmsford
MISONIX INC; Farmingdale
NATIONAL HOME HEALTH CARE CORP; Scarsdale
NATIONAL MEDICAL HEALTH CARD SYSTEMS INC; Port Washington
NEW YORK CITY HEALTH AND HOSPITALS CORPORATION; New York
NEW YORK HEALTH CARE INC; Brooklyn
NEW YORK-PRESBYTERIAN HEALTHCARE SYSTEM; New York
PAR PHARMACEUTICAL COMPANIES INC; Spring Valley
PFIZER INC; New York
SCHICK TECHNOLOGIES INC; Long Island City
WEIGHT WATCHERS INTERNATIONAL INC; Woodbury
WELCH ALLYN INC; Skaneateles Falls
WELLCHOICE INC; New York

NORTH CAROLINA
AAIPHARMA INC; Wilmington
BLUE CROSS AND BLUE SHIELD OF NORTH CAROLINA; Durham
LABORATORY CORP OF AMERICA HOLDINGS; Burlington
MEDCATH CORPORATION; Charlotte
PHARMACEUTICAL PRODUCT DEVELOPMENT INC; Wilmington
QUINTILES TRANSNATIONAL CORP; Durham
TRIPATH IMAGING INC; Burlington

OHIO
CARDINAL HEALTH INC; Dublin
CATHOLIC HEALTHCARE PARTNERS; Cincinnati
COLE NATIONAL CORPORATION; Twinsburg
INVACARE CORP; Elyria
KENDLE INTERNATIONAL INC; Cincinnati
LCA VISION INC; Cincinnati
MANOR CARE INC; Toledo
MEDICAL MUTUAL OF OHIO; Cleveland
MERIDIAN BIOSCIENCE INC; Cincinnati
OHIOHEALTH CORPORATION; Columbus
STERIS CORP; Mentor

OKLAHOMA
BLUE CROSS AND BLUE SHIELD OF OKLAHOMA; Tulsa
MARIAN HEALTH SYSTEMS; Tulsa
UROCOR INC; Oklahoma City

OREGON
REGENCE GROUP (THE); Portland
REGENT ASSISTED LIVING INC; Portland

PENNSYLVANIA
AMERISOURCEBERGEN CORP; Chesterbrook
ARROW INTERNATIONAL INC; Reading
BAYER CORP; Pittsburgh
CAPITAL BLUECROSS; Harrisburg
CEPHALON INC; West Chester
CIGNA CORP; Philadelphia
DENTSPLY INTERNATIONAL INC; York
ENDO PHARMACEUTICALS HOLDINGS INC; Chadds Ford
ENVIRONMENTAL TECTONICS CORP; Southampton
ERESEARCH TECHNOLOGY INC; Philadelphia
GENERAL NUTRITION COMPANIES INC; Pittsburgh
HIGHMARK INC; Pittsburg
JEFFERSON HEALTH SYSTEM INC; Radnor
MINE SAFETY APPLIANCES CO; Pittsburgh
MYLAN LABORATORIES INC; Canonsburg
OUTLOOK POINTE CORP; Mechanicsburg
RESPIRONICS INC; Murrysville
RITE AID CORPORATION; Camp Hill
UNIVERSAL HEALTH SERVICES INC; King of Prussia
UTI CORPORATION; Collegeville
VIASYS HEALTHCARE INC; Conshohocken
WEST PHARMACEUTICAL SERVICES INC; Lionville
ZLB BEHRING LLC; King of Prussia

RHODE ISLAND
CVS CORPORATION; Woonsocket

SOUTH CAROLINA
SPAN AMERICA MEDICAL SYSTEMS INC; Greenville

SOUTH DAKOTA
AVERA HEALTH; Sioux Falls

TENNESEE
ACCREDO HEALTH INC; Memphis
ADVOCAT INC; Franklin
AMERICA SERVICE GROUP INC; Brentwood
AMERICAN HEALTHWAYS INC; Nashville
AMERICAN HOMEPATIENT INC; Brentwood
AMERICAN RETIREMENT CORP; Brentwood

AMSURG CORP; Nashville
BLUE CROSS AND BLUE SHIELD OF TENNESSEE INC; Chattanooga
CAREMARK RX INC; Nashville
COMMUNITY HEALTH SYSTEMS INC; Brentwood
CTI MOLECULAR IMAGING; Knoxville
HCA INC; Nashville
HEALTHSTREAM INC; Nashville
LIFE CARE CENTERS OF AMERICA; Cleveland
MEDTRONIC SOFAMOR DANEK; Memphis
NATIONAL HEALTHCARE CORP; Murfreesboro
PROVINCE HEALTHCARE CO; Brentwood
PSYCHIATRIC SOLUTIONS INC; Franklin
RENAL CARE GROUP INC; Nashville
ST JUDE CHILDRENS RESEARCH HOSPITAL; Memphis
TEAM HEALTH; Knoxville
WRIGHT MEDICAL GROUP INC; Arlington

TEXAS
ADVANCEPCS INC; Irving
ASSISTED LIVING CONCEPTS INC; Dallas
ATRION CORPORATION; Allen
BLUE CROSS AND BLUE SHIELD OF TEXAS; Richardson
CAPITAL SENIOR LIVING CORP; Dallas
CASTLE DENTAL CENTERS INC; Houston
CHRISTUS HEALTH; Irving
CONCENTRA INC; Addision
CYBERONICS INC; Houston
DYNACQ HEALTHCARE INC; Pasadena
ENCORE MEDICAL CORPORATION; Austin
HEALTHAXIS INC; Irving
HEALTHTRONICS INC; Austin
HORIZON HEALTH CORPORATION; Lewisville
KIMBERLY CLARK CORP; Irving
KINETIC CONCEPTS INC; San Antonio
MEMORIAL HERMANN HEALTHCARE SYSTEM; Houston
MONARCH DENTAL CORP; Dallas
NOVATION LLC; Irving
ODYSSEY HEALTHCARE INC; Dallas
RADIOLOGIX INC; Dallas
TEXAS HEALTH RESOURCES; Arlington
TRIAD HOSPITALS INC; Plano
UNITED SURGICAL PARTNERS; Addison
US ONCOLOGY INC; Houston
US PHYSICAL THERAPY INC; Houston

UTAH
INTERMOUNTAIN HEALTH CARE; Salt Lake City
MERIT MEDICAL SYSTEMS INC; South Jordan
SONIC INNOVATIONS INC; Salt Lake City
UTAH MEDICAL PRODUCTS INC; Midvale

VIRGINIA
AMERICHOICE CORPORATION; Vienna
AMERIGROUP CORPORATION; Virginia Beach
OWENS & MINOR INC; Glen Allen
SENTARA HEALTHCARE; Norfolk
SUNRISE SENIOR LIVING; McLean

VERMONT
BLUE CROSS AND BLUE SHIELD OF VERMONT; Montpelier
IDX SYSTEMS CORP; Burlington

WASHINGTON
EMERITUS CORP; Seattle
FIRST CHOICE HEALTH NETWORK INC; Seattle
GROUP HEALTH COOPERATIVE OF PUGET SOUND; Seattle
PREMERA BLUE CROSS; Mountlake Terrace
PROVIDENCE HEALTH SYSTEM; Seattle

WISCONSIN
ALTERRA HEALTHCARE CORP; Milwaukee
AMERICAN MEDICAL SECURITY GROUP INC; Green Bay
ASSURANT HEALTH; Milwaukee
CRITICARE SYSTEMS INC; Waukesha
EPIC SYSTEMS CORPORATION; Madison

WYOMING
BLUE CROSS AND BLUE SHIELD OF WYOMING; Cheyenne

INDEX OF NON-U.S. HEADQUARTERS LOCATION BY COUNTRY

AUSTRALIA
ANSELL LIMITED COMPANY; Richmond
COCHLEAR LTD; Lane Cove

CANADA
AETERNA ZENTARIS INC; Quebec City
ART ADVANCED RESEARCH TECHNOLOGIES; Saint-Laurent
BIOVAIL CORPORATION; Mississauga
CEDARA SOFTWARE CORP; Mississauga
EXTENDICARE INC; Markham
MDS INC; Toronto
MIV THERAPEUTICS INC; Vancouver
TLC VISION CORPORATION; Mississauga

DENMARK
NOVO-NORDISK AS; Basgvaerd

FINLAND
INSTRUMENTARIUM CORPORATION; Helsinki

FRANCE
AVENTIS SA; Strasbourg
ESSILOR INTERNATIONAL SA; Charenton-le-Pont
SANOFI-SYNTHELABO; Paris

GERMANY
BAYER AG; Leverkusen
FRESENIUS AG; Bas Homburg
SCHERING AG; Berlin
SIEMENS MEDICAL SOLUTIONS; Erlangen

IRELAND
ELAN CORP PLC; Dublin
WARNER CHILCOTT PLC; Dublin

ISRAEL
LUMENIS LTD; Yokneam
SHL TELEMEDICINE; Tel Aviv
TEVA PHARMACEUTICAL INDUSTRIES; Petach Tikva

ITALY
LUXOTTICA GROUP SPA; Milan

JAPAN
FUJISAWA PHARMACEUTICALS COMPANY LTD; Osaka
TOSHIBA CORPORATION; Tokyo

NETHERLANDS ANTILLES
ORTHOFIX INTERNATIONAL NV; Curacao

SWEDEN
GAMBRO AB; Stockholm

SWITZERLAND
ALCON INC; Hunenberg
CENTERPULSE AG; Winterthur
INSTITUT STRAUMANN AG; Waldenburg
METTLER-TOLEDO INTERNATIONAL; Zurich
NOVARTIS AG; Basel
ROCHE GROUP; Basel
SERONO SA; Geneva

UNITED KINGDOM
AXA PPP HEALTHCARE; Tunbridge Wells
BESPAK PLC; Wolverton Mill South
BRITISH UNION PROVIDENT ASSOCIATION (BUPA); London
CELLTECH GROUP PLC; Slough
GE HEALTHCARE; Chalfont St. Giles
GLAXOSMITHKLINE PLC; Brentford
GYRUS GROUP; St. Mellons
HUNTLEIGH TECHNOLOGIES PLC; Luton
SHIRE PHARMACEUTICALS PLC; Basingstoke
SMITH & NEPHEW PLC; London
SSL INTERNATIONAL; London

INDEX BY REGIONS OF THE U.S. WHERE THE HEALTH CARE 500 FIRMS HAVE LOCATIONS

WEST

3M COMPANY
AAIPHARMA INC
ABBOTT LABORATORIES
ACCREDO HEALTH INC
ADVANCED BIONICS CORPORATION
ADVANCED MEDICAL OPTICS INC
ADVANCEPCS INC
ADVENTIST HEALTH SYSTEM
AETNA INC
AFLAC INC
ALCON INC
ALIGN TECHNOLOGY
ALLERGAN INC
ALLIANCE IMAGING INC
ALPHARMA INC
ALTERRA HEALTHCARE CORP
AMERICA SERVICE GROUP INC
AMERICAN HEALTHWAYS INC
AMERICAN HOMEPATIENT INC
AMERICAN MEDICAL SECURITY GROUP INC
AMERICAN PHARMACEUTICAL PARTNERS INC
AMERICAN RETIREMENT CORP
AMERICAN SHARED HOSPITAL SERVICES
AMERICHOICE CORPORATION
AMERIPATH INC
AMERISOURCEBERGEN CORP
AMGEN INC
AMSURG CORP
ANTHEM INC
AON CORPORATION
APOGENT TECHNOLOGIES INC
APPLERA CORPORATION
APPLIED BIOSYSTEMS GROUP
APRIA HEALTHCARE GROUP INC
ARADIGM CORPORATION
ARROW INTERNATIONAL INC
ARTHROCARE CORP
ASCENSION HEALTH
ASSISTED LIVING CONCEPTS INC
ASSURANT EMPLOYEE BENEFITS
ATC HEALTHCARE INC
ATRIA SENIOR LIVING GROUP
AVENTIS SA
BANNER HEALTH
BAUSCH & LOMB INC
BAXTER INTERNATIONAL INC
BAYER CORP
BECKMAN COULTER INC
BECTON DICKINSON & CO
BEVERLY ENTERPRISES INC
BIO RAD LABORATORIES INC
BIOMET INC
BLUE CROSS AND BLUE SHIELD ASSOCIATION
BLUE CROSS AND BLUE SHIELD OF MONTANA
BLUE CROSS AND BLUE SHIELD OF WYOMING
BLUE CROSS OF CALIFORNIA
BLUE CROSS OF IDAHO
BLUE SHIELD OF CALIFORNIA
BOSTON SCIENTIFIC CORP
BRISTOL MYERS SQUIBB CO
CAPITAL SENIOR LIVING CORP
CARDINAL HEALTH INC
CARDIOGENESIS CORP
CAREMARK RX INC
CASTLE DENTAL CENTERS INC
CATHOLIC HEALTH INITIATIVES
CATHOLIC HEALTHCARE WEST
CELERA GENOMICS GROUP
CENTENE CORPORATION
CENTERPULSE AG
CEPHALON INC
CERNER CORP
CHIRON CORP
CHOLESTECH CORP
CHRISTUS HEALTH
CIGNA CORP
COHERENT INC
COLE NATIONAL CORPORATION
COMMUNITY HEALTH SYSTEMS INC
CONCENTRA INC
CONMED CORP
COOPER COMPANIES INC
CORVEL CORP
COVANCE INC
CR BARD INC
CURATIVE HEALTH SERVICES INC
CVS CORPORATION
D & K HEALTHCARE RESOURCES INC
DADE BEHRING HOLDINGS INC
DATASCOPE CORP
DAVITA INC
DELTA DENTAL PLANS ASSOCIATION
DENTAL BENEFITS PROVIDERS
DENTSPLY INTERNATIONAL INC
DEPUY INC
DIAGNOSTIC PRODUCTS CORPORATION
DJ ORTHOPEDICS INC
ECLIPSYS CORPORATION
EDWARDS LIFESCIENCES CORP
ELAN CORP PLC
ELI LILLY & CO
EMERGENCY FILTRATION PRODUCTS INC
EMERGING VISION INC
EMERITUS CORP
ESSILOR INTERNATIONAL SA
EXCEL TECHNOLOGY INC
EXPRESS SCRIPTS INC
EXTENDICARE INC
FIRST CHOICE HEALTH NETWORK INC
FIRST CONSULTING GROUP INC
FIRST HEALTH GROUP CORP
FISCHER IMAGING CORP
FISHER SCIENTIFIC INTERNATIONAL INC
FRESENIUS AG
GAMBRO AB
GE COMMERCIAL FINANCE
GENENTECH INC
GENERAL NUTRITION COMPANIES INC
GENTIVA HEALTH SERVICES INC
GENZYME CORP
GISH BIOMEDICAL INC
GLAXOSMITHKLINE PLC
GROUP HEALTH COOPERATIVE OF PUGET SOUND
GSI LUMONICS INC
GUIDANT CORP
HANGER ORTHOPEDIC GROUP INC
HCA INC
HEALTH CARE SERVICE CORPORATION
HEALTH FITNESS CORP
HEALTH GRADES INC
HEALTH MANAGEMENT ASSOCIATES INC
HEALTH MANAGEMENT SYSTEMS INC
HEALTH NET INC
HEALTHSOUTH CORP
HEALTHSTREAM INC
HEARUSA INC
HEMACARE CORPORATION
HENRY SCHEIN INC
HOOPER HOLMES INC
HORIZON HEALTH CORPORATION
HOSPIRA INC
HUMANA INC
I FLOW CORPORATION
ICU MEDICAL INC
IDEXX LABORATORIES INC
IDX SYSTEMS CORP
IMPATH INC
IMS HEALTH INC
INAMED CORP
INSTITUT STRAUMANN AG
INTEGRA LIFESCIENCES HOLDINGS CORP
INTEGRAMED AMERICA INC
INTERMAGNETICS GENERAL CORP
INTERMOUNTAIN HEALTH CARE
INTERPORE CROSS INTERNATIONAL
INTUITIVE SURGICAL INC
INVACARE CORP
INVERNESS MEDICAL INNOVATIONS INC
IRIDEX CORP
IRIS INTERNATIONAL INC
JENNY CRAIG INC
JOHNSON & JOHNSON

KAISER PERMANENTE
KENDLE INTERNATIONAL INC
KIMBERLY CLARK CORP
KINDRED HEALTHCARE INC
KYPHON INC
LABORATORY CORP OF AMERICA HOLDINGS
LASERSCOPE
LCA VISION INC
LIFE CARE CENTERS OF AMERICA
LIFESCAN INC
LOGISTICARE INC
LONGS DRUG STORES CORPORATION
LUMENIS LTD
LUXOTTICA GROUP SPA
MAGELLAN HEALTH SERVICES INC
MALLINCKRODT INC
MANOR CARE INC
MARINER HEALTH CARE INC
MARSH & MCLENNAN COMPANIES INC
MATRIA HEALTHCARE INC
MAXYGEN INC
MCKESSON CORPORATION
MDS INC
MEDCATH CORPORATION
MEDCO HEALTH SOLUTIONS
MEDEX HOLDINGS CORPORATION
MEDQUIST INC
MEDTRONIC INC
MEDTRONIC MINIMED INC
MEDTRONIC VASCULAR
MEDTRONIC XOMED SURGICAL PRODUCTS INC
MENTOR CORP
MERCK & CO INC
MERIT MEDICAL SYSTEMS INC
METTLER-TOLEDO INTERNATIONAL
MILLENNIUM PHARMACEUTICALS INC
MINE SAFETY APPLIANCES CO
MISONIX INC
MOLECULAR DEVICES CORP
MONARCH DENTAL CORP
MOORE MEDICAL CORP
MORRISON MANAGEMENT SPECIALISTS INC
NATIONAL DENTEX CORP
NEIGHBORCARE INC
NEKTAR THERAPEUTICS
NOVAMED INC
NOVAMETRIX MEDICAL SYSTEMS INC
NOVATION LLC
NOVO-NORDISK AS
NYER MEDICAL GROUP INC
OCA INC
OCULAR SCIENCES INC
ODYSSEY HEALTHCARE INC
OMNICARE INC
OPTION CARE INC
ORTHOFIX INTERNATIONAL NV
OWENS & MINOR INC

PACIFICARE HEALTH SYSTEMS INC
PATTERSON COMPANIES INC
PDI INC
PEDIATRIC SERVICES OF AMERICA INC
PEDIATRIX MEDICAL GROUP INC
PERKINELMER INC
PETMED EXPRESS INC
PFIZER INC
PHARMACEUTICAL PRODUCT DEVELOPMENT INC
PHARMACOPEIA INC
PHC INC
PREMERA BLUE CROSS
PREMIER INC
PRIMEDEX HEALTH SYSTEMS INC
PRIORITY HEALTHCARE CORP
PROVIDENCE HEALTH SYSTEM
PROVINCE HEALTHCARE CO
PSS WORLD MEDICAL INC
PSYCHIATRIC SOLUTIONS INC
QUALITY SYSTEMS INC
QUEST DIAGNOSTICS INC
QUIDEL CORP
QUINTILES TRANSNATIONAL CORP
QUOVADX INC
RADIOLOGIX INC
REGENCE GROUP (THE)
REGENT ASSISTED LIVING INC
REHABCARE GROUP INC
RENAL CARE GROUP INC
RES CARE INC
RESMED INC
RESPIRONICS INC
RITA MEDICAL SYSTEMS INC
RITE AID CORPORATION
ROCHE GROUP
ROTECH HEALTHCARE INC
SAFEGUARD HEALTH ENTERPRISES INC
SCHERING-PLOUGH CORP
SEROLOGICALS CORP
SHIRE PHARMACEUTICALS PLC
SIERRA HEALTH SERVICES INC
SIGMA ALDRICH CORP
SIGNATURE EYEWEAR INC
SOLA INTERNATIONAL INC
SOLUCIENT LLC
SONIC INNOVATIONS INC
SPAN AMERICA MEDICAL SYSTEMS INC
SPECIALTY LABORATORIES INC
SPECTRANETICS CORP
SRI/SURGICAL EXPRESS INC
ST JUDE MEDICAL INC
STAAR SURGICAL CO
STERIS CORP
STRYKER CORP
SUN HEALTHCARE GROUP
SUNRISE MEDICAL INC
SUNRISE SENIOR LIVING
SUPERIOR CONSULTANT HOLDINGS CORP
SUTTER HEALTH
SYBRON DENTAL SPECIALTIES INC

TEAM HEALTH
TENET HEALTHCARE CORPORATION
TEVA PHARMACEUTICAL INDUSTRIES
TEXAS HEALTH RESOURCES
THERASENSE INC
THERMO ELECTRON CORP
THORATEC CORPORATION
TLC VISION CORPORATION
TOSHIBA CORPORATION
TRANSCEND SERVICES INC
TRIAD HOSPITALS INC
TRINITY HEALTH COMPANY
TRIPATH IMAGING INC
UNITED SURGICAL PARTNERS
UNITEDHEALTH GROUP INC
UNIVERSAL HEALTH SERVICES INC
UNIVERSAL HOSPITAL SERVICES INC
UROCOR INC
US ONCOLOGY INC
US PHYSICAL THERAPY INC
US VISION INC
UTAH MEDICAL PRODUCTS INC
UTI CORPORATION
VALEANT PHARMACEUTICALS INTERNATIONAL
VARIAN MEDICAL SYSTEMS INC
VCA ANTECH INC
VENTIV HEALTH INC
VIASYS HEALTHCARE INC
VISION SERVICE PLAN
VISX INC
VITAL SIGNS INC
VITALWORKS INC
WALGREEN CO
WATSON PHARMACEUTICALS INC
WEIGHT WATCHERS INTERNATIONAL INC
WELCH ALLYN INC
WELLPOINT HEALTH NETWORKS INC
WYETH
YOUNG INNOVATIONS INC
ZIMMER HOLDINGS INC
ZOLL MEDICAL CORP

SOUTHWEST
3M COMPANY
ABBOTT LABORATORIES
ACCREDO HEALTH INC
ADVANCEPCS INC
ADVENTIST HEALTH SYSTEM
ADVOCAT INC
AETNA INC
AFLAC INC
ALCON INC
ALLERGAN INC
ALLIANCE IMAGING INC
ALPHARMA INC
ALTERRA HEALTHCARE CORP
AMEDISYS INC
AMERICA SERVICE GROUP INC
AMERICAN HEALTHWAYS INC

AMERICAN HOMEPATIENT INC
AMERICAN MEDICAL SECURITY GROUP INC
AMERICAN RETIREMENT CORP
AMERICHOICE CORPORATION
AMERIGROUP CORPORATION
AMERIPATH INC
AMERISOURCEBERGEN CORP
AMSURG CORP
ANSELL LIMITED COMPANY
ANTHEM INC
AON CORPORATION
APOGENT TECHNOLOGIES INC
APPLERA CORPORATION
APRIA HEALTHCARE GROUP INC
ARKANSAS BLUE CROSS AND BLUE SHIELD
ARTHROCARE CORP
ASCENSION HEALTH
ASSISTED LIVING CONCEPTS INC
ASSURANT EMPLOYEE BENEFITS
ATC HEALTHCARE INC
ATRIA SENIOR LIVING GROUP
ATRION CORPORATION
AVENTIS SA
BANNER HEALTH
BAUSCH & LOMB INC
BAXTER INTERNATIONAL INC
BAYER CORP
BECKMAN COULTER INC
BECTON DICKINSON & CO
BEVERLY ENTERPRISES INC
BIOMET INC
BLUE CROSS AND BLUE SHIELD ASSOCIATION
BLUE CROSS AND BLUE SHIELD OF TEXAS
BOSTON SCIENTIFIC CORP
BRISTOL MYERS SQUIBB CO
CAPITAL SENIOR LIVING CORP
CARDINAL HEALTH INC
CAREMARK RX INC
CASTLE DENTAL CENTERS INC
CATHOLIC HEALTH INITIATIVES
CATHOLIC HEALTHCARE WEST
CENTENE CORPORATION
CENTERPULSE AG
CERNER CORP
CHIRON CORP
CHRISTUS HEALTH
CIGNA CORP
COLE NATIONAL CORPORATION
COMMUNITY HEALTH SYSTEMS INC
CONCENTRA INC
CONMED CORP
CORVEL CORP
COVANCE INC
COVENTRY HEALTH CARE INC
CR BARD INC
CURATIVE HEALTH SERVICES INC
CVS CORPORATION
CYBERONICS INC
D & K HEALTHCARE RESOURCES INC

DATASCOPE CORP
DAVITA INC
DELTA DENTAL PLANS ASSOCIATION
DENTAL BENEFITS PROVIDERS
DENTSPLY INTERNATIONAL INC
DEPUY INC
DYNACQ HEALTHCARE INC
ECLIPSYS CORPORATION
ELAN CORP PLC
ELI LILLY & CO
EMERGING VISION INC
EMERITUS CORP
ENCORE MEDICAL CORPORATION
ESSILOR INTERNATIONAL SA
ETHICON INC
EXPRESS SCRIPTS INC
EXTENDICARE INC
FIRST CONSULTING GROUP INC
FIRST HEALTH GROUP CORP
FISHER SCIENTIFIC INTERNATIONAL INC
FRESENIUS AG
GE COMMERCIAL FINANCE
GENERAL NUTRITION COMPANIES INC
GENTIVA HEALTH SERVICES INC
GENZYME CORP
GLAXOSMITHKLINE PLC
GUIDANT CORP
HANGER ORTHOPEDIC GROUP INC
HCA INC
HEALTH CARE SERVICE CORPORATION
HEALTH FITNESS CORP
HEALTH MANAGEMENT ASSOCIATES INC
HEALTH MANAGEMENT SYSTEMS INC
HEALTH NET INC
HEALTHAXIS INC
HEALTHSOUTH CORP
HEALTHTRONICS INC
HEMACARE CORPORATION
HENRY SCHEIN INC
HOOPER HOLMES INC
HORIZON HEALTH CORPORATION
HOSPIRA INC
HUMANA INC
IDEXX LABORATORIES INC
IDX SYSTEMS CORP
IMMUCOR INC
IMPATH INC
INTEGRAMED AMERICA INC
INVACARE CORP
IRIS INTERNATIONAL INC
JENNY CRAIG INC
JOHNSON & JOHNSON
KIMBERLY CLARK CORP
KINDRED HEALTHCARE INC
KINETIC CONCEPTS INC
LABORATORY CORP OF AMERICA HOLDINGS
LCA VISION INC
LIFE CARE CENTERS OF AMERICA

LOGISTICARE INC
LUXOTTICA GROUP SPA
MAGELLAN HEALTH SERVICES INC
MALLINCKRODT INC
MANOR CARE INC
MARIAN HEALTH SYSTEMS
MARINER HEALTH CARE INC
MARSH & MCLENNAN COMPANIES INC
MAYO FOUNDATION FOR MEDICAL EDUCATION AND RESEARCH
MCKESSON CORPORATION
MDS INC
MEDCATH CORPORATION
MEDCO HEALTH SOLUTIONS
MEDQUIST INC
MEDTRONIC INC
MEDTRONIC MINIMED INC
MEDTRONIC XOMED SURGICAL PRODUCTS INC
MEMORIAL HERMANN HEALTHCARE SYSTEM
MENTOR CORP
MERCK & CO INC
MERIT MEDICAL SYSTEMS INC
MICROTEK MEDICAL HOLDINGS INC
MONARCH DENTAL CORP
MORRISON MANAGEMENT SPECIALISTS INC
NATIONAL DENTEX CORP
NATIONAL MEDICAL HEALTH CARD SYSTEMS INC
NEIGHBORCARE INC
NOVAMED INC
NOVATION LLC
NOVO-NORDISK AS
OCA INC
OCULAR SCIENCES INC
ODYSSEY HEALTHCARE INC
OMNICARE INC
OPTION CARE INC
OWENS & MINOR INC
PACIFICARE HEALTH SYSTEMS INC
PATTERSON COMPANIES INC
PEDIATRIC SERVICES OF AMERICA INC
PEDIATRIX MEDICAL GROUP INC
PERKINELMER INC
PETMED EXPRESS INC
PFIZER INC
PRIORITY HEALTHCARE CORP
PROVINCE HEALTHCARE CO
PSS WORLD MEDICAL INC
PSYCHIATRIC SOLUTIONS INC
QUEST DIAGNOSTICS INC
QUINTILES TRANSNATIONAL CORP
QUOVADX INC
RADIOLOGIX INC
REGENT ASSISTED LIVING INC
REHABCARE GROUP INC
RENAL CARE GROUP INC
RES CARE INC
RESPIRONICS INC
RITE AID CORPORATION

ROTECH HEALTHCARE INC
SAFEGUARD HEALTH ENTERPRISES INC
SCHERING-PLOUGH CORP
SHIRE PHARMACEUTICALS PLC
SIERRA HEALTH SERVICES INC
SIGMA ALDRICH CORP
SISTERS OF MERCY HEALTH SYSTEMS
SRI/SURGICAL EXPRESS INC
ST JUDE MEDICAL INC
STERIS CORP
SUN HEALTHCARE GROUP
SUNRISE SENIOR LIVING
TEAM HEALTH
TENET HEALTHCARE CORPORATION
TEXAS HEALTH RESOURCES
THERMO ELECTRON CORP
TLC VISION CORPORATION
TOSHIBA CORPORATION
TRANSCEND SERVICES INC
TRIAD HOSPITALS INC
UNITED SURGICAL PARTNERS
UNITEDHEALTH GROUP INC
UNIVERSAL HEALTH SERVICES INC
UNIVERSAL HOSPITAL SERVICES INC
UROCOR INC
US ONCOLOGY INC
US PHYSICAL THERAPY INC
US VISION INC
UTI CORPORATION
VCA ANTECH INC
VENTANA MEDICAL SYSTEMS
VENTIV HEALTH INC
VISION SERVICE PLAN
WALGREEN CO
WEIGHT WATCHERS INTERNATIONAL INC
WELCH ALLYN INC
WELLPOINT HEALTH NETWORKS INC
WYETH
YOUNG INNOVATIONS INC
ZIMMER HOLDINGS INC

MIDWEST
3M COMPANY
AAIPHARMA INC
ABBOTT LABORATORIES
ACCREDO HEALTH INC
ADVANCEPCS INC
ADVENTIST HEALTH SYSTEM
ADVOCATE HEALTH CARE
AETNA INC
AFLAC INC
ALLERGAN INC
ALLIANCE IMAGING INC
ALLINA HOSPITALS AND CLINICS
ALPHARMA INC
ALTERRA HEALTHCARE CORP
AMERICA SERVICE GROUP INC
AMERICAN HEALTHWAYS INC
AMERICAN HOMEPATIENT INC

AMERICAN MEDICAL SECURITY GROUP INC
AMERICAN MEDICAL SYSTEMS HOLDINGS INC
AMERICAN PHARMACEUTICAL PARTNERS INC
AMERICAN RETIREMENT CORP
AMERICHOICE CORPORATION
AMERIGROUP CORPORATION
AMERIPATH INC
AMERISOURCEBERGEN CORP
AMGEN INC
AMSURG CORP
ANALOGIC CORP
ANDRX CORP
ANSELL LIMITED COMPANY
ANTHEM INC
AON CORPORATION
APOGENT TECHNOLOGIES INC
APRIA HEALTHCARE GROUP INC
ARKANSAS BLUE CROSS AND BLUE SHIELD
ASCENSION HEALTH
ASSISTED LIVING CONCEPTS INC
ASSURANT EMPLOYEE BENEFITS
ASSURANT HEALTH
ASSURANT INC
ATC HEALTHCARE INC
ATRIA SENIOR LIVING GROUP
ATS MEDICAL INC
AVENTIS SA
AVERA HEALTH
BANNER HEALTH
BARR LABORATORIES INC
BAUSCH & LOMB INC
BAXTER INTERNATIONAL INC
BAYER CORP
BECKMAN COULTER INC
BECTON DICKINSON & CO
BEVERLY ENTERPRISES INC
BIO RAD LABORATORIES INC
BIOMET INC
BJC HEALTHCARE
BLUE CARE NETWORK OF MICHIGAN
BLUE CROSS AND BLUE SHIELD ASSOCIATION
BLUE CROSS AND BLUE SHIELD OF KANSAS
BLUE CROSS AND BLUE SHIELD OF MICHIGAN
BLUE CROSS AND BLUE SHIELD OF MINNESOTA
BLUE CROSS AND BLUE SHIELD OF NEBRASKA
BLUE CROSS AND BLUE SHIELD OF OKLAHOMA
BON SECOURS HEALTH SYSTEM INC
BOSTON SCIENTIFIC CORP
BRISTOL MYERS SQUIBB CO
CAMBREX CORP
CANTEL MEDICAL CORP
CAPITAL SENIOR LIVING CORP
CARDINAL HEALTH INC

CARDINAL MEDICAL PRODUCTS AND SERVICES
CAREMARK RX INC
CATHOLIC HEALTH INITIATIVES
CATHOLIC HEALTHCARE PARTNERS
CENTENE CORPORATION
CENTERPULSE AG
CERNER CORP
CHIRON CORP
CHRISTUS HEALTH
CIGNA CORP
CIVCO MEDICAL INSTRUMENTS
CLARIAN HEALTH PARTNERS INC
CNS INC
COLE NATIONAL CORPORATION
COMMUNITY HEALTH SYSTEMS INC
COMPEX TECHNOLOGIES INC
CONCENTRA INC
CORVEL CORP
COVANCE INC
COVENTRY HEALTH CARE INC
CR BARD INC
CRITICARE SYSTEMS INC
CURATIVE HEALTH SERVICES INC
CVS CORPORATION
D & K HEALTHCARE RESOURCES INC
DADE BEHRING HOLDINGS INC
DATASCOPE CORP
DAVITA INC
DELTA DENTAL PLANS ASSOCIATION
DENTAL BENEFITS PROVIDERS
DENTSPLY INTERNATIONAL INC
DEPUY INC
DETROIT MEDICAL CENTER
DRUGMAX INC
ECLIPSYS CORPORATION
ELAN CORP PLC
ELI LILLY & CO
EMERGING VISION INC
EMERITUS CORP
EMPI INC
ENVIRONMENTAL TECTONICS CORP
EPIC SYSTEMS CORPORATION
ESSILOR INTERNATIONAL SA
EXPRESS SCRIPTS INC
EXTENDICARE INC
FAIRVIEW HEALTH SERVICES
FIRST CONSULTING GROUP INC
FIRST HEALTH GROUP CORP
FISHER SCIENTIFIC INTERNATIONAL INC
FOREST LABORATORIES INC
FUJISAWA PHARMACEUTICALS COMPANY LTD
GE COMMERCIAL FINANCE
GE HEALTHCARE
GENERAL NUTRITION COMPANIES INC
GENTIVA HEALTH SERVICES INC
GENZYME CORP

GLAXOSMITHKLINE PLC
GSI LUMONICS INC
GUIDANT CORP
GYRUS GROUP
HANGER ORTHOPEDIC GROUP INC
HARBORSIDE HEALTHCARE CORP
HCA INC
HEALTH CARE SERVICE CORPORATION
HEALTH FITNESS CORP
HEALTH MANAGEMENT ASSOCIATES INC
HEALTH MANAGEMENT SYSTEMS INC
HEALTHSOUTH CORP
HEALTHTRONICS INC
HEARUSA INC
HEMACARE CORPORATION
HENRY FORD HEALTH SYSTEMS
HENRY SCHEIN INC
HILLENBRAND INDUSTRIES
HILL-ROM COMPANY INC
HOOPER HOLMES INC
HORIZON HEALTH CORPORATION
HOSPIRA INC
HUMANA INC
I FLOW CORPORATION
IDEXX LABORATORIES INC
IDX SYSTEMS CORP
INSTRUMENTARIUM CORPORATION
INTEGRAMED AMERICA INC
INTERMAGNETICS GENERAL CORP
INVACARE CORP
JENNY CRAIG INC
JOHNSON & JOHNSON
KAISER PERMANENTE
KENDLE INTERNATIONAL INC
KIMBERLY CLARK CORP
KINDRED HEALTHCARE INC
LABONE INC
LABORATORY CORP OF AMERICA HOLDINGS
LCA VISION INC
LIFE CARE CENTERS OF AMERICA
LIFECORE BIOMEDICAL INC
LOGISTICARE INC
LUXOTTICA GROUP SPA
MAGELLAN HEALTH SERVICES INC
MALLINCKRODT INC
MANOR CARE INC
MARIAN HEALTH SYSTEMS
MARINER HEALTH CARE INC
MARSH & MCLENNAN COMPANIES INC
MAYO FOUNDATION FOR MEDICAL EDUCATION AND RESEARCH
MCKESSON CORPORATION
MDS INC
MEDCATH CORPORATION
MEDCO HEALTH SOLUTIONS
MEDEX HOLDINGS CORPORATION
MEDICAL MUTUAL OF OHIO
MEDICORE INC
MEDQUIST INC

MEDTRONIC INC
MEDTRONIC MINIMED INC
MEDTRONIC XOMED SURGICAL PRODUCTS INC
MENTOR CORP
MERCK & CO INC
MERIDIAN BIOSCIENCE INC
MERIDIAN MEDICAL TECHNOLOGIES INC
METTLER-TOLEDO INTERNATIONAL
MICROTEK MEDICAL HOLDINGS INC
MIM CORP
MINNTECH CORP
MONARCH DENTAL CORP
MORRISON MANAGEMENT SPECIALISTS INC
MYLAN LABORATORIES INC
NANOBIO CORPORATION
NATIONAL DENTEX CORP
NATIONAL HEALTHCARE CORP
NEIGHBORCARE INC
NOVAMED INC
NOVARTIS AG
NOVATION LLC
NOVO-NORDISK AS
OCA INC
OCCUPATIONAL HEALTH + REHABILITATION INC
ODYSSEY HEALTHCARE INC
OHIOHEALTH CORPORATION
OMNICARE INC
OPTION CARE INC
OUTLOOK POINTE CORP
OWENS & MINOR INC
PACIFICARE HEALTH SYSTEMS INC
PATIENT CARE INC
PATTERSON COMPANIES INC
PEDIATRIC SERVICES OF AMERICA INC
PEDIATRIX MEDICAL GROUP INC
PERKINELMER INC
PETMED EXPRESS INC
PFIZER INC
PHC INC
PREMIER INC
PRIORITY HEALTHCARE CORP
PROVINCE HEALTHCARE CO
PSS WORLD MEDICAL INC
PSYCHIATRIC SOLUTIONS INC
QUEST DIAGNOSTICS INC
QUINTILES TRANSNATIONAL CORP
RADIOLOGIX INC
REHABCARE GROUP INC
RENAL CARE GROUP INC
RES CARE INC
RITE AID CORPORATION
ROCHE GROUP
ROTECH HEALTHCARE INC
SCHERING-PLOUGH CORP
SEROLOGICALS CORP
SHIRE PHARMACEUTICALS PLC
SIGMA ALDRICH CORP

SISTERS OF MERCY HEALTH SYSTEMS
SOLA INTERNATIONAL INC
SOLUCIENT LLC
SONIC INNOVATIONS INC
SPECTRUM HEALTH
SRI/SURGICAL EXPRESS INC
SSM HEALTH CARE SYSTEM INC
ST JUDE MEDICAL INC
STERIS CORP
STRYKER CORP
SUN HEALTHCARE GROUP
SUNRISE MEDICAL INC
SUNRISE SENIOR LIVING
SUPERIOR CONSULTANT HOLDINGS CORP
SYBRON DENTAL SPECIALTIES INC
SYMMETRY MEDICAL INC
SYNOVIS LIFE TECHNOLOGIES INC
TEAM HEALTH
TECHNE CORP
TELEX COMMUNICATIONS INC
TENET HEALTHCARE CORPORATION
TEVA PHARMACEUTICAL INDUSTRIES
TEXAS HEALTH RESOURCES
THERMO ELECTRON CORP
TLC VISION CORPORATION
TRANSCEND SERVICES INC
TRIAD HOSPITALS INC
TRINITY HEALTH COMPANY
TRIPOS INC
UNITED SURGICAL PARTNERS
UNITEDHEALTH GROUP INC
UNIVERSAL HOSPITAL SERVICES INC
UROCOR INC
US ONCOLOGY INC
US PHYSICAL THERAPY INC
US VISION INC
UTI CORPORATION
VALEANT PHARMACEUTICALS INTERNATIONAL
VCA ANTECH INC
VENTANA MEDICAL SYSTEMS
VENTIV HEALTH INC
VIASYS HEALTHCARE INC
VISION SERVICE PLAN
VITAL SIGNS INC
VITALWORKS INC
WALGREEN CO
WATSON PHARMACEUTICALS INC
WEIGHT WATCHERS INTERNATIONAL INC
WELCH ALLYN INC
WELLCARE GROUP OF COMPANIES
WELLPOINT HEALTH NETWORKS INC
WEST PHARMACEUTICAL SERVICES INC
WRIGHT MEDICAL GROUP INC
WYETH
YOUNG INNOVATIONS INC
ZIMMER HOLDINGS INC

SOUTHEAST
3M COMPANY
AAIPHARMA INC
ABBOTT LABORATORIES
ACCREDO HEALTH INC
ADVANCEPCS INC
ADVENTIST HEALTH SYSTEM
ADVOCAT INC
AETNA INC
AFLAC INC
ALCON INC
ALLERGAN INC
ALLIANCE IMAGING INC
ALPHARMA INC
ALTERRA HEALTHCARE CORP
AMEDISYS INC
AMERICA SERVICE GROUP INC
AMERICAN HEALTHWAYS INC
AMERICAN HOMEPATIENT INC
AMERICAN MEDICAL SECURITY GROUP INC
AMERICAN RETIREMENT CORP
AMERICHOICE CORPORATION
AMERIGROUP CORPORATION
AMERIPATH INC
AMERISOURCEBERGEN CORP
AMGEN INC
AMSURG CORP
ANDRX CORP
ANTHEM INC
AON CORPORATION
APOGENT TECHNOLOGIES INC
APRIA HEALTHCARE GROUP INC
ARKANSAS BLUE CROSS AND BLUE SHIELD
ARTHROCARE CORP
ASCENSION HEALTH
ASSISTED LIVING CONCEPTS INC
ASSURANT EMPLOYEE BENEFITS
ASSURANT HEALTH
ASSURANT INC
ATC HEALTHCARE INC
ATRIA SENIOR LIVING GROUP
ATRION CORPORATION
AVENTIS SA
AVMED HEALTH PLAN
BAUSCH & LOMB INC
BAXTER INTERNATIONAL INC
BAYER CORP
BECKMAN COULTER INC
BECTON DICKINSON & CO
BEVERLY ENTERPRISES INC
BIOMET INC
BLUE CROSS AND BLUE SHIELD ASSOCIATION
BLUE CROSS AND BLUE SHIELD OF FLORIDA
BLUE CROSS AND BLUE SHIELD OF GEORGIA INC
BLUE CROSS AND BLUE SHIELD OF LOUISIANA
BLUE CROSS AND BLUE SHIELD OF TENNESSEE INC
BON SECOURS HEALTH SYSTEM INC
BOSTON SCIENTIFIC CORP
BRISTOL MYERS SQUIBB CO
CAPITAL SENIOR LIVING CORP
CARDINAL HEALTH INC
CAREMARK RX INC
CASTLE DENTAL CENTERS INC
CATHOLIC HEALTH INITIATIVES
CATHOLIC HEALTHCARE PARTNERS
CENTERPULSE AG
CERNER CORP
CHIRON CORP
CHRISTUS HEALTH
CIGNA CORP
CIVCO MEDICAL INSTRUMENTS
COAST DENTAL SERVICES INC
COLE NATIONAL CORPORATION
COMMUNITY HEALTH SYSTEMS INC
COMPEX TECHNOLOGIES INC
CONCENTRA INC
CONMED CORP
CONTINUCARE CORP
CORDIS CORP
CORVEL CORP
COVANCE INC
COVENTRY HEALTH CARE INC
CR BARD INC
CRYOLIFE INC
CTI MOLECULAR IMAGING
CURATIVE HEALTH SERVICES INC
CVS CORPORATION
D & K HEALTHCARE RESOURCES INC
DADE BEHRING HOLDINGS INC
DATASCOPE CORP
DAVITA INC
DELTA DENTAL PLANS ASSOCIATION
DENTAL BENEFITS PROVIDERS
DENTSPLY INTERNATIONAL INC
DEPUY INC
DRUGMAX INC
DYNACQ HEALTHCARE INC
ECLIPSYS CORPORATION
EDWARDS LIFESCIENCES CORP
ELAN CORP PLC
ELI LILLY & CO
EMERGING VISION INC
EMERITUS CORP
ENCORE MEDICAL CORPORATION
ESSILOR INTERNATIONAL SA
ETHICON INC
EXACTECH INC
EXCEL TECHNOLOGY INC
EXPRESS SCRIPTS INC
EXTENDICARE INC
FIRST CONSULTING GROUP INC
FIRST HEALTH GROUP CORP
FISHER SCIENTIFIC INTERNATIONAL INC
GE COMMERCIAL FINANCE
GENERAL NUTRITION COMPANIES INC
GENTIVA HEALTH SERVICES INC
GENZYME CORP
GLAXOSMITHKLINE PLC
GYRUS GROUP
HAEMONETICS CORPORATION
HANGER ORTHOPEDIC GROUP INC
HCA INC
HEALTH FITNESS CORP
HEALTH MANAGEMENT ASSOCIATES INC
HEALTH MANAGEMENT SYSTEMS INC
HEALTHSOUTH CORP
HEALTHSTREAM INC
HEALTHTRONICS INC
HEARUSA INC
HEMACARE CORPORATION
HENRY SCHEIN INC
HILLENBRAND INDUSTRIES
HOOPER HOLMES INC
HORIZON HEALTH CORPORATION
HOSPIRA INC
HUMANA INC
IDEXX LABORATORIES INC
IDX SYSTEMS CORP
IMMUCOR INC
INTEGRAMED AMERICA INC
INTERPORE CROSS INTERNATIONAL
INVACARE CORP
JENNY CRAIG INC
JOHNSON & JOHNSON
KAISER PERMANENTE
KIMBERLY CLARK CORP
KINDRED HEALTHCARE INC
LABORATORY CORP OF AMERICA HOLDINGS
LAKELAND INDUSTRIES INC
LCA VISION INC
LIFE CARE CENTERS OF AMERICA
LOGISTICARE INC
LUXOTTICA GROUP SPA
MAGELLAN HEALTH SERVICES INC
MALLINCKRODT INC
MANOR CARE INC
MARINER HEALTH CARE INC
MARSH & MCLENNAN COMPANIES INC
MATRIA HEALTHCARE INC
MAYO FOUNDATION FOR MEDICAL EDUCATION AND RESEARCH
MCKESSON CORPORATION
MDS INC
MEDCATH CORPORATION
MEDCO HEALTH SOLUTIONS
MEDEX HOLDINGS CORPORATION
MEDICAL ACTION INDUSTRIES INC
MEDICORE INC
MEDQUIST INC
MEDTRONIC INC
MEDTRONIC MINIMED INC
MEDTRONIC SOFAMOR DANEK
MEDTRONIC XOMED SURGICAL PRODUCTS INC
MERCK & CO INC
MERIDIAN BIOSCIENCE INC

METROPOLITAN HEALTH NETWORKS
METTLER-TOLEDO INTERNATIONAL
MICROTEK MEDICAL HOLDINGS INC
MID ATLANTIC MEDICAL SERVICES INC
MIM CORP
MINNTECH CORP
MONARCH DENTAL CORP
MOORE MEDICAL CORP
MORRISON MANAGEMENT SPECIALISTS INC
MYLAN LABORATORIES INC
NATIONAL DENTEX CORP
NATIONAL HEALTHCARE CORP
NATIONAL MEDICAL HEALTH CARD SYSTEMS INC
NEIGHBORCARE INC
NEKTAR THERAPEUTICS
NOVAMED INC
NOVARTIS AG
NOVATION LLC
NOVO-NORDISK AS
NOVOSTE CORPORATION
NYER MEDICAL GROUP INC
OCA INC
OCCUPATIONAL HEALTH + REHABILITATION INC
OCULAR SCIENCES INC
ODYSSEY HEALTHCARE INC
OMNICARE INC
OPTION CARE INC
ORTHOFIX INTERNATIONAL NV
OUTLOOK POINTE CORP
OWENS & MINOR INC
OXFORD HEALTH PLANS INC
PACIFICARE HEALTH SYSTEMS INC
PATIENT CARE INC
PATTERSON COMPANIES INC
PEDIATRIC SERVICES OF AMERICA INC
PEDIATRIX MEDICAL GROUP INC
PER SE TECHNOLOGIES INC
PERKINELMER INC
PETMED EXPRESS INC
PFIZER INC
PHARMACEUTICAL PRODUCT DEVELOPMENT INC
PLANVISTA CORP
POLYMEDICA CORPORATION
PREMIER INC
PRIORITY HEALTHCARE CORP
PROVINCE HEALTHCARE CO
PSS WORLD MEDICAL INC
PSYCHIATRIC SOLUTIONS INC
QUALITY SYSTEMS INC
QUEST DIAGNOSTICS INC
QUINTILES TRANSNATIONAL CORP
QUOVADX INC
RADIOLOGIX INC
REHABCARE GROUP INC
RENAL CARE GROUP INC
RES CARE INC

RESPIRONICS INC
RITA MEDICAL SYSTEMS INC
RITE AID CORPORATION
ROCHE GROUP
ROTECH HEALTHCARE INC
SAFEGUARD HEALTH ENTERPRISES INC
SCHERING-PLOUGH CORP
SEROLOGICALS CORP
SHIRE PHARMACEUTICALS PLC
SIGMA ALDRICH CORP
SISTERS OF MERCY HEALTH SYSTEMS
SMITH & NEPHEW PLC
SOLA INTERNATIONAL INC
SPAN AMERICA MEDICAL SYSTEMS INC
SRI/SURGICAL EXPRESS INC
SSM HEALTH CARE SYSTEM INC
ST JUDE CHILDRENS RESEARCH HOSPITAL
ST JUDE MEDICAL INC
STERIS CORP
STRYKER CORP
SUN HEALTHCARE GROUP
SUNRISE MEDICAL INC
SUNRISE SENIOR LIVING
SUPERIOR CONSULTANT HOLDINGS CORP
TEAM HEALTH
TELEX COMMUNICATIONS INC
TENET HEALTHCARE CORPORATION
TEXAS HEALTH RESOURCES
THERAGENICS CORP
THERMO ELECTRON CORP
TLC VISION CORPORATION
TRANSCEND SERVICES INC
TRIAD HOSPITALS INC
UNITED SURGICAL PARTNERS
UNITEDHEALTH GROUP INC
UNIVERSAL HOSPITAL SERVICES INC
UROCOR INC
US ONCOLOGY INC
US PHYSICAL THERAPY INC
US VISION INC
UTI CORPORATION
VCA ANTECH INC
VENTIV HEALTH INC
VISION SERVICE PLAN
VITAL SIGNS INC
VITALWORKS INC
WALGREEN CO
WATSON PHARMACEUTICALS INC
WEIGHT WATCHERS INTERNATIONAL INC
WELCH ALLYN INC
WELLCARE GROUP OF COMPANIES
WELLPOINT HEALTH NETWORKS INC
WEST PHARMACEUTICAL SERVICES INC
WRIGHT MEDICAL GROUP INC
WYETH

NORTHEAST
3M COMPANY
AAIPHARMA INC
ABBOTT LABORATORIES
ABIOMED INC
ACCREDO HEALTH INC
ADVANCEPCS INC
ADVENTIST HEALTH SYSTEM
AETNA INC
AFLAC INC
ALCON INC
ALLERGAN INC
ALLIANCE IMAGING INC
ALLIED HEALTHCARE INTERNATIONAL INC
ALPHARMA INC
ALTERRA HEALTHCARE CORP
AMEDISYS INC
AMERICA SERVICE GROUP INC
AMERICAN HEALTHWAYS INC
AMERICAN HOMEPATIENT INC
AMERICAN MEDICAL SECURITY GROUP INC
AMERICAN PHARMACEUTICAL PARTNERS INC
AMERICAN RETIREMENT CORP
AMERICHOICE CORPORATION
AMERIGROUP CORPORATION
AMERIPATH INC
AMERISOURCEBERGEN CORP
AMGEN INC
AMSURG CORP
ANALOGIC CORP
ANDRX CORP
ANSELL LIMITED COMPANY
ANTHEM INC
AON CORPORATION
APOGENT TECHNOLOGIES INC
APPLERA CORPORATION
APPLIED BIOSYSTEMS GROUP
APRIA HEALTHCARE GROUP INC
ARKANSAS BLUE CROSS AND BLUE SHIELD
ARQULE INC
ARROW INTERNATIONAL INC
ASCENSION HEALTH
ASPECT MEDICAL SYSTEMS INC
ASSISTED LIVING CONCEPTS INC
ASSURANT EMPLOYEE BENEFITS
ASSURANT INC
ATC HEALTHCARE INC
ATRIA SENIOR LIVING GROUP
AVENTIS SA
BARR LABORATORIES INC
BAUSCH & LOMB INC
BAXTER INTERNATIONAL INC
BAYER AG
BAYER CORP
BECKMAN COULTER INC
BECTON DICKINSON & CO
BESPAK PLC
BEVERLY ENTERPRISES INC
BIO RAD LABORATORIES INC
BIO REFERENCE LABORATORIES INC

BIOGEN IDEC INC
BIOMET INC
BIOPHAN TECHNOLOGIES INC
BIOVAIL CORPORATION
BLUE CROSS AND BLUE SHIELD ASSOCIATION
BLUE CROSS AND BLUE SHIELD OF MASSACHUSETTS
BLUE CROSS AND BLUE SHIELD OF NORTH CAROLINA
BLUE CROSS AND BLUE SHIELD OF VERMONT
BON SECOURS HEALTH SYSTEM INC
BOSTON SCIENTIFIC CORP
BRISTOL MYERS SQUIBB CO
CAMBREX CORP
CANDELA CORP
CANTEL MEDICAL CORP
CAPITAL BLUECROSS
CAPITAL SENIOR LIVING CORP
CARDINAL HEALTH INC
CAREFIRST INC
CAREMARK RX INC
CATHOLIC HEALTH INITIATIVES
CATHOLIC HEALTHCARE PARTNERS
CELERA GENOMICS GROUP
CELLTECH GROUP PLC
CENTENE CORPORATION
CENTERPULSE AG
CEPHALON INC
CERNER CORP
CHINDEX INTERNATIONAL INC
CHIRON CORP
CIGNA CORP
COAST DENTAL SERVICES INC
COHERENT INC
COLE NATIONAL CORPORATION
COMMUNITY HEALTH SYSTEMS INC
CONCENTRA INC
CONMED CORP
CONVATEC
COOPER COMPANIES INC
CORVEL CORP
COVANCE INC
COVENTRY HEALTH CARE INC
CR BARD INC
CURATIVE HEALTH SERVICES INC
CVS CORPORATION
DADE BEHRING HOLDINGS INC
DATASCOPE CORP
DAVITA INC
DELTA DENTAL PLANS ASSOCIATION
DENTAL BENEFITS PROVIDERS
DENTSPLY INTERNATIONAL INC
DEPUY INC
DIAGNOSTIC PRODUCTS CORPORATION
DIGENE CORPORATION
DRUGMAX INC
DUANE READE INC
ECLIPSYS CORPORATION

ELAN CORP PLC
ELI LILLY & CO
EMERGING VISION INC
EMERITUS CORP
ENDO PHARMACEUTICALS HOLDINGS INC
ENVIRONMENTAL TECTONICS CORP
EON LABS INC
ERESEARCH TECHNOLOGY INC
ESSILOR INTERNATIONAL SA
ETHICON INC
EXACTECH INC
EXCEL TECHNOLOGY INC
EXPRESS SCRIPTS INC
EXTENDICARE INC
E-Z-EM INC
FIRST CONSULTING GROUP INC
FIRST HEALTH GROUP CORP
FISHER SCIENTIFIC INTERNATIONAL INC
FOREST LABORATORIES INC
FRESENIUS AG
GE COMMERCIAL FINANCE
GENERAL NUTRITION COMPANIES INC
GENTIVA HEALTH SERVICES INC
GENZYME CORP
GLAXOSMITHKLINE PLC
GROUP HEALTH INCORPORATED
GSI LUMONICS INC
GTC BIOTHERAPEUTICS INC
HAEMONETICS CORPORATION
HANGER ORTHOPEDIC GROUP INC
HARBORSIDE HEALTHCARE CORP
HARVARD PILGRIM HEALTH CARE INC
HCA INC
HEALTH CARE SERVICE CORPORATION
HEALTH FITNESS CORP
HEALTH INSURANCE PLAN OF GREATER NEW YORK
HEALTH MANAGEMENT ASSOCIATES INC
HEALTH MANAGEMENT SYSTEMS INC
HEALTH NET INC
HEALTHNOW NEW YORK
HEALTHSOUTH CORP
HEARUSA INC
HEMACARE CORPORATION
HENRY SCHEIN INC
HIGHMARK INC
HILLENBRAND INDUSTRIES
HILL-ROM COMPANY INC
HOLOGIC INC
HOOPER HOLMES INC
HORIZON BLUE CROSS BLUE SHIELD OF NEW JERSEY
HORIZON HEALTH CORPORATION
HOSPIRA INC
HUMAN GENOME SCIENCES INC
HUMANA INC
HUNTLEIGH TECHNOLOGIES PLC

ICU MEDICAL INC
IDEXX LABORATORIES INC
IDX SYSTEMS CORP
IMPATH INC
IMS HEALTH INC
INCYTE CORP
INSTITUT STRAUMANN AG
INTEGRA LIFESCIENCES HOLDINGS CORP
INTEGRAMED AMERICA INC
INTERMAGNETICS GENERAL CORP
INTERPORE CROSS INTERNATIONAL
INVACARE CORP
INVERNESS MEDICAL INNOVATIONS INC
IRIS INTERNATIONAL INC
I-STAT CORP
JEFFERSON HEALTH SYSTEM INC
JENNY CRAIG INC
JOHNS HOPKINS MEDICINE
JOHNSON & JOHNSON
KAISER PERMANENTE
KENDLE INTERNATIONAL INC
KIMBERLY CLARK CORP
KINDRED HEALTHCARE INC
LABORATORY CORP OF AMERICA HOLDINGS
LAKELAND INDUSTRIES INC
LCA VISION INC
LIFE CARE CENTERS OF AMERICA
LIFECELL CORPORATION
LIFELINE SYSTEMS INC
LOGISTICARE INC
LUMENIS LTD
LUXOTTICA GROUP SPA
MAGELLAN HEALTH SERVICES INC
MALLINCKRODT INC
MANOR CARE INC
MARIAN HEALTH SYSTEMS
MARINER HEALTH CARE INC
MARSH & MCLENNAN COMPANIES INC
MATRIA HEALTHCARE INC
MCKESSON CORPORATION
MDS INC
MEDCATH CORPORATION
MEDCO HEALTH SOLUTIONS
MEDEX HOLDINGS CORPORATION
MEDICAL ACTION INDUSTRIES INC
MEDICAL MUTUAL OF OHIO
MEDICORE INC
MEDQUIST INC
MEDSTAR HEALTH
MEDTRONIC INC
MEDTRONIC MINIMED INC
MEDTRONIC SOFAMOR DANEK
MEDTRONIC XOMED SURGICAL PRODUCTS INC
MEMORIAL SLOAN KETTERING CANCER CENTER
MERCK & CO INC
MERIDIAN BIOSCIENCE INC
MERIDIAN MEDICAL TECHNOLOGIES INC

METROPOLITAN HEALTH NETWORKS
METTLER-TOLEDO INTERNATIONAL
MID ATLANTIC MEDICAL SERVICES
MILLENNIUM PHARMACEUTICALS
MIM CORP
MINE SAFETY APPLIANCES CO
MINNTECH CORP
MISONIX INC
MOORE MEDICAL CORP
MORRISON MANAGEMENT SPECIALISTS INC
MYLAN LABORATORIES INC
NATIONAL DENTEX CORP
NATIONAL HEALTHCARE CORP
NATIONAL HOME HEALTH CARE CORP
NATIONAL MEDICAL HEALTH CARD SYSTEMS INC
NEIGHBORCARE INC
NEW YORK CITY HEALTH AND HOSPITALS CORPORATION
NEW YORK HEALTH CARE INC
NEW YORK-PRESBYTERIAN HEALTHCARE SYSTEM
NMT MEDICAL INC
NOVAMED INC
NOVAMETRIX MEDICAL SYSTEMS INC
NOVARTIS AG
NOVATION LLC
NOVO-NORDISK AS
NYER MEDICAL GROUP INC
OCA INC
OCCUPATIONAL HEALTH + REHABILITATION INC
ODYSSEY HEALTHCARE INC
OMNICARE INC
OPTICARE HEALTH SYSTEMS
OPTION CARE INC
ORGANOGENESIS INC
ORTHOFIX INTERNATIONAL NV
OSTEOTECH INC
OUTLOOK POINTE CORP
OWENS & MINOR INC
OXFORD HEALTH PLANS INC
PALOMAR MEDICAL TECHNOLOGIES INC
PAR PHARMACEUTICAL COMPANIES INC
PARTNERS HEALTHCARE SYSTEM
PATIENT CARE INC
PATTERSON COMPANIES INC
PDI INC
PEDIATRIC SERVICES OF AMERICA INC
PEDIATRIX MEDICAL GROUP INC
PERKINELMER INC
PETMED EXPRESS INC
PFIZER INC
PHARMACEUTICAL PRODUCT DEVELOPMENT INC
PHARMACOPEIA INC
PHC INC
PHILIPS MEDICAL SYSTEMS
PLANVISTA CORP
POLYMEDICA CORPORATION
PRIORITY HEALTHCARE CORP
PROVINCE HEALTHCARE CO
PSS WORLD MEDICAL INC
PSYCHIATRIC SOLUTIONS INC
QUALITY SYSTEMS INC
QUEST DIAGNOSTICS INC
QUINTILES TRANSNATIONAL CORP
QUOVADX INC
RADIOLOGIX INC
REHABCARE GROUP INC
RENAL CARE GROUP INC
RES CARE INC
RESPIRONICS INC
RITE AID CORPORATION
ROCHE GROUP
ROTECH HEALTHCARE INC
SANOFI-SYNTHELABO
SCHERING AG
SCHERING-PLOUGH CORP
SCHICK TECHNOLOGIES INC
SENTARA HEALTHCARE
SEPRACOR INC
SEROLOGICALS CORP
SERONO SA
SHIRE PHARMACEUTICALS PLC
SIEMENS MEDICAL SOLUTIONS
SIGMA ALDRICH CORP
SMITH & NEPHEW PLC
SOLUCIENT LLC
SPAN AMERICA MEDICAL SYSTEMS INC
SPECIALTY LABORATORIES INC
SRI/SURGICAL EXPRESS INC
ST JUDE MEDICAL INC
STERIS CORP
STRYKER CORP
SUN HEALTHCARE GROUP
SUNRISE MEDICAL INC
SUNRISE SENIOR LIVING
SUPERIOR CONSULTANT HOLDINGS CORP
SYBRON DENTAL SPECIALTIES INC
TEAM HEALTH
TENET HEALTHCARE CORPORATION
TEVA PHARMACEUTICAL INDUSTRIES
TEXAS HEALTH RESOURCES
THERMO ELECTRON CORP
THORATEC CORPORATION
TLC VISION CORPORATION
TOSHIBA CORPORATION
TRANSCEND SERVICES INC
TRIAD HOSPITALS INC
TRINITY HEALTH COMPANY
TRIPATH IMAGING INC
TUFTS ASSOCIATED HEALTH PLANS
TYCO HEALTHCARE GROUP
UNIPRISE INCORPORATED
UNITED SURGICAL PARTNERS
UNITEDHEALTH GROUP INC
UNIVERSAL HEALTH SERVICES INC
UNIVERSAL HOSPITAL SERVICES INC
UROCOR INC
US ONCOLOGY INC
US PHYSICAL THERAPY INC
US VISION INC
UTI CORPORATION
VCA ANTECH INC
VENTIV HEALTH INC
VIASYS HEALTHCARE INC
VISION SERVICE PLAN
VITAL SIGNS INC
VITALWORKS INC
WALGREEN CO
WATSON PHARMACEUTICALS INC
WEBMD CORPORATION
WEIGHT WATCHERS INTERNATIONAL INC
WELCH ALLYN INC
WELLCARE GROUP OF COMPANIES
WELLCHOICE INC
WELLPOINT HEALTH NETWORKS INC
WEST PHARMACEUTICAL SERVICES INC
WYETH
ZIMMER HOLDINGS INC
ZLB BEHRING LLC
ZOLL MEDICAL CORP

INDEX OF FIRMS WITH OPERATIONS OUTSIDE THE U.S.

3M COMPANY
AAIPHARMA INC
ABBOTT LABORATORIES
ADVANCED BIONICS CORPORATION
ADVANCED MEDICAL OPTICS INC
AETERNA ZENTARIS INC
AFLAC INC
ALCON INC
ALiGN TECHNOLOGY
ALLERGAN INC
ALLIED HEALTHCARE INTERNATIONAL INC
ALPHARMA INC
AMERICAN MEDICAL SYSTEMS HOLDINGS INC
AMERICAN PHARMACEUTICAL PARTNERS INC
AMGEN INC
ANALOGIC CORP
ANSELL LIMITED COMPANY
AON CORPORATION
APOGENT TECHNOLOGIES INC
APPLERA CORPORATION
APPLIED BIOSYSTEMS GROUP
ARROW INTERNATIONAL INC
ART ADVANCED RESEARCH TECHNOLOGIES
ARTHROCARE CORP
ASPECT MEDICAL SYSTEMS INC
AVENTIS SA
AXA PPP HEALTHCARE
BAUSCH & LOMB INC
BAXTER INTERNATIONAL INC
BAYER AG
BECKMAN COULTER INC
BECTON DICKINSON & CO
BESPAK PLC
BIO RAD LABORATORIES INC
BIOGEN IDEC INC
BIOMET INC
BIOVAIL CORPORATION
BOSTON SCIENTIFIC CORP
BRISTOL MYERS SQUIBB CO
BRITISH UNION PROVIDENT ASSOCIATION (BUPA)
CAMBREX CORP
CANDELA CORP
CANTEL MEDICAL CORP
CARDINAL HEALTH INC
CARDINAL MEDICAL PRODUCTS AND SERVICES
CEDARA SOFTWARE CORP
CELLTECH GROUP PLC
CENTERPULSE AG
CEPHALON INC
CERNER CORP
CHINDEX INTERNATIONAL INC
CHIRON CORP
CHRISTUS HEALTH

CIGNA CORP
COCHLEAR LTD
COHERENT INC
COLE NATIONAL CORPORATION
COMPEX TECHNOLOGIES INC
CONMED CORP
CONVATEC
COOPER COMPANIES INC
COVANCE INC
CR BARD INC
CRYOLIFE INC
CTI MOLECULAR IMAGING
CYBERONICS INC
DADE BEHRING HOLDINGS INC
DATASCOPE CORP
DELTA DENTAL PLANS ASSOCIATION
DENTAL BENEFITS PROVIDERS
DENTSPLY INTERNATIONAL INC
DEPUY INC
DIAGNOSTIC PRODUCTS CORPORATION
DIGENE CORPORATION
DJ ORTHOPEDICS INC
DYNACQ HEALTHCARE INC
ECLIPSYS CORPORATION
EDWARDS LIFESCIENCES CORP
ELAN CORP PLC
ELI LILLY & CO
EMERGENCY FILTRATION PRODUCTS INC
EMERGING VISION INC
ENVIRONMENTAL TECTONICS CORP
ERESEARCH TECHNOLOGY INC
ESSILOR INTERNATIONAL SA
EXCEL TECHNOLOGY INC
EXPRESS SCRIPTS INC
EXTENDICARE INC
E-Z-EM INC
FIRST CONSULTING GROUP INC
FISCHER IMAGING CORP
FISHER SCIENTIFIC INTERNATIONAL INC
FOREST LABORATORIES INC
FRESENIUS AG
FUJISAWA PHARMACEUTICALS COMPANY LTD
GAMBRO AB
GE COMMERCIAL FINANCE
GE HEALTHCARE
GENENTECH INC
GENERAL NUTRITION COMPANIES INC
GENZYME CORP
GLAXOSMITHKLINE PLC
GSI LUMONICS INC
GUIDANT CORP
GYRUS GROUP
HAEMONETICS CORPORATION
HANGER ORTHOPEDIC GROUP INC
HCA INC
HEALTH FITNESS CORP
HEALTHSOUTH CORP
HEALTHSTREAM INC

HEARUSA INC
HENRY SCHEIN INC
HILLENBRAND INDUSTRIES
HILL-ROM COMPANY INC
HOLOGIC INC
HOOPER HOLMES INC
HOSPIRA INC
HUNTLEIGH TECHNOLOGIES PLC
I FLOW CORPORATION
ICU MEDICAL INC
IDEXX LABORATORIES INC
IMMUCOR INC
IMS HEALTH INC
INAMED CORP
INSTITUT STRAUMANN AG
INSTRUMENTARIUM CORPORATION
INTEGRA LIFESCIENCES HOLDINGS CORP
INTUITIVE SURGICAL INC
INVACARE CORP
INVERNESS MEDICAL INNOVATIONS INC
IRIS INTERNATIONAL INC
I-STAT CORP
JENNY CRAIG INC
JOHNS HOPKINS MEDICINE
JOHNSON & JOHNSON
KENDLE INTERNATIONAL INC
KIMBERLY CLARK CORP
KINETIC CONCEPTS INC
KYPHON INC
LABONE INC
LABORATORY CORP OF AMERICA HOLDINGS
LAKELAND INDUSTRIES INC
LCA VISION INC
LIFECORE BIOMEDICAL INC
LIFELINE SYSTEMS INC
LIFESCAN INC
LUMENIS LTD
LUXOTTICA GROUP SPA
MALLINCKRODT INC
MARSH & MCLENNAN COMPANIES INC
MAXYGEN INC
MCKESSON CORPORATION
MDS INC
MEDEX HOLDINGS CORPORATION
MEDTRONIC INC
MEDTRONIC MINIMED INC
MEDTRONIC SOFAMOR DANEK
MEDTRONIC XOMED SURGICAL PRODUCTS INC
MENTOR CORP
MERCK & CO INC
MERIDIAN BIOSCIENCE INC
MERIDIAN MEDICAL TECHNOLOGIES INC
MERIT MEDICAL SYSTEMS INC
METTLER-TOLEDO INTERNATIONAL
MICROTEK MEDICAL HOLDINGS INC

MILLENNIUM PHARMACEUTICALS INC
MINE SAFETY APPLIANCES CO
MINNTECH CORP
MISONIX INC
MIV THERAPEUTICS INC
MOLECULAR DEVICES CORP
MORRISON MANAGEMENT SPECIALISTS INC
NEKTAR THERAPEUTICS
NOVARTIS AG
NOVO-NORDISK AS
OCA INC
OCULAR SCIENCES INC
OMNICARE INC
ORTHOFIX INTERNATIONAL NV
OSTEOTECH INC
PACIFICARE HEALTH SYSTEMS INC
PAR PHARMACEUTICAL COMPANIES INC
PATTERSON COMPANIES INC
PEDIATRIX MEDICAL GROUP INC
PER SE TECHNOLOGIES INC
PERKINELMER INC
PFIZER INC
PHARMACEUTICAL PRODUCT DEVELOPMENT INC
PHARMACOPEIA INC
PHILIPS MEDICAL SYSTEMS
PSS WORLD MEDICAL INC
QUEST DIAGNOSTICS INC
QUIDEL CORP
QUINTILES TRANSNATIONAL CORP
QUOVADX INC

RES CARE INC
RESMED INC
RESPIRONICS INC
ROCHE GROUP
SANOFI-SYNTHELABO
SCHERING AG
SCHERING-PLOUGH CORP
SEPRACOR INC
SEROLOGICALS CORP
SERONO SA
SHIRE PHARMACEUTICALS PLC
SHL TELEMEDICINE
SIEMENS MEDICAL SOLUTIONS
SIGMA ALDRICH CORP
SIGNATURE EYEWEAR INC
SMITH & NEPHEW PLC
SOLA INTERNATIONAL INC
SOLUCIENT LLC
SONIC INNOVATIONS INC
SPECTRANETICS CORP
SSL INTERNATIONAL
ST JUDE MEDICAL INC
STAAR SURGICAL CO
STERIS CORP
STRYKER CORP
SUNRISE MEDICAL INC
SUNRISE SENIOR LIVING
SYBRON DENTAL SPECIALTIES INC
SYMMETRY MEDICAL INC
TECHNE CORP
TELEX COMMUNICATIONS INC
TEVA PHARMACEUTICAL INDUSTRIES
THERASENSE INC

THERMO ELECTRON CORP
THORATEC CORPORATION
TLC VISION CORPORATION
TOSHIBA CORPORATION
TRINITY HEALTH COMPANY
TRIPOS INC
TYCO HEALTHCARE GROUP
UNITED SURGICAL PARTNERS
UNIVERSAL HEALTH SERVICES INC
US VISION INC
UTAH MEDICAL PRODUCTS INC
UTI CORPORATION
VALEANT PHARMACEUTICALS INTERNATIONAL
VENTANA MEDICAL SYSTEMS
VENTIV HEALTH INC
VIASYS HEALTHCARE INC
VISX INC
VITAL SIGNS INC
WALGREEN CO
WARNER CHILCOTT PLC
WATSON PHARMACEUTICALS INC
WEIGHT WATCHERS INTERNATIONAL INC
WELCH ALLYN INC
WEST PHARMACEUTICAL SERVICES INC
WRIGHT MEDICAL GROUP INC
WYETH
YOUNG INNOVATIONS INC
ZIMMER HOLDINGS INC
ZLB BEHRING LLC
ZOLL MEDICAL CORP

Individual Profiles
On Each Of
THE HEALTH CARE 500

3M COMPANY

www.mmm.com

Industry Group Code: 339113 **Ranks within this company's industry group:** Sales: 1 Profits: 1

Insurance/HMO/PPO:	Drugs:	Equipment/Supplies:	Hospitals/Clinics:	Services:	Health Care:
Insurance:	Manufacturer: Y	Manufacturer: Y	Acute Care:	Diagnostics:	Home Health:
Managed Care:	Distributor:	Distributor:	Sub-Acute Care:	Labs/Testing:	Long-Term Care:
Utilization Mgmt.:	Specialty Pharm.:	Leasing/Finance:	Outpatient Surgery:	Staffing:	Physical Therapy:
Payment Proc.:	Vitamins/Nutri.:	Information Sys.: Y	Phys. Rehab. Center:	Waste Disposal:	Phys. Practice Mgmt.:
	Clinical Trials:		Psychiatric Clinics:	Specialty Services:	

TYPES OF BUSINESS:
Health Care Products
Industrial Products
Safety, Security & Protection Products
Display & Graphics Products
Consumer & Office Products
Electronic & Communications Products
Transportation Products
Fuel-Cell Technology

BRANDS/DIVISIONS/AFFILIATES:
Minnesota Mining and Manufacturing Company
Hornell International
GuardiaNet Systems, Inc.
Scotch-Brite
Filtek
Post-it
Scotch Tape
Scotchgard

CONTACTS:
Note: Officers with more than one job title may be intentionally listed here more than once.
W. James McNerney, Jr., CEO
Patrick D. Campbell, Sr. VP/CFO
David W. Powell, Sr. VP-Mktg.
M. Kay Grenz, Sr. VP-Human Resources
Jay V. Ihlenfeld, Sr. VP-Research & Dev.
David P. Drew, VP-IT
James T. Mahan, Sr. VP-Eng.
James T. Mahan, Sr. VP-Mfg. & Logistics
Richard F. Ziegler, Sr. VP/General Counsel
J. Mark Borseth, Exec. VP-Financial Svcs.
Steven J. Landwehr, Exec. VP-Transportation Bus.
Charles Reich, Exec. VP-Health Care Bus.
Moe S. Nozari, Exec. VP-Consumer & Office Bus.
Harold J. Wiens, Exec. VP-Industrial Bus.
W. James McNerney, Jr., Chmn.
Inge Thulin, Exec. VP-Int'l Oper.

Phone: 651-733-1110 **Fax:** 651-736-2133
Toll-Free: 800-364-3577
Address: 3M Center, Bldg. 220-11W-02, St. Paul, MN 55144-1000 US

GROWTH PLANS/SPECIAL FEATURES:
3M Company, originally known as Minnesota Mining and Manufacturing Company, is an integrated enterprise involved in the research, manufacture and marketing of a variety of products. 3M operates in more than 60 countries, and its products are sold in nearly 200 countries. The firm controls 40 business units organized into seven segments: health care products; industrial products; consumer and office products; display and graphics; electronics and communications products; transportation products; and safety, security and protection products. The company also produces apparel, bags and travel equipment, golf products and business products. Health care products (including medical and surgical supplies) generate the most revenues and profits. Industrial products (including tapes and adhesives), display and graphics products and consumer/office products are other top revenue generators. In addition, the firm develops technologies including fuel-cell components, light management, film solutions and light fiber. Among 3M's most recognizable brands are Post-it products and Scotch Tape, as well as Scotchgard, Thinsulate, Scotch-Brite, Filtrete, Dyneon and O-Cel-O. Because of the company's dedication to environmental safety, one out of every eight 3M scientists works with processes and chemicals aimed at minimizing impact on the environment. Via its technical collaboration with Nitto Denko, 3M has developed a two-in-one product that combines polarizing film with polarization conversion film for liquid crystal displays. 3M ESPE is the branch of 3M that manufactures and markets dental products. Some recent innovations in dentistry at 3M include Filtek technology, which uses nanoparticles and nanocluster fillers to create more natural-looking restorations. A divesture of 3M's fine particle pilot plant split-off to form a nanopowder company called Aveka, Inc. Recently, 3M completed the acquisition including related trademarks and patents of Hornell International, a global supplier of personal protective equipment for welding applications, based in Sweden.
Employees of 3M are offered medical, dental and life insurance as well as a gym.

FINANCIALS:
Sales and profits are in thousands of dollars—add 000 to get the full amount. Year 2004 note: Complete fiscal 2004 results were not available for all companies at press time. For this company, year 2004 is for 9 months.

2004 Sales: $14,920,000 (9 months)	2004 Profits: $2,270,000 (9 months)	**Stock Ticker:** MMM
2003 Sales: $18,232,000	2003 Profits: $2,403,000	**Employees:** 67,072
2002 Sales: $16,332,000	2002 Profits: $1,974,000	**Fiscal Year Ends:** 12/31
2001 Sales: $16,079,000	2001 Profits: $1,430,000	
2000 Sales: $16,724,000	2000 Profits: $1,782,000	

SALARIES/BENEFITS:
Pension Plan: Y	ESOP Stock Plan: Y	Profit Sharing:	Top Exec. Salary: $1,540,000	Bonus: $3,222,459
Savings Plan: Y	Stock Purch. Plan: Y		Second Exec. Salary: $618,512	Bonus: $406,147

OTHER THOUGHTS:
Apparent Top Female Officers: 1
Hot Spot for Advancement for Women/Minorities:

LOCATIONS: ("Y" = Yes)
West:	Southwest:	Midwest:	Southeast:	Northeast:	International:
Y	Y	Y	Y	Y	Y

AAIPHARMA INC

www.aaipharma.com

Industry Group Code: 541710 **Ranks within this company's industry group:** Sales: 5 Profits: 5

Insurance/HMO/PPO:	Drugs:		Equipment/Supplies:	Hospitals/Clinics:	Services:		Health Care:
Insurance:	Manufacturer:	Y	Manufacturer:	Acute Care:	Diagnostics:		Home Health:
Managed Care:	Distributor:		Distributor:	Sub-Acute Care:	Labs/Testing:	Y	Long-Term Care:
Utilization Mgmt.:	Specialty Pharm.:	Y	Leasing/Finance:	Outpatient Surgery:	Staffing:		Physical Therapy:
Payment Proc.:	Vitamins/Nutri.:		Information Sys.:	Phys. Rehab. Center:	Waste Disposal:		Phys. Practice Mgmt.:
	Clinical Trials:	Y		Psychiatric Clinics:	Specialty Services:	Y	

TYPES OF BUSINESS:
Research & Development Services-Pharmaceuticals
Pain Management and Critical Care Drugs

BRANDS/DIVISIONS/AFFILIATES:
Applied Analytical Industries, Inc.
AAI International
AAI Development Services
Darvocet
Darvon
Brethine
Ecabet
Azasan

CONTACTS:
Note: Officers with more than one job title may be intentionally listed here more than once.

Frederick Sancilio, CEO
Gregory Rayburn, Interim COO
Ginna Gutzeit, Interim CFO
Bowin Lindgren, Sr. VP-Human Resources
Vijay Aggarwal, Pres.-Research & Dev.
Gregory S. Bentley, Exec. VP/General Counsel
Bowin Lindgren, Sr. VP-Strategic Plans
Frederick D. Sancilio, Chmn.

Phone: 910-254-7000 **Fax:** 910-815-2300
Toll-Free: 800-575-4224
Address: 2320 Scientific Park Dr., Wilmington, NC 28405 US

GROWTH PLANS/SPECIAL FEATURES:
aaiPharma, Inc., formerly Applied Analytical Industries, Inc., is a specialty pharmaceutical and product development company with comprehensive drug development capabilities in the United States, Europe and Asia. The firm specializes in pain management and critical care drugs. Its pain management drug portfolio includes Darvocet A500, Oramorph SR, Roxicodone, Roxanol and Duraclon. Its critical care drug portfolio includes Brethine Injectable, Azathioprine 50 mg and Calcitriol Injection. The company partners with pharmaceutical companies on both a fee-for-service and royalty and milestone payment basis, providing the expertise and knowledge to create quality health care products. aaiPharma has earned a reputation for solving complex pharmaceutical challenges utilizing analytical testing and formulations development techniques, as well as validation and regulatory affairs support services. aaiPharma operates in three divisions: pharmaceuticals, research and development and AAI Development Services, formerly AAI International. The pharmaceuticals division acquires and commercializes branded pharmaceutical products in targeted therapeutic classes. The division has acquired the drugs Brethine, Darvon and Darvocet. The research and development division provides research and development expertise and maintains a portfolio of drug-delivery technologies and intellectual property rights, which the company uses to develop better and cheaper drugs. It currently has two pain management drugs in development, ProSorb-D in Phase III and Darvon/Darvocet L.E. in Phase I. In a break from its traditional focus on pain management and critical care, the company has developed a new gastroenterology drug, Ecabet, which is in Phase II trials. AAI Development Services offers a comprehensive range of pharmaceutical pre-clinical and clinical product development services to North American, European and Asian pharmaceutical, biotechnology and medical device companies. In recent news, aaiPharma received FDA approval for and launched Azasan, Calcitriol, Darvon Compound 32 and Darvocet A500. The firm acquired Oramorph SR, Roxicodone, Roxanol and Duraclon.

FINANCIALS:
Sales and profits are in thousands of dollars—add 000 to get the full amount. Year 2004 note: Complete fiscal 2004 results were not available for all companies at press time. For this company, year 2004 is for 9 months.

2004 Sales: $148,949 (9 months)	2004 Profits: $-39,180 (9 months)	**Stock Ticker: AAII**
2003 Sales: $282,700	2003 Profits: $34,300	Employees: 1,300
2002 Sales: $230,500	2002 Profits: $24,072	Fiscal Year Ends: 12/31
2001 Sales: $141,100	2001 Profits: $5,900	
2000 Sales: $104,245	2000 Profits: $-402	

SALARIES/BENEFITS:
Pension Plan:	ESOP Stock Plan:	Profit Sharing:	Top Exec. Salary: $400,000	Bonus: $287,000
Savings Plan:	Stock Purch. Plan:		Second Exec. Salary: $285,000	Bonus: $260,750

OTHER THOUGHTS:
Apparent Top Female Officers: 1
Hot Spot for Advancement for Women/Minorities:

LOCATIONS: ("Y" = Yes)
West:	Southwest:	Midwest:	Southeast:	Northeast:	International:
Y		Y	Y	Y	Y

ABBOTT LABORATORIES

www.abbott.com

Industry Group Code: 325412 Ranks within this company's industry group: Sales: 8 Profits: 6

Insurance/HMO/PPO:	Drugs:		Equipment/Supplies:		Hospitals/Clinics:	Services:	Health Care:
Insurance:	Manufacturer:	Y	Manufacturer:	Y	Acute Care:	Diagnostics:	Home Health:
Managed Care:	Distributor:		Distributor:		Sub-Acute Care:	Labs/Testing:	Long-Term Care:
Utilization Mgmt.:	Specialty Pharm.:		Leasing/Finance:		Outpatient Surgery:	Staffing:	Physical Therapy:
Payment Proc.:	Vitamins/Nutri.:	Y	Information Sys.:		Phys. Rehab. Center:	Waste Disposal:	Phys. Practice Mgmt.:
	Clinical Trials:				Psychiatric Clinics:	Specialty Services:	

TYPES OF BUSINESS:
Drugs-Antibiotics and Synthetic Hormones
Nutritional Products
Diagnostic Systems
Consumer Health Products
Hospital Products

BRANDS/DIVISIONS/AFFILIATES:
Hospira
AxSYM
Depakote
TAP Pharmaceutical Products
Flomax
Prevacid
Similac
TheraSense, Inc.

CONTACTS:
Note: Officers with more than one job title may be intentionally listed here more than once.

Miles D. White, CEO
Thomas C. Freyman, CFO
Thomas M. Wascoe, Sr. VP-Human Resources
Karen L. Miller, VP-IT
John C. Landgraf, VP-Corp. Eng.
Jose M. de Lasa, General Counsel
William G. Dempsey, Sr. VP-Pharma Oper.
Steven J. Weger, Jr., VP-Corp. Planning & Dev.
Catherine V. Babington, VP-Public Affairs
Catherine V. Babington, VP-Investor Rel.
Terrence C. Kearney, Treas.
Richard A. Gonzalez, Pres./COO-Medical Products
Joy A. Amundson, Sr. VP-Ross Products
Christopher B. Begley, Sr. VP-Hospital Products
Jeffrey M. Leiden, Pres./COO-Pharmaceutical Products
Miles D. White, Chmn.

Phone: 847-937-6100 Fax: 847-937-1511
Toll-Free:
Address: 100 Abbott Park Rd., Abbott Park, IL 60064-6400 US

GROWTH PLANS/SPECIAL FEATURES:

Abbott Laboratories' principal business is the discovery, development, manufacture and sale of a diversified line of health care products and services. The company operates through five major business segments: pharmaceutical products, diagnostic products, hospital products, Ross products and international. Principal pharmaceutical products include Depakote, which treats epilepsy, migraine and bipolar disorder; the anti-infective clarithromycin; various forms of erythromycin; and a broad line of cardiovascular products. The diagnostics segment markets systems for blood banks, hospitals, commercial laboratories, alternate-care testing sites and consumers. Hospital products include drugs and drug delivery systems, perioperative and intensive care products and cardiovascular, renal and oncology products. Ross products include a broad line of adult and pediatric nutritionals, specialty pharmaceuticals and consumer products. Ross brands include Similac and Isomil infant formulas, Ensure, Pedialyte, Selsun Blue and the Fact Plus line of pregnancy tests. The international segment markets a broad line of hospital, pharmaceutical and nutritional products outside the United States. Through a joint venture with TAP Pharmaceutical Products, Abbott makes the best-selling prostate cancer drug Lupron. Abbott Laboratories announced recently that it has started construction of a major biotechnology facility at its Murex manufacturing plant in the U.K. Abbott also completed the acquisition of TheraSense, Inc., a California-based company that manufactures blood glucose monitoring systems. TheraSense products include FreeStyle, a blood glucose self-monitoring system. In October 2004, the company agreed to acquire EAS, a national supplement manufacture, for $320 million dollars.

Abbott offers a full benefits package to its employees, including medical, dental, vision, life and accident insurance, retirement plans and tax-saving benefits. Fortune Magazine has ranked Abbott as one of the top 50 companies for minorities, and Working Mother magazine ranked it among the top 10 best companies for working mothers.

FINANCIALS:
Sales and profits are in thousands of dollars—add 000 to get the full amount. Year 2004 note: Complete fiscal 2004 results were not available for all companies at press time. For this company, year 2004 is for 9 months.

2004 Sales: $14,025,573 (9 months) 2004 Profits: $2,261,246 (9 months)
2003 Sales: $19,680,600 2003 Profits: $2,753,200
2002 Sales: $17,685,000 2002 Profits: $2,794,000
2001 Sales: $16,285,000 2001 Profits: $1,550,000
2000 Sales: $13,745,900 2000 Profits: $2,786,000

Stock Ticker: ABT
Employees: 72,200
Fiscal Year Ends: 12/31

SALARIES/BENEFITS:
Pension Plan: Y ESOP Stock Plan: Profit Sharing: Y Top Exec. Salary: $1,564,961 Bonus: $1,750,000
Savings Plan: Y Stock Purch. Plan: Second Exec. Salary: $882,692 Bonus: $970,000

OTHER THOUGHTS:
Apparent Top Female Officers: 3
Hot Spot for Advancement for Women/Minorities: Y

LOCATIONS: ("Y" = Yes)
West:	Southwest:	Midwest:	Southeast:	Northeast:	International:
Y	Y	Y	Y	Y	Y

ABIOMED INC

www.abiomed.com

Industry Group Code: 339113   Ranks within this company's industry group: Sales: 130   Profits: 129

Insurance/HMO/PPO:	Drugs:	Equipment/Supplies:	Hospitals/Clinics:	Services:	Health Care:
Insurance:	Manufacturer:	Manufacturer: Y	Acute Care:	Diagnostics:	Home Health:
Managed Care:	Distributor:	Distributor:	Sub-Acute Care:	Labs/Testing:	Long-Term Care:
Utilization Mgmt.:	Specialty Pharm.:	Leasing/Finance:	Outpatient Surgery:	Staffing:	Physical Therapy:
Payment Proc.:	Vitamins/Nutri.:	Information Sys.:	Phys. Rehab. Center:	Waste Disposal:	Phys. Practice Mgmt.:
	Clinical Trials:		Psychiatric Clinics:	Specialty Services:	

TYPES OF BUSINESS:
Equipment-Cardiac Assistance
Heart Replacement Technology

BRANDS/DIVISIONS/AFFILIATES:
Bi-Ventricular Support System
AbioCor
BVS-5000
AB500 Circulatory Support System

CONTACTS:
Note: Officers with more than one job title may be intentionally listed here more than once.

Michael R. Minogue, CEO
Michael R. Minogue, Pres.
Charles B. Haaser, Acting CFO
Christopher Macdonald, Sr. VP-Global Sales
Kimberley S. Rogers, Dir.-Human Resources
Robert T.V. Kung, Chief Scientific Officer
William J. Bolt, VP-Eng.
Karen A. Heffernan, Dir.-Mfg. Oper.
Tracy P. Berns, General Counsel
Javier Jimenez, VP-Oper.
Edward E. Berger, VP-Reimbursement & External Rel.
Farhad Zarinetchi, VP-Contract Research
Eugene D. Rabe, VP-Sales & Services
David M. Lederman, Chmn.

Phone: 978-777-5410   **Fax:** 978-777-8411
Toll-Free:
Address: 22 Cherry Hill Dr., Danvers, MA 01923 US

GROWTH PLANS/SPECIAL FEATURES:
ABIOMED, Inc. develops, manufactures and markets innovative cardiovascular products and is a leader in the research and development of advanced heart assistance and replacement systems. The company's Bi-Ventricular Support System (BVS-5000) is the most widely used FDA-approved advanced cardiac assist device for patients with reversible heart failure. The BVS has been used to support over 4,000 patients and is capable of taking over the full pumping function of both ventricles of a failing heart. ABIOMED's AbioCor implantable replacement heart is intended to replace a patient's irreparably damaged heart and take over its pumping function. AbioCor is currently in the clinical trial phase. In 2003, the company began selling the AB500 Circulatory Support System for patients needing circulatory support for longer periods of time than provided by the BVS-5000. In September 2004, ABIOMED began selling the AB500 in Europe.

FINANCIALS:
Sales and profits are in thousands of dollars—add 000 to get the full amount. Year 2004 note: Complete fiscal 2004 results were not available for all companies at press time. For this company, year 2004 is for 12 months.

2004 Sales: $25,739 (12 months)	2004 Profits: $-9,446 (12 months)	**Stock Ticker:** ABMD
2003 Sales: $23,300	2003 Profits: $-18,200	**Employees:** 239
2002 Sales: $26,900	2002 Profits: $-21,700	**Fiscal Year Ends:** 3/31
2001 Sales: $24,900	2001 Profits: $-11,400	
2000 Sales: $22,500	2000 Profits: $-10,500	

SALARIES/BENEFITS:
Pension Plan: ESOP Stock Plan: Profit Sharing: Top Exec. Salary: $312,000   Bonus: $156,000
Savings Plan: Y   Stock Purch. Plan: Second Exec. Salary: $208,000   Bonus: $75,000

OTHER THOUGHTS:
Apparent Top Female Officers: 3
Hot Spot for Advancement for Women/Minorities: Y

LOCATIONS: ("Y" = Yes)

West:	Southwest:	Midwest:	Southeast:	Northeast: Y	International:

ACCREDO HEALTH INC

www.accredohealth.com

Industry Group Code: 446110A Ranks within this company's industry group: Sales: 5 Profits: 5

Insurance/HMO/PPO:	Drugs:	Equipment/Supplies:	Hospitals/Clinics:	Services:	Health Care:
Insurance:	Manufacturer:	Manufacturer:	Acute Care:	Diagnostics:	Home Health:
Managed Care:	Distributor:	Distributor:	Sub-Acute Care:	Labs/Testing:	Long-Term Care:
Utilization Mgmt.:	Specialty Pharm.: Y	Leasing/Finance:	Outpatient Surgery:	Staffing:	Physical Therapy:
Payment Proc.:	Vitamins/Nutri.:	Information Sys.:	Phys. Rehab. Center:	Waste Disposal:	Phys. Practice Mgmt.:
	Clinical Trials:		Psychiatric Clinics:	Specialty Services: Y	

TYPES OF BUSINESS:
Drugs-Specialty Pharmacy
Contract Pharmaceutical Services

BRANDS/DIVISIONS/AFFILIATES:
AHI Pharmacies, Inc.
Hemophilia Health Services, Inc.
Nova Factor, Inc.
Sunrise Health Management
BioPartners In Care
Pharmacare Resources, Inc.
Hemophilia Resources of America, Inc.
HRA Holding Corporation

CONTACTS:
Note: Officers with more than one job title may be intentionally listed here more than once.

David D. Stevens, CEO
John R. Grow, Pres.
Joel R. Kimbrough, Sr. VP/CFO
Jill Stem, Dir.-Human Resources
Thomas W. Bell, Jr., General Counsel
Kery Finney, VP-Investor Rel.
Joel R. Kimbrough, Treas.
Thomas W. Bell, Jr., Corp. Sec.
David D. Stevens, Chmn.

Phone: 901-385-3688 Fax: 901-385-3689
Toll-Free: 877-222-7336
Address: 1640 Century Center Pkwy., Ste. 101, Memphis, TN 38134 US

GROWTH PLANS/SPECIAL FEATURES:

Accredo Health, Inc. and its subsidiaries, Hemophilia Health Services, Inc., Nova Factor, Inc. and Accredo, provide specialized contract pharmacy and related services pursuant to agreements with drug manufacturers. The company helps treat patients that have costly, chronic diseases, including growth hormone deficiency, Gaucher disease, hemophilia, multiple sclerosis, Crohn's disease, respiratory syncytial virus, rheumatoid arthritis, immune deficiencies and pulmonary arterial hypertension. Accredo's services include the collection of medication use and patient compliance information, patient education and monitoring, reimbursement expertise and overnight drug delivery. The company's Hemophilia Health Services and Nova Factor divisions are preferred distributors of injectable medications to Aetna U.S. Healthcare members and participating physicians. The firm has a number of other subsidiaries, including Sunrise Health Management, BioPartners In Care and Pharmacare Resources, Inc. These divisions are leading providers of pharmaceutical care for certain chronic, long-term patient populations, including those requiring the intravenous immunoglobulin (IVIG) clotting factor and growth hormone. Accredo anticipates that it will be able to offer its multiple sclerosis and rheumatoid arthritis patients access to an expanding utilization of IVIG combination therapy. The firm attributes its recent success to a continued, careful management of its product mix, strategically limiting the products that it provides under managed care contracts to its current product lines. Hemophilia Health Services recently acquired all of the outstanding stock of privately held HRA Holding Corporation and its wholly-owned subsidiary, Hemophilia Resources of America, Inc. (HRA). HRA is a leading full-service provider of hemophilia coagulation products and services for people with hemophilia and von Willebrand disease.

FINANCIALS:
Sales and profits are in thousands of dollars—add 000 to get the full amount. Year 2004 note: Complete fiscal 2004 results were not available for all companies at press time. For this company, year 2004 is for 12 months.

2004 Sales: $1,516,868 (12 months)   2004 Profits: $78,313 (12 months)
2003 Sales: $1,337,400   2003 Profits: $29,500
2002 Sales: $651,500   2002 Profits: $29,800
2001 Sales: $462,100   2001 Profits: $17,300
2000 Sales: $353,035   2000 Profits: $9,896

Stock Ticker: ACDO
Employees: 2,491
Fiscal Year Ends: 6/30

SALARIES/BENEFITS:
Pension Plan: ESOP Stock Plan: Y   Profit Sharing: Top Exec. Salary: $378,239   Bonus: $123,070
Savings Plan: Y Stock Purch. Plan: Second Exec. Salary: $244,281 Bonus: $58,753

OTHER THOUGHTS:
Apparent Top Female Officers: 2
Hot Spot for Advancement for Women/Minorities:

LOCATIONS: ("Y" = Yes)
West:	Southwest:	Midwest:	Southeast:	Northeast:	International:
Y	Y	Y	Y	Y	

ADVANCED BIONICS CORPORATION www.advancedbionics.com

Industry Group Code: 339113   Ranks within this company's industry group: Sales: Profits:

Insurance/HMO/PPO:	Drugs:	Equipment/Supplies:	Hospitals/Clinics:	Services:	Health Care:
Insurance:	Manufacturer:	Manufacturer: Y	Acute Care:	Diagnostics:	Home Health:
Managed Care:	Distributor:	Distributor:	Sub-Acute Care:	Labs/Testing:	Long-Term Care:
Utilization Mgmt.:	Specialty Pharm.:	Leasing/Finance:	Outpatient Surgery:	Staffing:	Physical Therapy:
Payment Proc.:	Vitamins/Nutri.:	Information Sys.:	Phys. Rehab. Center:	Waste Disposal:	Phys. Practice Mgmt.:
	Clinical Trials:		Psychiatric Clinics:	Specialty Services:	

TYPES OF BUSINESS:
Medical Equipment-Manufacturing
Bionic Devices
Cochlear Implant Technology

BRANDS/DIVISIONS/AFFILIATES:
CLARION CII Bionic Ear System
HiResolution Bionic Ear System

CONTACTS:
Note: Officers with more than one job title may be intentionally listed here more than once.
Al Mann, Co-CEO
Jeff Greiner, Pres./Co-CEO
Tom Santogrossi, VP-Mfg.
Al Mann, Chmn.

Phone: 661-362-1400   Fax: 661-362-1500
Toll-Free: 800-678-2575
Address: 12740 San Fernando Rd., Sylmar, CA 91342 US

GROWTH PLANS/SPECIAL FEATURES:
Advanced Bionics Corporation is a global leader in the development and marketing of implantable high-tech neurostimulation devices, or bionic technologies that treat neurological conditions. These technologies include treatments for deafness, urinary incontinence and chronic pain. Advanced Bionics was formed from two other highly successful companies that produced medical devices; one developed new-generation pacemakers and one developed novel micro-infusion systems (miniature drug-delivery pumps). Advanced Bionics emerged out of research conducted by the Alfred Mann Foundation for Scientific Research and MiniMed Technologies, Ltd. It is the only American company that develops cochlear implant technology. Advanced Bionics' primary product is the CLARION CII Bionic Ear System, one of the most electronically advanced medical implants in the world, which it markets with related sound processing devices as the HiResolution Bionic Ear System. The CLARION technology came from research at the University of California laboratory in San Francisco. Based in California, Advanced Bionics also has offices in France and Colombia.

Advanced Bionics offers a comprehensive benefits package including medical, dental and vision insurance for employees and family as well as disability and life insurance. Plus, the company sponsors an annual family picnic and holiday party. Volleyball, basketball and other outdoor activities are available at the firm's 63-acre campus in Valencia, California.

FINANCIALS:
Sales and profits are in thousands of dollars—add 000 to get the full amount. Year 2004 note: Complete fiscal 2004 results were not available for all companies at press time. For this company, year 2004 is for months.

2004 Sales: $ (months)   2004 Profits: $ (months)
2003 Sales: $ 2003 Profits: $
2002 Sales: $75,000   2002 Profits: $
2001 Sales: $ 2001 Profits: $
2000 Sales: $ 2000 Profits: $

Stock Ticker: Private
Employees: 500
Fiscal Year Ends: 12/31

SALARIES/BENEFITS:
Pension Plan: ESOP Stock Plan: Profit Sharing: Top Exec. Salary: $ Bonus: $
Savings Plan: Y   Stock Purch. Plan: Second Exec. Salary: $ Bonus: $

OTHER THOUGHTS:
Apparent Top Female Officers:
Hot Spot for Advancement for Women/Minorities:

LOCATIONS: ("Y" = Yes)
West:	Southwest:	Midwest:	Southeast:	Northeast:	International:
Y					Y

ADVANCED MEDICAL OPTICS INC

www.amo-inc.com

Industry Group Code: 339113 Ranks within this company's industry group: Sales: 35 Profits: 73

Insurance/HMO/PPO:	Drugs:	Equipment/Supplies:		Hospitals/Clinics:	Services:	Health Care:
Insurance: Managed Care: Utilization Mgmt.: Payment Proc.:	Manufacturer: Distributor: Specialty Pharm.: Vitamins/Nutri.: Clinical Trials:	Manufacturer: Distributor: Leasing/Finance: Information Sys.:	Y	Acute Care: Sub-Acute Care: Outpatient Surgery: Phys. Rehab. Center: Psychiatric Clinics:	Diagnostics: Labs/Testing: Staffing: Waste Disposal: Specialty Services:	Home Health: Long-Term Care: Physical Therapy: Phys. Practice Mgmt.:

TYPES OF BUSINESS:
Equipment/Supplies-Ophthalmic
Ophthalmic Surgical Supplies
Contact Lens Care Products

BRANDS/DIVISIONS/AFFILIATES:
Phacoflex II
OptiEdge
AMO Diplomax
Amadeu Microkeratome
Ultrazyme
AMO Gemini
ClariFlex
Sensar

CONTACTS:
Note: Officers with more than one job title may be intentionally listed here more than once.

James V. Mazzo, CEO
Richard A. Meier, CFO
C. Russell Trenary, VP/Chief Mktg. Officer
Francine D. Meza, Sr. VP-Human Resources
Jane E. Rady, VP-Tech.
Peter P. Nolan, Sr. VP-Mfg.
Aimee S. Weisner, VP/General Counsel
Richard A. Meier, Exec. VP-Oper.
Jane E. Rady, VP-Strategy
Sheree L. Aronson, VP-Corp. Comm.
Sheree L. Aronson, VP-Investor Rel.
Richard A. Meier, Exec. VP-Finance
Masatake Akedo, Pres.-Japan
Jim C. Cooke, VP-Asia Pacific

Phone: 714-247-8200 Fax: 714-247-8681
Toll-Free:
Address: 1700 E. St. Andrew Pl., Santa Ana, CA 92799-5162 US

GROWTH PLANS/SPECIAL FEATURES:
Advanced Medical Optics, Inc. (AMO) develops, manufactures and markets medical devices for the eye and eye care products. The company has two major product lines: ophthalmic surgical and eye care. The ophthalmic surgical product line includes foldable intraocular lenses implanted in the lens capsule to restore sight; phacoemulsification machines used to break up the cloudy human lens prior to its replacement with an intraocular lens; and related surgical accessories such as implantation systems, viscoelastics and disposables. Brand names in the foldable lenses product line include Phacoflex II, Sensar and ClariFlex. Both the ClariFlex and Sensar lenses have AMO's patented OptiEdge square edge, designed to reduce post-surgical posterior capsular opacification. This lessens the need for subsequent laser procedures and reduces the potential for glare and reflections following implantation. Brand names in the phacoemulsification line include Prestige, AMO Diplomax and Sovereign. AMO competes in the refractive surgery market with the Amadeu Microkeratome brand. Contact lens eye care products include single-bottle multi-purpose cleaning and disinfecting solutions, daily cleaners, enzymatic cleaners and contact lens rewetting drops. AMO's leading contact lens care brands include blink, Consept F and Ultrazyme. The company acquired the worldwide distribution rights to an AMO-branded vitreal retinal system, known as AMO Gemini, from Optikon. This system allows AMO to enter the market segment for treatment of the back of the eye. The firm's surgical products customers include surgeons who perform cataract surgeries, hospitals and ambulatory surgical centers. Eye care product customers include optometrists, opticians, ophthalmologists, retailers and clinics that sell directly to consumers. These retailers include mass merchandisers such as Wal-Mart and Walgreens as well as commercial optical chains and food stores. In recent news, AMO acquired Pfizer's ophthalmic surgical business for $450 million. In November 2004, the company agreed to acquire VISX for $1.27 billion.

FINANCIALS:
Sales and profits are in thousands of dollars—add 000 to get the full amount. Year 2004 note: Complete fiscal 2004 results were not available for all companies at press time. For this company, year 2004 is for 9 months.

2004 Sales: $517,414 (9 months)   2004 Profits: $9,074 (9 months)
2003 Sales: $601,453   2003 Profits: $10,357
2002 Sales: $538,087   2002 Profits: $25,910
2001 Sales: $ 2001 Profits: $
2000 Sales: $ 2000 Profits: $

Stock Ticker: AVO
Employees: 2,260
Fiscal Year Ends: 12/31

SALARIES/BENEFITS:
Pension Plan: ESOP Stock Plan: Profit Sharing: Top Exec. Salary: $475,000   Bonus: $500,000
Savings Plan: Y   Stock Purch. Plan: Y   Second Exec. Salary: $340,000   Bonus: $220,000

OTHER THOUGHTS:
Apparent Top Female Officers: 4
Hot Spot for Advancement for Women/Minorities: Y

LOCATIONS: ("Y" = Yes)
West	Southwest	Midwest	Southeast	Northeast	International
Y					Y

ADVANCEPCS INC

www.advparadigm.com

Industry Group Code: 522320A Ranks within this company's industry group: Sales: 2 Profits: 3

Insurance/HMO/PPO:	Drugs:	Equipment/Supplies:	Hospitals/Clinics:	Services:	Health Care:
Insurance:	Manufacturer:	Manufacturer:	Acute Care:	Diagnostics:	Home Health:
Managed Care:	Distributor:	Distributor:	Sub-Acute Care:	Labs/Testing:	Long-Term Care:
Utilization Mgmt.: Y	Specialty Pharm.: Y	Leasing/Finance:	Outpatient Surgery:	Staffing:	Physical Therapy:
Payment Proc.:	Vitamins/Nutri.:	Information Sys.:	Phys. Rehab. Center:	Waste Disposal:	Phys. Practice Mgmt.:
	Clinical Trials: Y		Psychiatric Clinics:	Specialty Services: Y	

TYPES OF BUSINESS:
Pharmacy Management
Online Pharmacy
Clinical Services
Clinical Trials Studies
Information Management
Prescription Discount Cards

BRANDS/DIVISIONS/AFFILIATES:
Caremark Rx, Inc.
PCS Health Systems
FFI Health Services
Advance Paradigm, Inc.
femScript
aVidaRx
MatureRx
MatureRx-Plus

CONTACTS:
Note: Officers with more than one job title may be intentionally listed here more than once.
David D. Halbert, CEO
David D. Halbert, Pres.
Yon Yoon Jorden, CFO
John H. Sattler, VP-Sales & Client Services
Alan T. Wright, Chief Science Officer
Ronald J. Merlino, VP-IT
Susan S. de Mars, General Counsel
Ernest Buys, VP-Oper. & Reengineering
Leslie Simmons, VP-Corp. Comm.
Rudy Mladenovic, VP-Manufacturer Contracting & Product Mgmt.
Ken Czarnecki, VP-Member Experience
Renwyck Elder, VP-Retail Network
Marsha Moore, VP-Medical Affairs
David D. Halbert, Chmn.

Phone: 469-524-4700 **Fax:** 469-524-4702
Toll-Free: 800-749-6199
Address: 750 W. John Carpenter Fwy., Ste. 1200, Irving, TX 75039 US

GROWTH PLANS/SPECIAL FEATURES:
AdvancePCS, Inc. (formerly Advance Paradigm, Inc.) is an independent provider of health improvement services. The firm is one of the largest pharmacy benefit management companies in the world, representing over 75 million Americans. Its portfolio of services includes prescription discount cards for the uninsured and under-insured, web-based programs, disease management, clinical trials and outcomes studies, integrated mail service and retail pharmacy networks, innovative clinical services, customized disease management programs, information management and other services. AdvancePCS is the result of a merger between Advance Paradigm, Inc. and PCS Health Systems. The firm also manages a group of affiliated, privately held companies, collectively known as FFI Health Services (FFI). FFI offers several pharmacy-related product lines under the names aVidaRx, femScript, MatureRx and MatureRx-Plus to under-insured or uninsured individuals, women and senior citizens, respectively. Also, the company has entered into a licensing agreement to provide its proprietary formulary data to ePocrates, the largest handheld network of physicians. The agreement allows physicians using ePocrates' clinical drug database software to immediately determine the formulary status of various drugs when prescribing medications for patients in drug benefit plans managed by AdvancePCS. The company currently manages 165 million pharmacy claims and $6 billion in drug expenditures annually for its clients, which include Blue Cross and Blue Shield organizations, Fortune 500 employers and state and local governments. The firm also operates buildingbetterhealth.com, which provides information on health issues, as well as AdvanceRx.com, an online pharmacy. In recent news, Caremark Rx, Inc., one of the other three major pharmacy benefits management companies, acquired AdvancePCS in an industry-changing decision. AdvancePCS is now a subsidiary of Caremark.

AdvancePCS offers its employees medical, life and dental coverage, a no-cost prescription drug card program, flexible spending accounts, adoption assistance and tuition reimbursement.

FINANCIALS:
Sales and profits are in thousands of dollars—add 000 to get the full amount. Year 2004 note: Complete fiscal 2004 results were not available for all companies at press time. For this company, year 2004 is for months.

2004 Sales: $ (months)   2004 Profits: $ (months)
2003 Sales: $14,110,900   2003 Profits: $168,400
2002 Sales: $13,107,000   2002 Profits: $116,000
2001 Sales: $7,024,300   2001 Profits: $22,700
2000 Sales: $1,833,888   2000 Profits: $20,876

Stock Ticker: Subsidiary
Employees: 6,500
Fiscal Year Ends: 3/31

SALARIES/BENEFITS:
Pension Plan: ESOP Stock Plan: Y   Profit Sharing: Top Exec. Salary: $ Bonus: $
Savings Plan: Y   Stock Purch. Plan: Second Exec. Salary: $ Bonus: $

OTHER THOUGHTS:
Apparent Top Female Officers: 3
Hot Spot for Advancement for Women/Minorities: Y

LOCATIONS: ("Y" = Yes)
West	Southwest	Midwest	Southeast	Northeast	International
Y	Y	Y	Y	Y	

Note: Financial information, benefits and other data can change quickly and may vary from those stated here.

ADVENTIST HEALTH SYSTEM

www.ahss.org

Industry Group Code: 622110 Ranks within this company's industry group: Sales: 4 Profits:

Insurance/HMO/PPO:	Drugs:	Equipment/Supplies:	Hospitals/Clinics:		Services:		Health Care:	
Insurance:	Manufacturer:	Manufacturer:	Acute Care:	Y	Diagnostics:		Home Health:	Y
Managed Care:	Distributor:	Distributor:	Sub-Acute Care:	Y	Labs/Testing:		Long-Term Care:	Y
Utilization Mgmt.:	Specialty Pharm.:	Leasing/Finance:	Outpatient Surgery:	Y	Staffing:		Physical Therapy:	
Payment Proc.:	Vitamins/Nutri.:	Information Sys.:	Phys. Rehab. Center:	Y	Waste Disposal:		Phys. Practice Mgmt.:	
	Clinical Trials:		Psychiatric Clinics:		Specialty Services:	Y		

TYPES OF BUSINESS:
Hospitals
Nursing Homes
Home Health Care Services
Information Management
Artificial Intelligence Research

BRANDS/DIVISIONS/AFFILIATES:
Florida Hospital
Sunbelt Home Health Care
Adventist Care Centers
Sunbelt Systems Concepts
MEDai

CONTACTS:
Note: Officers with more than one job title may be intentionally listed here more than once.
Thomas L. Werner, CEO
Thomas L. Werner, Pres.
Terry D. Shaw, Sr. VP/CFO
Donald G. Jones, VP-Human Resources
Brent G. Snyder, Sr. VP-Info. Services
Robert R. Henderschedt, Sr. VP-Admin.
T. L. Trimble, VP-Legal Services
Sandra K. Johnson, VP-Bus. Dev.
Paul Rathbun, VP-Finance
Donald L. Jernigan, Exec. VP
Gary Skilton, VP/Treas.
Loran D. Hauck, VP-Medical Affairs

Phone: 407-647-4400 **Fax:** 407-975-1469
Toll-Free:
Address: 111 N. Orlando Ave., Winter Park, FL 32789 US

GROWTH PLANS/SPECIAL FEATURES:
Adventist Health System (AHS), sponsored by the Seventh-Day Adventist Church, is the largest not-for-profit Protestant health care organization in the U.S. It operates 38 hospitals in 10 states, 23 nursing homes and over 20 home health care agencies, collectively serving more than 4 million patients annually. Its flagship organization, Florida Hospital, is the largest health care provider in central Florida and a national leader in cardiac care. It was recently ranked by the American Hospital Association as having the busiest community hospital emergency department in the country. The home health care division, Sunbelt Home Health Care (SHHC), manages 23 home health and hospice agencies. Adventist Care Centers (ACC) operates 24 extended care facilities and 23 nursing homes. AHS also manages Sunbelt Systems Concepts, an information management company, and MEDai, an artificial intelligence and outcome research company. Adventist Health Systems is guided by its Christian mission to extend the healing ministry of Christ, and by its combination of scientific treatment of disease with education in the prevention of disease and advocacy of a wholesome lifestyle.

FINANCIALS:
Sales and profits are in thousands of dollars—add 000 to get the full amount. Year 2004 note: Complete fiscal 2004 results were not available for all companies at press time. For this company, year 2004 is for months.

2004 Sales: $ (months)   2004 Profits: $ (months)
2003 Sales: $10,123,100   2003 Profits: $ **Stock Ticker: Nonprofit**
2002 Sales: $8,433,400   2002 Profits: $170,600   **Employees:** 44,000
2001 Sales: $ 2001 Profits: $ **Fiscal Year Ends:**
2000 Sales: $ 2000 Profits: $

SALARIES/BENEFITS:
| Pension Plan: | ESOP Stock Plan: | Profit Sharing: | Top Exec. Salary: $ | Bonus: $ |
| Savings Plan: | Stock Purch. Plan: | | Second Exec. Salary: $ | Bonus: $ |

OTHER THOUGHTS:
Apparent Top Female Officers: 2
Hot Spot for Advancement for Women/Minorities:

LOCATIONS: ("Y" = Yes)
West:	Southwest:	Midwest:	Southeast:	Northeast:	International:
Y	Y	Y	Y	Y	

ADVOCAT INC

www.irinfo.com/avc

Industry Group Code: 623110 Ranks within this company's industry group: Sales: 11 Profits: 10

Insurance/HMO/PPO:	Drugs:	Equipment/Supplies:	Hospitals/Clinics:	Services:	Health Care:
Insurance: Managed Care: Utilization Mgmt.: Payment Proc.:	Manufacturer: Distributor: Specialty Pharm.: Vitamins/Nutri.: Clinical Trials:	Manufacturer: Distributor: Leasing/Finance: Information Sys.:	Acute Care: Sub-Acute Care: Outpatient Surgery: Phys. Rehab. Center: Psychiatric Clinics:	Diagnostics: Labs/Testing: Staffing: Waste Disposal: Specialty Services:	Home Health: Long-Term Care: Y Physical Therapy: Phys. Practice Mgmt.:

TYPES OF BUSINESS:
Nursing Homes
Assisted Living Facilities

BRANDS/DIVISIONS/AFFILIATES:
Diversicare Canada Management Services Co., Inc.

CONTACTS:
Note: Officers with more than one job title may be intentionally listed here more than once.

William R. Council, III, CEO
William R. Council, III, Pres.
Raymond L. Tyler, Sr. VP/COO
L. Glynn Riddle, VP/CFO
Wallace E. Olson, Chmn.

Phone: 615-771-7575 **Fax:** 615-771-7409
Toll-Free:
Address: 277 Mallory Station Rd., Ste. 130, Franklin, TN 37067 US

GROWTH PLANS/SPECIAL FEATURES:

Advocat, Inc. provides long-term care services to nursing home patients and residents of assisted living facilities in nine states, primarily in the Southeast and three Canadian provinces. The company's total operations include 100 facilities, composed of 62 nursing homes containing 7,080 licensed beds and 38 assisted living facilities containing 3,965 units. Within its current portfolio, the firm manages 28 facilities on behalf of the owners, while its remaining facilities consist of 45 leased and 27 owned facilities that are operated by and for the company. In the U.S., Advocate operates 48 nursing homes and 14 assisted living facilities, while its Canadian subsidiary, Diversicare Canada Management Services Co., Inc. (DCM) operates 14 nursing homes and 24 assisted living facilities. The company's leased and managed homes provide a range of health care services to its residents. In addition to the nursing and social services usually provided in long-term care facilities, Advocat offers a variety of rehabilitative, nutritional, respiratory and other specialized ancillary services. The company plans to continue to focus on leasing or acquiring additional nursing and retirement centers, concentrating on rural markets in the southeastern U.S. In addition, where market conditions permit, Advocat intends to expand the operations of acquired facilities by offering more services, in an effort to increase the profitability of the facilities. Medicaid and Medicare payments make up approximately 75% of revenues. Increasing health care costs, combined with federal and state government budget cuts to Medicare and Medicaid programs, have had an adverse effect on the firm's financial position. Advocat has posted an operating loss for the past three years and has a working capital deficit of approximately $53 million. The company recently completed the sale of DCM and therefore only operates in the southeastern U.S.

FINANCIALS:
Sales and profits are in thousands of dollars—add 000 to get the full amount. Year 2004 note: Complete fiscal 2004 results were not available for all companies at press time. For this company, year 2004 is for 9 months.

2004 Sales: $158,751 (9 months)   2004 Profits: $6,946 (9 months)
2003 Sales: $195,750   2003 Profits: $-11,221
2002 Sales: $199,100   2002 Profits: $-13,000
2001 Sales: $206,200   2001 Profits: $-22,300
2000 Sales: $196,000   2000 Profits: $-3,900

Stock Ticker: AVCA
Employees: 5,579
Fiscal Year Ends: 12/31

SALARIES/BENEFITS:
| Pension Plan: | ESOP Stock Plan: | Profit Sharing: | Top Exec. Salary: $275,000 | Bonus: $225,000 |
| Savings Plan: | Stock Purch. Plan: | | Second Exec. Salary: $250,517 | Bonus: $ |

OTHER THOUGHTS:
Apparent Top Female Officers:
Hot Spot for Advancement for Women/Minorities:

LOCATIONS: ("Y" = Yes)
| West: | Southwest: Y | Midwest: | Southeast: Y | Northeast: | International: |

ADVOCATE HEALTH CARE

www.advocatehealth.com

Industry Group Code: 622110 Ranks within this company's industry group: Sales: 22 Profits: 11

Insurance/HMO/PPO:	Drugs:	Equipment/Supplies:	Hospitals/Clinics:		Services:		Health Care:	
Insurance:	Manufacturer:	Manufacturer:	Acute Care:	Y	Diagnostics:		Home Health:	Y
Managed Care:	Distributor:	Distributor:	Sub-Acute Care:		Labs/Testing:		Long-Term Care:	
Utilization Mgmt.:	Specialty Pharm.:	Leasing/Finance:	Outpatient Surgery:	Y	Staffing:		Physical Therapy:	
Payment Proc.:	Vitamins/Nutri.:	Information Sys.:	Phys. Rehab. Center:		Waste Disposal:		Phys. Practice Mgmt.:	Y
	Clinical Trials:		Psychiatric Clinics:		Specialty Services:			

TYPES OF BUSINESS:
Hospitals
Clinics & Outpatient Centers
Home Health Care
Physician Groups

BRANDS/DIVISIONS/AFFILIATES:
Advocate Hope Children's Hospital
Advocate Lutheran General Children's Hospital
Advocate Home Health Services
Advocate Good Samaritan Hospital
Advocate Bethany Hospital
Advocate Health Centers
Advocate Medical Group
Dreyer Medical Clinic

CONTACTS:
Note: Officers with more than one job title may be intentionally listed here more than once.
James H. Skogsbergh, CEO
James H. Skogsbergh, Pres.
William P. Santulli, Exec. VP/COO
Lawrence J. Majka, Sr. VP/CFO
Lee B. Sacks, Exec. VP/Chief Medical Officer
Daniel P. Schmidt, Pres., Advocate Health Centers
Debra A. Geihsler, Pres., Advocate Medical Group
Denise M. Keefe, Pres., Advocate Home Health Services

Phone: 630-572-9393 Fax: 630-572-9139
Toll-Free:
Address: 2025 Windsor Dr., Oak Brook, IL 60523-1586 US

GROWTH PLANS/SPECIAL FEATURES:
Advocate Health Care is a not-for-profit health care network that provides acute care and outpatient services at more than 200 sites in the Chicago area. The company's operations include eight hospitals with approximately 3,500 beds, two children's hospitals (Advocate Hope Children's Hospital and Advocate Lutheran General Children's Hospital) and Advocate Home Health Services, one of the state's largest full-service home health care companies. The firm's hospitals include Advocate Bethany Hospital, Advocate Christ Medical Center, Advocate Good Samaritan Hospital, Advocate Good Shepherd Hospital, Advocate Illinois Masonic Medical Center, Advocate Lutheran General Hospital, Advocate South Suburban Hospital and Advocate Trinity Hospital. The company has more than 4,600 affiliated physicians, including almost 2,000 in physician hospital organizations and approximately 475 from its three large physician groups (Advocate Health Centers, Advocate Medical Group and Dreyer Medical Clinic). Advocate's outpatient facilities include the sites run by its physician groups, as well as Advocate Medical Campus Southwest, Advocate Occupational Health, High Tech Medical Park, Midwest Center for Day Surgery, Naperville Surgical Center, Tinley Woods Surgery Center and the Center for Complementary Medicine. The company's primary academic and teaching affiliation is with the University of Illinois at Chicago Health Sciences Center.

FINANCIALS:
Sales and profits are in thousands of dollars—add 000 to get the full amount. Year 2004 note: Complete fiscal 2004 results were not available for all companies at press time. For this company, year 2004 is for months.

2004 Sales: $ (months)
2003 Sales: $2,715,900
2002 Sales: $2,603,600
2001 Sales: $
2000 Sales: $

2004 Profits: $ (months)
2003 Profits: $123,600
2002 Profits: $-6,800
2001 Profits: $
2000 Profits: $

Stock Ticker: Nonprofit
Employees: 25,000
Fiscal Year Ends: 12/31

SALARIES/BENEFITS:
Pension Plan: ESOP Stock Plan: Profit Sharing: Top Exec. Salary: $ Bonus: $
Savings Plan: Stock Purch. Plan: Second Exec. Salary: $ Bonus: $

OTHER THOUGHTS:
Apparent Top Female Officers: 2
Hot Spot for Advancement for Women/Minorities:

LOCATIONS: ("Y" = Yes)
West:	Southwest:	Midwest:	Southeast:	Northeast:	International:
		Y			

AETERNA ZENTARIS INC

www.aeternazentaris.com

Industry Group Code: 325412 Ranks within this company's industry group: Sales: 43 Profits: 32

Insurance/HMO/PPO:	Drugs:	Equipment/Supplies:	Hospitals/Clinics:	Services:	Health Care:
Insurance:	Manufacturer: Y	Manufacturer:	Acute Care:	Diagnostics:	Home Health:
Managed Care:	Distributor:	Distributor:	Sub-Acute Care:	Labs/Testing:	Long-Term Care:
Utilization Mgmt.:	Specialty Pharm.:	Leasing/Finance:	Outpatient Surgery:	Staffing:	Physical Therapy:
Payment Proc.:	Vitamins/Nutri.:	Information Sys.:	Phys. Rehab. Center:	Waste Disposal:	Phys. Practice Mgmt.:
	Clinical Trials:		Psychiatric Clinics:	Specialty Services:	

TYPES OF BUSINESS:
Drug Development
Oncology Products
Endocrine Therapy Products
Active Ingredients

BRANDS/DIVISIONS/AFFILIATES:
AEterna Laboratories
Zentaris GmbH
Atrium Biotechnologies, Inc.
Cetrotide
Impavido
Lobaplatin
Neovastat
Cetrorelix

CONTACTS:
Note: Officers with more than one job title may be intentionally listed here more than once.

Gilles R. Gagnon, CEO
Gilles R. Gagnon, Pres.
Jurgen Engel, COO
Dennis Turpin, VP/CFO
Jurgen Engel, Exec. VP-Global Research and Dev.
Jurgen Engel, CEO-Zentaris GmbH
Eckhard Gunther, VP-Drug Discovery
Matthias Rischer, VP-Pharmaceutical Dev.
Manfred Peukert, VP-Medical Affairs
Eric Dupont, Chmn.

Phone: 418-652-8525 Fax: 418-652-0881
Toll-Free:
Address: 1405 Parc-Technologique Blvd., Quebec City, Quebec G1P 4P5 Canada

GROWTH PLANS/SPECIAL FEATURES:

AEterna Zentaris, Inc., formerly AEterna Laboratories, is a biopharmaceutical company focused in oncology and endocrine therapy. The company owns 100% of Zentaris GmbH, a German biopharmaceutical company, and 60% of Atrium Biotechnologies, Inc. Atrium develops and markets active ingredients and specialty fine chemicals in the health and personal care industry for cosmetics, chemical, pharmaceutical and nutritional applications. The firm's marketed products include Cetrotide, which is marketed in Japan for in vitro fertilization; Impavido, which is marketed in Bangladesh and India for black fever, as well as for skin diseases in Brazil; and Lobaplatin, which is marketed for breast cancer, CML leukemia and small lung cancer in China. AEterna has several drugs in Phase III clinical trials, including Impavido for skin diseases in Pakistan, Afghanistan and Columbia; and Neovastat for lung cancer in Korea, Southern Europe, France, Belgium, South and Central America, Canada, Mexico, Australia and New Zealand. In addition, the firm has several drugs in Phase II clinical trials: Cetrorelix for endometriosis, uterine myoma and benign prostate hyperplasia worldwide (excluding Japan); D-63153 for prostate cancer worldwide; and Perifsoine for multiple cancers in the U.S., Canada, Mexico and the Netherlands. Teverelix is in Phase I clinical trials for prostate cancer worldwide, as is EP-1572, a growth hormone, for endocrine therapy worldwide. Solvay, an LHRH peptidomimetic for gynecology and prostate hyperplasia, is in the preclinical development phase.

FINANCIALS:
Sales and profits are in thousands of dollars—add 000 to get the full amount. Year 2004 note: Complete fiscal 2004 results were not available for all companies at press time. For this company, year 2004 is for 6 months.

2004 Sales: $93,900 (6 months)   2004 Profits: $2,000 (6 months)
2003 Sales: $128,587   2003 Profits: $-32,426
2002 Sales: $64,204   2002 Profits: $-16,748
2001 Sales: $27,523   2001 Profits: $-2,041
2000 Sales: $ 2000 Profits: $

Stock Ticker: Foreign
Employees: 259
Fiscal Year Ends: 12/31

SALARIES/BENEFITS:
Pension Plan: ESOP Stock Plan: Profit Sharing: Top Exec. Salary: $ Bonus: $
Savings Plan: Stock Purch. Plan: Second Exec. Salary: $ Bonus: $

OTHER THOUGHTS:
Apparent Top Female Officers:
Hot Spot for Advancement for Women/Minorities:

LOCATIONS: ("Y" = Yes)
West: Southwest: Midwest: Southeast: Northeast: International: Y

AETNA INC

www.aetna.com

Industry Group Code: 524114 Ranks within this company's industry group: Sales: 5 Profits: 3

Insurance/HMO/PPO:	Drugs:	Equipment/Supplies:	Hospitals/Clinics:	Services:	Health Care:
Insurance:	Manufacturer: Y	Manufacturer:	Acute Care:	Diagnostics:	Home Health:
Managed Care: Y	Distributor:	Distributor:	Sub-Acute Care:	Labs/Testing:	Long-Term Care:
Utilization Mgmt.:	Specialty Pharm.:	Leasing/Finance:	Outpatient Surgery:	Staffing:	Physical Therapy:
Payment Proc.:	Vitamins/Nutri.:	Information Sys.:	Phys. Rehab. Center:	Waste Disposal:	Phys. Practice Mgmt.:
	Clinical Trials:		Psychiatric Clinics:	Specialty Services:	

TYPES OF BUSINESS:
Health Insurance
HMO/PPO
Group Insurance
Pension Products
Dental Insurance
Disability Insurance
Life Insurance
Long-Term Care Insurance

BRANDS/DIVISIONS/AFFILIATES:
Aetna Life Insurance Company (ALIC)
intelihealth.com
ING Groep N.V.

CONTACTS: Note: Officers with more than one job title may be intentionally listed here more than once.
John W. Rowe, CEO
Ronald A. Williams, Pres.
Alan M. Bennett, Sr. VP/CFO
Elease E. Wright, Sr. VP-Human Resources
Wei-Tih Cheng, Sr. VP/CIO
Louis J. Briskman, Sr. VP/General Counsel
Craig R. Callen, Sr. VP-Strategic Planning & Bus. Dev.
Roger Bolton, Sr. VP-Comm.
David W. Entrekin, VP-Investor Rel.
Timothy A. Holt, Sr. VP/Chief Investment Officer
William C. Popik, Sr. VP/Chief Medical Officer
John W. Rowe, Chmn.

Phone: 860-273-0123   **Fax:** 860-273-3971
Toll-Free: 800-872-3862
Address: 151 Farmington Ave., Hartford, CT 06156 US

GROWTH PLANS/SPECIAL FEATURES:

Aetna, Inc. is one of the nation's largest health benefits companies, based on membership. Aetna's products fall into the categories of health care, group insurance and large case pensions. Health care products include HMO, point-of-service, PPO and indemnity products that offer both medical and dental insurance. Aetna insures 13.6 million people for medical coverage, 11.6 million for dental and 8.3 million for pharmaceuticals. The firm's group insurance products include life, disability and long-term care insurance policies, covering 13.3 million members. Insurees are covered by a network of 600,000 health care providers. Aetna's large case pension products are sold primarily in defined benefit and defined contribution plans. In addition to providing different insurance plans, Aetna provides health benefits products, patient management programs, health management programs and supplemental programs. Aetna also provides its members with access to health care services through networks of independent health care providers. Intelihealth.com, a web site partnership between Aetna, Johns Hopkins University and Health Systems, is a leading source for health information on the web. In 2000, Aetna's financial services and international businesses were merged with a subsidiary of ING Groep N.V.

Aetna provides comprehensive benefits to employees, including medical and life insurance and disability and retirement plans. Aetna has also been recognized as one of the most encouraging employers for minorities and women. Employment awards include being named to the 100 Best Corporate Citizens (Business Ethics Magazine), Top 30 Companies for Executive Women (National Association for Female Executives) and Top 50 List (Latina Style Magazine).

FINANCIALS:
Sales and profits are in thousands of dollars—add 000 to get the full amount. Year 2004 note: Complete fiscal 2004 results were not available for all companies at press time. For this company, year 2004 is for 9 months.

2004 Sales: $14,735,800 (9 months)	2004 Profits: $1,944,400 (9 months)	**Stock Ticker:** AET
2003 Sales: $17,976,400	2003 Profits: $933,800	**Employees:** 27,600
2002 Sales: $19,879,000	2002 Profits: $-2,522,000	**Fiscal Year Ends:** 12/31
2001 Sales: $25,191,000	2001 Profits: $-280,000	
2000 Sales: $26,818,900	2000 Profits: $127,100	

SALARIES/BENEFITS:
| Pension Plan: Y | ESOP Stock Plan: | Profit Sharing: | Top Exec. Salary: $1,042,146 | Bonus: $2,200,000 |
| Savings Plan: Y | Stock Purch. Plan: Y | | Second Exec. Salary: $914,943 | Bonus: $1,800,000 |

OTHER THOUGHTS:
Apparent Top Female Officers: 1
Hot Spot for Advancement for Women/Minorities:

LOCATIONS: ("Y" = Yes)

West:	Southwest:	Midwest:	Southeast:	Northeast:	International:
Y	Y	Y	Y	Y	

AFLAC INC

www.aflac.com

Industry Group Code: 524114A **Ranks within this company's industry group:** Sales: 1 Profits: 1

Insurance/HMO/PPO:	Drugs:	Equipment/Supplies:	Hospitals/Clinics:	Services:	Health Care:
Insurance: Y	Manufacturer:	Manufacturer:	Acute Care:	Diagnostics:	Home Health:
Managed Care:	Distributor:	Distributor:	Sub-Acute Care:	Labs/Testing:	Long-Term Care:
Utilization Mgmt.:	Specialty Pharm.:	Leasing/Finance:	Outpatient Surgery:	Staffing:	Physical Therapy:
Payment Proc.:	Vitamins/Nutri.:	Information Sys.:	Phys. Rehab. Center:	Waste Disposal:	Phys. Practice Mgmt.:
	Clinical Trials:		Psychiatric Clinics:	Specialty Services:	

TYPES OF BUSINESS:
Underwriting-Supplemental Medical
Life Insurance

BRANDS/DIVISIONS/AFFILIATES:
AFLAC Japan
AFLAC U.S.
American Family Life Assurance Company
Ever

CONTACTS:
Note: Officers with more than one job title may be intentionally listed here more than once.
Daniel P. Amos, CEO
Kriss Cloninger, III, Pres.
Kriss Cloninger, III, CFO
Bradley S. Jones, Sr. VP-Sales
Audrey B. Tillman, Sr. VP-Human Resources
James D. Lester, III, CIO
Rebecca C. Davis, Sr. VP/Chief Admin. Officer
Joey M. Loudermilk, Exec. VP/General Counsel
Kathleen V. Spencer, Dir.-Corp. Comm.
Kenneth S. Janke, Jr., Sr. VP-Investor Rel.
Ralph A. Rogers, Jr., Sr. VP-Financial Services
Joseph W. Smith, Jr., Sr. VP/Chief Investment Officer
Joey M. Loudermilk, Corp. Sec.
Hidefumi Matsui, Chmn.-AFLAC Japan
Daniel P. Amos, Chmn.
Akitoshi Kan, Exec. VP-Int'l Oper.

Phone: 706-323-3431 **Fax:** 706-324-6330
Toll-Free: 800-992-3522
Address: 1932 Wynnton Rd., Columbus, GA 31999 US

GROWTH PLANS/SPECIAL FEATURES:

AFLAC, Inc., a Fortune 500 company, is a holding company whose principle subsidiary, AFLAC (American Family Life Assurance Company), insures more than 40 million people worldwide. The subsidiary is a leading writer of supplemental insurance marketed at the worksite in the U.S., offering policies to employees at over 300,000 payroll accounts. Another subsidiary, AFLAC Japan, is the largest foreign-based insurer in that country, insuring one in four households. Ever, a whole life medical insurance policy sold in Japan, hit the 500,000 policy sales mark the year it was introduced. AFLAC Japan now accounts for about 75% of AFLAC, Inc.'s pretax insurance earnings. AFLAC's insurance is designed for people who already have major medical or primary insurance coverage. In the U.S., AFLAC sells 10 types of supplemental health insurance, including hospital intensive care, accident and disability, hospital confinement indemnity, long-term care, short-term disability, cancer treatment and dental plans. In addition, AFLAC offers specified health event coverage for major medical crises such as heart attack and stroke, among others.

AFLAC offers employees an on-site child care center (the largest in Georgia) and a choice of benefit programs, including medical, surgical, hospital, vision, prescription drug, behavioral health and wellness care. AFLAC also offers an on-site fitness center, extensive training and continuing education programs. In 2004, Fortune named AFLAC to its list of America's Most Admired Companies. AFLAC has also been named to Working Mother magazine's list of the 100 Best Companies for Working Mothers, as well as Hispanic magazine's Corporate 100 list for companies providing the most opportunities to Hispanics. AFLAC also strongly encourages its employees to participate in and support community service programs, such as Toys for Tots, Meals on Wheels and the American Cancer Society.

FINANCIALS:
Sales and profits are in thousands of dollars—add 000 to get the full amount. Year 2004 note: Complete fiscal 2004 results were not available for all companies at press time. For this company, year 2004 is for 9 months.

2004 Sales: $9,834,000 (9 months)   2004 Profits: $881,000 (9 months)
2003 Sales: $11,447,000   2003 Profits: $795,000
2002 Sales: $10,257,000   2002 Profits: $821,000
2001 Sales: $9,598,000   2001 Profits: $687,000
2000 Sales: $9,703,000   2000 Profits: $687,000

Stock Ticker: AFL
Employees: 6,186
Fiscal Year Ends: 12/31

SALARIES/BENEFITS:
| Pension Plan: Y | ESOP Stock Plan: | Profit Sharing: Y | Top Exec. Salary: $995,000 | Bonus: $2,170,593 |
| Savings Plan: Y | Stock Purch. Plan: Y | | Second Exec. Salary: $715,825 | Bonus: $1,222,630 |

OTHER THOUGHTS:
Apparent Top Female Officers: 3
Hot Spot for Advancement for Women/Minorities: Y

LOCATIONS: ("Y" = Yes)
West:	Southwest:	Midwest:	Southeast:	Northeast:	International:
Y	Y	Y	Y	Y	Y

ALCON INC

www.alconlabs.com

Industry Group Code: 325412 Ranks within this company's industry group: Sales: 18 Profits: 16

Insurance/HMO/PPO:	Drugs:	Equipment/Supplies:	Hospitals/Clinics:	Services:	Health Care:
Insurance:	Manufacturer: Y	Manufacturer: Y	Acute Care:	Diagnostics:	Home Health:
Managed Care:	Distributor:	Distributor:	Sub-Acute Care:	Labs/Testing:	Long-Term Care:
Utilization Mgmt.:	Specialty Pharm.:	Leasing/Finance:	Outpatient Surgery:	Staffing:	Physical Therapy:
Payment Proc.:	Vitamins/Nutri.:	Information Sys.: Y	Phys. Rehab. Center:	Waste Disposal:	Phys. Practice Mgmt.:
	Clinical Trials:		Psychiatric Clinics:	Specialty Services:	

TYPES OF BUSINESS:
Drugs-Eye Care
Ophthalmic Products and Equipment

BRANDS/DIVISIONS/AFFILIATES:
Opti-Free
Patanol
Brimonidine
AcrySof
Betoptic
RETAANE
Alcon Surgical
William C. Conner Research Center

CONTACTS: Note: Officers with more than one job title may be intentionally listed here more than once.
Cary Rayment, CEO
Cary Rayment, Pres.
Allen Baker, Exec. VP/COO
Jacqualyn Fouse, CFO
Gerald D. Cagle, Sr. VP-Research & Dev.
Andre Bens, Sr. VP-Global Mfg. & Tech. Support
Cary Rayment, Sr. VP-U.S. Oper.
Doug MacHatton, VP-Investor Rel.
Jacqualyn Fouse, Sr. VP-Finance
Cary Rayment, Chmn.
Fred Pettinato, Sr. VP-Int'l Oper.

Phone: 41-41-785-8888 Fax:
Toll-Free:
Address: Bosch 69, Hunenberg, 6331 Switzerland

GROWTH PLANS/SPECIAL FEATURES:
Alcon, Inc. is one of the largest eye care product companies in the world. It has specialized in the development, manufacture and marketing of ophthalmic products and instrumentation for over 50 years. Alcon maintains manufacturing plants, laboratories and offices in 50 countries, with products sold in over 75 countries. The company makes more than 10,000 unique products, including prescription and over-the-counter drugs, contact lens solutions, surgical instruments, intraocular lenses and office systems for ophthalmologists. Its brand names, such as Patanol solution for eye allergies, AcrySof intraocular lenses, Betoptic for glaucoma and the Opti-Free system for contact lens care, are known throughout the world. Housed at the company's research and development headquarters in Fort Worth is the 400,000-square-foot William C. Conner Research Center, the largest eye research center in the world. Alcon has several in-house divisions that handle e-business, information technology, implementation of new technology, human resources, finance and administration and legal services for all of the company's group members and subsidiaries. It also has a consumer products division, a pharmaceutical division and the Alcon Surgical division, which creates implantable lenses and viscoelastics and medical tools specifically made for ocular surgeons, including phacoemulsification instruments for cataract removal and absorbable sutures. In recent news, the company filed a new drug application with the FDA for RETAANE, an investigational treatment for preserving the vision of patients with all forms of wet age-related macular degeneration.

Alcon's U.S. employees receive heath care benefits, life insurance, disability benefits, wellness programs and educational training programs.

FINANCIALS:
Sales and profits are in thousands of dollars—add 000 to get the full amount. Year 2004 note: Complete fiscal 2004 results were not available for all companies at press time. For this company, year 2004 is for 9 months.

2004 Sales: $2,960,900 (9 months)	2004 Profits: $191,000 (9 months)	
2003 Sales: $3,406,900	2003 Profits: $595,400	Stock Ticker: Foreign
2002 Sales: $3,009,100	2002 Profits: $466,900	Employees: 12,000
2001 Sales: $2,747,700	2001 Profits: $315,600	Fiscal Year Ends: 12/31
2000 Sales: $2,553,600	2000 Profits: $331,700	

SALARIES/BENEFITS:
Pension Plan: Y	ESOP Stock Plan:	Profit Sharing:	Top Exec. Salary: $	Bonus: $
Savings Plan: Y	Stock Purch. Plan:		Second Exec. Salary: $	Bonus: $

OTHER THOUGHTS:
Apparent Top Female Officers: 1
Hot Spot for Advancement for Women/Minorities:

LOCATIONS: ("Y" = Yes)
West:	Southwest:	Midwest:	Southeast:	Northeast:	International:
Y	Y		Y	Y	Y

ALIGN TECHNOLOGY

www.invisalign.com

Industry Group Code: 339113 Ranks within this company's industry group: Sales: 81 Profits: 130

Insurance/HMO/PPO:	Drugs:	Equipment/Supplies:	Hospitals/Clinics:	Services:	Health Care:
Insurance: Managed Care: Utilization Mgmt.: Payment Proc.:	Manufacturer: Distributor: Specialty Pharm.: Vitamins/Nutri.: Clinical Trials:	Manufacturer: Y Distributor: Leasing/Finance: Information Sys.: Y	Acute Care: Sub-Acute Care: Outpatient Surgery: Phys. Rehab. Center: Psychiatric Clinics:	Diagnostics: Labs/Testing: Staffing: Waste Disposal: Specialty Services:	Home Health: Long-Term Care: Physical Therapy: Phys. Practice Mgmt.:

TYPES OF BUSINESS:
Orthodontic Equipment

BRANDS/DIVISIONS/AFFILIATES:
Invisalign
ClinCheck
Aligners

CONTACTS:
Note: Officers with more than one job title may be intentionally listed here more than once.

Thomas M. Prescott, CEO
Thomas M. Prescott, Pres.
Eldon M. Bullington, CFO
Robert D. Mitchell, VP-Worldwide Sales
Patricia Wadors, VP-Human Resources
Amir Abolfathi, VP-Research & Dev.
Cecilia Claudio, Chief Tech. Officer
Cecilia Claudio, VP-Eng.
Roger E. George, General Counsel/VP-Legal Affairs
Len Hedge, VP-Oper.
Eldon M. Bullington, VP-Finance
David S. Thrower, VP-Global Mktg.

Phone: 408-470-1000 Fax: 408-470-1010
Toll-Free:
Address: 881 Martin Ave., Santa Clara, CA 95050 US

GROWTH PLANS/SPECIAL FEATURES:
Align Technology, Inc. (ATI), founded in 1997, is engaged in the design, manufacture and marketing of Invisalign, a proprietary system for treating malocclusion, or the misalignment of teeth. The Invisalign system has two components: ClinCheck and Aligners. ClinCheck is an Internet-based application that allows dental professionals to simulate treatment, in three dimensions, by modeling two-week stages of tooth movement. Aligners are thin, clear plastic, removable dental appliances that are manufactured in a series to correspond to each two-week stage of the ClinCheck simulation. Aligners are customized to perform the treatment prescribed for an individual patient by dental professionals using ClinCheck. Two of the company's key production steps are performed outside the U.S. At ATI's facility in Costa Rica, technicians use a sophisticated, internally developed computer modeling program to prepare electronic treatment plans, which are transmitted electronically back to the U.S. These files form the basis of ClinCheck and are used in conjunction with stereolithography technology to manufacture Aligner molds. A third-party manufacturer in Mexico fabricates Aligners from the molds and ships the completed products to ATI's customers. Invisalign provides benefits to the dental professional, including ease of use, an expanded patient base, the ability to visualize treatment and likely outcomes, and decreased staff time; as well as benefits to the patient, including aesthetic benefits, comfort, improved oral hygiene, reduced overall treatment time and reduced incidence of emergencies. In recent news, the firm announced that the University of Illinois at Chicago is making Invisalign a part of its required undergraduate coursework in orthodontics.

FINANCIALS:
Sales and profits are in thousands of dollars—add 000 to get the full amount. Year 2004 note: Complete fiscal 2004 results were not available for all companies at press time. For this company, year 2004 is for 9 months.

2004 Sales: $129,175 (9 months)
2003 Sales: $122,725
2002 Sales: $69,698
2001 Sales: $
2000 Sales: $

2004 Profits: $7,647 (9 months)
2003 Profits: $-20,122
2002 Profits: $-72,819
2001 Profits: $
2000 Profits: $

Stock Ticker: ALGN
Employees: 741
Fiscal Year Ends: 12/31

SALARIES/BENEFITS:
Pension Plan: ESOP Stock Plan: Profit Sharing: Top Exec. Salary: $361,685 Bonus: $271,688
Savings Plan: Stock Purch. Plan: Second Exec. Salary: $212,503 Bonus: $83,921

OTHER THOUGHTS:
Apparent Top Female Officers: 2
Hot Spot for Advancement for Women/Minorities:

LOCATIONS: ("Y" = Yes)
West:	Southwest:	Midwest:	Southeast:	Northeast:	International:
Y					Y

Note: Financial information, benefits and other data can change quickly and may vary from those stated here.

ALLERGAN INC

www.allergan.com

Industry Group Code: 325412   Ranks within this company's industry group: Sales: 27   Profits: 33

Insurance/HMO/PPO:	Drugs:		Equipment/Supplies:		Hospitals/Clinics:	Services:	Health Care:
Insurance:	Manufacturer:	Y	Manufacturer:	Y	Acute Care:	Diagnostics:	Home Health:
Managed Care:	Distributor:		Distributor:		Sub-Acute Care:	Labs/Testing:	Long-Term Care:
Utilization Mgmt.:	Specialty Pharm.:		Leasing/Finance:		Outpatient Surgery:	Staffing:	Physical Therapy:
Payment Proc.:	Vitamins/Nutri.:		Information Sys.:		Phys. Rehab. Center:	Waste Disposal:	Phys. Practice Mgmt.:
	Clinical Trials:				Psychiatric Clinics:	Specialty Services:	

TYPES OF BUSINESS:
Supplies-Eye Care
Niche Pharmaceuticals
Skin Care Products
Neuromodulator Products

BRANDS/DIVISIONS/AFFILIATES:
Alphagan
Lumigan
Azelex
Tazorac
Botox
Oculex Pharmaceuticals, Inc
Posurdex
Restasis

CONTACTS:
Note: Officers with more than one job title may be intentionally listed here more than once.

David E.I. Pyott, CEO
David E.I. Pyott, Pres.
Eric Brandt, Exec. VP-Finance/CFO
Roy J. Wilson, Exec. VP-Human Resources
Lester J. Kaplan, Exec. VP-R&D
Jacqueline J. Schiavo, Exec. VP-Tech. Oper.
Douglas S. Ingram, Exec. VP/General Counsel & Sec.
Eric Brandt, Exec, VP-Strategy & Corp. Dev.
James F. Barlow, VP/Controller
F. Michael Ball, Exec. VP/Pres., Pharmaceuticals
David E.I. Pyott, Chmn.

Phone: 714-246-4500   **Fax:** 714-246-4971
Toll-Free: 800-347-4500
Address: 2525 Dupont Dr., Irvine, CA 92612-9534 US

GROWTH PLANS/SPECIAL FEATURES:
Allergan is a technology-driven global health care company that develops and commercializes specialty pharmaceutical products for the ophthalmic, neuromodulator, dermatological and other specialty markets. The company focuses on products for the treatment of a wide range of disease areas, including glaucoma and retinal disease, cataracts, dry eye, psoriasis, acne and neuromuscular disorders. The company's eye care pharmaceutical products, include Alphagan, Alphagan P and Lumigan ophthalmic solutions, which are used for the treatment of open-angle glaucoma and ocular hypertension; Acular LS, which reduces ocular pain; Pred Forte, a topical steroid; and Ocuflux, Oflox and Exocin ophthalmic anti-infective solution. The firm's neuromodulator products include Botox, which is used for more than 100 therapeutic and cosmetic treatments. Allergan's skin care product line is comprised of tazarotene products in cream and gel formulations for the treatment of acne, facial wrinkles and psoriasis marketed under the names Tazorac, Zorac and Avage; Azelex, an acne product; and M.D. Forte, a line of glycolic and alpha hydroxy acid based products. Recently, Allergan acquired Oculex Pharmaceuticals, Inc., which develops treatments for sight-threatening diseases of the eye, Posurdex, which delivers dexamethasone for the treatment of macular edema and will enter Phase III clinical trials in late 2004. In the U.S., the firm launched Restasis, a prescription only therapy for the treatment of chronic dry eye disease. Allergan received FDA approval for Zymar, an ophthalmic drug that treats bacterial conjunctivitis. The company filed a new drug application with the FDA for oral tazarotene for the treatment of psoriasis.

Allergen provides medical, dental and vision insurance, adoption assistance and education assistance. Its headquarters includes a gym, a company store, athletic fields, computer training facilities and a credit union.

FINANCIALS:
Sales and profits are in thousands of dollars—add 000 to get the full amount. Year 2004 note: Complete fiscal 2004 results were not available for all companies at press time. For this company, year 2004 is for 9 months.

2004 Sales: $1,489,400 (9 months)   2004 Profits: $264,600 (9 months)
2003 Sales: $1,171,400   2003 Profits: $-52,500
2002 Sales: $1,425,300   2002 Profits: $75,200
2001 Sales: $1,745,500   2001 Profits: $224,900
2000 Sales: $1,625,500   2000 Profits: $215,100

Stock Ticker: AGN
Employees: 4,930
Fiscal Year Ends: 12/31

SALARIES/BENEFITS:
| Pension Plan: | ESOP Stock Plan: | Profit Sharing: | Top Exec. Salary: $1,069,231 | Bonus: $1,075,000 |
| Savings Plan: Y | Stock Purch. Plan: Y | | Second Exec. Salary: $491,069 | Bonus: $273,600 |

OTHER THOUGHTS:
Apparent Top Female Officers: 1
Hot Spot for Advancement for Women/Minorities:

LOCATIONS: ("Y" = Yes)
West:	Southwest:	Midwest:	Southeast:	Northeast:	International:
Y	Y	Y	Y	Y	Y

ALLIANCE IMAGING INC

www.allianceimaging.com

Industry Group Code: 621511   Ranks within this company's industry group: Sales: 3   Profits: 9

Insurance/HMO/PPO:	Drugs:	Equipment/Supplies:	Hospitals/Clinics:	Services:		Health Care:
Insurance:	Manufacturer:	Manufacturer:	Acute Care:	Diagnostics:	Y	Home Health:
Managed Care:	Distributor:	Distributor:	Sub-Acute Care:	Labs/Testing:		Long-Term Care:
Utilization Mgmt.:	Specialty Pharm.:	Leasing/Finance:	Outpatient Surgery:	Staffing:		Physical Therapy:
Payment Proc.:	Vitamins/Nutri.:	Information Sys.:	Phys. Rehab. Center:	Waste Disposal:		Phys. Practice Mgmt.:
	Clinical Trials:		Psychiatric Clinics:	Specialty Services:	Y	

TYPES OF BUSINESS:
Diagnostic Imaging
Outsourcing and Support Services

BRANDS/DIVISIONS/AFFILIATES:

CONTACTS:
Note: Officers with more than one job title may be intentionally listed here more than once.

Paul S. Viviano, CEO
Andrew P. Hayek, Pres.
Andrew P. Hayek, COO
R. Brian Hanson, Exec. VP/CFO
Russell D. Phillips, Jr., General Counsel
Kenneth S. Ord, Investor Rel.
Paul S. Viviiano, Chmn.

Phone: 714-688-7100   Fax: 714-688-3333
Toll-Free: 800-544-3215
Address: 1900 S. State College Blvd., Ste. 600, Anaheim, CA 92806 US

GROWTH PLANS/SPECIAL FEATURES:
Alliance Imaging, Inc. provides outsourced diagnostic imaging services to small and mid-sized hospitals, helping its clients to avoid capital investment and financial risk associated with the purchase of equipment. The company concentrates mainly on magnetic resonance imaging, or MRI, but also offers positron emission tomography (PET), computed tomography (CT), x-ray, single photon emission computed tomography (SPECT) and ultrasound. The firm provides imaging and therapeutic services primarily to health care providers on a mobile, shared-services basis. Services normally include use of imaging or therapeutic systems, technologists to operate the systems, equipment maintenance and upgrades and management of day-to-day operations. Ancillary services, such as marketing support, education and training and billing assistance, are also available. Alliance Imaging has over 470 diagnostic imaging and therapeutic systems and serves over 1,300 clients in 42 states. It typically delivers service through exclusive, long-term contracts.

FINANCIALS:
Sales and profits are in thousands of dollars—add 000 to get the full amount. Year 2004 note: Complete fiscal 2004 results were not available for all companies at press time. For this company, year 2004 is for 9 months.

2004 Sales: $313,728 (9 months)   2004 Profits: $-38,143 (9 months)
2003 Sales: $415,283   2003 Profits: $-31,610
2002 Sales: $412,000   2002 Profits: $35,900
2001 Sales: $375,200   2001 Profits: $10,500
2000 Sales: $345,300   2000 Profits: $-2,200

Stock Ticker: AIQ
Employees: 2,224
Fiscal Year Ends: 12/31

SALARIES/BENEFITS:
Pension Plan: ESOP Stock Plan: Profit Sharing: Top Exec. Salary: $576,956   Bonus: $284,738
Savings Plan: Y Stock Purch. Plan: Second Exec. Salary: $396,923 Bonus: $384,750

OTHER THOUGHTS:
Apparent Top Female Officers:
Hot Spot for Advancement for Women/Minorities:

LOCATIONS: ("Y" = Yes)
West:	Southwest:	Midwest:	Southeast:	Northeast:	International:
Y	Y	Y	Y	Y	

ALLIED HEALTHCARE INTERNATIONAL INC

www.alliedhealthcare.com

Industry Group Code: 621610   Ranks within this company's industry group: Sales: 6   Profits: 7

Insurance/HMO/PPO:	Drugs:	Equipment/Supplies:	Hospitals/Clinics:	Services:	Health Care:
Insurance:	Manufacturer:	Manufacturer:	Acute Care:	Diagnostics:	Home Health: Y
Managed Care:	Distributor:	Distributor:	Sub-Acute Care:	Labs/Testing:	Long-Term Care:
Utilization Mgmt.:	Specialty Pharm.:	Leasing/Finance:	Outpatient Surgery:	Staffing: Y	Physical Therapy:
Payment Proc.:	Vitamins/Nutri.:	Information Sys.:	Phys. Rehab. Center:	Waste Disposal:	Phys. Practice Mgmt.:
	Clinical Trials:		Psychiatric Clinics:	Specialty Services: Y	

TYPES OF BUSINESS:
Home Health Care
Nursing and Para-Professional Services
Home Medical Equipment
Respiration Therapy
Medical Staffing

BRANDS/DIVISIONS/AFFILIATES:
Allied Oxycare
Medigas
Staffing Enterprise, Ltd.
Allied Healthcare, Ltd.
Nightingale Nursing Bureau, Ltd.
Balfor Medical, Ltd.
Medic-One Group

GROWTH PLANS/SPECIAL FEATURES:
Allied Healthcare International, Inc. provides health care services and products through its subsidiaries in the U.K. The company's offerings include nursing and para-professional services; medical staffing; respiratory therapy; and home medical equipment delivery. Allied's principal strategic focus is to become the leading provider of flexible staffing and services to the U.K. health care industry. The firm provides medical staff and services in the U.K. through Allied Healthcare, Nightingale Nursing Bureau, Balfor Medical, Staffing Enterprise and Medic-One Group. The group companies provide nursing and care staff services to a range of clients, particularly NHS trusts, nursing homes, private clients and local authority social services departments. Allied Oxycare and Medigas offer respiratory therapy, as well as supplying and maintaining respiratory equipment.

CONTACTS:
Note: Officers with more than one job title may be intentionally listed here more than once.
Sarah L. Eames, CEO
Sarah L. Eames, Pres.
Charles F. Murphy, Acting CFO
Leslie J. Levinson, Corp. Sec.
Timothy M. Aitken, Chmn.

Phone: 212-750-0064   Fax: 212-750-7221
Toll-Free:
Address: 555 Madison Ave., New York, NY 10022 US

FINANCIALS:
Sales and profits are in thousands of dollars—add 000 to get the full amount. Year 2004 note: Complete fiscal 2004 results were not available for all companies at press time. For this company, year 2004 is for 9 months.

2004 Sales: $240,624 (9 months)   2004 Profits: $7,704   (9 months)
2003 Sales: $294,400   2003 Profits: $8,000
2002 Sales: $259,900   2002 Profits: $4,800
2001 Sales: $154,600   2001 Profits: $-26,600
2000 Sales: $135,400   2000 Profits: $-24,900

Stock Ticker: AHCI
Employees: 705
Fiscal Year Ends: 9/30

SALARIES/BENEFITS:
| Pension Plan: | ESOP Stock Plan: | Profit Sharing: Y | Top Exec. Salary: $420,000 | Bonus: $230,000 |
| Savings Plan: | Stock Purch. Plan: | | Second Exec. Salary: $405,000 | Bonus: $270,000 |

OTHER THOUGHTS:
Apparent Top Female Officers: 1
Hot Spot for Advancement for Women/Minorities:

LOCATIONS: ("Y" = Yes)
West:	Southwest:	Midwest:	Southeast:	Northeast:	International:
				Y	Y

Plunkett's Health Care Industry Almanac 2005

ALLINA HOSPITALS AND CLINICS

www.allina.com

Industry Group Code: 622110 Ranks within this company's industry group: Sales: 32 Profits:

Insurance/HMO/PPO:	Drugs:	Equipment/Supplies:	Hospitals/Clinics:		Services:		Health Care:	
Insurance:	Manufacturer:	Manufacturer:	Acute Care:	Y	Diagnostics:		Home Health:	Y
Managed Care:	Distributor:	Distributor:	Sub-Acute Care:	Y	Labs/Testing:		Long-Term Care:	
Utilization Mgmt.:	Specialty Pharm.:	Leasing/Finance: Y	Outpatient Surgery:	Y	Staffing:		Physical Therapy:	
Payment Proc.:	Vitamins/Nutri.:	Information Sys.:	Phys. Rehab. Center:	Y	Waste Disposal:		Phys. Practice Mgmt.:	
	Clinical Trials:		Psychiatric Clinics:		Specialty Services:	Y		

TYPES OF BUSINESS:
Hospitals
Clinics & Ambulatory Care Centers
Medical Equipment Rental
Emergency Medical Transportation Services
Hospice Care
Pharmacies
Rehabilitation Services

BRANDS/DIVISIONS/AFFILIATES:
Allina Medical Clinic
Phillips Eye Institute
Sister Kenny Rehabilitation Insitute
Allina Home Oxygen & Medical Equipment
Allina Medical Transportation
medformation.com
Abbot Northwestern Hospital
Buffalo Hospital

CONTACTS:
Note: Officers with more than one job title may be intentionally listed here more than once.
Richard R. Pettingill, CEO
Richard R. Pettingill, Pres.
Mark G. Harrison, Exec. VP/CFO
Michael W. Howe, Exec. VP-Human Resources/Chief Talent Officer
Robert Plaszes, CIO
Mary P. Foarde, General Counsel/Corp. Sec.
Rickie Ressler, Exec. VP-Hospital & Specialty Oper.
Kendra Calhoun, Media Contact
Brian Anderson, Chief Medical Officer
Barbara Balik, Exec. VP-Safety & Quality Systems
Thomas Holets, Pres., Allina Medical Clinic
Laurel A. Krause, VP-Allina Medical Laboratories
Michael E. Dougherty, Chmn.

Phone: 612-775-5000 **Fax:** 612-863-5677
Toll-Free:
Address: 710 E. 24th St., Minneapolis, MN 55404-3840 US

GROWTH PLANS/SPECIAL FEATURES:

Allina Hospitals and Clinics (AH&C) is a nonprofit network of hospitals, clinics and other health care services located throughout Minnesota and western Wisconsin. The company owns and operates 11 hospitals, 42 Allina Medical Clinic sites, 23 hospital-based clinics, 12 community pharmacy sites and three ambulatory care centers. The firm's hospitals include Abbot Northwestern Hospital, Buffalo Hospital, Cambridge Medical Center, Mercy & Unity Hospitals, New Ulm Medical Center, Owatonna Hospital, River Falls Area Hospital, St. Francis Regional Medical Center, United Hospital and Phillips Eye Institute, the third-largest specialty hospital in the U.S. dedicated to eye diseases and disorders. Though Phillips is based in Minneapolis, it draws patients from a five-state region. Another specialized health care facility, Allina Hospice & Palliative Care, provides advanced illness or end-of-life care, while the Sister Kenny Rehabilitation Institute treats more than 60,000 patients each year for a variety of conditions, such as stroke and back pain, as well as sports-related, spinal cord and brain injuries. In addition, AH&C operates Allina Home Oxygen & Medical Equipment, which supplies oxygen, respiratory and other medical equipment and supplies to a patient's home; and Allina Medical Transportation, which provides pre-hospital emergency medical services, including advanced and basic life support, and scheduled transport in more than 75 Minnesota communities. The company also provides general medical information through its medformation.com web site.

FINANCIALS:
Sales and profits are in thousands of dollars—add 000 to get the full amount. Year 2004 note: Complete fiscal 2004 results were not available for all companies at press time. For this company, year 2004 is for months.

2004 Sales: $ (months)	2004 Profits: $ (months)	
2003 Sales: $1,940,000	2003 Profits: $	**Stock Ticker: Nonprofit**
2002 Sales: $1,800,000	2002 Profits: $	Employees: 22,583
2001 Sales: $	2001 Profits: $	Fiscal Year Ends: 12/31
2000 Sales: $	2000 Profits: $	

SALARIES/BENEFITS:
Pension Plan:	ESOP Stock Plan:	Profit Sharing:	Top Exec. Salary: $	Bonus: $
Savings Plan:	Stock Purch. Plan:		Second Exec. Salary: $	Bonus: $

OTHER THOUGHTS:
Apparent Top Female Officers: 4
Hot Spot for Advancement for Women/Minorities: Y

LOCATIONS: ("Y" = Yes)
West:	Southwest:	Midwest:	Southeast:	Northeast:	International:
		Y			

Note: Financial information, benefits and other data can change quickly and may vary from those stated here.

ALPHARMA INC

www.alpharma.com

Industry Group Code: 325416   Ranks within this company's industry group: Sales: 2 Profits: 4

Insurance/HMO/PPO:	Drugs:	Equipment/Supplies:	Hospitals/Clinics:	Services:	Health Care:
Insurance:	Manufacturer: Y	Manufacturer:	Acute Care:	Diagnostics:	Home Health:
Managed Care:	Distributor:	Distributor:	Sub-Acute Care:	Labs/Testing:	Long-Term Care:
Utilization Mgmt.:	Specialty Pharm.:	Leasing/Finance:	Outpatient Surgery:	Staffing:	Physical Therapy:
Payment Proc.:	Vitamins/Nutri.:	Information Sys.:	Phys. Rehab. Center:	Waste Disposal:	Phys. Practice Mgmt.:
	Clinical Trials:		Psychiatric Clinics:	Specialty Services:	

TYPES OF BUSINESS:
Drugs-Animal Health
Human Pharmaceuticals
Generic Pharmaceuticals
Active Pharmaceutical Ingredients

BRANDS/DIVISIONS/AFFILIATES:
Kadian
Serax
BMD
Aureomycin
Bovatec
Deccox
Avatec
Alpha-ject

CONTACTS:
Note: Officers with more than one job title may be intentionally listed here more than once.

Ingrid Wiik, CEO
Ingrid Wiik, Pres.
Matthew T. Farrell, Exec. VP/CFO
George P. Rose, Exec. VP-Human Resources
Ronald N. Warner, Exec. VP-Scientific Affairs & Compliance
Robert F. Wrobel, Exec. VP/Chief Legal Officer/Corp. Sec.
Kurt J. Orlofski, Sr. VP-Human Pharmaceuticals Bus. Dev.
George P. Rose, Exec. VP-Comm.
Carl-Ake Carlsson, Pres., API and Branded Products
Carol A. Wrenn, Exec. VP/Pres.-Animal Health Div.
Frederick J. Lynch, Pres., Generic Human Pharmaceuticals
Michael J. Nestor, Pres., U.S. Branded Human Pharmaceuticals
Einar W. Sissener, Chmn.
Frederick J. Lynch, Sr. VP-Human Pharmaceuticals Supply Chain

Phone: 201-947-7774   Fax: 201-947-4879
Toll-Free: 800-645-4216
Address: One Executive Dr., Fort Lee, NJ 07024 US

GROWTH PLANS/SPECIAL FEATURES:
Alpharma, Inc. is a multinational pharmaceutical company that develops, manufactures and markets specialty generic and proprietary human pharmaceutical and animal health products. The company is one of the largest manufacturers of generic liquid and topical pharmaceuticals in the United States and is a market leader in generic pharmaceutical products in Europe, with a growing presence in Southeast Asia as well. It is also one of the world's leading producers of important specialty antibiotics. The firm operates four businesses units: U.S. human pharmaceuticals, international generic, active pharmaceutical ingredients (API) and animal health. The company's U.S. human pharmaceuticals business is comprised of the generic and branded pharmaceuticals businesses, which provide over 200 generic and over-the-counter products in a number of therapeutic categories in most major dosage forms, including difficult-to-formulate products, such as extended-release, aerosol inhalants and nasal sprays. It also manufactures two branded products: Kadian and Serax. Alpharma's international business activities are comprised of its international generic and API businesses. The firm provides over 650 generic products and five key products/active pharmaceutical ingredients: Bacitracin, Polymyxin B, Vancomycin, Amphotericin B and Colistin. The company's key markets are in the U.K., Germany, Scandinavia, The Netherlands and Asia Pacific. Alpharma's animal health business unit is a leading provider of animal feed additives for poultry and livestock and vaccines for farmed fish. It provides over 100 animal health products, including antibiotics, antimicrobials and anticoccidials. Key products include BMD, Aureomycin, Bovatec, Deccox, Avatec and Alpha-ject vaccines. In recent news, Alpharma's three human pharmaceutical business segments (U.S. human pharmaceuticals, international generics and API) were aligned as one human pharmaceuticals organization divided into two operation units, each operated by separate management teams: human generic pharmaceuticals, and API and branded pharmaceuticals.

FINANCIALS:
Sales and profits are in thousands of dollars—add 000 to get the full amount. Year 2004 note: Complete fiscal 2004 results were not available for all companies at press time. For this company, year 2004 is for 9 months.

2004 Sales: $925,183 (9 months)   2004 Profits: $-7,215 (9 months)
2003 Sales: $1,297,285   2003 Profits: $16,936
2002 Sales: $1,238,000   2002 Profits: $-98,800
2001 Sales: $975,000   2001 Profits: $-37,900
2000 Sales: $919,523   2000 Profits: $61,143

Stock Ticker: ALO
Employees: 4,700
Fiscal Year Ends: 12/31

SALARIES/BENEFITS:
Pension Plan: Y   ESOP Stock Plan: Profit Sharing: Top Exec. Salary: $754,609   Bonus: $213,000
Savings Plan: Stock Purch. Plan: Second Exec. Salary: $467,308 Bonus: $115,000

OTHER THOUGHTS:
Apparent Top Female Officers: 2
Hot Spot for Advancement for Women/Minorities:

LOCATIONS: ("Y" = Yes)
West:	Southwest:	Midwest:	Southeast:	Northeast:	International:
Y	Y	Y	Y	Y	Y

ALTERRA HEALTHCARE CORP

www.assisted.com

Industry Group Code: 623110   Ranks within this company's industry group: Sales: Profits:

Insurance/HMO/PPO:	Drugs:	Equipment/Supplies:	Hospitals/Clinics:	Services:	Health Care:
Insurance:	Manufacturer:	Manufacturer:	Acute Care:	Diagnostics:	Home Health:
Managed Care:	Distributor:	Distributor:	Sub-Acute Care:	Labs/Testing:	Long-Term Care: Y
Utilization Mgmt.:	Specialty Pharm.:	Leasing/Finance:	Outpatient Surgery:	Staffing:	Physical Therapy:
Payment Proc.:	Vitamins/Nutri.:	Information Sys.:	Phys. Rehab. Center:	Waste Disposal:	Phys. Practice Mgmt.:
	Clinical Trials:		Psychiatric Clinics:	Specialty Services: Y	

TYPES OF BUSINESS:
Long-Term Health Care
Assisted Living Services
Pharmacy Services

BRANDS/DIVISIONS/AFFILIATES:
Clare Bridge
Clare Bridge Cottage
Wynwood
Alterra Villas
Sterling House
Crystal Health, LLC

CONTACTS:
Note: Officers with more than one job title may be intentionally listed here more than once.

Mark W. Ohlendorf, CEO
Mark W. Ohlendorf, Pres.
Kristin A. Ferge, CFO

Phone: 414-918-5000   Fax: 414-918-5050
Toll-Free: 888-780-1200
Address: 10000 Innovation Dr., Milwaukee, WI 53221 US

GROWTH PLANS/SPECIAL FEATURES:
Alterra Healthcare Corporation provides residential assisted care for the elderly and patients suffering from Alzheimer's disease who do not require nursing home care. The company operates over 300 facilities in 22 states. Alterra operates under several brand names, including dementia care models Clare Bridge and Clare Bridge Cottage; Wynwood, an upper-income frail elderly model; Sterling House, a moderate-income elderly model; and Alterra Villas, the company's independent living model. The company offers personal care, health care and support services in facilities designed for people suffering from a variety of diseases. Alterra's frail elderly care services include assistance with daily living, ongoing health assessments, organized social activities, meals, housekeeping and personal laundry services. The company's dementia services provide attention and personal care to help cognitively impaired residents maintain a higher quality of life. Alterra residents receive access to home health care, rehabilitation therapy and hospice care. Crystal Health, LLC, the company's joint venture, provides pharmacy services to residents. Alterra emerged from bankruptcy in December 2003.

Alterra provides an orientation process to help employees understand the company and its mission and role. It also has a hands-on training program for employees. The company offers a comprehensive benefits package including medical, dental, vision and life insurance, a disability plan, a legal assistance plan, flexible working hours and educational assistance. Most full-time benefits are available to part-time employees as well.

FINANCIALS:
Sales and profits are in thousands of dollars—add 000 to get the full amount. Year 2004 note: Complete fiscal 2004 results were not available for all companies at press time. For this company, year 2004 is for months.

2004 Sales: $ (months)   2004 Profits: $ (months)
2003 Sales: $ 2003 Profits: $
2002 Sales: $416,700   2002 Profits: $-222,000
2001 Sales: $502,700   2001 Profits: $-299,900
2000 Sales: $466,495   2000 Profits: $-117,806

Stock Ticker: Private
Employees: 11,800
Fiscal Year Ends: 12/31

SALARIES/BENEFITS:
Pension Plan: ESOP Stock Plan: Profit Sharing: Top Exec. Salary: $362,579   Bonus: $150,000
Savings Plan: Y   Stock Purch. Plan: Second Exec. Salary: $346,291 Bonus: $160,000

OTHER THOUGHTS:
Apparent Top Female Officers: 1
Hot Spot for Advancement for Women/Minorities:

LOCATIONS: ("Y" = Yes)
West:	Southwest:	Midwest:	Southeast:	Northeast:	International:
Y	Y	Y	Y	Y	

AMEDISYS INC

www.amedisys.com

Industry Group Code: 621610   Ranks within this company's industry group: Sales: 10   Profits: 2

Insurance/HMO/PPO:	Drugs:	Equipment/Supplies:	Hospitals/Clinics:	Services:	Health Care:
Insurance:	Manufacturer:	Manufacturer:	Acute Care:	Diagnostics:	Home Health: Y
Managed Care:	Distributor:	Distributor:	Sub-Acute Care:	Labs/Testing:	Long-Term Care:
Utilization Mgmt.:	Specialty Pharm.:	Leasing/Finance:	Outpatient Surgery:	Staffing:	Physical Therapy: Y
Payment Proc.:	Vitamins/Nutri.:	Information Sys.: Y	Phys. Rehab. Center:	Waste Disposal:	Phys. Practice Mgmt.:
	Clinical Trials:		Psychiatric Clinics:	Specialty Services:	

TYPES OF BUSINESS:
Home Health Care
Medical Software

BRANDS/DIVISIONS/AFFILIATES:
Partners in Wound Care Program
River Region Home Health
Freedom Home Health

CONTACTS:
Note: Officers with more than one job title may be intentionally listed here more than once.

William F. Borne, CEO
Larry R. Graham, Pres.
Larry R. Graham, COO
Gregory H. Browne, CFO
Patty Graham, Sr. VP-Mktg.
Cindy Phillips, Sr. VP-Human Resources
Alice Ann Schwartz, CIO
Jeffrey D. Jeter, Corporate Counsel/VP-Compliance
Jill Cannon, Sr. VP-Oper.
Ric Pritchard, Sr. VP-Bus. Dev.
Scott Bozzell, Sr. VP-Finance
Dorrie Rambo, Sr. VP-Acct./Controller
Pete Hartley, Sr. VP-MIS
William F. Borne, Chmn.

Phone: 225-292-2031   Fax: 225-295-9624
Toll-Free: 800-467-2662
Address: 11100 Mead Rd., Ste. 300, Baton Rouge, LA 70816 US

GROWTH PLANS/SPECIAL FEATURES:
Amedisys, Inc. is a leading multi-regional provider of home health care nursing services. The company operates 64 home care nursing offices and two corporate offices in the southern and southeastern United States. Home health care, in addition to providing patient comfort and convenience, can usually provide lower costs as an alternative to traditional institutional settings. Amedisys's services include skilled nursing; physical, occupational and speech therapy; infusion therapy; oncology and psychiatric services; diabetes assistance; pain management; and hospice care. The company has successfully consolidated its assets in a usually fragmented industry through various measures including the implementation of internally developed clinical management software now licensed to CareSouth Home Health Services, Inc. In addition, the Medicare Prospective Payment System (PPS) places a greater emphasis upon wound care and stasis ulcers in the clinical scoring process, which validates Amedisys's Partners in Wound Care Program. The program integrates the firm's expert clinical and support services with ConvaTec, a Bristol-Myers Squibb company, MeadJohnson Nutritionals and Hill-Rom, a leader in specialty medical beds and other therapeutic support surfaces. Amedisys has made several smaller acquisitions in the past year, including River Region Home Health in Mississippi, Freedom Home Health in Virginia, and two home health agencies in Georgia and South Carolina from Winyah Health Care Group.

FINANCIALS:
Sales and profits are in thousands of dollars—add 000 to get the full amount. Year 2004 note: Complete fiscal 2004 results were not available for all companies at press time. For this company, year 2004 is for 6 months.

2004 Sales: $104,235 (6 months)   2004 Profits: $9,182 (6 months)
2003 Sales: $142,500   2003 Profits: $84,800
2002 Sales: $129,400   2002 Profits: $800
2001 Sales: $110,200   2001 Profits: $5,400
2000 Sales: $90,755   2000 Profits: $6,370

Stock Ticker: AMED
Employees: 2,520
Fiscal Year Ends: 12/31

SALARIES/BENEFITS:
Pension Plan: ESOP Stock Plan: Profit Sharing: Top Exec. Salary: $350,000   Bonus: $375,000
Savings Plan: Y   Stock Purch. Plan: Y   Second Exec. Salary: $220,385   Bonus: $137,500

OTHER THOUGHTS:
Apparent Top Female Officers: 5
Hot Spot for Advancement for Women/Minorities: Y

LOCATIONS: ("Y" = Yes)
West:	Southwest:	Midwest:	Southeast:	Northeast:	International:
	Y		Y	Y	

AMERICA SERVICE GROUP INC

www.asgr.com

Industry Group Code: 621490   Ranks within this company's industry group: Sales: 5   Profits: 9

Insurance/HMO/PPO:	Drugs:	Equipment/Supplies:	Hospitals/Clinics:		Services:		Health Care:
Insurance:	Manufacturer:	Manufacturer:	Acute Care:		Diagnostics:	Y	Home Health:
Managed Care:	Distributor:	Distributor:	Sub-Acute Care:	Y	Labs/Testing:		Long-Term Care:
Utilization Mgmt.:	Specialty Pharm.:	Leasing/Finance:	Outpatient Surgery:		Staffing:		Physical Therapy:
Payment Proc.:	Vitamins/Nutri.:	Information Sys.:	Phys. Rehab. Center:		Waste Disposal:		Phys. Practice Mgmt.:
	Clinical Trials:		Psychiatric Clinics:		Specialty Services:	Y	

TYPES OF BUSINESS:
Diversified Health Care Services-Prisons
Military Health Care
Administrative Support Services

BRANDS/DIVISIONS/AFFILIATES:
EMSA Military Services, Inc.

CONTACTS:
Note: Officers with more than one job title may be intentionally listed here more than once.
Michael Catalano, CEO
Michael Catalano, Pres.
Michael W. Taylor, CFO
Lawrence H. Pomeroy, Sr. VP/Chief Dev. Officer
Eric W. Thrailkill, CIO
T. Scott Hoffman, Chief Admin. Officer
Jean L. Byassee, General Counsel
Richard D. Wright, VP-Oper.
Lawrence H. Pomeroy, Sr. VP/Chief Dev. Officer
Carl J. Keldie, Corp. Medical Dir.
Jean L. Byassee, Corp. Sec.
Richard D. Wright, Pres./CEO-Prison Health Services
Benjamin S. Purser, Jr., VP-Ethics & Compliance
Michael Catalano, Chmn.

Phone: 615-373-3100   Fax: 615-376-1350
Toll-Free: 800-729-0069
Address: 105 Westpark Dr., Ste. 200, Brentwood, TN 37027 US

GROWTH PLANS/SPECIAL FEATURES:
America Service Group, Inc. (ASG) is a leading national provider of health care services to correctional facilities in the U.S. The company contracts with state, county and local government agencies to provide a wide range of on-site health care programs as well as off-site hospitalization and specialty outpatient care. The firm's clinics emphasize inmate treatment during the initial stages of incarceration in order to identify illness. Medical services provided on-site include physical and mental health screening upon intake. After initial screening, the company may provide regular physical and dental screening and care, psychiatric care, OB-GYN screening and care and diagnostic testing. It holds sick call on a regular basis and provides infirmary bed care in some facilities. Medical services ASG provides off-site include specialty outpatient diagnostic testing and care, emergency room care, surgery and hospitalization. In addition, ASG provides administrative support services both on-site and at its headquarters and regional offices. Administrative programs include on-site medical records and management and employee education and licensing. Central and regional offices provide quality assurance, medical audits, credentialing, continuing education and clinical program development activities. Aside from correctional facility-based health care, ASG provides emergency medicine and primary health care services to active and retired military personnel through EMSA Military Services.

FINANCIALS:
Sales and profits are in thousands of dollars—add 000 to get the full amount. Year 2004 note: Complete fiscal 2004 results were not available for all companies at press time. For this company, year 2004 is for 9 months.

2004 Sales: $502,723 (9 months)	2004 Profits: $4,238 (9 months)	**Stock Ticker: ASGR**
2003 Sales: $549,257	2003 Profits: $11,875	Employees: 6,650
2002 Sales: $481,500	2002 Profits: $11,900	Fiscal Year Ends: 12/31
2001 Sales: $552,500	2001 Profits: $-44,800	
2000 Sales: $381,946	2000 Profits: $7,807	

SALARIES/BENEFITS:
Pension Plan: ESOP Stock Plan: Profit Sharing: Top Exec. Salary: $474,779   Bonus: $19,108
Savings Plan: Y   Stock Purch. Plan: Y   Second Exec. Salary: $254,039   Bonus: $10,856

OTHER THOUGHTS:
Apparent Top Female Officers: 1
Hot Spot for Advancement for Women/Minorities:

LOCATIONS: ("Y" = Yes)

West:	Southwest:	Midwest:	Southeast:	Northeast:	International:
Y	Y	Y	Y	Y	

AMERICAN HEALTHWAYS INC
www.americanhealthways.com

Industry Group Code: 621490   Ranks within this company's industry group: Sales: 10   Profits: 7

Insurance/HMO/PPO:	Drugs:	Equipment/Supplies:	Hospitals/Clinics:		Services:		Health Care:	
Insurance:	Manufacturer:	Manufacturer:	Acute Care:		Diagnostics:		Home Health:	
Managed Care:	Distributor:	Distributor:	Sub-Acute Care:	Y	Labs/Testing:		Long-Term Care:	
Utilization Mgmt.:	Specialty Pharm.:	Leasing/Finance:	Outpatient Surgery:	Y	Staffing:		Physical Therapy:	
Payment Proc.:	Vitamins/Nutri.:	Information Sys.:	Phys. Rehab. Center:	Y	Waste Disposal:		Phys. Practice Mgmt.:	
	Clinical Trials:		Psychiatric Clinics:		Specialty Services:	Y		

TYPES OF BUSINESS:
Outsourced Diabetes Treatment Programs
Ambulatory Surgery Centers
Arthritis Care
Osteoporosis Care
Cardiac Disease Management Services
Respiratory Disease Management Services
Online Disease Management

BRANDS/DIVISIONS/AFFILIATES:
CentreVu Customer Care Solution
Cardiac Healthways
Respiratory Healthways
Diabetes Healthways
MyHealthways

GROWTH PLANS/SPECIAL FEATURES:
American Healthways provides specialized, comprehensive disease management services to health plans, physicians and hospitals. Through its three product lines, Diabetes Healthways, Cardiac Healthways and Respiratory Healthways, the company provides disease management programs in more than 65 hospitals in 20 states. Its programs are designed to improve health care quality at a lower cost for people with chronic diseases. MyHealthways is a new web-based application that allows physicians, patients and care coordinators to actively monitor a chronic disease, receive customized plans of action or identify at-risk individuals through predictive modeling technology. The firm uses customer relationship management solutions from Avaya, a leading provider of communications systems, to support its disease management programs. Avaya's CentreVu Customer Care Solution routes calls to the American Healthways professional most familiar with the patient's case and most appropriate for the patient's current needs.

CONTACTS:
Note: Officers with more than one job title may be intentionally listed here more than once.

Ben R. Leedle, CEO
Ben R. Leedle, Pres.
Donald B. Taylor, COO
Mary Chaput, Exec. VP/CFO
Henry D. Herr, Exec. VP-Admin.
Thomas G. Cigarran, Chmn.

Phone: 615-665-1122   Fax: 615-665-7697
Toll-Free:
Address: 3841 Green Hills Village Dr., Nashville, TN 37215-6104 US

FINANCIALS:
Sales and profits are in thousands of dollars—add 000 to get the full amount. Year 2004 note: Complete fiscal 2004 results were not available for all companies at press time. For this company, year 2004 is for 9 months.

2004 Sales: $173,600 (9 months)	2004 Profits: $17,000 (9 months)	
2003 Sales: $165,500	2003 Profits: $18,500	Stock Ticker: AMHC
2002 Sales: $122,800	2002 Profits: $10,400	Employees: 1,017
2001 Sales: $75,100	2001 Profits: $3,200	Fiscal Year Ends: 8/31
2000 Sales: $53,030	2000 Profits: $148	

SALARIES/BENEFITS:
Pension Plan:	ESOP Stock Plan:	Profit Sharing:	Top Exec. Salary: $435,000	Bonus: $154,561
Savings Plan: Y	Stock Purch. Plan:		Second Exec. Salary: $347,000	Bonus: $122,945

OTHER THOUGHTS:
Apparent Top Female Officers: 1
Hot Spot for Advancement for Women/Minorities:

LOCATIONS: ("Y" = Yes)
West:	Southwest:	Midwest:	Southeast:	Northeast:	International:
Y	Y	Y	Y	Y	

AMERICAN HOMEPATIENT INC

www.ahom.com

Industry Group Code: 621610 **Ranks within this company's industry group:** Sales: 3 Profits: 5

Insurance/HMO/PPO:	Drugs:	Equipment/Supplies:	Hospitals/Clinics:	Services:	Health Care:
Insurance: Managed Care: Utilization Mgmt.: Payment Proc.:	Manufacturer: Distributor: Specialty Pharm.: Vitamins/Nutri.: Clinical Trials:	Manufacturer: Distributor: Leasing/Finance: Y Information Sys.: Y	Acute Care: Sub-Acute Care: Outpatient Surgery: Phys. Rehab. Center: Psychiatric Clinics:	Diagnostics: Labs/Testing: Staffing: Waste Disposal: Specialty Services: Y	Home Health: Y Long-Term Care: Physical Therapy: Phys. Practice Mgmt.:

TYPES OF BUSINESS:
Health Care-Home Health
Respiratory Therapy Services
Infusion Therapy Services
Equipment Leasing
Home Health Supplies

BRANDS/DIVISIONS/AFFILIATES:

GROWTH PLANS/SPECIAL FEATURES:
American HomePatient, Inc. provides respiratory and infusion therapies and rents and sells home medical equipment and home health care supplies. The company runs 286 centers in 35 states. Revenues come primarily from Medicare, Medicaid and other third parties. The firm's respiratory services include oxygen systems to assist in breathing, nebulizers, home ventilators, non-invasive positive-pressure ventilation masks, continuous and bi-level positive airway pressure therapies, apnea monitors and home sleep screenings and studies. Home infusion therapies include enteral nutrition, antibiotic therapy, total parenteral nutrition and pain management. The company also rents and sells wheelchairs, hospital beds, ambulatory aids, bathroom aids and safety and rehabilitation equipment. The company recently emerged from Chapter 11 bankruptcy according to an approved plan of reorganization.

CONTACTS:
Note: Officers with more than one job title may be intentionally listed here more than once.
Joseph F. Furlong, III, CEO
Joseph F. Furlong, III, Pres.
Thomas E. Mills, Exec. VP/COO

Phone: 615-221-8884 **Fax:** 615-373-9932
Toll-Free: 800-890-7271
Address: 5200 Maryland Way, Ste. 400, Brentwood, TN 37027-5018 US

FINANCIALS:
Sales and profits are in thousands of dollars—add 000 to get the full amount. Year 2004 note: Complete fiscal 2004 results were not available for all companies at press time. For this company, year 2004 is for 9 months.

2004 Sales: $251,587 (9 months)	2004 Profits: $5,005 (9 months)	
2003 Sales: $336,181	2003 Profits: $14,025	**Stock Ticker:** AHOM
2002 Sales: $319,797	2002 Profits: $-61,154	**Employees:** 3,451
2001 Sales: $352,600	2001 Profits: $-11,500	**Fiscal Year Ends:** 12/31
2000 Sales: $363,400	2000 Profits: $-31,700	

SALARIES/BENEFITS:
Pension Plan:	ESOP Stock Plan:	Profit Sharing:	Top Exec. Salary: $485,000	Bonus: $679,000
Savings Plan: Y	Stock Purch. Plan: Y		Second Exec. Salary: $250,000	Bonus: $200,000

OTHER THOUGHTS:
Apparent Top Female Officers:
Hot Spot for Advancement for Women/Minorities:

LOCATIONS: ("Y" = Yes)
West:	Southwest:	Midwest:	Southeast:	Northeast:	International:
Y	Y	Y	Y	Y	

AMERICAN MEDICAL SECURITY GROUP INC

www.eams.com

Industry Group Code: 524114 **Ranks within this company's industry group:** Sales: 50 Profits: 38

Insurance/HMO/PPO:	Drugs:	Equipment/Supplies:	Hospitals/Clinics:	Services:	Health Care:
Insurance:	Manufacturer: Y	Manufacturer:	Acute Care:	Diagnostics:	Home Health:
Managed Care: Y	Distributor: Y	Distributor:	Sub-Acute Care:	Labs/Testing:	Long-Term Care:
Utilization Mgmt.:	Specialty Pharm.:	Leasing/Finance:	Outpatient Surgery:	Staffing:	Physical Therapy:
Payment Proc.:	Vitamins/Nutri.:	Information Sys.:	Phys. Rehab. Center:	Waste Disposal:	Phys. Practice Mgmt.:
	Clinical Trials:		Psychiatric Clinics:	Specialty Services: Y	

TYPES OF BUSINESS:
HMO/PPO
Health Care Benefits and Insurance Products
Health Information Line

BRANDS/DIVISIONS/AFFILIATES:
GroupMedChoice
MedOne
AMSMedOne
Nurse Healthline, Inc.
PacifiCare Health Systems

CONTACTS:
Note: Officers with more than one job title may be intentionally listed here more than once.

Samuel V. Miller, CEO
Samuel V. Miller, Pres.
John R. Lombardi, Exec. VP/CFO
Timothy O'Keefe, Sr. VP/Chief Mktg. Officer
John R. Wirch, VP-Human Resources
Penny Paque, VP/CIO
Timothy J. Moore, Sr. VP/General Counsel
Thomas G. Zielinski, Exec. VP-Oper.
Clifford A. Bowers, VP-Corp. Comm.
John R. Lombardi, Treas.
James C. Modaff, Exec. VP/Chief Actuary
Timothy J. Moore, Corp. Sec.
Samuel V. Miller, Chmn.

Phone: 920-661-1111 **Fax:** 920-661-2222
Toll-Free: 800-232-5432
Address: 3100 AMS Blvd., Green Bay, WI 54307-9032 US

GROWTH PLANS/SPECIAL FEATURES:
American Medical Security Group, through its operating subsidiaries, markets health care benefits and insurance products to small businesses, families and individuals. The PPO serves customers in 32 states and the District of Columbia through partnerships with professionals, independent agents and quality health care providers. GroupMedChoice is the company's primary small group product. It allows a business to offer a variety of health care plans to each employee. Although premiums may vary between the plans, the employer's cost does not. The firm's MedOne product line for individuals and families offers selection and flexibility through plans that are affordable and easy to comprehend. Clients are allowed to choose from a variety of options, customizing coverage for their specific needs. MedOne membership constitutes 45% of American Medical's business. The firm's AMSMedOne product is designed for cost-conscious consumers and features more attractive premium rates, protection from catastrophic medical costs and more patient responsibility for routine health care expenses. One of American Medical's subsidiaries, Nurse Healthline, Inc., provides a 24-hour-a-day health information line. Recently, American Medical agreed to sell its Accountable Health Plans of America, Inc. subsidiary to IPACQ, Inc. for $3.5 million. In September 2004, the company agreed to be acquired by PacifiCare Health Systems for $502 million.

FINANCIALS:
Sales and profits are in thousands of dollars—add 000 to get the full amount. Year 2004 note: Complete fiscal 2004 results were not available for all companies at press time. For this company, year 2004 is for 9 months.

2004 Sales: $552,993 (9 months)	2004 Profits: $23,996 (9 months)	**Stock Ticker:** AMZ
2003 Sales: $743,716	2003 Profits: $29,310	Employees: 1,444
2002 Sales: $789,500	2002 Profits: $-37,600	Fiscal Year Ends: 12/31
2001 Sales: $876,600	2001 Profits: $4,200	
2000 Sales: $989,900	2000 Profits: $2,700	

SALARIES/BENEFITS:
Pension Plan:	ESOP Stock Plan:	Profit Sharing:	Top Exec. Salary: $700,000	Bonus: $490,000
Savings Plan: Y	Stock Purch. Plan:		Second Exec. Salary: $310,154	Bonus: $222,400

OTHER THOUGHTS:
Apparent Top Female Officers: 1
Hot Spot for Advancement for Women/Minorities:

LOCATIONS: ("Y" = Yes)
West:	Southwest:	Midwest:	Southeast:	Northeast:	International:
Y	Y	Y	Y	Y	

AMERICAN MEDICAL SYSTEMS HOLDINGS INC   www.visitams.com

Industry Group Code: 339113   Ranks within this company's industry group: Sales: 69   Profits: 44

Insurance/HMO/PPO:	Drugs:	Equipment/Supplies:		Hospitals/Clinics:	Services:	Health Care:
Insurance:	Manufacturer:	Manufacturer:	Y	Acute Care:	Diagnostics:	Home Health:
Managed Care:	Distributor:	Distributor:		Sub-Acute Care:	Labs/Testing:	Long-Term Care:
Utilization Mgmt.:	Specialty Pharm.:	Leasing/Finance:		Outpatient Surgery:	Staffing:	Physical Therapy:
Payment Proc.:	Vitamins/Nutri.:	Information Sys.:		Phys. Rehab. Center:	Waste Disposal:	Phys. Practice Mgmt.:
	Clinical Trials:			Psychiatric Clinics:	Specialty Services:	

TYPES OF BUSINESS:
Urological Devices Manufacturing
Erectile Dysfunction Products
Incontinence Products
Prostate Disease Products

BRANDS/DIVISIONS/AFFILIATES:
TherMatrx, Inc.

CONTACTS: Note: Officers with more than one job title may be intentionally listed here more than once.
Douglas W. Kohrs, CEO
Martin J. Emerson, Pres.
Martin J. Emerson, COO
Carmen L. Diersen, Exec. VP/CFO
Martin J. Emerson, VP-Global Mktg. & Sales
Janet L. Dick, VP-Human Resources
Ross Longhini, Exec. VP/Chief Tech. Officer
M. James Call, Exec. VP-Planning & Dev.
Lawrence W. Getlin, VP-Regulatory, Medical Affairs & Quality Assurance
Douglas W. Kohrs, Chmn.

Phone: 952-930-6000   **Fax:** 952-930-6157
Toll-Free: 800-328-3881
Address: 10700 Bren Rd. W., Minnetonka, MN 55343 US

GROWTH PLANS/SPECIAL FEATURES:
American Medical Systems, Inc. (AMS) supplies medical devices for treating urological and gynecological disorders. The company manufactures and markets a broad and well-established line of proprietary products, focusing on three major urological disorders: incontinence, erectile dysfunction and prostate disease. AMS offers a broad line of products designed to treat men and women suffering from urinary and fecal incontinence. Products include artificial sphincters, male and female sling systems, a vaginal vault prolapse system and graft materials. The firm is the market leader in the surgical erectile dysfunction market, holding about 70% of the market share. Products include a full line of inflatable and malleable penile prostheses and accessories used in the diagnosis and treatment of erectile dysfunction. Erectile dysfunction products represent half of AMS's sales. The company also offers prostatic stents and resection loops for sufferers of prostate disease. Outside the U.S., the company markets a minimally invasive ethanol injection system for the treatment of benign prostatic hyperplasia. AMS has acquired rights to a number of less invasive or less expensive technologies treating urological disorders. In July 2004, American Medical Systems acquired TherMatrx, Inc., a corporation that manufactures and markets the TMx 2000, a benign prostatic hyperplasia therapy.

FINANCIALS:
Sales and profits are in thousands of dollars—add 000 to get the full amount. Year 2004 note: Complete fiscal 2004 results were not available for all companies at press time. For this company, year 2004 is for 6 months.

2004 Sales: $96,406 (6 months)	2004 Profits: $16,456 (6 months)	
2003 Sales: $168,283	2003 Profits: $29,050	**Stock Ticker:** AMMD
2002 Sales: $141,600	2002 Profits: $24,900	Employees: 587
2001 Sales: $117,900	2001 Profits: $6,500	Fiscal Year Ends: 12/31
2000 Sales: $100,300	2000 Profits: $100	

SALARIES/BENEFITS:
Pension Plan:	ESOP Stock Plan:	Profit Sharing:	Top Exec. Salary: $304,039	Bonus: $134,618
Savings Plan:	Stock Purch. Plan:		Second Exec. Salary: $23,500	Bonus: $86,130

OTHER THOUGHTS:
Apparent Top Female Officers: 2
Hot Spot for Advancement for Women/Minorities:

LOCATIONS: ("Y" = Yes)
West:	Southwest:	Midwest:	Southeast:	Northeast:	International:
		Y			Y

AMERICAN PHARMACEUTICAL PARTNERS INC
www.appdrugs.com

Industry Group Code: 325412   Ranks within this company's industry group: Sales: 40   Profits: 28

Insurance/HMO/PPO:	Drugs:		Equipment/Supplies:	Hospitals/Clinics:	Services:	Health Care:
Insurance: Managed Care: Utilization Mgmt.: Payment Proc.:	Manufacturer: Distributor: Specialty Pharm.: Vitamins/Nutri.: Clinical Trials:	Y	Manufacturer: Distributor: Leasing/Finance: Information Sys.:	Acute Care: Sub-Acute Care: Outpatient Surgery: Phys. Rehab. Center: Psychiatric Clinics:	Diagnostics: Labs/Testing: Staffing: Waste Disposal: Specialty Services:	Home Health: Long-Term Care: Physical Therapy: Phys. Practice Mgmt.:

TYPES OF BUSINESS:
Drugs-Manufacturing
Injectables

BRANDS/DIVISIONS/AFFILIATES:
Mesna
Pamidronate
Doxycycline
Ifosfamide
Cisplatin
Cystosar-U
Pipracil
Gentamicin

CONTACTS:
Note: Officers with more than one job title may be intentionally listed here more than once.

Patrick Soon-Shiong, CEO
Patrick Soon-Shiong, Pres.
Derek J. Brown, Co-COO/Corp. Sec.
Nicole S. Williams, Exec. VP/CFO
Lorin Drake, VP-Sales
Mia Igyarto, VP-Human Resources
Sam Trippie, VP-Mfg.
Jack C. Silhavy, VP/General Counsel
Donna Felch, VP/Treas.
Jeffrey M. Yordon, Co-COO
Shahid Ahmed, VP-Regulatory Affairs
Thomas Shea, VP-Corp. Mktg.
Deen Reyes, VP-Mktg.
Patrick Soon-Shiong, Chmn.

Phone: 847-969-2700   Fax: 800-743-7082
Toll-Free: 888-391-6300
Address: 1101 Perimeter Dr., Ste. 300, Schaumburg, IL 60173-5837 US

GROWTH PLANS/SPECIAL FEATURES:

American Pharmaceutical Partners, Inc. (APP) is a specialty drug company that develops, manufactures and markets injectable pharmaceutical products in each of the three basic forms sold: liquid, powder and lyophilized or freeze-dried. The company focuses on the oncology, anti-infective and critical care markets of the pharmaceutical industry. APP is one of the largest producers of injectables, producing approximately 130 generic products in over 350 dosages and formulations. It currently has over 50 product candidates under development and manufactures and markets 13 proprietary injectable oncology products in 30 dosages and formulations; 15 proprietary injectable anti-infective products; and more than 50 proprietary injectable critical care products. The company's products include Pamidronate, Mesna, Cisplatin and Ifosfamide for the oncology market; Cefoxitin, Vancomycin, Doxycycline, Cefotaxime and Gentamicin for the anti-infective market; and Heparin, Oxytocin and Haloperidol Lactate for the critical care market. APP has the exclusive North American rights to manufacture and market ABRAXANE, a proprietary injectable oncology product that was formerly known as ABI-007. In recent news, ABRAXANE completed Phase III clinical trials for metastatic breast cancer. The FDA granted it fast-track status to speed product development. The FDA also approved ciprofloxacin, an anti-infective that will be marketed as Cipro in 2006; cytarabine, an oncology product marketed as Cytosar-U; piperacillin, an anti-infective marketed as Pipracil; fluconazole, a critical care product marketed as Diflucan; carboplatin, an oncology product marketed as Paraplatin; and Bacitracin, an anti-infective. In other news, the company recently acquired a manufacturing facility and injectable oncology products from Switzerland-based Bigmar, giving the company its first presence in Europe.

APP offers a competitive benefits and compensation package including health, dental and life insurance and tuition assistance.

FINANCIALS:
Sales and profits are in thousands of dollars—add 000 to get the full amount. Year 2004 note: Complete fiscal 2004 results were not available for all companies at press time. For this company, year 2004 is for 9 months.

2004 Sales: $282,456 (9 months)	2004 Profits: $34,827 (9 months)	**Stock Ticker:** APPX
2003 Sales: $351,315	2003 Profits: $71,693	Employees: 1,212
2002 Sales: $277,474	2002 Profits: $45,199	Fiscal Year Ends: 12/31
2001 Sales: $192,029	2001 Profits: $12,628	
2000 Sales: $	2000 Profits: $	

SALARIES/BENEFITS:
Pension Plan:	ESOP Stock Plan: Y	Profit Sharing:	Top Exec. Salary: $366,231	Bonus: $405,000
Savings Plan: Y	Stock Purch. Plan: Y		Second Exec. Salary: $294,039	Bonus: $325,000

OTHER THOUGHTS:
Apparent Top Female Officers: 5
Hot Spot for Advancement for Women/Minorities: Y

LOCATIONS: ("Y" = Yes)
West:	Southwest:	Midwest:	Southeast:	Northeast:	International:
Y		Y		Y	Y

Plunkett's Health Care Industry Almanac 2005

AMERICAN RETIREMENT CORP
www.arclp.com

Industry Group Code: 623110   Ranks within this company's industry group: Sales: 9   Profits: 12

Insurance/HMO/PPO:	Drugs:	Equipment/Supplies:	Hospitals/Clinics:	Services:	Health Care:
Insurance: Managed Care: Utilization Mgmt.: Payment Proc.:	Manufacturer: Distributor: Specialty Pharm.: Vitamins/Nutri.: Clinical Trials:	Manufacturer: Distributor: Leasing/Finance: Information Sys.:	Acute Care: Sub-Acute Care: Outpatient Surgery: Phys. Rehab. Center: Psychiatric Clinics:	Diagnostics: Labs/Testing: Staffing: Waste Disposal: Specialty Services:	Home Health: Y Long-Term Care: Y Physical Therapy: Y Phys. Practice Mgmt.:

TYPES OF BUSINESS:
Long-Term Health Care
Home Health Care
Assisted Living Services

BRANDS/DIVISIONS/AFFILIATES:

CONTACTS: Note: Officers with more than one job title may be intentionally listed here more than once.
W. E. Sheriff, CEO
W. E. Sheriff, Pres.
Gregory B. Richard, Exec VP/COO
Bryan Richardson, Exec. VP/CFO
James T. Money, Exec. VP-Mktg.
Terry Frisby, Sr. VP-Human Resources & Corp. Compliance
Fred Ewing, VP-Oper.
H. Todd Kaestner, Exec. VP-Corp. Dev.
Matt Fontana, VP-Public Rel.
Ross Roadman, Sr. VP-Investor Rel. & Strategic Planning
George T. Hicks, Exec. VP-Finance
W. E. Sheriff, Chmn.
Richard Raessler, VP-Asset Mgmt. & Purchasing

Phone: 615-221-2250   Fax: 615-221-2269
Toll-Free:
Address: 111 Westwood Pl., Ste. 202, Brentwood, TN 37027 US

GROWTH PLANS/SPECIAL FEATURES:
American Retirement Corp. offers a broad range of care and services to seniors, including independent living, assisted living, therapy services, skilled nursing and Alzheimer's care. The company currently operates 66 senior living communities in 14 states with an aggregate capacity of approximately 14,600 residents. The firm's strategy is to develop senior living networks in major metropolitan regions. These networks are made up of large continuing care retirement communities and freestanding assisted living residences located in the same markets, with skilled nursing capabilities at one or more of the network communities. Continuing care retirement communities offer a wide array of services, including independent living, assisted living and skilled nursing care in large, often campus-style settings. The company's retirement centers are established communities with strong reputations within their respective markets and generally maintain high and consistent occupancy levels. These retirement centers form the core segment of the firm's business. They comprise 32 of the 66 communities that the firm operates, representing approximately 77% of the total resident capacity. Freestanding assisted living residencies are much smaller than retirement centers and are generally stand-alone communities that are not located on a retirement center campus. Most provide specialized care such as Alzheimer's, memory enhancement and other dementia programs. American Retirement currently operates 33 freestanding assisted living residencies.

FINANCIALS:
Sales and profits are in thousands of dollars—add 000 to get the full amount. Year 2004 note: Complete fiscal 2004 results were not available for all companies at press time. For this company, year 2004 is for 9 months.

2004 Sales: $331,341 (9 months)   2004 Profits: $-14,290 (9 months)
2003 Sales: $368,096   2003 Profits: $-17,314
2002 Sales: $331,900   2002 Profits: $-94,800
2001 Sales: $256,200   2001 Profits: $-34,900
2000 Sales: $206,100   2000 Profits: $-5,846

Stock Ticker: ACR
Employees: 8,700
Fiscal Year Ends: 12/31

SALARIES/BENEFITS:
Pension Plan: ESOP Stock Plan: Profit Sharing: Top Exec. Salary: $271,500   Bonus: $101,590
Savings Plan: Y   Stock Purch. Plan: Second Exec. Salary: $202,000   Bonus: $21,985

OTHER THOUGHTS:
Apparent Top Female Officers: 1
Hot Spot for Advancement for Women/Minorities:

LOCATIONS: ("Y" = Yes)
West:	Southwest:	Midwest:	Southeast:	Northeast:	International:
Y	Y	Y	Y	Y	

Note: Financial information, benefits and other data can change quickly and may vary from those stated here.

AMERICAN SHARED HOSPITAL SERVICES

www.ashs.com

Industry Group Code: 621490 Ranks within this company's industry group: Sales: 19 Profits: 15

Insurance/HMO/PPO:	Drugs:	Equipment/Supplies:	Hospitals/Clinics:	Services:	Health Care:
Insurance:	Manufacturer:	Manufacturer:	Acute Care:	Diagnostics:	Home Health:
Managed Care:	Distributor:	Distributor:	Sub-Acute Care:	Labs/Testing:	Long-Term Care:
Utilization Mgmt.:	Specialty Pharm.:	Leasing/Finance: Y	Outpatient Surgery: Y	Staffing:	Physical Therapy:
Payment Proc.:	Vitamins/Nutri.:	Information Sys.:	Phys. Rehab. Center:	Waste Disposal:	Phys. Practice Mgmt.:
	Clinical Trials:		Psychiatric Clinics:	Specialty Services: Y	

TYPES OF BUSINESS:
Hospitals/Clinics-Outpatient & Surgery
Radiosurgery Services
Equipment Financing

BRANDS/DIVISIONS/AFFILIATES:
GK Financing, LLC
Operating Room for the 21st Century (The)

CONTACTS: Note: Officers with more than one job title may be intentionally listed here more than once.
Ernest A. Bates, CEO
Craig K. Tagawa, COO
Craig K. Tagawa, CFO
Ernest A. Bates, Chmn.

Phone: 415-788-5300 Fax: 415-788-5660
Toll-Free: 800-735-0641
Address: 4 Embarcadero Ctr., Ste. 3700, San Francisco, CA 94111 US

GROWTH PLANS/SPECIAL FEATURES:
American Shared Hospital Services (ASHS) is a medical services company with interests in radiosurgery devices and a program called The Operating Room for the 21st-Century (OR21), which offers turnkey development of surgical suites to medical centers. The company provides its services through its majority-owned GK Financing, LLC (GKF) subsidiary. GKF provides Leksell Gamma Knife radiosurgery equipment, manufactured by Elekta, to medical centers and offers gamma knife stereotactic radiosurgery services worldwide. Gamma knife radiosurgery is an alternative to conventional brain surgery. The procedure has been in use in the United States for over 10 years, with an excess of 250,000 procedures performed worldwide. It has proved itself as a highly effective treatment of certain malignant and benign brain tumors and other brain conditions. Treatment of Parkinson's disease, epilepsy and intractable pain also show promising results. Because it is a non-invasive procedure, gamma knife radiosurgery reduces surgical risk and patient discomfort, shortens hospital stays and lowers the risk of complications. In the majority of cases, patients resume normal activities within days of treatment, compared to the weeks or months of recovery time needed after conventional surgery. ASHS's 18th gamma knife unit recently opened at Lehigh Valley Hospital-Muhlenberg in Bethlehem, Pennsylvania. In other news, the company signed a contract for its 21st gamma knife center with Mercy Health Center in Oklahoma City, Oklahoma.

FINANCIALS:
Sales and profits are in thousands of dollars—add 000 to get the full amount. Year 2004 note: Complete fiscal 2004 results were not available for all companies at press time. For this company, year 2004 is for 6 months.

2004 Sales: $8,348 (6 months)   2004 Profits: $759 (6 months)
2003 Sales: $16,178   2003 Profits: $1,382
2002 Sales: $13,400   2002 Profits: $1,100
2001 Sales: $11,800   2001 Profits: $1,100
2000 Sales: $9,300   2000 Profits: $1,300

Stock Ticker: AMS
Employees: 8
Fiscal Year Ends: 12/31

SALARIES/BENEFITS:
| Pension Plan: | ESOP Stock Plan: | Profit Sharing: | Top Exec. Salary: $432,443 | Bonus: $55,770 |
| Savings Plan: | Stock Purch. Plan: | | Second Exec. Salary: $250,875 | Bonus: $100,000 |

OTHER THOUGHTS:
Apparent Top Female Officers:
Hot Spot for Advancement for Women/Minorities:

LOCATIONS: ("Y" = Yes)
West:	Southwest:	Midwest:	Southeast:	Northeast:	International:
Y					

AMERICHOICE CORPORATION

www.americhoice.com

Industry Group Code: 524114   Ranks within this company's industry group: Sales: Profits:

Insurance/HMO/PPO:	Drugs:	Equipment/Supplies:	Hospitals/Clinics:	Services:	Health Care:
Insurance:	Manufacturer:	Manufacturer:	Acute Care:	Diagnostics:	Home Health:
Managed Care: Y	Distributor:	Distributor:	Sub-Acute Care:	Labs/Testing:	Long-Term Care:
Utilization Mgmt.: Y	Specialty Pharm.:	Leasing/Finance:	Outpatient Surgery:	Staffing:	Physical Therapy:
Payment Proc.:	Vitamins/Nutri.:	Information Sys.:	Phys. Rehab. Center:	Waste Disposal:	Phys. Practice Mgmt.:
	Clinical Trials:		Psychiatric Clinics:	Specialty Services: Y	

TYPES OF BUSINESS:
Health Insurance
Management Services
IT Services

BRANDS/DIVISIONS/AFFILIATES:
AmeriChoice Personal Care Model
Telemedicine
Healthy First Steps
UnitedHealth Group

CONTACTS:
Note: Officers with more than one job title may be intentionally listed here more than once.
Anthony Welters, CEO
Anthony Welters, Pres.
Jess E. Sweely, COO
Eric Settle, Sr. VP/General Counsel
Anthony Welters, Chmn.

Phone: 703-506-3555   Fax: 703-506-3556
Toll-Free:
Address: 8045 Leesburg Pike, Ste. 650, Vienna, VA 22182 US

GROWTH PLANS/SPECIAL FEATURES:
AmeriChoice Corporation, a UnitedHealth Group company, is committed to serving recipients of government health care programs. The company operates its own government program health insurance plans and provides management and information technology services to other managed care organizations, serving over 1 million members in more than a dozen states. AmeriChoice features community-based networks, a focus on preventative services, outreach and intensive case management. It targets the most frequent causes of severe illness in its service areas, addressing conditions such as asthma, diabetes, sickle cell disease and high-risk pregnancies. The AmeriChoice Personal Care Model assigns members to nurses and social workers who build a support network involving family, physicians, ancillary providers and government and community-based organizations and resources. Its Telemedicine program uses video units in members' homes, allowing case managers to monitor certain vital signs and check medications over the phone. The company's Healthy First Steps maternal and obstetrical care program helps women schedule prenatal doctor visits, select a pediatrician and get health services for the baby. AmeriChoice tries to promote prevention through health education and programs. The company sends reminders to members encouraging them to get annual physicals and routine diagnostic and screening tests, and often makes special arrangements, including door-to-door transportation, child care and private appointments, for groups of women to receive mammograms and for children to be immunized. AmeriChoice physicians receive extra compensation for routine preventive care, and those who exceed state averages for certain procedures are eligible for significant cash bonuses.

AmeriChoice offers medical, dental and vision benefits, education reimbursement, adoption assistance and employee assistance.

FINANCIALS:
Sales and profits are in thousands of dollars—add 000 to get the full amount. Year 2004 note: Complete fiscal 2004 results were not available for all companies at press time. For this company, year 2004 is for   months.

2004 Sales: $ (months)   2004 Profits: $ (months)
2003 Sales: $ 2003 Profits: $
2002 Sales: $ 2002 Profits: $
2001 Sales: $ 2001 Profits: $
2000 Sales: $ 2000 Profits: $

Stock Ticker: Subsidiary
Employees:
Fiscal Year Ends: 12/31

SALARIES/BENEFITS:
Pension Plan: ESOP Stock Plan: Profit Sharing: Top Exec. Salary: $ Bonus: $
Savings Plan: Y   Stock Purch. Plan: Y   Second Exec. Salary: $ Bonus: $

OTHER THOUGHTS:
Apparent Top Female Officers:
Hot Spot for Advancement for Women/Minorities:

LOCATIONS: ("Y" = Yes)
West	Southwest	Midwest	Southeast	Northeast	International
Y	Y	Y	Y	Y	

AMERIGROUP CORPORATION

www.amerigrp.com

Industry Group Code: 524114   Ranks within this company's industry group: Sales: 38   Profits: 28

Insurance/HMO/PPO:	Drugs:	Equipment/Supplies:	Hospitals/Clinics:	Services:	Health Care:
Insurance: Managed Care: Y Utilization Mgmt.: Payment Proc.:	Manufacturer: Distributor: Specialty Pharm.: Vitamins/Nutri.: Clinical Trials:	Manufacturer: Distributor: Leasing/Finance: Information Sys.:	Acute Care: Sub-Acute Care: Outpatient Surgery: Phys. Rehab. Center: Psychiatric Clinics:	Diagnostics: Labs/Testing: Staffing: Waste Disposal: Specialty Services:	Home Health: Long-Term Care: Physical Therapy: Phys. Practice Mgmt.:

TYPES OF BUSINESS:
HMO
Managed Health Care

BRANDS/DIVISIONS/AFFILIATES:
AMERICAID
AMERIKIDS
AMERIPLUS
AMERIFAM
CarePlus Health Plan

CONTACTS:
Note: Officers with more than one job title may be intentionally listed here more than once.

Jeffrey L. McWaters, CEO
James G. Carlson, Pres.
James G. Carlson, COO
E. Paul Dunn, Jr., Exec. VP/CFO
Richard C. Zoretic, Sr. VP/Chief Mktg. Officer
Lorenzo Childress, Jr., Exec. VP/Chief Medical Officer
Leon A. Root, Jr., Exec. VP/CIO
Stanley F. Baldwin, Exec. VP/General Counsel
James E. Hargroves, VP-Corp. Dev.
John E. Little, Sr. VP-Gov't Rel.
Sherri E. Lee, Sr. VP/Treas.
Janet M. Brashear, Exec. VP-Strategic Planning
Nancy L. Groden, Exec. VP-Planning & Dev.
Kathleen K. Toth, Exec. VP/Chief Acct. Officer
Catherine S. Callahan, Exec. VP-Associate Services
Jeffrey L. McWaters, Chmn.

Phone: 757-490-6900   Fax: 757-490-7152
Toll-Free: 800-600-4441
Address: 4425 Corporation Ln., Virginia Beach, VA 23462 US

GROWTH PLANS/SPECIAL FEATURES:
AMERIGROUP Corporation is a managed health care company focused exclusively on serving people who receive health care benefits through state-sponsored programs, including Medicaid, the State Children's Health Insurance Program (SCHIP) and FamilyCare. Since the company does not offer Medicare or commercial products, people served by AMERIGROUP are generally younger. These customers also tend to access health care in an inefficient manner and have a greater percentage of medical expenses related to obstetrics, diabetes and circulatory and respiratory conditions; therefore the company designs its programs to focus on these conditions. In addition, because AMERIGROUP's new members typically use the emergency room as a primary care provider, the firm reduces costs for families and state governments by combining social and behavioral health services to help members obtain quality health care in an efficient and cost-effective manner. AMERIGROUP currently enrolls members in Texas, Florida, New Jersey, Maryland, the District of Columbia and Illinois, serving approximately 857,000 members. The firm offers a variety of insurance products, including AMERICAID, a Medicaid product designed for low-income children and pregnant women; AMERIKIDS, an SCHIP product for uninsured children not eligible for Medicaid; AMERIPLUS, a product for the low-income aged, blind and disabled who receive Social Security; and AMERIFAM, designed for uninsured parents of SCHIP and Medicaid children. The plans all include some combination of primary and specialty physician care, inpatient and outpatient hospital care, emergency care, prenatal care, laboratory and x-ray services, home health and medical equipment, behavioral health services, substance abuse, long-term and nursing home care, vision care, dental care, chiropractic care and prescription coverage. In October 2004, AMERIGROUP announced that it would purchase CarePlus Health Plan from CarePlus, LLC, a Medicaid managed care company serving approximately 114,000 members in New York City.

FINANCIALS:
Sales and profits are in thousands of dollars—add 000 to get the full amount. Year 2004 note: Complete fiscal 2004 results were not available for all companies at press time. For this company, year 2004 is for 9 months.

2004 Sales: $1,333,408 (9 months)   2004 Profits: $63,617 (9 months)
2003 Sales: $1,622,234   2003 Profits: $67,324
2002 Sales: $1,160,700   2002 Profits: $47,000
2001 Sales: $891,200   2001 Profits: $36,100
2000 Sales: $659,500   2000 Profits: $26,100

Stock Ticker: AMG
Employees: 2,100
Fiscal Year Ends: 12/31

SALARIES/BENEFITS:
Pension Plan: ESOP Stock Plan: Profit Sharing: Top Exec. Salary: $612,462   Bonus: $1,225,181
Savings Plan: Y   Stock Purch. Plan: Y   Second Exec. Salary: $344,658   Bonus: $416,667

OTHER THOUGHTS:
Apparent Top Female Officers: 5
Hot Spot for Advancement for Women/Minorities: Y

LOCATIONS: ("Y" = Yes)
West:	Southwest:	Midwest:	Southeast:	Northeast:	International:
	Y	Y	Y	Y	

AMERIPATH INC

www.ameripath.com

Industry Group Code: 621111   Ranks within this company's industry group: Sales: 4   Profits: 6

Insurance/HMO/PPO:	Drugs:	Equipment/Supplies:	Hospitals/Clinics:	Services:		Health Care:	
Insurance: Managed Care: Utilization Mgmt.: Payment Proc.:	Manufacturer: Distributor: Specialty Pharm.: Vitamins/Nutri.: Clinical Trials:	Manufacturer: Distributor: Leasing/Finance: Information Sys.:	Acute Care: Sub-Acute Care: Outpatient Surgery: Phys. Rehab. Center: Psychiatric Clinics:	Diagnostics: Labs/Testing: Staffing: Waste Disposal: Specialty Services:	Y Y Y Y	Home Health: Long-Term Care: Physical Therapy: Phys. Practice Mgmt.:	Y

TYPES OF BUSINESS:
Anatomic Pathology Practice Management
Cancer Diagnostic Services
Staffing Services
Operations Management
Health Care Information Services

BRANDS/DIVISIONS/AFFILIATES:
Dermpath Diagnostics
AmeriPath Institute of Gastrointestinal Pathology
Center for Advanced Diagnostics
Welsh, Carson, Anderson & Rowe

CONTACTS:
Note: Officers with more than one job title may be intentionally listed here more than once.
Donald E. Steen, CEO
Joseph A. Sonnier, Pres.
Martin J. Stefanelli, Exec. VP/COO
David L. Redmond, CFO
Bruce C. Walton, VP-Mktg. & Sales
Stephen V. Fuller, Sr. VP-Human Resources
Bob J. Copeland, VP/CIO
Steven Casper, VP-Bus. Dev.
Jeffrey A. Mossler, Chief Medical Officer
Clay J. Cockerell, Medical Dir.-Dermpath Diagnostics
Donald E. Steen, Chmn.

Phone: 561-845-1850   Fax: 561-845-0129
Toll-Free: 800-330-6565
Address: 7289 Garden Rd., Ste. 200, Riviera Beach, FL 33404 US

GROWTH PLANS/SPECIAL FEATURES:

AmeriPath is one of the nation's leading providers of anatomic pathology services, cancer diagnostic and health care information services to physicians, hospitals, national clinical laboratories and managed care organizations. The company provides services at 200 hospitals and more than 50 outpatient laboratories. AmeriPath's primary business is developing, staffing and operating clinical laboratories, which includes providing staffing, equipment, courier services and administrative services. In addition, AmeriPath's Dermpath Diagnostics division is entirely committed to dermatological diagnosis. The AmeriPath Insitute of Gastrointestinal Pathology and Digestive Disease specializaes in rendering specific diagnoses on gastrointestinal biopsy specimens and in providing second-opinion surgical pathology interpretations. The Center for Advanced Diagnostics, in Orlando, Florida, provides worldwide access to diagnostic technologies, pathology specialists, educational services and disease management programs. AmeriPath was acquired in March 2003 by the private New York-based equity firm of Welsh, Carson, Anderson & Stowe.

AmeriPath offers its employees comprehensive medical, dental and life insurance. In addition, the company offers tuition reimbursement and child and dependant care.

FINANCIALS:
Sales and profits are in thousands of dollars—add 000 to get the full amount. Year 2004 note: Complete fiscal 2004 results were not available for all companies at press time. For this company, year 2004 is for months.

2004 Sales: $ (months)   2004 Profits: $ (months)
2003 Sales: $485,000   2003 Profits: $23,400
2002 Sales: $478,800   2002 Profits: $44,600
2001 Sales: $418,700   2001 Profits: $23,300
2000 Sales: $330,100   2000 Profits: $13,100

Stock Ticker: Subsidiary
Employees: 2,685
Fiscal Year Ends: 12/31

SALARIES/BENEFITS:
Pension Plan: ESOP Stock Plan: Profit Sharing: Top Exec. Salary: $425,000   Bonus: $255,000
Savings Plan: Y   Stock Purch. Plan: Second Exec. Salary: $348,769 Bonus: $100,000

OTHER THOUGHTS:
Apparent Top Female Officers:
Hot Spot for Advancement for Women/Minorities:

LOCATIONS: ("Y" = Yes)
West:	Southwest:	Midwest:	Southeast:	Northeast:	International:
Y	Y	Y	Y	Y	

AMERISOURCEBERGEN CORP

www.amerisourcebergen.net

Industry Group Code: 422210 Ranks within this company's industry group: Sales: 3 Profits: 3

Insurance/HMO/PPO:	Drugs:		Equipment/Supplies:		Hospitals/Clinics:	Services:		Health Care:	
Insurance:	Manufacturer:		Manufacturer:	Y	Acute Care:	Diagnostics:		Home Health:	
Managed Care:	Distributor:	Y	Distributor:	Y	Sub-Acute Care:	Labs/Testing:		Long-Term Care:	
Utilization Mgmt.:	Specialty Pharm.:	Y	Leasing/Finance:		Outpatient Surgery:	Staffing:		Physical Therapy:	
Payment Proc.:	Vitamins/Nutri.:		Information Sys.:	Y	Phys. Rehab. Center:	Waste Disposal:		Phys. Practice Mgmt.:	
	Clinical Trials:				Psychiatric Clinics:	Specialty Services:	Y		

TYPES OF BUSINESS:
Distribution-Drugs
Alternate Care Distribution
Infusion Therapy Services
Online Ordering Systems
Mail-Order Pharmacy Services
Management and Consulting Services
Cosmetics Distribution
Contract Pharmaceutical Packaging

BRANDS/DIVISIONS/AFFILIATES:
PharMerica, Inc.
AmerisourceBergen Drug Corporation
AmerisourceBergen Specialty Group
American Health Packaging
Pharmacy Healthcare Solutions
AutoMed Technologies
iECHO
Rita Ann

CONTACTS: Note: Officers with more than one job title may be intentionally listed here more than once.
R. David Yost, CEO
Kurt J. Hilzinger, Pres.
Kurt J. Hilzinger, COO
Michael D. DiCandilo, Sr. VP/CFO
Thomas P. Connolly, Sr. VP-Mktg. & Sales
Jeanne Fisher, Sr. VP-Human Resources
Thomas H. Murphy, Sr. VP/CIO
William D. Sprague, Sr. VP/General Counsel/Corp. Sec.
David M. Senior, VP-Bus. Dev.
Michael Kilpatric, VP-Corp. Rel.
Michael Kilpatric, VP-Investor Rel.
J.F. Quinn, VP/Treas.
David W. Neu, Sr. VP-Retail Sales & Mktg.
Tim G. Guttman, VP/Corp. Controller
Steven H. Collis, Sr. VP/Pres., AmerisourceBergen Specialty Group
Terrance P. Hass, Sr. VP/Pres., AmerisourceBergen Drug Corp.
James R. Mellor, Chmn.
Len DeCandia, Sr. VP-Supply Chain Mgmt.

Phone: 610-727-7000 Fax: 610-727-3600
Toll-Free: 800-829-3132
Address: 1300 Morris Dr., Ste. 100, Chesterbrook, PA 19087-5594 US

GROWTH PLANS/SPECIAL FEATURES:
AmerisourceBergen Corp. is one of the nation's largest wholesale distributors of pharmaceutical products and services to health care providers and pharmaceutical manufacturers. The firm operates through two business segments: pharmaceutical distribution and PharMerica. The pharmaceutical distribution division includes AmerisourceBergen Drug Corporation (ADC) and AmerisourceBergen Specialty Group (ASG). ADC is the firm's wholesale drug distribution business, which also provides promotion, packaging, inventory management, pharmacy automation, bedside medication safety software and information services through its subsidiaries and affiliates (American Health Packaging, Anderson Packaging, AutoMed Technologies, Bridge Medical and Pharmacy Healthcare Solutions). ASG sells specialty pharmaceutical products to physicians, clinics, patients and other providers primarily in the oncology, nephrology, plasma and vaccine sectors. It also provides third-party logistics, reimbursement consulting services and physician education consulting. PharMerica is a national provider of institutional pharmacy products and services through a network of 125 pharmacies to patients in long-term care and alternate care settings. It also provides mail-order and online pharmacy services to chronically ill patients under workers' compensation programs, as well as providing pharmaceutical claims administration services for payors. In addition, AmerisourceBergen offers several specialty programs, including iECHO, a proprietary online ordering system; Family Pharmacy and Good Neighbor Pharmacy, which enable independent community pharmacies and small chain drug stores to compete more effectively; Pharmacy Healthcare Solutions, which provides hospital pharmacy consulting services; and Rita Ann, the firm's cosmetics distributor. The company acquired Imedex, Inc., an accredited provider of physician continuing medical education, and MedSelect, Inc., a provider of automated medication and supply dispensing cabinets. The firm launched the AutoMed Efficiency Pharmacy H750, the first radio frequency identification (RFID) enabled hospital pharmacy automation and barcoding system for all types of orders and dosage forms.

FINANCIALS: Sales and profits are in thousands of dollars—add 000 to get the full amount. Year 2004 note: Complete fiscal 2004 results were not available for all companies at press time. For this company, year 2004 is for 9 months.

2004 Sales: $39,790,280 (9 months)   2004 Profits: $376,401 (9 months)
2003 Sales: $49,657,300   2003 Profits: $441,200
2002 Sales: $45,235,000   2002 Profits: $345,000
2001 Sales: $16,191,400   2001 Profits: $125,100
2000 Sales: $11,645,000   2000 Profits: $99,000

Stock Ticker: ABC
Employees: 14,800
Fiscal Year Ends: 9/30

SALARIES/BENEFITS:
Pension Plan: ESOP Stock Plan: Profit Sharing: Top Exec. Salary: $960,350   Bonus: $995,000
Savings Plan: Y   Stock Purch. Plan: Y   Second Exec. Salary: $549,077   Bonus: $562,000

OTHER THOUGHTS:
Apparent Top Female Officers: 1
Hot Spot for Advancement for Women/Minorities:

LOCATIONS: ("Y" = Yes)
West:	Southwest:	Midwest:	Southeast:	Northeast:	International:
Y	Y	Y	Y	Y	

Note: Financial information, benefits and other data can change quickly and may vary from those stated here.

AMGEN INC

www.amgen.com

Industry Group Code: 325412 **Ranks within this company's industry group:** Sales: 14 Profits: 11

Insurance/HMO/PPO:	Drugs:	Equipment/Supplies:	Hospitals/Clinics:	Services:	Health Care:
Insurance:	Manufacturer: Y	Manufacturer:	Acute Care:	Diagnostics:	Home Health:
Managed Care:	Distributor:	Distributor:	Sub-Acute Care:	Labs/Testing:	Long-Term Care:
Utilization Mgmt.:	Specialty Pharm.:	Leasing/Finance:	Outpatient Surgery:	Staffing:	Physical Therapy:
Payment Proc.:	Vitamins/Nutri.:	Information Sys.:	Phys. Rehab. Center:	Waste Disposal:	Phys. Practice Mgmt.:
	Clinical Trials:		Psychiatric Clinics:	Specialty Services:	

TYPES OF BUSINESS:
Drugs-Diversified

BRANDS/DIVISIONS/AFFILIATES:
Neupogen
Epogen
Aranesp
Enbrel
Kineret
Tularik, Inc.
Immunex Corp.
Sensipar

CONTACTS:
Note: Officers with more than one job title may be intentionally listed here more than once.
Kevin W. Sharer, CEO
Kevin W. Sharer, Pres.
Richard D. Nanula, CFO/Exec. VP
Brian McNamee, Sr. VP-Human Resources
Roger Perlmutter, Exec. VP-Research & Dev.
Hassan Dayem, CIO/Sr. VP
Fabrizio Bonanni, Sr. VP-Mfg.
David J. Scott, General Counsel/Sec./Sr. VP
Dennis M. Fenton, Exec. VP-Oper.
Marie Kennedy, VP-Corp. Comm.
Beth C. Seidenberg, Sr. VP-Dev.
Joseph Miletich, Sr. VP-Research and Pre-clinical Dev.
Kevin W. Sharer, Chmn.
George Morrow, Exec. VP-Global Commercial Oper.

Phone: 805-447-1000 **Fax:** 805-447-1010
Toll-Free:
Address: One Amgen Center Dr., Thousand Oaks, CA 91320-1799 US

GROWTH PLANS/SPECIAL FEATURES:
Amgen, Inc. is a global biotechnology company that develops, manufactures and markets human therapeutics based on advanced cellular and molecular biology. Its products are used for the treatment of nephrology, oncology, inflammation, neurology and metabolic disorders. Amgen manufactures and markets a line of human therapeutic products including Neupogen, Epogen, Aranesp, Enbrel, Kineret and Neulasta and Sensipar. Neupogen and Neulasta selectively stimulate the growth of infection-fighting white blood cells (known as neutrophils). Kineret and Enbrel reduce the signs and symptoms of moderately to severely active rheumatoid arthritis. Epogen and Aranesp stimulate the production of red blood cells. In 2002, the firm acquired Immunex Corporation, a leading biotechnology company dedicated to developing immune system science to protect human health. The acquisition enhanced Amgen's strategic position within the biotechnology industry by strengthening and diversifying its product base and product pipeline in key therapeutic areas and discovery research capabilities in proteins and antibodies. Amgen's research and development efforts are focused on human therapeutics delivered in the form of proteins, monoclonal antibodies and small molecules in the areas of hematology, oncology, inflammation, metabolic and bone disorders and neuroscience. Sensipar is Amgen's first small molecule drug (chemically synthesized drugs that interact with molecular targets, including those within human cells). It is used to treat forms of hyperparathyroidsm and is licensed from NPS Pharmaceuticals Inc. In recent news, Amgen announced that it would buy Tularik, Inc. for $1.3 billion dollars. Tularik is focused on drug discovery related to cell signaling and the control of gene expression, and adds five clinical programs and 300 research scientists to Amgen's organization.

Employee benefits include dental and vision insurance, tuition reimbursement, relocation benefits, child care assistance, a fitness program and team-building events. Amgen's MBA Leadership Program offers career opportunities in finance and marketing for MBA students.

FINANCIALS:
Sales and profits are in thousands of dollars—add 000 to get the full amount. Year 2004 note: Complete fiscal 2004 results were not available for all companies at press time. For this company, year 2004 is for 9 months.

2004 Sales: $7,641,000 (9 months) 2004 Profits: $1,674,000 (9 months)
2003 Sales: $8,356,000 2003 Profits: $2,259,500
2002 Sales: $5,523,000 2002 Profits: $-1,392,000
2001 Sales: $3,763,000 2001 Profits: $1,119,700
2000 Sales: $3,629,400 2000 Profits: $1,138,500

Stock Ticker: AMGN
Employees: 12,900
Fiscal Year Ends: 12/31

SALARIES/BENEFITS:
Pension Plan: Y ESOP Stock Plan: Profit Sharing: Y Top Exec. Salary: $1,098,333 Bonus: $2,475,000
Savings Plan: Y Stock Purch. Plan: Y   Second Exec. Salary: $756,011 Bonus: $1,390,000

OTHER THOUGHTS:
Apparent Top Female Officers: 2
Hot Spot for Advancement for Women/Minorities:

LOCATIONS: ("Y" = Yes)
West	Southwest	Midwest	Southeast	Northeast	International
Y		Y	Y	Y	Y

Note: Financial information, benefits and other data can change quickly and may vary from those stated here.

AMSURG CORP

www.amsurg.com

Industry Group Code: 621490 Ranks within this company's industry group: Sales: 6 Profits: 5

Insurance/HMO/PPO:	Drugs:	Equipment/Supplies:	Hospitals/Clinics:		Services:		Health Care:	
Insurance:	Manufacturer:	Manufacturer:	Acute Care:		Diagnostics:		Home Health:	
Managed Care:	Distributor:	Distributor:	Sub-Acute Care:		Labs/Testing:		Long-Term Care:	
Utilization Mgmt.:	Specialty Pharm.:	Leasing/Finance:	Outpatient Surgery:	Y	Staffing:		Physical Therapy:	
Payment Proc.:	Vitamins/Nutri.:	Information Sys.:	Phys. Rehab. Center:		Waste Disposal:		Phys. Practice Mgmt.:	
	Clinical Trials:		Psychiatric Clinics:		Specialty Services:			

TYPES OF BUSINESS:
Practice-Based Ambulatory Surgery Centers

BRANDS/DIVISIONS/AFFILIATES:

CONTACTS:
Note: Officers with more than one job title may be intentionally listed here more than once.

Ken P. McDonald, CEO
Ken P. McDonald, Pres.
Claire M. Gulmi, Sr. VP/CFO
David L. Manning, Sr. VP-Dev.
Royce D. Harrell, Sr. VP-Corp. Services
Claire M. Gulmi, Corp. Sec.
Thomas G. Cigarran, CEO-American Healthways

Phone: 615-665-1283   Fax: 615-665-0755
Toll-Free: 800-945-2301
Address: 20 Burton Hills Blvd., Ste. 500, Nashville, TN 37215 US

GROWTH PLANS/SPECIAL FEATURES:

AmSurg is a leader in the development, acquisition and management of practice-based ambulatory surgery centers and specialty physician networks for partnership with other medical practices. The practice-based ambulatory surgery centers are licensed outpatient facilities equipped and staffed for a single medical specialty. The centers are usually located in or near a physician group practice, as the firm's objective is to form partnerships with physicians. The company has targeted ownership in centers that perform gastrointestinal endoscopy, ophthalmology, urology, orthopedics or otolaryngology procedures. These centers perform many high-volume, lower-risk procedures that are appropriate for the practice-based setting. The focus at each center on procedures in a single specialty results in these centers generally having significantly lower capital and operating costs than hospitals, which are designed to provide more intensive services in a broader array of surgical specialties. The types of procedures performed at each center depend on the specialty of the resident physicians. Those most often performed include laser eye surgery, carpal tunnel repair, colonoscopy and knee surgery. AmSurg provides services to its business partners that include coordinating with the architect, providing operation and procedure manuals, all transfer services, state licensing procedures and obtaining all necessary permits needed to operate the facility. The company has a significant stake in more than 100 centers across the U.S. In recent news, AmSurg was named to Forbes' 200 Best Small Companies list for the fifth consecutive year.

FINANCIALS:
Sales and profits are in thousands of dollars—add 000 to get the full amount. Year 2004 note: Complete fiscal 2004 results were not available for all companies at press time. For this company, year 2004 is for 9 months.

2004 Sales: $245,988 (9 months)	2004 Profits: $31,020 (9 months)	
2003 Sales: $301,408	2003 Profits: $30,126	Stock Ticker: AMSG
2002 Sales: $251,500	2002 Profits: $24,000	Employees: 1,110
2001 Sales: $202,300	2001 Profits: $14,900	Fiscal Year Ends: 12/31
2000 Sales: $143,300	2000 Profits: $9,100	

SALARIES/BENEFITS:
Pension Plan:	ESOP Stock Plan:	Profit Sharing:	Top Exec. Salary: $400,000	Bonus: $149,000
Savings Plan: Y	Stock Purch. Plan:		Second Exec. Salary: $250,000	Bonus: $53,625

OTHER THOUGHTS:
Apparent Top Female Officers: 1
Hot Spot for Advancement for Women/Minorities:

LOCATIONS: ("Y" = Yes)
West:	Southwest:	Midwest:	Southeast:	Northeast:	International:
Y	Y	Y	Y	Y	

ANALOGIC CORP

www.analogic.com

Industry Group Code: 339113 Ranks within this company's industry group: Sales: 42 Profits: 33

Insurance/HMO/PPO:	Drugs:	Equipment/Supplies:	Hospitals/Clinics:	Services:	Health Care:
Insurance:	Manufacturer:	Manufacturer: Y	Acute Care:	Diagnostics:	Home Health:
Managed Care:	Distributor:	Distributor:	Sub-Acute Care:	Labs/Testing:	Long-Term Care:
Utilization Mgmt.:	Specialty Pharm.:	Leasing/Finance:	Outpatient Surgery:	Staffing:	Physical Therapy:
Payment Proc.:	Vitamins/Nutri.:	Information Sys.:	Phys. Rehab. Center:	Waste Disposal:	Phys. Practice Mgmt.:
	Clinical Trials:		Psychiatric Clinics:	Specialty Services:	

TYPES OF BUSINESS:
Equipment-Medical Image Processing
Signal Processing Equipment
Patient Monitoring Equipment
Computed Tomography Imaging Systems
Portable, Multi-Functional Patient Monitors
Explosive Detection Security Systems

BRANDS/DIVISIONS/AFFILIATES:
Anexa
Anrad
B-K Medical A/S
Camtronics Medical Systems
Sound Technology
SKY Computers
EXACT

CONTACTS:
Note: Officers with more than one job title may be intentionally listed here more than once.
John W. Wood, Jr., CEO
John W. Wood, Jr., Pres.
John J. Millerick, Sr. VP/CFO
Julian Soshnick, VP/General Counsel/Corp. Sec.
Paul M. Roberts, Dir.-Corp. Comm.
John J. Millerick, Treas.
John A. Torello, Chmn.

Phone: 978-977-3000 Fax: 978-977-6809
Toll-Free:
Address: 8 Centennial Dr., Peabody, MA 01960 US

GROWTH PLANS/SPECIAL FEATURES:

Analogic Corporation designs, manufactures and sells advanced health and security systems and subsystems to be utilized in medical, industrial and scientific applications. Analogic's divisions specialize in computed tomography, digital radiography systems, life care systems, medical imaging components, test and measurement, ultrasound systems and customer service. Its subsidiaries include Anexa, Anrad, B-K Medical, Camtronics, SKY Computers and Sound Technology. The company is a leader in precision analog-to-digital and digital-to-analog signals, such as those representing temperature, pressure, voltage, weight, velocity, ultrasound and x-ray intensity into the numeric form required by data processing equipment. Analogic's medical imaging data acquisition systems and related computing equipment are incorporated into computer assisted tomography scanners that generate images of the internal anatomy to diagnose medical conditions. The company also manufactures a lightweight, portable, multi-functional, custom patient monitor instrument, used in a variety of hospital settings, that acquires, calculates and displays combinations of the five most common vital sign parameters: ECG, respiration, temperature, NIBP and SpO2. Analogic also manufactures the EXACT system, an advanced computed tomography imaging system capable of providing data for full 3-D images of every object in a package, parcel or bag. Additionally, the company entered into an agreement with Sanders Design International to develop, manufacture and deploy an aircraft infrared countermeasures system for commercial airlines. Analogic also formed a strategic marketing agreement with Lockheed Martin to market threat detection products.

Employee benefits include medical and dental insurance and tuition reimbursement.

FINANCIALS:
Sales and profits are in thousands of dollars—add 000 to get the full amount. Year 2004 note: Complete fiscal 2004 results were not available for all companies at press time. For this company, year 2004 is for 12 months.

2004 Sales: $370,766 (12 months)	2004 Profits: $11,630 (12 months)	Stock Ticker: ALOGE
2003 Sales: $471,500	2003 Profits: $49,500	Employees: 1,800
2002 Sales: $313,600	2002 Profits: $3,300	Fiscal Year Ends: 7/31
2001 Sales: $360,600	2001 Profits: $15,200	
2000 Sales: $297,619	2000 Profits: $14,108	

SALARIES/BENEFITS:

Pension Plan:	ESOP Stock Plan:	Profit Sharing:	Top Exec. Salary: $366,300	Bonus: $50,000
Savings Plan: Y	Stock Purch. Plan: Y		Second Exec. Salary: $215,100	Bonus: $25,000

OTHER THOUGHTS:
Apparent Top Female Officers:
Hot Spot for Advancement for Women/Minorities:

LOCATIONS: ("Y" = Yes)

West:	Southwest:	Midwest: Y	Southeast:	Northeast: Y	International: Y

ANDRX CORP

www.andrx.com

Industry Group Code: 325416 Ranks within this company's industry group: Sales: 4 Profits: 3

Insurance/HMO/PPO:	Drugs:		Equipment/Supplies:	Hospitals/Clinics:	Services:	Health Care:
Insurance: Managed Care: Utilization Mgmt.: Payment Proc.:	Manufacturer: Distributor: Specialty Pharm.: Vitamins/Nutri.: Clinical Trials:	Y	Manufacturer: Distributor: Leasing/Finance: Information Sys.:	Acute Care: Sub-Acute Care: Outpatient Surgery: Phys. Rehab. Center: Psychiatric Clinics:	Diagnostics: Labs/Testing: Staffing: Waste Disposal: Specialty Services:	Home Health: Long-Term Care: Physical Therapy: Phys. Practice Mgmt.:

TYPES OF BUSINESS:
Drugs-Controlled Release
Drug Delivery Technologies

BRANDS/DIVISIONS/AFFILIATES:
Andrx Laboratories
Andrx Pharmaceuticals
Anda, Inc.
ANCIRC Pharmaceuticals
Altoprev
Entex LA
Fortamet

CONTACTS:
Note: Officers with more than one job title may be intentionally listed here more than once.

Thomas P. Rice, CEO
Angelo C. Malahias, Pres.
John M. Hanson, CFO/Sr. VP
Ian J. Watkins, Sr. VP-Human Resources
Thomas R. Giordano, CIO/Sr. VP
Scott Lodin, General Counsel/Exec. VP
Daniel H. Movens, Pres., Anda, Inc.
Lawrence J. Rosenthal, Pres., Andrx Pharmaceuticals, Inc.
Sylvia S. McBrinn, Exec. VP-Andrx Laboratories, Inc.
Elliot F. Hahn, Chmn.

Phone: 954-584-0300 Fax:
Toll-Free:
Address: 4955 Orange Dr., Davie, FL 33314 US

GROWTH PLANS/SPECIAL FEATURES:

Andrx Corporation formulates and commercializes controlled-release oral pharmaceuticals using proprietary drug delivery technologies. Andrx also markets and distributes generic drugs manufactured by third parties. The company has 96 patents issued, allowed or pending in the U.S. and 127 internationally. Andrx believes that its technologies are flexible and can be modified to apply to a variety of pharmaceutical products. Through Andrx Pharmaceuticals and Andrx Laboratories, the company is applying proprietary drug delivery technologies and formulation skills, either directly or through collaborative arrangements, to the development of generic versions of select brand-name pharmaceuticals. Among the drugs Andrx currently manufactures and sells are bioequivalent versions of Cardizem CD, Dilacor XR, Ventolin, Glucophage, K-Dur and Naprelan. The company also manufactures and sells a bioequivalent version of Oruvail, which was developed through Andrx's ANCIRC Pharmaceuticals joint venture with Watson and is used for the treatment of patients with rheumatoid arthritis and osteoarthritis. Through its brand program, Andrx sells and markets internally developed products including Altoprev, Entex LA and Fortamet. Anda, a unit of the company, purchases products directly from manufactures and wholesalers and markets them through its telemarketing staff and sales representatives. In 2003, the company signed a multi-year agreement with L. Perrigo Company to manufacture bioequivalent versions of Claritin-D 12 Hour, Claritin Reditabs and Claritin-D 24 Hour, which Perrigo markets as over-the-counter products. Recently, Andx has received exclusive U.S. marketing rights from Genpharm, Inc. to market bioequivalent versions of Paxil.
Employees receive health insurance, disability benefits, educational assistance and credit union membership.

FINANCIALS:
Sales and profits are in thousands of dollars—add 000 to get the full amount. Year 2004 note: Complete fiscal 2004 results were not available for all companies at press time. For this company, year 2004 is for 9 months.

2004 Sales: $855,045 (9 months)   2004 Profits: $44,907 (9 months)
2003 Sales: $1,046,300   2003 Profits: $48,200
2002 Sales: $771,000   2002 Profits: $-91,800
2001 Sales: $749,000   2001 Profits: $37,500
2000 Sales: $520,000   2000 Profits: $58,500

Stock Ticker: ADRX
Employees: 2,100
Fiscal Year Ends: 12/31

SALARIES/BENEFITS:
Pension Plan: ESOP Stock Plan: Profit Sharing: Top Exec. Salary: $624,900   Bonus: $218,700
Savings Plan: Y   Stock Purch. Plan: Y   Second Exec. Salary: $418,500   Bonus: $104,600

OTHER THOUGHTS:
Apparent Top Female Officers: 1
Hot Spot for Advancement for Women/Minorities

LOCATIONS: ("Y" = Yes)

West:	Southwest:	Midwest:	Southeast:	Northeast:	International:
		Y	Y	Y	

ANSELL LIMITED COMPANY

www.ansell.com

Industry Group Code: 339113   **Ranks within this company's industry group:** Sales: 30   Profits: 40

Insurance/HMO/PPO:	Drugs:	Equipment/Supplies:		Hospitals/Clinics:		Services:		Health Care:	
Insurance:	Manufacturer:	Manufacturer:	Y	Acute Care:		Diagnostics:		Home Health:	
Managed Care:	Distributor:	Distributor:	Y	Sub-Acute Care:		Labs/Testing:		Long-Term Care:	
Utilization Mgmt.:	Specialty Pharm.:	Leasing/Finance:		Outpatient Surgery:		Staffing:		Physical Therapy:	
Payment Proc.:	Vitamins/Nutri.:	Information Sys.:		Phys. Rehab. Center:		Waste Disposal:		Phys. Practice Mgmt.:	
	Clinical Trials:			Psychiatric Clinics:		Specialty Services:			

TYPES OF BUSINESS:
Latex Gloves
Condoms
Protective Clothing
Tires

BRANDS/DIVISIONS/AFFILIATES:
Pacific Dunlop Limited
Ansell
Ansell Perry
Gammex
NuTex
LifeStyles
AnsellCares
South Pacific Tyres

CONTACTS:
Note: Officers with more than one job title may be intentionally listed here more than once.

Douglas D. Tough, CEO/Managing Dir.
Rustom Jilla, CFO
Phil Corke, Sr. VP-Human Resources
Mike Zedalis, Sr. VP-Science
Peter Soszyn, Sr. VP/CIO
Mike Zedalis, Sr. VP-Tech.
Rainer Wolf, Head-Global Mfg.
Bill Reilly, Sr. VP/General Counsel
David Graham, General Mgr.-Finance & Acct.
Bill Reed, Sr. VP/Regional Dir.-Americas
Neil O'Donnell, Sr. VP/Regional Dir.-Asia Pacific
Werner Heintz, Sr. VP/Regional Dir.-Europe
Rob Bartlett, General Mgr./Corp. Sec.
Scott Papier, VP-Global Supply & Logistics

Phone: 61-3-9270-7270   **Fax:** 61-3-9270-7300
Toll-Free:
Address: 678 Victoria St., Level 3, Richmond, Victoria 3121 Australia

GROWTH PLANS/SPECIAL FEATURES:

Ansell Limited Company, formerly Pacific Dunlop Limited, is a leading global manufacturer of synthetic and natural latex gloves, condoms and protective wear through 18 factories in seven countries. The company's professional health care division is a leading global manufacturer of surgical and medical examination gloves under the umbrella brand names Ansell and Ansell Perry. It also manufactures other latex products, such as tubing and wall brackets, under product-specific brand names, including Gammex, Conform, Encore, NuTex, MicrOptic, X-AM, Synsation, Dermaclean and Nitratouch. The company's consumer health care division manufactures and distributes a variety of condom lines around the world under the LifeStyles, Mates, Manix, Contempo and Kama Sutra brand names, including condoms with flavors, colors, spermicide, studded and ribbed features. It also makes and distributes Medi-Touch gloves and personal lubricants. Ansell's occupational division manufactures and markets a wide range of industrial and consumer gloves, as well as protective clothing (rainwear, aprons, sleeves and vests). Its products include critical environment gloves, which are used by companies in the semiconductor, electronics and other high-technology markets to both protect workers from the manufacturing process, as well as protect the manufactured product from contamination. The division also offers a full line of gloves developed for the food-processing and foodservice industry, which includes the packing, processing, preparation and serving of various food products. However, its core market is the automotive and durable-goods industry, which uses chemical-resistant, cut-resistant and special-purpose gloves. The company's AnsellCares program is a global, multifaceted research and education program directed by an independent scientific advisory board that addresses latex allergies and barrier protection issues. Approximately 56% of Ansell's total sales come from North America. The company also owns a major interest in South Pacific Tyres, which manufactures and distributes Dunlop and Goodyear tires for passenger vehicles and trucks and for agricultural and industrial purposes in Australia and New Zealand.

FINANCIALS:
Sales and profits are in thousands of dollars—add 000 to get the full amount. Year 2004 note: Complete fiscal 2004 results were not available for all companies at press time. For this company, year 2004 is for months.

2004 Sales: $ (months)	2004 Profits: $ (months)	**Stock Ticker:** Foreign
2003 Sales: $862,961	2003 Profits: $37,291	**Employees:** 12,013
2002 Sales: $797,185	2002 Profits: $-103,495	**Fiscal Year Ends:** 6/30
2001 Sales: $	2001 Profits: $	
2000 Sales: $	2000 Profits: $	

SALARIES/BENEFITS:
Pension Plan:	ESOP Stock Plan:	Profit Sharing:	Top Exec. Salary: $	Bonus: $
Savings Plan:	Stock Purch. Plan:		Second Exec. Salary: $	Bonus: $

OTHER THOUGHTS:
Apparent Top Female Officers:
Hot Spot for Advancement for Women/Minorities:

LOCATIONS: ("Y" = Yes)
West:	Southwest:	Midwest:	Southeast:	Northeast:	International:
	Y	Y		Y	Y

ANTHEM INC

www.anthem-inc.com

Industry Group Code: 524114 Ranks within this company's industry group: Sales: 6 Profits: 4

Insurance/HMO/PPO:		Drugs:		Equipment/Supplies:		Hospitals/Clinics:		Services:		Health Care:	
Insurance:	Y	Manufacturer:		Manufacturer:		Acute Care:		Diagnostics:		Home Health:	
Managed Care:	Y	Distributor:		Distributor:		Sub-Acute Care:		Labs/Testing:		Long-Term Care:	
Utilization Mgmt.:		Specialty Pharm.:		Leasing/Finance:		Outpatient Surgery:		Staffing:		Physical Therapy:	
Payment Proc.:		Vitamins/Nutri.:		Information Sys.:		Phys. Rehab. Center:		Waste Disposal:		Phys. Practice Mgmt.:	
		Clinical Trials:				Psychiatric Clinics:		Specialty Services:	Y		

TYPES OF BUSINESS:
Underwriting-Health & Medical Insurance
Medicare HMO
Medicaid HMO
Prescription Benefits Management
Managed Care Services
Life Insurance

BRANDS/DIVISIONS/AFFILIATES:
WellPoint Health Networks, Inc.

CONTACTS: Note: Officers with more than one job title may be intentionally listed here more than once.
Larry C. Glasscock, CEO
Larry C. Glasscock, Pres.
Michael L. Smith, Exec. VP/CFO
Mark Boxer, Exec. VP/CIO
David R. Frick, Exec. VP/Chief Admin. Officer
David R. Frick, Chief Legal Officer
Mark Boxer, Chief Strategy & Bus. Dev. Officer
Tami Durle, Investor Rel.
Samuel R. Nussbaum, Exec. VP/Chief Medical Officer
Michael L. Smith, Pres.-Anthem Nat'l Accounts
Thomas R. Byrd, Pres.-Anthem Specialty Bus.
Larry C. Glasscock, Chmn.

Phone: 317-488-6000	Fax: 317-488-6028
Toll-Free:	
Address: 120 Monument Cir., Indianapolis, IN 46204 US	

GROWTH PLANS/SPECIAL FEATURES:

Anthem, Inc. is a leading health care benefits company, providing benefits plans and management services to more than 11.9 million members, primarily in Indiana, Kentucky, Ohio, Connecticut, New Hampshire, Maine, Colorado, Nevada and Virginia. The company markets its services using the Blue Cross and Blue Shield names. Its product portfolio includes a mix of preferred provider organizations (PPOs), health maintenance organizations (HMOs) and point-of-service plans, as well as traditional indemnity products. Anthem also offers administrative and managed care services and partially insured products for employer self-funded plans, including claims processing, stop loss insurance, actuarial services, provider network access and medical cost management. In addition, the company offers specialty products, such as group life and disability insurance benefits, pharmacy benefit management and dental, vision and behavioral health benefits services. Anthem's customers are large and small employers, federal employees, individuals and Medicare supplement customers. In July 2004, the company received approval from the California Department of Managed Health Care to complete its acquisition of WellPoint Health Networks, Inc. The merger, which will combine the nation's two largest Blue Cross providers, creating a firm that will cover 26 million people in 13 states, is still awaiting approval by the California Department of Insurance.

Anthem offers its employees medical, dental and vision coverage, a wellness program, education assistance, flexible work schedules and on-site cafeterias and fitness centers.

FINANCIALS: Sales and profits are in thousands of dollars—add 000 to get the full amount. Year 2004 note: Complete fiscal 2004 results were not available for all companies at press time. For this company, year 2004 is for 9 months.

2004 Sales: $12,577,500 (9 months)	2004 Profits: $775,600 (9 months)	
2003 Sales: $16,771,400	2003 Profits: $774,300	Stock Ticker: ATH
2002 Sales: $13,282,000	2002 Profits: $549,000	Employees: 20,130
2001 Sales: $10,445,000	2001 Profits: $342,000	Fiscal Year Ends: 12/31
2000 Sales: $8,771,000	2000 Profits: $226,000	

SALARIES/BENEFITS:

Pension Plan: Y	ESOP Stock Plan:	Profit Sharing:	Top Exec. Salary: $1,040,000	Bonus: $2,311,845
Savings Plan: Y	Stock Purch. Plan: Y		Second Exec. Salary: $500,000	Bonus: $777,720

OTHER THOUGHTS:
Apparent Top Female Officers: 1
Hot Spot for Advancement for Women/Minorities:

LOCATIONS: ("Y" = Yes)

West:	Southwest:	Midwest:	Southeast:	Northeast:	International:
Y	Y	Y	Y	Y	

AON CORPORATION

www.aon.com

Industry Group Code: 524210 Ranks within this company's industry group: Sales: 2 Profits: 2

Insurance/HMO/PPO:	Drugs:	Equipment/Supplies:	Hospitals/Clinics:	Services:	Health Care:
Insurance: Y	Manufacturer:	Manufacturer:	Acute Care:	Diagnostics:	Home Health:
Managed Care:	Distributor:	Distributor:	Sub-Acute Care:	Labs/Testing:	Long-Term Care:
Utilization Mgmt.:	Specialty Pharm.:	Leasing/Finance:	Outpatient Surgery:	Staffing:	Physical Therapy:
Payment Proc.:	Vitamins/Nutri.:	Information Sys.:	Phys. Rehab. Center:	Waste Disposal:	Phys. Practice Mgmt.:
	Clinical Trials:		Psychiatric Clinics:	Specialty Services: Y	

TYPES OF BUSINESS:
Insurance Brokerage and Consulting
Consumer Insurance Underwriting
Risk Management
Online Business Services
Outsourcing

BRANDS/DIVISIONS/AFFILIATES:
AonLine
Aon Market Exhange
Aon Risk Monitor
Aon Re Worldwide

CONTACTS:
Note: Officers with more than one job title may be intentionally listed here more than once.
Patrick G. Ryan, CEO
Michael D. O'Halleran, Pres.
Michael D. O'Halleran, COO
David P. Bolger, Exec. VP/CFO
Jeremy G.O. Farmer, Sr. VP-Human Resources
D. Cameron Findlay, Exec. VP/General Counsel
Craig Streem, VP-Investor Rel.
Diane M. Aigotti, Treas.
Michael A. Conway, Sr. VP/Sr. Investment Officer
Kevann M. Cooke, VP/Corp. Sec.
Vaughn Hooks, VP-Taxes
Carl J. Bleecher, VP-Internal Audit
Patrick G. Ryan, Chmn.

Phone: 312-381-1000 **Fax:** 312-381-6032
Toll-Free:
Address: 200 E. Randolph St., Chicago, IL 60601 US

GROWTH PLANS/SPECIAL FEATURES:

Aon Corporation, one of the world's largest insurance brokerages, is a holding company engaged in three major business segments: commercial brokerage, consulting services and consumer insurance underwriting. Other services include risk management, human capital consulting, outsourcing and warranty services. The firm offers many of its services online, including AonLine, Aon Market Exchange and Aon Risk Monitor. The human capital consulting services segment provides solutions that help clients with employee benefits, compensation, management consulting and human resources outsourcing. Aon's subsidiary Aon Re Worldwide provides services in the design, structure and implementation of its risk-transfer (reinsurance) programs. Aon offers companies help in addressing the risks they take in conducting business across geographic, cultural and legal lines. The firm also offers terrorism and natural disaster risk consultation. It analyzes its clients' businesses through a variety of risk management processes such as enterprise risk management. Aon's brokerage operations consist of retail and wholesale insurance for groups and businesses, while its insurance underwriting segment offers supplementary health, accident and life insurance and extended warranties for consumer goods. The firm operates in more than 120 countries around the world through more than 600 offices.

Aon and its subsidiaries provide employees with medical, vision and dental coverage, an employee assistance program and matching gifts for charitable contributions.

FINANCIALS:
Sales and profits are in thousands of dollars—add 000 to get the full amount. Year 2004 note: Complete fiscal 2004 results were not available for all companies at press time. For this company, year 2004 is for 9 months.

2004 Sales: $7,510,000 (9 months)	2004 Profits: $465,000 (9 months)	**Stock Ticker:** AOC
2003 Sales: $9,810,000	2003 Profits: $628,000	Employees: 54,000
2002 Sales: $8,822,000	2002 Profits: $466,000	Fiscal Year Ends: 12/31
2001 Sales: $7,676,000	2001 Profits: $203,000	
2000 Sales: $7,375,000	2000 Profits: $474,000	

SALARIES/BENEFITS:
Pension Plan: Y   ESOP Stock Plan: Profit Sharing: Top Exec. Salary: $1,125,000   Bonus: $1,250,000
Savings Plan: Stock Purch. Plan: Second Exec. Salary: $1,000,000   Bonus: $900,000

OTHER THOUGHTS:
Apparent Top Female Officers: 2
Hot Spot for Advancement for Women/Minorities:

LOCATIONS: ("Y" = Yes)
West:	Southwest:	Midwest:	Southeast:	Northeast:	International:
Y	Y	Y	Y	Y	Y

APOGENT TECHNOLOGIES INC

www.apogent.com

Industry Group Code: 339113   Ranks within this company's industry group: Sales: 23   Profits: 126

Insurance/HMO/PPO:	Drugs:	Equipment/Supplies:		Hospitals/Clinics:	Services:	Health Care:
Insurance: Managed Care: Utilization Mgmt.: Payment Proc.:	Manufacturer: Distributor: Specialty Pharm.: Vitamins/Nutri.: Clinical Trials:	Manufacturer: Distributor: Leasing/Finance: Information Sys.:	Y	Acute Care: Sub-Acute Care: Outpatient Surgery: Phys. Rehab. Center: Psychiatric Clinics:	Diagnostics: Labs/Testing: Staffing: Waste Disposal: Specialty Services:	Home Health: Long-Term Care: Physical Therapy: Phys. Practice Mgmt.:

TYPES OF BUSINESS:
Equipment-Laboratory
Diagnostic Products
Life Science Products

BRANDS/DIVISIONS/AFFILIATES:
Fisher Scientific International, Inc.
Microgenics Corp.
Capitol Vial, Inc.
Barnstead International
Genevac, Ltd.
Chromacol, Ltd.
Separation Technology, Inc.
Lab-Line Instruments, Inc.

CONTACTS:
Note: Officers with more than one job title may be intentionally listed here more than once.
Frank H. Jellinek, Jr., CEO
Frank H. Jellinek, Jr., Pres.
Jan Kuhlmann, VP-Int'l Sales & Mktg.

Phone: 603-433-6131   Fax: 603-431-0860
Toll-Free: 800-327-9970
Address: 30 Penhallow St., Portsmouth, NH 03801 US

GROWTH PLANS/SPECIAL FEATURES:
Apogent Technologies, Inc., a wholly-owned subsidiary of Fisher Scientific International, Inc., designs, manufactures and markets laboratory, diagnostic and life science products for health care diagnostics and scientific research. Over 80% of its products are consumable. The company operates through two business groups, clinical and research, each of which is organized based on the market it serves. The firm markets its products to distributors, pharmaceutical and biotechnology companies, original equipment manufacturers and clinical, research and industrial laboratories mostly in the U.S., Europe and Japan. The clinical group offers products geared toward diagnostic testing and screening services such as specimen collection, drug testing and pregnancy testing. Products include microscope slides, cover glass, glass tubes, diagnostic test kits, stains and reagents, culture media and other products used in detecting causes of various diseases and conditions. The research group produces reusable labware, consumables and high-end instrumentation for life science and research applications. These products are used in areas such as combinatorial chemistry, chromatography, laboratory safety and packaging applications. Products include reusable and disposable plastic and glass products, products for critical packaging applications, environmental and safety containers and instruments used in drug discovery. In addition, the segment provides a broad range of laboratory equipment for research, industrial, clinical and general laboratory applications. Products include hot plates, stirrers and shakers, systems for producing ultra-pure water, bottle top dispensers, furnaces and fluorometers and solvent evaporation technology.

FINANCIALS:
Sales and profits are in thousands of dollars—add 000 to get the full amount. Year 2004 note: Complete fiscal 2004 results were not available for all companies at press time. For this company, year 2004 is for 9 months.

2004 Sales: $884,290 (9 months)	2004 Profits: $96,949 (9 months)	
2003 Sales: $1,097,487	2003 Profits: $-11,746	Stock Ticker: Subsidiary
2002 Sales: $1,074,600	2002 Profits: $121,100	Employees: 7,000
2001 Sales: $984,500	2001 Profits: $96,000	Fiscal Year Ends: 9/30
2000 Sales: $863,600	2000 Profits: $128,300	

SALARIES/BENEFITS:
Pension Plan: Y	ESOP Stock Plan:	Profit Sharing:	Top Exec. Salary: $751,384	Bonus: $126,042
Savings Plan: Y	Stock Purch. Plan: Y		Second Exec. Salary: $348,010	Bonus: $800,000

OTHER THOUGHTS:
Apparent Top Female Officers: 1
Hot Spot for Advancement for Women/Minorities:

LOCATIONS: ("Y" = Yes)
West:	Southwest:	Midwest:	Southeast:	Northeast:	International:
Y	Y	Y	Y	Y	Y

APPLERA CORPORATION

www.applera.com

Industry Group Code: 339113   Ranks within this company's industry group: Sales: 16   Profits: 19

Insurance/HMO/PPO:	Drugs:	Equipment/Supplies:		Hospitals/Clinics:		Services:		Health Care:	
Insurance:	Manufacturer:	Manufacturer:	Y	Acute Care:		Diagnostics:		Home Health:	
Managed Care:	Distributor:	Distributor:		Sub-Acute Care:		Labs/Testing:		Long-Term Care:	
Utilization Mgmt.:	Specialty Pharm.:	Leasing/Finance:		Outpatient Surgery:		Staffing:		Physical Therapy:	
Payment Proc.:	Vitamins/Nutri.:	Information Sys.:	Y	Phys. Rehab. Center:		Waste Disposal:		Phys. Practice Mgmt.:	
	Clinical Trials:			Psychiatric Clinics:		Specialty Services:	Y		

TYPES OF BUSINESS:
Equipment-Life Sciences and Genomics
Genetic Database Management
Proteomics
Medical Software
Microbial Populations
DNA Sequencing
Organic Synthesis
High-Throughput Screening

BRANDS/DIVISIONS/AFFILIATES:
Applied Biosystems
Celera Genomics
Celera Diagnostics
ViroSeq

CONTACTS:
Note: Officers with more than one job title may be intentionally listed here more than once.
Tony L. White, CEO
Tony L. White, Pres.
Dennis L. Winger, Sr. VP/CFO
Barbara J. Kerr, VP-Human Resources
William B. Sawch, Sr. VP/General Counsel
Michael W. Hunkapiller, Sr. VP/Pres., Applied Biosystems
Catherine M. Burzik, Exec. VP-Applied Biosystems
Kathy P. Ordonez, Pres., Celera Genomics and Celera Diagnostics
Robert F.G. Booth, Chief Scientific Officer, Celera Genomics
Tony L. White, Chmn.

Phone: 203-840-2000   Fax: 203-840-2312
Toll-Free: 800-761-5381
Address: 301 Merritt 7, Norwalk, CT 06856-5435 US

GROWTH PLANS/SPECIAL FEATURES:

Applera Corporation provides technology and information solutions that help biologists understand and use the power of life. Applera operates three divisions, Applied Biosystems, Celera Genomics and Celera Diagnostics, a separate joint venture between the two. Applied Biosystems develops, manufactures, sells and services instrument systems and associated consumable products for life science research and related applications. Its products find use in applications including the synthesis, amplification, purification, isolation, analysis and sequencing of nucleic acids, proteins and other biological molecules. Celera Genomics operates online information databases and therapeutic discovery research projects. Pharmaceutical, biotechnology and academic customers use Celera's information, along with the firm's customized information technology solutions, to facilitate life science, pharmaceutical and diagnostic research and development. Celera Genomics intends to identify drug targets and diagnostic markers and to discover and develop novel therapeutic candidates, both in internal programs and through collaborations. Celera Diagnostics focuses on discovering, developing and commercializing diagnostic tests for diagnosing and treating disease. Its ViroSeq HIV-1 Genotyping system tests human blood samples for specific mutations in the HIV-1 genome that correlate with drug resistance. In recent news Celera Genomics began collaborating with Seattle Genetics, Inc. in order to discover and develop antibody-based therapies for cancer.

Applera offers its workforce an educational assistance plan, travel accident insurance, basic and supplemental life insurance and an adoption assistance program.

FINANCIALS:
Sales and profits are in thousands of dollars—add 000 to get the full amount. Year 2004 note: Complete fiscal 2004 results were not available for all companies at press time. For this company, year 2004 is for months.

2004 Sales: $ (months)   2004 Profits: $ (months)
2003 Sales: $1,777,232   2003 Profits: $118,480
2002 Sales: $1,701,218   2002 Profits: $-40,581
2001 Sales: $1,644,100   2001 Profits: $27,200
2000 Sales: $1,371,000   2000 Profits: $95,500

Stock Ticker: Private
Employees: 5,360
Fiscal Year Ends: 6/30

SALARIES/BENEFITS:
Pension Plan: ESOP Stock Plan: Profit Sharing: Top Exec. Salary: $1,000,000   Bonus: $1,300,000
Savings Plan: Y   Stock Purch. Plan: Y   Second Exec. Salary: $560,504   Bonus: $517,104

OTHER THOUGHTS:
Apparent Top Female Officers: 4
Hot Spot for Advancement for Women/Minorities: Y

LOCATIONS: ("Y" = Yes)
West:	Southwest:	Midwest:	Southeast:	Northeast:	International:
Y	Y			Y	Y

APPLIED BIOSYSTEMS GROUP   www.appliedbiosystems.com

Industry Group Code: 541710   Ranks within this company's industry group: Sales: 2   Profits: 2

Insurance/HMO/PPO:	Drugs:	Equipment/Supplies:		Hospitals/Clinics:	Services:		Health Care:	
Insurance:	Manufacturer:	Manufacturer:	Y	Acute Care:	Diagnostics:		Home Health:	
Managed Care:	Distributor:	Distributor:		Sub-Acute Care:	Labs/Testing:		Long-Term Care:	
Utilization Mgmt.:	Specialty Pharm.:	Leasing/Finance:		Outpatient Surgery:	Staffing:		Physical Therapy:	
Payment Proc.:	Vitamins/Nutri.:	Information Sys.:	Y	Phys. Rehab. Center:	Waste Disposal:		Phys. Practice Mgmt.:	
	Clinical Trials:			Psychiatric Clinics:	Specialty Services:	Y		

TYPES OF BUSINESS:
Research & Development Services
Instrument-Based Systems
Life Science Software

BRANDS/DIVISIONS/AFFILIATES:
Applera Corp.
Celera Diagnostics
ABI PRISM Genetic Analyzer
TaqMan
Voyager Biospectrometry Workstation
QSTAR
Q TRAP

CONTACTS: Note: Officers with more than one job title may be intentionally listed here more than once.
Catherine M. Burzik, Pres.
Catherine M. Burzik, COO
Scott Jenkins, VP-Mktg.
Dennis A. Gilbert, VP-Advanced Research
Dennis A. Gilbert, VP-Tech.
Robert P. Ragusa, Sr. VP-Global Oper.
Susan L. Koppy, VP-Strategy & Planning
Sandeep Nayyar, VP-Finance
Paul D. Grossman, VP-Intellectual Property
Michael G. Schneider, Pres.-Service
Laura Lauman, Pres.-Proteomics & Small-Molecule
Deborah A. Smeltzer, VP/Mgr.-Genetic Analysis Bus.
Masahide Habu, Pres., Applied Biosystems Japan, Ltd.

Phone: 650-638-5800   Fax: 650-638-5884
Toll-Free: 800-327-3002
Address: 850 Lincoln Centre Dr., Foster City, CA 94404 US

GROWTH PLANS/SPECIAL FEATURES:

Applied Biosystems Group, a subsidiary of Applera Corp., is involved in the development, manufacture, sale and service of instrument-based systems, reagents and software for life science and related applications. Products developed by Applied Biosystems facilitate the synthesis, amplification, purification, isolation, analysis and sequencing of nucleic acids, proteins and other biological molecules. These are used in basic human disease research and genetic analysis performed by universities, government agencies and other nonprofit organizations; pharmaceutical drug discovery, development and manufacturing; human identification; agriculture; biosecurity; and food and environmental testing. Products include the ABI PRISM Genetic Analyzer, TaqMan gene expression and genotyping assays, the Voyager Biospectrometry Workstation and QSTAR and Q TRAP systems. Its next-generation systems are significant in that they improve data quality and increase productivity by a factor of two or more compared to current technology platforms, introducing new tools for rapid, accurate and cost-effective DNA analysis to researchers worldwide that study human and other genomes. Applied Biosystems also oversees the licensing of sister subsidiary Celera Genomics Group's Celera Discovery System. Celera Diagnostics, a joint venture between Applied Biosystems and Celera Genomics, researches, develops and manufactures products for diagnosing, monitoring and treating diseases and some genetic conditions.

Applied Biosystems offers its employees medical, dental and vision insurance, an education assistance plan and adoption assistance.

FINANCIALS: Sales and profits are in thousands of dollars—add 000 to get the full amount. Year 2004 note: Complete fiscal 2004 results were not available for all companies at press time. For this company, year 2004 is for 12 months.

2004 Sales: $1,741,100 (12 months)   2004 Profits: $182,900 (12 months)
2003 Sales: $1,682,900   2003 Profits: $183,200
2002 Sales: $1,604,000   2002 Profits: $168,500
2001 Sales: $1,619,500   2001 Profits: $212,400
2000 Sales: $1,388,100   2000 Profits: $186,247

Stock Ticker: ABI
Employees: 5,360
Fiscal Year Ends: 6/30

SALARIES/BENEFITS:
Pension Plan: ESOP Stock Plan: Profit Sharing: Top Exec. Salary: $625,385   Bonus: $538,650
Savings Plan: Y   Stock Purch. Plan: Y   Second Exec. Salary: $529,307   Bonus: $462,977

OTHER THOUGHTS:
Apparent Top Female Officers: 4
Hot Spot for Advancement for Women/Minorities: Y

LOCATIONS: ("Y" = Yes)

West:	Southwest:	Midwest:	Southeast:	Northeast:	International:
Y				Y	Y

APRIA HEALTHCARE GROUP INC

www.apria.com

Industry Group Code: 621610   Ranks within this company's industry group: Sales: 1   Profits: 1

Insurance/HMO/PPO:	Drugs:	Equipment/Supplies:	Hospitals/Clinics:	Services:	Health Care:
Insurance:	Manufacturer:	Manufacturer:	Acute Care:	Diagnostics:	Home Health: Y
Managed Care:	Distributor:	Distributor:	Sub-Acute Care:	Labs/Testing:	Long-Term Care:
Utilization Mgmt.:	Specialty Pharm.:	Leasing/Finance:	Outpatient Surgery:	Staffing:	Physical Therapy:
Payment Proc.:	Vitamins/Nutri.:	Information Sys.:	Phys. Rehab. Center:	Waste Disposal:	Phys. Practice Mgmt.:
	Clinical Trials:		Psychiatric Clinics:	Specialty Services: Y	

TYPES OF BUSINESS:
Home Health Care
Home Medical Equipment
Respiratory Therapy
Infusion Therapy
Patient Travel Programs

BRANDS/DIVISIONS/AFFILIATES:
Great Escapes Travel Program

CONTACTS:
Note: Officers with more than one job title may be intentionally listed here more than once.

Lawrence M. Higby, CEO
Lawrence A. Mastrovich, Pres.
Lawrence A. Mastrovich, COO
Amin I. Khalifa, Exec. VP/CFO
Anthony S. Domenico, Exec. VP-Sales
Frank C. Bianchi, Sr. VP-Human Resources
George J. Suda, Exec. VP-Info. Services
Robert S. Holcombe, Exec. VP/General Counsel
Daniel J. Starck, Exec. VP-Bus. Oper.
Robert G. Abood, Sr. VP-Acquisitions
Lisa M. Getson, Exec. VP-Gov't Rel.
Lisa M. Getson, Exec. VP-Investor Services
James E. Baker, Exec. VP/Treas.
Kimberlie Rogers-Bowers, Sr. VP-Regulatory Affairs & Acquisitions
Ralph V. Whitworth, Chmn.
John J. McDowell, Exec. VP-Logistics

Phone: 949-639-2094   **Fax:** 949-639-2900
Toll-Free: 800-277-4288
Address: 26220 Enterprise Ct., Lake Forest, CA 92630 US

GROWTH PLANS/SPECIAL FEATURES:

Apria Healthcare Group, Inc. is one of the largest providers of home health care services in the U.S., offering home respiratory therapy, home infusion and home medical equipment through 455 branches serving patients across 50 states. The home respiratory division provides oxygen systems, stationary and portable ventilators, obstructive sleep apnea equipment, nebulizers and respiratory medications. Home infusion therapy consists of the intravenous administration of anti-infectives, pain management, chemotherapy, nutrients, immune globulin and other medications. The company's home medical equipment unit provides patients with safety items, ambulatory aids and in-home equipment such as wheelchairs and hospital beds. In each of its service lines, Apria provides patients with a variety of clinical and ancillary services in addition to products and supplies, most of which are prescribed by a physician as part of a care plan. These services include in-home care, pharmacy management, patient and caregiver education and training, monitoring of patients' treatment plans, reporting patient progress and status to the physician, maintaining and repairing equipment and processing claims to third-party payors. Through its field sales force, Apria markets its services primarily to managed care organizations, physicians, hospitals, medical groups, home health agencies and case managers. Apria also offers its Great Escapes Travel Program for patients who wish to travel but have special needs such as oxygen, infusion or other therapy.

FINANCIALS:
Sales and profits are in thousands of dollars—add 000 to get the full amount. Year 2004 note: Complete fiscal 2004 results were not available for all companies at press time. For this company, year 2004 is for 9 months.

2004 Sales: $1,075,012 (9 months)   2004 Profits: $86,741 (9 months)
2003 Sales: $1,380,900   2003 Profits: $116,000
2002 Sales: $1,252,200   2002 Profits: $115,600
2001 Sales: $1,131,900   2001 Profits: $71,900
2000 Sales: $1,014,201   2000 Profits: $57,006

Stock Ticker: AHG
Employees: 10,582
Fiscal Year Ends: 12/31

SALARIES/BENEFITS:
Pension Plan: ESOP Stock Plan: Profit Sharing: Top Exec. Salary: $687,479   Bonus: $700,000
Savings Plan: Y   Stock Purch. Plan: Second Exec. Salary: $438,214   Bonus: $450,000

OTHER THOUGHTS:
Apparent Top Female Officers: 2
Hot Spot for Advancement for Women/Minorities:

LOCATIONS: ("Y" = Yes)
West	Southwest	Midwest	Southeast	Northeast	International
Y	Y	Y	Y	Y	

Note: Financial information, benefits and other data can change quickly and may vary from those stated here.

ARADIGM CORPORATION

www.aradigm.com

Industry Group Code: 339113   Ranks within this company's industry group: Sales: 122   Profits: 131

Insurance/HMO/PPO:	Drugs:	Equipment/Supplies:	Hospitals/Clinics:	Services:	Health Care:
Insurance: Managed Care: Utilization Mgmt.: Payment Proc.:	Manufacturer: Distributor: Specialty Pharm.: Vitamins/Nutri.: Clinical Trials:	Manufacturer: Y Distributor: Leasing/Finance: Information Sys.:	Acute Care: Sub-Acute Care: Outpatient Surgery: Phys. Rehab. Center: Psychiatric Clinics:	Diagnostics: Labs/Testing: Staffing: Waste Disposal: Specialty Services:	Home Health: Long-Term Care: Physical Therapy: Phys. Practice Mgmt.:

TYPES OF BUSINESS:
Equipment-Handheld Electronic Inhalers
Pulmonary Drug Delivery Systems

BRANDS/DIVISIONS/AFFILIATES:
AERx Pulmonary Drug Delivery System
AERx Pain Management System
AERx Insulin Diabetes Management System
Intraject

CONTACTS: Note: Officers with more than one job title may be intentionally listed here more than once.
Richard P. Thompson, CEO
V. Bryan Lawlis, Pres.
V. Bryan Lawlis, COO
Thomas C. Chesterman, Sr. VP/CFO
Norma L. Milligin, VP-Human Resources
Stephen J. Farr, Sr. VP/Chief Scientific Officer
Bobba Venkatadri, Sr. VP-Oper.
John Turanin, VP-Corp. Planning & Program Mgmt.
Klaus Kohl, Sr. VP-Quality/Tech. Dir.-iDMS Program
Babatunde A. Otulana, VP-Clinical & Regulatory Affairs
Richard P. Thompson, Chmn.

Phone: 510-265-9000   **Fax:** 510-265-0277
Toll-Free:
Address: 3929 Point Eden Way, Hayward, CA 94545 US

GROWTH PLANS/SPECIAL FEATURES:
Aradigm Corporation develops advanced pulmonary drug delivery systems for the treatment of systemic conditions and lung diseases. The company is focused on improving the quality and cost-effectiveness of medical treatment by enabling patients to self-administer drugs without needles or lengthy nebulizer treatments. Consequently, the firm is currently developing novel drug delivery systems that exploit the lungs' natural ability to absorb and rapidly transfer molecules into the bloodstream. The firm's operations are centered around its AERx Pulmonary Drug Delivery System, which creates aerosols from liquid drug formulations. The AERx system is the only pulmonary delivery system that allows accurate and reproducible pulmonary drug delivery. The system has the potential to be used for both inpatient and outpatient services, due to the fact that it is handheld and can be self-administered. It also has a wide array of possible applications, including diabetes management (AERx insulin) and pain management (AERx morphine). AERx interferon is approved for the treatment of hepatitis C and B, as well as some cancers, and AERx testosterone is a treatment for postmenopausal women. In recent news, Aradigm and Novo Nordisk's joint-venture Type 2 diabetes treatment, AERx Insulin Diabetes Management System, is undergoing Phase III trials. The company and GlaxoSmitheKline currently have the AERx Pain Management System in Phase II studies. The results have shown that the system delivers morphine as quickly as intravenous administration. The firm acquired Weston Medical's proprietary Intraject technology, a single-use, pen-sized, needle-free alternative to conventional injections that delivers a variety of liquid formulations to subcutaneous tissue. It is currently under development to deliver biotherapeutics including monoclonal antibodies, proteins and small-molecule drugs.

FINANCIALS: Sales and profits are in thousands of dollars—add 000 to get the full amount. Year 2004 note: Complete fiscal 2004 results were not available for all companies at press time. For this company, year 2004 is for 6 months.

2004 Sales: $13,721 (6 months)	2004 Profits: $-15,181 (6 months)	**Stock Ticker:** ARDM
2003 Sales: $33,857	2003 Profits: $-25,970	Employees: 242
2002 Sales: $29,000	2002 Profits: $-35,900	Fiscal Year Ends: 12/31
2001 Sales: $28,900	2001 Profits: $-32,300	
2000 Sales: $20,300	2000 Profits: $-35,600	

SALARIES/BENEFITS:
Pension Plan:	ESOP Stock Plan: Y	Profit Sharing: Y	Top Exec. Salary: $345,000	Bonus: $69,000
Savings Plan: Y	Stock Purch. Plan: Y		Second Exec. Salary: $280,000	Bonus: $56,000

OTHER THOUGHTS:
Apparent Top Female Officers: 2
Hot Spot for Advancement for Women/Minorities:

LOCATIONS: ("Y" = Yes)
West:	Southwest:	Midwest:	Southeast:	Northeast:	International:
Y					

ARKANSAS BLUE CROSS AND BLUE SHIELD
www.arkbluecross.com

Industry Group Code: 524114   Ranks within this company's industry group: Sales: 47   Profits: 33

Insurance/HMO/PPO:	Drugs:	Equipment/Supplies:	Hospitals/Clinics:	Services:	Health Care:
Insurance:	Manufacturer:	Manufacturer:	Acute Care:	Diagnostics:	Home Health:
Managed Care: Y	Distributor:	Distributor:	Sub-Acute Care:	Labs/Testing:	Long-Term Care:
Utilization Mgmt.:	Specialty Pharm.:	Leasing/Finance:	Outpatient Surgery:	Staffing:	Physical Therapy:
Payment Proc.:	Vitamins/Nutri.:	Information Sys.:	Phys. Rehab. Center:	Waste Disposal:	Phys. Practice Mgmt.:
	Clinical Trials:		Psychiatric Clinics:	Specialty Services:	

TYPES OF BUSINESS:
Health Insurance
PPO

BRANDS/DIVISIONS/AFFILIATES:
Arkansas FirstSource PPO
DentalBlue
BasicBlue
USAble MCO
MyChoice Blue
Health Advantage
BlueCard Program

CONTACTS:
Note: Officers with more than one job title may be intentionally listed here more than once.

Robert L. Shoptaw, CEO
Sharon Allen, Pres.
Sharon Allen, COO
Mark White, Exec. VP/CFO
Richard Cooper, VP-Human Resources
Charles Clem, VP-Info. Systems
Robert Cabe, Exec. VP-Legal
Reggie Favors, VP-Oper. & Public Programs
Patrick O'Sullivan, VP-Advertising & Comm.
James Adamson, VP/Chief Medical Officer
David Bridges, Sr. VP-Customer Services
Mike Brown, Sr. VP-Enterprise Networks
Lee Douglass, VP-Law & Gov't Rel.
Hays C. McClerkin, Chmn.

Phone: 501-378-2000   Fax: 501-378-3258
Toll-Free:
Address: 601 S. Gaines St., Little Rock, AR 72201 US

GROWTH PLANS/SPECIAL FEATURES:
Arkansas Blue Cross and Blue Shield is a nonprofit mutual insurance company providing comprehensive health insurance and related services to a membership of more than 962,000 spread throughout Arkansas. As an independent licensee of the Blue Cross and Blue Shield name and service mark, the company's board of directors is required to consist of a majority of public members, meaning people from the community not employed by the health care industry. As a result, Blue Cross and Blue Shield health plans maintain a commitment to local communities and customers not necessarily shared by commercial insurance companies. Arkansas Blue Cross and Blue Shield provides health insurance through a variety of subsidiaries and plans, including Arkansas FirstSource PPO, DentalBlue, BasicBlue, USAble MCO, MyChoice Blue and Health Advantage. The BlueCard Program allows members to submit claims while traveling outside of their plan's area, including a network of participating hospitals around the world. The company acts as a Medicare Part B (physicians' benefits) contractor for Louisiana, Oklahoma, Missouri and New Mexico, and as such maintains offices in those states. Likewise, the company is a Medicare Part A (hospital benefits) contractor for Rhode Island and maintains an office there as well.

Arkansas Blue Cross and Blue Shield provides comprehensive employee benefits, including dental and health insurance, employee assistance and tuition reimbursement.

FINANCIALS:
Sales and profits are in thousands of dollars—add 000 to get the full amount. Year 2004 note: Complete fiscal 2004 results were not available for all companies at press time. For this company, year 2004 is for months.

2004 Sales: $ (months)   2004 Profits: $ (months)
2003 Sales: $907,100   2003 Profits: $52,400
2002 Sales: $848,500   2002 Profits: $
2001 Sales: $ 2001 Profits: $
2000 Sales: $ 2000 Profits: $

Stock Ticker: Nonprofit
Employees: 2,300
Fiscal Year Ends: 12/31

SALARIES/BENEFITS:
Pension Plan: ESOP Stock Plan: Profit Sharing: Top Exec. Salary: $ Bonus: $
Savings Plan: Y   Stock Purch. Plan: Second Exec. Salary: $ Bonus: $

OTHER THOUGHTS:
Apparent Top Female Officers: 1
Hot Spot for Advancement for Women/Minorities:

LOCATIONS: ("Y" = Yes)
West	Southwest	Midwest	Southeast	Northeast	International
	Y	Y	Y	Y	

ARQULE INC

www.arqule.com

Industry Group Code: 541710 Ranks within this company's industry group: Sales: 9 Profits: 8

Insurance/HMO/PPO:	Drugs:	Equipment/Supplies:	Hospitals/Clinics:	Services:	Health Care:
Insurance:	Manufacturer:	Manufacturer:	Acute Care:	Diagnostics:	Home Health:
Managed Care:	Distributor:	Distributor:	Sub-Acute Care:	Labs/Testing: Y	Long-Term Care:
Utilization Mgmt.:	Specialty Pharm.:	Leasing/Finance:	Outpatient Surgery:	Staffing:	Physical Therapy:
Payment Proc.:	Vitamins/Nutri.:	Information Sys.: Y	Phys. Rehab. Center:	Waste Disposal:	Phys. Practice Mgmt.:
	Clinical Trials:		Psychiatric Clinics:	Specialty Services: Y	

TYPES OF BUSINESS:
Research-Drug Discovery
Small-Molecule Compounds
Systems and Software
Predictive Modeling

BRANDS/DIVISIONS/AFFILIATES:
AIMS/PCMS
AMAP Chemistry Operating System
Optimal Chemical Entities
Activated Checkpoint Therapy
Camitro Corporation
ADME/Tox

CONTACTS:
Note: Officers with more than one job title may be intentionally listed here more than once.

Stephen A. Hill, CEO
Stephen A. Hill, Pres.
Andrew C.G. Uprichard, COO
Louise A. Mawhinney, CFO
Anthony S. Messina, VP-Human Dev.
Chiang J. Li, Chief Scientific Officer
Alan L. Hillyard, CIO/VP-IT
J. David Jacobs, VP-Legal/General Counsel
John M. Sorvillo, VP-Bus. Dev.
Jean M. Devine, Dir.-Investor Rel.
Louise A. Mawhinny, VP-Finance
Carmen M. Baldino, VP-Chemistry
Adam R. Craig, VP-Clinical Dev.
James N. Kyranos, VP-Chemical Tech.
Patrick J. Zenner, Chmn.

Phone: 781-994-0300 Fax: 781-376-6019
Toll-Free:
Address: 19 Presidential Way, Woburn, MA 01801 US

GROWTH PLANS/SPECIAL FEATURES:

ArQule, Inc. seeks to bring together genomics and clinical development by applying its proprietary technology platform and world-class chemistry capabilities to drug discovery. The company designs small-molecule compounds called Optimal Chemical Entities, which in theory have a greater chance of success in clinical trials. ArQule engages in research and development of small-molecule cancer therapeutics based on its Activated Checkpoint Therapy (ACT). ACT compounds selectively kill cancer cells by restoring and activating cellular checkpoints that are defective in them. The firm's chief compounds under investigation are ARQ 501 for solid tumors and ARQ 101, an optimized small-molecule compound aimed at treating rheumatoid arthritis. ArQule's AMAP Chemistry Operating System allows it to perform high-throughput, automated production of new chemical compounds. The AMAP system forms the foundation of the company's parallel synthesis approach to combinatorial chemistry. AMAP consists of an integrated series of automated workstations that perform tasks such as weighing and dissolution, chemical synthesis, thermally controlled agitation and reaction process development. ArQule's proprietary Array Information Management and Process Control Management System (AIMS/PCMS) software allows the firm to capture information about every compound in its library, as well as to process this information and audit test data. The firm's subsidiary, Camitro Corporation, is a predictive modeling company that produces computational models and a predictive ADME/Tox platform. In April 2004, Roche and ArQule announced a partnership to discover and develop drug candidates targeting a new pathway in order to selectively kill cancer cells.

ArQule offers its employees counseling, legal services, tuition reimbursement, college savings plans, aid in seeking permanent resident status for foreign nationals, dry cleaning services, mortgage services and discounted ski vouchers, yoga classes and movie passes.

FINANCIALS:
Sales and profits are in thousands of dollars—add 000 to get the full amount. Year 2004 note: Complete fiscal 2004 results were not available for all companies at press time. For this company, year 2004 is for 9 months.

2004 Sales: $40,367 (9 months) 2004 Profits: $-3,912 (9 months)
2003 Sales: $65,500 2003 Profits: $-34,800
2002 Sales: $62,800 2002 Profits: $-77,900
2001 Sales: $58,400 2001 Profits: $-41,000
2000 Sales: $50,300 2000 Profits: $3,900

Stock Ticker: ARQL
Employees: 257
Fiscal Year Ends: 12/31

SALARIES/BENEFITS:
Pension Plan: Y ESOP Stock Plan: Profit Sharing: Top Exec. Salary: $410,616 Bonus: $226,600
Savings Plan: Y Stock Purch. Plan: Y Second Exec. Salary: $297,696 Bonus: $14,000

OTHER THOUGHTS:
Apparent Top Female Officers: 3
Hot Spot for Advancement for Women/Minorities: Y

LOCATIONS: ("Y" = Yes)
| West: | Southwest: | Midwest: | Southeast: | Northeast: Y | International: |

ARROW INTERNATIONAL INC

www.arrowintl.com

Industry Group Code: 339113 Ranks within this company's industry group: Sales: 48 Profits: 36

Insurance/HMO/PPO:	Drugs:	Equipment/Supplies:	Hospitals/Clinics:	Services:	Health Care:
Insurance:	Manufacturer:	Manufacturer: Y	Acute Care:	Diagnostics:	Home Health:
Managed Care:	Distributor:	Distributor:	Sub-Acute Care:	Labs/Testing:	Long-Term Care:
Utilization Mgmt.:	Specialty Pharm.:	Leasing/Finance:	Outpatient Surgery:	Staffing:	Physical Therapy:
Payment Proc.:	Vitamins/Nutri.:	Information Sys.:	Phys. Rehab. Center:	Waste Disposal:	Phys. Practice Mgmt.:
	Clinical Trials:		Psychiatric Clinics:	Specialty Services:	

TYPES OF BUSINESS:
Equipment-Catheters and Related Products
Cardiac Assistance Devices

BRANDS/DIVISIONS/AFFILIATES:
Arrow-Howes
ARROWguard
FlexTip Plus
AutoCAT
Berman
Arrow LionHeart
Super Arrow-Flex
Magnaflow

CONTACTS: Note: Officers with more than one job title may be intentionally listed here more than once.
Carl G. Anderson, Jr., CEO
Philip B. Fleck, Pres.
Philip B. Fleck, COO
Frederick J. Hirt, CFO
Christopher Mennone, VP-Int'l Sales & Mktg.
Carl W. Staples, VP-Human Resources
Carl N. Botterbusch, VP-Research
Carl N. Botterbusch, VP-Eng.
Paul Frankhouser, Exec. VP-Bus. Dev.
John C. Long, VP/Treas.
Paul A. Cornelison, VP-Regulatory Affairs & Quality Assurance
Carl N. Botterbusch, VP-Cardiac Assist Div.
Carl G. Anderson, Jr., Chmn.

Phone: 610-378-0131 Fax: 610-374-5360
Toll-Free: 800-233-3187
Address: 2400 Bernville Rd., Reading, PA 19605 US

GROWTH PLANS/SPECIAL FEATURES:
Arrow International, Inc. develops, manufactures and markets a broad range of clinically advanced disposable catheters and related products for critical care medicine and interventional cardiology and radiology. The company's critical care catheterization products are used to access the central vascular system for administration of fluids, drugs and blood products. Arrow's cardiac care products are used for the diagnosis and treatment of patients with heart and vascular disease. Anesthesiologists, critical care specialists, surgeons, cardiologists, nephrologists, emergency and trauma physicians and other health care providers use the company's products. Arrow's critical care products include the Arrow-Howes multi-lumen catheter, a catheter equipped with three or four channels that enables the simultaneous administration of multiple critical care therapies through a single puncture site; FlexTip Plus epidural catheters, which are designed to minimize in-dwelling complications associated with conventional epidural catheters; and percutaneous thrombolytic devices, which are designed for clearance of thrombosed hemodialysis grafts in chronic hemodialysis patients. Cardiac care products include intra-aortic balloon (IAB) pumps and catheters, used primarily to temporarily augment the pumping capability of the heart following cardiac surgery, serious heart attack or balloon angioplasty; AutoCAT, an advanced automatic IAB pump that continuously monitors and selects the best signal from multiple electrocardiogram and arterial pressure sources to automatically adjust balloon inflation; the Berman angiographic catheter, used for pediatric cardiac angiographic procedures; and the Super Arrow-Flex, a sheath that provides a kink-resistant passageway for the introduction of catheters into the vascular system.

The firm offers its employees a continuing education program, an incentive commission program, matching gift donations and a fitness center.

FINANCIALS: Sales and profits are in thousands of dollars—add 000 to get the full amount. Year 2004 note: Complete fiscal 2004 results were not available for all companies at press time. For this company, year 2004 is for 9 months.

2004 Sales: $320,174 (9 months)   2004 Profits: $41,534 (9 months)
2003 Sales: $380,400   2003 Profits: $45,700
2002 Sales: $340,800   2002 Profits: $39,000
2001 Sales: $334,000   2001 Profits: $46,500
2000 Sales: $320,300   2000 Profits: $46,200

Stock Ticker: ARRO
Employees: 3,005
Fiscal Year Ends: 8/31

SALARIES/BENEFITS:
Pension Plan: Y   ESOP Stock Plan: Profit Sharing: Top Exec. Salary: $463,500   Bonus: $254,925
Savings Plan: Y   Stock Purch. Plan: Second Exec. Salary: $294,784   Bonus: $145,918

OTHER THOUGHTS:
Apparent Top Female Officers:
Hot Spot for Advancement for Women/Minorities:

LOCATIONS: ("Y" = Yes)
West:	Southwest:	Midwest:	Southeast:	Northeast:	International:
Y				Y	Y

Note: Financial information, benefits and other data can change quickly and may vary from those stated here.

ART ADVANCED RESEARCH TECHNOLOGIES

www.art.ca

Industry Group Code: 334500 **Ranks within this company's industry group:** Sales: 4 Profits: 2

Insurance/HMO/PPO:	Drugs:	Equipment/Supplies:	Hospitals/Clinics:	Services:	Health Care:
Insurance: Managed Care: Utilization Mgmt.: Payment Proc.:	Manufacturer: Distributor: Specialty Pharm.: Vitamins/Nutri.: Clinical Trials:	Manufacturer: Y Distributor: Leasing/Finance: Information Sys.:	Acute Care: Sub-Acute Care: Outpatient Surgery: Phys. Rehab. Center: Psychiatric Clinics:	Diagnostics: Labs/Testing: Staffing: Waste Disposal: Specialty Services:	Home Health: Long-Term Care: Physical Therapy: Phys. Practice Mgmt.:

TYPES OF BUSINESS:
Equipment-Optical Imaging Technology
Diagnostic Equipment

BRANDS/DIVISIONS/AFFILIATES:
eXplore Optix
SoftScan

GROWTH PLANS/SPECIAL FEATURES:
ART Advanced Research Technologies, Inc. researches, designs, develops and markets optical imaging technologies used to detect biological anomalies and visualize processes in living systems. The company's products are based on its time domain (TD) optical imaging. TD measures light absorption and scatter characteristics in the visible and near-infrared region of the spectrum to provide detailed profiles of biological tissues. These profiles allow the characterization of diseases like cancer. They also allow the user to analyze the molecular pathways leading to disease. ART's eXplore Optix, a pre-clinical optical molecular imager, provides in vivo pharmacokinetics and biodistribution. The company is in the process of launching SoftScan, a digital imagining device developed to detect and diagnose breast cancer. SoftScan will be introduced as a diagnostic technology, able to complement standard diagnostic technologies like x-ray.

CONTACTS:
Note: Officers with more than one job title may be intentionally listed here more than once.

Micheline Bouchard, CEO
Micheline Bouchard, Pres.
Warren Baker, COO
Jacques Bedard, CFO
Pierre Couture, VP-Mktg. & Sales
Sebastien Gignac, General Counsel
Joseph Kozikowski, Chief Medical Officer

Phone: 514-832-0777 **Fax:** 514-832-0778
Toll-Free:
Address: 2300 Alfred-Nobel Blvd., Saint-Laurent, Quebec H4S 2A4 Canada

FINANCIALS:
Sales and profits are in thousands of dollars—add 000 to get the full amount. Year 2004 note: Complete fiscal 2004 results were not available for all companies at press time. For this company, year 2004 is for months.

2004 Sales: $ (months)
2003 Sales: $1,003,100
2002 Sales: $
2001 Sales: $
2000 Sales: $

2004 Profits: $ (months)
2003 Profits: $148,100
2002 Profits: $
2001 Profits: $
2000 Profits: $

Stock Ticker: Foreign
Employees:
Fiscal Year Ends: 4/30

SALARIES/BENEFITS:
Pension Plan: ESOP Stock Plan: Profit Sharing: Top Exec. Salary: $ Bonus: $
Savings Plan: Stock Purch. Plan: Second Exec. Salary: $ Bonus: $

OTHER THOUGHTS:
Apparent Top Female Officers: 1
Hot Spot for Advancement for Women/Minorities:

LOCATIONS: ("Y" = Yes)
West:	Southwest:	Midwest:	Southeast:	Northeast:	International: Y

ARTHROCARE CORP

www.arthrocare.com

Industry Group Code: 339113   Ranks within this company's industry group: Sales: 84   Profits: 78

Insurance/HMO/PPO:	Drugs:	Equipment/Supplies:	Hospitals/Clinics:	Services:	Health Care:
Insurance:	Manufacturer:	Manufacturer: Y	Acute Care:	Diagnostics:	Home Health:
Managed Care:	Distributor:	Distributor:	Sub-Acute Care:	Labs/Testing:	Long-Term Care:
Utilization Mgmt.:	Specialty Pharm.:	Leasing/Finance:	Outpatient Surgery:	Staffing:	Physical Therapy:
Payment Proc.:	Vitamins/Nutri.:	Information Sys.:	Phys. Rehab. Center:	Waste Disposal:	Phys. Practice Mgmt.:
	Clinical Trials:		Psychiatric Clinics:	Specialty Services:	

TYPES OF BUSINESS:
Equipment-Tissue Removal Systems
Cosmetic & Dermatologic Surgery Products
Advanced Radiofrequency Devices

BRANDS/DIVISIONS/AFFILIATES:
Coblation
VersiTor
Medical Device Alliance, Inc.
Opus Medical

CONTACTS:
Note: Officers with more than one job title may be intentionally listed here more than once.

Michael A. Baker, CEO
Michael A. Baker, Pres.
Fernando V. Sanchez, Sr. VP/CFO
John R. Tighe, Sr. VP-Mktg. & Sales
Jean Woloszko, Chief Science Officer
Jean Woloszko, Chief Tech. Officer
John T. Raffle, VP-Legal Affairs
Richard Christensen, Sr. VP-Oper.
John T. Raffle, VP-Corp. Dev.
Bruce Prothro, VP-Regulatory Affairs/Mgr.-Coblation Tech.
Sten I. Dahlborg, VP/Mgr.-ArthroCare Europe
David Applegate, VP/Mgr.-ArthroCare Spine
Jack Giroux, Sr. VP-Surgical Bus. Units

Phone: 408-736-0224   Fax: 408-736-0226
Toll-Free: 800-348-8929
Address: 680 Vaqueros Ave., Sunnyvale, CA 94085 US

GROWTH PLANS/SPECIAL FEATURES:
ArthroCare Corp. is a medical device company that develops, manufactures and markets products based on its patented Coblation technology. Coblation is a unique process that employs radiofrequency energy for soft tissue removal with minimal damage to surrounding tissue. The firm's products operate at lower temperatures than traditional electrosurgical or laser surgery tools and enable surgeons to ablate, shrink, sculpt, cut, aspirate and suction soft tissue and to seal small bleeding vessels. The company believes its Coblation technology can replace the multiple surgical tools traditionally used in soft tissue surgery with one multi-purpose surgical system. The firm's strategy includes applying its patented technology to a wide range of soft tissue surgical markets, including arthroscopic surgery, spinal surgery, neurosurgery, cosmetic surgery, urologic surgery, various cardiology applications, gynecological surgery, laproscopic/general surgical procedures and ear, nose and throat procedures. The company has FDA approval to specifically label its Coblation-based systems for use in neurosurgery; arthroscopic surgery of the knee, shoulder, ankle, elbow, wrist and hip; and for general dermatologic procedures. In addition, ArthroCare manufactures other disposable devices for spinal surgery, which are designed to improve the ease of use and functionality of the company's Coblation-based spinal surgery system. For example, VersiTor is a precise tissue-cutting tool with a longer shaft for improved access to the surgical area. Recently, ArthroCare acquired Medical Device Alliance, Inc., a subsidiary of Parallax Medical, which makes products for bone access, bone augmentation and the injection of bone cement. It also expanded its sport medicine product lines through a distribution agreement with Biocomposites, a company that designs, makes and distributes sports medicine and bone grating devices. In addition, the company agreed to acquire Opus Medical, a maker of soft tissue orthopedic repair systems, for a total of $90 million in cash and stock.

ArthroCare offers its employees medical, dental and vision insurance, flexible spending accounts, performance-based bonuses and tuition reimbursement.

FINANCIALS:
Sales and profits are in thousands of dollars—add 000 to get the full amount. Year 2004 note: Complete fiscal 2004 results were not available for all companies at press time. For this company, year 2004 is for 6 months.

2004 Sales: $48,307 (6 months)   2004 Profits: $4,716 (6 months)
2003 Sales: $118,900   2003 Profits: $7,500
2002 Sales: $88,800   2002 Profits: $1,100
2001 Sales: $83,300   2001 Profits: $10,100
2000 Sales: $67,600   2000 Profits: $11,500

Stock Ticker: ARTC
Employees: 565
Fiscal Year Ends: 12/31

SALARIES/BENEFITS:
Pension Plan: ESOP Stock Plan: Profit Sharing: Top Exec. Salary: $395,000   Bonus: $252,405
Savings Plan: Y   Stock Purch. Plan: Y   Second Exec. Salary: $215,476   Bonus: $119,019

OTHER THOUGHTS:
Apparent Top Female Officers: 1
Hot Spot for Advancement for Women/Minorities:

LOCATIONS: ("Y" = Yes)
West	Southwest	Midwest	Southeast	Northeast	International
Y	Y		Y		Y

Note: Financial information, benefits and other data can change quickly and may vary from those stated here.

ASCENSION HEALTH

www.ascensionhealth.org

Industry Group Code: 622110 Ranks within this company's industry group: Sales: 5 Profits:

Insurance/HMO/PPO:	Drugs:	Equipment/Supplies:	Hospitals/Clinics:		Services:		Health Care:	
Insurance:	Manufacturer:	Manufacturer:	Acute Care:	Y	Diagnostics:		Home Health:	
Managed Care:	Distributor:	Distributor:	Sub-Acute Care:	Y	Labs/Testing:		Long-Term Care:	Y
Utilization Mgmt.:	Specialty Pharm.:	Leasing/Finance:	Outpatient Surgery:		Staffing:		Physical Therapy:	
Payment Proc.:	Vitamins/Nutri.:	Information Sys.:	Phys. Rehab. Center:	Y	Waste Disposal:		Phys. Practice Mgmt.:	
	Clinical Trials:		Psychiatric Clinics:		Specialty Services:			

TYPES OF BUSINESS:
Hospitals
Acute Care Hospitals
Rehabilitation Hospitals
Psychiatric Hospitals

BRANDS/DIVISIONS/AFFILIATES:
Daughters of Charity National Health System
Sisters of St. Joseph Health System
Sisters of St. Joseph of Carondelet
Ascension Health Ventures
Radianse, Inc.

CONTACTS:
Note: Officers with more than one job title may be intentionally listed here more than once.

Anthony R. Tersigni, CEO
Anthony R. Tersigni, Pres.
Robert J. Henkel, COO
Anthony Speranzo, Sr. VP/CFO
Sherry L. Browne, Sr. VP/CIO
Deborah A. Proctor, Chief Admin. Officer
Rex P. Killian, Sr. VP/General Counsel
John D. Doyle, Chief Strategy Officer
Trudy Barthels, Dir.-Comm.
Susan N. Levy, Sr. VP-Advocacy & External Rel.
Maureen McGuire, Sr. VP-Mission Integration
David Pryor, Sr. VP-Clinical Excellences
Andrew Allen, Pres.-Western & Southern States Oper. Group
John O. Mudd, Chmn.

Phone: 314-733-8000 Fax: 314-733-8013
Toll-Free:
Address: 4600 Edmundson Rd., St. Louis, MO 63134 US

GROWTH PLANS/SPECIAL FEATURES:
Ascension Health is the largest not-for-profit health system in the country, with 63 general acute care hospitals in 20 states, four long-term acute care hospitals, four rehabilitation hospitals, four psychiatric hospitals and 16,727 licensed beds. The Catholic organization was formed in 1999 from the union of the Daughters of Charity National Health System based in St. Louis, Missouri and the Sisters of St. Joseph Health System based in Ann Arbor, Michigan. In 2002, Ascension Health added the hospitals and health facilities of the Sisters of St. Joseph of Carondelet, also based in St. Louis, Missouri. Ascension Health Ventures, the organization's investment subsidiary, identifies and supports companies that offer potential breakthroughs in health-care-related products, services and technologies. Most recently it invested $2.5 million in Radianse, Inc., a startup company that helps health care organizations track people and equipment with radio frequency identification technology. Ascension Health has a strong commitment to assisting uninsured and underinsured patients as part of its mission to affect the transformation of health care in the U.S. into a more just and compassionate system.

Ascension Health provides employees with medical, dental and life insurance, tuition reimbursement and an employee assistance program.

FINANCIALS:
Sales and profits are in thousands of dollars—add 000 to get the full amount. Year 2004 note: Complete fiscal 2004 results were not available for all companies at press time. For this company, year 2004 is for months.

2004 Sales: $ (months)	2004 Profits: $ (months)	**Stock Ticker:** Nonprofit
2003 Sales: $9,054,300	2003 Profits: $	Employees: 87,469
2002 Sales: $7,666,100	2002 Profits: $111,100	Fiscal Year Ends:
2001 Sales: $	2001 Profits: $	
2000 Sales: $	2000 Profits: $	

SALARIES/BENEFITS:
Pension Plan: Y ESOP Stock Plan: Profit Sharing: Top Exec. Salary: $ Bonus: $
Savings Plan: Stock Purch. Plan: Second Exec. Salary: $ Bonus: $

OTHER THOUGHTS:
Apparent Top Female Officers: 5
Hot Spot for Advancement for Women/Minorities: Y

LOCATIONS: ("Y" = Yes)
West:	Southwest:	Midwest:	Southeast:	Northeast:	International:
Y	Y	Y	Y	Y	

ASPECT MEDICAL SYSTEMS INC

www.aspectms.com

Industry Group Code: 339113 Ranks within this company's industry group: Sales: 115 Profits: 120

Insurance/HMO/PPO:	Drugs:	Equipment/Supplies:	Hospitals/Clinics:	Services:	Health Care:
Insurance:	Manufacturer:	Manufacturer: Y	Acute Care:	Diagnostics:	Home Health:
Managed Care:	Distributor:	Distributor:	Sub-Acute Care:	Labs/Testing:	Long-Term Care:
Utilization Mgmt.:	Specialty Pharm.:	Leasing/Finance:	Outpatient Surgery:	Staffing:	Physical Therapy:
Payment Proc.:	Vitamins/Nutri.:	Information Sys.:	Phys. Rehab. Center:	Waste Disposal:	Phys. Practice Mgmt.:
	Clinical Trials:		Psychiatric Clinics:	Specialty Services:	

TYPES OF BUSINESS:
Equipment-Anesthesia Monitoring Systems
Patient Monitoring Systems

BRANDS/DIVISIONS/AFFILIATES:
Bispectral Index
BIS System
BIS Module Kit
BIS Sensors
BIS Sensor Plus
BIS Pediatric Sensor

CONTACTS: Note: Officers with more than one job title may be intentionally listed here more than once.
Nassib G. Chamoun, CEO
Nassib G. Chamoun, Pres.
J. Neal Armstrong, VP/CFO
William Floyd, VP-Mktg. & Sales
Philip H. Devlin, VP-Tech.
Marc Davidson, VP-Eng.
John Coolidge, VP-Mfg.
Eliot Daley, VP-Strategy
Michael Falvey, VP-Finance
Paul J. Manberg, VP-Clinical, Regulatory & Quality Assurance
Scott D. Kelley, VP/Dir.-Medical
Philip H. Devlin, VP/Mgr.-Neuroscience
J. Breckenridge Eagle, Chmn.
Boudewijn L.P.M. Bollen, Pres.-Int'l Oper.

Phone: 617-559-7000   Fax: 619-559-7400
Toll-Free:
Address: 141 Needham St., Newton, MA 02464-1505 US

GROWTH PLANS/SPECIAL FEATURES:
Aspect Medical Systems, Inc. develops, manufactures and markets the BIS System, an anesthesia monitoring system. The BIS System enables anesthesia providers to assess and manage a patient's level of consciousness during surgery. Patient monitoring with the BIS System provides several benefits, such as reducing the amount of anesthetics used and lessening the risk of surgical awareness, which is the unintentional regaining of consciousness during surgery. The BIS System is based on the firm's patented core technology, the Bispectral Index, commonly known as the BIS Index. The BIS Index is a numerical index that correlates with levels of consciousness and is displayed as a number between 0 and 100. The BIS System includes the BIS Monitor or BIS Module Kit and single-use, disposable BIS Sensors. The BIS Sensor is applied to a patient's forehead to measure the electrical activity of the brain, which is then analyzed by the BIS Monitor or BIS Module Kit to produce the BIS Index. The firm's product line includes the BIS Pediatric Sensor, a smaller sensor designed to visually appeal to children. More than 19,000 BIS monitors and modules have been installed worldwide. Aspect markets its products in the U.S. through direct sales organizations and specialty distributors. Internationally, the firm sells the BIS System through distributors and several marketing partners, including Nihon Kohden and Instrumentarium's Datex-Ohmeda division. Aspect also has original equipment manufacturer (OEM) relationships with several patient monitoring and anesthesia equipment companies. In recent news, Aspect has secured exclusive rights to commercialize brain monitoring technology for neurodegenerative diseases, such as Alzheimer's disease and depression, developed by the Neuropsychiatric Institute and David Geffen School of Medicine at UCLA.

FINANCIALS: Sales and profits are in thousands of dollars—add 000 to get the full amount. Year 2004 note: Complete fiscal 2004 results were not available for all companies at press time. For this company, year 2004 is for 9 months.

2004 Sales: $39,848 (9 months)   2004 Profits: $-652 (9 months)
2003 Sales: $44,091   2003 Profits: $-6,523
2002 Sales: $39,800   2002 Profits: $-15,300
2001 Sales: $35,800   2001 Profits: $-17,700
2000 Sales: $36,000   2000 Profits: $-5,300

Stock Ticker: ASPM
Employees: 198
Fiscal Year Ends: 12/31

SALARIES/BENEFITS:
Pension Plan: ESOP Stock Plan: Profit Sharing: Top Exec. Salary: $326,114   Bonus: $150,000
Savings Plan: Y   Stock Purch. Plan: Y   Second Exec. Salary: $250,000 Bonus: $200,000

OTHER THOUGHTS:
Apparent Top Female Officers:
Hot Spot for Advancement for Women/Minorities:

LOCATIONS: ("Y" = Yes)
West:	Southwest:	Midwest:	Southeast:	Northeast:	International:
				Y	Y

Note: Financial information, benefits and other data can change quickly and may vary from those stated here.

ASSISTED LIVING CONCEPTS INC

www.alcco.com

Industry Group Code: 623110 Ranks within this company's industry group: Sales: 12 Profits: 8

Insurance/HMO/PPO:	Drugs:	Equipment/Supplies:	Hospitals/Clinics:	Services:	Health Care:
Insurance: Managed Care: Utilization Mgmt.: Payment Proc.:	Manufacturer: Distributor: Specialty Pharm.: Vitamins/Nutri.: Clinical Trials:	Manufacturer: Distributor: Leasing/Finance: Information Sys.:	Acute Care: Sub-Acute Care: Outpatient Surgery: Phys. Rehab. Center: Psychiatric Clinics:	Diagnostics: Labs/Testing: Staffing: Waste Disposal: Specialty Services:	Home Health: Long-Term Care: Y Physical Therapy: Phys. Practice Mgmt.:

TYPES OF BUSINESS:
Long-Term Health Care
Assisted Living Residences

BRANDS/DIVISIONS/AFFILIATES:

CONTACTS:
Note: Officers with more than one job title may be intentionally listed here more than once.
Steven L. Vick, CEO
Steven L. Vick, Pres.
Linda Martin, COO
Edward Barnes, Sr. VP/CFO
Edward Barnes, Treas./Chief Acct. Officer
Sandra Petersen, Sr. VP-Quality & Clinical Services
W. Andrew Adams, Chmn.

Phone: 214-424-4000 Fax:
Toll-Free: 800-881-0678
Address: 1349 Empire Central, Ste. 900, Dallas, TX 75247 US

GROWTH PLANS/SPECIAL FEATURES:
Assisted Living Concepts, Inc. owns and operates assisted living residences for older adults who need help with the activities of everyday life, such as bathing and dressing. In addition to housing, the company provides personal care, support services and nursing services according to the individual needs of its residents. These services include meals, activities, laundry, housekeeping, assistance with medication, coordination of transportation and grooming. In addition, Assisted Living Concepts can provide or arrange for other services, including physical therapy, hospice and pharmacy services. This grouping of housing and services provides a cost-effective alternative and an independent lifestyle for individuals who do not require the broader array of medical and health services provided by nursing facilities. Increases in the country's elderly population are accompanied by a rising demand in the less costly, more appealing residential options that the firm offers. Assisted Living Concepts focuses on providing assisted living services to moderate-income elderly Americans in rural and suburban communities, a market which is both larger and less competitive than the wealthy elderly segment targeted by most assisted living companies. The firm operates 6,838 units in 177 assisted living residences, 122 of which it owns. The company tries to balance its revenue between private pay residents and Medicaid payment in states with favorable regulatory and reimbursement climates.

FINANCIALS:
Sales and profits are in thousands of dollars—add 000 to get the full amount. Year 2004 note: Complete fiscal 2004 results were not available for all companies at press time. For this company, year 2004 is for 9 months.

2004 Sales: $125,519 (9 months)   2004 Profits: $2,770 (9 months)
2003 Sales: $168,012   2003 Profits: $ 157
2002 Sales: $146,300   2002 Profits: $-4,400
2001 Sales: $150,700   2001 Profits: $-63,900
2000 Sales: $139,400   2000 Profits: $-25,800

Stock Ticker: ASLC
Employees: 3,462
Fiscal Year Ends: 12/31

SALARIES/BENEFITS:
Pension Plan: ESOP Stock Plan: Profit Sharing: Top Exec. Salary: $275,000   Bonus: $477,750
Savings Plan: Y   Stock Purch. Plan: Second Exec. Salary: $180,356   Bonus: $238,875

OTHER THOUGHTS:
Apparent Top Female Officers: 2
Hot Spot for Advancement for Women/Minorities:

LOCATIONS: ("Y" = Yes)
West:	Southwest:	Midwest:	Southeast:	Northeast:	International:
Y	Y	Y	Y	Y	

Note: Financial information, benefits and other data can change quickly and may vary from those stated here.

ASSURANT EMPLOYEE BENEFITS
www.assurantemployeebenefits.com

Industry Group Code: 524113   Ranks within this company's industry group: Sales: 1   Profits:

Insurance/HMO/PPO:	Drugs:	Equipment/Supplies:	Hospitals/Clinics:	Services:	Health Care:
Insurance: Y	Manufacturer:	Manufacturer:	Acute Care:	Diagnostics:	Home Health:
Managed Care:	Distributor:	Distributor:	Sub-Acute Care:	Labs/Testing:	Long-Term Care:
Utilization Mgmt.:	Specialty Pharm.:	Leasing/Finance:	Outpatient Surgery:	Staffing:	Physical Therapy:
Payment Proc.:	Vitamins/Nutri.:	Information Sys.:	Phys. Rehab. Center:	Waste Disposal:	Phys. Practice Mgmt.:
	Clinical Trials:		Psychiatric Clinics:	Specialty Services:	

TYPES OF BUSINESS:
Underwriting-Diversified Insurance

BRANDS/DIVISIONS/AFFILIATES:
American Bankers Insurance Group, Inc.
Fortis Benefits Insurance Company
Assurant, Inc.
Assurant Group

CONTACTS:
Note: Officers with more than one job title may be intentionally listed here more than once.
Robert B. Pollock, CEO
Robert B. Pollock, Pres.
Floyd F. Chadee, Sr. VP/CFO
Mark J. Bohen, Sr. VP-Mktg.
Sylvia R. Wagner, Sr. VP-Human Resources
Karla J. Schacht, Sr. VP/CIO
Kenneth D. Bowen, General Counsel
Mark A. Andruss, VP-Corp. Dev.
Larry M. Cains, Treas.
Michael J. Peninger, Exec. VP/Pres.-Non-Medical Group
Miles B. Yakre, VP/Corp. Actuary
Clifford S. Korte, Sr. VP-Risk & Claims
James R. Logan, Sr. VP-Mortgage

Phone: 816-474-2345   Fax: 816-881-8996
Toll-Free: 800-733-7879
Address: 2323 Grand Blvd., Kansas City, MO 64108 US

GROWTH PLANS/SPECIAL FEATURES:
Assurant Employee Benefits, formerly Fortis Benefits Insurance Company, a subsidiary of Assurant, Inc., provides specialty insurance and investment products to businesses and is one of the major providers in the insurance marketplace. It is licensed in all 50 states except New York and the District of Colombia. The company offers health insurance, long- and short-term disability insurance, accidental death and dismemberment insurance, term life and dental insurance. The firm also provides a series of voluntary benefits, the premiums of which are paid 100% by employees. Voluntary benefits include additional long- and short-term disability, life and dental; a self-funded disability plan; work and family benefits, such as child and elder care; and a special premium plan. Parent company Assurant, Inc., formerly Fortis, Inc., has divisions across the United States as well as in Belgium and the Netherlands. Assurant recently acquired American Bankers Insurance Group, Inc. and merged it with its own subsidiaries to create Assurant Group.

Fortis offers its employees flexible work hours and training opportunities and an on-site cafeteria, health center and fitness center (with paid work-out time). Generous vacation policies, free employee parking and employee club discounts are also available. Children of employees are eligible for scholarships. For working students, the company offers tuition reimbursement.

FINANCIALS:
Sales and profits are in thousands of dollars—add 000 to get the full amount. Year 2004 note: Complete fiscal 2004 results were not available for all companies at press time. For this company, year 2004 is for months.

2004 Sales: $ (months)   2004 Profits: $ (months)
2003 Sales: $1,450,000   2003 Profits: $
2002 Sales: $ 2002 Profits: $
2001 Sales: $161,500   2001 Profits: $32,700
2000 Sales: $ 2000 Profits: $

Stock Ticker: Subsidiary
Employees: 2,000
Fiscal Year Ends: 12/31

SALARIES/BENEFITS:
Pension Plan: ESOP Stock Plan: Profit Sharing: Top Exec. Salary: $375,000   Bonus: $155,025
Savings Plan: Y   Stock Purch. Plan: Second Exec. Salary: $282,500   Bonus: $101,264

OTHER THOUGHTS:
Apparent Top Female Officers: 2
Hot Spot for Advancement for Women/Minorities:

LOCATIONS: ("Y" = Yes)
West	Southwest	Midwest	Southeast	Northeast	International
Y	Y	Y	Y	Y	

ASSURANT HEALTH

www.assuranthealth.com

Industry Group Code: 524114   Ranks within this company's industry group: Sales: 33   Profits:

Insurance/HMO/PPO:	Drugs:	Equipment/Supplies:	Hospitals/Clinics:	Services:	Health Care:
Insurance:	Manufacturer: Y	Manufacturer:	Acute Care:	Diagnostics:	Home Health:
Managed Care:	Distributor:	Distributor:	Sub-Acute Care:	Labs/Testing:	Long-Term Care:
Utilization Mgmt.:	Specialty Pharm.:	Leasing/Finance:	Outpatient Surgery:	Staffing:	Physical Therapy:
Payment Proc.:	Vitamins/Nutri.:	Information Sys.:	Phys. Rehab. Center:	Waste Disposal:	Phys. Practice Mgmt.:
	Clinical Trials:		Psychiatric Clinics:	Specialty Services:	

TYPES OF BUSINESS:
Insurance Brokerage-Health Care
Student Health Insurance
Short-Term Medical Insurance
Health Savings Accounts
Small-Group Insurance

BRANDS/DIVISIONS/AFFILIATES:
Fortis Health
Fortis Insurance Co.
John Alden Life Insurance Co.
Fortis Benefits Insurance Co.

CONTACTS:
Note: Officers with more than one job title may be intentionally listed here more than once.
Don Hamm, CEO
Don Hamm, Pres.
Steve Keller, Dir.-Mktg.
Tim Bireley, VP-Small Group Product Mgmt.
Scott Krienke, VP-Individual Medical Product Mgmt.

Phone: 414-271-3011   Fax: 414-224-0472
Toll-Free: 800-800-1212
Address: 501 W. Michigan, Milwaukee, WI 53201-0624 US

GROWTH PLANS/SPECIAL FEATURES:
Assurant Health, formerly Fortis Health, is a national provider of health insurance, focusing on individual, small-group, short-term and specialty insurance products. The company provides coverage to over 1 million people and is one of the top sellers of temporary health insurance in the U.S. Its individual major medical product is targeted at those that are not offered health insurance by their workplace; small-group insurance is designed for small businesses that are looking for a flexible, appropriate health plan for their employees; and short-term medical is a plan made for people between jobs that still want coverage during interim periods. The company's student select plan covers college students not covered by their parents' insurance plans. Assurant's insurance plans are issued and underwritten by Fortis Insurance Co., John Alden Life Insurance Co. and Fortis Benefits Insurance Co. In addition to these lines of insurance, Assurant Health offers health savings accounts, accounts set up specifically for individuals to plan for future medical expenses and to pay for health care expenses not covered by insurance, using pre-taxed dollars. It also provides health reimbursement arrangements, which are employer-sponsored accounts used for employee reimbursement.

Assurant Health offers medical, dental and vision insurance, tuition reimbursement, an employee assistance program, employee wellness program and parking and bus subsidies.

FINANCIALS:
Sales and profits are in thousands of dollars—add 000 to get the full amount. Year 2004 note: Complete fiscal 2004 results were not available for all companies at press time. For this company, year 2004 is for months.

2004 Sales: $ (months)	2004 Profits: $ (months)	Stock Ticker: Subsidiary
2003 Sales: $2,091,000	2003 Profits: $	Employees: 3,000
2002 Sales: $	2002 Profits: $	Fiscal Year Ends: 12/31
2001 Sales: $	2001 Profits: $	
2000 Sales: $	2000 Profits: $	

SALARIES/BENEFITS:
Pension Plan: Y   ESOP Stock Plan: Profit Sharing: Top Exec. Salary: $ Bonus: $
Savings Plan: Y   Stock Purch. Plan: Second Exec. Salary: $ Bonus: $

OTHER THOUGHTS:
Apparent Top Female Officers:
Hot Spot for Advancement for Women/Minorities:

LOCATIONS: ("Y" = Yes)
West:	Southwest:	Midwest:	Southeast:	Northeast:	International:
		Y	Y		

ASSURANT INC

www.assurant.com

Industry Group Code: 524114   Ranks within this company's industry group: Sales: 15 Profits: 19

Insurance/HMO/PPO:	Drugs:	Equipment/Supplies:	Hospitals/Clinics:	Services:	Health Care:
Insurance: Y	Manufacturer:	Manufacturer:	Acute Care:	Diagnostics:	Home Health:
Managed Care: Y	Distributor:	Distributor:	Sub-Acute Care:	Labs/Testing:	Long-Term Care:
Utilization Mgmt.:	Specialty Pharm.:	Leasing/Finance:	Outpatient Surgery:	Staffing:	Physical Therapy:
Payment Proc.:	Vitamins/Nutri.:	Information Sys.:	Phys. Rehab. Center:	Waste Disposal:	Phys. Practice Mgmt.:
	Clinical Trials:		Psychiatric Clinics:	Specialty Services:	

TYPES OF BUSINESS:
PPO
Health and Dental Insurance
Life Insurance
Funeral Insurance
Homeowners' Insurance
Credit Insurance
Warranties
Debt Protection Administration

BRANDS/DIVISIONS/AFFILIATES:
Assurant Employee Benefits
Assurant Health
Assurant PreNeed
Assurant Solutions
Fortis, Inc.

CONTACTS:
Note: Officers with more than one job title may be intentionally listed here more than once.
J. Kerry Clayton, CEO
J. Kerry Clayton, Pres.
Robert B. Pollock, Exec. VP/CFO
Lance R. Wilson, Sr. VP/CIO
Katherine Greenzang, Sr. VP/General Counsel/Corp. Sec.
Lucinda Landreth, Chief Investment Officer-Assurant Asset Mgmt.
Edwin L. Harper, Sr. VP-Public Affairs & Gov't Rel.
Larry M. Cains, Sr. VP-Investor Rel.
Barbara R. Hege, Sr. VP-Finance
Lesley Silver, Exec. VP
Michael J. Peninger, Exec. VP/CEO-Assurant Employee Benefits
Donald Hamm, Exec. VP/CEO-Assurant Health
Philip Bruce Camacho, Exec. VP/CEO-Assurant Solutions
John Michael Palms, Chmn.

Phone: 212-859-7000   Fax: 212-859-7010
Toll-Free:
Address: One Chase Manhattan Plaza, New York, NY 10005 US

GROWTH PLANS/SPECIAL FEATURES:

Assurant, Inc., formerly Fortis, Inc., is a leading provider of insurance products and services in North America and selected other markets. The firm provides creditor-placed homeowners' insurance, manufactured housing homeowners' insurance, debt protection administration, credit insurance, warranties and extended service contracts, individual health and small employer group health insurance, group dental insurance, group disability insurance, group life insurance and pre-funded funeral insurance. The markets Assurant targets are generally complex, have a relatively limited number of competitors and offer attractive profit opportunities. In its Assurant Solutions business, the company has leadership positions or is aligned with clients who are leaders in creditor-placed homeowners' insurance, manufactured housing homeowners' insurance and debt protection administration. This segment also provides credit insurance and warranties for products including appliances, automobiles and recreational vehicles, consumer electronics and wireless devices. In its Assurant Employee Benefits business, Assurant is a leading writer of group dental plans sponsored by employers. It also provides group disability and term life insurance. In its Assurant PreNeed business, the firm is the largest writer of pre-funded funeral insurance. In addition, the company's Assurant Health business, a preferred provider organization (PPO), provides individual health insurance, including short-term medical and student medical insurance, and small employer group health insurance. After operating as an arm of Fortis Insurance N.V. for the past 25 years, Assurant launched its new brand identity in March 2004.

Assurant provides employees with medical, dental, life and long- and short-term disability insurance, as well as flexible spending accounts, tuition assistance, a matching gift program and a work/life balance program.

FINANCIALS:
Sales and profits are in thousands of dollars—add 000 to get the full amount. Year 2004 note: Complete fiscal 2004 results were not available for all companies at press time. For this company, year 2004 is for 9 months.

2004 Sales: $5,536,001 (9 months)	2004 Profits: $264,432 (9 months)	Stock Ticker: AIZ
2003 Sales: $7,066,213	2003 Profits: $185,652	Employees: 12,200
2002 Sales: $6,532,200	2002 Profits: $-1,001,199	Fiscal Year Ends: 12/31
2001 Sales: $	2001 Profits: $	
2000 Sales: $	2000 Profits: $	

SALARIES/BENEFITS:
| Pension Plan: Y | ESOP Stock Plan: | Profit Sharing: | Top Exec. Salary: $811,200 | Bonus: $1,622,400 |
| Savings Plan: Y | Stock Purch. Plan: | | Second Exec. Salary: $649,000 | Bonus: $1,103,300 |

OTHER THOUGHTS:
Apparent Top Female Officers: 4
Hot Spot for Advancement for Women/Minorities: Y

LOCATIONS: ("Y" = Yes)
West:	Southwest:	Midwest:	Southeast:	Northeast:	International:
		Y	Y	Y	

ATC HEALTHCARE INC

www.atchealthcare.com

Industry Group Code: 621610 **Ranks within this company's industry group:** Sales: 9 Profits: 12

Insurance/HMO/PPO:	Drugs:	Equipment/Supplies:	Hospitals/Clinics:	Services:	Health Care:
Insurance:	Manufacturer:	Manufacturer:	Acute Care:	Diagnostics:	Home Health:
Managed Care:	Distributor:	Distributor:	Sub-Acute Care:	Labs/Testing:	Long-Term Care:
Utilization Mgmt.:	Specialty Pharm.:	Leasing/Finance:	Outpatient Surgery:	Staffing: Y	Physical Therapy:
Payment Proc.:	Vitamins/Nutri.:	Information Sys.:	Phys. Rehab. Center:	Waste Disposal:	Phys. Practice Mgmt.:
	Clinical Trials:		Psychiatric Clinics:	Specialty Services: Y	

TYPES OF BUSINESS:
Supplemental Staffing for the Health Care Industry
Management Consulting Services

BRANDS/DIVISIONS/AFFILIATES:

CONTACTS:
Note: Officers with more than one job title may be intentionally listed here more than once.
David Savitsky, CEO
Stephen Savitsky, Pres.
Andrew Rieben, Sr. VP/CFO
Stephen Savitsky, Chmn.

Phone: 516-750-1600   **Fax:** 516-750-1755
Toll-Free:
Address: 1983 Marcus Ave., Ste. E122, Lake Success, NY 11042 US

GROWTH PLANS/SPECIAL FEATURES:
ATC Healthcare, Inc. is a national provider of supplemental staffing and management consulting services to health care institutions through its network of 52 owned and franchised offices in 23 states. The company's supplemental staffing operations provide clients with registered nurses, licensed practical nurses and certified nursing assistants in over 60 job categories, including critical care, neonatal, labor and delivery, as well as administrative assistants, collection personnel and medical records clerks. It also offers allied health staffing, which includes mental health technicians, radiology technicians, phlebotomists and speech, occupational and physical therapists. Health care institutions use supplemental staffing to cover permanent positions for which they have openings, for peak periods, vacations and emergencies and to accommodate periodic increases in the number of patients. ATC Healthcare takes care of the payment of wages, benefits, payroll taxes, workers' compensation and unemployment insurance. The company also operates a travel nurse program whereby nurses and physical and occupational therapists are recruited from the U.S. and other countries to perform services on a long-term basis in the U.S.

FINANCIALS:
Sales and profits are in thousands of dollars—add 000 to get the full amount. Year 2004 note: Complete fiscal 2004 results were not available for all companies at press time. For this company, year 2004 is for 12 months.

2004 Sales: $130,401 (12 months)	2004 Profits: $-6,180 (12 months)	**Stock Ticker:** AHN
2003 Sales: $148,700	2003 Profits: $-2,800	**Employees:** 15,154
2002 Sales: $149,400	2002 Profits: $3,600	**Fiscal Year Ends:** 2/28
2001 Sales: $120,700	2001 Profits: $-1,100	
2000 Sales: $114,994	2000 Profits: $-3,240	

SALARIES/BENEFITS:
Pension Plan:	ESOP Stock Plan:	Profit Sharing:	Top Exec. Salary: $412,880	Bonus: $10,000
Savings Plan: Y	Stock Purch. Plan: Y		Second Exec. Salary: $310,043	Bonus: $

OTHER THOUGHTS:
Apparent Top Female Officers:
Hot Spot for Advancement for Women/Minorities:

LOCATIONS: ("Y" = Yes)
West:	Southwest:	Midwest:	Southeast:	Northeast:	International:
Y	Y	Y	Y	Y	

ATRIA SENIOR LIVING GROUP

www.arvi.com

Industry Group Code: 623110 Ranks within this company's industry group: Sales: Profits:

Insurance/HMO/PPO:	Drugs:	Equipment/Supplies:	Hospitals/Clinics:	Services:	Health Care:
Insurance:	Manufacturer:	Manufacturer:	Acute Care:	Diagnostics:	Home Health:
Managed Care:	Distributor:	Distributor:	Sub-Acute Care:	Labs/Testing:	Long-Term Care: Y
Utilization Mgmt.:	Specialty Pharm.:	Leasing/Finance:	Outpatient Surgery:	Staffing:	Physical Therapy:
Payment Proc.:	Vitamins/Nutri.:	Information Sys.:	Phys. Rehab. Center:	Waste Disposal:	Phys. Practice Mgmt.:
	Clinical Trials:		Psychiatric Clinics:	Specialty Services:	

TYPES OF BUSINESS:
Long-Term Health Care
Assisted Living Centers

BRANDS/DIVISIONS/AFFILIATES:
Prometheus Assisted Living, LLC

CONTACTS:
Note: Officers with more than one job title may be intentionally listed here more than once.
John A. Moore, CEO
John A. Moore, Pres.
Mark Jessee, CFO

Phone: 502-719-1600 Fax: 502-719-1699
Toll-Free: 888-287-4201
Address: 501 S. 4th Ave., Ste. 140, Louisville, KY 40202 US

GROWTH PLANS/SPECIAL FEATURES:
Atria Senior Living Group, a subsidiary of Prometheus Assisted Living, LLC, is one of the nation's largest operators of facilities providing assisted living services for the country's burgeoning senior population. The company currently operates 132 communities across 28 states, which provide support for day-to-day activities and chores, such as shopping and cleaning, but exclude any sort of acute care such as would be found in a nursing home. Atria's special retirement living program focuses on making its residents as independent as possible, encouraging them to engage in activities and hobbies and allowing them to choose their own degree of privacy or sociability. Each program is tailored to the individual, with residents free to bring their own furnishings and even pets. Atria also offers the Atria Author Series, which allows residents to write for publications that are available to families, organizations, schools and churches. In addition to basic assisted living, Atria offers programs for those with Alzheimer's disease and other forms of dementia, making special provisions for memory retention and close family contact.

FINANCIALS:
Sales and profits are in thousands of dollars—add 000 to get the full amount. Year 2004 note: Complete fiscal 2004 results were not available for all companies at press time. For this company, year 2004 is for months.

2004 Sales: $ (months)	2004 Profits: $ (months)	
2003 Sales: $	2003 Profits: $	Stock Ticker: Subsidiary
2002 Sales: $158,400	2002 Profits: $-3,300	Employees: 3,070
2001 Sales: $145,400	2001 Profits: $1,000	Fiscal Year Ends: 12/31
2000 Sales: $138,900	2000 Profits: $6,500	

SALARIES/BENEFITS:
| Pension Plan: | ESOP Stock Plan: | Profit Sharing: | Top Exec. Salary: $350,000 | Bonus: $210,000 |
| Savings Plan: Y | Stock Purch. Plan: | | Second Exec. Salary: $225,000 | Bonus: $110,000 |

OTHER THOUGHTS:
Apparent Top Female Officers:
Hot Spot for Advancement for Women/Minorities:

LOCATIONS: ("Y" = Yes)
West:	Southwest:	Midwest:	Southeast:	Northeast:	International:
Y	Y	Y	Y	Y	

ATRION CORPORATION

www.atrioncorp.com

Industry Group Code: 339113   Ranks within this company's industry group: Sales: 107   Profits: 86

Insurance/HMO/PPO:	Drugs:	Equipment/Supplies:		Hospitals/Clinics:	Services:	Health Care:
Insurance:	Manufacturer:	Manufacturer:	Y	Acute Care:	Diagnostics:	Home Health:
Managed Care:	Distributor:	Distributor:		Sub-Acute Care:	Labs/Testing:	Long-Term Care:
Utilization Mgmt.:	Specialty Pharm.:	Leasing/Finance:		Outpatient Surgery:	Staffing:	Physical Therapy:
Payment Proc.:	Vitamins/Nutri.:	Information Sys.:		Phys. Rehab. Center:	Waste Disposal:	Phys. Practice Mgmt.:
	Clinical Trials:			Psychiatric Clinics:	Specialty Services:	

TYPES OF BUSINESS:
Equipment-Ophthalmic, Diagnostic & Cardiovascular
Fluid Delivery Devices
Medical Device Components
Contract Manufacturing

BRANDS/DIVISIONS/AFFILIATES:
Atrion Medical Products
Halkey-Roberts Corp.
Quest Medical, Inc.
MPS Myocardial Protection System

CONTACTS:
Note: Officers with more than one job title may be intentionally listed here more than once.
Emile A. Battat, CEO
Emile A. Battat, Pres.
Jeffery Strickland, VP/CFO
Emile A. Battat, Chmn.

Phone: 972-390-9800   Fax: 972-396-7581
Toll-Free:
Address: One Allentown Pkwy., Allen, TX 75002-4211 US

GROWTH PLANS/SPECIAL FEATURES:

Atrion Corporation designs, develops, manufactures, markets, sells and distributes products and components, primarily for the medical and health care industry. It markets components to other equipment manufacturers for incorporation in their products and sells finished devices to physicians, hospitals, clinics and other treatment centers. Products and services range from cardiovascular products to fluid delivery devices and contract manufacturing services. A large portion of profits come from international sales, with approximately 26% of total revenues generated from sales to parties outside the U.S. Current operations are conducted through three subsidiaries: Atrion Medical Products, Inc., Halkey-Roberts Corporation and Quest Medical, Inc. Atrion Medical's products are used in ophthalmic, diagnostic and cardiovascular procedures and are sold primarily to major health care companies which market and distribute the products to hospitals, clinics, surgical centers, physicians and other health care providers. Halkey-Roberts designs, develops, manufactures and sells proprietary medical device components used to control the flow of fluids and gases. Its valves and clamps are used in a wide variety of hospital and outpatient care products, such as Foley catheters, pressure cuffs, dialysis and blood collection sets and drug delivery systems. Quest Medical manufactures and sells the MPS myocardial protection system, an innovative and sophisticated system for the delivery of solutions to the heart during open-heart surgery. It is the only device used in open-heart surgery that allows for the mixing of drugs into the bloodstream without diluting the blood.

Atrion provides employees with medical, dental, prescription drug and life coverage.

FINANCIALS:
Sales and profits are in thousands of dollars—add 000 to get the full amount. Year 2004 note: Complete fiscal 2004 results were not available for all companies at press time. For this company, year 2004 is for 6 months.

2004 Sales: $33,200 (6 months)	2004 Profits: $2,800 (6 months)	**Stock Ticker:** ATRI
2003 Sales: $62,800	2003 Profits: $5,100	Employees: 427
2002 Sales: $59,500	2002 Profits: $2,700	Fiscal Year Ends: 12/31
2001 Sales: $57,600	2001 Profits: $9,800	
2000 Sales: $51,400	2000 Profits: $2,800	

SALARIES/BENEFITS:
Pension Plan: Y   ESOP Stock Plan: Profit Sharing: Top Exec. Salary: $500,000   Bonus: $100,000
Savings Plan: Stock Purch. Plan: Second Exec. Salary: $180,000   Bonus: $68,220

OTHER THOUGHTS:
Apparent Top Female Officers:
Hot Spot for Advancement for Women/Minorities:

LOCATIONS: ("Y" = Yes)
West:	Southwest:	Midwest:	Southeast:	Northeast:	International:
	Y		Y		

Note: Financial information, benefits and other data can change quickly and may vary from those stated here.

ATS MEDICAL INC

www.atsmedical.com

Industry Group Code: 339113 **Ranks within this company's industry group:** Sales: 132 Profits: 127

Insurance/HMO/PPO:	Drugs:	Equipment/Supplies:		Hospitals/Clinics:	Services:	Health Care:
Insurance:	Manufacturer:	Manufacturer:	Y	Acute Care:	Diagnostics:	Home Health:
Managed Care:	Distributor:	Distributor:	Y	Sub-Acute Care:	Labs/Testing:	Long-Term Care:
Utilization Mgmt.:	Specialty Pharm.:	Leasing/Finance:		Outpatient Surgery:	Staffing:	Physical Therapy:
Payment Proc.:	Vitamins/Nutri.:	Information Sys.:		Phys. Rehab. Center:	Waste Disposal:	Phys. Practice Mgmt.:
	Clinical Trials:			Psychiatric Clinics:	Specialty Services:	

TYPES OF BUSINESS:
Equipment-Mechanical Heart Valves
Cardiovascular Accessories

BRANDS/DIVISIONS/AFFILIATES:
ATS Open Pivot

CONTACTS:
Note: Officers with more than one job title may be intentionally listed here more than once.

Michael D. Dale, CEO
Michael D. Dale, Pres.
Jack Judd, CFO
Richard A. Curtis, VP-Mktg.
Richard A. Curtis, VP-Bus. Dev.
Marc P. Sportsman, VP-Worldwide Sales
Michael D. Dale, Chmn.

Phone: 763-553-7736 **Fax:** 763-553-2244
Toll-Free: 800-399-1381
Address: 3905 Annapolis Ln., Ste. 105, Minneapolis, MN 55447 US

GROWTH PLANS/SPECIAL FEATURES:

ATS Medical, Inc. is a leading device manufacturer specializing in mechanical heart valves, aortic valve graft prostheses and related cardiovascular accessories. The company has FDA approval to sell the ATS Open Pivot bileaflet heart valve for the treatment of heart valve failure caused by the natural aging process, rheumatic heart disease, prosthetic valve failure and congenital defects. The Open Pivot valve has been designed to eliminate the cavity associated with the pivot of other bileaflet valves and to improve the ability of the blood to flow through the valve without forming clots. The company markets the ATS Open Pivot valve in the U.S. through a sales organization divided into four regions and 28 sales territories. It focuses its sales and marketing efforts on developing awareness of the pivot valve in approximately 970 U.S. open heart centers. ATS Medical currently works with cardiac surgeons in approximately 170 of these centers. The firm sells its products through an independent distribution network in all of its international markets except France, where it has a direct sales organization. In recent news, ATS Medical reached an agreement to purchase the exclusive development, licensing and marketing rights of a new ultrasound-based technology for blood filtration during cardiac surgery from ErySave AB, a research firm based in Sweden.

The company offers its employees health coverage, flexible spending accounts, educational assistance and health club reimbursement.

FINANCIALS:
Sales and profits are in thousands of dollars—add 000 to get the full amount. Year 2004 note: Complete fiscal 2004 results were not available for all companies at press time. For this company, year 2004 is for 9 months.

2004 Sales: $20,789 (9 months)   2004 Profits: $-11,199   (9 months)
2003 Sales: $18,484   2003 Profits: $-13,292
2002 Sales: $13,300   2002 Profits: $-18,200
2001 Sales: $15,100   2001 Profits: $-6,800
2000 Sales: $14,600   2000 Profits: $ 500

Stock Ticker: ATSI
Employees: 87
Fiscal Year Ends: 12/31

SALARIES/BENEFITS:
Pension Plan:	ESOP Stock Plan:	Profit Sharing:	Top Exec. Salary: $250,000	Bonus: $100,000
Savings Plan: Y	Stock Purch. Plan: Y		Second Exec. Salary: $185,000	Bonus: $49,256

OTHER THOUGHTS:
Apparent Top Female Officers:
Hot Spot for Advancement for Women/Minorities:

LOCATIONS: ("Y" = Yes)
West:	Southwest:	Midwest:	Southeast:	Northeast:	International:
		Y			

AVENTIS SA

www.aventis.com

Industry Group Code: 325412 **Ranks within this company's industry group:** Sales: 6 Profits: 10

Insurance/HMO/PPO:	Drugs:		Equipment/Supplies:	Hospitals/Clinics:	Services:	Health Care:
Insurance:	Manufacturer:	Y	Manufacturer:	Acute Care:	Diagnostics:	Home Health:
Managed Care:	Distributor:		Distributor:	Sub-Acute Care:	Labs/Testing:	Long-Term Care:
Utilization Mgmt.:	Specialty Pharm.:		Leasing/Finance:	Outpatient Surgery:	Staffing:	Physical Therapy:
Payment Proc.:	Vitamins/Nutri.:		Information Sys.:	Phys. Rehab. Center:	Waste Disposal:	Phys. Practice Mgmt.:
	Clinical Trials:			Psychiatric Clinics:	Specialty Services:	

TYPES OF BUSINESS:
Drugs-Diversified
Pharmaceutical Manufacturing
Drug Research and Development
Animal Health Products
Vaccines
Skin Care Treatments

BRANDS/DIVISIONS/AFFILIATES:
Aventis Pharma
Aventis Pasteur
Ketek
Merial
Allegra
Lovenox
Taxotere
Sanofi-Synthelabo

CONTACTS:
Note: Officers with more than one job title may be intentionally listed here more than once.
Igor Landau, Chmn.-Mgmt. Board
Richard J. Markham, COO
Patrick Langlois, CFO
Heinz-Werner Meier, Exec. VP-Human Resources
Dirk Oldenburg, Exec. VP/General Counsel
Thierry Soursac, Exec. VP-Commercial Oper.
Frank L. Douglas, Exec. VP-Drug Innovation & Approval
Jurgen Dormann, Chmn.-Supervisory Board

Phone: 33-3-88-99-1100	Fax: 33-3-88-99-1101
Toll-Free:	
Address: 16 Ave. de l'Europe, Strasbourg, 67917 France	

GROWTH PLANS/SPECIAL FEATURES:
Aventis SA, a global leader in the pharmaceutical industry, offers a wide assortment of patented prescription drugs and human vaccines through its many subsidiaries, including Aventis Pharma, which accounts for approximately 85% of revenues. The firm has a commercial presence in 85 countries, with products available in more than 170. Aventis has leading positions in several therapeutic areas, including cardiology, oncology, diabetes and respiratory. The firm's core businesses are prescription drugs, human vaccines through Aventis Pasteur and animal health through Merial, its joint venture with Merck and Co. The company's primary drug products are Allegra and Telfast for the treatment of seasonal allergies, Lovenox and Clexane for the treatment of deep vein thrombosis and heart attacks, Taxotere for the treatment of breast cancer, Delix and Tritace for the treatment of hypertension, Actonel for the treatment of osteoporosis, the antibiotic Ketek and Lantus for the treatment of diabetes. Its primary markets are the United States, France, Germany and Japan. The U.S. accounts for about 38% of sales in Aventis's strategic brands. Aventis is continually developing therapeutic innovations, including compounds for the treatment of diabetes, cancer, cardiovascular diseases and respiratory problems. Other research and development efforts include progress in AIDS vaccines, Alzheimer's treatments and Parkinson's care. In recent news, Aventis agreed to be acquired by Sanofi-Synthelabo, if the transaction is completed, the combined company would be the world's third largest pharmaceutical company.

FINANCIALS:
Sales and profits are in thousands of dollars—add 000 to get the full amount. Year 2004 note: Complete fiscal 2004 results were not available for all companies at press time. For this company, year 2004 is for months.

2004 Sales: $ (months)	2004 Profits: $ (months)	
2003 Sales: $22,397,000	2003 Profits: $2,390,000	**Stock Ticker:** Foreign
2002 Sales: $21,659,000	2002 Profits: $2,285,000	Employees: 75,000
2001 Sales: $20,447,000	2001 Profits: $1,455,000	Fiscal Year Ends: 12/31
2000 Sales: $21,006,000	2000 Profits: $-27,000	

SALARIES/BENEFITS:
Pension Plan: Y	ESOP Stock Plan: Y	Profit Sharing: Y	Top Exec. Salary: $	Bonus: $
Savings Plan:	Stock Purch. Plan:		Second Exec. Salary: $	Bonus: $

OTHER THOUGHTS:
Apparent Top Female Officers:
Hot Spot for Advancement for Women/Minorities:

LOCATIONS: ("Y" = Yes)
West:	Southwest:	Midwest:	Southeast:	Northeast:	International:
Y	Y	Y	Y	Y	Y

AVERA HEALTH

www.avera.org

Industry Group Code: 622110   Ranks within this company's industry group: Sales: Profits:

Insurance/HMO/PPO:	Drugs:	Equipment/Supplies:	Hospitals/Clinics:		Services:	Health Care:	
Insurance:	Manufacturer:	Manufacturer:	Acute Care:	Y	Diagnostics:	Home Health:	Y
Managed Care: Y	Distributor:	Distributor:	Sub-Acute Care:	Y	Labs/Testing:	Long-Term Care:	Y
Utilization Mgmt.:	Specialty Pharm.:	Leasing/Finance:	Outpatient Surgery:		Staffing:	Physical Therapy:	
Payment Proc.:	Vitamins/Nutri.:	Information Sys.:	Phys. Rehab. Center:		Waste Disposal:	Phys. Practice Mgmt.:	
	Clinical Trials:		Psychiatric Clinics:		Specialty Services:		

TYPES OF BUSINESS:
Hospitals
Nursing Homes
Insurance

BRANDS/DIVISIONS/AFFILIATES:
Avera McKennan
Avera Sacred Heart
Avera Queen of Peace
Avera St. Luke's
Avera Marshall
Avera Health Plans
Avera Select
Avera Health Foundation

GROWTH PLANS/SPECIAL FEATURES:
Avera Health was created in 2000 by an agreement between the Benedictine Sisters of Yankton, South Dakota and the Presentation Sisters of Aberdeen, South Dakota. The partnership combined independent hospitals, nursing homes, clinics and other health services at over 100 locations in South Dakota, Minnesota, Iowa and Nebraska. The organization is divided into five regions: Avera McKennan, Avera Sacred Heart, Avera Queen of Peace, Avera St. Luke's and Avera Marshall. Avera Health operates through several subsidiaries, including Avera Health Plans, offering an array of employer-sponsored health plans; Avera Center for Public Policy, which seeks to influence state and federal legislation; Avera Select, which offers Medicare supplement insurance; and Avera Health Foundation, which coordinates charitable giving programs and fundraising.

CONTACTS:
Note: Officers with more than one job title may be intentionally listed here more than once.

John T. Porter, CEO
John T. Porter, Pres.
Richard Thompson, Sr. VP-Mktg.
Jim Breckenridge, Sr. VP-Finance

Phone: 605-322-4700   **Fax:** 605-322-4666
Toll-Free:
Address: 3900 W. Avera Dr., Sioux Falls, SD 57108 US

FINANCIALS:
Sales and profits are in thousands of dollars—add 000 to get the full amount. Year 2004 note: Complete fiscal 2004 results were not available for all companies at press time. For this company, year 2004 is for months.

2004 Sales: $ (months)   2004 Profits: $ (months)
2003 Sales: $ 2003 Profits: $
2002 Sales: $ 2002 Profits: $
2001 Sales: $ 2001 Profits: $
2000 Sales: $ 2000 Profits: $

Stock Ticker: Nonprofit
Employees:
Fiscal Year Ends:

SALARIES/BENEFITS:
Pension Plan: ESOP Stock Plan: Profit Sharing: Top Exec. Salary: $ Bonus: $
Savings Plan: Stock Purch. Plan: Second Exec. Salary: $ Bonus: $

OTHER THOUGHTS:
Apparent Top Female Officers:
Hot Spot for Advancement for Women/Minorities:

LOCATIONS: ("Y" = Yes)
West:	Southwest:	Midwest:	Southeast:	Northeast:	International:
		Y			

… 244

AVMED HEALTH PLAN

www.avmed.com

Industry Group Code: 524114   Ranks within this company's industry group: Sales: Profits:

Insurance/HMO/PPO:	Drugs:	Equipment/Supplies:	Hospitals/Clinics:	Services:	Health Care:
Insurance:	Manufacturer:	Manufacturer:	Acute Care:	Diagnostics:	Home Health:
Managed Care: Y	Distributor:	Distributor:	Sub-Acute Care:	Labs/Testing:	Long-Term Care:
Utilization Mgmt.:	Specialty Pharm.:	Leasing/Finance:	Outpatient Surgery:	Staffing:	Physical Therapy:
Payment Proc.:	Vitamins/Nutri.:	Information Sys.:	Phys. Rehab. Center:	Waste Disposal:	Phys. Practice Mgmt.:
	Clinical Trials:		Psychiatric Clinics:	Specialty Services: Y	

TYPES OF BUSINESS:
Insurance
HMO & POS Plans
Health Education Services
Disease Management

BRANDS/DIVISIONS/AFFILIATES:
On Call

GROWTH PLANS/SPECIAL FEATURES:
AvMed Health Plan is a statewide not-for-profit and one of Florida's leading HMO providers, serving nearly 300,000 members. The firm's policies include employer group HMO, Medicare HMO, POS and self-funded plans. In addition, the company offers health promotion opportunities, smoking cessation programs and a number of on-site health-related seminars. The firm's disease management program provides assistance to members with congestive heart problems, asthma and high-risk pregnancies. In addition, it provides On Call, a free, 24-hour phone service that provides health information to its members.

CONTACTS:
Note: Officers with more than one job title may be intentionally listed here more than once.
Robert C. Hudson, CEO
Robert C. Hudson, Pres.
Douglas G. Cueny, COO
Joe G. Dunlop, Chmn.

Phone: 352-372-8400   Fax: 352-337-8521
Toll-Free: 800-346-0231
Address: 4300 NW 89th Blvd., Gainesville, FL 32606 US

FINANCIALS:
Sales and profits are in thousands of dollars—add 000 to get the full amount. Year 2004 note: Complete fiscal 2004 results were not available for all companies at press time. For this company, year 2004 is for months.

2004 Sales: $ (months)   2004 Profits: $ (months)
2003 Sales: $ 2003 Profits: $
2002 Sales: $ 2002 Profits: $
2001 Sales: $ 2001 Profits: $
2000 Sales: $ 2000 Profits: $

Stock Ticker: Nonprofit
Employees:
Fiscal Year Ends: 12/31

SALARIES/BENEFITS:
Pension Plan: ESOP Stock Plan: Profit Sharing: Top Exec. Salary: $ Bonus: $
Savings Plan: Stock Purch. Plan: Second Exec. Salary: $ Bonus: $

OTHER THOUGHTS:
Apparent Top Female Officers:
Hot Spot for Advancement for Women/Minorities:

LOCATIONS: ("Y" = Yes)
| West: | Southwest: | Midwest: | Southeast: Y | Northeast: | International: |

Note: Financial information, benefits and other data can change quickly and may vary from those stated here.

AXA PPP HEALTHCARE

www.axappphealthcare.co.uk

Industry Group Code: 524114   Ranks within this company's industry group: Sales: 42   Profits:

Insurance/HMO/PPO:	Drugs:	Equipment/Supplies:	Hospitals/Clinics:	Services:	Health Care:
Insurance:	Manufacturer:	Manufacturer:	Acute Care:	Diagnostics:	Home Health:
Managed Care: Y	Distributor:	Distributor:	Sub-Acute Care:	Labs/Testing:	Long-Term Care:
Utilization Mgmt.:	Specialty Pharm.:	Leasing/Finance:	Outpatient Surgery:	Staffing:	Physical Therapy:
Payment Proc.:	Vitamins/Nutri.:	Information Sys.:	Phys. Rehab. Center:	Waste Disposal:	Phys. Practice Mgmt.:
	Clinical Trials:		Psychiatric Clinics:	Specialty Services:	

TYPES OF BUSINESS:
Health & Occupational Insurance
HMO
Dental & Travel Insurance

BRANDS/DIVISIONS/AFFILIATES:
AXA Group
CashBack

CONTACTS:
Note: Officers with more than one job title may be intentionally listed here more than once.

Dennis Holt, CEO-AXA U.K.

Phone: 44-870-608-0850   Fax: 44-1892-515143
Toll-Free:
Address: Phillips House, Crescent Rd., Tunbridge Wells, Kent TN1 2PL UK

GROWTH PLANS/SPECIAL FEATURES:
AXA PPP Healthcare, a subsidiary of the AXA Group, is one of the U.K.'s largest managed care companies. The company's U.K. health care products include employer medical insurance for different sizes of businesses, voluntary employee-paid medical insurance and an employee support program, which offers professional counseling and stress management to employees. In addition, its occupational health insurance services include a fixed-cost package of occupational health and safety services, on-call expert support, executive care health assessment for key employees, safety services that manage the risk of work-related accidents or illnesses, a free health information service, a tailored package of health and fitness services for employees, an independent referral review service for patients with long-term health problems, attendance management and pre-employment medical clearance services. AXA also provides dental and travel insurance, as well as its CashBack program, which provides money back on the cost of everyday health care, such as optical and dental bills. In addition, the company provides international health insurance plans to expatriates that live or work outside of their own country for more than six months a year. The firm provides three health insurance plans (standard, comprehensive and prestige) for three geographical areas: worldwide cover, worldwide cover except the U.S. and Canada, and European coverage. In addition, it provides tailor-made health plans in Malta, Cyprus, United Arab Emirates, Saudi Arabia and Bahrain, as well as health insurance plans for people living in the Channel Islands.

FINANCIALS:
Sales and profits are in thousands of dollars—add 000 to get the full amount. Year 2004 note: Complete fiscal 2004 results were not available for all companies at press time. For this company, year 2004 is for months.

2004 Sales: $ (months)	2004 Profits: $ (months)	**Stock Ticker:** Subsidiary
2003 Sales: $1,200,100	2003 Profits: $	Employees:
2002 Sales: $	2002 Profits: $	Fiscal Year Ends: 12/31
2001 Sales: $	2001 Profits: $	
2000 Sales: $	2000 Profits: $	

SALARIES/BENEFITS:
Pension Plan: ESOP Stock Plan: Profit Sharing: Top Exec. Salary: $ Bonus: $
Savings Plan: Stock Purch. Plan: Second Exec. Salary: $ Bonus: $

OTHER THOUGHTS:
Apparent Top Female Officers:
Hot Spot for Advancement for Women/Minorities:

LOCATIONS: ("Y" = Yes)
West:	Southwest:	Midwest:	Southeast:	Northeast:	International: Y

ns
BANNER HEALTH

www.bannerhealth.com

Industry Group Code: 622110   Ranks within this company's industry group: Sales: Profits:

Insurance/HMO/PPO:	Drugs:	Equipment/Supplies:	Hospitals/Clinics:		Services:		Health Care:	
Insurance:	Manufacturer:	Manufacturer:	Acute Care:	Y	Diagnostics:		Home Health:	Y
Managed Care:	Distributor:	Distributor:	Sub-Acute Care:	Y	Labs/Testing:		Long-Term Care:	Y
Utilization Mgmt.:	Specialty Pharm.:	Leasing/Finance:	Outpatient Surgery:		Staffing:		Physical Therapy:	
Payment Proc.:	Vitamins/Nutri.:	Information Sys.:	Phys. Rehab. Center:	Y	Waste Disposal:		Phys. Practice Mgmt.:	
	Clinical Trials:		Psychiatric Clinics:		Specialty Services:	Y		

TYPES OF BUSINESS:
Hospitals
Long-Term Care Centers
Home Care Services
Home Medical Equipment Services
Family Clinics
Nursing Registry

BRANDS/DIVISIONS/AFFILIATES:

CONTACTS: Note: Officers with more than one job title may be intentionally listed here more than once.
Peter S. Fine, CEO
Peter S. Fine, Pres.
Ron Bunnel, Sr. VP/CFO
Daniel J. Snyder, Pres.-Western Region
Susan Edwards, Pres.-Arizona Region
Thomas F. Madison, Chmn.

Phone: 602-495-4000   Fax: 602-495-4559
Toll-Free:
Address: 1441 N. 12th St., Phoenix, AZ 85006 US

GROWTH PLANS/SPECIAL FEATURES:

Banner Health, based in Phoenix, Arizona, is one of the nation's largest nonprofit health care systems, with 19 hospitals and six long-term care centers located in Alaska, Arizona, California, Colorado, Kansas, Nebraska, Nevada and Wyoming. Banner Health offers an array of services including home care, home medical equipment services, family clinics and a nursing registry. In addition to basic medical and emergency services, the firm's hospitals provide specialized services including heart care, organ transplants, cancer treatment, multiple-birth deliveries, rehabilitation services and behavioral health services. The company is also involved in research in areas including Alzheimer's disease and spinal cord injuries. With yearly revenues of $2.1 billion, Banner Health's annual charitable care and community service contributions amount to $49.5 million. Recently, the firm completed construction of a new cardiology center at Banner Good Samaritan Medical Center in Phoenix.

Employee benefits at Banner Health include medical, dental and vision insurance, legal plans, flexible spending accounts and an employee assistance program. The company also provides benefits for domestic partners, child and elderly dependent care and educational support.

FINANCIALS: Sales and profits are in thousands of dollars—add 000 to get the full amount. Year 2004 note: Complete fiscal 2004 results were not available for all companies at press time. For this company, year 2004 is for months.

2004 Sales: $ (months)   2004 Profits: $ (months)
2003 Sales: $ 2003 Profits: $ Stock Ticker: Nonprofit
2002 Sales: $ 2002 Profits: $ Employees:
2001 Sales: $ 2001 Profits: $ Fiscal Year Ends: 12/31
2000 Sales: $ 2000 Profits: $

SALARIES/BENEFITS:
Pension Plan: ESOP Stock Plan: Profit Sharing: Top Exec. Salary: $ Bonus: $
Savings Plan: Y   Stock Purch. Plan: Second Exec. Salary: $ Bonus: $

OTHER THOUGHTS:
Apparent Top Female Officers: 1
Hot Spot for Advancement for Women/Minorities:

LOCATIONS: ("Y" = Yes)
West:	Southwest:	Midwest:	Southeast:	Northeast:	International:
Y	Y	Y			

ns
BARR LABORATORIES INC

www.barrlabs.com

Industry Group Code: 325412 Ranks within this company's industry group: Sales: 28 Profits: 24

Insurance/HMO/PPO:	Drugs:		Equipment/Supplies:	Hospitals/Clinics:	Services:	Health Care:
Insurance:	Manufacturer:	Y	Manufacturer:	Acute Care:	Diagnostics:	Home Health:
Managed Care:	Distributor:		Distributor:	Sub-Acute Care:	Labs/Testing:	Long-Term Care:
Utilization Mgmt.:	Specialty Pharm.:		Leasing/Finance:	Outpatient Surgery:	Staffing:	Physical Therapy:
Payment Proc.:	Vitamins/Nutri.:		Information Sys.:	Phys. Rehab. Center:	Waste Disposal:	Phys. Practice Mgmt.:
	Clinical Trials:			Psychiatric Clinics:	Specialty Services:	

TYPES OF BUSINESS:
Drugs-Generic Pharmaceuticals
Female Health Care Products
Cardiovascular Drugs
Pain Management Products
Psychotherapeutics
Anti-Infectives and Antibiotics
Oncology Drugs

BRANDS/DIVISIONS/AFFILIATES:
Barr Research, Inc.
SEASONALE
Cenestine
ViaSpan
Trexell
Tamoxifen
Aviane
Claravis

CONTACTS:
Note: Officers with more than one job title may be intentionally listed here more than once.

Bruce L. Downey, CEO
Paul M. Bisaro, Pres.
Paul M. Bisaro, COO
William T. McKee, Sr. VP/CFO
Timothy P. Catlett, VP-Sales & Mktg.
Catherine F. Higgins, Sr. VP-Human Resources
Salah U. Ahmed, Sr. VP-Product Dev.
Michael J. Bogda, Sr. VP-Eng.
Michael J. Bogda, Sr. VP-Mfg.
Fredrick J. Killion, Sr. VP/General Counsel/Corp. Sec.
Martin Zeiger, Sr. VP-Strategic Bus. Dev.
William T. McKee, Treas.
Carole S. Ben-Maimon, Pres., Barr Research, Inc.
Christine Mundkur, VP-Quality and Regulatory Counsel
Bruce L. Downey, Chmn.

Phone: 845-362-1100 Fax: 845-362-2774
Toll-Free: 800-222-0190
Address: 2 Quaker Rd., Pomona, NY 10970-0519 US

GROWTH PLANS/SPECIAL FEATURES:
Barr Laboratories, Inc. is an established pharmaceutical company engaged in the development, manufacture and marketing of generic and proprietary prescription pharmaceuticals. The company currently manufactures and distributes more than 100 different dosage forms and strengths of pharmaceutical products. The firm's product line is concentrated primarily on six core therapeutic categories: oncology, female health care (including oral contraceptives and hormone replacements), cardiovascular, anti-infectives and antibiotics, pain management, and psychotherapeutics for such disorders as anxiety and depression. Barr's business strategy has three core components: the development and marketing of proprietary pharmaceuticals; the development and marketing of generic pharmaceuticals that have one or more barriers to entry; and developing the generic version and then challenging patents protecting select brand pharmaceuticals where the company believes that such patents are either invalid, unenforceable or not infringed by the company's product. The company currently makes a total of 10 proprietary products, including SEASONALE extended-cycle oral contraceptive, Cenestine (synthetic conjugated estrogens), Plan B emergency oral contraceptive, ViaSpan transplant preservation agent, Trexall tablets (for rheumatoid arthritis) and Aygestin (for secondary amenorrhea). The firm's generic products include Claravis, a generic form of Accutane, which is used to treat cystic acne; Tamoxifen Citrate (Tamoxifen), a generic form of Nolvadex, which is used to treat advanced breast cancer, as well as to impede the recurrence of tumors following surgery; Aviane, a generic form of Alesse, for female health care; Dipyridamole, a generic form of Persantine, a cardiovascular drug; Methotrexate, a generic form of Rheumatrex, for rheumatoid arthritis; and Dextroamphetamine Sulfate, a generic form of Dexedrine Spansule, a psychotherapeutic. Recently, Barr acquired the rights to four products marketed by Wyeth: Diamox Sequels, Zebeta, Ziac and Aygestin.

Barr Laboratories provides employees with a full benefits package and tuition reimbursement programs.

FINANCIALS:
Sales and profits are in thousands of dollars—add 000 to get the full amount. Year 2004 note: Complete fiscal 2004 results were not available for all companies at press time. For this company, year 2004 is for 12 months.

2004 Sales: $1,309,088 (12 months) 2004 Profits: $123,103 (12 months)
2003 Sales: $902,900 2003 Profits: $167,600
2002 Sales: $1,189,000 2002 Profits: $212,200
2001 Sales: $509,700 2001 Profits: $62,500
2000 Sales: $482,278 2000 Profits: $42,342

Stock Ticker: BRL
Employees: 1,500
Fiscal Year Ends: 6/30

SALARIES/BENEFITS:
Pension Plan: Y ESOP Stock Plan: Profit Sharing: Top Exec. Salary: $846,154 Bonus: $500,000
Savings Plan: Y Stock Purch. Plan: Y Second Exec. Salary: $448,077 Bonus: $250,000

OTHER THOUGHTS:
Apparent Top Female Officers: 3
Hot Spot for Advancement for Women/Minorities: Y

LOCATIONS: ("Y" = Yes)
West:	Southwest:	Midwest:	Southeast:	Northeast:	International:
		Y		Y	

BAUSCH & LOMB INC

www.bausch.com

Industry Group Code: 339113   Ranks within this company's industry group: Sales: 13   Profits: 18

Insurance/HMO/PPO:	Drugs:		Equipment/Supplies:		Hospitals/Clinics:	Services:	Health Care:
Insurance:	Manufacturer:	Y	Manufacturer:	Y	Acute Care:	Diagnostics:	Home Health:
Managed Care:	Distributor:	Y	Distributor:		Sub-Acute Care:	Labs/Testing:	Long-Term Care:
Utilization Mgmt.:	Specialty Pharm.:		Leasing/Finance:		Outpatient Surgery:	Staffing:	Physical Therapy:
Payment Proc.:	Vitamins/Nutri.:		Information Sys.:		Phys. Rehab. Center:	Waste Disposal:	Phys. Practice Mgmt.:
	Clinical Trials:				Psychiatric Clinics:	Specialty Services:	

TYPES OF BUSINESS:
Supplies-Eye Care
Generic & Prescription Pharmaceuticals
Surgical Products

BRANDS/DIVISIONS/AFFILIATES:
LENSender Direct Lens Delivery
ReNu
Boston
SofLens
SofPort
Ocuvite
Alrex
PreserVision

CONTACTS:
Note: Officers with more than one job title may be intentionally listed here more than once.
Ronald L. Zarrella, CEO
Stephen C. McCluski, Sr. VP/CFO
David R. Nachbar, Sr. VP-Human Resources
Praveen Tyle, Sr. VP-Research & Dev./Chief Scientific Officer
Marie L. Smith, VP/CIO
Gary M. Aron, Sr. VP-Eng., Research & Dev.
Robert B. Stiles, Sr. VP/General Counsel
Barbara M. Kelley, VP-Corp. Comm.
Barbara M. Kelley, VP-Investor Rel.
Jurij Z. Kushner, VP/Controller
Brian Levy, VP/Chief Medical Officer
Gary M. Phillips, VP-Global Pharmaceuticals
Angela J. Panzarella, VP-Global Vision Care
Kamal K. Sarbadhikari, VP-Global Surgical
Ronald L. Zarrella, Chmn.
Alan H. Farnsworth, Sr. VP/Pres., Europe, Middle East & Africa
Dwaine L. Hahs, Sr. VP-Global Supply Chain Mgmt.

Phone: 585-338-6000   Fax: 585-338-6007
Toll-Free: 800-344-8815
Address: One Bausch & Lomb Pl., Rochester, NY 14604-2701 US

GROWTH PLANS/SPECIAL FEATURES:
Bausch & Lomb (B&L), Inc. is a world leader in the development, manufacture and marketing of health care products for the eye. Its products are marketed in over 100 countries. B&L has three product lines: vision care, pharmaceuticals and surgical. The company's vision care division includes contact lenses, lens care products and the vision accessories business. Vision care products include soft and gas permeable (GP) contact lenses; lens care products for soft and GP contact lenses; eye care products, such as eye drops and ointments; and vision accessories, such as magnifiers and eyeglass accessories. They are marketed to licensed eye care professionals, health products retailers, independent pharmacies, drug stores, food stores and mass merchandisers by the company's sales force and distributors. The pharmaceutical division manufactures and sells generic and proprietary prescription pharmaceuticals with a strategic emphasis in the ophthalmic field and over-the-counter ophthalmic medications. Its products treat a wide range of eye conditions, including glaucoma, eye allergies, conjunctivitis and dry eyes. The surgical sector manufactures and sells products and equipment for cataract, refractive and retinal surgery. Some of B&L's brands include ReNu, Boston, SofLens, SofPort, Optima, Ocuvite, Alrex and Opcon. The company offers its customers the LENSender Direct Lens Delivery service in which the company ships the contact lenses directly to the customers' homes or offices. Recently, B&L launched its SofLens One Day lens in Japan. It also plans to launch the next generation of its ReNu line of multi-purpose lens care solutions in the U.S. The company launched PreserVision, a formulation of vitamins and minerals shown to reduce the risk of blindness for patients with high risk of developing age-related macular degeneration.

FINANCIALS:
Sales and profits are in thousands of dollars—add 000 to get the full amount. Year 2004 note: Complete fiscal 2004 results were not available for all companies at press time. For this company, year 2004 is for 9 months.

2004 Sales: $1,625,700 (9 months)   2004 Profits: $108,100 (9 months)
2003 Sales: $2,019,500   2003 Profits: $125,500
2002 Sales: $1,816,700   2002 Profits: $72,500
2001 Sales: $1,711,900   2001 Profits: $21,500
2000 Sales: $1,772,400   2000 Profits: $83,400

Stock Ticker: BOL
Employees: 11,600
Fiscal Year Ends: 12/31

SALARIES/BENEFITS:
Pension Plan: Y   ESOP Stock Plan: Profit Sharing: Top Exec. Salary: $413,259   Bonus: $340,000
Savings Plan: Y   Stock Purch. Plan: Second Exec. Salary: $403,685   Bonus: $315,000

OTHER THOUGHTS:
Apparent Top Female Officers: 3
Hot Spot for Advancement for Women/Minorities: Y

LOCATIONS: ("Y" = Yes)

West:	Southwest:	Midwest:	Southeast:	Northeast:	International:
Y	Y	Y	Y	Y	Y

BAXTER INTERNATIONAL INC

www.baxter.com

Industry Group Code: 339113 Ranks within this company's industry group: Sales: 3 Profits: 3

Insurance/HMO/PPO:	Drugs:	Equipment/Supplies:	Hospitals/Clinics:	Services:	Health Care:
Insurance: Managed Care: Utilization Mgmt.: Payment Proc.:	Manufacturer: Y Distributor: Specialty Pharm.: Vitamins/Nutri.: Clinical Trials:	Manufacturer: Y Distributor: Leasing/Finance: Information Sys.:	Acute Care: Sub-Acute Care: Outpatient Surgery: Phys. Rehab. Center: Psychiatric Clinics:	Diagnostics: Labs/Testing: Staffing: Waste Disposal: Specialty Services:	Home Health: Long-Term Care: Physical Therapy: Phys. Practice Mgmt.:

TYPES OF BUSINESS:
Supplies-Intravenous and Renal Dialysis Systems
Tissue Heart Valves
Medication Delivery Products
Biopharmaceutical Products
Biosurgery Products
Vaccines

BRANDS/DIVISIONS/AFFILIATES:
ASTA Medica Oncology
Ceprotin

CONTACTS:
Note: Officers with more than one job title may be intentionally listed here more than once.
Robert L. Parkinson, CEO
John Greisch, CFO
Karen J. May, VP-Human Resources
Norbert G. Riedel, Chief Scientific Officer
John Moon, CIO
J. Michael Gatling, VP-Global Mfg. Oper.
Marla Persky, General Counsel
Neville J. Jeharajah, VP-Investor Rel. & Financial Planning
Steven J. Meyer, Treas.
David F. Drohan, VP/Pres.-Medication Delivery
James R. Hurley, VP-Integration and Alliance Mgmt.
Carlos del Salto, VP/Pres.-International/Asia/Rental
Robert L. Parkinson, Chmn.

Phone: 847-948-2000   Fax: 847-948-3642
Toll-Free: 800-422-9837
Address: One Baxter Pkwy., Deerfield, IL 60015-4633 US

GROWTH PLANS/SPECIAL FEATURES:
Baxter International, Inc. develops, manufactures and distributes its medical products in 29 countries and sells them in over 100 countries. Its products are used by hospitals, clinical and medical research labs, blood and blood dialysis centers, rehab facilities, nursing homes, doctor's offices and patients undergoing supervised home care. The company operates in three segments: medication delivery, which provides a range of intravenous solutions and specialty products that are used in combination for fluid replenishment, nutrition therapy, pain management, antibiotic therapy and chemotherapy; BioScience, which develops biopharmaceuticals, biosurgery products, vaccines and blood collection, processing and storage products and technologies; and renal, which develops products and provides services to treat end-stage kidney disease. The medication delivery segment includes ASTA Medica Oncology, a German-based manufacturer of chemotherapy drugs. The BioScience division is known as a leading producer of both plasma-based and recombinant clotting factors for hemophilia, as well as biopharmaceuticals used to treat immune deficiencies, cancer and other disorders. The company has a European licensure for Ceprotin, a new protein C concentrate used to treat congenital protein C deficiency. Baxter has been growing its presence in renal care by addressing the needs of kidney-disease patients from initial diagnosis through dialysis and organ replacement. Baxter is pursuing nanotechnology applications through a partnership with Northwestern University. Northwestern will receive the patent rights, while Baxter will be able to exclusively license the technology.

Baxter is committed to maintaining a highly diverse workforce. The company offers employees a relaxed work environment with business casual dress.

FINANCIALS:
Sales and profits are in thousands of dollars—add 000 to get the full amount. Year 2004 note: Complete fiscal 2004 results were not available for all companies at press time. For this company, year 2004 is for 9 months.

2004 Sales: $6,908,000 (9 months)   2004 Profits: $282,000 (9 months)
2003 Sales: $8,916,000   2003 Profits: $881,000
2002 Sales: $8,110,000   2002 Profits: $778,000
2001 Sales: $7,663,000   2001 Profits: $612,000
2000 Sales: $6,896,000   2000 Profits: $740,000

Stock Ticker: BAX
Employees: 51,300
Fiscal Year Ends: 12/31

SALARIES/BENEFITS:
Pension Plan: Y   ESOP Stock Plan: Profit Sharing: Top Exec. Salary: $925,000   Bonus: $647,500
Savings Plan: Stock Purch. Plan: Y   Second Exec. Salary: $625,000 Bonus: $140,000

OTHER THOUGHTS:
Apparent Top Female Officers: 2
Hot Spot for Advancement for Women/Minorities:

LOCATIONS: ("Y" = Yes)
West:	Southwest:	Midwest:	Southeast:	Northeast:	International:
Y	Y	Y	Y	Y	Y

BAYER AG

www.bayer.de

Industry Group Code: 325000 Ranks within this company's industry group: Sales: 1 Profits: 2

Insurance/HMO/PPO:	Drugs:		Equipment/Supplies:	Hospitals/Clinics:	Services:	Health Care:
Insurance:	Manufacturer:	Y	Manufacturer:	Acute Care:	Diagnostics:	Home Health:
Managed Care:	Distributor:		Distributor:	Sub-Acute Care:	Labs/Testing:	Long-Term Care:
Utilization Mgmt.:	Specialty Pharm.:		Leasing/Finance:	Outpatient Surgery:	Staffing:	Physical Therapy:
Payment Proc.:	Vitamins/Nutri.:	Y	Information Sys.:	Phys. Rehab. Center:	Waste Disposal:	Phys. Practice Mgmt.:
	Clinical Trials:			Psychiatric Clinics:	Specialty Services:	

TYPES OF BUSINESS:
Chemical Manufacturing
Health Care
Crop Science
Synthetic Materials
Business Services
Technology Services
Industry Services

BRANDS/DIVISIONS/AFFILIATES:
LANXESS
Bayer CropScience
Bayer HealthCare
Bayer MaterialScience
Bayer Chemicals
Bayer Industry Services
Bayer Technology Services
Bayer Corporation

CONTACTS:
Note: Officers with more than one job title may be intentionally listed here more than once.
Werner Wenning, Chmn.-Mgmt. Board
Klaus Kuhn, CFO
Richard Pott, Human Resources
Udo Oels, Tech. and Environment
Richard Pott, Strategy
Manfred Schneider, Chmn.-Supervisory Board

Phone: 49-214-30-1   Fax: 49-214-30-66328
Toll-Free:
Address: D-51368, Leverkusen, Germany

GROWTH PLANS/SPECIAL FEATURES:
The Bayer Group is a German holding company represented by some 350 individual companies on all five continents. Its seven business subgroups cover an array of industries, operating under the names Bayer Chemicals, Bayer CropScience, Bayer HealthCare, Bayer MaterialScience, Bayer Business Services, Bayer Industry Services and Bayer Technology Services. Bayer Chemicals' products are essential to the electronic, optics, metal processing, food, coatings, textile, leather, paper, plastics, rubber, building materials and engineering ceramics industries. In addition to producing basic chemicals for industrial and laboratory work, inorganic pigments and ion exchange resins, the company has a wide range of chemical products available for the manufacture and treatment of leather, including tanning agents and dyestuffs. As a leading world supplier in the textile processing industry, Bayer Chemicals offers products for the process of pretreatment and auxiliaries for dyeing, finishing and printing textiles. Bayer CropScience is one of the world's leading innovative enterprises in the areas of crop protection, seeds, biotechnology and non-agricultural pest control. Through plant biotechnology and modern breeding methods, the company's BioScience business group researches ways to increase the quantity and quality of food, feed and fibers. Best known for producing pharmaceuticals and non-prescription drugs, most notably Aspirin, the company's Bayer HealthCare division also provides veterinary drugs and biological products such as synthetic proteins. Bayer Material Science produces plastics and rubbers. Following its successful reorganization, the Bayer Group intends to maintain focus on its core businesses, in the future concentrating on health care, nutrition and innovative materials. For this reason, Bayer will combine most of its chemicals activities with certain business units from the materials segment to form the new company LANXESS, to be listed on the stock exchange by 2005. In July 2004, Bayer agreed to buy the over-the-counter drug unit of Roche.

Bayer offers its employees individual training and development opportunities, sports amenities, flexible work schedules and a varied program of cultural events.

FINANCIALS:
Sales and profits are in thousands of dollars—add 000 to get the full amount. Year 2004 note: Complete fiscal 2004 results were not available for all companies at press time. For this company, year 2004 is for 3 months.

2004 Sales: $9,059,000 (3 months)   2004 Profits: $500,000 (3 months)
2003 Sales: $35,914,000   2003 Profits: $-1,585,000
2002 Sales: $32,172,327   2002 Profits: $1,338,679
2001 Sales: $25,639,068   2001 Profits: $708,800
2000 Sales: $ 2000 Profits: $

Stock Ticker: Foreign
Employees: 118,280
Fiscal Year Ends: 12/31

SALARIES/BENEFITS:
Pension Plan: Y   ESOP Stock Plan: Profit Sharing: Top Exec. Salary: $1,001,375   Bonus: $949,592
Savings Plan: Stock Purch. Plan: Second Exec. Salary: $587,716   Bonus: $537,442

OTHER THOUGHTS:
Apparent Top Female Officers:
Hot Spot for Advancement for Women/Minorities:

LOCATIONS: ("Y" = Yes)
West:	Southwest:	Midwest:	Southeast:	Northeast:	International:
				Y	Y

BAYER CORP

www.bayerus.com

Industry Group Code: 325412   Ranks within this company's industry group: Sales: 12   Profits:

Insurance/HMO/PPO:	Drugs:	Equipment/Supplies:	Hospitals/Clinics:	Services:	Health Care:
Insurance:	Manufacturer: Y	Manufacturer:	Acute Care:	Diagnostics: Y	Home Health:
Managed Care:	Distributor:	Distributor:	Sub-Acute Care:	Labs/Testing: Y	Long-Term Care:
Utilization Mgmt.:	Specialty Pharm.:	Leasing/Finance:	Outpatient Surgery:	Staffing:	Physical Therapy:
Payment Proc.:	Vitamins/Nutri.:	Information Sys.:	Phys. Rehab. Center:	Waste Disposal:	Phys. Practice Mgmt.:
	Clinical Trials:		Psychiatric Clinics:	Specialty Services:	

TYPES OF BUSINESS:
Drugs
Animal Health
Consumer Care Products
Diagnostic Testing
Chemicals
Herbicides, Fungicides and Insecticides
Coatings, Adhesives and Sealants

BRANDS/DIVISIONS/AFFILIATES:
Bayer Group
Bayer HealthCare
Bayer MaterialSciences, LLC
Bayer CropScience, LP
Bayer Chemicals Corp.
Bayer Polymers
LANXESS Corp.
Aleve

GROWTH PLANS/SPECIAL FEATURES:
Bayer Corporation is the U.S. subsidiary of chemical and pharmaceutical giant the Bayer Group. The company operates through four operating subsidiaries. Bayer HealthCare operates through six divisions: animal health, biological products, consumer care, diagnostics professional testing, diagnostics self-testing systems and pharmaceuticals. Bayer MaterialScience, LLC produces coatings, adhesives and sealant raw materials; inorganic basic chemicals; polycarbonates; polyurethanes; and thermoplastic polyurethane. Bayer CropScience, LP makes herbicides, fungicides and insecticides, including NoBugs, Bayleton, Home Health Total Termite Control, Provado Insectecide and Sencor. Bayer Chemicals Corporation manufactures basic chemicals, pigments and fine chemicals that are used in pharmaceuticals. Bayer's popular brands include Bayer Aspirin, Aleve, Alka-Seltzer and Phillips' Milk of Magnesia. In recent news, Bayer is combining most of Bayer Chemicals and portions of Bayer MaterialSciences to form a new company, LANXESS Corporation. LANXESS will produce rubber, rubber chemicals, styrenics, semi-crystalline products, Dorlastan fibers, the polymer additives of Rheine Chemie and a wide array of fine, basic and specialty chemicals.

CONTACTS:
Note: Officers with more than one job title may be intentionally listed here more than once.

Attila Molnar, CEO
Attila Molnar, Pres.
Mark A. Ryan, Head-Corp. Comm.
Joseph A. Akers, General Mgr.-Biological Products Div.
Gary S. Balkema, General Mgr.-Consumer Care Div.
Esmail Zirakparvar, Pres./CEO-Bayer CropScience, LP
Gregory S. Babe, Pres./CEO-Bayer MaterialScience, LLC

Phone: 412-777-2000   **Fax:** 412-777-2034
Toll-Free:
Address: 100 Bayer Rd., Pittsburgh, PA 15205-9741 US

FINANCIALS:
Sales and profits are in thousands of dollars—add 000 to get the full amount. Year 2004 note: Complete fiscal 2004 results were not available for all companies at press time. For this company, year 2004 is for months.

2004 Sales: $ (months)   2004 Profits: $ (months)
2003 Sales: $10,999,300   2003 Profits: $
2002 Sales: $9,424,500   2002 Profits: $
2001 Sales: $8,686,200   2001 Profits: $
2000 Sales: $ 2000 Profits: $

Stock Ticker: Subsidiary
Employees: 23,300
Fiscal Year Ends: 12/31

SALARIES/BENEFITS:
Pension Plan: ESOP Stock Plan: Profit Sharing: Top Exec. Salary: $ Bonus: $
Savings Plan: Stock Purch. Plan: Second Exec. Salary: $ Bonus: $

OTHER THOUGHTS:
Apparent Top Female Officers:
Hot Spot for Advancement for Women/Minorities:

LOCATIONS: ("Y" = Yes)

West:	Southwest:	Midwest:	Southeast:	Northeast:	International:
Y	Y	Y	Y	Y	

Note: Financial information, benefits and other data can change quickly and may vary from those stated here.

BECKMAN COULTER INC

www.beckmancoulter.com

Industry Group Code: 339113   Ranks within this company's industry group: Sales: 10   Profits: 14

Insurance/HMO/PPO:	Drugs:	Equipment/Supplies:	Hospitals/Clinics:	Services:	Health Care:
Insurance: Managed Care: Utilization Mgmt.: Payment Proc.:	Manufacturer: Distributor: Specialty Pharm.: Vitamins/Nutri.: Clinical Trials:	Manufacturer: Y Distributor: Leasing/Finance: Information Sys.:	Acute Care: Sub-Acute Care: Outpatient Surgery: Phys. Rehab. Center: Psychiatric Clinics:	Diagnostics: Labs/Testing: Staffing: Waste Disposal: Specialty Services:	Home Health: Long-Term Care: Physical Therapy: Phys. Practice Mgmt.:

TYPES OF BUSINESS:
Equipment-Laboratory Instruments
Laboratory Test Kits

BRANDS/DIVISIONS/AFFILIATES:
Coulter Corporation
Beckman Instruments, Inc.
Biomec 3000
Biomek NX
GI Monitor
Access BR Monitor
GenomeLab SNPstream Genotyping System

CONTACTS:
Note: Officers with more than one job title may be intentionally listed here more than once.

John P. Wareham, CEO
Scott Garrett, Pres.
Scott Garrett, COO
James T. Glover, Interim CFO
Fidencio M. Mares, VP-Human Resources
William H. May, VP/General Counsel/Corp. Sec.
Edgar E. Vivanco, VP-Oper.
Fidencio M. Mares, VP-Corp. Comm.
Jeanie Herbert, Dir.-Investor Rel.
James T. Glover, VP/Controller/Chief Acct. Officer
Elias Caro, Pres.-Biomedical Research Div.
Scott Garrett, Pres.-Clinical Diagnostics Div.
Paul Glyer, VP/Treas.
John P. Wareham, Chmn.

Phone: 714-871-4848   Fax: 714-773-8283
Toll-Free: 800-233-4685
Address: 4300 N. Harbor Blvd., Fullerton, CA 92834-3100 US

GROWTH PLANS/SPECIAL FEATURES:

Beckman Coulter designs, manufactures and markets systems that consist of instruments, chemistries, software and supplies that simplify and automate a variety of laboratory processes. It operates through two divisions: clinical diagnostics and biomedical research. The company's products have a range of applications, from instruments used for pioneering medical research and drug discovery to diagnostic tools found in hospitals and physicians' offices. Beckman's product lines include virtually all blood tests routinely performed in hospital laboratories and a range of systems for medical and pharmaceutical research. The organization has approximately 200,000 installed systems operating in laboratories around the world, with 64% of its annual revenues coming from sales of reagents and kits, supplies and services for its installed systems. Beckman markets its products in approximately 130 countries, with approximately 44% of its revenues coming from outside the U.S. The firm's customers include hospital clinical laboratories, physicians' offices, group practices, commercial reference laboratories, universities, medical research laboratories, pharmaceutical companies and biotechnology firms. In recent news, Beckman introduced two new laboratory automation workstations, the Biomec 3000 and the Biomek NX. The company also launched GI Monitor, a new pancreatic cancer test, and Access BR Monitor, a new breast cancer test. In addition, the firm began shipping its new GenomeLab SNPstream Genotyping System, which is capable of performing 4,600 to over 800,000 genotypes per day.

The company offers jobs in all aspects of its worldwide operations, including customer service, communications, administration and legal divisions. Beckman offers tuition reimbursement to qualified employees.

FINANCIALS:
Sales and profits are in thousands of dollars—add 000 to get the full amount. Year 2004 note: Complete fiscal 2004 results were not available for all companies at press time. For this company, year 2004 is for 9 months.

2004 Sales: $1,715,300 (9 months)   2004 Profits: $151,100 (9 months)
2003 Sales: $2,192,500   2003 Profits: $207,200
2002 Sales: $2,059,400   2002 Profits: $135,500
2001 Sales: $1,984,000   2001 Profits: $138,400
2000 Sales: $1,886,900   2000 Profits: $125,500

Stock Ticker: BEC
Employees: 9,900
Fiscal Year Ends: 12/31

SALARIES/BENEFITS:
Pension Plan: Y   ESOP Stock Plan: Profit Sharing: Top Exec. Salary: $775,000   Bonus: $706,880
Savings Plan: Y   Stock Purch. Plan: Second Exec. Salary: $425,000 Bonus: $259,500

OTHER THOUGHTS:
Apparent Top Female Officers: 1
Hot Spot for Advancement for Women/Minorities:

LOCATIONS: ("Y" = Yes)
West:	Southwest:	Midwest:	Southeast:	Northeast:	International:
Y	Y	Y	Y	Y	Y

BECTON DICKINSON & CO

www.bd.com

Industry Group Code: 339113 Ranks within this company's industry group: Sales: 5 Profits: 4

Insurance/HMO/PPO:	Drugs:	Equipment/Supplies:		Hospitals/Clinics:	Services:	Health Care:
Insurance:	Manufacturer:	Manufacturer:	Y	Acute Care:	Diagnostics:	Home Health:
Managed Care:	Distributor:	Distributor:		Sub-Acute Care:	Labs/Testing:	Long-Term Care:
Utilization Mgmt.:	Specialty Pharm.:	Leasing/Finance:		Outpatient Surgery:	Staffing:	Physical Therapy:
Payment Proc.:	Vitamins/Nutri.:	Information Sys.:		Phys. Rehab. Center:	Waste Disposal:	Phys. Practice Mgmt.:
	Clinical Trials:			Psychiatric Clinics:	Specialty Services:	

TYPES OF BUSINESS:
Equipment-Injection/Infusion
Prefillable Drug Delivery Systems
Vascular Access Products
Specialty and Surgical Blades
Disposable Scrubs
Test Kits

BRANDS/DIVISIONS/AFFILIATES:
Becton Dickinson Medical
Becton Dickinson Biosciences
Becton Dickinson Diagnostics
Vacutainer
Hypak

CONTACTS:
Note: Officers with more than one job title may be intentionally listed here more than once.

Edward J. Ludwig, CEO
Edward J. Ludwig, Pres.
John R. Considine, CFO
Jean-Marc Dageville, VP-Human Resources
Vincent A. Forlenza, Sr. VP-Tech.
Bridget M. Healy, General Counsel
William A. Kozy, Sr. VP-Oper.
Vincent A. Forlenza, Sr. VP-Strategy & Dev.
Vincent A. Forlenza, Pres., Becton Dickinson Biosciences
Gary M. Cohen, Pres., Becton Dickinson Medical
William A. Kozy, Pres., Becton Dickinson Diagnostics
Bridget M. Healy, Corp. Sec.
Edward J. Ludwig, Chmn.

Phone: 201-847-6800 **Fax:** 201-847-6475
Toll-Free: 800-284-6845
Address: 1 Becton Dr., Franklin Lakes, NJ 07417-1880 US

GROWTH PLANS/SPECIAL FEATURES:

Becton, Dickinson & Company (BD) manufactures and sells a broad line of medical supplies, devices and diagnostic systems used by health care professionals, medical research institutions and the general public. The company operates in three segments: BD Medical, BD Biosciences and BD Diagnostics. BD Medical offers hypodermic products, specially designed devices for diabetes care, prefillable drug delivery systems and infusion therapy products. It also offers anesthesia and surgical products, ophthalmic surgery devices; critical care systems, elastic support products and thermometers. BD Biosciences offers industrial microbiology products, cellular analysis systems, research and clinical reagents for cellular and nucleic acid analysis, cell culture lab ware and growth media, hematology instruments and other diagnostic systems, including immunodiagnostic test kits. BD Diagnostics offers are specimen collection products and services, consulting services and customized, automated bar-code systems for patient identification and point-of-care data capture. Two of BD's most popular products are Hypak prefillable syringes and Vacutainer blood-collection products. Outside of the U.S., BD's products are manufactured and sold in Europe, Japan, Mexico, Asia Pacific, Canada and Brazil. BD Biosciences and NuGenesis Technologies are currently working to provide a productivity solution that creates an easy-to-use data management and archival system for flow cytometry data. The company recently announced the discontinuation of sales of many conventional needles across a range of product categories, reflecting an industry focus on creating safer alternatives to protect healthcare workers from accidental injury. In other news, the company is researching lab-on-a-chip nanotechnology for the identification of proteins and enzymes, nano-drug delivery systems and nano-tagging systems for biological research.

The firm offers employees fitness centers, an employee assistance program and adoption assistance, as well as stock options and scholarship programs. The company's LifeWorks program provides employees and families with information on topics ranging from retirement to adoption. Larger facilities have heath centers offering preventive health screenings and routine examinations.

FINANCIALS:
Sales and profits are in thousands of dollars—add 000 to get the full amount. Year 2004 note: Complete fiscal 2004 results were not available for all companies at press time. For this company, year 2004 is for 9 months.

2004 Sales: $3,727,809 (9 months)	2004 Profits: $399,958 (9 months)	**Stock Ticker:** BDX
2003 Sales: $4,527,940	2003 Profits: $547,056	**Employees:** 24,783
2002 Sales: $4,033,100	2002 Profits: $480,000	**Fiscal Year Ends:** 9/30
2001 Sales: $3,754,300	2001 Profits: $401,600	
2000 Sales: $3,618,300	2000 Profits: $392,900	

SALARIES/BENEFITS:
Pension Plan: Y ESOP Stock Plan: Profit Sharing: Top Exec. Salary: $850,000 Bonus: $750,000
Savings Plan: Y Stock Purch. Plan: Second Exec. Salary: $535,000 Bonus: $410,000

OTHER THOUGHTS:
Apparent Top Female Officers: 1
Hot Spot for Advancement for Women/Minorities:

LOCATIONS: ("Y" = Yes)
West:	Southwest:	Midwest:	Southeast:	Northeast:	International:
Y	Y	Y	Y	Y	Y

Note: Financial information, benefits and other data can change quickly and may vary from those stated here.

BESPAK PLC

www.bespak.com

Industry Group Code: 339113 **Ranks within this company's industry group:** Sales: 75 Profits: 90

Insurance/HMO/PPO:	Drugs:	Equipment/Supplies:		Hospitals/Clinics:	Services:		Health Care:
Insurance:	Manufacturer:	Manufacturer:	Y	Acute Care:	Diagnostics:		Home Health:
Managed Care:	Distributor:	Distributor:		Sub-Acute Care:	Labs/Testing:		Long-Term Care:
Utilization Mgmt.:	Specialty Pharm.:	Leasing/Finance:		Outpatient Surgery:	Staffing:		Physical Therapy:
Payment Proc.:	Vitamins/Nutri.:	Information Sys.:		Phys. Rehab. Center:	Waste Disposal:		Phys. Practice Mgmt.:
	Clinical Trials:			Psychiatric Clinics:	Specialty Services:	Y	

TYPES OF BUSINESS:
Drug Delivery Technologies
Medical Devices
Development and Manufacturing Services

BRANDS/DIVISIONS/AFFILIATES:
Diskus

CONTACTS:
Note: Officers with more than one job title may be intentionally listed here more than once.

Mark C. Throdahl, Chief Exec.
Martin P. Hopcroft, Group Finance Dir.
Chris Halling, Mktg. Mgr.
Ginny Hargrove, Head-Human Resources
Tom Hawkins, Media Contact
Louise Scott, Corp. Sec.
John Robinson, Chmn.

Phone: 44-1908-552-600 **Fax:** 44-1908-552-613
Toll-Free:
Address: Blackhill Dr., Featherstone Rd., Wolverton Mill South, Milton Keynes MK12 5TS UK

GROWTH PLANS/SPECIAL FEATURES:

Bespak plc is a leading developer, manufacturer and supplier of drug delivery technologies, medical devices and associated services to pharmaceutical, drug delivery and biotechnology companies. The firm's proprietary drug delivery devices and technologies include pressurized metered-dose inhalers and actuators, dose counters, breath-coordinated and breath-activated devices, dry powder inhalers and electrostatic atomization, as well as a range of unit and multi-dose, liquid and dry powder nasal devices. The company's devices enable patients to take their medications without using needle injections or having to swallow a pill. In addition, Bespak provides complete medical device development services to other companies, from prototyping and testing to clinical trials and regulatory compliance to industrialization and full-scale manufacture. The firm also offers access to its range of proprietary drug delivery devices. In recent news, Bespak announced a co-marketing agreement with Cardinal Health, Inc., a leading provider of products and services that support the health care industry. The FDA approved GlaxoSmithKline's Advair Diskus 250/50 asthma inhaler, utilizing the company's Diskus drug delivery device. The firm also agreed to develop, at its own expense, the delivery device for Britannia Pharmaceuticals' AdSurf, which is now in Phase III clinical trials for the prevention of surgical adhesions.

FINANCIALS:
Sales and profits are in thousands of dollars—add 000 to get the full amount. Year 2004 note: Complete fiscal 2004 results were not available for all companies at press time. For this company, year 2004 is for months.

2004 Sales: $ (months)	2004 Profits: $ (months)	
2003 Sales: $140,800	2003 Profits: $4,400	**Stock Ticker:** Foreign
2002 Sales: $146,300	2002 Profits: $	**Employees:** 826
2001 Sales: $	2001 Profits: $	**Fiscal Year Ends:** 4/30
2000 Sales: $	2000 Profits: $	

SALARIES/BENEFITS:
Pension Plan:	ESOP Stock Plan:	Profit Sharing:	Top Exec. Salary: $	Bonus: $
Savings Plan:	Stock Purch. Plan:		Second Exec. Salary: $	Bonus: $

OTHER THOUGHTS:
Apparent Top Female Officers: 2
Hot Spot for Advancement for Women/Minorities:

LOCATIONS: ("Y" = Yes)
West:	Southwest:	Midwest:	Southeast:	Northeast:	International:
				Y	Y

BEVERLY ENTERPRISES INC

www.beverlycares.com

Industry Group Code: 623110   Ranks within this company's industry group: Sales: 3   Profits: 2

Insurance/HMO/PPO:	Drugs:	Equipment/Supplies:	Hospitals/Clinics:		Services:		Health Care:	
Insurance:	Manufacturer:	Manufacturer:	Acute Care:		Diagnostics:		Home Health:	Y
Managed Care:	Distributor:	Distributor:	Sub-Acute Care:		Labs/Testing:		Long-Term Care:	Y
Utilization Mgmt.:	Specialty Pharm.:	Leasing/Finance:	Outpatient Surgery:		Staffing:		Physical Therapy:	Y
Payment Proc.:	Vitamins/Nutri.:	Information Sys.:	Phys. Rehab. Center:	Y	Waste Disposal:		Phys. Practice Mgmt.:	
	Clinical Trials:		Psychiatric Clinics:		Specialty Services:	Y		

TYPES OF BUSINESS:
Long-Term Health Care/Nursing Homes
Web-Based Procurement Management
Assisted Living Centers
Rehabilitation Therapy Services
Outpatient Therapy Clinics
Hospice Centers
Home Care Services
Case Management Services

BRANDS/DIVISIONS/AFFILIATES:
Ceres Purchasing Solutions
Aegis Therapies, Inc.

CONTACTS: Note: Officers with more than one job title may be intentionally listed here more than once.
William R. Floyd, CEO
William R. Floyd, Pres.
Jeffrey P. Freimark, Exec. VP/CFO
Blaise J. Mercadante, VP-Mktg. & New Bus. Innovation
Lawrence Deans, Sr. VP-Human Resources
Jeffrey P. Freimark, CIO
Douglas J. Babb, Exec. VP/Chief Admin. Officer
Douglas J. Babb, Chief Legal Officer/Corp. Sec.
Harold A. Price, VP-Bus. Dev. & Sales
James M. Griffith, VP-Corp. Comm.
James M. Griffith, VP-Investor Rel.
Pamela H. Daniels, Sr. VP/Controller/Chief Acct. Officer
David R. Devereaux, COO-Nursing Facilities
Cindy H. Susienka, Pres., AEGIS Therapies, Inc. & Home Care
Chris W. Roussos, Pres., Ceres Purchasing Solutions
Barbara R. Paul, Sr. VP/Chief Medical Officer
William R. Floyd, Chmn.

Phone: 479-201-2000   Fax: 479-201-1101
Toll-Free: 877-823-8375
Address: 1000 Beverly Way, Ft. Smith, AR 72919 US

GROWTH PLANS/SPECIAL FEATURES:
Beverly Enterprises, Inc. provides long-term health care services, including the operation of nursing facilities, assisted living centers, hospice and home care centers, outpatient therapy clinics and rehabilitation therapy services. The company is one of the largest operators of nursing facilities in the U.S., with 368 facilities with a total of 38,781 licensed beds in 23 states and the District of Columbia. Beverly owns 19 assisted living centers containing 526 units, 10 outpatient therapy clinics and 25 hospice and home care centers. In addition, it provides rehabilitation therapy services in 35 states and D.C. The company operates through three primary segments: nursing facilities, Aegis Therapies and home care. Beverly's nursing facilities segment offers long-term care, skilled nursing and assisted living services. Long-term care services include daily nursing, dietary, social and recreational services and a full range of pharmacy services and medical supplies. Aegis Therapies, a leading contract rehabilitation company, serves Beverly and non-Beverly businesses and offers physical, occupational and speech therapy. The home care segment offers hospice care, home health services, infusion therapy and home medical equipment.

Beverly provides employees with health insurance, child care assistance and paid time off.

FINANCIALS:
Sales and profits are in thousands of dollars—add 000 to get the full amount. Year 2004 note: Complete fiscal 2004 results were not available for all companies at press time. For this company, year 2004 is for 9 months.

2004 Sales: $1,486,304 (9 months)	2004 Profits: $21,916 (9 months)	**Stock Ticker:** BEV
2003 Sales: $1,996,981	2003 Profits: $80,468	Employees: 36,300
2002 Sales: $2,419,900	2002 Profits: $-146,100	Fiscal Year Ends: 12/31
2001 Sales: $2,709,900	2001 Profits: $-301,300	
2000 Sales: $2,628,260	2000 Profits: $-54,502	

SALARIES/BENEFITS:
Pension Plan:	ESOP Stock Plan:	Profit Sharing:	Top Exec. Salary: $834,591	Bonus: $1,337,414
Savings Plan: Y	Stock Purch. Plan: Y		Second Exec. Salary: $427,786	Bonus: $420,949

OTHER THOUGHTS:
Apparent Top Female Officers: 3
Hot Spot for Advancement for Women/Minorities: Y

LOCATIONS: ("Y" = Yes)
West:	Southwest:	Midwest:	Southeast:	Northeast:	International:
Y	Y	Y	Y	Y	

BIO RAD LABORATORIES INC

www.bio-rad.com

Industry Group Code: 339113 **Ranks within this company's industry group:** Sales: 27 Profits: 22

Insurance/HMO/PPO:	Drugs:	Equipment/Supplies:		Hospitals/Clinics:	Services:		Health Care:	
Insurance:	Manufacturer:	Manufacturer:	Y	Acute Care:	Diagnostics:	Y	Home Health:	
Managed Care:	Distributor:	Distributor:		Sub-Acute Care:	Labs/Testing:	Y	Long-Term Care:	
Utilization Mgmt.:	Specialty Pharm.:	Leasing/Finance:		Outpatient Surgery:	Staffing:		Physical Therapy:	
Payment Proc.:	Vitamins/Nutri.:	Information Sys.:	Y	Phys. Rehab. Center:	Waste Disposal:		Phys. Practice Mgmt.:	
	Clinical Trials:			Psychiatric Clinics:	Specialty Services:			

TYPES OF BUSINESS:
Equipment-Life Sciences Research
Clinical Diagnostics Products
Analytical Instruments
Laboratory Devices
Biomaterials
Imaging Products
Assays
Software

BRANDS/DIVISIONS/AFFILIATES:
PhD Workstation
Hematronix, Inc.
VersArray
SmartSpec Plus
PowerPac HC
Rapid D-10
Osiris
Evolis

CONTACTS:
Note: Officers with more than one job title may be intentionally listed here more than once.

Norman Schwartz, CEO
Norman Schwartz, Pres.
James J. Bennett, COO
Christine Tsingos, VP/CFO
Sanford S. Wadler, VP/General Counsel
James R. Stark, Corp. Controller
John Goetz, VP/Group Mgr.
Sanford S. Wadler, Corp. Sec.
David Schwartz, Chmn.

Phone: 510-724-7000	Fax: 510-741-5817
Toll-Free: 800-224-6723	
Address: 1000 Alfred Nobel Dr., Hercules, CA 94547 US	

GROWTH PLANS/SPECIAL FEATURES:
Bio-Rad Laboratories supplies the life science research, health care and analytical chemistry markets with a broad range of products and systems used to separate complex chemical and biological materials and to identify, analyze and purify their components. The firm's life science division develops laboratory devices, biomaterials, imaging products and microscopy systems. The division uses electrophoresis, image analysis and microplate readers, chromatography, gene transfer and sample preparation and amplification as its primary technological applications. Bio-Rad provides its services to universities and medical schools, industrial research organizations, government agencies, pharmaceutical manufacturers and biotechnology researchers. The company's clinical diagnostics division encompasses a broad array of technologies incorporated into a variety of tests used to detect, identify and quantify substances in blood or other bodily fluids and tissues. The test results are used as aids for medical diagnosis, detection, evaluation, monitoring and treatment of diseases and other medical conditions. In addition, Bio-Rad is a leading provider of bovine spongiform encephalopathy (BSE) or mad cow tests throughout the world. Recently, Bio-Rad sold its Confocal Microscopy business to Carl Zeiss. The company acquired the majority of assets of Hematronix, Inc., a full-line manufacturer of hematology and urine controls, hematology reagents and regulatory products and services. The firm's life science division launched its new VersArray hybridization chamber, SmartSpec Plus spectrophotometer, PowerPac HC power supply and the Quick Start Bradford Protein Assay products. The clinical diagnostics division introduced its Rapid D-10 Dual Assay Program, Osiris data management software, PhD Workstation and the Evolis fully automated microplate processing system. In addition, Bio-Rad began marketing a new salmonella culture media and a new BSE testing system used in Europe.

Bio-Rad provides tuition reimbursement and dental and vision insurance to its employees.

FINANCIALS:
Sales and profits are in thousands of dollars—add 000 to get the full amount. Year 2004 note: Complete fiscal 2004 results were not available for all companies at press time. For this company, year 2004 is for 9 months.

2004 Sales: $782,144 (9 months)	2004 Profits: $51,131 (9 months)	
2003 Sales: $1,003,382	2003 Profits: $76,171	**Stock Ticker:** BIO
2002 Sales: $892,700	2002 Profits: $67,900	Employees: 4,800
2001 Sales: $817,500	2001 Profits: $44,200	Fiscal Year Ends: 12/31
2000 Sales: $725,884	2000 Profits: $31,100	

SALARIES/BENEFITS:
Pension Plan:	ESOP Stock Plan:	Profit Sharing: Y	Top Exec. Salary: $509,440	Bonus: $166,248
Savings Plan: Y	Stock Purch. Plan: Y		Second Exec. Salary: $455,414	Bonus: $150,082

OTHER THOUGHTS:
Apparent Top Female Officers: 1
Hot Spot for Advancement for Women/Minorities:

LOCATIONS: ("Y" = Yes)
West:	Southwest:	Midwest:	Southeast:	Northeast:	International:
Y		Y		Y	Y

BIO REFERENCE LABORATORIES INC

www.bio-referencelabs.com

Industry Group Code: 621511   Ranks within this company's industry group: Sales: 9   Profits: 5

Insurance/HMO/PPO:	Drugs:	Equipment/Supplies:	Hospitals/Clinics:	Services:	Health Care:
Insurance:	Manufacturer:	Manufacturer:	Acute Care:	Diagnostics:	Home Health:
Managed Care:	Distributor:	Distributor:	Sub-Acute Care:	Labs/Testing: Y	Long-Term Care:
Utilization Mgmt.:	Specialty Pharm.:	Leasing/Finance:	Outpatient Surgery:	Staffing:	Physical Therapy:
Payment Proc.:	Vitamins/Nutri.:	Information Sys.:	Phys. Rehab. Center:	Waste Disposal:	Phys. Practice Mgmt.:
	Clinical Trials:		Psychiatric Clinics:	Specialty Services: Y	

TYPES OF BUSINESS:
Services-Laboratories & Testing
Clinical Laboratory Services
Clinical Knowledge Database
Physician-Based Health Portal

BRANDS/DIVISIONS/AFFILIATES:
PSIMedica
careevolve.com

CONTACTS:
Note: Officers with more than one job title may be intentionally listed here more than once.

Marc D. Grodman, CEO
Marc D. Grodman, Pres.
Howard Dubinett, Exec. VP/COO
Sam Singer, VP/CFO
Charles T. Todd, Sr. VP-Mktg. & Sales
Richard L. Faherty, CIO
Kara Kelly, Investor Rel. Coordinator
Nicholas Papazicos, VP-Financial Oper.
Richard L. Faherty, CEO-PSIMedica & careevolve.com
Warren Erdmann, VP/General Mgr.
Nick Cetani, VP/Lab Mgr.
Bader Maria Pedemonte-Coira, Chief Medical Officer
Marc D. Grodman, Chmn.

Phone: 201-791-2186   **Fax:**
Toll-Free: 800-229-5227
Address: 481 Edward H. Ross Dr., Elmwood Park, NJ 07407 US

GROWTH PLANS/SPECIAL FEATURES:

Bio-Reference Laboratories, Inc. is a regional clinical laboratory offering services to clients in most parts of New York and New Jersey. Serving health care providers in these areas, Bio-Reference offers testing services utilized in detection, diagnosis, evaluation, monitoring and treatment of diseases. Tests are performed at processing facilities in Elmwood Park, New Jersey and Valley Cottage, New York, with samples taken at 52 small draw stations in the New York metropolitan area. Routine tests, which account for approximately 72% of the company's clinical business, include blood cell counts, cholesterol level testing, HIV-related tests, pap smears, pregnancy tests, urinalysis and drug trace testing. The company also performs specialized testing in medical fields such as endocrinology, genetics, immunology, microbiology, oncology, serology and toxicology. The firm's primary source of business is from physicians, though it also provides testing for government agencies, large employer groups and correctional facilities. Bio-Reference's PSIMedica division operates a clinical knowledge management system that analyses enrollment, claims, pharmacy, laboratory results and other data, providing administrative and clinical analysis of a population. In addition, the company hosts careevolve.com, a physician-based health portal that seeks to enhance physician-to-patient and physician-to-payer electronic communications. These communications include secure notification of lab results, e-mail prescriptions, payer verification and eligibility, as well as other Internet-based services. In 2004, Bio-Reference acquired the molecular and cytogenetics facilities of Cancer Genetics, Inc., including commercial diagnostic laboratory facilities in Milford, Massachusetts.

FINANCIALS:
Sales and profits are in thousands of dollars—add 000 to get the full amount. Year 2004 note: Complete fiscal 2004 results were not available for all companies at press time. For this company, year 2004 is for 9 months.

2004 Sales: $98,440 (9 months)   2004 Profits: $5,203 (9 months)
2003 Sales: $109,033   2003 Profits: $6,539
2002 Sales: $96,600   2002 Profits: $4,900
2001 Sales: $80,600   2001 Profits: $2,400
2000 Sales: $66,460   2000 Profits: $ 105

Stock Ticker: BRLI
Employees: 828
Fiscal Year Ends: 10/31

SALARIES/BENEFITS:
| Pension Plan: | ESOP Stock Plan: | Profit Sharing: | Top Exec. Salary: $499,750 | Bonus: $125,000 |
| Savings Plan: | Stock Purch. Plan: | | Second Exec. Salary: $240,000 | Bonus: $60,000 |

OTHER THOUGHTS:
Apparent Top Female Officers: 2
Hot Spot for Advancement for Women/Minorities:

LOCATIONS: ("Y" = Yes)
| West: | Southwest: | Midwest: | Southeast: | Northeast: Y | International: |

BIOGEN IDEC INC

www.biogenidec.com

Industry Group Code: 325412 **Ranks within this company's industry group:** Sales: 33 Profits: 42

Insurance/HMO/PPO:	Drugs:	Equipment/Supplies:	Hospitals/Clinics:	Services:	Health Care:
Insurance:	Manufacturer: Y	Manufacturer:	Acute Care:	Diagnostics:	Home Health:
Managed Care:	Distributor:	Distributor:	Sub-Acute Care:	Labs/Testing:	Long-Term Care:
Utilization Mgmt.:	Specialty Pharm.:	Leasing/Finance:	Outpatient Surgery:	Staffing:	Physical Therapy:
Payment Proc.:	Vitamins/Nutri.:	Information Sys.:	Phys. Rehab. Center:	Waste Disposal:	Phys. Practice Mgmt.:
	Clinical Trials:		Psychiatric Clinics:	Specialty Services:	

TYPES OF BUSINESS:
Drugs-Multiple Sclerosis
Psoriasis Treatments
Genetic Engineering
Vaccines

BRANDS/DIVISIONS/AFFILIATES:
AVONEX
AMEVIVE
ANTEGREN

CONTACTS:
Note: Officers with more than one job title may be intentionally listed here more than once.

James C. Mullen, CEO
James C. Mullen, Pres.
William R. Rohn, COO
Peter N. Kellogg, CFO
Craig E. Schneier, VP-Human Resources
Michael Gilman, Exec. VP-Research
Thomas J. Bucknum, General Counsel
Mark Wiggins, Exec. VP-Bus. Dev.
Connie L. Matsui, VP-Corp. Comm.
John M. Dunn, Exec. VP-New Ventures
William H. Rastetter, Chmn.

Phone: 617-679-2000 **Fax:** 617-679-2617
Toll-Free:
Address: 14 Cambridge Ctr., Cambridge, MA 02142-1481 US

GROWTH PLANS/SPECIAL FEATURES:
Ranking near the top of all biotech firms, Biogen IDEC, Inc. develops, manufactures and markets novel therapeutic products. AVONEX is used to decrease the frequency of neurological attacks in patients with relapsing forms of multiple sclerosis (MS). For adults with moderate to severe chronic plaque psoriasis who are candidates for systemic therapy or phototherapy, Biogen produces the biologic therapy AMEVIVE. Biogen is conducting clinical studies of a number of drugs, including ANTEGREN, which the company developed in collaboration with Elan Corporation. ANTEGREN, a humanized monoclonal antibody, has the potential to treat MS and Crohn's disease. Biogen also generates revenue by licensing drugs it has developed to other companies, including Schering-Plough, Merck and Abbott Laboratories. The company's licensed products include alpha interferon and hepatitis B vaccines. In addition to its drug portfolio, Biogen operates three licensed and dedicated bulk biological manufacturing facilities, including one of the world's largest cell culture facilities. In June 2004, Biogen IDEC announced that its license application for ANTEGREN earned priority review and accelerated approval designation from the FDA. In July, the company officially began operating its new international headquarters in Zug, Switzerland.

Biogen offers its employees dental insurance, tuition reimbursement, referral bonuses and on-site fitness centers at some locations.

FINANCIALS:
Sales and profits are in thousands of dollars—add 000 to get the full amount. Year 2004 note: Complete fiscal 2004 results were not available for all companies at press time. For this company, year 2004 is for 9 months.

2004 Sales: $1,623,782 (9 months)   2004 Profits: $-3,603 (9 months)
2003 Sales: $679,183   2003 Profits: $-875,097
2002 Sales: $404,222   2002 Profits: $148,090
2001 Sales: $ 2001 Profits: $
2000 Sales: $ 2000 Profits: $

Stock Ticker: BGEN
Employees: 3,727
Fiscal Year Ends: 12/31

SALARIES/BENEFITS:
Pension Plan: Y   ESOP Stock Plan: Profit Sharing: Top Exec. Salary: $691,846   Bonus: $465,000
Savings Plan: Y   Stock Purch. Plan: Y   Second Exec. Salary: $445,571   Bonus: $211,012

OTHER THOUGHTS:
Apparent Top Female Officers: 1
Hot Spot for Advancement for Women/Minorities:

LOCATIONS: ("Y" = Yes)
West:	Southwest:	Midwest:	Southeast:	Northeast:	International:
				Y	Y

ent
BIOMET INC

www.biomet.com

Industry Group Code: 339113 **Ranks within this company's industry group:** Sales: 20 Profits: 10

Insurance/HMO/PPO:	Drugs:	Equipment/Supplies:	Hospitals/Clinics:	Services:	Health Care:
Insurance:	Manufacturer:	Manufacturer: Y	Acute Care:	Diagnostics:	Home Health:
Managed Care:	Distributor:	Distributor:	Sub-Acute Care:	Labs/Testing:	Long-Term Care:
Utilization Mgmt.:	Specialty Pharm.:	Leasing/Finance:	Outpatient Surgery:	Staffing:	Physical Therapy:
Payment Proc.:	Vitamins/Nutri.:	Information Sys.:	Phys. Rehab. Center:	Waste Disposal:	Phys. Practice Mgmt.:
	Clinical Trials:		Psychiatric Clinics:	Specialty Services:	

TYPES OF BUSINESS:
Supplies-Orthopedic
Electrical Bone Growth Stimulators
Orthopedic Support Devices
Operating Room Supplies
Powered Surgical Instruments
Arthroscopy Products
Imaging Equipment
Human Bone Joint Replacement Systems

BRANDS/DIVISIONS/AFFILIATES:
Anthrotek, Inc.
Walter Lorenz Surgical, Inc.
EBI, LP
Biomet Merck Group
3i
Interpore International
Maxim Total Knee System
Finn Knee Replacement System

CONTACTS:
Note: Officers with more than one job title may be intentionally listed here more than once.

Dane A. Miller, CEO
Dane A. Miller, Pres.
Gregory D. Hartman, CFO
William C. Kolter, VP-Mktg.
Darlene K. Whaley, VP-Human Resources
Anthony L. Flemming, VP-R&D
Richard J. Borror, Jr., VP-Mfg.
Daniel P. Hann, General Counsel
Thomas R. Allen, VP-Oper., Americas & Asia Pacific
Greg W. Sasso, VP-Corp. Dev.
Greg W. Sasso, VP-Corp. Comm.
Gregory D. Hartman, Sr. VP-Finance/Treas.
Garry L. England, Sr. VP-Warsaw Oper.
Craig Blaschke, VP-Biomaterials Tech.
David L. Montgomery, VP-Sales, Biomet Orthopedics, Inc.
James W. Haller, VP-Finance, Biomet Orthopedics, Inc.
Niles L. Noblitt, Chmn.
Charles E. Niemier, Sr. VP-Int'l Oper.

Phone: 574-267-6639 **Fax:** 574-267-8137
Toll-Free: 800-348-9500
Address: 56 E. Bell Dr., Warsaw, IN 46582 US

GROWTH PLANS/SPECIAL FEATURES:

Biomet, Inc. designs, manufactures and markets products used primarily by musculoskeletal medical specialists in both surgical and non-surgical therapies. Products include reconstructive and fixation devices, electrical bone growth stimulators, orthopedic support devices, operating room supplies, general surgical instruments, arthroscopy products, spinal products, bone cements and accessories, bone substitute materials, craniomaxillofacial implants and instruments and dental reconstructive implants and associated instrumentation. Biomet manufactures numerous knee systems, including the Maxim Total Knee System, the Finn Knee Replacement System and the AGC Total Knee System. The firm also manufactures several hip and shoulder replacement systems. Biomet's Arthrotek, Inc. subsidiary manufactures surgical systems, pumps, shavers, cameras, arthroscopic imagers and bone cement removal systems, while its Walter Lorenz Surgical, Inc. subsidiary manufactures orthopedic equipment. The firm's other subsidiaries are Biomet Merck Group; EBI, LP, formerly Electro-Biology, Inc.; and 3i, formerly Implant Innovations, Inc. Biomet recently completed its acquisition of Interpore International, a maker of spinal surgery products, and has signed an agreement with Diamicron, Inc. to distribute its diamond articulation technology for total hip arthroplasty worldwide.

Biomet invests in the communities where it conducts business and encourages employees to participate in nonprofit, charitable, educational, civic, cultural and service organizations.

FINANCIALS:
Sales and profits are in thousands of dollars—add 000 to get the full amount. Year 2004 note: Complete fiscal 2004 results were not available for all companies at press time. For this company, year 2004 is for 12 months.

2004 Sales: $1,615,751 (12 months)   2004 Profits: $325,627 (12 months)
2003 Sales: $1,390,300   2003 Profits: $286,700
2002 Sales: $1,191,900   2002 Profits: $239,700
2001 Sales: $1,030,700   2001 Profits: $197,500
2000 Sales: $923,600   2000 Profits: $173,771

Stock Ticker: BMET
Employees: 3,620
Fiscal Year Ends: 5/31

SALARIES/BENEFITS:
Pension Plan: ESOP Stock Plan: Profit Sharing: Top Exec. Salary: $279,700   Bonus: $230,000
Savings Plan: Y   Stock Purch. Plan: Second Exec. Salary: $273,800   Bonus: $209,000

OTHER THOUGHTS:
Apparent Top Female Officers: 1
Hot Spot for Advancement for Women/Minorities:

LOCATIONS: ("Y" = Yes)
West:	Southwest:	Midwest:	Southeast:	Northeast:	International:
Y	Y	Y	Y	Y	Y

Note: Financial information, benefits and other data can change quickly and may vary from those stated here.

BIOPHAN TECHNOLOGIES INC

www.biophan.com

Industry Group Code: 339113 Ranks within this company's industry group: Sales: Profits: 117

Insurance/HMO/PPO:	Drugs:	Equipment/Supplies:	Hospitals/Clinics:	Services:	Health Care:
Insurance:	Manufacturer:	Manufacturer: Y	Acute Care:	Diagnostics:	Home Health:
Managed Care:	Distributor:	Distributor:	Sub-Acute Care:	Labs/Testing:	Long-Term Care:
Utilization Mgmt.:	Specialty Pharm.:	Leasing/Finance:	Outpatient Surgery:	Staffing:	Physical Therapy:
Payment Proc.:	Vitamins/Nutri.:	Information Sys.:	Phys. Rehab. Center:	Waste Disposal:	Phys. Practice Mgmt.:
	Clinical Trials:		Psychiatric Clinics:	Specialty Services:	

TYPES OF BUSINESS:

Medical Equipment-Manufacturing
MRI Products and Contrast Agents
Biomedical Coatings
Polymer Composites
Photonics

BRANDS/DIVISIONS/AFFILIATES:

NanoView

CONTACTS: Note: Officers with more than one job title may be intentionally listed here more than once.

Michael L. Weiner, CEO
Robert J. Wood, CFO
Stuart G. MacDonald, VP-Research and Dev.
Jeffrey L. Helfer, VP-Eng.
Racquel Rivera, VP-Investor Rel.
Robert J. Wood, VP/Treas.
Guenter Jaensch, Chmn.

Phone: 585-214-2441 **Fax:** 585-427-2433
Toll-Free:
Address: 150 Lucius Gordon Dr., Ste. 215, West Henrietta, NY 14586 US

GROWTH PLANS/SPECIAL FEATURES:

Biophan Technologies, Inc. is developing products to make biomedical devices, such as pacemakers, other implanted devices and devices used in surgical and diagnostic procedures, safe and compatible with MRI equipment. The firm is also using its technology to create enhanced MRI contrast agents. The company currently has four issued U.S. patents and over 50 patents pending, in areas including nanomagnetic particle coatings, radio frequency filters, polymer composites and photonics. The firm's nanoparticle-based biomedical coating, NanoView, significantly reduces tissue damage, interference in image quality and other problems caused by medical implants during MRI scans. Nanomagnetic coating shields the strong electromagnetic radio waves that are generated when the EM fields created during an MRI scan interacts with implanted medical devices. Without such shielding, the EM fields could heat the metal implants and damage tissues surrounding them, which could prove fatal. Other medical devices such as guide wires, catheters and endoscopes can also utilize NanoView for shielding. In addition to coating capabilities, these nanomaterials can be employed as MRI contrast agents that highlight specific tissues that may be infected or malfunctioning. In recent news, Biophan secured up to $25 million in additional funding from SBI-Brightline.

FINANCIALS: Sales and profits are in thousands of dollars—add 000 to get the full amount. Year 2004 note: Complete fiscal 2004 results were not available for all companies at press time. For this company, year 2004 is for 12 months.

2004 Sales: $ 75 (12 months)   2004 Profits: $-3,718 (12 months)
2003 Sales: $ 2003 Profits: $-3,438
2002 Sales: $ 75   2002 Profits: $-3,706
2001 Sales: $ 2001 Profits: $- 729
2000 Sales: $ 2000 Profits: $

Stock Ticker: BIPH
Employees: 11
Fiscal Year Ends: 2/28

SALARIES/BENEFITS:

Pension Plan: ESOP Stock Plan: Profit Sharing: Top Exec. Salary: $175,000   Bonus: $
Savings Plan: Stock Purch. Plan: Second Exec. Salary: $116,057 Bonus: $

OTHER THOUGHTS:

Apparent Top Female Officers: 1
Hot Spot for Advancement for Women/Minorities:

LOCATIONS: ("Y" = Yes)

West:	Southwest:	Midwest:	Southeast:	Northeast: Y	International:

BIOVAIL CORPORATION

www.biovail.com

Industry Group Code: 325412 Ranks within this company's industry group: Sales: 29 Profits: 31

Insurance/HMO/PPO:	Drugs:		Equipment/Supplies:	Hospitals/Clinics:	Services:	Health Care:
Insurance: Managed Care: Utilization Mgmt.: Payment Proc.:	Manufacturer: Distributor: Specialty Pharm.: Vitamins/Nutri.: Clinical Trials:	Y	Manufacturer: Distributor: Leasing/Finance: Information Sys.:	Acute Care: Sub-Acute Care: Outpatient Surgery: Phys. Rehab. Center: Psychiatric Clinics:	Diagnostics: Labs/Testing: Staffing: Waste Disposal: Specialty Services:	Home Health: Long-Term Care: Physical Therapy: Phys. Practice Mgmt.:

TYPES OF BUSINESS:
Drugs-Hypertension
Generic Drugs
Drug Delivery Technologies
Nutraceuticals

BRANDS/DIVISIONS/AFFILIATES:
Biovail Pharmaceuticals, Inc.
Biovail Pharmaceuticals Canada
FlashDose
SportSafe
Wellbutrin XL
Nutravail Technologies, Inc.
Biovail Ventures
Cardizem LA

CONTACTS:
Note: Officers with more than one job title may be intentionally listed here more than once.
Eugene N. Melnyk, CEO
Brian H. Crombie, Sr. VP/CFO
Mark Durham, VP-Corp. Human Resources
Gregory J. Szpunar, Sr. VP/Chief Scientific Officer
Patrick Dwyer, VP-Mfg.
Kenneth C. Cancellara, Sr. VP/Chief Legal Officer/Corp. Sec.
Kris Peterson, Sr. VP-Commercial Oper.
Rolf K. Reininghaus, Sr. VP-Corp. & Strategic Dev.
Kenneth G. Howling, VP-Finance
John Miszuk, VP/Controller
John Sebben, VP-Global Mfg.
Eugene N. Melnyk, Chmn.

Phone: 905-286-3000 Fax: 905-286-3050
Toll-Free:
Address: 7150 Mississauga Rd., Mississauga, Ontario L5N8M5 Canada

GROWTH PLANS/SPECIAL FEATURES:
Biovail Corp. is a full-service pharmaceutical company involved in the development, testing, registration, manufacturing, sale and marketing of pharmaceutical products that make use of its oral controlled-release and FlashDose technologies. Biovail markets its own and other select licensed products directly to health care professionals through its North American sales operations at Biovail Pharmaceuticals, Inc. and Biovail Pharmaceuticals Canada. The company develops and markets products in the areas of cardiovascular disease, pain management and central nervous system therapy, with an emphasis on chronic care medications. In addition, Biovail Ventures invests in strategic technology partnerships, early-stage development companies and acquisitions that will strengthen its core competencies. Its most famous drug, marketed worldwide through GlaxoSmithKline, is antidepressant Wellbutrin XL. The company also owns Nutravail Technologies, Inc., which specializes in the development of innovative nutraceuticals, nutritional products and functional foods, with over 80 patents, including the SportSafe line of products. In recent news, the firm received FDA approval for Cardizem LA, for the treatment of chronic stable angina.

FINANCIALS:
Sales and profits are in thousands of dollars—add 000 to get the full amount. Year 2004 note: Complete fiscal 2004 results were not available for all companies at press time. For this company, year 2004 is for 6 months.

2004 Sales: $392,900 (6 months)	2004 Profits: $65,300 (6 months)	Stock Ticker: Foreign
2003 Sales: $823,700	2003 Profits: $-27,300	Employees: 1,322
2002 Sales: $788,000	2002 Profits: $87,800	Fiscal Year Ends: 12/31
2001 Sales: $583,300	2001 Profits: $87,400	
2000 Sales: $309,200	2000 Profits: $-148,000	

SALARIES/BENEFITS:
Pension Plan: ESOP Stock Plan: Y Profit Sharing: Top Exec. Salary: $668,699 Bonus: $219,793
Savings Plan: Stock Purch. Plan: Y Second Exec. Salary: $412,923 Bonus: $219,793

OTHER THOUGHTS:
Apparent Top Female Officers:
Hot Spot for Advancement for Women/Minorities:

LOCATIONS: ("Y" = Yes)
West:	Southwest:	Midwest:	Southeast:	Northeast:	International:
				Y	Y

BJC HEALTHCARE

www.bjc.org

Industry Group Code: 622110   Ranks within this company's industry group: Sales: 27   Profits:

Insurance/HMO/PPO:	Drugs:	Equipment/Supplies:	Hospitals/Clinics:		Services:		Health Care:	
Insurance:	Manufacturer:	Manufacturer:	Acute Care:	Y	Diagnostics:		Home Health:	Y
Managed Care:	Distributor:	Distributor:	Sub-Acute Care:	Y	Labs/Testing:		Long-Term Care:	Y
Utilization Mgmt.:	Specialty Pharm.:	Leasing/Finance:	Outpatient Surgery:		Staffing:		Physical Therapy:	
Payment Proc.:	Vitamins/Nutri.:	Information Sys.:	Phys. Rehab. Center:	Y	Waste Disposal:		Phys. Practice Mgmt.:	Y
	Clinical Trials:		Psychiatric Clinics:		Specialty Services:	Y		

TYPES OF BUSINESS:

Hospitals
Home Health Services
Physical Rehab Center
Physician Groups
Long-Term Health Care
Occupational Health Services
Hospice Services

BRANDS/DIVISIONS/AFFILIATES:

Barnes-Jewish Hospital
St. Louis Children's Hospital
Rehabilitation Institute of St. Louis (The)
BJC Home Care Services
BJC Corporate Health Services
BarnesCare
OccuMed
BJC Medical Group

CONTACTS:
Note: Officers with more than one job title may be intentionally listed here more than once.

Steven H. Lipstein, CEO
Steven H. Lipstein, Pres.
Patrick Dupuis, VP/CFO
Paul McKee, Jr., Chmn.

Phone: 314-286-2000   **Fax:** 314-286-2060
Toll-Free:
Address: 4444 Forest Park Ave., St. Louis, MO 63108 US

GROWTH PLANS/SPECIAL FEATURES:

BJC Healthcare is one of the largest nonprofit health care organizations in the U.S. The firm operates 13 hospitals and approximately 100 primary care and home health facilities in the greater St. Louis, southern Illinois and mid-Missouri regions, with 4,321 licensed beds. Two of the company's hospitals, Barnes-Jewish Hospital and St. Louis Children's Hospital, are ranked highly among America's elite medical centers and teaching hospitals. Both hospitals are affiliated with Washington University School of Medicine, which is considered one of the best medical schools in the nation. The firm also operates the only freestanding rehabilitation hospital in the region, the Rehabilitation Institute of St. Louis. BJC's services include inpatient and outpatient care, primary care, community health and wellness, corporate health, home health, long-term care and hospice care. BJC Home Care Services offers patients a wide range of in-home services, including skilled nursing, adult and pediatric supportive care, rehabilitation therapy, home respiratory care, home infusion therapy and hospice services. Through BJC Corporate Health Services, the company provides occupational health services through five locations run by BarnesCare; access to OccuMed, a comprehensive occupational medicine network that helps companies control workers' compensation costs; the mammography van, which offers convenient screenings at worksites; Travelers' Health Service, which provides immunizations and information on international health risks to patients, prior to flying; and BJC Employee Assistance Program, which assists in the identification and resolution of health, behavioral and productivity problems. One of BarnesCare's newest services is the Corporate Health Nurse Program, which allows local employers to contract for workplace nursing services on a full- or part-time basis. The BJC Medical Group was established to help grow the physician base in the St. Louis metropolitan region by recruiting doctors, establishing practices and providing administrative support. Recently, BJC broke ground on a new hospital, Progressive West HealthCare Center, in southern St. Charles County, Missouri.

FINANCIALS:
Sales and profits are in thousands of dollars—add 000 to get the full amount. Year 2004 note: Complete fiscal 2004 results were not available for all companies at press time. For this company, year 2004 is for months.

2004 Sales: $ (months)	2004 Profits: $ (months)	**Stock Ticker:** Nonprofit
2003 Sales: $2,500,000	2003 Profits: $	Employees: 25,525
2002 Sales: $2,400,000	2002 Profits: $	Fiscal Year Ends: 12/31
2001 Sales: $	2001 Profits: $	
2000 Sales: $	2000 Profits: $	

SALARIES/BENEFITS:

Pension Plan:	ESOP Stock Plan:	Profit Sharing:	Top Exec. Salary: $	Bonus: $
Savings Plan:	Stock Purch. Plan:		Second Exec. Salary: $	Bonus: $

OTHER THOUGHTS:

Apparent Top Female Officers:
Hot Spot for Advancement for Women/Minorities:

LOCATIONS: ("Y" = Yes)

West:	Southwest:	Midwest: Y	Southeast:	Northeast:	International:

BLUE CARE NETWORK OF MICHIGAN

www.bcbsm.com/bcn_hp

Industry Group Code: 524114   Ranks within this company's industry group: Sales: 41   Profits: 32

Insurance/HMO/PPO:		Drugs:		Equipment/Supplies:		Hospitals/Clinics:		Services:		Health Care:	
Insurance:		Manufacturer:		Manufacturer:		Acute Care:		Diagnostics:		Home Health:	
Managed Care:	Y	Distributor:		Distributor:		Sub-Acute Care:		Labs/Testing:		Long-Term Care:	
Utilization Mgmt.:	Y	Specialty Pharm.:		Leasing/Finance:		Outpatient Surgery:		Staffing:		Physical Therapy:	
Payment Proc.:	Y	Vitamins/Nutri.:		Information Sys.:		Phys. Rehab. Center:		Waste Disposal:		Phys. Practice Mgmt.:	
		Clinical Trials:				Psychiatric Clinics:		Specialty Services:	Y		

TYPES OF BUSINESS:
Health Insurance
HMO
Disease Management

BRANDS/DIVISIONS/AFFILIATES:
Blue Cross Blue Shield of Michigan
Health e-Blue
BlueHealthConnection

GROWTH PLANS/SPECIAL FEATURES:
Blue Care Network of Michigan (BCN), a subsidiary of Blue Cross Blue Shield of Michigan, is the largest HMO network in the state. It provides health coverage to over 600,000 members. The company also offers traditional indemnity and Medicare, as well as supplementary management and care services. BCN works closely with its physician network and provides services and tools, such as its Health e-Blue software, to support its partners. Its BlueHealthConnection service, in collaboration with Blue Cross Blue Shield of Michigan, combines diverse programs to assist members with chronic or complex illnesses. BCN has an ongoing partnership with Accordant Health Services, Inc. that provides specialized care for members with rare, chronic and progressive diseases, including multiple sclerosis and Parkinson's disease.

CONTACTS:
Note: Officers with more than one job title may be intentionally listed here more than once.

Kevin Seitz, CEO
Kevin Seitz, Pres.
Jeanne Carlson, COO
Susan A. Kluge, Sr. VP/CFO
Sandra Boozer, VP-Human Resources
Janet MacQueen, VP/CIO
Susan Kozik, VP-Product & Process Improvement
Patricia Turner, VP-Finance
Douglas R. Woll, Sr. VP/Chief Medical Officer
David R. Nelson, Sr. VP/Chief Actuarial Officer
Janie Flemming, VP-Quality Improvement Programs
Kevin Klobucar, VP-Health Centers
Frank Garrison, Chmn.

Phone: 248-354-7450   **Fax:** 248-799-6979
Toll-Free: 800-848-5101
Address: 25925 Telegraph Rd., Southfield, MI 48086 US

FINANCIALS:
Sales and profits are in thousands of dollars—add 000 to get the full amount. Year 2004 note: Complete fiscal 2004 results were not available for all companies at press time. For this company, year 2004 is for months.

2004 Sales: $ (months)   2004 Profits: $ (months)
2003 Sales: $1,400,000   2003 Profits: $53,100
2002 Sales: $1,314,400   2002 Profits: $
2001 Sales: $ 2001 Profits: $
2000 Sales: $ 2000 Profits: $

Stock Ticker: Subsidiary
Employees: 1,000
Fiscal Year Ends: 12/31

SALARIES/BENEFITS:
| Pension Plan: | ESOP Stock Plan: | Profit Sharing: | Top Exec. Salary: $ | Bonus: $ |
| Savings Plan: | Stock Purch. Plan: | | Second Exec. Salary: $ | Bonus: $ |

OTHER THOUGHTS:
Apparent Top Female Officers: 7
Hot Spot for Advancement for Women/Minorities: Y

LOCATIONS: ("Y" = Yes)
West:	Southwest:	Midwest:	Southeast:	Northeast:	International:
		Y			

BLUE CROSS AND BLUE SHIELD ASSOCIATION   www.bcbs.com

Industry Group Code: 524114   **Ranks within this company's industry group:** Sales: 1   Profits:

Insurance/HMO/PPO:	Drugs:	Equipment/Supplies:	Hospitals/Clinics:	Services:	Health Care:
Insurance: Y	Manufacturer:	Manufacturer:	Acute Care:	Diagnostics:	Home Health:
Managed Care: Y	Distributor:	Distributor:	Sub-Acute Care:	Labs/Testing:	Long-Term Care:
Utilization Mgmt.: Y	Specialty Pharm.:	Leasing/Finance:	Outpatient Surgery:	Staffing:	Physical Therapy:
Payment Proc.: Y	Vitamins/Nutri.:	Information Sys.:	Phys. Rehab. Center:	Waste Disposal:	Phys. Practice Mgmt.:
	Clinical Trials:		Psychiatric Clinics:	Specialty Services:	

TYPES OF BUSINESS:
Health Insurance
HMO/PPO

BRANDS/DIVISIONS/AFFILIATES:
Blue Cross and Blue Shield System
Blue Cross Association
National Association of Blue Shield Plans
BlueCard

CONTACTS:
Note: Officers with more than one job title may be intentionally listed here more than once.
Scott Serota, CEO
Scott Serota, Pres.
Ralph Rambach, VP-Admin.
Maureen Sullivan, Sr. VP-Strategic Services
Ralph Rambach, VP-Finance
Allan Korn, Sr. VP/Chief Medical Officer

Phone: 312-297-6000   **Fax:** 312-297-6609
Toll-Free:
Address: 225 N. Michigan Ave., Chicago, IL 60601-7680 US

GROWTH PLANS/SPECIAL FEATURES:
Blue Cross and Blue Shield Association (BCBSA) coordinates 41 independent and locally operated Blue Cross and Blue Shield Plans across America. Together these health insurance and care providers constitute the Blue Cross and Blue Shield System, the oldest and largest group of health care companies in the country. BCBSA Plans provide health care for more than 88 million people, or roughly 30% of all Americans, in every state, the District of Columbia and Puerto Rico. The association was formed in 1982 from the merger of the Blue Cross Association and the National Association of Blue Shield Plans, two companies whose roots form the foundation of prepaid health care in America. Blue Cross was formed in 1929 by an official at Baylor University in Texas who guaranteed schoolteachers 21 days of hospital care for $6 per year. Blue Shield grew out of turn-of-the-century lumber and mining camps in the Pacific Northwest, from employers wishing to provide medical care for their workers. Of the 88 million members of BCBSA, 43.3 million belong to PPOs, 16.6 million belong to HMOs, 6.8 million belong to POSs and 19.7 million belong to traditional, fee-for-service plans. Nationwide, more than 80% of hospitals and nearly 90% of physicians contract with BCBSA plans. Blue Cross and Blue Shield's Federal Employee Program, which enrolls more than 4.1 million federal employees, is the largest privately underwritten health insurance contract in the world. The Association's BlueCard program electronically links independent Blue Plans across the country through a single electronic network for claims processing and reimbursement, allowing employees of nationwide corporations to participate as well as allowing individuals with local plans to file claims while traveling outside their region. In the first six months of 2004, BCBSA companies paid out more than $100 billion in health care claims.

As could be expected, BCBSA provides its employees with the option for every health care benefit under the sun. The company's BluePrint program gives employees credit dollars, allowing them to choose for themselves the combination of benefits that best meet their individual needs.

FINANCIALS:
Sales and profits are in thousands of dollars—add 000 to get the full amount. Year 2004 note: Complete fiscal 2004 results were not available for all companies at press time. For this company, year 2004 is for months.

2004 Sales: $ (months)   2004 Profits: $ (months)
2003 Sales: $182,700,000   2003 Profits: $
2002 Sales: $162,800,000   2002 Profits: $
2001 Sales: $ 2001 Profits: $
2000 Sales: $ 2000 Profits: $

Stock Ticker: Nonprofit
Employees: 150,000
Fiscal Year Ends: 12/31

SALARIES/BENEFITS:
Pension Plan: ESOP Stock Plan: Profit Sharing: Top Exec. Salary: $ Bonus: $
Savings Plan: Y   Stock Purch. Plan: Second Exec. Salary: $ Bonus: $

OTHER THOUGHTS:
Apparent Top Female Officers: 1
Hot Spot for Advancement for Women/Minorities:

LOCATIONS: ("Y" = Yes)
West:	Southwest:	Midwest:	Southeast:	Northeast:	International:
Y	Y	Y	Y	Y	

BLUE CROSS AND BLUE SHIELD OF FLORIDA   www.bcbsfl.com

Industry Group Code: 524114   Ranks within this company's industry group: Sales: 18   Profits: 10

Insurance/HMO/PPO:	Drugs:	Equipment/Supplies:	Hospitals/Clinics:	Services:	Health Care:
Insurance: Y	Manufacturer:	Manufacturer:	Acute Care:	Diagnostics:	Home Health:
Managed Care: Y	Distributor:	Distributor:	Sub-Acute Care:	Labs/Testing:	Long-Term Care:
Utilization Mgmt.: Y	Specialty Pharm.:	Leasing/Finance:	Outpatient Surgery:	Staffing:	Physical Therapy:
Payment Proc.: Y	Vitamins/Nutri.:	Information Sys.:	Phys. Rehab. Center:	Waste Disposal:	Phys. Practice Mgmt.:
	Clinical Trials:		Psychiatric Clinics:	Specialty Services: Y	

TYPES OF BUSINESS:
Health Insurance
HMO/PPO
Dental Insurance
Life Insurance

BRANDS/DIVISIONS/AFFILIATES:
RelayHealth
Availity, Inc.
TriCenturion, Inc.
Navigy, Inc
Incepture, Inc.
Florida Combined Life Insurance Company, Inc.
First Coast Service Options, Inc.
Health Options, Inc.

CONTACTS: Note: Officers with more than one job title may be intentionally listed here more than once.
Robert I. Lufrano, CEO
R. Chris Doerr, Sr. VP/CFO
Barbara Hunter, Interim Chief Human Resources Officer
Duke Livermore, Sr. VP/CIO
Bruce N. Bagni, General Counsel
L. Joseph Grantham, Sr. VP/Chief Strategy Officer
Bruce N. Bagni, Sr. VP-Public Affairs
Cyrus M. Jollivette, Group VP-Public Affairs
Robert I. Lufrano, Chmn.

Phone: 904-791-6111   Fax: 904-905-4486
Toll-Free: 800-477-3736
Address: 4800 Deerwood Campus Pkwy., Jacksonville, FL 32246 US

GROWTH PLANS/SPECIAL FEATURES:
Blue Cross Blue Shield of Florida is a nonprofit mutual health insurance company providing comprehensive health insurance and related services to a membership of approximately 3.5 million. BlueChoice and BlueCare are the company's PPO and HMO group health care plans for both small and large companies. For individuals under 65, the company provides the BlueOptions PPO or the BlueChoice PPO. Individuals over 65 have several plans to choose from involving a combination of Medicare supplements, HMOs and other services. The company also provides multiple options for pharmacy coverage, dental coverage (DentalBlue), life insurance (LifeEssentials), accidental death and dismemberment, disability, long-term care and workers' compensation. The Health Dialog program provides resources for health information and support to help members make educated health care choices. Hospital Advisor, a web-based utility, gives members access to detailed information about hospitals, such as success rates in medical procedures, complication and infection rates and technological capabilities. Blue Cross Blue Shield of Florida operates through a number of subsidiaries, including Health Options, Inc., a combination individual practice association and network model HMO; Florida Combined Life Insurance Company, Inc.; First Coast Service Options, Inc., a Medicare administrator for more than 3 million people in Florida and Connecticut; Incepture, Inc., a company dedicated to increasing efficiency and lowering health care costs through services such as staffing, training, print-mail services and software solutions; Navigy, Inc., likewise focused on increasing the efficiency of health care administration; TriCenturion, Inc., a contractor for Medicare and Medicaid services; and Availity, Inc., committed to improving administrative efficiency primarily through information technology solutions. In recent news, Blue Cross Blue Shield of Florida has introduced RelayHealth, a service allowing online medical consultations for patients seeking non-urgent care.

Blue Cross Blue Shield of Florida provides its employees with health, dental and vision plans, long-term care, life insurance, flexible spending accounts, an employee assistance program and tuition reimbursement.

FINANCIALS: Sales and profits are in thousands of dollars—add 000 to get the full amount. Year 2004 note: Complete fiscal 2004 results were not available for all companies at press time. For this company, year 2004 is for months.

2004 Sales: $ (months)   2004 Profits: $ (months)
2003 Sales: $5,991,000   2003 Profits: $281,000
2002 Sales: $ 2002 Profits: $
2001 Sales: $ 2001 Profits: $
2000 Sales: $ 2000 Profits: $

Stock Ticker: Nonprofit
Employees: 9,200
Fiscal Year Ends: 12/31

SALARIES/BENEFITS:
Pension Plan: Y   ESOP Stock Plan: Profit Sharing: Top Exec. Salary: $ Bonus: $
Savings Plan: Y   Stock Purch. Plan: Second Exec. Salary: $ Bonus: $

OTHER THOUGHTS:
Apparent Top Female Officers: 1
Hot Spot for Advancement for Women/Minorities:

LOCATIONS: ("Y" = Yes)
| West: | Southwest: | Midwest: | Southeast: Y | Northeast: | International: |

Note: Financial information, benefits and other data can change quickly and may vary from those stated here.

BLUE CROSS AND BLUE SHIELD OF GEORGIA INC
www.bcbsga.com

Industry Group Code: 524114   Ranks within this company's industry group: Sales: Profits:

Insurance/HMO/PPO:	Drugs:	Equipment/Supplies:	Hospitals/Clinics:	Services:	Health Care:
Insurance: Y	Manufacturer:	Manufacturer:	Acute Care:	Diagnostics:	Home Health:
Managed Care: Y	Distributor:	Distributor:	Sub-Acute Care:	Labs/Testing:	Long-Term Care:
Utilization Mgmt.: Y	Specialty Pharm.:	Leasing/Finance:	Outpatient Surgery:	Staffing:	Physical Therapy:
Payment Proc.: Y	Vitamins/Nutri.:	Information Sys.:	Phys. Rehab. Center:	Waste Disposal:	Phys. Practice Mgmt.:
	Clinical Trials:		Psychiatric Clinics:	Specialty Services: Y	

TYPES OF BUSINESS:
Health Insurance
HMO/PPO
Dental and Vision Plans

BRANDS/DIVISIONS/AFFILIATES:
Cerulean Companies, Inc.
Group Benefits of Georgia, Inc.
Greater Georgia Life Insurance Company, Inc.
WellPoint Health Networks, Inc.
Blue Value
FlexPlus
BlueChoice Vision
Healthy Extensions

CONTACTS: Note: Officers with more than one job title may be intentionally listed here more than once.
John Watts, CEO
John Watts, Pres.
Gregg Chandler, CFO
Ken Goulet, Sr. VP-Sales
Debbie Lane, VP-Human Resources
Douglas Brown, VP-Info. Services
Joseph Feuer, VP-Legal
Kevin Lenihan, VP-Oper.
Charlie Harman, VP-Public Affairs
Gregg Chandler, VP-Finance
Vincent Barksdale, VP-Provider Network
Pam Bell, VP-Gov't Services
Mike Burks, VP-Actuarial

Phone: 404-842-8000   Fax: 404-842-8100
Toll-Free:
Address: 3350 Peachtree Rd. NE, Atlanta, GA 30326 US

GROWTH PLANS/SPECIAL FEATURES:
Blue Cross Blue Shield of Georgia provides comprehensive health insurance and related services to a membership of more than 2.2 million, making it the largest heath care coverage provider in the state. The company is a subsidiary of Cerulean Companies, Inc., a holding company created in 1996 for the Blue Cross Blue Shield branded affiliates, which include Blue Cross and Blue Shield Healthcare Plan of Georgia, Inc., a health maintenance organization; Group Benefits of Georgia, Inc., a general insurance agency; and Greater Georgia Life Insurance Company, a life insurer. In March 2001, Cerulean Companies merged with WellPoint Health Networks, Inc., one of the nation's largest publicly traded health care companies. Blue Cross Blue Shield of Georgia offers a range of plans for individuals, seniors and small and large groups to choose from. Its individual plans are offered under the names Blue Value, a range of PPO offerings, and FlexPlus, an array of traditional plans. For seniors, Blue Cross Blue Shield of Georgia offers Medicare supplements, dental plans, BlueChoice Vision (which provides discounts on eye exams, glasses, contact lenses and LASIK eye surgery) and Healthy Extensions, a program for discounts in vitamins, wellness books, videos and yoga, among other things. For small and large groups, the company offers HMO, POS, PPO, dental plans, pharmacy programs and a range of life insurance options.

FINANCIALS: Sales and profits are in thousands of dollars—add 000 to get the full amount. Year 2004 note: Complete fiscal 2004 results were not available for all companies at press time. For this company, year 2004 is for months.

2004 Sales: $ (months)   2004 Profits: $ (months)
2003 Sales: $ 2003 Profits: $
2002 Sales: $ 2002 Profits: $
2001 Sales: $ 2001 Profits: $
2000 Sales: $ 2000 Profits: $

Stock Ticker: Subsidiary
Employees:
Fiscal Year Ends: 12/31

SALARIES/BENEFITS:
Pension Plan: Y   ESOP Stock Plan: Profit Sharing: Top Exec. Salary: $ Bonus: $
Savings Plan: Y   Stock Purch. Plan: Second Exec. Salary: $ Bonus: $

OTHER THOUGHTS:
Apparent Top Female Officers: 2
Hot Spot for Advancement for Women/Minorities:

LOCATIONS: ("Y" = Yes)
West:	Southwest:	Midwest:	Southeast:	Northeast:	International:
			Y		

BLUE CROSS AND BLUE SHIELD OF KANSAS   www.bcbsks.com

Industry Group Code: 524114   Ranks within this company's industry group: Sales: 43   Profits: 26

Insurance/HMO/PPO:	Drugs:	Equipment/Supplies:	Hospitals/Clinics:	Services:	Health Care:
Insurance:	Manufacturer:	Manufacturer:	Acute Care:	Diagnostics:	Home Health:
Managed Care: Y	Distributor:	Distributor:	Sub-Acute Care:	Labs/Testing:	Long-Term Care:
Utilization Mgmt.: Y	Specialty Pharm.:	Leasing/Finance:	Outpatient Surgery:	Staffing:	Physical Therapy:
Payment Proc.: Y	Vitamins/Nutri.:	Information Sys.:	Phys. Rehab. Center:	Waste Disposal:	Phys. Practice Mgmt.:
	Clinical Trials:		Psychiatric Clinics:	Specialty Services:	

TYPES OF BUSINESS:
Health Insurance
HMO
Life, Disability & Accidental Death Insurance
Medicare Claims Processing Service
Electronic Claims Clearinghouse

BRANDS/DIVISIONS/AFFILIATES:
Premier Health, Inc.
Premier Blue
Advance Insurance Company of Kansas
Administrative Services of Kansas, Inc.
EDI Midwest

CONTACTS:
Note: Officers with more than one job title may be intentionally listed here more than once.

Michael M. Mattox, CEO
Michael M. Mattox, Pres.
Andrew C. Corbin, VP-External Sales & Provider Affairs
Gerald F. Weigel, VP-Info. Services & Claims
Jane C. Holt, VP/General Counsel
S. Graham Bailey, VP-Corp. Comm. & Public Rel.
Donald R. Lynn, VP-Finance
William H. Pitsenberger, Sr. VP
Shelley Pittman, VP-Internal Sales & Member Rel.
Ralph H. Weber, VP-Medical Affairs
Robin R. LacKamp, Chmn.

Phone: 785-291-7000   **Fax:** 785-290-0711
Toll-Free: 800-432-3990
Address: 1133 SW Topeka Blvd., Topeka, KS 66629-0001 US

GROWTH PLANS/SPECIAL FEATURES:
Blue Cross and Blue Shield of Kansas, Inc. (BCBSK), an independent member of the Blue Cross and Blue Shield Association, is one of Kansas's largest health insurance providers, serving more than 750,000 members. The company also provides Medicare claims processing services to Kansas, Missouri and Nebraska. In addition, the company is a subcontractor in Kansas for TRICARE, the U.S. military health system. BCBSK operates three subsidiaries: Premier Health, Inc. (d.b.a. Premier Blue), Advance Insurance Company of Kansas (AICK) and Administrative Services of Kansas, Inc. (ASK). Premier Blue is a for-profit HMO with more than 40,000 members in Kansas. AICK underwrites ancillary coverage, such as group term life, disability and accidental death, in the firm's service area. ASK leases and sells computer hardware and software for the company's paperless claims network. A subsidiary of ASK, EDI Midwest, is an electronic claims clearinghouse used by more than 800 insurance carriers.

FINANCIALS:
Sales and profits are in thousands of dollars—add 000 to get the full amount. Year 2004 note: Complete fiscal 2004 results were not available for all companies at press time. For this company, year 2004 is for months.

2004 Sales: $ (months)   2004 Profits: $ (months)
2003 Sales: $1,125,400   2003 Profits: $100,600
2002 Sales: $ 2002 Profits: $
2001 Sales: $ 2001 Profits: $
2000 Sales: $ 2000 Profits: $

Stock Ticker: Nonprofit
Employees: 1,850
Fiscal Year Ends: 12/31

SALARIES/BENEFITS:
Pension Plan:	ESOP Stock Plan:	Profit Sharing:	Top Exec. Salary: $	Bonus: $
Savings Plan:	Stock Purch. Plan:		Second Exec. Salary: $	Bonus: $

OTHER THOUGHTS:
Apparent Top Female Officers: 2
Hot Spot for Advancement for Women/Minorities

LOCATIONS: ("Y" = Yes)
West:	Southwest:	Midwest:	Southeast:	Northeast:	International:
		Y			

BLUE CROSS AND BLUE SHIELD OF LOUISIANA www.bcbsla.com

Industry Group Code: 524114 **Ranks within this company's industry group:** Sales: Profits:

Insurance/HMO/PPO:		Drugs:		Equipment/Supplies:		Hospitals/Clinics:		Services:		Health Care:	
Insurance:	Y	Manufacturer:		Manufacturer:		Acute Care:		Diagnostics:		Home Health:	
Managed Care:	Y	Distributor:		Distributor:		Sub-Acute Care:		Labs/Testing:		Long-Term Care:	
Utilization Mgmt.:		Specialty Pharm.:		Leasing/Finance:		Outpatient Surgery:		Staffing:		Physical Therapy:	
Payment Proc.:		Vitamins/Nutri.:		Information Sys.:		Phys. Rehab. Center:		Waste Disposal:		Phys. Practice Mgmt.:	
		Clinical Trials:				Psychiatric Clinics:		Specialty Services:	Y		

TYPES OF BUSINESS:

Health Insurance
HMO
POS Plans
Life Insurance

BRANDS/DIVISIONS/AFFILIATES:

HMO Louisiana, Inc.
Southern National Life Insurance Company, Inc.
BlueSelect

GROWTH PLANS/SPECIAL FEATURES:

Blue Cross and Blue Shield of Louisiana and its subsidiary, HMO Louisiana, Inc., provide health insurance and services to more than 1 million members in Louisiana. The company also provides life insurance through Southern National Life Insurance Company, Inc. Blue Cross and Blue Shield of Louisiana offers a diverse range of coverage options, including HMO, point-of-service (POS) and small group coverage. Its newest coverage plan, BlueSelect, features basic catastrophic coverage as well as inpatient and outpatient rehabilitation benefits, with a wide variety of deductibles.

CONTACTS: *Note: Officers with more than one job title may be intentionally listed here more than once.*

Gerry J. Barry, CEO
Gerry J. Barry, Pres.
Mark Rishell, Sr. VP/CFO
Mike Reitz, Sr. VP/Chief Mktg. Officer
Sandra Smith, VP-Human Resources
Worachote Soonthornsima, Sr. VP/CIO
Sam Griffin, VP-IT
Michele Calandro, Sr. VP/General Counsel
Tony Wittmann, VP/Chief Actuary
James J. Carney, VP/Chief Medical Officer
Dean Simon, VP-Underwriting, Membership & Billing
Allison Young, VP-Benefits Admin.

Phone: 225-295-3307 **Fax:** 225-295-2054
Toll-Free: 800-599-2583
Address: 5525 Reitz Ave., Baton Rouge, LA 70809 US

FINANCIALS: **Sales and profits are in thousands of dollars—add 000 to get the full amount. Year 2004 note: Complete fiscal 2004 results were not available for all companies at press time. For this company, year 2004 is for months.**

2004 Sales: $ (months) 2004 Profits: $ (months)
2003 Sales: $ 2003 Profits: $
2002 Sales: $1,226,900 2002 Profits: $
2001 Sales: $ 2001 Profits: $
2000 Sales: $ 2000 Profits: $

Stock Ticker: Nonprofit
Employees:
Fiscal Year Ends: 12/31

SALARIES/BENEFITS:

Pension Plan: ESOP Stock Plan: Profit Sharing: Top Exec. Salary: $ Bonus: $
Savings Plan: Stock Purch. Plan: Second Exec. Salary: $ Bonus: $

OTHER THOUGHTS:

Apparent Top Female Officers: 3
Hot Spot for Advancement for Women/Minorities: Y

LOCATIONS: ("Y" = Yes)

West:	Southwest:	Midwest:	Southeast:	Northeast:	International:
			Y		

BLUE CROSS AND BLUE SHIELD OF MASSACHUSETTS
www.bcbsma.com

Industry Group Code: 524114   **Ranks within this company's industry group:** Sales: 24   Profits: 15

Insurance/HMO/PPO:	Drugs:	Equipment/Supplies:	Hospitals/Clinics:	Services:	Health Care:
Insurance:	Manufacturer:	Manufacturer:	Acute Care:	Diagnostics:	Home Health:
Managed Care: Y	Distributor:	Distributor:	Sub-Acute Care:	Labs/Testing:	Long-Term Care:
Utilization Mgmt.:	Specialty Pharm.:	Leasing/Finance:	Outpatient Surgery:	Staffing:	Physical Therapy:
Payment Proc.:	Vitamins/Nutri.:	Information Sys.:	Phys. Rehab. Center:	Waste Disposal:	Phys. Practice Mgmt.:
	Clinical Trials:		Psychiatric Clinics:	Specialty Services:	

Insurance: Y (Insurance/HMO/PPO)

TYPES OF BUSINESS:
Insurance-Health
HMO/PPO
Dental Plans
Indemnity Insurance

BRANDS/DIVISIONS/AFFILIATES:
Associated Hospital Service Corp. of Massachusetts
HMO Blue
HMO Blue New England
Blue Choice New England
Medex
MedsInfo-ED

CONTACTS:
Note: Officers with more than one job title may be intentionally listed here more than once.
William C. Van Faasen, CEO
Cleve Killingsworth, Jr., Pres.
Cleve Killingsworth, Jr., COO
Allen Maltz, CFO
Carl Ascenzo, CIO
Sandra Jesse, Chief Legal Officer
John A. Fallon, Chief Physician Exec.
William C. Van Faasen, Chmn.

Phone: 617-246-5000   **Fax:**
Toll-Free: 800-262-2583
Address: Landmark Center, 401 Park Dr., Boston, MA 00215-3326 US

GROWTH PLANS/SPECIAL FEATURES:
Blue Cross and Blue Shield of Massachusetts (BCBSMA) is an independent, not-for-profit health care company that provides health services and insurance in Massachusetts. The firm began as the Associated Hospital Service Corporation of Massachusetts in 1937 and is now New England's largest health plan provider, with 2.5 million members, providing a wide range of health care programs, educational services and insurance plans. Insurance plans include indemnity insurance, dental plans, HMOs, PPOs and Medicare extension programs under the names HMO Blue, HMO Blue New England, Blue Choice New England and Medex. Customers receive health care coverage through a range of employer-sponsored group plans, non-group and senior citizen programs and individual and family plans. The company has joined with other regional Blue Cross and Blue Shield companies to offer additional plans through HMO Blue New England and Blue Choice New England, which include discounts for healthy living and some health clubs. In recent news, the firm announced a new patient safety tool called MedsInfo-ED, an electronic health information exchange project with hospitals and emergency medical teams, for patient information.

FINANCIALS:
Sales and profits are in thousands of dollars—add 000 to get the full amount. Year 2004 note: Complete fiscal 2004 results were not available for all companies at press time. For this company, year 2004 is for months.

2004 Sales: $ (months)   2004 Profits: $ (months)
2003 Sales: $4,300,000   2003 Profits: $232,300
2002 Sales: $4,043,000   2002 Profits: $104,000
2001 Sales: $ 2001 Profits: $
2000 Sales: $ 2000 Profits: $

Stock Ticker: Nonprofit
Employees: 3,545
Fiscal Year Ends: 12/31

SALARIES/BENEFITS:
Pension Plan: ESOP Stock Plan: Profit Sharing: Top Exec. Salary: $ Bonus: $
Savings Plan: Stock Purch. Plan: Second Exec. Salary: $ Bonus: $

OTHER THOUGHTS:
Apparent Top Female Officers: 1
Hot Spot for Advancement for Women/Minorities:

LOCATIONS: ("Y" = Yes)
West: Southwest: Midwest: Southeast: Northeast: Y   International:

BLUE CROSS AND BLUE SHIELD OF MICHIGAN www.bcbsm.com

Industry Group Code: 524114   Ranks within this company's industry group: Sales: 7 Profits: 7

Insurance/HMO/PPO:	Drugs:	Equipment/Supplies:	Hospitals/Clinics:	Services:	Health Care:
Insurance: Y	Manufacturer:	Manufacturer:	Acute Care:	Diagnostics:	Home Health:
Managed Care: Y	Distributor:	Distributor:	Sub-Acute Care:	Labs/Testing:	Long-Term Care:
Utilization Mgmt.: Y	Specialty Pharm.:	Leasing/Finance:	Outpatient Surgery:	Staffing:	Physical Therapy:
Payment Proc.:	Vitamins/Nutri.:	Information Sys.:	Phys. Rehab. Center:	Waste Disposal:	Phys. Practice Mgmt.:
	Clinical Trials:		Psychiatric Clinics:	Specialty Services:	

TYPES OF BUSINESS:
Health Insurance
HMO, PPO & POS
Dental, Vision & Prescription Coverage
Health Care Management Services

BRANDS/DIVISIONS/AFFILIATES:
Blue Care Network of Michigan
Preferred Provider Organization of Michigan
Blue Care Network HMO
Blue Traditional
Blue Prefferred PPO
Blue Choice POS
Blue Vision PPO
Blue MedSave

CONTACTS: Note: Officers with more than one job title may be intentionally listed here more than once.
Richard E. Whitmer, CEO
Richard E. Whitmer, Pres.
Mark R. Bartlett, Exec. VP/CFO
J. Paul Austin, VP-Michigan Sales & Services
George F. Francis, III, Sr. VP/Chief Admin. Officer
Lisa S. DeMoss, Sr. VP/General Counsel/Corp. Sec.
Daniel Loepp, Sr. VP-Corp. Comm./Chief-Staff
Carolynn Walton, VP/Treas.
Kevin L. Seitz, Pres./CEO-Blue Care Network of Michigan
Marianne Udow, Sr. VP-Health Care Products & Provider Services
Thomas L. Simmer, Sr. VP/Chief Medical Officer
Leslie A. Viegas, Sr. VP-Auto/Nat'l Bus. Unit
Greg A. Sudderth, Chmn.

Phone: 313-225-9000   Fax: 313-225-5629
Toll-Free:
Address: 600 E. Lafayette Blvd., Detroit, MI 48226-2998 US

GROWTH PLANS/SPECIAL FEATURES:
Blue Cross Blue Shield of Michigan (BCBSM) is a not-for-profit organization and one of the nation's top Blue Cross Blue Shield health insurance associations, serving nearly 4.8 million members. The firm's insurance plans include Blue Traditional, Blue Preferred and Community Blue PPOs, Blue Choice POS and BCN HMO. Blue Care Network of Michigan (BCNM) is one of the largest statewide HMO networks in Michigan. It operates the company's BCN (Blue Care Network) HMO, which encompasses more than 3,100 primary care physicians, 7,600 specialists and 110 hospitals, serving more than 500,000 members. BCNM also provides traditional indemnity and supplemental Medicare, as well as wellness and disease management services to its members. In addition, BCBSM offers Community, Traditional and Exclusive Dental; Blue Vision PPO; Preferred Rx, Traditional Rx and Blue MedSave; and Medicare supplement coverage, as well as workers' compensation insurance, health assessment and health care management services. The firm's wholly-owned for-profit subsidiary, Preferred Provider Organization of Michigan (PPOM), provides private health care management services and maintains one of the largest Midwest access PPO networks. Its network includes more than 380 hospitals and 55,000 physicians, as well as other health care providers in Michigan, Ohio and Indiana. Its services include the development and maintenance of health care provider networks for group health, workers' compensation and automotive/personal injury protection benefits, as well as other administrative services. In recent news, BCBSM expanded its product portfolio to include new PPO, HMO and Health Savings Account products. In addition, BCNM introduced Weigh to Go, a new weight management and lifestyle modification program for obese adults. The company agreed to sell PPOM to HMS Healthcare, Inc.

FINANCIALS: Sales and profits are in thousands of dollars—add 000 to get the full amount. Year 2004 note: Complete fiscal 2004 results were not available for all companies at press time. For this company, year 2004 is for months.

2004 Sales: $ (months)   2004 Profits: $ (months)
2003 Sales: $13,716,000   2003 Profits: $367,700
2002 Sales: $12,510,500   2002 Profits: $161,400
2001 Sales: $ 2001 Profits: $
2000 Sales: $ 2000 Profits: $

Stock Ticker: Nonprofit
Employees: 8,500
Fiscal Year Ends: 12/31

SALARIES/BENEFITS:
Pension Plan: ESOP Stock Plan: Profit Sharing: Top Exec. Salary: $ Bonus: $
Savings Plan: Stock Purch. Plan: Second Exec. Salary: $ Bonus: $

OTHER THOUGHTS:
Apparent Top Female Officers: 4
Hot Spot for Advancement for Women/Minorities: Y

LOCATIONS: ("Y" = Yes)
West:	Southwest:	Midwest:	Southeast:	Northeast:	International:
		Y			

BLUE CROSS AND BLUE SHIELD OF MINNESOTA
www.bluecrossmn.com

Industry Group Code: 524114 **Ranks within this company's industry group:** Sales: 19 Profits: 24

Insurance/HMO/PPO:		Drugs:	Equipment/Supplies:	Hospitals/Clinics:	Services:		Health Care:
Insurance:		Manufacturer:	Manufacturer:	Acute Care:	Diagnostics:		Home Health:
Managed Care:	Y	Distributor:	Distributor:	Sub-Acute Care:	Labs/Testing:		Long-Term Care:
Utilization Mgmt.:		Specialty Pharm.:	Leasing/Finance:	Outpatient Surgery:	Staffing:		Physical Therapy:
Payment Proc.:		Vitamins/Nutri.:	Information Sys.:	Phys. Rehab. Center:	Waste Disposal:		Phys. Practice Mgmt.:
		Clinical Trials:		Psychiatric Clinics:	Specialty Services:	Y	

TYPES OF BUSINESS:
Health Insurance
Managed Care
Life Insurance
Investment Management
Pharmacy Benefit Management
Behavioral Health Services
Workers' Compensation

BRANDS/DIVISIONS/AFFILIATES:
Blue Plus
Aware
Cross and Blue Shield Associati

GROWTH PLANS/SPECIAL FEATURES:
Blue Cross Blue Shield of Minnesota (BCBSM) is the largest and oldest health plan in Minnesota, with more than 2.6 million members. The firm is a member of the Blue Cross Blue Shield Association and offers medical, dental, life, indemnity and short-term insurance. Insurance plans include HMOs, such as Blue Plus; PPOs; and Medicare supplementals for corporations, groups and individuals. BCBSM customers include General Mills/Pillsbury, Northwest Airlines, Target Corp. and several organized labor groups. In addition, BCBSM covers employees of more than 315 public schools and 345 city, county and other government agencies. The company also has a number of affiliates not licensed by the Blue
Cross and Blue Shield Association that cover behavioral health services, fixed-income investment management, health insurance, life insurance/long-term care, pharmacy benefits management and workers' compensation.

CONTACTS:
Note: Officers with more than one job title may be intentionally listed here more than once.
Mark W. Banks, CEO
Mark W. Banks, Pres.
Timothy M. Peterson, CFO
Colleen F. Reitan, VP-Oper.

Phone: 615-662-8000 **Fax:** 615-622-2777
Toll-Free: 800-382-2000
Address: 3535 Blue Cross Rd., Eagan, MN 55122-1154 US

FINANCIALS:
Sales and profits are in thousands of dollars—add 000 to get the full amount. Year 2004 note: Complete fiscal 2004 results were not available for all companies at press time. For this company, year 2004 is for months.

2004 Sales: $ (months)   2004 Profits: $ (months)
2003 Sales: $5,983,900   2003 Profits: $149,500
2002 Sales: $ 2002 Profits: $
2001 Sales: $ 2001 Profits: $
2000 Sales: $ 2000 Profits: $

Stock Ticker: Nonprofit
Employees: 3,500
Fiscal Year Ends: 12/31

SALARIES/BENEFITS:
Pension Plan: ESOP Stock Plan: Profit Sharing: Top Exec. Salary: $ Bonus: $
Savings Plan: Stock Purch. Plan: Second Exec. Salary: $ Bonus: $

OTHER THOUGHTS:
Apparent Top Female Officers: 1
Hot Spot for Advancement for Women/Minorities:

LOCATIONS: ("Y" = Yes)
West:	Southwest:	Midwest:	Southeast:	Northeast:	International:
		Y			

BLUE CROSS AND BLUE SHIELD OF MONTANA   www.bcbsmt.com

Industry Group Code: 524114   **Ranks within this company's industry group:** Sales: 53   Profits: 40

Insurance/HMO/PPO:	Drugs:	Equipment/Supplies:	Hospitals/Clinics:	Services:	Health Care:
Insurance:	Manufacturer: Y	Manufacturer:	Acute Care:	Diagnostics:	Home Health:
Managed Care: Y	Distributor:	Distributor:	Sub-Acute Care:	Labs/Testing:	Long-Term Care:
Utilization Mgmt.:	Specialty Pharm.:	Leasing/Finance:	Outpatient Surgery:	Staffing:	Physical Therapy:
Payment Proc.:	Vitamins/Nutri.:	Information Sys.:	Phys. Rehab. Center:	Waste Disposal:	Phys. Practice Mgmt.:
	Clinical Trials:		Psychiatric Clinics:	Specialty Services:	

TYPES OF BUSINESS:
Health Insurance

BRANDS/DIVISIONS/AFFILIATES:
Caring Foundation of Montana, Inc.
Combined Benefits Management, Inc.
bluecrossmontana.com
Blue Club

CONTACTS:
Note: Officers with more than one job title may be intentionally listed here more than once.
Peter J. Babin, CEO
Peter J. Babin, Pres.
Wayne K. Knutson, VP/CFO
Sherry L. Cladouhos, Sr. VP-Mktg.
Sherry L. Cladouhos, Sr. VP-Oper.
Michael S. Wagner, Treas.
Dennis H. Toussaint, Sr. VP-Subsidiary Oper.
Roy M. Arnold, Corp. Medical Dir.
Peter J. Babin, Chmn.

Phone: 406-444-8200   **Fax:** 406-447-3454
Toll-Free: 800-447-7828
Address: 560 N. Park Ave., Helena, MT 59604-4309 US

GROWTH PLANS/SPECIAL FEATURES:
Blue Cross Blue Shield of Montana (BCBSMT) provides 240,000 members with a full spectrum of health care coverage, including prepaid health plans that cover hospital expenses and plans to cover physician services. More than 1,700 licensed physicians are BCBSMT providers. In addition, 2,300 health care professionals and 250 hospitals are associated with the firm. Subsidiaries include the Caring Foundation of Montana, which offers health coverage for children and mammograms/prostate screening for the adults in low-income families, and Combined Benefits Management. Through partnerships with community-based health care providers in western, north-central and wouthwestern Montana, BCBSMT members can choose their own primary care doctor. Montana Health and MontanaCare are two partnerships the company has established with doctors and hospitals, which give its members a choice of physicians that offer personalized health care. In recent news, the firm formed an agreement with Health Advocate, Inc. (HA) to provide HA personalized advocacy services to BCBSMT members. The services will help members navigate the health care system through assistance with medical and administration issues. Also in recent news, members now have expanded access to over 2,400 Blue Club discounted health products and services through BCBSMT's bluecrossmontana.com web site.

BCBSMT offers its employees health benefits, life insurance, short- and long-term disability, tuition reimbursement and employee assistance.

FINANCIALS:
Sales and profits are in thousands of dollars—add 000 to get the full amount. Year 2004 note: Complete fiscal 2004 results were not available for all companies at press time. For this company, year 2004 is for months.

2004 Sales: $ (months)	2004 Profits: $ (months)	**Stock Ticker:** Nonprofit
2003 Sales: $478,300	2003 Profits: $17,800	Employees: 1,000
2002 Sales: $	2002 Profits: $	Fiscal Year Ends: 12/31
2001 Sales: $	2001 Profits: $	
2000 Sales: $	2000 Profits: $	

SALARIES/BENEFITS:
Pension Plan: Y   ESOP Stock Plan: Profit Sharing: Top Exec. Salary: $ Bonus: $
Savings Plan: Y   Stock Purch. Plan: Second Exec. Salary: $ Bonus: $

OTHER THOUGHTS:
Apparent Top Female Officers: 1
Hot Spot for Advancement for Women/Minorities: Y

LOCATIONS: ("Y" = Yes)
West	Southwest	Midwest	Southeast	Northeast	International
Y					

BLUE CROSS AND BLUE SHIELD OF NEBRASKA
www.bcbsne.com

Industry Group Code: 524114 **Ranks within this company's industry group:** Sales: 51 Profits: 34

Insurance/HMO/PPO:		Drugs:	Equipment/Supplies:	Hospitals/Clinics:	Services:	Health Care:
Insurance:	Y	Manufacturer:	Manufacturer:	Acute Care:	Diagnostics:	Home Health:
Managed Care:	Y	Distributor:	Distributor:	Sub-Acute Care:	Labs/Testing:	Long-Term Care:
Utilization Mgmt.:		Specialty Pharm.:	Leasing/Finance:	Outpatient Surgery:	Staffing:	Physical Therapy:
Payment Proc.:		Vitamins/Nutri.:	Information Sys.:	Phys. Rehab. Center:	Waste Disposal:	Phys. Practice Mgmt.:
		Clinical Trials:		Psychiatric Clinics:	Specialty Services:	

TYPES OF BUSINESS:
Health Insurance
HMO
PPO

BRANDS/DIVISIONS/AFFILIATES:
BluePreferred
Rx Nebraska
BluePrime
BlueClassic
BlueChoice
NaturalBlue

CONTACTS:
Note: Officers with more than one job title may be intentionally listed here more than once.

Steven S. Martin, CEO
Steven S. Martin, Pres.
Celann LaGreca, Sr. VP-Comm.
Jack D. Mills, Chmn.

Phone: 402-390-1820 **Fax:** 402-398-3736
Toll-Free: 800-642-8980
Address: 7261 Mercy Rd., Omaha, NE 68180 US

GROWTH PLANS/SPECIAL FEATURES:
BlueCross BlueShield of Nebraska (BCBSN) provides health services to nearly 620,000 Nebraskans, representing over one-third of the state's population. Its network of BluePreferred hospitals, physicians and other health care professionals is the state's largest, encompassing every non-governmental acute care hospital in the state and 94% of physicians. The company's Rx Nebraska network includes 448 pharmacies statewide and 55,468 nationwide. BCBSN offers a number of health plans, including its BluePrime HMO, BlueClassic traditional major medical and BlueChoice POS plans, dental and Medicare supplemental plans. It also provides plans designed specifically for Nebraska Farm Bureau members and Comprehensive Health Insurance Pool plans for individuals who have difficulty purchasing a policy because of medical problems. In addition, its NaturalBlue discount program provides reduced-rate massages, acupuncture, wellness products and fitness club memberships.

FINANCIALS:
Sales and profits are in thousands of dollars—add 000 to get the full amount. Year 2004 note: Complete fiscal 2004 results were not available for all companies at press time. For this company, year 2004 is for months.

2004 Sales: $ (months)   2004 Profits: $ (months)
2003 Sales: $705,600   2003 Profits: $45,800
2002 Sales: $ 2002 Profits: $
2001 Sales: $ 2001 Profits: $
2000 Sales: $ 2000 Profits: $

Stock Ticker: Nonprofit
Employees: 985
Fiscal Year Ends: 12/31

SALARIES/BENEFITS:
Pension Plan: ESOP Stock Plan: Profit Sharing: Top Exec. Salary: $ Bonus: $
Savings Plan: Stock Purch. Plan: Second Exec. Salary: $ Bonus: $

OTHER THOUGHTS:
Apparent Top Female Officers: 1
Hot Spot for Advancement for Women/Minorities:

LOCATIONS: ("Y" = Yes)
West:	Southwest:	Midwest:	Southeast:	Northeast:	International:
		Y			

BLUE CROSS AND BLUE SHIELD OF NORTH CAROLINA
www.bcbsnc.com

Industry Group Code: 524114 Ranks within this company's industry group: Sales: 26 Profits: 18

Insurance/HMO/PPO:	Drugs:	Equipment/Supplies:	Hospitals/Clinics:	Services:	Health Care:
Insurance: Y	Manufacturer:	Manufacturer:	Acute Care:	Diagnostics:	Home Health:
Managed Care: Y	Distributor:	Distributor:	Sub-Acute Care:	Labs/Testing:	Long-Term Care:
Utilization Mgmt.:	Specialty Pharm.:	Leasing/Finance:	Outpatient Surgery:	Staffing:	Physical Therapy:
Payment Proc.:	Vitamins/Nutri.:	Information Sys.:	Phys. Rehab. Center:	Waste Disposal:	Phys. Practice Mgmt.:
	Clinical Trials:		Psychiatric Clinics:	Specialty Services:	

TYPES OF BUSINESS:
Health Insurance
HMO/PPO
Dental Insurance
Life Insurance

BRANDS/DIVISIONS/AFFILIATES:
BlueAdvantage
DentalBlue
BlueCare
BlueOptions
ClassicBlue
Partners National Health Plans of North Carolina
Group Insurance Services, Inc.
Behavioral Health Resources, Inc.

CONTACTS:
Note: Officers with more than one job title may be intentionally listed here more than once.

Robert Greczyn, Jr., CEO
Robert Greczyn, Jr., Pres.
Daniel E. Glaser, CFO
John T. Roos, Sr. VP-Sales & Mktg.
Robert T. Vavrina, Sr. VP-Human Resources
John Sternbergh, Sr. VP/CIO
J. Bradley Wilson, Sr. VP/General Counsel
Frederick Goldwater, Sr. VP-Strategic Dev. & Services
Daniel E. Glaser, Sr. VP-Finance
James J. Broderick, Pres./CEO-Partners
Robert T. Harris, Sr. VP-Health Care Services/Chief Medical Officer
J. Bradley Wilson, Corp. Sec.

Phone: 919-489-7431 Fax: 919-765-4837
Toll-Free: 800-250-3630
Address: 5901 Chapel Hill Rd., Durham, NC 27707 US

GROWTH PLANS/SPECIAL FEATURES:
Blue Cross Blue Shield of North Carolina is a nonprofit mutual insurance company providing comprehensive health insurance and related services to a membership of more than 2.9 million spread across all 100 North Carolina counties. The company offers short- and long-term care; Medicare supplement; BlueAdvantage, for individuals under 65, providing the freedom to choose your own doctor; DentalBlue, allowing the freedom to choose any North Carolina dentist; BlueCare, an HMO with flexible benefit plan design; BlueOptions, a PPO; ClassicBlue, a comprehensive major medical plan; small group coverage; and life insurance and other ancillary plans. The BlueExtras program provides members with a variety of services at no added cost, including discounts on medicine services, hearing aids and vitamin supplements; cash back on online shopping; discounts on corrective laser eye surgery, nutrition and fitness information resources; and discounts and information on cosmetic surgery, to name a few. The BlueCard Program allows members to submit claims while traveling outside of their plan's area, including a network of participating hospitals around the world. Blue Cross Blue Shield of North Carolina also operates three subsidiaries that sell their own health insurance: Partners National Health Plans of North Carolina, Inc., Group Insurance Services, Inc. and Behavioral Health Resources, Inc.

Blue Cross Blue Shield of North Carolina offers its employees a comprehensive benefits package, including health, dental, vision and prescription drug plans, as well as life insurance, paid leave for completion of a college degree, tuition assistance, adoption assistance and numerous employee development, recreation and wellness programs.

FINANCIALS:
Sales and profits are in thousands of dollars—add 000 to get the full amount. Year 2004 note: Complete fiscal 2004 results were not available for all companies at press time. For this company, year 2004 is for months.

2004 Sales: $ (months)
2003 Sales: $3,153,900
2002 Sales: $
2001 Sales: $
2000 Sales: $

2004 Profits: $ (months)
2003 Profits: $196,300
2002 Profits: $
2001 Profits: $
2000 Profits: $

Stock Ticker: Nonprofit
Employees: 3,000
Fiscal Year Ends: 12/31

SALARIES/BENEFITS:
Pension Plan: ESOP Stock Plan: Profit Sharing: Top Exec. Salary: $ Bonus: $
Savings Plan: Y Stock Purch. Plan: Second Exec. Salary: $ Bonus: $

OTHER THOUGHTS:
Apparent Top Female Officers:
Hot Spot for Advancement for Women/Minorities:

LOCATIONS: ("Y" = Yes)
West:	Southwest:	Midwest:	Southeast:	Northeast:	International:
				Y	

BLUE CROSS AND BLUE SHIELD OF OKLAHOMA
www.bcbsok.com

Industry Group Code: 524114   Ranks within this company's industry group: Sales: 44   Profits:

Insurance/HMO/PPO:	Drugs:	Equipment/Supplies:	Hospitals/Clinics:	Services:	Health Care:
Insurance: Y	Manufacturer:	Manufacturer:	Acute Care:	Diagnostics:	Home Health:
Managed Care: Y	Distributor:	Distributor:	Sub-Acute Care:	Labs/Testing:	Long-Term Care:
Utilization Mgmt.:	Specialty Pharm.:	Leasing/Finance:	Outpatient Surgery:	Staffing:	Physical Therapy:
Payment Proc.:	Vitamins/Nutri.:	Information Sys.:	Phys. Rehab. Center:	Waste Disposal:	Phys. Practice Mgmt.:
	Clinical Trials:		Psychiatric Clinics:	Specialty Services:	

TYPES OF BUSINESS:
Health Insurance
Managed Care
Life Insurance
Property and Casualty Insurance

BRANDS/DIVISIONS/AFFILIATES:
GHS Holding Company, Inc.
Member Service Life Insurance Company
Group Health Service of Oklahoma, Inc.
GHS Property and Casualty Insurance Company
GHS General Insurance Agency
Oklahoma Caring Foundation (The)
BlueLincs HMO

GROWTH PLANS/SPECIAL FEATURES:
Blue Cross and Blue Shield of Oklahoma (BCBSO), also known as Group Health Service of Oklahoma, Inc., is Oklahoma's oldest and largest private health insurer, with 833,000 customers. The firm has been operating for 64 years as a nonprofit insurance company and a member of the Blue Cross and Blue Shield Association. BCBSO offers health, life, prescription and dental insurances as well as Medicare supplemental insurance for corporations, groups and individuals. The firm also offers hearing aid, laser vision correction and child proofing discounts with membership. The firm runs all subsidiary operations through GHS Holding Company, Inc. Subsidiaries include Member Service Life Insurance Company, BlueLincs HMO, GHS Property and Casualty Insurance Company, GHS General Insurance Agency and The Oklahoma Caring Foundation, Inc.

CONTACTS:
Note: Officers with more than one job title may be intentionally listed here more than once.

Ronald F. King, CEO
Ronald F. King, Pres.
C. Wyndham Kidd, Jr., CFO
C. Wyndham Kidd, Jr., VP-Oper.
Jon Polcha, VP-Planning
Mike Edmondson, Chief Learning Officer
Ronald F. King, Chmn.

Phone: 918-560-3500   Fax: 918-560-3060
Toll-Free:
Address: P.O. Box 3283, Tulsa, OK 74102-3283 US

FINANCIALS:
Sales and profits are in thousands of dollars—add 000 to get the full amount. Year 2004 note: Complete fiscal 2004 results were not available for all companies at press time. For this company, year 2004 is for months.

2004 Sales: $ (months)   2004 Profits: $ (months)
2003 Sales: $1,063,900   2003 Profits: $
2002 Sales: $ 2002 Profits: $
2001 Sales: $ 2001 Profits: $
2000 Sales: $ 2000 Profits: $

Stock Ticker: Nonprofit
Employees: 1,300
Fiscal Year Ends: 12/31

SALARIES/BENEFITS:
Pension Plan: ESOP Stock Plan: Profit Sharing: Top Exec. Salary: $ Bonus: $
Savings Plan: Y   Stock Purch. Plan: Second Exec. Salary: $ Bonus: $

OTHER THOUGHTS:
Apparent Top Female Officers:
Hot Spot for Advancement for Women/Minorities:

LOCATIONS: ("Y" = Yes)
West:	Southwest:	Midwest:	Southeast:	Northeast:	International:
	Y				

BLUE CROSS AND BLUE SHIELD OF TENNESSEE INC
www.bcbst.com

Industry Group Code: 524114   Ranks within this company's industry group: Sales: 35   Profits: 25

Insurance/HMO/PPO:	Drugs:	Equipment/Supplies:	Hospitals/Clinics:	Services:	Health Care:
Insurance:	Manufacturer:	Manufacturer:	Acute Care:	Diagnostics:	Home Health:
Managed Care: Y	Distributor:	Distributor:	Sub-Acute Care:	Labs/Testing:	Long-Term Care:
Utilization Mgmt.:	Specialty Pharm.:	Leasing/Finance:	Outpatient Surgery:	Staffing:	Physical Therapy:
Payment Proc.:	Vitamins/Nutri.:	Information Sys.:	Phys. Rehab. Center:	Waste Disposal:	Phys. Practice Mgmt.:
	Clinical Trials:		Psychiatric Clinics:	Specialty Services:	

Insurance: Y (Managed Care: Y)

TYPES OF BUSINESS:
Health Insurance
HMO
PPO

BRANDS/DIVISIONS/AFFILIATES:
Blue Perks
Blue Network P
Demand Generics

CONTACTS:
Note: Officers with more than one job title may be intentionally listed here more than once.

Vicky Gregg, CEO
Vicky Gregg, Pres.
David Deal, Sr. VP/CFO
Joan Harp, Sr. VP/Chief Mktg. Officer
Dan Blomberg, Sr. VP/Chief Human Resources Officer
Bill Everley, Sr. VP-Benefit Admin.
Bill Young, Sr. VP/General Counsel
Bob Worthington, Sr. VP-Bus. Oper.
Bill Steverson, Dir.-Comm.
Steven Coulter, Sr. VP/Chief Medical Officer
Ron Harr, Sr. VP-Gov't Programs
Mark Austin, Sr. VP-Network Mgmt.
Herbert H. Hilliard, Chmn.

Phone: 423-755-5600   Fax: 800-292-5311
Toll-Free: 800-565-9140
Address: 801 Pine St., Chattanooga, TN 37402 US

GROWTH PLANS/SPECIAL FEATURES:
BlueCross BlueShield of Tennessee, Inc. (BCBST) is the largest health benefits company in the state. As part of the nationwide BlueCross BlueShield Association, it offers customers the full range of Blue Cross and Blue Shield insurance products. The firm serves over 4.6 million people, paying approximately 44.5 million claims per year. Its Blue Network P includes more than 130 hospitals, 15,000 physicians and 2,000 pharmacies. BCBST works hard to keep costs down, and as a result was able to lower the base rate for fully insured group coverage in 2003 and pay back over $67 million in returned premiums. Its Demand Generics cost-cutting program reduces or eliminates co-pays for customers who choose generic over name-brand drugs. The company also offers Blue Perks, a program featuring discounts for members on massages, alternative medicine, fitness centers, LASIK and PRK vision surgery and other services.

BCBST provides employees with health benefits, bonus and advancement opportunities, tuition reimbursement and flexible work hours.

FINANCIALS:
Sales and profits are in thousands of dollars—add 000 to get the full amount. Year 2004 note: Complete fiscal 2004 results were not available for all companies at press time. For this company, year 2004 is for   months.

2004 Sales: $ (months)
2003 Sales: $1,965,300
2002 Sales: $
2001 Sales: $
2000 Sales: $

2004 Profits: $ (months)
2003 Profits: $101,000
2002 Profits: $
2001 Profits: $
2000 Profits: $

Stock Ticker: Nonprofit
Employees: 4,200
Fiscal Year Ends: 12/31

SALARIES/BENEFITS:
Pension Plan: ESOP Stock Plan: Profit Sharing: Top Exec. Salary: $ Bonus: $
Savings Plan: Stock Purch. Plan: Second Exec. Salary: $ Bonus: $

OTHER THOUGHTS:
Apparent Top Female Officers: 2
Hot Spot for Advancement for Women/Minorities:

LOCATIONS: ("Y" = Yes)
West	Southwest	Midwest	Southeast	Northeast	International
			Y		

BLUE CROSS AND BLUE SHIELD OF TEXAS   www.bcbstx.com

Industry Group Code: 524114   Ranks within this company's industry group: Sales: 29   Profits:

Insurance/HMO/PPO:	Drugs:	Equipment/Supplies:	Hospitals/Clinics:	Services:	Health Care:
Insurance: Y	Manufacturer:	Manufacturer:	Acute Care:	Diagnostics:	Home Health:
Managed Care: Y	Distributor:	Distributor:	Sub-Acute Care:	Labs/Testing:	Long-Term Care:
Utilization Mgmt.:	Specialty Pharm.:	Leasing/Finance:	Outpatient Surgery:	Staffing:	Physical Therapy:
Payment Proc.:	Vitamins/Nutri.:	Information Sys.:	Phys. Rehab. Center:	Waste Disposal:	Phys. Practice Mgmt.:
	Clinical Trials:		Psychiatric Clinics:	Specialty Services:	

TYPES OF BUSINESS:
Health Insurance
HMO, PPO & POS
Behavioral Health & Dental Insurance
Medicare Supplement Plan

BRANDS/DIVISIONS/AFFILIATES:
Health Care Service Corporation
HMO Blue Texas
Magellan Behavioral Health
BlueEdge PPO
Select Blue Advantage PPO
SelecTEMP
Select Saver
Dental Indemnity USA

GROWTH PLANS/SPECIAL FEATURES:
Blue Cross and Blue Shield of Texas, a division of Health Care Service Corporation, is a not-for-profit insurer serving more than 3 million members throughout all 254 Texas counties. The company's health care provider network consists of more than 27,000 physicians and 400 hospitals across Texas. The firm places great emphasis on preventive medicine in order to control operating costs. Its group health insurance products include HMO Blue Texas, a PPO plan, a POS plan, Magellan Behavioral Health plan, consumer choice plans and BlueEdge PPO, while its individual health insurance products include Select Blue Advantage PPO, Select Choice PPO, Select Saver, SelecTEMP, Medicare Supplement Plan and Dental Indemnity USA.

CONTACTS:
Note: Officers with more than one job title may be intentionally listed here more than once.
Patricia A. Hemingway Hall, Pres.
Margaret Jarvis, Media Contact

Phone: 972-766-6900   Fax: 972-766-6234
Toll-Free:
Address: 901 S. Central Expy., Richardson, TX 75080 US

FINANCIALS:
Sales and profits are in thousands of dollars—add 000 to get the full amount. Year 2004 note: Complete fiscal 2004 results were not available for all companies at press time. For this company, year 2004 is for months.

2004 Sales: $ (months)   2004 Profits: $ (months)
2003 Sales: $2,549,000   2003 Profits: $
2002 Sales: $ 2002 Profits: $
2001 Sales: $ 2001 Profits: $
2000 Sales: $ 2000 Profits: $

Stock Ticker: Subsidiary
Employees: 4,400
Fiscal Year Ends: 12/31

SALARIES/BENEFITS:
Pension Plan: ESOP Stock Plan: Profit Sharing: Top Exec. Salary: $ Bonus: $
Savings Plan: Stock Purch. Plan: Second Exec. Salary: $ Bonus: $

OTHER THOUGHTS:
Apparent Top Female Officers: 2
Hot Spot for Advancement for Women/Minorities:

LOCATIONS: ("Y" = Yes)
West	Southwest	Midwest	Southeast	Northeast	International
	Y				

BLUE CROSS AND BLUE SHIELD OF VERMONT www.bcbsvt.com

Industry Group Code: 524114   Ranks within this company's industry group: Sales: Profits:

Insurance/HMO/PPO:	Drugs:	Equipment/Supplies:	Hospitals/Clinics:	Services:	Health Care:
Insurance: Y	Manufacturer:	Manufacturer:	Acute Care:	Diagnostics:	Home Health:
Managed Care: Y	Distributor:	Distributor:	Sub-Acute Care:	Labs/Testing:	Long-Term Care:
Utilization Mgmt.: Y	Specialty Pharm.:	Leasing/Finance:	Outpatient Surgery:	Staffing:	Physical Therapy:
Payment Proc.: Y	Vitamins/Nutri.:	Information Sys.:	Phys. Rehab. Center:	Waste Disposal:	Phys. Practice Mgmt.:
	Clinical Trials:		Psychiatric Clinics:	Specialty Services:	

TYPES OF BUSINESS:
Health Insurance
HMO, PPO & POS
Administrative Services

BRANDS/DIVISIONS/AFFILIATES:
Vermont Freedom Plan
Vermont Health Partnership Plan
Vermont Health Plan
Comprehensive Benefits Administrators
Blue HealthSolutions
Heathwise Knowledgebase

GROWTH PLANS/SPECIAL FEATURES:
Blue Cross and Blue Shield of Vermont, a nonprofit organization, is the largest health insurance provider in Vermont and the only health insurance provider based in the state, serving more than 200,000 members. In addition to offering Medicare supplement, vision and dental plans, Blue Cross and Blue Shield of Vermont offers the Vermont Freedom Plan, a PPO, the Vermont Health Partnership Plan, a POS, and the Vermont Health Plan, an HMO. Subsidiary Comprehensive Benefits Administrators offers third-party administrative services. The company's Blue HealthSolutions division focuses on reducing health care costs through specialty case management, focused inpatient review, tiered and incentive programs for purchasing pharmacy drugs and decision support, among other things. The Healthwise Knowledgebase is an online resource center for members only, offering up-to-date medical information.

CONTACTS:
Note: Officers with more than one job title may be intentionally listed here more than once.
William R. Milnes, CEO
William R. Milnes, Pres.
Walter Merrow, COO
Deborah Grandquist, Chmn.

Phone: 802-223-6131   Fax: 802-223-4229
Toll-Free: 800-255-4550
Address: 445 Industrial Ln., Montpelier, VT 05601 US

FINANCIALS:
Sales and profits are in thousands of dollars—add 000 to get the full amount. Year 2004 note: Complete fiscal 2004 results were not available for all companies at press time. For this company, year 2004 is for months.

2004 Sales: $ (months)   2004 Profits: $ (months)
2003 Sales: $ 2003 Profits: $
2002 Sales: $ 2002 Profits: $
2001 Sales: $ 2001 Profits: $
2000 Sales: $ 2000 Profits: $

Stock Ticker: Nonprofit
Employees:
Fiscal Year Ends: 12/31

SALARIES/BENEFITS:
Pension Plan: ESOP Stock Plan: Profit Sharing: Top Exec. Salary: $ Bonus: $
Savings Plan: Stock Purch. Plan: Second Exec. Salary: $ Bonus: $

OTHER THOUGHTS:
Apparent Top Female Officers: 1
Hot Spot for Advancement for Women/Minorities:

LOCATIONS: ("Y" = Yes)
West:	Southwest:	Midwest:	Southeast:	Northeast: Y	International:

BLUE CROSS AND BLUE SHIELD OF WYOMING
www.bcbswy.com

Industry Group Code: 524114   Ranks within this company's industry group: Sales: Profits:

Insurance/HMO/PPO:		Drugs:		Equipment/Supplies:	Hospitals/Clinics:	Services:	Health Care:	
Insurance:	Y	Manufacturer:		Manufacturer:	Acute Care:	Diagnostics:	Home Health:	
Managed Care:	Y	Distributor:		Distributor:	Sub-Acute Care:	Labs/Testing:	Long-Term Care:	
Utilization Mgmt.:		Specialty Pharm.:		Leasing/Finance:	Outpatient Surgery:	Staffing:	Physical Therapy:	
Payment Proc.:		Vitamins/Nutri.:		Information Sys.:	Phys. Rehab. Center:	Waste Disposal:	Phys. Practice Mgmt.:	
		Clinical Trials:			Psychiatric Clinics:	Specialty Services:		

TYPES OF BUSINESS:
Health Insurance
Life Insurance
Annuities

BRANDS/DIVISIONS/AFFILIATES:
Employer Plan Services

CONTACTS:
Note: Officers with more than one job title may be intentionally listed here more than once.

Tim J. Crilly, CEO
Tim J. Crilly, Pres.
Cliff Kirk, Vice-Chmn.
Tim Crilly, Corp. Sec.
Dave Bonner, Chmn.

Phone: 307-634-1393   Fax: 307-634-5742
Toll-Free: 800-442-2376
Address: P.O. Box 2266, Cheyenne, WY 82003 US

GROWTH PLANS/SPECIAL FEATURES:
Blue Cross Blue Shield of Wyoming (BCBSWY) is a nonprofit insurance company and a Blue Cross Blue Shield Association member serving a quarter of the population of Wyoming. The firm provides medical, vision and dental insurance to groups and individuals as well as Medicare supplemental coverage, group life insurance, cancer and dread disease coverage, annuities, flexible benefits administration, worksite benefits and a prescription drug program. Employer Plan Services, a subsidiary of the company, offers allied health and accident coverage. The company is the TriCare Provider for Wyoming, which covers military retirees and dependents of active duty personnel. BCBSWY covers all administrative costs for the Caring Foundation, which provides basic health care services to uninsured children, meets the health care needs of uninsured women and aids in the prevention of domestic violence.

Employees at BCBSWY are offered health and life insurance along with an extended illness time bank and educational assistance.

FINANCIALS:
Sales and profits are in thousands of dollars—add 000 to get the full amount. Year 2004 note: Complete fiscal 2004 results were not available for all companies at press time. For this company, year 2004 is for months.

2004 Sales: $ (months)   2004 Profits: $ (months)
2003 Sales: $ 2003 Profits: $
2002 Sales: $ 2002 Profits: $
2001 Sales: $ 2001 Profits: $
2000 Sales: $ 2000 Profits: $

Stock Ticker: Nonprofit
Employees:
Fiscal Year Ends: 12/31

SALARIES/BENEFITS:
Pension Plan: Y   ESOP Stock Plan: Profit Sharing: Top Exec. Salary: $ Bonus: $
Savings Plan: Y   Stock Purch. Plan: Second Exec. Salary: $ Bonus: $

OTHER THOUGHTS:
Apparent Top Female Officers:
Hot Spot for Advancement for Women/Minorities:

LOCATIONS: ("Y" = Yes)
West:	Southwest:	Midwest:	Southeast:	Northeast:	International:
Y					

BLUE CROSS OF CALIFORNIA

www.bluecrossca.com

Industry Group Code: 524114   Ranks within this company's industry group: Sales: 9   Profits:

Insurance/HMO/PPO:	Drugs:	Equipment/Supplies:	Hospitals/Clinics:	Services:	Health Care:
Insurance: Y	Manufacturer:	Manufacturer:	Acute Care:	Diagnostics:	Home Health:
Managed Care: Y	Distributor:	Distributor:	Sub-Acute Care:	Labs/Testing:	Long-Term Care:
Utilization Mgmt.:	Specialty Pharm.:	Leasing/Finance:	Outpatient Surgery:	Staffing:	Physical Therapy:
Payment Proc.: Y	Vitamins/Nutri.:	Information Sys.:	Phys. Rehab. Center:	Waste Disposal:	Phys. Practice Mgmt.:
	Clinical Trials:		Psychiatric Clinics:	Specialty Services:	

TYPES OF BUSINESS:
Health Insurance
HMO, PPO & POS

BRANDS/DIVISIONS/AFFILIATES:
Medi-Cal
WellPoint Health Networks
Healthy Families Program

GROWTH PLANS/SPECIAL FEATURES:
Blue Cross of California, a subsidiary of WellPoint Health Networks, provides health insurance and related care services to more than 6.8 million members in California. The company provides HMO, PPO and point-of-service plans, as well as Medicare and Medicaid. Blue Cross of California is the largest health plan provider of state-managed programs in California, with more than 811,000 Medi-Cal (Medicaid) members in 13 counties and more than 244,000 children in all 58 California counties in the Healthy Families Program.

Employees of Blue Cross of California receive medical, dental and vision coverage; life and accidental death insurance; and tuition assistance. Company offices have a business-casual dress policy.

CONTACTS:
Note: Officers with more than one job title may be intentionally listed here more than once.

David S. Helwig, CEO
David S. Helwig, Pres.
Alan Katz, Sr. VP-Sales, Individual & Small Group Div.
Josh Valdez, Sr. VP-Network Dev.
Gregory B. Baird, Sr. VP-Large Group Div.
Ivan J. Kamil, VP/Dir.-Medical, Medical Policy & Quality

Phone: 805-557-6655   Fax: 805-557-6872
Toll-Free: 800-333-0912
Address: One WellPoint Way, Thousand Oaks, CA 91362 US

FINANCIALS:
Sales and profits are in thousands of dollars—add 000 to get the full amount. Year 2004 note: Complete fiscal 2004 results were not available for all companies at press time. For this company, year 2004 is for months.

2004 Sales: $ (months)   2004 Profits: $ (months)
2003 Sales: $11,808,600   2003 Profits: $
2002 Sales: $ 2002 Profits: $
2001 Sales: $ 2001 Profits: $
2000 Sales: $ 2000 Profits: $

Stock Ticker: Nonprofit
Employees: 7,000
Fiscal Year Ends: 12/31

SALARIES/BENEFITS:
Pension Plan: Y   ESOP Stock Plan: Profit Sharing: Top Exec. Salary: $ Bonus: $
Savings Plan: Y   Stock Purch. Plan: Second Exec. Salary: $ Bonus: $

OTHER THOUGHTS:
Apparent Top Female Officers:
Hot Spot for Advancement for Women/Minorities:

LOCATIONS: ("Y" = Yes)
West	Southwest	Midwest	Southeast	Northeast	International
Y					

BLUE CROSS OF IDAHO

www.bcidaho.com

Industry Group Code: 524114 **Ranks within this company's industry group:** Sales: 52 Profits:

Insurance/HMO/PPO:	Drugs:	Equipment/Supplies:	Hospitals/Clinics:	Services:	Health Care:
Insurance:	Manufacturer:	Manufacturer:	Acute Care:	Diagnostics:	Home Health:
Managed Care: Y	Distributor:	Distributor:	Sub-Acute Care:	Labs/Testing:	Long-Term Care:
Utilization Mgmt.:	Specialty Pharm.:	Leasing/Finance:	Outpatient Surgery:	Staffing:	Physical Therapy:
Payment Proc.:	Vitamins/Nutri.:	Information Sys.:	Phys. Rehab. Center:	Waste Disposal:	Phys. Practice Mgmt.:
	Clinical Trials:		Psychiatric Clinics:	Specialty Services:	

Insurance: Y (Note: Insurance row — Insurance: Y, Managed Care: Y)

TYPES OF BUSINESS:
Health Insurance
PPO
HMO
Dental & Vision Insurance
Life Insurance
Health Savings Accounts

BRANDS/DIVISIONS/AFFILIATES:
BlueCare
HMOBlue
AccessBlue
PersonalBlue
DentalBlue
ClassicBlue
True Blue
My Health Plan

CONTACTS:
Note: Officers with more than one job title may be intentionally listed here more than once.

Ray Flachbart, CEO
Ray Flachbart, Pres.
Jack A. Myers, CFO
Richard M. Armstrong, Sr. VP-Mktg. & Sales
Debra M. Henry, VP-Human Resources
Michael D. Cannon, VP-Info. Services
Debra M. Henry, VP-Admin. Services
Thomas B. Bassler, Sr. VP/General Counsel
Jack A. Myers, Sr. VP-Finance
Gary M. Dyer, Exec. VP
Douglas W. Dammrose, Sr. VP/Medical Dir.
Drew S. Forney, VP-Benefits Mgmt. & Member Services
David J. Hutchins, VP-Actuarial Services
Jack Gustavel, Chmn.

Phone: 208-345-4550 **Fax:** 208-331-7311
Toll-Free: 800-274-4018
Address: 3000 E. Pine Ave., Meridian, ID 83642 US

GROWTH PLANS/SPECIAL FEATURES:
Blue Cross of Idaho (BCI) is Idaho's oldest health insurer, with approximately 317,000 people, or one-quarter of the state's population, enrolled in its traditional, PPO and managed care programs. Every hospital and 96% of Idaho physicians participate in its traditional network, and 98% of hospitals and 88% of physicians contract in its BlueCare PPO network. The company's HMOBlue managed care product is the largest in the state. In addition, it offers AccessBlue, a lower-cost plan for small businesses; PersonalBlue for individuals; a DentalBlue PPO; ClassicBlue and True Blue Medicare Advantage plans; and health savings accounts, as well as other group products including dental, vision, life, accidental death and disability coverage. Through My Health Plan, customers can obtain personalized health insurance information via the company's web site.

BCI offers its employees group health care, tuition reimbursement, opportunities for advancement and on-site cafeterias and fitness centers.

FINANCIALS:
Sales and profits are in thousands of dollars—add 000 to get the full amount. Year 2004 note: Complete fiscal 2004 results were not available for all companies at press time. For this company, year 2004 is for months.

2004 Sales: $ (months)	2004 Profits: $ (months)
2003 Sales: $660,300	2003 Profits: $
2002 Sales: $	2002 Profits: $
2001 Sales: $	2001 Profits: $
2000 Sales: $	2000 Profits: $

Stock Ticker: Nonprofit
Employees: 650
Fiscal Year Ends: 12/31

SALARIES/BENEFITS:
Pension Plan: Y   ESOP Stock Plan: Profit Sharing: Top Exec. Salary: $ Bonus: $
Savings Plan: Y   Stock Purch. Plan: Second Exec. Salary: $ Bonus: $

OTHER THOUGHTS:
Apparent Top Female Officers: 1
Hot Spot for Advancement for Women/Minorities:

LOCATIONS: ("Y" = Yes)
West	Southwest	Midwest	Southeast	Northeast	International
Y					

BLUE SHIELD OF CALIFORNIA

www.mylifepath.com

Industry Group Code: 524114 Ranks within this company's industry group: Sales: 17 Profits: 9

Insurance/HMO/PPO:	Drugs:	Equipment/Supplies:	Hospitals/Clinics:	Services:	Health Care:
Insurance: Y	Manufacturer:	Manufacturer:	Acute Care:	Diagnostics:	Home Health:
Managed Care: Y	Distributor:	Distributor:	Sub-Acute Care:	Labs/Testing:	Long-Term Care:
Utilization Mgmt.:	Specialty Pharm.:	Leasing/Finance:	Outpatient Surgery:	Staffing:	Physical Therapy:
Payment Proc.:	Vitamins/Nutri.:	Information Sys.:	Phys. Rehab. Center:	Waste Disposal:	Phys. Practice Mgmt.:
	Clinical Trials:		Psychiatric Clinics:	Specialty Services:	

TYPES OF BUSINESS:
Health Insurance
Managed Care
Life Insurance

BRANDS/DIVISIONS/AFFILIATES:
California Physician's Service
TriWest
Blue Shield of California Life & Health Insurance
Blue Shield of California Foundation

CONTACTS:
Note: Officers with more than one job title may be intentionally listed here more than once.

Bruce G. Bodaken, CEO
Bruce G. Bodaken, Pres.
Kenneth F. Wood, Exec. VP/COO
Heidi Kunz, Exec. VP/CFO
Brian Clinch, VP-Direct Sales
Marianne Jackson, VP-Human Resources
David Bowen, CIO
Seth A. Jacobs, General Counsel
Bob Novelli, VP-Oper.
Patrice Smith, VP-Corp. Comm.
Kirk Clove, VP-Finance
Eric Book, Chief Medical Officer
Peter G. Duncan, VP-Group Sales
Charles Sweeris, Chief Compliance Officer
Robert Clifton, VP-Life Companies
Bruce G. Bodaken, Chmn.

Phone: 415-229-5000 Fax:
Toll-Free:
Address: 50 Beale St., San Francisco, CA 94105-1808 US

GROWTH PLANS/SPECIAL FEATURES:

Blue Shield of California (BSC), the operating subsidiary of California Physician's Service, is a not-for-profit Blue Cross Blue Shield Association member with more than 3 million customers. The firm offers insurance packages including HMOs, PPOs, dental, Medicare supplemental and TriWest through 20 offices in California. BSC also offers executive medical reimbursement, life and vision insurance and short-term health plans through Blue Shield of California Life and Health Insurance. Additionally, the Blue Shield of California Foundation, another subsidiary, provides charitable contributions, conducts research and supports programs with an emphasis on domestic violence prevention and medical technology assessments. BSC achieves approximately $6 billion in revenues annually.

BSC offers its employees health, dental, vision, life and disability insurance, as well as tuition reimbursement, the Blue Shield Scholarship Program for dependants, employee assistance plans, pre-tax commuter benefits and flexible spending accounts.

FINANCIALS:
Sales and profits are in thousands of dollars—add 000 to get the full amount. Year 2004 note: Complete fiscal 2004 results were not available for all companies at press time. For this company, year 2004 is for months.

2004 Sales: $ (months)   2004 Profits: $ (months)
2003 Sales: $6,000,000   2003 Profits: $314,300
2002 Sales: $4,624,400   2002 Profits: $
2001 Sales: $ 2001 Profits: $
2000 Sales: $ 2000 Profits: $

Stock Ticker: Nonprofit
Employees: 4,200
Fiscal Year Ends: 12/31

SALARIES/BENEFITS:
Pension Plan: Y   ESOP Stock Plan: Profit Sharing: Top Exec. Salary: $ Bonus: $
Savings Plan: Y   Stock Purch. Plan: Second Exec. Salary: $ Bonus: $

OTHER THOUGHTS:
Apparent Top Female Officers: 3
Hot Spot for Advancement for Women/Minorities: Y

LOCATIONS: ("Y" = Yes)
West: Y   Southwest: Midwest: Southeast: Northeast: International:

BON SECOURS HEALTH SYSTEM INC

www.bshsi.com

Industry Group Code: 622110   **Ranks within this company's industry group:** Sales: 25   Profits:

Insurance/HMO/PPO:	Drugs:	Equipment/Supplies:	Hospitals/Clinics:		Services:		Health Care:	
Insurance:	Manufacturer:	Manufacturer:	Acute Care:	Y	Diagnostics:		Home Health:	Y
Managed Care:	Distributor:	Distributor:	Sub-Acute Care:	Y	Labs/Testing:		Long-Term Care:	Y
Utilization Mgmt.:	Specialty Pharm.:	Leasing/Finance:	Outpatient Surgery:		Staffing:		Physical Therapy:	
Payment Proc.:	Vitamins/Nutri.:	Information Sys.:	Phys. Rehab. Center:		Waste Disposal:		Phys. Practice Mgmt.:	
	Clinical Trials:		Psychiatric Clinics:		Specialty Services:			

TYPES OF BUSINESS:
Hospitals
Assisted Living Facilities
Psychiatric Facilities
Hospice Care

BRANDS/DIVISIONS/AFFILIATES:
Sisters of Bon Secours

CONTACTS:
Note: Officers with more than one job title may be intentionally listed here more than once.
Christopher M. Carney, CEO
Christopher M. Carney, Pres.
Anne Lutz, Sr. VP-Sponsorship
Patricia A. Eck, Chmn.

Phone: 410-442-5511   **Fax:** 410-442-1082
Toll-Free:
Address: 1505 Marriottsville Rd., Marriottsville, MD 21104 US

GROWTH PLANS/SPECIAL FEATURES:
Bon Secours Health System, Inc. (BSHSI) is a Catholic health care ministry operated by the Sisters of Bon Secours. Its system includes 24 acute-care hospitals, one psychiatric hospital, nine nursing care facilities, numerous ambulatory sites, eight assisted living facilities, two retirement communities, home health services and hospice care, with a total of nearly 7,000 beds and 750 assisted living units. Its facilities comprise 15 regional health systems in Michigan, New York, New Jersey, Pennsylvania, Maryland, Virginia, Kentucky, South Carolina and Florida. BSHSI also has strategic relationships with the Henry Ford Health System, Conemaugh Health System, Health Corporation of Virginia, Medical Society of South Carolina, Carolinas Health Care System, Life Care Services and Manor House. In recent news, the company agreed to sell its Florida hospitals, Bon Secours Venice Hospital and Bon Secours St. Joseph Hospital, to Health Management Associates, Inc.

FINANCIALS:
Sales and profits are in thousands of dollars—add 000 to get the full amount. Year 2004 note: Complete fiscal 2004 results were not available for all companies at press time. For this company, year 2004 is for months.

2004 Sales: $ (months)	2004 Profits: $ (months)	**Stock Ticker:** Nonprofit
2003 Sales: $2,523,400	2003 Profits: $	Employees: 34,512
2002 Sales: $2,305,000	2002 Profits: $	Fiscal Year Ends: 8/31
2001 Sales: $	2001 Profits: $	
2000 Sales: $	2000 Profits: $	

SALARIES/BENEFITS:
Pension Plan:	ESOP Stock Plan:	Profit Sharing:	Top Exec. Salary: $	Bonus: $
Savings Plan:	Stock Purch. Plan:		Second Exec. Salary: $	Bonus: $

OTHER THOUGHTS:
Apparent Top Female Officers: 2
Hot Spot for Advancement for Women/Minorities:

LOCATIONS: ("Y" = Yes)
West:	Southwest:	Midwest:	Southeast:	Northeast:	International:
		Y	Y	Y	

BOSTON SCIENTIFIC CORP

www.bostonscientific.com

Industry Group Code: 339113   Ranks within this company's industry group: Sales: 8 Profits: 5

Insurance/HMO/PPO:	Drugs:	Equipment/Supplies:	Hospitals/Clinics:	Services:	Health Care:
Insurance:	Manufacturer:	Manufacturer: Y	Acute Care:	Diagnostics:	Home Health:
Managed Care:	Distributor:	Distributor:	Sub-Acute Care:	Labs/Testing:	Long-Term Care:
Utilization Mgmt.:	Specialty Pharm.:	Leasing/Finance:	Outpatient Surgery:	Staffing:	Physical Therapy:
Payment Proc.:	Vitamins/Nutri.:	Information Sys.:	Phys. Rehab. Center:	Waste Disposal:	Phys. Practice Mgmt.:
	Clinical Trials:		Psychiatric Clinics:	Specialty Services:	

TYPES OF BUSINESS:
Supplies-Surgery
Interventional Medical Products
Catheters
Guidewires
Stents

BRANDS/DIVISIONS/AFFILIATES:
Advanced Bionics Corp.
IQ Guide Wire
Taxus

CONTACTS: Note: Officers with more than one job title may be intentionally listed here more than once.
James R. Tobin, CEO
James R. Tobin, Pres.
Lawrence C. Best, CFO
Robert G. MacLean, Sr. VP-Human Resources
Fred A. Colen, Chief Tech. Officer
Lawrence C. Best, Sr. VP-Admin.
Paul W. Sandman, General Counsel/Corp. Sec.
James H. Taylor, Jr., Sr. VP-Oper.
Paul Donovan, VP-Corp. Comm.
Milan Kofol, VP-Investor Rel.
Lawrence C. Best, Sr. VP-Finance
Stephen F. Moreci, Group Pres.-Endosurgery
Paul A. LaViolette, Group Pres.-Cardiovascular
Peter M. Nicholas, Chmn.

Phone: 508-650-8000   **Fax:** 508-647-2393
Toll-Free:
Address: One Boston Scientific Pl., Natick, MA 01760-1537 US

GROWTH PLANS/SPECIAL FEATURES:
Boston Scientific Corporation, with offices in over 30 countries, develops, manufactures and markets minimally invasive medical devices. The company's products are used in a wide range of interventional medical applications, including cardiology, electrophysiology, gastroenterology, neuro-endovascular therapy, pulmonary medicine, radiology, urology and vascular surgery. Products include steerable catheters, micro-guidewires, polypectomy snares and stents. Stents, flexible metal tubes used to open arteries, account for 20% of sales. The company sells its products to over 10,000 hospitals, clinics, outpatient facilities and medical offices. Boston Scientifc's electrophysiology division is currently investigating advanced modalities for arrhythmia diagnosis and treatment of atrial flutter and atrial fibrillation. Additionally, the firm's oncology division is studying technologies intended to treat kidney disease and symptomatic uterine fibroids. In June 2004, the company announced plans to purchase Advanced Bionics Corp. for $740 million. The firm is suffering from the FDA's limited recall of the Taxus stent, which may present some problems during the surgical implantation stage. The FDA began conducting a broad review of the product as of mid-2004. Meanwhile, many hospitals curtailed use of the Taxus, at least temporarily. The FDA has, however, recently approved the company's new coronary IQ Guide Wire, used to facilitate the placement of balloon catheters.
Boston Scientific offers its employees dental and vision insurance, tuition reimbursement and adoption assistance.

FINANCIALS: Sales and profits are in thousands of dollars—add 000 to get the full amount. Year 2004 note: Complete fiscal 2004 results were not available for all companies at press time. For this company, year 2004 is for 9 months.

2004 Sales: $4,024,000 (9 months)   2004 Profits: $675,000 (9 months)
2003 Sales: $3,476,000   2003 Profits: $472,000
2002 Sales: $2,919,000   2002 Profits: $373,000
2001 Sales: $2,673,000   2001 Profits: $-54,000
2000 Sales: $2,664,000   2000 Profits: $373,000

Stock Ticker: BSX
Employees: 13,900
Fiscal Year Ends: 12/31

SALARIES/BENEFITS:
Pension Plan:	ESOP Stock Plan: Y	Profit Sharing:	Top Exec. Salary: $824,395	Bonus: $1,098,666
Savings Plan: Y	Stock Purch. Plan:		Second Exec. Salary: $575,016	Bonus: $527,196

OTHER THOUGHTS:
Apparent Top Female Officers:
Hot Spot for Advancement for Women/Minorities:

LOCATIONS: ("Y" = Yes)
West:	Southwest:	Midwest:	Southeast:	Northeast:	International:
Y	Y	Y	Y	Y	Y

BRISTOL MYERS SQUIBB CO

www.bms.com

Industry Group Code: 325412   Ranks within this company's industry group: Sales: 7   Profits: 5

Insurance/HMO/PPO:	Drugs:	Equipment/Supplies:	Hospitals/Clinics:	Services:	Health Care:
Insurance:	Manufacturer: Y	Manufacturer: Y	Acute Care:	Diagnostics:	Home Health:
Managed Care:	Distributor:	Distributor:	Sub-Acute Care:	Labs/Testing:	Long-Term Care:
Utilization Mgmt.:	Specialty Pharm.:	Leasing/Finance:	Outpatient Surgery:	Staffing:	Physical Therapy:
Payment Proc.:	Vitamins/Nutri.:	Information Sys.:	Phys. Rehab. Center:	Waste Disposal:	Phys. Practice Mgmt.:
	Clinical Trials:		Psychiatric Clinics:	Specialty Services:	

TYPES OF BUSINESS:
Drugs-Cardiovascular
Medical Devices
Nutritional Products
Beauty Aids
Personal Care Products

BRANDS/DIVISIONS/AFFILIATES:
ConvaTec
Clairol, Inc.
Mead Johnson Nutritionals
Excedrin
Nice n' Easy
Boost
NanoCrystal
Cre Lox Technology

CONTACTS: *Note: Officers with more than one job title may be intentionally listed here more than once.*
Peter R. Dolan, CEO
Andrew R. J. Bonfield, Sr. VP/CFO
Wendy L. Dixon, Pres., Global Mktg./Chief Mktg. Officer
Stephen E. Bear, Sr. VP-Human Resources
James B. D. Palmer, Chief Scientific Officer
John L. McGoldrick, Exec. VP/General Counsel
Tamar D. Howson, Sr. VP-Corp. & Bus. Dev.
Robert T. Zito, Sr. VP-Corp. Affairs
Anthony C. Hooper, Pres., US Pharmaceuticals
Elliott Sigal, Sr. VP-Global Clinical Pharma. Dev.
Donald J. Hayden, Jr., Exec. VP/Pres. Americas
Andrew G. Bodnar, Sr. VP-Strategy & External Affairs
Peter R. Dolan, Chmn.
Lamberto Andreotti, Sr. VP/Pres. Intl.

Phone: 212-546-4000   **Fax:** 212-546-4020
Toll-Free:
Address: 345 Park Ave., New York, NY 10154-0037 US

GROWTH PLANS/SPECIAL FEATURES:
Bristol-Myers Squibb is one of the largest health and personal care companies in the world. Highly diversified, Bristol Myers produces and distributes pharmaceuticals, infant formulas and nutritional products, ostomy & advanced wound care, cardiovascular imaging and over-the-counter products. Bristol-Myers is a leader in providing drugs for anti-cancer therapies and treatments for heart disease, high blood pressure, stroke, type-2 diabetes, HIV/AIDS, depression, anxiety and pain. Some well-known products include Pravachol, a cholesterol-reduction drug; TAXOL, a cancer treatment drug; and Excedrin, a headache drug. Its Clairol group, the number one hair products company in the U.S., produces hair care, skin care and hair color items, with such products as Nice n' Easy, Infusium 23, Loving Care and Herbal Essences. Mead Johnson Nutritionals, a subsidiary of the company, offers nutritional products for infants and adults, including energy drinks and bars, beverages, infant formula and vitamins such as Boost, Enfamil and Poly-Vi-Sol. Another subsidiary, ConvaTec, offers ostomy care and modern wound care products such as Active Life, a one-piece ostomy system; DuiDERM, a hydroactive gel; and SAF-Clens, a chronic wound cleanser. The company's acquisition of DuPont Pharmaceuticals Company has strengthened its virology and cardiovascular franchises, as well as its research and development labs which now hold the rights to Cre-Lox DNA technologies. Bristol-Myers Squibb's drug discovery program includes about 50 biotechnology alliances and collaborative agreements including several associations with various nanotech and biotech companies. For instance, Elan Corporation recently announced that its drug delivery business unit, NanoSystems, has signed a license agreement with Bristol-Myers Squibb for NanoCrystal technology.

Bristol-Myers offers a choice of comprehensive medical plans, with pharmacy benefits, dental plan and employee and dependent life insurance. Some facilities offer child-care services and the firm sends baby formula to an employee's home for a newborn's first year.

FINANCIALS:
Sales and profits are in thousands of dollars—add 000 to get the full amount. Year 2004 note: Complete fiscal 2004 results were not available for all companies at press time. For this company, year 2004 is for 9 months.

2004 Sales: $16,038,000 (9 months)   2004 Profits: $2,249,000 (9 months)
2003 Sales: $20,671,000   2003 Profits: $2,952,000
2002 Sales: $18,119,000   2002 Profits: $2,066,000
2001 Sales: $19,423,000   2001 Profits: $5,245,000
2000 Sales: $18,216,000   2000 Profits: $4,711,000

Stock Ticker: BMY
Employees: 44,000
Fiscal Year Ends: 12/31

SALARIES/BENEFITS:
Pension Plan: Y   ESOP Stock Plan: Profit Sharing: Y   Top Exec. Salary: $1,100,000   Bonus: $2,125,000
Savings Plan: Y   Stock Purch. Plan: Y   Second Exec. Salary: $725,000   Bonus: $554,495

OTHER THOUGHTS:
Apparent Top Female Officers: 1
Hot Spot for Advancement for Women/Minorities:

LOCATIONS: ("Y" = Yes)
West:	Southwest:	Midwest:	Southeast:	Northeast:	International:
Y	Y	Y	Y	Y	Y

Note: Financial information, benefits and other data can change quickly and may vary from those stated here.

BRITISH UNION PROVIDENT ASSOCIATION (BUPA)

www.bupa.co.uk

Industry Group Code: 524114   Ranks within this company's industry group: Sales: Profits:

Insurance/HMO/PPO:	Drugs:	Equipment/Supplies:	Hospitals/Clinics:		Services:		Health Care:	
Insurance: Y	Manufacturer:	Manufacturer:	Acute Care:	Y	Diagnostics:		Home Health:	
Managed Care:	Distributor:	Distributor:	Sub-Acute Care:	Y	Labs/Testing:		Long-Term Care:	Y
Utilization Mgmt.:	Specialty Pharm.:	Leasing/Finance:	Outpatient Surgery:	Y	Staffing:	Y	Physical Therapy:	
Payment Proc.:	Vitamins/Nutri.:	Information Sys.:	Phys. Rehab. Center:		Waste Disposal:		Phys. Practice Mgmt.:	
	Clinical Trials:		Psychiatric Clinics:		Specialty Services:	Y		

TYPES OF BUSINESS:
Health Insurance
Life & Disability Insurance
Long-Term Health Care
Hospitals, Clinics & Health Screening Centers
Travel Insurance
Day Care Services
Staffing Services

BRANDS/DIVISIONS/AFFILIATES:
BUPA
BUPA Health Insurance
BUPA International
BUPA Heartbeat
BUPA TravelCover
BUPA Care Homes
BUPA Childcare
Sanitas

CONTACTS:
Note: Officers with more than one job title may be intentionally listed here more than once.

Val Gooding, CEO
Ray King, Dir.-Finance
Paula Covey, Head-Mktg., BUPA Int'l
Dean Pollard, Dir.-Dev., BUPA Int'l
Pablo J. Azpilicueta, Managing Dir.-Sanitas
Chris Dark, Clinical Dir.
Bryan Sanderson, Chmn.
Bill Ward, Managing Dir.-BUPA Int'l

Phone: 44-20-7656-2000   Fax: 44-20-7656-2700
Toll-Free:
Address: BUPA House, 15-19 Bloomsbury Way, London, WC1A 2BA UK

GROWTH PLANS/SPECIAL FEATURES:

British Union Provident Association, also known as BUPA, is the U.K.'s leading private health care insurer, with an estimated 40% market share. It is a global organization with over 3 million medical insurance customers in the U.K. and more than 7.5 million worldwide. BUPA Health Insurance provides medical insurance in the U.K., while BUPA International covers U.K. expatriates and other customers in Australia, Hong Kong, Ireland, Thailand, Saudi Arabia and over 180 other countries. The company's primary health insurance plan is BUPA Heartbeat, with the BUPA Cash Plan available for everyday health expenses. In addition, the company provides critical illness and other long-term insurance protection products, including Life Cover, Critical Illness Cover and Lifestyle and Income Protection, while BUPA TravelCover offers travel insurance. In the U.K., BUPA owns and operates 34 hospitals and three outpatient clinics, 34 health screening centers with three more on the way, and 299 retirement and care homes through BUPA Care Homes, the U.K.'s largest long-term care provider. The association's hospitals are open to all, with fees agreed upon before treatment for those who are paying their own way. BUPA Childcare owns and operates 44 Teddies Nurseries for children between three months and five years of age, as well as providing day care services to employers and nanny placement services to individuals through Children@work. BUPA Healthcare Professionals and Strand Nurses Bureau provide doctors and nurses for long- and short-term work. Sanitas, BUPA's Spanish health care business, provides medical insurance to over 1 million members and owns and operates two hospitals, 17 day centers and a chain of care homes.

FINANCIALS:
Sales and profits are in thousands of dollars—add 000 to get the full amount. Year 2004 note: Complete fiscal 2004 results were not available for all companies at press time. For this company, year 2004 is for months.

2004 Sales: $ (months)   2004 Profits: $ (months)
2003 Sales: $ 2003 Profits: $
2002 Sales: $ 2002 Profits: $
2001 Sales: $ 2001 Profits: $
2000 Sales: $ 2000 Profits: $

Stock Ticker: Nonprofit
Employees:
Fiscal Year Ends: 12/31

SALARIES/BENEFITS:
Pension Plan: ESOP Stock Plan: Profit Sharing: Top Exec. Salary: $ Bonus: $
Savings Plan: Stock Purch. Plan: Second Exec. Salary: $ Bonus: $

OTHER THOUGHTS:
Apparent Top Female Officers: 1
Hot Spot for Advancement for Women/Minorities:

LOCATIONS: ("Y" = Yes)
West: Southwest: Midwest: Southeast: Northeast: International: Y

Note: Financial information, benefits and other data can change quickly and may vary from those stated here.

CAMBREX CORP

www.cambrex.com

Industry Group Code: 325412   Ranks within this company's industry group: Sales: 39   Profits: 34

Insurance/HMO/PPO:	Drugs:		Equipment/Supplies:	Hospitals/Clinics:	Services:		Health Care:
Insurance:	Manufacturer:	Y	Manufacturer:	Acute Care:	Diagnostics:		Home Health:
Managed Care:	Distributor:		Distributor:	Sub-Acute Care:	Labs/Testing:		Long-Term Care:
Utilization Mgmt.:	Specialty Pharm.:		Leasing/Finance:	Outpatient Surgery:	Staffing:		Physical Therapy:
Payment Proc.:	Vitamins/Nutri.:		Information Sys.:	Phys. Rehab. Center:	Waste Disposal:		Phys. Practice Mgmt.:
	Clinical Trials:			Psychiatric Clinics:	Specialty Services:	Y	

TYPES OF BUSINESS:
Drug Ingredients for Over-the-Counter & Prescription Drugs
Contract Research and Manufacturing Services
Bioproducts
Bulk Biopharmaceuticals

BRANDS/DIVISIONS/AFFILIATES:

CONTACTS:
Note: Officers with more than one job title may be intentionally listed here more than once.
James A. Mack, CEO
James A. Mack, Pres.
James A. Mack, COO
Luke M. Beshar, Exec. VP/CFO
Robert J. Congiusti, VP-IT Services
Ron D. Carroll, VP-Pharmaceutical Tech.
Steven M. Klosk, Exec. VP-Admin.
Peter E. Thauer, Sr. VP-Law/General Counsel/Corp. Sec.
Salvatore J. Guccione, Exec. VP-Corp. Strategy & Dev.
Greg Sargen, VP-Finance
Peter van Hoorn, Pres., Biopharmaceutical Bus.
Daniel R. Marshak, VP-Biotech.
Garly L. Mossman, Pres./CEO-Pharma & Biopharma Bus.
Steven M. Klosk, COO-Pharma & Biopharma Bus.
James A. Mack, Chmn.

Phone: 201-804-3000   **Fax:** 201-804-9852
Toll-Free:
Address: One Meadowlands Plaza, East Rutherford, NJ 07073 US

GROWTH PLANS/SPECIAL FEATURES:
Cambrex Corporation primarily provides products and services to the worldwide life sciences industry, operating in three segments: human health, bioproducts and biopharma. The firm manufactures more than 1,800 products, which are sold to more than 14,000 customers worldwide. Currently, the company's overall strategy for these segments is to focus on niche markets that have global opportunities, build on strong customer relations to enhance its new products pipeline and support state-of-the-art technology. The human health segment primarily manufactures active pharmaceutical ingredients and pharmaceutical intermediates used in prescription and over-the-counter drugs that treat gastrointestinal, cardiovascular, endocrine, central nervous system, respiratory, infective and various other problems. It also provides custom development, custom manufacturing, contract research, route selection, process development and analytical services to pharmaceutical companies. This segment constitutes the largest portion of the company's revenue. The bioproducts segment consists of products and services applied to the life sciences market to support drug discovery and disease research, drug development and the production of biopharmaceuticals. It is organized into three product categories: cells and media; endotoxin detection; and electrophoresis, chromatography and other. The biopharma segment develops and manufactures bulk biopharmaceuticals under contract for biopharmaceutical companies. Biopharmaceuticals are therapeutics that are produced using biotechnology and include recombinant proteins, monoclonal antibodies, vaccines, recombinant enzymes and peptides. The segment provides services from strain and process development through Phase III clinical and commercial production, including access to Cambrex's full range of development and manufacturing services. Recently, Cambrex sold its Rutherford Chemicals segment, which had operations in animal health, agriculture and specialty and fine chemicals.

Cambrex provides its workforce with a health plan, awards, tuition reimbursement and scholarship programs, all of which begin on the first day of employment.

FINANCIALS:
Sales and profits are in thousands of dollars—add 000 to get the full amount. Year 2004 note: Complete fiscal 2004 results were not available for all companies at press time. For this company, year 2004 is for 9 months.

2004 Sales: $319,515 (9 months)   2004 Profits: $-30,865   (9 months)
2003 Sales: $405,600   2003 Profits: $-54,100
2002 Sales: $526,900   2002 Profits: $36,200
2001 Sales: $498,900   2001 Profits: $26,600
2000 Sales: $484,246   2000 Profits: $49,605

Stock Ticker: CBM
Employees: 1,861
Fiscal Year Ends: 12/31

SALARIES/BENEFITS:
Pension Plan: Y   ESOP Stock Plan: Profit Sharing: Top Exec. Salary: $650,000   Bonus: $100,000
Savings Plan: Y   Stock Purch. Plan: Second Exec. Salary: $325,000 Bonus: $90,000

OTHER THOUGHTS:
Apparent Top Female Officers:
Hot Spot for Advancement for Women/Minorities:

LOCATIONS: ("Y" = Yes)

West:	Southwest:	Midwest:	Southeast:	Northeast:	International:
		Y		Y	Y

Note: Financial information, benefits and other data can change quickly and may vary from those stated here.

CANDELA CORP

www.clzr.com

Industry Group Code: 339113 Ranks within this company's industry group: Sales: 99 Profits: 79

Insurance/HMO/PPO:	Drugs:	Equipment/Supplies:		Hospitals/Clinics:	Services:	Health Care:
Insurance:	Manufacturer:	Manufacturer:	Y	Acute Care:	Diagnostics:	Home Health:
Managed Care:	Distributor:	Distributor:		Sub-Acute Care:	Labs/Testing:	Long-Term Care:
Utilization Mgmt.:	Specialty Pharm.:	Leasing/Finance:		Outpatient Surgery:	Staffing:	Physical Therapy:
Payment Proc.:	Vitamins/Nutri.:	Information Sys.:		Phys. Rehab. Center:	Waste Disposal:	Phys. Practice Mgmt.:
	Clinical Trials:			Psychiatric Clinics:	Specialty Services:	

TYPES OF BUSINESS:
Equipment-Laser Systems
Cosmetic Clinical Solutions

BRANDS/DIVISIONS/AFFILIATES:
ALEXLAZR
GentleLASE
C-beam
GentleYAG
Skintonic
YAGLAZR
Smoothbeam
Vbeam

CONTACTS: Note: Officers with more than one job title may be intentionally listed here more than once.
Gerard E. Puorro, CEO
Gerard E. Puorro, Pres.
F. Paul Broyer, Sr. VP/CFO
David A. Davis, VP-Global Mktg.
Kathleen McMillan, VP-Research
James C. Hsia, Chief Tech. Officer
F. Paul Broyer, Sr. VP-Finance & Admin.
William H. McGrail, VP-Oper. & Dev.
Catherine Kniker, VP-Corp. Dev.
Robert E. Quinn, Treas.
Dennis S. Herman, VP-North American Sales
Robert J. Wilber, VP-European Oper.
Toshio Mori, Pres., Candela K.K.
Antony Shaw, Pres.-Asia-Pacific Sales & Mktg.
Kenneth D. Roberts, Chmn.

Phone: 508-358-7400 Fax: 508-358-5602
Toll-Free: 800-799-8550
Address: 530 Boston Post Rd., Wayland, MA 01778 US

GROWTH PLANS/SPECIAL FEATURES:
Candela Corporation develops, manufactures and distributes clinical solutions that enable physicians, surgeons and personal care practitioners to treat selected cosmetic and medical conditions using lasers, aesthetic laser systems and other advanced technologies. The company markets and services its products in over 60 countries from offices in the United States, Europe, Japan and other Asian locations. The firm was a pioneer in the aesthetic laser market 14 years ago and has installed over 6,500 lasers worldwide. The Smoothbeam diode laser helps reduce wrinkles and treat both back acne scars and atrophic acne scars. Vbeam with the DCD Cool Comfort system works on vascular lesions and wrinkles. The GentleLASE family treats vascular lesions, pigmented lesions and wrinkles and removes hair. ALEXLAZR removes pigmented lesions and unwanted tattoos. The C-beam treats psoriasis and surgical scars. GentleYAG removes facial wrinkles and ingrown hairs. Candela plans to capitalize on the expansion in the aesthetic and cosmetic laser surgery industry and intends to establish itself as an industry leader by using its proprietary technology and expertise in light and tissue interaction, as well as by developing market-oriented products that utilize related technologies. In recent news, Candela announced a partnership with Chindex International, Inc., the leading American provider of western health care products to China, whereby Chindex will market and distribute Candela's line of aesthetic laser systems to dermatologists, plastic surgeons, family practitioners and general and vascular surgeons throughout the country.

FINANCIALS: Sales and profits are in thousands of dollars—add 000 to get the full amount. Year 2004 note: Complete fiscal 2004 results were not available for all companies at press time. For this company, year 2004 is for 12 months.

2004 Sales: $104,438 (12 months)   2004 Profits: $8,119 (12 months)
2003 Sales: $80,800   2003 Profits: $6,800
2002 Sales: $61,500   2002 Profits: $-2,200
2001 Sales: $64,800   2001 Profits: $2,500
2000 Sales: $75,390   2000 Profits: $14,563

Stock Ticker: CLZR
Employees: 290
Fiscal Year Ends: 6/30

SALARIES/BENEFITS:
Pension Plan:	ESOP Stock Plan:	Profit Sharing:	Top Exec. Salary: $841,164	Bonus: $47,390
Savings Plan: Y	Stock Purch. Plan:		Second Exec. Salary: $347,607	Bonus: $154,505

OTHER THOUGHTS:
Apparent Top Female Officers: 2
Hot Spot for Advancement for Women/Minorities:

LOCATIONS: ("Y" = Yes)
West:	Southwest:	Midwest:	Southeast:	Northeast:	International:
				Y	Y

CANTEL MEDICAL CORP

www.cantelmedical.com

Industry Group Code: 339113 Ranks within this company's industry group: Sales: 80 Profits: 76

Insurance/HMO/PPO:	Drugs:	Equipment/Supplies:		Hospitals/Clinics:	Services:		Health Care:
Insurance:	Manufacturer:	Manufacturer:	Y	Acute Care:	Diagnostics:		Home Health:
Managed Care:	Distributor:	Distributor:	Y	Sub-Acute Care:	Labs/Testing:		Long-Term Care:
Utilization Mgmt.:	Specialty Pharm.:	Leasing/Finance:		Outpatient Surgery:	Staffing:		Physical Therapy:
Payment Proc.:	Vitamins/Nutri.:	Information Sys.:		Phys. Rehab. Center:	Waste Disposal:		Phys. Practice Mgmt.:
	Clinical Trials:			Psychiatric Clinics:	Specialty Services:	Y	

TYPES OF BUSINESS:
Equipment-Disinfection and Disposable Equipment
Infection Control Products
Diagnostic Medical Equipment
Precision Instruments
Industrial Equipment
Photographic Equipment
Maintenance Services
Water Treatment Equipment and Services

BRANDS/DIVISIONS/AFFILIATES:
Biolab Group (The)
Carsen Group, Inc.
Minntech Corp.
Endoscope Reprocessing System
Mar Cor Services

GROWTH PLANS/SPECIAL FEATURES:
Cantel Medical Corp. provides products and services for the control and prevention of infection. Through its Canadian subsidiary, Carsen Group, Inc., the firm markets and distributes medical equipment, precision instruments and industrial equipment. In addition, Carsen distributes a full range of photographic equipment and supplies. Cantel's subsidiaries provide technical maintenance services for their own products as well as for selected competitors' products. Subsidiary Minntech Corp. develops, manufactures and markets disinfection and reprocessing systems for renal dialysis, as well as filtration and separation products for medical and non-medical applications. Minntech recently acquired the state-of-the-art Endoscope Reprocessing System and accessory infection control technologies of Netherlands-based Dyped Medical BV. Cantel also owns water treatment companies Mar Cor Services and the Biolab Group. Operating in 12 U.S. cities, Mar Cor provides water treatment equipment design, project management, installation, maintenance, service deionization and mixing systems to the medical community. Biolab produces water purification systems for the medical, pharmaceutical, biotechnology and semiconductor industries.

CONTACTS:
Note: Officers with more than one job title may be intentionally listed here more than once.

James P. Reilly, CEO
James P. Reilly, Pres.
Andrew A. Krakauer, Exec. VP/COO
Craig A. Sheldon, CFO
Serth R. Segel, VP-Corp. Dev.
Charles M. Diker, Chmn.

Phone: 973-890-7220 Fax: 973-890-7270
Toll-Free:
Address: 150 Clove Rd., Little Falls, NJ 07424-2139 US

FINANCIALS:
Sales and profits are in thousands of dollars—add 000 to get the full amount. Year 2004 note: Complete fiscal 2004 results were not available for all companies at press time. For this company, year 2004 is for 12 months.

2004 Sales: $170,000 (12 months)	2004 Profits: $10,700 (12 months)	
2003 Sales: $129,300	2003 Profits: $7,900	Stock Ticker: CMN
2002 Sales: $120,000	2002 Profits: $7,200	Employees: 701
2001 Sales: $49,000	2001 Profits: $4,400	Fiscal Year Ends: 7/31
2000 Sales: $40,988	2000 Profits: $2,684	

SALARIES/BENEFITS:
Pension Plan:	ESOP Stock Plan:	Profit Sharing: Y	Top Exec. Salary: $350,000	Bonus: $47,250
Savings Plan: Y	Stock Purch. Plan:		Second Exec. Salary: $293,750	Bonus: $150,822

OTHER THOUGHTS:
Apparent Top Female Officers:
Hot Spot for Advancement for Women/Minorities:

LOCATIONS: ("Y" = Yes)
West:	Southwest:	Midwest:	Southeast:	Northeast:	International:
		Y		Y	Y

Note: Financial information, benefits and other data can change quickly and may vary from those stated here.

CAPITAL BLUECROSS

www.capbluecross.com

Industry Group Code: 524114   Ranks within this company's industry group: Sales: 37   Profits:

Insurance/HMO/PPO:	Drugs:	Equipment/Supplies:	Hospitals/Clinics:	Services:	Health Care:
Insurance: Y	Manufacturer:	Manufacturer:	Acute Care:	Diagnostics:	Home Health:
Managed Care: Y	Distributor:	Distributor:	Sub-Acute Care:	Labs/Testing:	Long-Term Care:
Utilization Mgmt.:	Specialty Pharm.:	Leasing/Finance:	Outpatient Surgery:	Staffing:	Physical Therapy:
Payment Proc.:	Vitamins/Nutri.:	Information Sys.:	Phys. Rehab. Center:	Waste Disposal:	Phys. Practice Mgmt.:
	Clinical Trials:		Psychiatric Clinics:	Specialty Services:	

TYPES OF BUSINESS:
Health Insurance
HMO/PPO
Administrative Services

BRANDS/DIVISIONS/AFFILIATES:
adultBasic
Consolidated Benefits, Inc.
Capital Administrative Services
Capital Advantage Insurance Company
Keystone Health Plan Central
CHIP

CONTACTS: Note: Officers with more than one job title may be intentionally listed here more than once.
Anita M. Smith, CEO
Anita M. Smith, Pres.
Vincent R. Burke, Sr. VP-Finance
Vincent R. Burke, Treas.
William Lehr, Jr., Chmn.

Phone: 717-541-7000   Fax: 717-541-6915
Toll-Free: 800-962-2242
Address: 2500 Elmerton Ave., Harrisburg, PA 17110 US

GROWTH PLANS/SPECIAL FEATURES:
Capital BlueCross provides health insurance and related services to nearly 1 million members spread through 21 counties in central Pennsylvania and the Lehigh Valley. The company has a physician network of more than 8,300 and works with 37 hospitals in the region to provide care. Capital BlueCross has a comprehensive range of products for groups and individuals, including a choice of several PPOs and dental, vision and pharmacy benefit programs. The state of Pennsylvania, in partnership with Capital BlueCross, offers the adultBasic program, providing low-cost health insurance for those who either do not have health care coverage or do not qualify for other programs. The program is funded from the National Tobacco Settlement monies. CHIP (Children's Health Insurance Program) is Capital BlueCross's low-cost or free health insurance program for uninsured children and adolescents who do not qualify for medical assistance through the Department of Public Welfare and who meet certain guidelines with respect to family size and income. Capital Administrative Services, a wholly-owned subsidiary, operates as a third-party administrator for self-funded customers. Capital Advantage Insurance Company, also a wholly-owned subsidiary, offers comprehensive health coverage alone or in combination with Capital BlueCross. Keystone Health Plan Central is Capital BlueCross's HMO subsidiary. Consolidated Benefits, Inc., the only subsidiary not licensed under the Blue Cross name, offers life, short-term disability and accidental death and dismemberment coverage.

Capital BlueCross provides its roughly 2,000 employees with an excellent benefits package, including tuition reimbursement, employee assistance, wellness activities, flexible spending accounts and health education, as well as medical, short- and long-term disability, travel accident insurance and prescription drug coverage.

FINANCIALS: Sales and profits are in thousands of dollars—add 000 to get the full amount. Year 2004 note: Complete fiscal 2004 results were not available for all companies at press time. For this company, year 2004 is for months.

2004 Sales: $ (months)   2004 Profits: $ (months)
2003 Sales: $1,675,000   2003 Profits: $
2002 Sales: $ 2002 Profits: $
2001 Sales: $ 2001 Profits: $
2000 Sales: $ 2000 Profits: $

Stock Ticker: Nonprofit
Employees: 2,000
Fiscal Year Ends: 12/31

SALARIES/BENEFITS:
Pension Plan: Y   ESOP Stock Plan: Profit Sharing: Top Exec. Salary: $ Bonus: $
Savings Plan: Stock Purch. Plan: Second Exec. Salary: $ Bonus: $

OTHER THOUGHTS:
Apparent Top Female Officers: 1
Hot Spot for Advancement for Women/Minorities:

LOCATIONS: ("Y" = Yes)
West:	Southwest:	Midwest:	Southeast:	Northeast:	International:
				Y	

CAPITAL SENIOR LIVING CORP

www.capitalsenior.com

Industry Group Code: 623110   Ranks within this company's industry group: Sales: 13   Profits: 6

Insurance/HMO/PPO:	Drugs:	Equipment/Supplies:	Hospitals/Clinics:	Services:	Health Care:	
Insurance:	Manufacturer:	Manufacturer:	Acute Care:	Diagnostics:	Home Health:	Y
Managed Care:	Distributor:	Distributor:	Sub-Acute Care:	Labs/Testing:	Long-Term Care:	Y
Utilization Mgmt.:	Specialty Pharm.:	Leasing/Finance:	Outpatient Surgery:	Staffing:	Physical Therapy:	
Payment Proc.:	Vitamins/Nutri.:	Information Sys.:	Phys. Rehab. Center:	Waste Disposal:	Phys. Practice Mgmt.:	
	Clinical Trials:		Psychiatric Clinics:	Specialty Services:		

TYPES OF BUSINESS:
Long-Term Health Care/Nursing Homes
Assisted Living Services
Home Care Services

BRANDS/DIVISIONS/AFFILIATES:
CGI Management, Inc.

CONTACTS:
Note: Officers with more than one job title may be intentionally listed here more than once.
Lawrence A. Cohen, CEO
Keith N. Johannessen, Pres.
Keith N. Johannessen, COO
Ralph Beattie, Exec. VP/CFO
David R. Brickman, VP/General Counsel
James A. Stroud, Corp. Sec.
James A. Stroud, Chmn.

Phone: 972-770-5600   Fax: 972-770-5666
Toll-Free:
Address: 14160 Dallas Pkwy., Ste. 300, Dallas, TX 75240 US

GROWTH PLANS/SPECIAL FEATURES:
Capital Senior Living Corporation is one of the nation's largest operators and developers of residential communities for seniors. The firm operates 56 communities in 20 states with an aggregate capacity of approximately 8,700 residents, including 41 communities that it owns or has an ownership interest in. The company's operating philosophy emphasizes a continuum of care, which integrates independent living, assisted living and home care services, in order to provide residents with the opportunity to age with minimal disruption to their home lives. Approximately 85% of its residents live independently, while the remaining 15% require some assistance. Each Capital community offers a relaxed atmosphere of warmth and caring that promotes companionship among residents and staff. These communities feature social and recreational programs, maid service, restaurant-quality meals and complimentary laundry rooms. Capital has formed a joint venture with Blackstone Real Estate Advisors, an affiliate of The Blackstone Group, through which the two firms will acquire senior housing properties worth over $200 million, with Capital retaining a 10% stake in the venture. The joint venture currently collectively owns and operates six senior living communities. In recent news, Capital acquired CGI Management, Inc., which operates 13 senior independent and assisted living communities in the Southwest, with a resident capacity of approximately 1,600.

FINANCIALS:
Sales and profits are in thousands of dollars—add 000 to get the full amount. Year 2004 note: Complete fiscal 2004 results were not available for all companies at press time. For this company, year 2004 is for 6 months.

2004 Sales: $45,643 (6 months)	2004 Profits: $-3,642 (6 months)	Stock Ticker: CSU
2003 Sales: $66,325	2003 Profits: $4,990	Employees: 2,336
2002 Sales: $61,500	2002 Profits: $4,700	Fiscal Year Ends: 12/31
2001 Sales: $70,500	2001 Profits: $2,700	
2000 Sales: $59,654	2000 Profits: $1,239	

SALARIES/BENEFITS:
Pension Plan: ESOP Stock Plan: Profit Sharing: Top Exec. Salary: $352,647   Bonus: $254,262
Savings Plan: Y   Stock Purch. Plan: Second Exec. Salary: $293,872   Bonus: $197,756

OTHER THOUGHTS:
Apparent Top Female Officers:
Hot Spot for Advancement for Women/Minorities:

LOCATIONS: ("Y" = Yes)

West:	Southwest:	Midwest:	Southeast:	Northeast:	International:
Y	Y	Y	Y	Y	

CARDINAL HEALTH INC

www.cardinal-health.com

Industry Group Code: 422210 Ranks within this company's industry group: Sales: 2 Profits: 1

Insurance/HMO/PPO:	Drugs:		Equipment/Supplies:		Hospitals/Clinics:	Services:		Health Care:
Insurance:	Manufacturer:		Manufacturer:		Acute Care:	Diagnostics:		Home Health:
Managed Care:	Distributor:	Y	Distributor:	Y	Sub-Acute Care:	Labs/Testing:		Long-Term Care:
Utilization Mgmt.:	Specialty Pharm.:	Y	Leasing/Finance:		Outpatient Surgery:	Staffing:		Physical Therapy:
Payment Proc.:	Vitamins/Nutri.:		Information Sys.:	Y	Phys. Rehab. Center:	Waste Disposal:		Phys. Practice Mgmt.:
	Clinical Trials:				Psychiatric Clinics:	Specialty Services:	Y	

TYPES OF BUSINESS:
Distribution-Drugs
Surgical/Hospital Supplies
Pharmaceutical Services
Automation & Information Services
Retail Pharmacies
Nuclear Medicine Services
Drug Delivery Technologies
Consulting Services

BRANDS/DIVISIONS/AFFILIATES:
cardinal.com
Medicine Shoppe International, Inc.
Zydis
ALARIS Medical Systems, Inc.

CONTACTS:
Note: Officers with more than one job title may be intentionally listed here more than once.

Robert D. Walter, CEO
George Fotiades, Pres.
George Fotiades, COO
Michael Losh, CFO
Carole S. Watkins, Exec. VP-Human Resources
Jody Davids, Exec. VP/CIO
Dave Schlotterbeck, CEO-Clinical Tech. & Services
Anthony J. Rucci, Chief Admin. Officer
Paul S. Williams, Chief Legal Officer
Brendan A. Ford, Exec. VP-Corp. Dev.
Mark Parrish, Exec. VP/Pres.-Pharmaceutical Distribution
Dwight Winstead, Pres./COO-Clinical Tech. & Services
Gary Dolch, Exec. VP-Quality & Regulatory Affairs
Tony Rucci, Exec. VP-Strategic Corp. Resources
Robert D. Walter, Chmn.
Ron Labrum, CEO-Cardinal Health Int'l

Phone: 614-757-5000 Fax: 614-757-8871
Toll-Free: 800-234-8701
Address: 7000 Cardinal Pl., Dublin, OH 43017 US

GROWTH PLANS/SPECIAL FEATURES:
Cardinal Health, Inc., through its subsidiaries, provides value-added services in support of the health care industry. Its pharmaceutical distribution and provider services segment is a wholesale distributor of pharmaceutical and related products to independent and chain drug stores, hospitals, alternate care centers and the pharmacy departments of supermarkets and mass merchandisers throughout the U.S. and the U.K. This segment also provides support services to pharmacies, including online procurement, fulfillment and information through cardinal.com; computerized order entry and confirmation systems; generic sourcing; product movement and management reports; and customer training. Cardinal also franchises its apothecary-style retail pharmacies through Medicine Shoppe International. The company's medical products and services segment offers a range of medical and laboratory products to hospitals and other health care providers. It manufactures sterile and non-sterile procedure kits; single-use surgical drapes, gowns and apparel; exam and surgical gloves; fluid suction and collection systems; respiratory therapy products; surgical instruments; and special procedure products. Cardinal's pharmaceutical technologies and services segment provides proprietary drug delivery technologies, including softgel capsules, controlled-release forms and Zydis fast-dissolving wafers; aseptic blow/fill/seal technology, drug lyophilization and manufacturing for sterile dose forms; and pharmaceutical packaging services including cartons, inserts and labels, with proprietary expertise in child-resistant and unit dose/compliance package design. It also offers consulting for drug development and medical education and operates nuclear pharmacies that prepare and deliver radiopharmaceuticals for use in nuclear imaging and other procedures. Finally, its automation and information services segment develops, manufactures, leases, sells and services point-of-use systems that automate the distribution and management of medications and supplies. In June 2004, the company acquired ALARIS Medical Systems, Inc., a developer of products for safe delivery of IV medications, for $2 billion in cash and stocks.

FINANCIALS:
Sales and profits are in thousands of dollars—add 000 to get the full amount. Year 2004 note: Complete fiscal 2004 results were not available for all companies at press time. For this company, year 2004 is for 12 months.

2004 Sales: $65,053,500 (12 months) 2004 Profits: $1,474,500 (12 months)
2003 Sales: $56,737,000 2003 Profits: $1,405,800
2002 Sales: $51,136,000 2002 Profits: $1,056,000
2001 Sales: $47,947,600 2001 Profits: $857,400
2000 Sales: $38,349,900 2000 Profits: $717,800

Stock Ticker: CAH
Employees: 55,000
Fiscal Year Ends: 6/30

SALARIES/BENEFITS:
Pension Plan: ESOP Stock Plan: Profit Sharing: Top Exec. Salary: $1,037,500 Bonus: $2,112,135
Savings Plan: Y Stock Purch. Plan: Y   Second Exec. Salary: $622,692 Bonus: $387,412

OTHER THOUGHTS:
Apparent Top Female Officers: 2
Hot Spot for Advancement for Women/Minorities:

LOCATIONS: ("Y" = Yes)
West:	Southwest:	Midwest:	Southeast:	Northeast:	International:
Y	Y	Y	Y	Y	Y

Note: Financial information, benefits and other data can change quickly and may vary from those stated here.

CARDINAL MEDICAL PRODUCTS AND SERVICES

www.cardinal.com/mps

Industry Group Code: 421450   Ranks within this company's industry group: Sales: Profits:

Insurance/HMO/PPO:	Drugs:	Equipment/Supplies:		Hospitals/Clinics:		Services:		Health Care:	
Insurance:	Manufacturer:	Manufacturer:	Y	Acute Care:		Diagnostics:		Home Health:	
Managed Care:	Distributor:	Distributor:	Y	Sub-Acute Care:		Labs/Testing:		Long-Term Care:	
Utilization Mgmt.:	Specialty Pharm.:	Leasing/Finance:		Outpatient Surgery:		Staffing:		Physical Therapy:	
Payment Proc.:	Vitamins/Nutri.:	Information Sys.:		Phys. Rehab. Center:		Waste Disposal:		Phys. Practice Mgmt.:	
	Clinical Trials:			Psychiatric Clinics:		Specialty Services:	Y		

TYPES OF BUSINESS:
Health Care Supplies, Manufacturing & Distribution
Medical Equipment Repair

BRANDS/DIVISIONS/AFFILIATES:
Cardinal Health
OnSite

CONTACTS:
Note: Officers with more than one job title may be intentionally listed here more than once.
Ronald K. Labrum, CEO
Ronald K. Labrum, Pres.
Jo Anne Fasetti, Sr. VP-Human Resources
Richard Gius, Sr. VP-IT
Jerry C. Webb, Sr. VP-Tech. Affairs
Elizabeth E. Ford, Sr. VP/General Counsel
Steven J. Adams, Sr. VP-Finance

Phone: 847-689-8410   **Fax:** 847-578-4437
Toll-Free: 800-964-5227
Address: 1430 Waukegan Rd., McGaw Park, IL 60085-6787 US

GROWTH PLANS/SPECIAL FEATURES:
Cardinal Medical Products and Services (CM), a subsidiary of Cardinal Health, distributes more than 300,000 medical laboratory and surgical products to hospitals, surgery centers, laboratories, clinics, long-term care facilities, home health agencies, physicians offices and ambulatory care centers. The company manufactures many of the products it distributes, including drapes, gowns, masks and gloves used in surgery; surgical scrubs and prep products; and tubing and canisters to drain fluids from the surgical field. The rest of the products the firm sells come from other leading health and medical companies around the world. In addition, the company's procedure kits and services group designs and delivers procedure-specific products and services for all areas of the hospital, outpatient surgery centers and surgeons' offices. Its equipment management services group offers solutions and repairs for the surgical equipment and instruments used in operating rooms, GI labs, surgery centers and physicians' offices. OnSite vans perform repairs right at the hospital, while clients can also mail-in repairs off-site at a number of national facilities. CM delivers approximately 1 million cases of products per day to more than 6,000 patient care sites across the country. Its distribution services are provided through four main points of care: hospital supply distribution, which provides supply chain solutions and logistics management to all acute-care hospitals, including group purchasing organizations, integrated delivery networks and health systems; physician products and services, providing physician office practices with more than 35,000 medical, laboratory and pharmaceutical products; scientific products distribution, marketing a broad offering of diagnostic tests, equipment and supplies to clinical and reference laboratories nationwide; and surgery center products and services, offering medical, surgical and pharmacology products and services to more than 10,000 freestanding surgery centers.

FINANCIALS:
Sales and profits are in thousands of dollars—add 000 to get the full amount. Year 2004 note: Complete fiscal 2004 results were not available for all companies at press time. For this company, year 2004 is for months.

2004 Sales: $ (months)   2004 Profits: $ (months)
2003 Sales: $ 2003 Profits: $
2002 Sales: $6,255,500   2002 Profits: $
2001 Sales: $ 2001 Profits: $
2000 Sales: $ 2000 Profits: $

Stock Ticker: Subsidiary
Employees:
Fiscal Year Ends: 6/30

SALARIES/BENEFITS:
| Pension Plan: | ESOP Stock Plan: | Profit Sharing: | Top Exec. Salary: $ | Bonus: $ |
| Savings Plan: | Stock Purch. Plan: | | Second Exec. Salary: $ | Bonus: $ |

OTHER THOUGHTS:
Apparent Top Female Officers: 2
Hot Spot for Advancement for Women/Minorities:

LOCATIONS: ("Y" = Yes)
| West: | Southwest: | Midwest: Y | Southeast: | Northeast: | International: Y |

CARDIOGENESIS CORP

www.cardiogenesis.com

Industry Group Code: 339113 Ranks within this company's industry group: Sales: 134 Profits: 105

Insurance/HMO/PPO:	Drugs:	Equipment/Supplies:		Hospitals/Clinics:	Services:	Health Care:
Insurance:	Manufacturer:	Manufacturer:	Y	Acute Care:	Diagnostics:	Home Health:
Managed Care:	Distributor:	Distributor:	Y	Sub-Acute Care:	Labs/Testing:	Long-Term Care:
Utilization Mgmt.:	Specialty Pharm.:	Leasing/Finance:		Outpatient Surgery:	Staffing:	Physical Therapy:
Payment Proc.:	Vitamins/Nutri.:	Information Sys.:		Phys. Rehab. Center:	Waste Disposal:	Phys. Practice Mgmt.:
	Clinical Trials:			Psychiatric Clinics:	Specialty Services:	

TYPES OF BUSINESS:
Equipment-Laser & Fiber-Optic Systems
Laser-Based Surgical Products
Disposable Fiber-Optic Accessories
Cardiovascular Surgical Products

BRANDS/DIVISIONS/AFFILIATES:
TMR 2000
New Star PMR
Axcis
Sologrip III

CONTACTS: Note: Officers with more than one job title may be intentionally listed here more than once.
Michael J. Quinn, CEO
Michael J. Quinn, Pres.
Christine Ocampo, CFO
Richard P. Lanigan, Sr. VP-Mktg.
Marvin J. Slepian, Chief Scientific Officer
Christine Ocampo, Chief Acct. Officer/Treas./Corp. Sec.
Hank Rossell, Sr. VP/General Mgr.-Atlantic Div.
Gerard A. Arthur, VP/General Mgr.-Worldwide Service Div.
Joseph R. Kletzel II, Sr. VP/General Mgr.-Pacific Div.
Janet M. Fauls, VP-Regulatory, Quality & Clinical Affairs
Michael J. Quinn, Chmn.

Phone: 714-649-5000 Fax: 714-649-5103
Toll-Free: 800-238-2205
Address: 26632 Towne Centre Dr., Ste. 320, Foothill Ranch, CA 92610 US

GROWTH PLANS/SPECIAL FEATURES:
CardioGenesis Corporation designs, develops, manufactures and distributes medical devices for the treatment of cardiovascular disease and is a leader in devices that stimulate cardiac angiogenesis, the growth of new blood vessels. The company's main products, the YAG laser system and its disposable fiber-optic accessories, are used to perform transmyocardial revascularization (TMR) to treat patients suffering from angina. The firm's newest procedure, percutaneous transluminal myocardial revascularization (PMR), is currently being marketed in Europe and other international markets but is still under review by the FDA. TMR and PMR are recent laser-based heart treatments in which channels are made in the heart muscle. In the TMR procedure, the surgeon inserts a laser device through the myocardium to create a new pathway into the heart. This procedure can be done through open chest surgery or less invasive methods. The PMR procedure is less invasive than TMR, in that a catheter is inserted in the femoral artery in the leg. CardioGenesis products include the TMR 2000 laser system and Sologrip III laser delivery system for TMR, which are sold in the U.S., as well as the New Star PMR laser system and Axcis laser catheter for PMR, which are sold internationally, pending FDA approval.

FINANCIALS:
Sales and profits are in thousands of dollars—add 000 to get the full amount. Year 2004 note: Complete fiscal 2004 results were not available for all companies at press time. For this company, year 2004 is for 6 months.

2004 Sales: $7,417 (6 months)	2004 Profits: $ 3 (6 months)
2003 Sales: $13,518	2003 Profits: $- 348
2002 Sales: $13,000	2002 Profits: $- 500
2001 Sales: $14,200	2001 Profits: $-10,200
2000 Sales: $22,200	2000 Profits: $-14,600

Stock Ticker: CGCP
Employees: 31
Fiscal Year Ends: 12/31

SALARIES/BENEFITS:
Pension Plan: ESOP Stock Plan: Profit Sharing: Top Exec. Salary: $388,400 Bonus: $80,000
Savings Plan: Y Stock Purch. Plan: Second Exec. Salary: $259,200 Bonus: $40,000

OTHER THOUGHTS:
Apparent Top Female Officers: 2
Hot Spot for Advancement for Women/Minorities:

LOCATIONS: ("Y" = Yes)
West:	Southwest:	Midwest:	Southeast:	Northeast:	International:
Y					

CAREFIRST INC

www.carefirst.com

Industry Group Code: 524114   **Ranks within this company's industry group:** Sales: 14   Profits: 20

Insurance/HMO/PPO:		Drugs:		Equipment/Supplies:		Hospitals/Clinics:		Services:		Health Care:	
Insurance:		Manufacturer:		Manufacturer:		Acute Care:		Diagnostics:		Home Health:	
Managed Care:	Y	Distributor:		Distributor:		Sub-Acute Care:		Labs/Testing:		Long-Term Care:	
Utilization Mgmt.:		Specialty Pharm.:		Leasing/Finance:		Outpatient Surgery:		Staffing:		Physical Therapy:	
Payment Proc.:		Vitamins/Nutri.:		Information Sys.:		Phys. Rehab. Center:		Waste Disposal:		Phys. Practice Mgmt.:	
		Clinical Trials:				Psychiatric Clinics:		Specialty Services:	Y		

TYPES OF BUSINESS:
Health Insurance
HMO
Claims Processing
Administrative Services

BRANDS/DIVISIONS/AFFILIATES:
CareFirst BlueCross BlueShield
CareFirst of Maryland, Inc.
Group Hospitalization and Medical Services, Inc.
BlueCross BlueShield of Delaware
CareFirst BlueChoice

CONTACTS:
Note: Officers with more than one job title may be intentionally listed here more than once.
G. Mark Chaney, Exec. VP/CFO
Gregory A. Devou, Exec. VP/Chief Mktg. Officer
Sharon J. Vecchioni, Exec. VP/Chief of Staff
John A. Picciotto, Exec. VP/General Counsel/Corp. Sec.
Leon Kaplan, Exec. VP-Oper.
David D. Wolf, Exec. VP-Corp. Dev. & Medical Systems
William L. Jews, Pres./CEO-CareFirst BlueCross BlueShield
Michael R. Merson, Chmn.

Phone: 410-581-3000   **Fax:** 410-998-5351
Toll-Free: 800-321-3497
Address: 10455 Mill Run Cir., Owings Mills, MD 21117 US

GROWTH PLANS/SPECIAL FEATURES:
CareFirst, Inc., with operations in Maryland, Delaware, northern Virginia and the District of Columbia, is the nonprofit parent company of Group Hospitalization and Medical Services, Inc. and CareFirst of Maryland, Inc., which do business as CareFirst BlueCross BlueShield. Another affiliate does business as BlueCross BlueShield of Delaware. CareFirst is the largest health care insurer in the Mid-Atlantic, with over 3.2 million members, and is affiliated with 165 hospitals in the region. Over 80% of health care providers in its operating region participate in one or more of its provider networks. Through a third-party administrator, the company also offers administrative services to self-insured employers. In addition, CareFirst operates a for-profit regional HMO subsidiary, CareFirst BlueChoice, with more than 3,500 primary care physicians. The firm also owns a West Virginia-based subsidiary that processes over 5 million claims annually for Federal Government subscribers and dependents. In recent news, CareFirst ended its ownership of Patuxent Medical Group, a money-losing group of 47 physicians and 180 support personnel.

FINANCIALS:
Sales and profits are in thousands of dollars—add 000 to get the full amount. Year 2004 note: Complete fiscal 2004 results were not available for all companies at press time. For this company, year 2004 is for months.

2004 Sales: $ (months)	2004 Profits: $ (months)	
2003 Sales: $7,292,300	2003 Profits: $171,300	**Stock Ticker:** Nonprofit
2002 Sales: $	2002 Profits: $	Employees: 6,500
2001 Sales: $	2001 Profits: $	Fiscal Year Ends: 12/31
2000 Sales: $	2000 Profits: $	

SALARIES/BENEFITS:
Pension Plan:	ESOP Stock Plan:	Profit Sharing:	Top Exec. Salary: $	Bonus: $
Savings Plan:	Stock Purch. Plan:		Second Exec. Salary: $	Bonus: $

OTHER THOUGHTS:
Apparent Top Female Officers: 1
Hot Spot for Advancement for Women/Minorities:

LOCATIONS: ("Y" = Yes)
West:	Southwest:	Midwest:	Southeast:	Northeast:	International:
				Y	

CARAMARK RX INC

www.caremark.com

Industry Group Code: 446110A   Ranks within this company's industry group: Sales: 1   Profits: 1

Insurance/HMO/PPO:	Drugs:	Equipment/Supplies:	Hospitals/Clinics:	Services:	Health Care:
Insurance:	Manufacturer:	Manufacturer:	Acute Care:	Diagnostics:	Home Health:
Managed Care:	Distributor:	Distributor:	Sub-Acute Care:	Labs/Testing:	Long-Term Care:
Utilization Mgmt.:	Specialty Pharm.: Y	Leasing/Finance:	Outpatient Surgery:	Staffing:	Physical Therapy:
Payment Proc.: Y	Vitamins/Nutri.:	Information Sys.:	Phys. Rehab. Center:	Waste Disposal:	Phys. Practice Mgmt.:
	Clinical Trials:		Psychiatric Clinics:	Specialty Services: Y	

TYPES OF BUSINESS:
Drugs-Specialty Pharmacy
Prescription Benefit Management Programs
Disease Management Programs

BRANDS/DIVISIONS/AFFILIATES:
AdvancePCS

CONTACTS: Note: Officers with more than one job title may be intentionally listed here more than once.
Mac Crawford, CEO
Mac Crawford, Pres.
Howard A. McLure, Exec. VP/CFO
David Joyner, Exec. VP-Sales
Kirk McConnell, Exec. VP-Human Resources
Kirk McConnell, Exec. VP/Chief Admin. Officer
Edward L. Hardin, Jr., Exec. VP/General Counsel
Rich Scardina, Exec. VP-Oper.
Brad Karro, Exec. VP-Corp. Dev.
Peter J. Clemens, IV, Sr. VP-Finance/Treas.
Sara J. Finley, Sr. VP/Corp. Sec.
Rudy Mladenovic, Exec. VP-Industry Rel.
Diane Nobles, Exec. VP-Compliance & Integrity
David Golding, Sr. VP-Specialty Pharmacy
Mac Crawford, Chmn.

Phone: 615-743-6600   Fax: 205-733-9780
Toll-Free:
Address: 211 Commerce St., Ste. 800, Nashville, TN 37201 US

GROWTH PLANS/SPECIAL FEATURES:
Caremark Rx is a leading prescription benefit manager that provides comprehensive drug benefit services to over 1,200 health-plan sponsors. Annually, over 23 million U.S. participants receive more than 90 million prescriptions via Caremark. The company's clients include managed care organizations, insurance companies, corporate health plans, unions, government agencies and other funded benefit plans. The firm manages the entire spectrum of drug benefit plans and therapies to ensure appropriate and cost-effective pharmaceutical selection, prescribing, dispensing and reimbursement, helping plan sponsors meet their financial and quality objectives. Caremark operates a national retail pharmacy benefit management network with over 55,000 participating pharmacies, four automated mail-service pharmacies, 19 smaller mail-order pharmacies and an FDA-regulated repackaging plant. The company is also engaged in disorder and disease management programs that target complex, high-cost conditions. In March 2004, Caremark completed a merger with AdvancePCS, one of the three other major pharmacy benefit management companies, to form a new company with combined revenues of $23 billion. In other news, the company relocated its corporate headquarters to Nashville, Tennessee, from its previous location in Birmingham, Alabama.

Caremark provides a comprehensive benefits program, including vision and dental insurance, employee assistance, adoption assistance, an incentive salary program and various professional development training programs.

FINANCIALS: Sales and profits are in thousands of dollars—add 000 to get the full amount. Year 2004 note: Complete fiscal 2004 results were not available for all companies at press time. For this company, year 2004 is for 9 months.

2004 Sales: $17,788,277 (9 months)	2004 Profits: $395,226 (9 months)	Stock Ticker: CMX
2003 Sales: $9,067,291	2003 Profits: $290,838	Employees: 4,870
2002 Sales: $6,805,000	2002 Profits: $791,000	Fiscal Year Ends: 12/31
2001 Sales: $5,614,000	2001 Profits: $190,000	
2000 Sales: $4,480,100	2000 Profits: $-163,300	

SALARIES/BENEFITS:
Pension Plan: ESOP Stock Plan: Profit Sharing: Top Exec. Salary: $1,500,000   Bonus: $500,000
Savings Plan: Y   Stock Purch. Plan: Y   Second Exec. Salary: $1,000,000   Bonus: $450,000

OTHER THOUGHTS:
Apparent Top Female Officers: 2
Hot Spot for Advancement for Women/Minorities:

LOCATIONS: ("Y" = Yes)
West:	Southwest:	Midwest:	Southeast:	Northeast:	International:
Y	Y	Y	Y	Y	

CASTLE DENTAL CENTERS INC

www.castledental.com

Industry Group Code: 621111 Ranks within this company's industry group: Sales: 8 Profits: 5

Insurance/HMO/PPO:	Drugs:	Equipment/Supplies:	Hospitals/Clinics:	Services:	Health Care:
Insurance:	Manufacturer:	Manufacturer:	Acute Care:	Diagnostics:	Home Health:
Managed Care:	Distributor:	Distributor:	Sub-Acute Care:	Labs/Testing:	Long-Term Care:
Utilization Mgmt.:	Specialty Pharm.:	Leasing/Finance:	Outpatient Surgery:	Staffing:	Physical Therapy:
Payment Proc.:	Vitamins/Nutri.:	Information Sys.:	Phys. Rehab. Center:	Waste Disposal:	Phys. Practice Mgmt.: Y
	Clinical Trials:		Psychiatric Clinics:	Specialty Services:	

TYPES OF BUSINESS:
Dental Practice Management

BRANDS/DIVISIONS/AFFILIATES:
Bright Now! Dental, Inc.

CONTACTS:
Note: Officers with more than one job title may be intentionally listed here more than once.

John M. Slack, Acting CEO
Joseph P. Keane, Sr. VP/CFO
James M. Slack, Chief Admin. Officer
David S. Lober, Chmn.

Phone: 713-490-8400   Fax: 713-490-8415
Toll-Free: 800-867-6453
Address: 3701 Kirby Dr., Ste. 550, Houston, TX 77098 US

GROWTH PLANS/SPECIAL FEATURES:

Castle Dental Centers, Inc. develops, manages and operates integrated dental networks through contracts with general, orthodontic and multi-specialty dental practices in the United States. The company manages approximately 74 dental centers with approximately 158 affiliated dentists, orthodontists and specialists in Texas, Florida, Tennessee and California. The prototypical Castle Dental Center provides general dentistry as well as a full range of dental specialties including orthodontics, pedodontics, periodontics, endodontics, oral surgery and implantology. Bringing together multi-specialty dental services within a single practice allows Castle to operate more efficiently, use facilities more completely and share dental specialists among multiple locations. This practice model also incorporates quality assurance and quality control programs, such as peer review and continuing education. Castle establishes regional dental care networks in order to centralize its advertising, billing and collections, payroll and accounting systems. In recent news, Castle became a subsidiary of Bright Now! Dental, Inc., a dental practice management service provider serving 300 offices in 19 states.

Castle Dental offers its employees medical and dental coverage as well as career development opportunities.

FINANCIALS:
Sales and profits are in thousands of dollars—add 000 to get the full amount. Year 2004 note: Complete fiscal 2004 results were not available for all companies at press time. For this company, year 2004 is for 3 months.

2004 Sales: $25,291 (3 months)	2004 Profits: $ 740 (3 months)	
2003 Sales: $93,889	2003 Profits: $26,104	Stock Ticker: Subsidiary
2002 Sales: $100,900	2002 Profits: $-29,600	Employees: 1,025
2001 Sales: $97,900	2001 Profits: $-14,800	Fiscal Year Ends: 12/31
2000 Sales: $106,023	2000 Profits: $-19,124	

SALARIES/BENEFITS:
Pension Plan:	ESOP Stock Plan:	Profit Sharing:	Top Exec. Salary: $249,722	Bonus: $63,334
Savings Plan: Y	Stock Purch. Plan:		Second Exec. Salary: $237,138	Bonus: $61,584

OTHER THOUGHTS:
Apparent Top Female Officers:
Hot Spot for Advancement for Women/Minorities:

LOCATIONS: ("Y" = Yes)

West:	Southwest:	Midwest:	Southeast:	Northeast:	International:
Y	Y		Y		

CATHOLIC HEALTH INITIATIVES

www.catholichealthinit.org

Industry Group Code: 622110 Ranks within this company's industry group: Sales: 7 Profits: 7

Insurance/HMO/PPO:	Drugs:	Equipment/Supplies:	Hospitals/Clinics:		Services:		Health Care:	
Insurance:	Manufacturer:	Manufacturer:	Acute Care:	Y	Diagnostics:		Home Health:	Y
Managed Care:	Distributor:	Distributor:	Sub-Acute Care:	Y	Labs/Testing:		Long-Term Care:	Y
Utilization Mgmt.:	Specialty Pharm.:	Leasing/Finance:	Outpatient Surgery:		Staffing:		Physical Therapy:	
Payment Proc.:	Vitamins/Nutri.:	Information Sys.:	Phys. Rehab. Center:		Waste Disposal:		Phys. Practice Mgmt.:	
	Clinical Trials:		Psychiatric Clinics:		Specialty Services:	Y		

TYPES OF BUSINESS:
Hospitals
Long-Term Care
Assisted and Independent Living Services
Community Health Organizations
Home Care Services
Occupational Health Clinic
Cancer Prevention Institute

BRANDS/DIVISIONS/AFFILIATES:
Centura Health
CARITAS Health Services
Alegant Health
Good Samaritan Health Systems
Premier Health Partners
Franciscan Health System

CONTACTS:
Note: Officers with more than one job title may be intentionally listed here more than once.
Kevin E. Lofton, CEO
Kevin E. Lofton, Pres.
Michael T. Rowan, Exec. VP/COO
Geraldine Hoyler, Sr. VP-Finance/Treas.

Phone: 303-298-9100 Fax: 303-298-9690
Toll-Free:
Address: 1999 Broadway, Ste. 2600, Denver, CO 80202-4004 US

GROWTH PLANS/SPECIAL FEATURES:

Catholic Health Initiatives (CHI), formed in 1996 with the purpose of strengthening and advancing the Catholic health ministry into the 21st century, is a national not-for-profit health care organization encompassing 68 hospitals; 44 long-term care, assisted and independent living residential facilities; and six community health organizations, across 19 states. CHI has several major affiliates. Centura Health, based in Colorado and jointly operated between CHI and PorterCare Adventist Health Care, is one of the state's largest private employers, with 12 hospitals and eight senior residences and home care and hospice services. CARITAS Health Services, based in Kentucky, is committed to the well-being of the body, mind and spirit and is anchored by its flagship facility, CARITAS Medical Center, a 331-bed primary care hospital offering cancer treatment, surgery and emergency services. Alegent Health, jointly operated with Immanuel Healthcare System and based in Nebraska, is made up of seven acute care hospitals with 1,433 beds, two long-term care facilities and a primary care physician network. Good Samaritan Health Systems, also based in Nebraska, is a network of hospitals and services serving more than 350,000 customers in the region. Premier Health Partners, based in Ohio and jointly operated with MedAmerica Health Systems, includes three hospitals, one assisted living community, a home health care service and a cancer prevention institute. The Franciscan Health System in Washington includes three full-service hospitals, a long-term care facility, a women's health center and midwives service and an occupational health clinic, among other services. In the near future, CHI will try to centralize business processes and streamline costs while attempting to maintain high-quality, safe and state-of-the-art local health ministries.

FINANCIALS:
Sales and profits are in thousands of dollars—add 000 to get the full amount. Year 2004 note: Complete fiscal 2004 results were not available for all companies at press time. For this company, year 2004 is for months.

2004 Sales: $ (months)	2004 Profits: $ (months)	Stock Ticker: Nonprofit
2003 Sales: $6,071,600	2003 Profits: $202,900	Employees: 67,000
2002 Sales: $5,900,200	2002 Profits: $117,100	Fiscal Year Ends:
2001 Sales: $	2001 Profits: $	
2000 Sales: $	2000 Profits: $	

SALARIES/BENEFITS:
Pension Plan:	ESOP Stock Plan:	Profit Sharing:	Top Exec. Salary: $	Bonus: $
Savings Plan:	Stock Purch. Plan:		Second Exec. Salary: $	Bonus: $

OTHER THOUGHTS:
Apparent Top Female Officers: 1
Hot Spot for Advancement for Women/Minorities:

LOCATIONS: ("Y" = Yes)
West:	Southwest:	Midwest:	Southeast:	Northeast:	International:
Y	Y	Y	Y	Y	

CATHOLIC HEALTHCARE PARTNERS   www.health-partners.org

Industry Group Code: 622110   Ranks within this company's industry group: Sales: 18   Profits:

Insurance/HMO/PPO:	Drugs:	Equipment/Supplies:	Hospitals/Clinics:		Services:		Health Care:	
Insurance:	Manufacturer:	Manufacturer:	Acute Care:	Y	Diagnostics:		Home Health:	Y
Managed Care:	Distributor:	Distributor:	Sub-Acute Care:	Y	Labs/Testing:		Long-Term Care:	Y
Utilization Mgmt.:	Specialty Pharm.:	Leasing/Finance:	Outpatient Surgery:		Staffing:		Physical Therapy:	
Payment Proc.:	Vitamins/Nutri.:	Information Sys.:	Phys. Rehab. Center:		Waste Disposal:		Phys. Practice Mgmt.:	
	Clinical Trials:		Psychiatric Clinics:		Specialty Services:	Y		

TYPES OF BUSINESS:
Hospitals
Long-Term Care
Hospice Programs
Home Health Services
Low-Income Housing

BRANDS/DIVISIONS/AFFILIATES:
Mercy Health Partners
Community Health Partners
West Central Ohio Health Partners
Humility of Mary Health Partners
Community Mercy Health Partners
St. Elizabeth Health Partners
St. Mary's Health Partners
Laurel Lake Retirement Community

CONTACTS:
Note: Officers with more than one job title may be intentionally listed here more than once.
Michael D. Connelly, CEO
Michael D. Connelly, Pres.
William Shuttleworth, Sr. VP/CFO
Jon C. Abeles, Sr. VP-Human Resources
Rebecca Sykes, Sr. VP/CIO
Michael A. Bezney, Sr. VP/General Counsel
Doris Gottenmoeller, Sr. VP-Mission & Values Integration
Donald E. Casey, Jr., Sr. VP/Chief Medical Officer
R. Jeffrey Copeland, Sr. VP-Insurance & Physician Services
Mildred Ely, Chmn.

Phone: 513-639-2800   Fax: 513-639-2700
Toll-Free:
Address: 615 Elsinore Pl., Cincinnati, OH 45202 US

GROWTH PLANS/SPECIAL FEATURES:
Catholic Healthcare Partners (CHP) is a not-for-profit health system consisting of more than 100 corporations in Ohio, Indiana, Kentucky, Pennsylvania and Tennessee. The organization has a total of 32 hospitals, 19 of which have long-term care beds, 14 long-term care facilities, 581 HUD housing units, 442 low-income tax credit housing units, 12 hospice programs, 11 home health agencies and 9,173 affiliated physicians. The organization was originally founded in 1986 by the Sisters of Mercy, Regional Community of Cincinnati and has since grown to include the sponsorship of four other congregations. It is separated into 11 main divisions, each exercising considerable autonomy, yet still profiting from improved strategic, operational and organizational benefits as a result its partnership in CHP: Mercy Health Partners (with northern, northeast, southwest Ohio and Kentucky/Indiana regions), Community Health Partners, West Central Ohio Health Partners, Humility of Mary Health Partners, Community Mercy Health Partners, St. Elizabeth Health Partners, St. Mary's Health Partners and Laurel Lake Retirement Community. Together these divisions have as their mission the extension of the healing ministry of Jesus with emphasis on people who are poor and under-served.

FINANCIALS:
Sales and profits are in thousands of dollars—add 000 to get the full amount. Year 2004 note: Complete fiscal 2004 results were not available for all companies at press time. For this company, year 2004 is for months.

2004 Sales: $ (months)   2004 Profits: $ (months)
2003 Sales: $2,874,300   2003 Profits: $
2002 Sales: $2,714,800   2002 Profits: $-122,200
2001 Sales: $ 2001 Profits: $
2000 Sales: $ 2000 Profits: $

Stock Ticker: Nonprofit
Employees:
Fiscal Year Ends:

SALARIES/BENEFITS:
Pension Plan: ESOP Stock Plan: Profit Sharing: Top Exec. Salary: $ Bonus: $
Savings Plan: Stock Purch. Plan: Second Exec. Salary: $ Bonus: $

OTHER THOUGHTS:
Apparent Top Female Officers: 3
Hot Spot for Advancement for Women/Minorities: Y

LOCATIONS: ("Y" = Yes)
West:	Southwest:	Midwest:	Southeast:	Northeast:	International:
		Y	Y	Y	

CATHOLIC HEALTHCARE WEST

www.chwhealth.org

Industry Group Code: 622110   Ranks within this company's industry group: Sales: 9   Profits: 15

Insurance/HMO/PPO:	Drugs:	Equipment/Supplies:	Hospitals/Clinics:		Services:	Health Care:
Insurance:	Manufacturer:	Manufacturer:	Acute Care:	Y	Diagnostics:	Home Health:
Managed Care:	Distributor:	Distributor:	Sub-Acute Care:		Labs/Testing:	Long-Term Care:
Utilization Mgmt.:	Specialty Pharm.:	Leasing/Finance:	Outpatient Surgery:		Staffing:	Physical Therapy:
Payment Proc.:	Vitamins/Nutri.:	Information Sys.:	Phys. Rehab. Center:		Waste Disposal:	Phys. Practice Mgmt.:
	Clinical Trials:		Psychiatric Clinics:		Specialty Services:	

TYPES OF BUSINESS:
Hospitals

BRANDS/DIVISIONS/AFFILIATES:
Mercy Healthcare Sacramento

CONTACTS:
Note: Officers with more than one job title may be intentionally listed here more than once.

Lloyd H. Dean, CEO
Lloyd H. Dean, Pres.
Michael Erne, Exec. VP/COO
Michael D. Blaszyk, Exec. VP/CFO
Ernest H. Urquhart, Sr. VP-Human Resources
Elizabeth Shih, Sr. VP-Admin.
Derek F. Covert, Sr. VP/General Counsel
Charles P. Francis, Sr. VP-Strategy
George Bo-Linn, Sr. VP/Chief Medical Officer
Bernita McTernan, Sr. VP-Sponsorship & Mission Integration
John Wray, Sr. VP-Managed Care
Diane Grassilli, Chmn.

Phone: 415-438-5500   **Fax:** 415-438-5724
Toll-Free:
Address: 185 Berry St., Ste. 300, San Francisco, CA 94107-1739 US

GROWTH PLANS/SPECIAL FEATURES:

Catholic Healthcare West (CHW), based in San Francisco, comprises 42 acute-care hospitals, skilled nursing facilities and medical centers, totaling 8,071 beds, located in California, Arizona and Nevada. It is the eighth-largest hospital system in the country and the largest not-for-profit system in California. The organization remains committed to compassionate and affordable health care services to all, without regard to financial resources, providing roughly $422 million in charity care in 2003. CHW was founded in 1986 by the Sisters of Mercy Burlingame Regional Community and the Sisters of Mercy Auburn Regional Community when the two congregations merged their respective health care ministries into one. Since then six other congregations have joined the organization. Mercy Healthcare Sacramento is one of CHW's largest divisions, consisting of six hospitals in Sacramento County. In recent news, CHW assumed ownership of two hospitals from Universal Health Services, Inc., Arroyo Grande Community Hospital and French Hospital Medical Center, both in California.

FINANCIALS:
Sales and profits are in thousands of dollars—add 000 to get the full amount. Year 2004 note: Complete fiscal 2004 results were not available for all companies at press time. For this company, year 2004 is for 12 months.

2004 Sales: $5,396,800 (12 months)   2004 Profits: $246,100 (12 months)
2003 Sales: $4,989,100   2003 Profits: $50,700
2002 Sales: $4,501,500   2002 Profits: $-50,600
2001 Sales: $ 2001 Profits: $
2000 Sales: $ 2000 Profits: $

Stock Ticker: Nonprofit
Employees: 40,000
Fiscal Year Ends: 6/30

SALARIES/BENEFITS:
| Pension Plan: | ESOP Stock Plan: | Profit Sharing: | Top Exec. Salary: $ | Bonus: $ |
| Savings Plan: | Stock Purch. Plan: | | Second Exec. Salary: $ | Bonus: $ |

OTHER THOUGHTS:
Apparent Top Female Officers: 3
Hot Spot for Advancement for Women/Minorities: Y

LOCATIONS: ("Y" = Yes)
West:	Southwest:	Midwest:	Southeast:	Northeast:	International:
Y	Y				

CEDARA SOFTWARE CORP

www.cedara.com

Industry Group Code: 511200   Ranks within this company's industry group: Sales: 12   Profits: 10

Insurance/HMO/PPO:	Drugs:	Equipment/Supplies:		Hospitals/Clinics:		Services:		Health Care:	
Insurance:	Manufacturer:	Manufacturer:	Y	Acute Care:		Diagnostics:		Home Health:	
Managed Care:	Distributor:	Distributor:		Sub-Acute Care:		Labs/Testing:		Long-Term Care:	
Utilization Mgmt.:	Specialty Pharm.:	Leasing/Finance:		Outpatient Surgery:		Staffing:		Physical Therapy:	
Payment Proc.:	Vitamins/Nutri.:	Information Sys.:	Y	Phys. Rehab. Center:		Waste Disposal:		Phys. Practice Mgmt.:	
	Clinical Trials:			Psychiatric Clinics:		Specialty Services:			

TYPES OF BUSINESS:
Software-Medical Imaging
Custom-Designed Medical Products

BRANDS/DIVISIONS/AFFILIATES:
Cedara Imaging Application Platform
Cedara OpenEyes
Cedara OrthoWorks
Cedara Vivace
eMed Technologies Corporation

CONTACTS:
Note: Officers with more than one job title may be intentionally listed here more than once.
Abe Schwartz, CEO
Abe Schwartz, Pres.
Brian Pedlar, CFO
Jacques Cornet, VP-Mktg.
Manu Mahbubani, VP-Eng.
Jacques Cornet, VP-Oper.
Loris Sartor, VP-Sales
Peter J. Cooper, Chmn.

Phone: 905-672-2100   **Fax:** 905-672-2307
Toll-Free: 800-724-5970
Address: 6509 Airport Rd., Mississauga, Ontario L4V 1S7 Canada

GROWTH PLANS/SPECIAL FEATURES:
Cedara Software Corp. is engaged in the development and manufacturing of medical imaging software and support systems, as well as the licensing and development of custom-designed medical products for its clients. The firm uses three software development models, which include turnkey applications, platform toolkits and custom engineering. The Cedara Imaging Application Platform (IAP) is part of 30% of MRIs shipped annually and 82% of all PET-CT systems installed in the U.S. The application is used for advanced 3-D processing, computed tomography (CT), digital x-rays, mammography, fluoroscopy, nuclear medicine and ultrasound. The company's imaging and information solutions division focuses on outsourcing intellectual property in imaging software applications, components, platforms and toolkits, as well as specialized development and custom engineering projects. Some examples of Cedara's software products are Cedara OpenEyes, the world's first open health care imaging platform, which enables health care providers to significantly reduce product development time; Cedara OrthoWorks, a suite of desktop and web server software designed for orthopedic surgeons; and Cedara Vivace, a suite of 3-D software plug-in components for examining images acquired from CT and MRI scanners. The company's clients include GE, Philips Medical Systems, Hitachi and Toshiba. In recent news, Cedara acquired eMed Technologies Corporation, a private company providing web-based medical imaging radiology software and picture archiving and communications systems (PACS). eMed has a broad base of hospital and imaging centers across the U.S., which will provide Cedara with a sales force to promote its clinical applications and technologies. Also in recent news, the company opened a new office in Shanghai, China.

The firm offers its employees flexible work hours, an in-house massage therapist, vision insurance, departmental events and discounted tickets to recreation sites and entertainment events.

FINANCIALS:
Sales and profits are in thousands of dollars—add 000 to get the full amount. Year 2004 note: Complete fiscal 2004 results were not available for all companies at press time. For this company, year 2004 is for months.

2004 Sales: $ (months)   2004 Profits: $ (months)
2003 Sales: $22,992   2003 Profits: $-10,152
2002 Sales: $30,000   2002 Profits: $1,000
2001 Sales: $30,900   2001 Profits: $-44,800
2000 Sales: $36,200   2000 Profits: $-4,300

Stock Ticker: CDSW
Employees: 234
Fiscal Year Ends: 6/30

SALARIES/BENEFITS:
Pension Plan: ESOP Stock Plan: Profit Sharing: Top Exec. Salary: $ Bonus: $
Savings Plan: Stock Purch. Plan: Second Exec. Salary: $ Bonus: $

OTHER THOUGHTS:
Apparent Top Female Officers:
Hot Spot for Advancement for Women/Minorities:

LOCATIONS: ("Y" = Yes)
West: Southwest: Midwest: Southeast: Northeast: International: Y

CELERA GENOMICS GROUP

www.celera.com

Industry Group Code: 541710 Ranks within this company's industry group: Sales: 8 Profits: 10

Insurance/HMO/PPO:	Drugs:	Equipment/Supplies:	Hospitals/Clinics:	Services:	Health Care:
Insurance:	Manufacturer:	Manufacturer:	Acute Care:	Diagnostics:	Home Health:
Managed Care:	Distributor:	Distributor:	Sub-Acute Care:	Labs/Testing: Y	Long-Term Care:
Utilization Mgmt.:	Specialty Pharm.:	Leasing/Finance:	Outpatient Surgery:	Staffing:	Physical Therapy:
Payment Proc.:	Vitamins/Nutri.:	Information Sys.: Y	Phys. Rehab. Center:	Waste Disposal:	Phys. Practice Mgmt.:
	Clinical Trials:		Psychiatric Clinics:	Specialty Services: Y	

TYPES OF BUSINESS:
Research-Human Genome Mapping
Information Management and Analysis Software
Consulting, Research and Development Services
Discovery, Validation and Licensing

BRANDS/DIVISIONS/AFFILIATES:
Celera Discovery System
Applera Corp.
Celera Diagnostics
Applied Biosystems

CONTACTS: Note: Officers with more than one job title may be intentionally listed here more than once.
Kathy Ordonez, Pres.
Peter Chambre, COO/VP-Applera
Bridgette Robinson, VP-Human Resources
Robert Booth, Chief Scientific Officer
John Reynders, VP-Informatics
Steven M. Ruben, VP-Protein Therapeutics
James Yee, VP-Dev.
Vikram Jog, VP-Finance
Samuel Broder, Chief Medical Officer
Paulette Dillon, Chief Bus. Officer
Michael J. Green, VP-Chemistry
Robert R. Young, VP-Biology

Phone: 240-453-3000 Fax: 240-453-4000
Toll-Free: 877-235-3721
Address: 45 W. Gude Dr., Rockville, MD 20850 US

GROWTH PLANS/SPECIAL FEATURES:
Celera Genomics Group, a division of Applera Corporation, generates, compiles, sells and supports genomic information as well as related information management and analysis software. The company also provides discovery, validation and licensing of proprietary gene products, genetic markers and information concerning genetic variability and related consulting, contract research and development services. It assists pharmaceutical, biotechnology and life science research entities in areas of research, including new drugs and improved drug development processes; novel genes and factors that regulate and control gene expression; and interrelationships between genetic variability, disease and drug response. Celera completed mapping the human genome ahead of the government-sponsored Human Genome Project and ahead of its own expectations. The underlying human genetic sequence provides the basis for Celera's development of a value-added, integrated information and discovery system. The system includes increasing layers of functional information such as gene expression data, comparative data from other model organisms (such as the fruit fly Drosophila Melanogaster and mouse), genetic variation and ultimately, gene function. Celera also operates the Celera Discovery System, a web-based resource that catalogues and regularly updates genomic information from mouse and human genomes. The company collaborates in drug discovery and development with Aventis Pharma, Merck, Maxim Pharmaceuticals, Isis Pharmaceuticals and SomaLogic. Paracel, a subsidiary of Celera, develops genomic data for pharmaceutical, biotechnology, information services and government markets. In July 2004, Celera announced a joint research collaboration with GE Global Research under which the companies will seek to understand and differentiate disease at the molecular level. Also in July, Celera began collaborating with Seattle Genetics, Inc. in order to discover and develop antibody-based therapies for cancer.

Every business in the Applera family provides a comprehensive benefits package; employee, education and adoption assistance programs; and three weeks of paid vacation per year.

FINANCIALS: Sales and profits are in thousands of dollars—add 000 to get the full amount. Year 2004 note: Complete fiscal 2004 results were not available for all companies at press time. For this company, year 2004 is for 12 months.

2004 Sales: $60,100 (12 months) 2004 Profits: $-57,500 (12 months)
2003 Sales: $88,300 2003 Profits: $-81,900
2002 Sales: $120,900 2002 Profits: $-211,800
2001 Sales: $89,400 2001 Profits: $-186,200
2000 Sales: $42,700 2000 Profits: $-92,700

Stock Ticker: CRA
Employees: 530
Fiscal Year Ends: 6/30

SALARIES/BENEFITS:
Pension Plan: ESOP Stock Plan: Profit Sharing: Top Exec. Salary: $468,077 Bonus: $451,250
Savings Plan: Y Stock Purch. Plan: Y   Second Exec. Salary: $484,069 Bonus: $258,851

OTHER THOUGHTS:
Apparent Top Female Officers: 2
Hot Spot for Advancement for Women/Minorities:

LOCATIONS: ("Y" = Yes)
West	Southwest	Midwest	Southeast	Northeast	International
Y				Y	

CELLTECH GROUP PLC

www.celltechgroup.com

Industry Group Code: 325412 **Ranks within this company's industry group:** Sales: 35 Profits: 38

Insurance/HMO/PPO:	Drugs:		Equipment/Supplies:	Hospitals/Clinics:	Services:	Health Care:
Insurance:	Manufacturer:	Y	Manufacturer:	Acute Care:	Diagnostics:	Home Health:
Managed Care:	Distributor:		Distributor:	Sub-Acute Care:	Labs/Testing:	Long-Term Care:
Utilization Mgmt.:	Specialty Pharm.:		Leasing/Finance:	Outpatient Surgery:	Staffing:	Physical Therapy:
Payment Proc.:	Vitamins/Nutri.:		Information Sys.:	Phys. Rehab. Center:	Waste Disposal:	Phys. Practice Mgmt.:
	Clinical Trials:			Psychiatric Clinics:	Specialty Services:	

TYPES OF BUSINESS:
Drugs-Diversified
Pain Therapies
Cancer Therapies
Autoimmune Therapies
Vaccines

BRANDS/DIVISIONS/AFFILIATES:
UCB SA
Celltech Pharmaceuticals
Celltech R&D
Zavesca

CONTACTS: Note: Officers with more than one job title may be intentionally listed here more than once.
Goran A. Ando, Group Chief Exec.
Melanie G. Lee, Dir.-Research & Discovery
Peter V. Allen, Dir.-Finance
Ingelise Saunders, CEO-Celltech Pharmaceuticals
Peter J. Fellner, Chmn.

Phone: 44-1753-534-655 **Fax:** 44-1753-536-632
Toll-Free:
Address: 208 Bath Rd., Slough, Berkshire SL1 3WE UK

GROWTH PLANS/SPECIAL FEATURES:
Celltech Group is a leading European biotechnology company involved in the discovery, development, marketing, distribution and manufacturing of innovative drugs for a wide range of applications. The company consists of two operating companies: Celltech R&D and Celltech Pharmaceuticals. Celltech R&D, the discovery and development arm, focuses on autoimmune and inflammatory disorders and cancer. Key products in its development pipeline include CDP 870 for the treatment of rheumatoid arthritis and Crohn's disease and PDE 4 for asthma. Zavesca, for the treatment of Gaucher's disease, recently secured approval. The company has formed strategic partnerships with Pharmacia, Merck & Co., Bristol-Myers Squibb, Schering Plough, American Home Products, AstraZeneca, Johnson & Johnson, Biogen, Abgenix, Neogenesis and Targeted Genetics. Celltech Pharmaceuticals is the firm's international pharmaceutical business, with operations in the U.S. and Europe. The company's portfolio of over 60 products includes treatments for disorders of the central nervous system, skin, gastrointestinal system, respiratory system and circulation, as well as inflammatory conditions and rheumatoid arthritis. In July 2004, Celltech partnered with scientists at Pembroke College, Cambridge, in a diverse set of research projects. In other news, Celltech accepted UCB SA's May 2004 offer to acquire the company for approximately $2.8 billion in cash.

FINANCIALS:
Sales and profits are in thousands of dollars—add 000 to get the full amount. Year 2004 note: Complete fiscal 2004 results were not available for all companies at press time. For this company, year 2004 is for months.

2004 Sales: $ (months)   2004 Profits: $ (months)
2003 Sales: $630,100   2003 Profits: $-96,100
2002 Sales: $517,999   2002 Profits: $369,169
2001 Sales: $441,400   2001 Profits: $-80,800
2000 Sales: $329,800   2000 Profits: $-601,500

Stock Ticker: Foreign
Employees: 2,029
Fiscal Year Ends: 6/30

SALARIES/BENEFITS:
Pension Plan: ESOP Stock Plan: Profit Sharing: Top Exec. Salary: $ Bonus: $
Savings Plan: Stock Purch. Plan: Second Exec. Salary: $ Bonus: $

OTHER THOUGHTS:
Apparent Top Female Officers: 2
Hot Spot for Advancement for Women/Minorities:

LOCATIONS: ("Y" = Yes)

West:	Southwest:	Midwest:	Southeast:	Northeast:	International:
				Y	Y

CENTENE CORPORATION

www.centene.com

Industry Group Code: 524114 Ranks within this company's industry group: Sales: 49 Profits: 37

Insurance/HMO/PPO:		Drugs:		Equipment/Supplies:		Hospitals/Clinics:		Services:		Health Care:	
Insurance:		Manufacturer:		Manufacturer:		Acute Care:		Diagnostics:		Home Health:	
Managed Care:	Y	Distributor:		Distributor:		Sub-Acute Care:		Labs/Testing:		Long-Term Care:	
Utilization Mgmt.:		Specialty Pharm.:		Leasing/Finance:		Outpatient Surgery:		Staffing:		Physical Therapy:	
Payment Proc.:		Vitamins/Nutri.:		Information Sys.:		Phys. Rehab. Center:		Waste Disposal:		Phys. Practice Mgmt.:	
		Clinical Trials:				Psychiatric Clinics:		Specialty Services:			

TYPES OF BUSINESS:
Managed Care
Life Insurance
Health Insurance
Medicare HMO
Medicaid HMO

BRANDS/DIVISIONS/AFFILIATES:
Cenpatico Behavior Health
Group Practice Affiliates, LLC
NurseWise
ScriptAssist
CenCorp Health Solutions

CONTACTS: Note: Officers with more than one job title may be intentionally listed here more than once.
Michael F. Neidorff, CEO
Michael F. Neidorff, Pres.
Karey L. Witty, Sr. VP/CFO
Brian G. Spanel, Sr. VP/CIO
James D. Donovan, Jr., Sr. VP-Product Dev.
Carol E. Goldman, Sr. VP/Chief Admin. Officer
Joseph P. Drozda, Jr., Exec. VP-Oper.
Cary D. Hobbs, Sr. VP-Strategy & Bus.
Lisa M. Wilson, VP-Investor Rel.
Marie J. Glancy, VP-Gov't Rel.
Daniel R. Paquin, Sr. VP-New Plan Implementation & Dev.
John D. Tadich, Sr. VP-Specialty Companies
Patricia J. Darnley, Pres./CEO-University Health Plans
Michael F. Neidorff, Chmn.

Phone: 314-725-4477 **Fax:** 314-725-2065
Toll-Free: 800-225-2573
Address: 7711 Carondelet Ave., Ste. 800, St Louis, MO 63105 US

GROWTH PLANS/SPECIAL FEATURES:
CENTENE Corporation is a government services managed health care company. The firm focuses on providing managed care programs to individuals entitled to benefits under Medicaid, including Supplemental Security Income and the State Children's Health Insurance Program (SCHIP). The company has health plans in Wisconsin, Texas, Indiana, New Jersey and Ohio and provides specialty services in Texas, California, Arizona, Colorado, Wisconsin and Indiana. The firm focuses on a local approach to managing health plans, which includes providing member services and culturally sensitive health care services to its members. CENTENE recently announced plans to realign its specialty companies, Cenpatico Behavior Health (formerly Group Practice Affiliates, LLC), NurseWise and ScriptAssist, into a subsidiary called CenCorp Health Solutions. CenCorp will be a Medicaid-focused specialty platform concentrated on behavioral health, nurse triage and pharmacy compliance. Also in recent news, the company plans to establish a 50,000-square-foot processing facility in Great Falls, Montana.

CENTENE offers its employees tuition reimbursement, vision insurance, business travel accident coverage and an employee assistance program.

FINANCIALS: Sales and profits are in thousands of dollars—add 000 to get the full amount. Year 2004 note: Complete fiscal 2004 results were not available for all companies at press time. For this company, year 2004 is for 9 months.

2004 Sales: $712,876 (9 months)   2004 Profits: $32,302 (9 months)
2003 Sales: $769,730   2003 Profits: $33,270
2002 Sales: $461,500   2002 Profits: $25,600
2001 Sales: $326,600   2001 Profits: $12,900
2000 Sales: $221,400   2000 Profits: $7,700

Stock Ticker: CNC
Employees: 950
Fiscal Year Ends: 12/31

SALARIES/BENEFITS:
| Pension Plan: | ESOP Stock Plan: | Profit Sharing: | Top Exec. Salary: $500,000 | Bonus: $1,200,000 |
| Savings Plan: Y | Stock Purch. Plan: | | Second Exec. Salary: $285,000 | Bonus: $90,000 |

OTHER THOUGHTS:
Apparent Top Female Officers: 5
Hot Spot for Advancement for Women/Minorities: Y

LOCATIONS: ("Y" = Yes)
West:	Southwest:	Midwest:	Southeast:	Northeast:	International:
Y	Y	Y		Y	

CENTERPULSE AG

www.centerpulse.com

Industry Group Code: 339113 **Ranks within this company's industry group:** Sales: Profits:

Insurance/HMO/PPO:	Drugs:	Equipment/Supplies:		Hospitals/Clinics:		Services:		Health Care:	
Insurance:	Manufacturer:	Manufacturer:	Y	Acute Care:		Diagnostics:		Home Health:	
Managed Care:	Distributor:	Distributor:	Y	Sub-Acute Care:		Labs/Testing:		Long-Term Care:	
Utilization Mgmt.:	Specialty Pharm.:	Leasing/Finance:		Outpatient Surgery:		Staffing:		Physical Therapy:	
Payment Proc.:	Vitamins/Nutri.:	Information Sys.:		Phys. Rehab. Center:		Waste Disposal:		Phys. Practice Mgmt.:	
	Clinical Trials:			Psychiatric Clinics:		Specialty Services:			

TYPES OF BUSINESS:
Artificial Joints & Implants
Dental Implants
Tissue Regeneration Materials

GROWTH PLANS/SPECIAL FEATURES:
Centerpulse Orthopedics AG, formerly Sulzer Medical and now a subsidiary of Zimmer Holdings, Inc., is one of Europe's leading reconstructive orthopedic companies. The company operates through three business divisions: dental, which operates as Zimmer Dental, Inc.; orthopedics, which operates as Centerpulse Orthopedics, Ltd. in Europe and Centerpulse Orthopedics, Inc. in the U.S.; and spine-tech, which operates as Centerpulse Spine-Tech, Inc. The firm offers a wide range of products, including tissue regeneration materials, artificial joints, mechanical and biological implants for meniscus and ligament repair, pates and screws for treatment of bone fractures, dental implants, and hip, joint and spinal implants.

BRANDS/DIVISIONS/AFFILIATES:
Sulzer Medical
Zimmer Holdings, Inc.
Zimmer Dental, Inc.
Centerpulse Orthopedics, Ltd.
Centerpulse Orthopedics, Inc.
Centerpulse Spine-Tech, Inc.

CONTACTS:
Note: Officers with more than one job title may be intentionally listed here more than once.
Max E. Link, CEO
Urs Kamber, CFO
Beatrice Tschanz, VP-Corp. Comm.
Max E. Link, Chmn.

Phone: 41-52-262-60-70   **Fax:** 41-52-262-01-39
Toll-Free:
Address: Sulzer-Allee 8, Winterthur, CH-8405 Switzerland

FINANCIALS:
Sales and profits are in thousands of dollars—add 000 to get the full amount. Year 2004 note: Complete fiscal 2004 results were not available for all companies at press time. For this company, year 2004 is for   months.

2004 Sales: $ (months)   2004 Profits: $ (months)
2003 Sales: $ 2003 Profits: $
2002 Sales: $ 2002 Profits: $
2001 Sales: $ 2001 Profits: $
2000 Sales: $ 2000 Profits: $

Stock Ticker: Subsidiary
Employees:
Fiscal Year Ends: 12/31

SALARIES/BENEFITS:
Pension Plan: ESOP Stock Plan: Profit Sharing: Top Exec. Salary: $ Bonus: $
Savings Plan: Stock Purch. Plan: Second Exec. Salary: $ Bonus: $

OTHER THOUGHTS:
Apparent Top Female Officers: 1
Hot Spot for Advancement for Women/Minorities:

LOCATIONS: ("Y" = Yes)
West	Southwest	Midwest	Southeast	Northeast	International
Y	Y	Y	Y	Y	Y

Note: Financial information, benefits and other data can change quickly and may vary from those stated here.

CEPHALON INC

www.cephalon.com

Industry Group Code: 325412   **Ranks within this company's industry group:** Sales: 31   Profits: 27

Insurance/HMO/PPO:	Drugs:		Equipment/Supplies:	Hospitals/Clinics:	Services:	Health Care:
Insurance:	Manufacturer:	Y	Manufacturer:	Acute Care:	Diagnostics:	Home Health:
Managed Care:	Distributor:		Distributor:	Sub-Acute Care:	Labs/Testing:	Long-Term Care:
Utilization Mgmt.:	Specialty Pharm.:		Leasing/Finance:	Outpatient Surgery:	Staffing:	Physical Therapy:
Payment Proc.:	Vitamins/Nutri.:		Information Sys.:	Phys. Rehab. Center:	Waste Disposal:	Phys. Practice Mgmt.:
	Clinical Trials:			Psychiatric Clinics:	Specialty Services:	

TYPES OF BUSINESS:
Drugs-Sleep-Related Disorders
Neurological Disorder Treatments
Cancer Treatments
Pain Medications

BRANDS/DIVISIONS/AFFILIATES:
PROVIGIL
Actiq
GABRITRIL
CIMA Labs, Inc.

CONTACTS: Note: Officers with more than one job title may be intentionally listed here more than once.
Frank Baldino, Jr., CEO
J. Kevin Buchi, Sr. VP/CFO
Carl A. Savini, Sr. VP-Human Resources
Jeffry L. Vaught, Sr. VP-Research & Dev.
Peter E. Grebow, Sr. VP-Worldwide Tech. Oper.
John E. Osborn, Sr. VP/General Counsel
Robert P. Roche, Jr., Sr. VP-Pharmaceutical Oper.
Paul Blake, Sr. VP-Clinical Research and Regulatory Affairs
John E. Osborn, Corp. Sec.
Kenneth J. Fiorelli, VP-Global Process Dev.
Frank Baldino, Jr., Chmn.

Phone: 610-344-0200   **Fax:** 610-738-6590
Toll-Free:
Address: 145 Brandywine Pkwy., West Chester, PA 19380 US

GROWTH PLANS/SPECIAL FEATURES:
Cephalon, Inc. is a biopharmaceutical company that is engaged in the discovery, development and marketing of products to treat sleep disorders, neurological and psychiatric disorders, cancer and pain. The company markets more than 20 products internationally and three in the U.S. PROVIGIL increases wakefulness in patients that suffer from abnormal daytime sleepiness due to obstructive sleep apnea. The drug is designed as a wake-promoting agent for sleep disorders related to narcolepsy. Actiq is a treatment breakthrough for cancer pain, and GABRITRIL is used for the treatment of epilepsy. Cephalon's foreign products include treatments for depression, obsessive compulsive disorder, Parkinson's disease, cardiovascular disorders, bipolar disease and epilepsy. It also markets the popular drug Ritalin for attention deficit hyperactivity disorder in the U.K. In addition, three more drugs are in clinical trials for the treatment of Parkinson's disease, leukemia, prostate cancer and solid tumors. The company will acquire CIMA Labs, Inc. during 2004.

Employees at Cephalon receive a full benefits package that includes flexible spending accounts.

FINANCIALS: Sales and profits are in thousands of dollars—add 000 to get the full amount. Year 2004 note: Complete fiscal 2004 results were not available for all companies at press time. For this company, year 2004 is for 9 months.

2004 Sales: $716,426 (9 months)	2004 Profits: $151,918 (9 months)	**Stock Ticker:** CEPH
2003 Sales: $714,800	2003 Profits: $83,900	Employees: 1,646
2002 Sales: $506,897	2002 Profits: $171,528	Fiscal Year Ends: 12/31
2001 Sales: $226,100	2001 Profits: $-55,500	
2000 Sales: $111,790	2000 Profits: $-101,200	

SALARIES/BENEFITS:
Pension Plan:	ESOP Stock Plan:	Profit Sharing:	Top Exec. Salary: $880,000	Bonus: $880,000
Savings Plan: Y	Stock Purch. Plan:		Second Exec. Salary: $400,000	Bonus: $160,000

OTHER THOUGHTS:
Apparent Top Female Officers:
Hot Spot for Advancement for Women/Minorities:

LOCATIONS: ("Y" = Yes)
West:	Southwest:	Midwest:	Southeast:	Northeast:	International:
Y				Y	Y

CERNER CORP

www.cerner.com

Industry Group Code: 511200   Ranks within this company's industry group: Sales: 2   Profits: 3

Insurance/HMO/PPO:	Drugs:	Equipment/Supplies:	Hospitals/Clinics:	Services:	Health Care:
Insurance:	Manufacturer:	Manufacturer:	Acute Care:	Diagnostics:	Home Health:
Managed Care:	Distributor:	Distributor:	Sub-Acute Care:	Labs/Testing:	Long-Term Care:
Utilization Mgmt.:	Specialty Pharm.:	Leasing/Finance:	Outpatient Surgery:	Staffing:	Physical Therapy:
Payment Proc.:	Vitamins/Nutri.:	Information Sys.: Y	Phys. Rehab. Center:	Waste Disposal:	Phys. Practice Mgmt.:
	Clinical Trials:		Psychiatric Clinics:	Specialty Services: Y	

TYPES OF BUSINESS:
Software-Clinical
Medical Information Systems
Application Hosting
Integrated Delivery Networks
Access Management
Consulting Services

BRANDS/DIVISIONS/AFFILIATES:
Cerner Millennium
PowerInsight

CONTACTS: Note: Officers with more than one job title may be intentionally listed here more than once.
Neal L. Patterson, CEO
Trace Devanny, Pres.
Glenn P. Tobin, Exec. VP/COO
Marc G. Naughton, Sr. VP/CFO
Don Trigg, Sr. VP/Chief Mktg. Officer
David McCallie, Jr., Chief Scientist & Medical Informatics Officer
Randy Sims, Chief Legal Officer
Jack A. Newman, Jr., Exec. VP
Paul Gorup, Sr. VP-Knowledge & Discovery
Douglas M. Krebs, Pres.-Global Organization
Jeffrey S. Rose, Chief Medical Officer
Neal L. Patterson, Chmn.

Phone: 816-221-1024   Fax: 816-474-1742
Toll-Free:
Address: 2800 Rockcreek Pkwy., Ste. 601, Kansas City, MO 64117 US

GROWTH PLANS/SPECIAL FEATURES:

Cerner Corporation, with more than 1,500 clients worldwide, designs, develops, installs and supports information technology and content solutions for health care organizations, consumers and physicians. Cerner's solutions are designed to help eliminate error, variance and waste in the care process, as well as provide appropriate health information and knowledge to care givers, clinicians and consumers and appropriate management information to health care administrations. The firm allows secure access to data by users in organized care settings and by general consumers from their homes. The Cerner Millennium platform of applications is a single-architecture health care information system capable of both retrieving and disseminating information across an entire health system. Cerner also markets more than 200 solutions options that complement its major information systems. In addition, Cerner offers comprehensive consulting services including readiness assessments, transition management and process redesign and learning services. Cerner's new health care intelligence solution, PowerInsight, provides health care organizations with a single data warehouse of resources and information regarding data collection, decision-making and scientific content.

The company offers employees a fitness center as well as immunizations and health screenings for them and their dependents. Employees also enjoy flexible work schedules and an on-site Montessori school.

FINANCIALS: Sales and profits are in thousands of dollars—add 000 to get the full amount. Year 2004 note: Complete fiscal 2004 results were not available for all companies at press time. For this company, year 2004 is for 9 months.

2004 Sales: $678,184 (9 months)	2004 Profits: $43,222 (9 months)	Stock Ticker: CERN
2003 Sales: $839,587	2003 Profits: $42,791	Employees: 5,077
2002 Sales: $751,900	2002 Profits: $48,000	Fiscal Year Ends: 12/30
2001 Sales: $542,600	2001 Profits: $-42,400	
2000 Sales: $404,504	2000 Profits: $105,300	

SALARIES/BENEFITS:
Pension Plan: Y   ESOP Stock Plan: Profit Sharing: Top Exec. Salary: $569,903   Bonus: $137,579
Savings Plan: Y   Stock Purch. Plan: Second Exec. Salary: $412,788   Bonus: $228,808

OTHER THOUGHTS:
Apparent Top Female Officers: 1
Hot Spot for Advancement for Women/Minorities:

LOCATIONS: ("Y" = Yes)

West:	Southwest:	Midwest:	Southeast:	Northeast:	International:
Y	Y	Y	Y	Y	Y

CHINDEX INTERNATIONAL INC

www.chindex.com

Industry Group Code: 421450   Ranks within this company's industry group: Sales: Profits:

Insurance/HMO/PPO:	Drugs:	Equipment/Supplies:	Hospitals/Clinics:	Services:	Health Care:
Insurance:	Manufacturer:	Manufacturer:	Acute Care: Y	Diagnostics:	Home Health:
Managed Care:	Distributor:	Distributor: Y	Sub-Acute Care:	Labs/Testing:	Long-Term Care:
Utilization Mgmt.:	Specialty Pharm.:	Leasing/Finance:	Outpatient Surgery:	Staffing:	Physical Therapy:
Payment Proc.:	Vitamins/Nutri.:	Information Sys.:	Phys. Rehab. Center:	Waste Disposal:	Phys. Practice Mgmt.:
	Clinical Trials:		Psychiatric Clinics:	Specialty Services: Y	

TYPES OF BUSINESS:
Health Care Products Distribution
Marketing, Sales and Technical Services
Private Hospitals

BRANDS/DIVISIONS/AFFILIATES:
U.S.-China Industrial Exchange, Inc.
Beijing United Family Hospital and Clinics
Shanghai United Family Hospital and Clinics

CONTACTS:
Note: Officers with more than one job title may be intentionally listed here more than once.
Roberta Lipson, CEO
Roberta Lipson, Pres.
Robert C. Goodwin, Jr., General Counsel
Robert C. Goodwin, Jr., Exec. VP-Oper.
Lawrence Pemble, Exec. VP-Bus. Dev.
Lawrence Pemble, Exec. VP-Finance
Elyse B. Siverberg, Exec. VP/Corp. Sec.
Roberta Lipson, Chmn.

Phone: 301-215-7777   **Fax:** 301-215-7719
Toll-Free:
Address: 7201 Wisconsin Ave., Ste 703, Bethesda, MD 20814 US

GROWTH PLANS/SPECIAL FEATURES:

Chindex, Inc., formerly U.S.-China Industrial Exchange, Inc., provides U.S., European and other manufacturers of health care products with access to the Chinese marketplace. The company also offers a wide range of marketing, sales and technical services for its products. The company operates in three segments. Through the capital medical equipment division, Chindex markets, sells and facilitates the export of select capital health care equipment and instrumentation throughout China on the basis of exclusive agreements with the manufacturers of these products. Chindex is the largest independent U.S. distributor of health care equipment in China. Second, the company's health care products distribution division, through a network of foreign-owned subsidiaries, imports and distributes off-the-shelf health care instrumentation and health-related consumable products. Finally, the health care services division operates the company's private hospitals, Beijing United Family Hospital and Clinics and Shanghai United Family Hospital and Clinics, which opened in 2003. In recent news, Chindex announced an agreement with Candela Corporation to distribute Candela's extensive line of aesthetic laser systems throughout the health care industry in China.

Almost all of Chindex's employees live in China and Hong Kong.

FINANCIALS:
Sales and profits are in thousands of dollars—add 000 to get the full amount. Year 2004 note: Complete fiscal 2004 results were not available for all companies at press time. For this company, year 2004 is for 12 months.

2004 Sales: $88,183 (12 months)   2004 Profits: $-1,987 (12 months)
2003 Sales: $ 2003 Profits: $
2002 Sales: $70,600   2002 Profits: $ 300
2001 Sales: $56,100   2001 Profits: $ 400
2000 Sales: $45,100   2000 Profits: $ 600

Stock Ticker: CHDX
Employees: 759
Fiscal Year Ends: 3/31

SALARIES/BENEFITS:
Pension Plan: ESOP Stock Plan: Profit Sharing: Top Exec. Salary: $184,437   Bonus: $25,000
Savings Plan: Stock Purch. Plan: Second Exec. Salary: $177,606   Bonus: $25,000

OTHER THOUGHTS:
Apparent Top Female Officers: 2
Hot Spot for Advancement for Women/Minorities:

LOCATIONS: ("Y" = Yes)

West:	Southwest:	Midwest:	Southeast:	Northeast:	International:
				Y	Y

Note: Financial information, benefits and other data can change quickly and may vary from those stated here.

CHIRON CORP

www.chiron.com

Industry Group Code: 325412 Ranks within this company's industry group: Sales: 23 Profits: 22

Insurance/HMO/PPO:	Drugs:	Equipment/Supplies:	Hospitals/Clinics:	Services:	Health Care:
Insurance:	Manufacturer: Y	Manufacturer:	Acute Care:	Diagnostics: Y	Home Health:
Managed Care:	Distributor:	Distributor:	Sub-Acute Care:	Labs/Testing: Y	Long-Term Care:
Utilization Mgmt.:	Specialty Pharm.:	Leasing/Finance:	Outpatient Surgery:	Staffing:	Physical Therapy:
Payment Proc.:	Vitamins/Nutri.:	Information Sys.:	Phys. Rehab. Center:	Waste Disposal:	Phys. Practice Mgmt.:
	Clinical Trials:		Psychiatric Clinics:	Specialty Services: Y	

TYPES OF BUSINESS:
Drugs-Cancer
Biopharmaceuticals
Vaccines
Blood Screening Assays

BRANDS/DIVISIONS/AFFILIATES:
TOBI
Proleukin
Betaseron
Fluad
Menjugate
Chiron Blood Testing
Chiron Biopharmaceuticals
Chiron Vaccines

CONTACTS:
Note: Officers with more than one job title may be intentionally listed here more than once.

Howard Pien, CEO
Howard Pien, Pres.
David V. Smith, VP/CFO
Rino Rappuoli, VP/Chief Scientific Officer
William G. Green, Sr. VP/General Counsel
Kevin Bryett, VP-Oper., Chiron Vaccines
Bryan Walser, VP-Strategy
Craig A. Wheeler, Pres., Chiron Biopharmaceuticals
Linda W. Short, VP-Corp. Resources
Jack Goldstein, Pres., Chiron Blood Testing
John A. Lambert, Pres., Chiron Vaccines
Howard Pein, Chmn.

Phone: 510-655-8730 Fax: 510-655-9910
Toll-Free:
Address: 4560 Horton St., Emeryville, CA 94608-2916 US

GROWTH PLANS/SPECIAL FEATURES:
Chiron is a biotechnology company that participates in three global health care businesses: biopharmaceuticals, vaccines and blood testing. The company applies a broad and integrated scientific approach to the development of innovative products for preventing and treating cancer, infectious diseases and cardiovascular disease. Chiron Biopharmaceuticals discovers, develops, manufactures and markets a range of therapeutic products, including TOBI for pseudomonal lung infections in cystic fibrosis patients, Betaseron for multiple sclerosis and Proleukin for cancer. Chiron Vaccines, the fifth-largest vaccines business in the world, currently offers more than 30 vaccines. Its vaccines include Menjugate for meningococcal meningitis, Fluad for influenza, Encepur for tick-borne encephalitis and Rabipur/RabAvert for rabies. Menjugate has not been approved for use in the U.S. Chiron Blood Testing provides products used by the blood banking industry. Its nucleic acid testing blood screening assays include the Procleix HIV-1/HCV assay. The company began clinical trials in 2003 for its Ultrio assay, designed to detect HIV and hepatitis C and B viruses. Through the company's joint business with Ortho-Clinical Diagnostics, Inc., a Johnson & Johnson company, it develops and markets a line of immunodiagnostic screening and supplemental tests for infectious diseases. In July 2004, Chiron initiated a clinical trial of its Procleix West Nile virus blood screening assay. In October 2004, the company announced that it will be unable to deliver half of the flu vaccine needed in the U.S. because of contamination at its processing plant in the U.K.

The company offers its employees educational assistance, credit union membership and access to prepaid legal services, as well as discounted auto and home insurance. The firm also has a LifeCare service that provides information and support on topics such as adoption, prenatal planning and child care.

FINANCIALS:
Sales and profits are in thousands of dollars—add 000 to get the full amount. Year 2004 note: Complete fiscal 2004 results were not available for all companies at press time. For this company, year 2004 is for 9 months.

2004 Sales: $1,297,262 (9 months)   2004 Profits: $107,822 (9 months)
2003 Sales: $1,776,361   2003 Profits: $227,313
2002 Sales: $972,900   2002 Profits: $180,800
2001 Sales: $1,140,700   2001 Profits: $180,100
2000 Sales: $972,119   2000 Profits: $8,500

Stock Ticker: CHIR
Employees: 5,332
Fiscal Year Ends: 12/31

SALARIES/BENEFITS:
Pension Plan: Y   ESOP Stock Plan: Profit Sharing: Top Exec. Salary: $800,000   Bonus: $897,293
Savings Plan: Y   Stock Purch. Plan: Y   Second Exec. Salary: $552,461 Bonus: $1,500,000

OTHER THOUGHTS:
Apparent Top Female Officers: 1
Hot Spot for Advancement for Women/Minorities:

LOCATIONS: ("Y" = Yes)
West:	Southwest:	Midwest:	Southeast:	Northeast:	International:
Y	Y	Y	Y	Y	Y

CHOLESTECH CORP

www.cholestech.com

Industry Group Code: 339113 **Ranks within this company's industry group:** Sales: 112 Profits: 89

Insurance/HMO/PPO:	Drugs:	Equipment/Supplies:		Hospitals/Clinics:	Services:	Health Care:
Insurance:	Manufacturer:	Manufacturer:	Y	Acute Care:	Diagnostics:	Home Health:
Managed Care:	Distributor:	Distributor:	Y	Sub-Acute Care:	Labs/Testing:	Long-Term Care:
Utilization Mgmt.:	Specialty Pharm.:	Leasing/Finance:		Outpatient Surgery:	Staffing:	Physical Therapy:
Payment Proc.:	Vitamins/Nutri.:	Information Sys.:		Phys. Rehab. Center:	Waste Disposal:	Phys. Practice Mgmt.:
	Clinical Trials:			Psychiatric Clinics:	Specialty Services:	

TYPES OF BUSINESS:
Equipment-Blood Diagnostic Test Systems

BRANDS/DIVISIONS/AFFILIATES:
LDX System
GDX System
LDX Analyzer
Aspartate Aminotransferase Test

CONTACTS:
Note: Officers with more than one job title may be intentionally listed here more than once.
Warren E. Pinckert, II, CEO
Warren E. Pinckert, II, Pres.
John Glenn, CFO
Kenneth F. Miller, VP-Mktg. & Sales
Terry Wassmann, VP-Human Resources
Donald P. Wood, VP-Oper.
Thomas E. Worthy, VP-Dev. & Regulatory Affairs
John Glenn, VP-Finance
John H. Landon, Chmn.

Phone: 510-732-7200 **Fax:** 510-732-7227
Toll-Free: 800-733-0404
Address: 3347 Investment Blvd., Hayward, CA 94545-3808 US

GROWTH PLANS/SPECIAL FEATURES:
Cholestech provides diagnostic tools for immediate risk assessment and monitoring of heart disease and diabetes. It currently manufactures the LDX System, which includes the LDX Analyzer and a variety of single-use test cassettes. The company markets the LDX System in the United States, Europe, Asia, Australia and South America. The LDX System, waived under the Clinical Laboratory Improvement Amendments (CLIA), allows health care providers to perform individual tests or combinations of tests with a single drop of blood within five minutes. Cholestech also markets and distributes the GDX System under a multi-year global distribution agreement with Provalis Diagnostics, Ltd. The GDX is a hemoglobin A1C (A1C) testing system that is also waived under CLIA. Unlike daily glucose monitoring, which provides a snapshot of a patient's glucose level at the time of testing, A1C provides an average glucose level over the previous 90 days. A1C levels indicate the long-term progress of a patient's diabetes and therapy management. The firm's primary market is the physician office laboratory market, but it also sells its products to the health promotion market, which includes a variety of venues such as corporate wellness programs, fitness centers, health promotion service providers, community health centers, public health programs, the United States military and other independent screeners. Recently, Cholestech agreed to distribute Itamar Medical's Endo-Pat 2000, an assessment system for vascular endothelial dysfunction. The Endo-Pat measures peripheral arterial tone (PAT), a neurovascular signal that provides a non-invasive way of monitoring autonomic nervous system and arterial health. Also in recent news, the company has begun shipment of its CLIA-waived Aspartate Aminotransferase (AST) Test for monitoring the effects of various drugs on the liver.

Cholestech offers its employees medical, dental and life insurance as well as product training and usage.

FINANCIALS:
Sales and profits are in thousands of dollars—add 000 to get the full amount. Year 2004 note: Complete fiscal 2004 results were not available for all companies at press time. For this company, year 2004 is for 12 months.

2004 Sales: $52,376 (12 months)   2004 Profits: $8,707 (12 months)
2003 Sales: $48,500   2003 Profits: $4,900
2002 Sales: $47,400   2002 Profits: $5,600
2001 Sales: $37,003   2001 Profits: $-2,606
2000 Sales: $27,549   2000 Profits: $3,261

Stock Ticker: CTEC
Employees: 199
Fiscal Year Ends: 3/31

SALARIES/BENEFITS:
| Pension Plan: | ESOP Stock Plan: Y | Profit Sharing: | Top Exec. Salary: $369,465 | Bonus: $33,750 |
| Savings Plan: Y | Stock Purch. Plan: | | Second Exec. Salary: $220,390 | Bonus: $15,053 |

OTHER THOUGHTS:
Apparent Top Female Officers: 1
Hot Spot for Advancement for Women/Minorities:

LOCATIONS: ("Y" = Yes)
West:	Southwest:	Midwest:	Southeast:	Northeast:	International:
Y					

CHRISTUS HEALTH

www.christushealth.org

Industry Group Code: 622110 **Ranks within this company's industry group:** Sales: 29 Profits: 17

Insurance/HMO/PPO:	Drugs:	Equipment/Supplies:	Hospitals/Clinics:		Services:		Health Care:	
Insurance:	Manufacturer:	Manufacturer:	Acute Care:	Y	Diagnostics:		Home Health:	
Managed Care:	Distributor:	Distributor:	Sub-Acute Care:	Y	Labs/Testing:		Long-Term Care:	Y
Utilization Mgmt.:	Specialty Pharm.:	Leasing/Finance:	Outpatient Surgery:		Staffing:		Physical Therapy:	
Payment Proc.:	Vitamins/Nutri.:	Information Sys.:	Phys. Rehab. Center:		Waste Disposal:		Phys. Practice Mgmt.:	
	Clinical Trials:		Psychiatric Clinics:		Specialty Services:			

TYPES OF BUSINESS:
Hospitals

GROWTH PLANS/SPECIAL FEATURES:
CHRISTUS Health System is a faith-based, not-for-profit organization formed in 1999 by the combination of two Catholic charities, Sisters of Charity of the Incarnate Word in Houston and Sisters of Charity of the Incarnate Word in San Antonio. Today, CHRISTUS is one of the top 10 Catholic health systems in the U.S., with more than 40 hospitals, inpatient and long-term care facilities, dozens of clinics and physician offices and roughly 8,000 physicians in more than 70 cities in Texas, Arkansas, Louisiana, Oklahoma, Utah and Mexico. Its web site provides information on healthy recipes, health news and information and a section for testimony of miracles connected with the organization. The mission of CHRISTUS is to extend the healing ministry of Jesus Christ.

CHRISTUS provides dental and vision coverage, a prescription drug plan, day care, tuition reimbursement and various career development programs.

BRANDS/DIVISIONS/AFFILIATES:
Sisters of Charity of the Incarnate Word

CONTACTS:
Note: Officers with more than one job title may be intentionally listed here more than once.

Thomas C. Royer, CEO
Thomas C. Royer, Pres.
Linda McClung, Sr. VP-Comm. & Public Affairs
Richard S. Blair, Chmn.

Phone: 214-492-8500 **Fax:** 214-492-8540
Toll-Free:
Address: 6363 N. Hwy. 161, Ste. 450, Irving, TX 75038 US

FINANCIALS:
Sales and profits are in thousands of dollars—add 000 to get the full amount. Year 2004 note: Complete fiscal 2004 results were not available for all companies at press time. For this company, year 2004 is for months.

2004 Sales: $ (months)   2004 Profits: $ (months)
2003 Sales: $2,302,400   2003 Profits: $20,000
2002 Sales: $2,377,500   2002 Profits: $
2001 Sales: $ 2001 Profits: $
2000 Sales: $ 2000 Profits: $

Stock Ticker: Nonprofit
Employees: 8,000
Fiscal Year Ends: 6/30

SALARIES/BENEFITS:
Pension Plan: Y   ESOP Stock Plan: Profit Sharing: Top Exec. Salary: $ Bonus: $
Savings Plan: Stock Purch. Plan: Second Exec. Salary: $ Bonus: $

OTHER THOUGHTS:
Apparent Top Female Officers: 1
Hot Spot for Advancement for Women/Minorities:

LOCATIONS: ("Y" = Yes)
West:	Southwest:	Midwest:	Southeast:	Northeast:	International:
Y	Y	Y	Y		Y

CIGNA CORP

www.cigna.com

Industry Group Code: 524114 **Ranks within this company's industry group:** Sales: 4 Profits: 5

Insurance/HMO/PPO:		Drugs:		Equipment/Supplies:		Hospitals/Clinics:		Services:		Health Care:	
Insurance:	Y	Manufacturer:		Manufacturer:		Acute Care:		Diagnostics:		Home Health:	
Managed Care:	Y	Distributor:		Distributor:		Sub-Acute Care:		Labs/Testing:		Long-Term Care:	
Utilization Mgmt.:		Specialty Pharm.:		Leasing/Finance:		Outpatient Surgery:		Staffing:		Physical Therapy:	
Payment Proc.:		Vitamins/Nutri.:		Information Sys.:		Phys. Rehab. Center:		Waste Disposal:		Phys. Practice Mgmt.:	
		Clinical Trials:				Psychiatric Clinics:		Specialty Services:	Y		

TYPES OF BUSINESS:
Underwriting-Health Care Plans
Indemnity Insurance
Investment Management Services

BRANDS/DIVISIONS/AFFILIATES:
CIGNA International
CIGNA Group Insurance
CIGNA HealthCare
CIGNA Pharmacy Management
CIGNA Behavioral Health
CIGNA Dental & Vision Care

CONTACTS:
Note: Officers with more than one job title may be intentionally listed here more than once.
H. Edward Hanway, CEO
H. Edward Hanway, Pres.
Michael W. Bell, CFO
David M. Cordani, Sr. VP-Customer Segments & Mktg.
John Murabito, Exec. VP-Human Resources & Services
Andrea Anania, Exec. VP/CIO
Judith E. Sotlz, Exec. VP/General Counsel
Scott A. Storrer, Sr. VP-Service Oper., CIGNA HealthCare
John Cannon, III, Sr. VP-Public Affairs
Keith Dixon, Pres., CIGNA Behavioral Health
Karen S. Rohan, Pres., CIGNA Dental & Vision Care
Gregory H. Wolf, Pres., CIGNA Group Insurance
James H. Bryant, III, Pres., CIGNA Pharmacy Management
H. Edward Hanway, Chmn.
Terry Kendall, Pres., CIGNA International

Phone: 215-761-1000 **Fax:** 215-761-5515
Toll-Free:
Address: One Liberty Pl., 1650 Market St., Philadelphia, PA 19192 US

GROWTH PLANS/SPECIAL FEATURES:
CIGNA Corporation and its subsidiaries constitute one of the largest investor-owned employee benefits organizations in the U.S. Its subsidiaries are major providers of employee benefits offered through the workplace, including health care products and services, group life, accident and disability insurance, retirement products and services and investment management. CIGNA HealthCare offers a wide range of medical insurance plans, including point-of-service plans, open access, preferred provider plans, HMOs, indemnity plans and many other programs. Its plans cover approximately 11.5 million members for medical needs, 12.1 million for dental and nearly 9 million for prescriptions. CIGNA Group Insurance markets benefits packages to employers that include life insurance, accident insurance, disability insurance and specialty programs. CIGNA International services clients in Asia, Europe and the Americas. The company's other operations consist of deferred gains recognized from the sale of its individual life insurance and annuity business, corporate life insurance on which policy loans are outstanding, its settlement annuity business and investment management services. As part of CIGNA's strategy to focus more on its health care business, the firm announced the sale of its CIGNA Retirement & Investment Services to Prudential in November 2003.

Employees of CIGNA enjoy medical, dental, disability, life and mental health coverage, in addition to flexible work arrangements, elder and child care assistance, adoption assistance, tuition reimbursement, fitness programs and retail discounts. CIGNA has been named to Working Mother Magazine's Top 100 Employers for Working Mothers as well as to LATINA Style Magazine's Top 50 Companies for Latinas to Work For.

FINANCIALS:
Sales and profits are in thousands of dollars—add 000 to get the full amount. Year 2004 note: Complete fiscal 2004 results were not available for all companies at press time. For this company, year 2004 is for 9 months.

2004 Sales: $13,834,000 (9 months)	2004 Profits: $913,000 (9 months)	
2003 Sales: $18,808,000	2003 Profits: $668,000	**Stock Ticker:** CI
2002 Sales: $19,348,000	2002 Profits: $-398,000	Employees: 32,700
2001 Sales: $19,115,000	2001 Profits: $989,000	Fiscal Year Ends: 12/31
2000 Sales: $19,994,000	2000 Profits: $987,000	

SALARIES/BENEFITS:
Pension Plan: Y	ESOP Stock Plan:	Profit Sharing:	Top Exec. Salary: $1,030,000	Bonus: $2,100,000
Savings Plan: Y	Stock Purch. Plan:		Second Exec. Salary: $600,000	Bonus: $1,560,000

OTHER THOUGHTS:
Apparent Top Female Officers: 3
Hot Spot for Advancement for Women/Minorities: Y

LOCATIONS: ("Y" = Yes)
West:	Southwest:	Midwest:	Southeast:	Northeast:	International:
Y	Y	Y	Y	Y	Y

CIVCO MEDICAL INSTRUMENTS   www.ultrasoundsupplies.com

Industry Group Code: 339113   Ranks within this company's industry group: Sales: Profits:

Insurance/HMO/PPO:	Drugs:	Equipment/Supplies:	Hospitals/Clinics:	Services:	Health Care:
Insurance: Managed Care: Utilization Mgmt.: Payment Proc.:	Manufacturer: Distributor: Specialty Pharm.: Vitamins/Nutri.: Clinical Trials:	Manufacturer: Distributor: Leasing/Finance: Information Sys.: Y	Acute Care: Sub-Acute Care: Outpatient Surgery: Phys. Rehab. Center: Psychiatric Clinics:	Diagnostics: Labs/Testing: Staffing: Waste Disposal: Specialty Services:	Home Health: Long-Term Care: Physical Therapy: Phys. Practice Mgmt.:

TYPES OF BUSINESS:
Equipment-Diagnostic & Therapeutic Medical Products
Ultrasound Products
Minimally Invasive Surgical Products
Medical Monitors
Needle & Biopsy Instruments
Disinfectants
Medical Printers & Print Supplies

BRANDS/DIVISIONS/AFFILIATES:
KRG Capital Partners
Ultra-Pro II Needle Guide

GROWTH PLANS/SPECIAL FEATURES:
CIVCO Medical Instruments, a subsidiary of KRG Capital Partners, is a designer and manufacturer of ultrasound and minimally invasive surgical products. The company primarily manufactures cardiology products, disinfectants, needle and biopsy instruments, medical monitors, transducer covers, positioners and stabilizers. Cardiology products include disposable electrodes, bite blocks and instrument accessories. The company also produces a respiration monitor that is compatible with ECGs and ultrasound systems. In addition, CIVCO produces medical printers, print media and associated supplies. The company's biopsy supplies are mostly a variety of disposable and reusable needles. These products are sold to more than 7,500 hospitals and clinics in the U.S. and distributed worldwide through CIVCO's partners in Europe, Asia, Australia, the Middle East and Central and South America. In recent news, the company's Ultra-Pro II Needle Guide is being used in the new GE Healthcare 8L-RS Transducer. The transducer is used primarily in arterial and vascular applications.

CONTACTS: Note: Officers with more than one job title may be intentionally listed here more than once.

Phone: 319-656-4447   Fax:
Toll-Free:
Address: 102 First St. S., Kalona, IA 52247-9589 US

FINANCIALS:
Sales and profits are in thousands of dollars—add 000 to get the full amount. Year 2004 note: Complete fiscal 2004 results were not available for all companies at press time. For this company, year 2004 is for months.

2004 Sales: $ (months)   2004 Profits: $ (months)
2003 Sales: $ 2003 Profits: $
2002 Sales: $70,700   2002 Profits: $-3,100
2001 Sales: $77,200   2001 Profits: $-2,700
2000 Sales: $74,003   2000 Profits: $2,991

Stock Ticker: Subsidiary
Employees: 360
Fiscal Year Ends: 12/31

SALARIES/BENEFITS:
Pension Plan: ESOP Stock Plan: Profit Sharing: Top Exec. Salary: $205,891   Bonus: $142,439
Savings Plan: Stock Purch. Plan: Second Exec. Salary: $162,293   Bonus: $107,043

OTHER THOUGHTS:
Apparent Top Female Officers:
Hot Spot for Advancement for Women/Minorities:

LOCATIONS: ("Y" = Yes)

West:	Southwest:	Midwest:	Southeast:	Northeast:	International:
		Y	Y		

CLARIAN HEALTH PARTNERS INC

www.clarian.org

Industry Group Code: 622110 Ranks within this company's industry group: Sales: 31 Profits: 13

Insurance/HMO/PPO:	Drugs:	Equipment/Supplies:	Hospitals/Clinics:		Services:		Health Care:	
Insurance:	Manufacturer:	Manufacturer:	Acute Care:	Y	Diagnostics:		Home Health:	
Managed Care:	Distributor:	Distributor:	Sub-Acute Care:	Y	Labs/Testing:		Long-Term Care:	
Utilization Mgmt.:	Specialty Pharm.:	Leasing/Finance:	Outpatient Surgery:		Staffing:		Physical Therapy:	
Payment Proc.:	Vitamins/Nutri.:	Information Sys.:	Phys. Rehab. Center:		Waste Disposal:		Phys. Practice Mgmt.:	
	Clinical Trials:		Psychiatric Clinics:		Specialty Services:			

TYPES OF BUSINESS:
Hospitals

BRANDS/DIVISIONS/AFFILIATES:
Methodist Hospital
Indiana University Hospital
Riley Hospital for Children
Riley Children's Foundaton
Methodist Health Foundation
Camp Riley
James Whitcomb Riley Museum Home
Clarian West Medical Center

CONTACTS: *Note: Officers with more than one job title may be intentionally listed here more than once.*
Daniel F. Evans, Jr., CEO
Daniel F. Evans, Jr., Pres.
Marvin Pember, Exec. VP/CFO
Daniel F. Evans, Jr., Chmn.

Phone: 317-962-2000 Fax: 317-962-4533
Toll-Free:
Address: 1701 N. Senate Ave., Indianapolis, IN 46202 US

GROWTH PLANS/SPECIAL FEATURES:
Clarian Health Partners was formed in 1997 from the union of Methodist Hospital, Indiana University Hospital and Riley Hospital for Children, all located in Indianapolis. The hospitals have 1,319 beds in total, the largest being Methodist with 763, next Indiana University with 317 and finally Riley with 239. Clarian had 55,579 total inpatient visits last year and 877,363 total outpatient visits, 95% of which came from Indiana. Two foundations raise funds for Clarian, Riley Children's Foundation and Methodist Health Foundation. Riley Children's Foundation provides support and philanthropic leadership for Riley Hospital for Children; Camp Riley, an outdoor recreation camp for children with physical disabilities; and the James Whitcomb Riley Museum Home, the Victorian house of poet James Whitcomb Riley, for whom the foundation, hospital and camp are named. The Methodist Health Foundation supports Methodist Hospital's research and education initiatives as well as various clinical services and programs. Construction is currently underway for two new hospitals: Clarian West Medical Center and Clarian North Medical Center, both of which will serve expanding communities in the Indianapolis area. All three Clarian hospitals enjoy an excellent reputation in Indiana and have been named to the U.S. News & World Report list of Best Hospitals for the past several years running.

FINANCIALS: Sales and profits are in thousands of dollars—add 000 to get the full amount. Year 2004 note: Complete fiscal 2004 results were not available for all companies at press time. For this company, year 2004 is for months.

2004 Sales: $ (months)   2004 Profits: $ (months)
2003 Sales: $2,102,200   2003 Profits: $89,000
2002 Sales: $1,659,800   2002 Profits: $
2001 Sales: $ 2001 Profits: $
2000 Sales: $ 2000 Profits: $

Stock Ticker: Nonprofit
Employees: 11,088
Fiscal Year Ends: 12/31

SALARIES/BENEFITS:
Pension Plan: ESOP Stock Plan: Profit Sharing: Top Exec. Salary: $ Bonus: $
Savings Plan: Stock Purch. Plan: Second Exec. Salary: $ Bonus: $

OTHER THOUGHTS:
Apparent Top Female Officers:
Hot Spot for Advancement for Women/Minorities:

LOCATIONS: ("Y" = Yes)

West:	Southwest:	Midwest:	Southeast:	Northeast:	International:
		Y			

Note: Financial information, benefits and other data can change quickly and may vary from those stated here.

CNS INC

www.cns.com

Industry Group Code: 339113 **Ranks within this company's industry group:** Sales: 100 Profits: 81

Insurance/HMO/PPO:	Drugs:	Equipment/Supplies:	Hospitals/Clinics:	Services:	Health Care:
Insurance: Managed Care: Utilization Mgmt.: Payment Proc.:	Manufacturer: Distributor: Specialty Pharm.: Vitamins/Nutri.: Clinical Trials:	Manufacturer: Y Distributor: Leasing/Finance: Information Sys.:	Acute Care: Sub-Acute Care: Outpatient Surgery: Phys. Rehab. Center: Psychiatric Clinics:	Diagnostics: Labs/Testing: Staffing: Waste Disposal: Specialty Services:	Home Health: Long-Term Care: Physical Therapy: Phys. Practice Mgmt.:

TYPES OF BUSINESS:
Supplies-Nasal Products
Consumer Health Products
Breathing Aids

BRANDS/DIVISIONS/AFFILIATES:
Breathe Right Nasal Strips
Breathe Right Vapor Shot!
FiberChoice

CONTACTS:
Note: Officers with more than one job title may be intentionally listed here more than once.

Marti Morfitt, CEO
Marti Morfitt, Pres.
Samuel E. Reinkensmeyer, CFO
John J. Keppeler, VP-Worldwide Sales
Larry Muma, VP-Oper.
Linda J. Kollofski, VP-Domestic Mktg.
Carol J. Watzke, VP-Consumer Strategy
Daniel E. Cohen, Chmn.
Kevin McKenna, VP-Int'l

Phone: 952-229-1500 **Fax:** 952-229-1700
Toll-Free:
Address: 7615 Smetana Ln., Minneapolis, MN 55344 US

GROWTH PLANS/SPECIAL FEATURES:

CNS, Inc. develops and markets consumer health care products, including Breathe Right nasal strips, Breathe Right Vapor Shot! personal vaporizers and FiberChoice chewable fiber tablets. The company focuses on products that address the aging and self-care market, including better breathing and digestive health products. The firm's principal product, the Breathe Right nasal strip, improves breathing by reducing nasal airflow resistance. Nasal strips provide drug-free temporary relief from nasal congestion, reduce snoring and reduce breathing difficulties due to a deviated nasal septum. The Breathe Right Vapor Shot! personal vaporizer is designed to relieve day-time congestion related to colds, flu and allergies. This product builds on the existing line of Breathe Right mentholated vapor strips, which are primarily used to relieve night-time congestion. The company maintains four strategic business teams: the Breathe Right brand team, which is responsible for the strategic development and management of products that carry the Breathe Right brand name; the FiberChoice team, which is responsible for the FiberChoice fiber supplement business, including new product development related to the digestive health product platform; the international team, which is responsible for the company's overseas markets and its relationships with international distributors and representatives; and the new business development team, which is responsible for identifying and evaluating potential new products, inventions and other business prospects. CNS subcontracts with multiple manufacturers to produce its products and has multi-year contracts with manufacturers that purchase most of the major components for the Breath Right nasal strips directly from 3M. In recent news, the company expanded distribution of its Breath Right Tan and Clear nasal strips to Mexico through a three-year exclusive agreement with Grisi Hnos, S.A. de C.V., a consumer products manufacturer, marketer and distributor based in Mexico City.

CNS offers its employees training, tuition reimbursement and a casual dress policy.

FINANCIALS:
Sales and profits are in thousands of dollars—add 000 to get the full amount. Year 2004 note: Complete fiscal 2004 results were not available for all companies at press time. For this company, year 2004 is for 12 months.

2004 Sales: $86,980 (12 months)   2004 Profits: $8,547 (12 months)
2003 Sales: $79,100   2003 Profits: $6,500
2002 Sales: $ 2002 Profits: $
2001 Sales: $83,900   2001 Profits: $ 100
2000 Sales: $68,892   2000 Profits: $-15,660

Stock Ticker: CNXS
Employees: 57
Fiscal Year Ends: 3/31

SALARIES/BENEFITS:
Pension Plan: ESOP Stock Plan: Profit Sharing: Top Exec. Salary: $425,000   Bonus: $301,300
Savings Plan: Y   Stock Purch. Plan: Second Exec. Salary: $213,600   Bonus: $97,313

OTHER THOUGHTS:
Apparent Top Female Officers: 2
Hot Spot for Advancement for Women/Minorities:

LOCATIONS: ("Y" = Yes)

West:	Southwest:	Midwest:	Southeast:	Northeast:	International:
		Y			

COAST DENTAL SERVICES INC

www.coastdental.com

Industry Group Code: 621111   Ranks within this company's industry group: Sales: 10   Profits: 9

Insurance/HMO/PPO:	Drugs:	Equipment/Supplies:	Hospitals/Clinics:	Services:	Health Care:
Insurance: Managed Care: Utilization Mgmt.: Payment Proc.:	Manufacturer: Distributor: Specialty Pharm.: Vitamins/Nutri.: Clinical Trials:	Manufacturer: Distributor: Leasing/Finance: Information Sys.:	Acute Care: Sub-Acute Care: Outpatient Surgery: Phys. Rehab. Center: Psychiatric Clinics:	Diagnostics: Labs/Testing: Staffing: Waste Disposal: Specialty Services:	Home Health: Long-Term Care: Physical Therapy: Phys. Practice Mgmt.: Y

TYPES OF BUSINESS:
Dental Practice Management

BRANDS/DIVISIONS/AFFILIATES:

CONTACTS: Note: Officers with more than one job title may be intentionally listed here more than once.
Terek Diasti, CEO
Adam Diasti, Pres.
Thomas J. Marler, COO
Michael T. Smith, VP-IT
Timothy G. Merrick, VP-Finance
Adam Diasti, Dir.-Dental
Terek Diasti, Chmn.

Phone: 813-288-1999   **Fax:** 813-281-9284
Toll-Free:
Address: 2502 Rocky Point Dr. N., Ste. 1000, Tampa, FL 33607 US

GROWTH PLANS/SPECIAL FEATURES:

Coast Dental Services, Inc. is a leading provider of management services to one of the largest teams of affiliated general dentists and support staffs in the southeastern United States. It serves more than 500,000 customers through 109 dental centers in Florida, Georgia, Tennessee and Virginia. The company's operating model allows dentists to focus on providing quality dentistry, while the firm's system takes care of the important aspects of office administration, including human resources, training, insurance processing and marketing. Coast Dental also has a revolving credit program for its patients, which has the backing of a financial institution. In addition, the firm has multiple 40-year evergreen dental services agreements with Coast Florida P.A., whereby it receives fees for services provided for Coast Florida. The company continues to focus on the internal development of its existing dental centers by strengthening operations and providing the resources necessary for these operations to mature. In recent news, Coast Dental has decided to terminate its status as a public company due to the costs of auditing fees, board fees and insurance premiums.

The firm offers its employees comprehensive medical coverage, life insurance and tuition reimbursement. Employees also receive a dependent care spending account and dental discounts.

FINANCIALS: Sales and profits are in thousands of dollars—add 000 to get the full amount. Year 2004 note: Complete fiscal 2004 results were not available for all companies at press time. For this company, year 2004 is for months.

2004 Sales: $ (months)   2004 Profits: $ (months)
2003 Sales: $56,416   2003 Profits: $-2,986   **Stock Ticker:** CDEN
2002 Sales: $56,000   2002 Profits: $-3,900   Employees: 677
2001 Sales: $43,600   2001 Profits: $-9,300   Fiscal Year Ends: 12/31
2000 Sales: $45,826   2000 Profits: $-1,264

SALARIES/BENEFITS:

Pension Plan:	ESOP Stock Plan:	Profit Sharing:	Top Exec. Salary: $273,077	Bonus: $
Savings Plan: Y	Stock Purch. Plan:		Second Exec. Salary: $219,231	Bonus: $

OTHER THOUGHTS:
Apparent Top Female Officers:
Hot Spot for Advancement for Women/Minorities:

LOCATIONS: ("Y" = Yes)

West:	Southwest:	Midwest:	Southeast: Y	Northeast: Y	International:

Plunkett's Health Care Industry Almanac 2005　　317

COCHLEAR LTD
www.cochlear.com

Industry Group Code: 339113　**Ranks within this company's industry group:** Sales:　Profits:

Insurance/HMO/PPO:	Drugs:	Equipment/Supplies:		Hospitals/Clinics:	Services:	Health Care:
Insurance:	Manufacturer:	Manufacturer:	Y	Acute Care:	Diagnostics:	Home Health:
Managed Care:	Distributor:	Distributor:		Sub-Acute Care:	Labs/Testing:	Long-Term Care:
Utilization Mgmt.:	Specialty Pharm.:	Leasing/Finance:		Outpatient Surgery:	Staffing:	Physical Therapy:
Payment Proc.:	Vitamins/Nutri.:	Information Sys.:		Phys. Rehab. Center:	Waste Disposal:	Phys. Practice Mgmt.:
	Clinical Trials:			Psychiatric Clinics:	Specialty Services:	

TYPES OF BUSINESS:
Hearing Implants

BRANDS/DIVISIONS/AFFILIATES:
Nucleus 3
SPrint
ESPrit 3G

CONTACTS: Note: Officers with more than one job title may be intentionally listed here more than once.
Chris Roberts, CEO
Chris Roberts, Pres.
Tommie C.E. Bergman, Chmn.

Phone: 61-2-9428-6555	Fax: 61-2-9428-6353
Toll-Free:	
Address: 14 Mars Rd., Lane Cove, NSW 2066 Australia	

GROWTH PLANS/SPECIAL FEATURES:
Cochlear is the world leader in cochlear implants, the breakthrough technology that has enabled tens of thousands of severe to profoundly hearing-impaired people to hear. The company was formed in 1982 to build on the unique work of Australian Professor Graeme Clark, inventor of the multi-channel implant. The firm has created electronic ear implants as a medical option for individuals with severe to profound sensorineural hearing loss in both ears. The firm is the innovator and manufacturer of the Nucleus 3 cochlear implant system. The Nucleus 3 is a safe, reliable and effective treatment for severe-to-profound hearing loss in adults and for profound hearing loss in children. Designed to let implant users experience sounds as they occur, this electronic device can enhance communication abilities with better hearing and speaking potential for implant recipients. The device consists of an internal implant and two choices of external speech processor: the body-worn SPrint or the revolutionary behind-the-ear ESPrit 3G. Supporting over 50,000 Nucleus recipients, Cochlear continues to innovate. Its research program is extensive, with the company participating in more than 90 collaborative research programs with university and research hospitals in more than 35 countries. The company's research efforts are closely linked to those of the Bionic Ear Institute, the University of Melbourne and the Cooperative Research Centre for Cochlear Implants and Hearing Innovation. Cochlear continues to expand its export base throughout the Americas, Asia Pacific, Europe and the Middle East.

FINANCIALS: Sales and profits are in thousands of dollars—add 000 to get the full amount. Year 2004 note: Complete fiscal 2004 results were not available for all companies at press time. For this company, year 2004 is for months.

2004 Sales: $ (months)	2004 Profits: $ (months)	
2003 Sales: $	2003 Profits: $	Stock Ticker: Foreign
2002 Sales: $	2002 Profits: $	Employees:
2001 Sales: $	2001 Profits: $	Fiscal Year Ends:
2000 Sales: $	2000 Profits: $	

SALARIES/BENEFITS:
Pension Plan:	ESOP Stock Plan:	Profit Sharing:	Top Exec. Salary: $	Bonus: $
Savings Plan:	Stock Purch. Plan:		Second Exec. Salary: $	Bonus: $

OTHER THOUGHTS:
Apparent Top Female Officers:
Hot Spot for Advancement for Women/Minorities:

LOCATIONS: ("Y" = Yes)
West:	Southwest:	Midwest:	Southeast:	Northeast:	International: Y

Note: Financial information, benefits and other data can change quickly and may vary from those stated here.

COHERENT INC

www.cohr.com

Industry Group Code: 339113   Ranks within this company's industry group: Sales: 44   Profits: 133

Insurance/HMO/PPO:	Drugs:	Equipment/Supplies:	Hospitals/Clinics:	Services:	Health Care:
Insurance:	Manufacturer:	Manufacturer: Y	Acute Care:	Diagnostics:	Home Health:
Managed Care:	Distributor:	Distributor:	Sub-Acute Care:	Labs/Testing:	Long-Term Care:
Utilization Mgmt.:	Specialty Pharm.:	Leasing/Finance:	Outpatient Surgery:	Staffing:	Physical Therapy:
Payment Proc.:	Vitamins/Nutri.:	Information Sys.:	Phys. Rehab. Center:	Waste Disposal:	Phys. Practice Mgmt.:
	Clinical Trials:		Psychiatric Clinics:	Specialty Services:	

TYPES OF BUSINESS:
Equipment-Lasers & Laser Systems
Precision Optics
Research Services

BRANDS/DIVISIONS/AFFILIATES:
Lambda Physik
Electro-Optics

CONTACTS: Note: Officers with more than one job title may be intentionally listed here more than once.
John R. Ambroseo, CEO
John R. Ambroseo, Pres.
Helene Simonet, CFO
Vittorio Fossati-Bellani, Exec. VP/Chief Mktg. Officer
Ron A. Victor, Exec. VP-Human Resources
Luis Spinelli, Exec. VP/Chief Tech. Officer
Michael J. Cumbo, Exec. VP-Optical Tech.
Paul L. Meissner, Exec. VP-Laser Systems
Bernard J. Couillaud, Chmn.

Phone: 408-764-4000   Fax: 408-764-4800
Toll-Free:
Address: 5100 Patrick Henry Dr., Santa Clara, CA 95054 US

GROWTH PLANS/SPECIAL FEATURES:

Coherent, Inc. designs, manufactures and sells lasers, laser systems, precision optics and related accessories for both the commercial and medical markets. The company sells products in over 80 countries and has production, research and service facilities worldwide. Coherent's two main operating subsidiaries are Electro-Optics and Lambda Physik. Electro-Optics specializes in semiconductors and engages in materials processing, OEM laser components, scientific research, government programs and graphic arts. Lambda Physik, based in Gottingden, Germany, manufactures lasers for thin-film transistors used in flat-panel displays, microlithography applications in the semiconductor industry, ink-jet printers, automotive, environmental research, scientific research, medical OEMs, materials processing and micro-machining applications. The company's products are used in a range of scientific research programs, for everything from cell sorting and DNA sequencing to quantum control spectroscopy. Avidly engaging in research and development, Coherent spends about 12% of its budget on new products.

The company offers employees tuition reimbursement, a computer purchase plan, credit union membership, discounted entertainment tickets and a variety of recreational events. Additionally, the firm has on-site fitness centers at its two facilities in California.

FINANCIALS: Sales and profits are in thousands of dollars—add 000 to get the full amount. Year 2004 note: Complete fiscal 2004 results were not available for all companies at press time. For this company, year 2004 is for 9 months.

2004 Sales: $361,710 (9 months)   2004 Profits: $7,951 (9 months)
2003 Sales: $406,235   2003 Profits: $-45,891
2002 Sales: $397,300   2002 Profits: $-68,900
2001 Sales: $477,900   2001 Profits: $100,800
2000 Sales: $568,272   2000 Profits: $69,937

Stock Ticker: COHR
Employees: 2,136
Fiscal Year Ends: 9/30

SALARIES/BENEFITS:
Pension Plan: ESOP Stock Plan: Profit Sharing: Y   Top Exec. Salary: $520,000   Bonus: $229,429
Savings Plan: Y   Stock Purch. Plan: Y   Second Exec. Salary: $431,853   Bonus: $95,014

OTHER THOUGHTS:
Apparent Top Female Officers: 1
Hot Spot for Advancement for Women/Minorities:

LOCATIONS: ("Y" = Yes)
West:	Southwest:	Midwest:	Southeast:	Northeast:	International:
Y				Y	Y

COLE NATIONAL CORPORATION

www.colenational.com

Industry Group Code: 446130   Ranks within this company's industry group: Sales: 1 Profits: 2

Insurance/HMO/PPO:	Drugs:	Equipment/Supplies:		Hospitals/Clinics:		Services:		Health Care:	
Insurance:	Manufacturer:	Manufacturer:	Y	Acute Care:		Diagnostics:		Home Health:	
Managed Care:	Distributor:	Distributor:	Y	Sub-Acute Care:		Labs/Testing:		Long-Term Care:	
Utilization Mgmt.:	Specialty Pharm.:	Leasing/Finance:		Outpatient Surgery:		Staffing:		Physical Therapy:	
Payment Proc.:	Vitamins/Nutri.:	Information Sys.:		Phys. Rehab. Center:		Waste Disposal:		Phys. Practice Mgmt.:	
	Clinical Trials:			Psychiatric Clinics:		Specialty Services:	Y		

TYPES OF BUSINESS:
Eyeglasses & Related Products, Retail
Optometry Services
Managed Vision Care Services
Gift Stores

BRANDS/DIVISIONS/AFFILIATES:
Cole Vision Corp.
Sears Optical
Pearle Vision
Things Remembered
BJ's Wholesale Club
Target Optical
Cole Managed Vision
Luxottica Group SpA

CONTACTS:
Note: Officers with more than one job title may be intentionally listed here more than once.
Larry Pollock, CEO
Larry Pollock, Pres.
Lawrence E. Hyatt, Exec. VP/CFO
Patricia Luzier, Sr. VP/Chief Admin. Officer
Leslie Dunn, Sr. VP/General Counsel
Joseph Gaglioti, VP/Treas.
David Holmberg, Pres.-Licensed Brands
Suzanne Sutter, Pres., Things Remembered
Terry J. Hanson, Pres., Pearle Vision
Steve Holden, Pres., Cole Managed Vision
Walter J. Salmon, Chmn.

Phone: 330-486-3100   Fax: 330-486-3596
Toll-Free:
Address: 1925 Enterprise Pkwy., Twinsburg, OH 44087 US

GROWTH PLANS/SPECIAL FEATURES:
Cole National Corporation is a leading provider of eyewear products, optometry services and personalized gifts. Through its subsidiaries, the company operates retail establishments under names including Sears Optical, Pearle Vision, BJ's Wholesale Club and Target Optical. Cole Managed Vision, a subsidiary created in 1988, develops, markets and administers group vision benefit programs for employers, health plans, trust funds and associations nationwide. In conjunction with its Pearle franchisees, Cole National has 2,925 locations in the U.S., Canada, Puerto Rico and the Virgin Islands. The firm also has a 21% interest in Pearle Europe, which operates over 1,460 optical stores in the Netherlands, Belgium, Germany, Austria, Italy, Portugal, Sweden, Norway, Denmark and Poland. Subsidiary Things Remembered operates nearly 750 gift stores and kiosks located in large enclosed shopping malls in 47 states and accounts for approximately 24% of Cole National's revenue. Things Remembered also generates sales through an Internet web site and a mail-order catalog. The company announced in early 2004 that it plans to be acquired by Luxottica Group SpA, based in Italy, for $441 million.

Cole National has locations all over the country and offers its employees competitive benefits packages.

FINANCIALS:
Sales and profits are in thousands of dollars—add 000 to get the full amount. Year 2004 note: Complete fiscal 2004 results were not available for all companies at press time. For this company, year 2004 is for 12 months.

2004 Sales: $1,201,800 (12 months)   2004 Profits: $-10,683 (12 months)
2003 Sales: $1,148,100   2003 Profits: $-5,100
2002 Sales: $1,101,300   2002 Profits: $5,200
2001 Sales: $1,077,147   2001 Profits: $2,229
2000 Sales: $1,040,426   2000 Profits: $2,008

Stock Ticker: Subsidiary
Employees: 13,709
Fiscal Year Ends: 1/31

SALARIES/BENEFITS:
Pension Plan: ESOP Stock Plan: Profit Sharing: Top Exec. Salary: $738,942   Bonus: $126,875
Savings Plan: Stock Purch. Plan: Second Exec. Salary: $320,192 Bonus: $65,625

OTHER THOUGHTS:
Apparent Top Female Officers: 3
Hot Spot for Advancement for Women/Minorities: Y

LOCATIONS: ("Y" = Yes)
West:	Southwest:	Midwest:	Southeast:	Northeast:	International:
Y	Y	Y	Y	Y	Y

COMMUNITY HEALTH SYSTEMS INC

www.chs.net

Industry Group Code: 622110   Ranks within this company's industry group: Sales: 19   Profits: 10

Insurance/HMO/PPO:	Drugs:	Equipment/Supplies:	Hospitals/Clinics:		Services:	Health Care:
Insurance:	Manufacturer:	Manufacturer:	Acute Care:	Y	Diagnostics:	Home Health:
Managed Care:	Distributor:	Distributor:	Sub-Acute Care:		Labs/Testing:	Long-Term Care:
Utilization Mgmt.:	Specialty Pharm.:	Leasing/Finance:	Outpatient Surgery:		Staffing:	Physical Therapy:
Payment Proc.:	Vitamins/Nutri.:	Information Sys.:	Phys. Rehab. Center:		Waste Disposal:	Phys. Practice Mgmt.:
	Clinical Trials:		Psychiatric Clinics:		Specialty Services:	

TYPES OF BUSINESS:
Hospitals
Surgical & Emergency Services
Acute Care Facilities

BRANDS/DIVISIONS/AFFILIATES:
Pottstown Memorial Medical Center
Brandywine Hospital
Easton Hospital
Gateway Regional Medical Center
Dyersburg Regional Medical Center
Springs Memorial Hospital
Phoenixville Hospital
Galesburg Cottage Hospital

CONTACTS:
Note: Officers with more than one job title may be intentionally listed here more than once.

Wayne T. Smith, CEO
Wayne T. Smith, Pres.
W. Larry Cash, Exec. VP/CFO
Linda K. Parsons, VP-Human Resources
J. Gary Seay, VP/CIO
Robert A. Horrar, VP-Admin.
Rachel A. Seifert, Sr. VP/General Counsel/Corp. Sec.
Martin G. Schweinhart, Sr. VP-Oper.
Kenneth D. Hawkins, Sr. VP-Dev. & Acquisitions
James W. Doucette, VP-Finance/Treas.
Jerry A. Weissman, VP-Medical Staff Dev.
T. Mark Buford, VP/Corp. Controller/Chief Acct. Officer
Carolyn S. Lipp, Sr. VP-Quality & Resource Mgmt.
William S. Hussey, Sr. VP-Group Oper.
Wayne T. Smith, Chmn.

Phone: 615-373-9600   Fax: 615-371-1068
Toll-Free:
Address: 155 Franklin Rd., Ste. 400, Brentwood, TN 37027-4600 US

GROWTH PLANS/SPECIAL FEATURES:
Community Health Systems, Inc. is one of the largest rural providers of hospital health care services in the United States. The firm owns, operates or leases 72 hospitals across 22 states with approximately 8,025 licensed beds. The company continues to expand based on a selective acquisition strategy of primarily targeting municipally owned or not-for-profit hospitals. Community Health focuses its operations on rural areas that usually have a small but growing population base and that generally have a lack of community health services. Some of the company's hospitals offer personalized home and nursing care, and they all offer a full range of services that include surgical and emergency provision. Community Health's hospitals gain a competitive advantage by benefiting from the larger corporate structure that they fall under. These advantages include greater purchasing efficiencies, optimized resource allocation and inter-hospital collaboration that leads to more efficient, standardized operations. In recent news, Community Health divested two smaller 50-bed hospitals, the Randolph County Medical Center in Pocahontas, Arkansas and the Sabine Medical Center in Many, Louisiana. The company also acquired Phoenixville Hospital, a 143-bed acute care general hospital outside of Philadelphia, and the Galesburg Cottage Hospital, a 170-bed acute care general hospital outside of Peoria, Illinois.

FINANCIALS:
Sales and profits are in thousands of dollars—add 000 to get the full amount. Year 2004 note: Complete fiscal 2004 results were not available for all companies at press time. For this company, year 2004 is for 9 months.

2004 Sales: $2,460,968 (9 months)   2004 Profits: $111,204 (9 months)
2003 Sales: $2,834,624   2003 Profits: $131,472   **Stock Ticker:** CYH
2002 Sales: $2,200,400   2002 Profits: $100,000   Employees: 30,500
2001 Sales: $1,693,600   2001 Profits: $44,700   Fiscal Year Ends: 12/31
2000 Sales: $1,337,500   2000 Profits: $9,600

SALARIES/BENEFITS:
| Pension Plan: | ESOP Stock Plan: | Profit Sharing: | Top Exec. Salary: $700,000 | Bonus: $637,000 |
| Savings Plan: Y | Stock Purch. Plan: | | Second Exec. Salary: $500,000 | Bonus: $455,000 |

OTHER THOUGHTS:
Apparent Top Female Officers: 3
Hot Spot for Advancement for Women/Minorities: Y

LOCATIONS: ("Y" = Yes)
West:	Southwest:	Midwest:	Southeast:	Northeast:	International:
Y	Y	Y	Y	Y	

COMPEX TECHNOLOGIES INC
www.compextechnologies.com

Industry Group Code: 339113 Ranks within this company's industry group: Sales: 103 Profits: 87

Insurance/HMO/PPO:	Drugs:	Equipment/Supplies:		Hospitals/Clinics:	Services:	Health Care:
Insurance:	Manufacturer:	Manufacturer:	Y	Acute Care:	Diagnostics:	Home Health:
Managed Care:	Distributor:	Distributor:	Y	Sub-Acute Care:	Labs/Testing:	Long-Term Care:
Utilization Mgmt.:	Specialty Pharm.:	Leasing/Finance:		Outpatient Surgery:	Staffing:	Physical Therapy:
Payment Proc.:	Vitamins/Nutri.:	Information Sys.:		Phys. Rehab. Center:	Waste Disposal:	Phys. Practice Mgmt.:
	Clinical Trials:			Psychiatric Clinics:	Specialty Services:	

TYPES OF BUSINESS:
Equipment-Rehabilitation & Pain Management
Electrical Stimulation Products
Athletic Training Products

BRANDS/DIVISIONS/AFFILIATES:
Rehabilicare
Ortho DX
Compex Sport

CONTACTS:
Note: Officers with more than one job title may be intentionally listed here more than once.
Dan W. Gladney, CEO
Dan W. Gladney, Pres.
Scott P. Youngstrom, CFO
Gary Goodpaster, VP-Sales
Wayne K. Chrystal, VP-Mfg. Oper.
Marshall Masko, VP-U.S. Consumer Oper.
Scott P. Youngstrom, VP-Finance
Serge Darcy, CEO-Compex SA
Gary Goodpaster, VP-Managed Care

Phone: 612-631-0590 Fax:
Toll-Free:
Address: 1811 Old Hwy. 8, New Brighton, MN 55112 US

GROWTH PLANS/SPECIAL FEATURES:
Compex Technologies, Inc. designs, manufactures and sells electrical stimulation products for use in clinical, home health care, sports and occupational medicine settings in the U.S. and Europe. The company offers a number of electrotherapy devices for rehabilitation, acute pain management and athletic training, consisting of small, portable, battery-powered electrical pulse generators, which are connected by wires to electrodes placed on the skin. Rehabilitation products include neuromuscular stimulators, which facilitate faster recovery and function in diseased or injured muscles and soft tissue; and pulsed direct current devices, which reduce pain and swelling, influence local blood circulation and increase range of motion. The Ortho DX electrotherapy system, designed for post-surgical knee rehabilitation, combines both these forms into one stimulator. Pain management products include transcutaneous electrical nerve stimulation, interferential stimulators and iontophoresis devices. In addition, the firm sells various accessories and supplies, such as self-adhesive electrode pads, lead wires, batteries and power packs. Athletic products include the Compex Sport, a high-precision muscle stimulator designed to improve the performance of high-level athletes through strengthening and encouraging muscle recovery after strenuous workouts. The company's consumer products and European medical devices are sold under the Compex name, while U.S. prescription medical devices are sold primarily under the Rehabilicare name. Compex also distributes products manufactured by others under other name brands, such as Slendertone.

FINANCIALS:
Sales and profits are in thousands of dollars—add 000 to get the full amount. Year 2004 note: Complete fiscal 2004 results were not available for all companies at press time. For this company, year 2004 is for 12 months.

2004 Sales: $85,960 (12 months) 2004 Profits: $3,050 (12 months)
2003 Sales: $75,500 2003 Profits: $5,000
2002 Sales: $72,500 2002 Profits: $4,900
2001 Sales: $62,000 2001 Profits: $3,300
2000 Sales: $58,800 2000 Profits: $2,200

Stock Ticker: CMPX
Employees: 432
Fiscal Year Ends: 6/30

SALARIES/BENEFITS:
Pension Plan: ESOP Stock Plan: Profit Sharing: Top Exec. Salary: $336,705 Bonus: $52,905
Savings Plan: Y Stock Purch. Plan: Y   Second Exec. Salary: $259,809 Bonus: $23,331

OTHER THOUGHTS:
Apparent Top Female Officers:
Hot Spot for Advancement for Women/Minorities:

LOCATIONS: ("Y" = Yes)
West:	Southwest:	Midwest:	Southeast:	Northeast:	International:
		Y	Y		Y

ns
CONCENTRA INC

www.concentra.com

Industry Group Code: 524114   Ranks within this company's industry group: Sales: 45   Profits: 36

Insurance/HMO/PPO:	Drugs:	Equipment/Supplies:	Hospitals/Clinics:	Services:	Health Care:
Insurance:	Manufacturer:	Manufacturer:	Acute Care:	Diagnostics:	Home Health:
Managed Care:	Distributor:	Distributor:	Sub-Acute Care:	Labs/Testing: Y	Long-Term Care:
Utilization Mgmt.: Y	Specialty Pharm.:	Leasing/Finance:	Outpatient Surgery:	Staffing:	Physical Therapy: Y
Payment Proc.:	Vitamins/Nutri.:	Information Sys.:	Phys. Rehab. Center:	Waste Disposal:	Phys. Practice Mgmt.:
	Clinical Trials:		Psychiatric Clinics:	Specialty Services: Y	

TYPES OF BUSINESS:
Workers' Compensation & Occupational Health Services
Insurance Services
Physical Therapy
Drug & Alcohol Testing

BRANDS/DIVISIONS/AFFILIATES:
CONCENTRA Managed Care
Concentra Operating Corporation

CONTACTS:
Note: Officers with more than one job title may be intentionally listed here more than once.

Daniel J. Thomas, CEO
Thomas E. Kiraly, Exec. VP/CFO
Andrew R. Daniels, Chief Mktg. Officer/Sr. VP-Bus. Dev.
Tammy S. Steele, Sr. VP-Human Resources & Compliance
Laura Ciavola, Sr. VP/CIO
Richard A. Parr, II, Exec. VP/General Counsel/Corp. Sec.
James M. Greenwood, Exec. VP-Corp. Dev.
Thomas E. Kiraly, Treas.
W. Tom Fogarty, Sr. VP/Chief Medical Officer

Phone: 972-364-8000	Fax: 972-381-1938
Toll-Free: 800-232-3550	
Address: 5080 Spectrum Dr., W. Tower, Ste. 400, Addision, TX 75001 US	

GROWTH PLANS/SPECIAL FEATURES:
Concentra, Inc., formerly CONCENTRA Managed Care, is a leading national provider of workers' compensation and occupational health care services, as well as group health and auto liability. Concentra Operating Corporation, a wholly-owned subsidiary, manages the firm's operations, which encompass three business segments: health services, network services and care management services. The health services segment treats workplace injuries and illnesses, provides physical therapy, pre-placement physicals and drug and alcohol screening. It operates through 259 owned and managed centers in 34 states and approximately 569 affiliated primary care physicians, as well as affiliated physical therapists, nurses and other health care providers. The network services segment assists insurance companies and other payors in reviewing, repricing and reducing the out-of-network bills they receive from medical providers. It attempts to increase customer savings through fee negotiations, bill repricing and access to provider networks. The care management services segment offers services designed to monitor cases and facilitate the return to work of injured employees who have been out of work for an extended period of time due primarily to a work-related illness or injury. The company has partnerships with 13 hospital systems throughout the U.S., including Vanderbilt University Medical Center, University of Pittsburgh Medical Center, Wake Forest University Baptist Medical Center and Colmubia's Trident Medical Center in Charleston, South Carolina.

FINANCIALS:
Sales and profits are in thousands of dollars—add 000 to get the full amount. Year 2004 note: Complete fiscal 2004 results were not available for all companies at press time. For this company, year 2004 is for months.

2004 Sales: $ (months)
2003 Sales: $1,050,700
2002 Sales: $999,000
2001 Sales: $
2000 Sales: $

2004 Profits: $ (months)
2003 Profits: $43,300
2002 Profits: $-3,600
2001 Profits: $
2000 Profits: $

Stock Ticker: Private
Employees: 10,000
Fiscal Year Ends: 12/31

SALARIES/BENEFITS:
Pension Plan:	ESOP Stock Plan:	Profit Sharing:	Top Exec. Salary: $	Bonus: $
Savings Plan:	Stock Purch. Plan:		Second Exec. Salary: $	Bonus: $

OTHER THOUGHTS:
Apparent Top Female Officers: 2
Hot Spot for Advancement for Women/Minorities:

LOCATIONS: ("Y" = Yes)
West:	Southwest:	Midwest:	Southeast:	Northeast:	International:
Y	Y	Y	Y	Y	

CONMED CORP

www.conmed.com

Industry Group Code: 339113   **Ranks within this company's industry group:** Sales: 39   Profits: 42

Insurance/HMO/PPO:	Drugs:	Equipment/Supplies:		Hospitals/Clinics:	Services:	Health Care:
Insurance: Managed Care: Utilization Mgmt.: Payment Proc.:	Manufacturer: Distributor: Specialty Pharm.: Vitamins/Nutri.: Clinical Trials:	Manufacturer: Distributor: Leasing/Finance: Information Sys.:	Y Y	Acute Care: Sub-Acute Care: Outpatient Surgery: Phys. Rehab. Center: Psychiatric Clinics:	Diagnostics: Labs/Testing: Staffing: Waste Disposal: Specialty Services:	Home Health: Long-Term Care: Physical Therapy: Phys. Practice Mgmt.:

TYPES OF BUSINESS:
Equipment-Surgical & Medical Procedure
Patient Care Products
Sports Medicine Equipment

BRANDS/DIVISIONS/AFFILIATES:
Hall Surgical
Linvatec Corporation
Reflex
Universal
Trogard Finesse

CONTACTS:
Note: Officers with more than one job title may be intentionally listed here more than once.
Eugene R. Corasanti, CEO
Joseph J. Corasanti, Pres.
Joseph J. Corasanti, COO
Robert D. Shallish, Jr., CFO
Chip Jones, VP-Corp. Mktg. & Sales
Daniel S. Jonas, VP-Legal Affairs/General Counsel
Thomas M. Acey, Treas.
William W. Abraham, Sr. VP
John J. Stotts, VP-Patient Care
Luke A. Pomilio, VP
Frank R. Williams, VP-Endosurgery
Eugene R. Corasanti, Chmn.
Alan Fink, VP-Int'l

Phone: 315-797-8375   **Fax:** 315-797-0321
Toll-Free:
Address: 525 French Rd., Utica, NY 13502 US

GROWTH PLANS/SPECIAL FEATURES:
Conmed Corporation is a leading developer, manufacturer and supplier of a broad range of medical instruments and systems used in surgical and other medical procedures. The firm specializes in instruments and implants for arthroscopic sports medicine and powered surgical instruments for orthopedic surgery and neurosurgery. In addition, Conmed has broadened its product offerings to include arthroscopic surgery devices and products and imaging products for minimally invasive surgery. Its new products include arthroscopes, reconstructive systems, tissue repair sets, fluid management systems, imaging products, metal and bioabsorbable implants and related disposable products. Conmed's powered surgical instruments division sells tools for cutting, drilling and reaming, primarily under the Hall Surgical brand. Its Linvatec subsidiary is developing a technology base for large-bone, small-bone, arthroscopic, neurosurgical and spine instruments that can be adapted and modified for new procedures. The firm's radio frequency electrosurgery products are used in general, dermatologic, thoracic, orthopedic, urologic, neurosurgical, gynecological, laparoscopic, arthroscopic and endoscopic procedures and include electrosurgical pencils and blades, ground pads, generators, the argon-beam coagulation system and related disposable products. Its endoscopy products include the Reflex clip applier, Universal laparoscopic instruments, surgical staplers and the Trogard Finesse, which incorporates a blunt-tipped trocar, resulting in smaller wounds and less bleeding. The company also produces patient care products for monitoring cardiac rhythms, wound care management and intravenous therapy, including ECG electrodes and cables, wound dressings, catheter stabilization dressings, disposable surgical suction instruments and connecting tubing. Conmed's product breadth has enhanced its ability to market to hospitals, surgery centers, group purchasing organizations and other customers, particularly as institutions seek to reduce costs and minimize the number of suppliers. In October 2004, the company acquired CR Bard's endoscopic unit for $80 million in cash.

FINANCIALS:
Sales and profits are in thousands of dollars—add 000 to get the full amount. Year 2004 note: Complete fiscal 2004 results were not available for all companies at press time. For this company, year 2004 is for 9 months.

2004 Sales: $363,321 (9 months)   2004 Profits: $19,137 (9 months)
2003 Sales: $497,100   2003 Profits: $32,100
2002 Sales: $453,100   2002 Profits: $34,200
2001 Sales: $428,700   2001 Profits: $24,400
2000 Sales: $392,200   2000 Profits: $19,300

Stock Ticker: CNMD
Employees: 2,600
Fiscal Year Ends: 12/31

SALARIES/BENEFITS:
Pension Plan: Y   ESOP Stock Plan: Profit Sharing: Top Exec. Salary: $387,307   Bonus: $120,000
Savings Plan: Y   Stock Purch. Plan: Second Exec. Salary: $292,308   Bonus: $91,500

OTHER THOUGHTS:
Apparent Top Female Officers:
Hot Spot for Advancement for Women/Minorities:

LOCATIONS: ("Y" = Yes)
West:	Southwest:	Midwest:	Southeast:	Northeast:	International:
Y	Y		Y	Y	Y

CONTINUCARE CORP

www.continucare.com

Industry Group Code: 621610   Ranks within this company's industry group: Sales: 11   Profits: 11

Insurance/HMO/PPO:	Drugs:	Equipment/Supplies:	Hospitals/Clinics:		Services:		Health Care:	
Insurance:	Manufacturer:	Manufacturer:	Acute Care:		Diagnostics:		Home Health:	
Managed Care:	Distributor:	Distributor:	Sub-Acute Care:	Y	Labs/Testing:		Long-Term Care:	
Utilization Mgmt.: Y	Specialty Pharm.:	Leasing/Finance:	Outpatient Surgery:	Y	Staffing:		Physical Therapy:	
Payment Proc.:	Vitamins/Nutri.:	Information Sys.:	Phys. Rehab. Center:		Waste Disposal:		Phys. Practice Mgmt.:	Y
	Clinical Trials:		Psychiatric Clinics:		Specialty Services:			

TYPES OF BUSINESS:
Home Health Care
Managed Health Care
Practice Management

BRANDS/DIVISIONS/AFFILIATES:

GROWTH PLANS/SPECIAL FEATURES:
Continucare Corporation is a provider of outpatient health care and practice management services in the Florida market. The company's network of 15 medical centers provides primary health care services throughout Miami-Dade, Broward and Hillsborough counties. In addition, the firm provides financial reports and assistance with medical utilization management, pharmacy management and specialist network development to 31 independent physician affiliates in the same area. Continucare serves over 28,000 patients, most of whom are participants in the Medicare Advantage program. The company has managed care agreements with Humana, Vista and Wellcare, which together account for substantially all of its revenue. The firm's growth strategy is to increase patient volume at its existing medical centers, expand its network to include additional medical centers and further develop its management activities.

CONTACTS:
Note: Officers with more than one job title may be intentionally listed here more than once.

Richard C. Pfenniger, Jr., CEO
Richard C. Pfenniger, Jr., Pres.
Fernando Fernandez, CFO
Luis H. Izquierdo, Sr. VP-Mktg.
Frank Houston, Dir.-IT
Patrick M. Healy, Exec. VP-Oper.
Luis H. Izquierdo, Sr. VP-Bus. Dev.
Janet Holt, Controller
Michael Cavanaugh, Sr. Chief Medical Officer
Mark Stern, Chief Medical Officer
Stephanie Moss, Dir.-Oper.
Deborah Meck, Dir.-Clinical Compliance
Richard C. Pfenniger, Jr., Chmn.

Phone: 305-500-2000   **Fax:** 305-500-2142
Toll-Free:
Address: 7200 Corporate Center Dr., Ste. 600, Miami, FL 33126 US

FINANCIALS:
Sales and profits are in thousands of dollars—add 000 to get the full amount. Year 2004 note: Complete fiscal 2004 results were not available for all companies at press time. For this company, year 2004 is for 12 months.

2004 Sales: $102,459 (12 months)	2004 Profits: $5,288 (12 months)	**Stock Ticker:** CNU
2003 Sales: $101,400	2003 Profits: $ 100	**Employees:** 248
2002 Sales: $105,500	2002 Profits: $-3,600	**Fiscal Year Ends:** 6/30
2001 Sales: $112,600	2001 Profits: $- 100	
2000 Sales: $116,583	2000 Profits: $14,118	

SALARIES/BENEFITS:
| Pension Plan: | ESOP Stock Plan: | Profit Sharing: | Top Exec. Salary: $226,154 | Bonus: $25,000 |
| Savings Plan: Y | Stock Purch. Plan: | | Second Exec. Salary: $137,415 | Bonus: $ |

OTHER THOUGHTS:
Apparent Top Female Officers: 3
Hot Spot for Advancement for Women/Minorities: Y

LOCATIONS: ("Y" = Yes)
| West: | Southwest: | Midwest: | Southeast: Y | Northeast: | International: |

CONVATEC

www.convatec.com

Industry Group Code: 339113   Ranks within this company's industry group: Sales: Profits:

Insurance/HMO/PPO:	Drugs:	Equipment/Supplies:		Hospitals/Clinics:	Services:	Health Care:
Insurance:	Manufacturer:	Manufacturer:	Y	Acute Care:	Diagnostics:	Home Health:
Managed Care:	Distributor:	Distributor:		Sub-Acute Care:	Labs/Testing:	Long-Term Care:
Utilization Mgmt.:	Specialty Pharm.:	Leasing/Finance:		Outpatient Surgery:	Staffing:	Physical Therapy:
Payment Proc.:	Vitamins/Nutri.:	Information Sys.:		Phys. Rehab. Center:	Waste Disposal:	Phys. Practice Mgmt.:
	Clinical Trials:			Psychiatric Clinics:	Specialty Services:	

TYPES OF BUSINESS:
Wound Care Products
Ostomy Products
Skin Care Products

BRANDS/DIVISIONS/AFFILIATES:
Bristol-Myers Squibb
AQUACEL
DuoDerm
SAF-Clens
ActiveLife
Little Ones
Aloe Vesta
Septi-Soft

CONTACTS: Note: Officers with more than one job title may be intentionally listed here more than once.
Gary C. Restani, Pres.
Francis Royle, Press Officer
Henry A. Holzapfel, VP/General Mgr.-Professional Health Care

Phone: 908-904-2500   Fax: 908-904-2780
Toll-Free: 800-422-8811
Address: 200 Headquarters Park Dr., Skillman, NJ 08558 US

GROWTH PLANS/SPECIAL FEATURES:
ConvaTec, a subsidiary of Bristol-Myers Squibb, is a leading manufacturer of wound care, ostomy care and skin care products for the health care industry. The company's wound care products include wound cleansers, wound dressings, bandages and wound hydration products sold under the AQUACEL, CarboFlex, DuoDerm, Hyalofill, KALTOSTAT, LYOFOAM, OPTIPORE, SurePress, SAF-Clens, SAF-GEL, Shur-Clens, Tubifast, Tubigrip, Tubipad and UNNA-FLEX brand names. The newest wound care products are SAF-Clens AF dermal wound cleanser; Versiva, an advanced wound dressing that combines three proven technologies; and AQUACEL Ag, an antimicrobial wound dressing for acute and chronic wounds. The firm's ostomy care products include Stomahesive and Durahesive skin barriers, as well as Esteem Synergy, SUR-FIT Natura and SUR-FIT AutoLock two-piece pouching systems; ActiveLife one-piece pouching systems; and Little Ones pediatric pouching systems. Pouching systems allow patients with stomas (artificial openings) to dispose of bodily waste into an attachable pouch. ConvaTec's newest ostomy products include Durahesive and Moldable Convex Skin Barrier with flange, a customizable skin barrier for difficult-to-manage stomas. In addition, the company offers a range of skin care products, including skin cleansers, moisturizers, barriers, bathing and antifungal products, under the Aloe Vesta, Sensi-Care and Septi-Soft brand names. Aloe Vesta bathing cloths are its newest skin care product.

FINANCIALS: Sales and profits are in thousands of dollars—add 000 to get the full amount. Year 2004 note: Complete fiscal 2004 results were not available for all companies at press time. For this company, year 2004 is for months.

2004 Sales: $ (months)   2004 Profits: $ (months)
2003 Sales: $ 2003 Profits: $
2002 Sales: $ 2002 Profits: $ Stock Ticker: Subsidiary
2001 Sales: $ 2001 Profits: $ Employees:
2000 Sales: $ 2000 Profits: $ Fiscal Year Ends: 12/31

SALARIES/BENEFITS:
Pension Plan: ESOP Stock Plan: Profit Sharing: Top Exec. Salary: $ Bonus: $
Savings Plan: Stock Purch. Plan: Second Exec. Salary: $ Bonus: $

OTHER THOUGHTS:
Apparent Top Female Officers:
Hot Spot for Advancement for Women/Minorities:

LOCATIONS: ("Y" = Yes)
West:	Southwest:	Midwest:	Southeast:	Northeast:	International:
				Y	Y

COOPER COMPANIES INC

www.coopercos.com

Industry Group Code: 339113 **Ranks within this company's industry group:** Sales: 43 Profits: 24

Insurance/HMO/PPO:	Drugs:	Equipment/Supplies:	Hospitals/Clinics:	Services:	Health Care:
Insurance:	Manufacturer:	Manufacturer: Y	Acute Care:	Diagnostics:	Home Health:
Managed Care:	Distributor:	Distributor:	Sub-Acute Care:	Labs/Testing:	Long-Term Care:
Utilization Mgmt.:	Specialty Pharm.:	Leasing/Finance:	Outpatient Surgery:	Staffing:	Physical Therapy:
Payment Proc.:	Vitamins/Nutri.:	Information Sys.:	Phys. Rehab. Center:	Waste Disposal:	Phys. Practice Mgmt.:
	Clinical Trials:		Psychiatric Clinics:	Specialty Services:	

TYPES OF BUSINESS:
Supplies-Contact Lenses
Disposable Medical Products
Gynecological Instruments
Diagnostic Products

BRANDS/DIVISIONS/AFFILIATES:
CooperVision, Inc.
CooperSurgical, Inc.
Cerveillance Scope

CONTACTS:
Note: Officers with more than one job title may be intentionally listed here more than once.
A. Thomas Bender, CEO
A. Thomas Bender, Pres.
Robert S. Weiss, Exec. VP/CFO
Carol R. Kaufman, Chief Admin. Officer
Carol R. Kaufman, VP-Legal Affairs
B. Norris Battin, VP-Investor Rel.
David G. Acosta, Treas./Tax Dir.
Gregory A. Fryling, COO-CooperVision, Inc.
Nicholas J. Pichotta, Pres./CEO-CooperSurgical, Inc.
Paul L. Remmell, COO-CooperSurgical, Inc.
Rodney E. Folden, Corp. Controller
A. Thomas Bender, Chmn.

Phone: 925-460-3600	Fax: 925-460-3649
Toll-Free:	
Address: 6140 Stoneridge Mall Rd., Ste. 590, Pleasanton, CA 94588 US	

GROWTH PLANS/SPECIAL FEATURES:

The Cooper Companies, Inc. is a specialty health care company that conducts business through its two subsidiaries: CooperVision, Inc. and CooperSurgical, Inc. CooperVision markets a broad range of contact lenses throughout the world, and CooperSurgical markets diagnostic products, surgical instruments and accessories for the women's health care market. CooperVision has developed a niche market in the contact lens industry by acquiring certain patents that allow it to make exclusive claims about the comfort of its contact lenses. CooperSurgical has produced a number of innovative products for in-office practices where physicians screen, diagnose and treat commonly occurring gynecological conditions. One such product is the innovative digital colposcopy system, Cerveillance Scope. Using Cerveillance Scope, physicians can examine the cervix and then document, store and recall digital images of their findings. CooperSurgical anticipates strong growth due to an increased number of women using their gynecologist as their general practitioner.

The firm offers a retirement income plan to all full-time employees with 30 years of service.

FINANCIALS:
Sales and profits are in thousands of dollars—add 000 to get the full amount. Year 2004 note: Complete fiscal 2004 results were not available for all companies at press time. For this company, year 2004 is for 9 months.

2004 Sales: $359,365 (9 months)	2004 Profits: $64,102 (9 months)	**Stock Ticker:** COO
2003 Sales: $411,790	2003 Profits: $68,770	Employees: 3,500
2002 Sales: $315,300	2002 Profits: $48,900	Fiscal Year Ends: 10/31
2001 Sales: $234,600	2001 Profits: $37,100	
2000 Sales: $197,317	2000 Profits: $28,968	

SALARIES/BENEFITS:
| Pension Plan: Y | ESOP Stock Plan: | Profit Sharing: | Top Exec. Salary: $461,300 | Bonus: $393,258 |
| Savings Plan: Y | Stock Purch. Plan: | | Second Exec. Salary: $244,000 | Bonus: $177,875 |

OTHER THOUGHTS:
Apparent Top Female Officers: 1
Hot Spot for Advancement for Women/Minorities:

LOCATIONS: ("Y" = Yes)
West:	Southwest:	Midwest:	Southeast:	Northeast:	International:
Y				Y	Y

Note: Financial information, benefits and other data can change quickly and may vary from those stated here.

CORDIS CORP

www.cordis.com

Industry Group Code: 339113   Ranks within this company's industry group: Sales: Profits:

Insurance/HMO/PPO:	Drugs:	Equipment/Supplies:	Hospitals/Clinics:	Services:	Health Care:
Insurance:	Manufacturer:	Manufacturer: Y	Acute Care:	Diagnostics:	Home Health:
Managed Care:	Distributor:	Distributor:	Sub-Acute Care:	Labs/Testing:	Long-Term Care:
Utilization Mgmt.:	Specialty Pharm.:	Leasing/Finance:	Outpatient Surgery:	Staffing:	Physical Therapy:
Payment Proc.:	Vitamins/Nutri.:	Information Sys.:	Phys. Rehab. Center:	Waste Disposal:	Phys. Practice Mgmt.:
	Clinical Trials:		Psychiatric Clinics:	Specialty Services:	

TYPES OF BUSINESS:
Vascular Treatment Products
Stents & Catheters
Guidewires & Balloons

BRANDS/DIVISIONS/AFFILIATES:
Johnson & Johnson
Cordis Neurovascular, Inc.
Carmeda End-Point Attached Heparin
VISTA BRITE TIP Guiding Catheter
Bx SONIC Stent
CYPHER

CONTACTS:
Note: Officers with more than one job title may be intentionally listed here more than once.

Guy J. Lebeau, Worldwide Pres.
Rick Anderson, U.S. Pres.-Cordis Cardiology Div.
Carol L. Zilm, Worldwide Pres.-Cordis Endovascular Div.
Carol L. Zilm, Worldwide Pres., Cordis Neurovascular, Inc.
Robert W. Croce, Worldwide Franchise Chmn.

Phone: 786-313-2000   **Fax:** 786-313-2440
Toll-Free: 800-327-7714
Address: 14201 NW 60th Ave., Miami Lakes, FL 33014 US

GROWTH PLANS/SPECIAL FEATURES:
Cordis Corp., a subsidiary of Johnson & Johnson, develops less-invasive products to treat vascular disease. The firm operates through two divisions, Cordis Cardiology and Cordis Endovascular, as well as one subsidiary, Cordis Neurovascular, Inc. Its business units focus on developing cardiological, endovascular, neurological and electrophysiological uses for its products. The firm's products include guidewires, balloons, catheters and stents. The company's newest products include the Bx SONIC Stent with HEPACOAT, Carmeda End-Point Attached Heparin and the VISTA BRITE TIP Guiding Catheter. In recent news, Cordis gained FDA approval for the CYPHER Sirolimus-Eluting Coronary Stent, a drug-eluting stent that delivers sirolimus, which can be used to treat a broad range of conditions, including diabetes and restenosis (the constriction of a duct or passage after corrective surgery on a heart valve). In addition, the company entered into a strategic alliance with Guidant Corporation for the co-promotion of their drug-eluting stents, including the CYPHER, as well as the option to co-promote bioabsorbable vascular products. They also agreed to develop a CYPHER stent that uses Guidant's Multi-Link Vision Stent Delivery System.

FINANCIALS:
Sales and profits are in thousands of dollars—add 000 to get the full amount. Year 2004 note: Complete fiscal 2004 results were not available for all companies at press time. For this company, year 2004 is for months.

2004 Sales: $ (months)   2004 Profits: $ (months)
2003 Sales: $ 2003 Profits: $
2002 Sales: $ 2002 Profits: $
2001 Sales: $ 2001 Profits: $
2000 Sales: $ 2000 Profits: $

Stock Ticker: Subsidiary
Employees:
Fiscal Year Ends: 12/31

SALARIES/BENEFITS:
Pension Plan: ESOP Stock Plan: Profit Sharing: Top Exec. Salary: $ Bonus: $
Savings Plan: Stock Purch. Plan: Second Exec. Salary: $ Bonus: $

OTHER THOUGHTS:
Apparent Top Female Officers: 1
Hot Spot for Advancement for Women/Minorities:

LOCATIONS: ("Y" = Yes)

West:	Southwest:	Midwest:	Southeast: Y	Northeast:	International:

Note: Financial information, benefits and other data can change quickly and may vary from those stated here.

CORVEL CORP

www.corvel.com

Industry Group Code: 621999   Ranks within this company's industry group: Sales: 1   Profits: 1

Insurance/HMO/PPO:	Drugs:	Equipment/Supplies:	Hospitals/Clinics:	Services:	Health Care:
Insurance:	Manufacturer:	Manufacturer:	Acute Care:	Diagnostics: Y	Home Health:
Managed Care:	Distributor:	Distributor:	Sub-Acute Care:	Labs/Testing:	Long-Term Care:
Utilization Mgmt.: Y	Specialty Pharm.:	Leasing/Finance:	Outpatient Surgery:	Staffing:	Physical Therapy:
Payment Proc.: Y	Vitamins/Nutri.:	Information Sys.: Y	Phys. Rehab. Center:	Waste Disposal:	Phys. Practice Mgmt.:
	Clinical Trials:		Psychiatric Clinics:	Specialty Services: Y	

TYPES OF BUSINESS:
Utilization Management
Managed Care Services
Preferred Provider Networks
Payment Processing

BRANDS/DIVISIONS/AFFILIATES:
CoreCare
CareMC
caremc.com
Scan One
Advocacy

CONTACTS: Note: Officers with more than one job title may be intentionally listed here more than once.
V. Gordon Clemons, CEO
V. Gordon Clemons, Pres.
Richard J. Schweppe, CFO
Peter E. Flynn, VP-Bus. Dev.
Richard J. Schweppe, Corp. Sec.
V. Gordon Clemons, Chmn.

Phone: 949-851-1473   Fax: 949-851-1469
Toll-Free:
Address: 2010 Main St., Ste. 600, Irvine, CA 92614 US

GROWTH PLANS/SPECIAL FEATURES:
CorVel Corporation is an independent nationwide provider of managed care services designed to address the escalating medical costs of workers' compensation and other health care benefits, primarily coverage under group health and auto policies. The company offers services in two general categories: network solutions, which assists customers in managing the increasing medical costs of workers' compensation, group health and auto insurance; and patient management services, which monitor the quality of care provided to claimants. The firm's network solutions services include automated medical fee auditing, preferred provider networks and utilization review. Its patient management services, otherwise known as CorCase, provide a suite of services including first notice of loss, early intervention, utilization management, telephonic case management, on-site case management, peer review, vocational rehabilitation, Medicare set-asides and life care planning. CorCase uses CorVel's proprietary Advocacy software to determine available indemnity payments from the employer and coordinate case management information and issues. The firm provides its services to insurance companies, government entities, third-party administrators and self-administered employers. Through its CareMC web site, caremc.com, CorVel serves the health care and claims needs of insurers and employers managing employee absences and disability insurance losses. In addition, the site provides direct access to the firm's managed care services. It also functions as an application service provider through which other managed care providers can supply their services to major employers and insurers nationwide. The service allows physicians to obtain real-time confirmation of the acceptance and review of invoices for service. In recent news, CorVel acquired Scan One, a provider of scanning, optical character recognition and document management services.

FINANCIALS:
Sales and profits are in thousands of dollars—add 000 to get the full amount. Year 2004 note: Complete fiscal 2004 results were not available for all companies at press time. For this company, year 2004 is for 12 months.

2004 Sales: $305,279 (12 months)   2004 Profits: $16,013 (12 months)
2003 Sales: $282,800   2003 Profits: $16,600
2002 Sales: $235,900   2002 Profits: $23,900
2001 Sales: $209,554   2001 Profits: $13,200
2000 Sales: $186,765   2000 Profits: $12,000

Stock Ticker: CRVL
Employees: 3,215
Fiscal Year Ends: 3/31

SALARIES/BENEFITS:
Pension Plan: ESOP Stock Plan: Profit Sharing: Top Exec. Salary: $291,938   Bonus: $16,000
Savings Plan: Y   Stock Purch. Plan: Y   Second Exec. Salary: $120,000 Bonus: $19,163

OTHER THOUGHTS:
Apparent Top Female Officers:
Hot Spot for Advancement for Women/Minorities:

LOCATIONS: ("Y" = Yes)
West:	Southwest:	Midwest:	Southeast:	Northeast:	International:
Y	Y	Y	Y	Y	

COVANCE INC

www.covance.com

Industry Group Code: 541710 **Ranks within this company's industry group:** Sales: 3 Profits: 3

Insurance/HMO/PPO:	Drugs:	Equipment/Supplies:	Hospitals/Clinics:	Services:		Health Care:	
Insurance:	Manufacturer:	Manufacturer:	Acute Care:	Diagnostics:	Y	Home Health:	
Managed Care:	Distributor:	Distributor:	Sub-Acute Care:	Labs/Testing:	Y	Long-Term Care:	
Utilization Mgmt.:	Specialty Pharm.:	Leasing/Finance:	Outpatient Surgery:	Staffing:		Physical Therapy:	
Payment Proc.:	Vitamins/Nutri.:	Information Sys.:	Phys. Rehab. Center:	Waste Disposal:		Phys. Practice Mgmt.:	
	Clinical Trials: Y		Psychiatric Clinics:	Specialty Services:	Y		

TYPES OF BUSINESS:
Research & Development-Drug Preclinical/Clinical Trials
Laboratory Testing & Analysis
Drug Approval Assistance Services
Health Economics & Outcomes Services

BRANDS/DIVISIONS/AFFILIATES:
Study Tracker
LabLink
Trial Tracker
Covance Clinical Research Unit, Inc.
Covance Pharmaceutical Packaging Services, Inc.
BioLink

CONTACTS:
Note: Officers with more than one job title may be intentionally listed here more than once.

Christopher A. Kuebler, CEO
Joseph L. Herring, Pres.
Joseph L. Herring, COO
William Klitgaard, Sr. VP/CFO
Donald Kraft, Sr. VP-Human Resources
Howard Moody, Sr. VP/CIO
Jeffrey S. Hurwitz, Sr. VP/General Counsel
Michael Giannetto, Controller
Stephen J. Sullivan, Sr. VP/Pres.,Global Central Laboratory Services
James A. Bannon, Sr. VP/Pres.,Clinical & Periapproval Services
William Klitgaard, Treas.
Jeffrey S. Hurwitz, Sec.
Christopher A. Kuebler, Chmn.

Phone: 609-452-4440 **Fax:** 609-452-9375
Toll-Free: 888-268-2623
Address: 210 Carnegie Ctr., Princeton, NJ 08540-6233 US

GROWTH PLANS/SPECIAL FEATURES:

Covance, Inc. is a leading drug development services company providing a wide range of product development services on a worldwide basis to pharmaceutical, biotechnology and medical device industries. The company also provides laboratory testing services to the chemical, agrochemical and food industries. In addition, the firm provides early development services and late-stage development services. Early development services include pre-clinical services (toxicology, pharmaceutical development, research products and BioLink, a bioanalytical testing service) and Phase I clinical services. Late-stage development services include clinical development services, clinical support services, commercialization services (periapproval services, and health economics and outcome services), central laboratory services and central ECG diagnostic services. Covance has also introduced several Internet-based products. Study Tracker is an Internet-based client access product, which permits customers of toxicology services to review study data and schedules on a near real-time basis. LabLink is a client access program that allows customers of central laboratory services to review and query lab data on a near real-time basis. Trial Tracker is a web-enabled clinical trial project management and tracking tool intended to allow both employees and customers of its late-stage clinical business to review and manage all aspects of clinical trial projects. Digitography in the company's central diagnostics business allows on-screen digital ECG waveform measurement with resolution unmatched in the industry. In recent news, Covance expanded its clinical trail operations in China through a collaboration with Excel PharmaStudies, Inc., the largest domestic research organization in China providing full clinical development services.

FINANCIALS:
Sales and profits are in thousands of dollars—add 000 to get the full amount. Year 2004 note: Complete fiscal 2004 results were not available for all companies at press time. For this company, year 2004 is for 9 months.

2004 Sales: $774,053 (9 months)
2003 Sales: $974,210
2002 Sales: $924,700
2001 Sales: $855,900
2000 Sales: $868,087

2004 Profits: $70,637 (9 months)
2003 Profits: $76,136
2002 Profits: $63,800
2001 Profits: $47,900
2000 Profits: $15,236

Stock Ticker: CVD
Employees: 6,500
Fiscal Year Ends: 12/31

SALARIES/BENEFITS:
Pension Plan: ESOP Stock Plan: Profit Sharing: Top Exec. Salary: $588,584   Bonus: $378,431
Savings Plan: Stock Purch. Plan: Second Exec. Salary: $416,666   Bonus: $214,317

OTHER THOUGHTS:
Apparent Top Female Officers:
Hot Spot for Advancement for Women/Minorities:

LOCATIONS: ("Y" = Yes)

West:	Southwest:	Midwest:	Southeast:	Northeast:	International:
Y	Y	Y	Y	Y	Y

Note: Financial information, benefits and other data can change quickly and may vary from those stated here.

COVENTRY HEALTH CARE INC

www.coventryhealthcare.com

Industry Group Code: 524114 Ranks within this company's industry group: Sales: 23 Profits: 12

Insurance/HMO/PPO:	Drugs:	Equipment/Supplies:	Hospitals/Clinics:	Services:	Health Care:
Insurance: Managed Care: Y Utilization Mgmt.: Payment Proc.:	Manufacturer: Distributor: Specialty Pharm.: Vitamins/Nutri.: Clinical Trials:	Manufacturer: Distributor: Leasing/Finance: Information Sys.:	Acute Care: Sub-Acute Care: Outpatient Surgery: Phys. Rehab. Center: Psychiatric Clinics:	Diagnostics: Labs/Testing: Staffing: Waste Disposal: Specialty Services:	Home Health: Long-Term Care: Physical Therapy: Phys. Practice Mgmt.:

TYPES OF BUSINESS:
HMO/PPO
Managed Care Products and Services

BRANDS/DIVISIONS/AFFILIATES:
First Health Group
Coventry Health and Life
Carelink Health Plans
Southern Health
HealthAmerica
HealthAssurance
HealthCare USA
WellPath

CONTACTS:
Note: Officers with more than one job title may be intentionally listed here more than once.

Dale B. Wolf, CEO
Thomas P. McDonough, Pres.
Shawn Guertin, CFO
J. Stewart Lavelle, Sr. VP-Mktg. & Sales
Harvey C. DeMovick, Jr., CIO
Thomas C. Zielinski, General Counsel
Harvey C. DeMovick, Jr., Sr. VP-Customer Service Oper.
Shawn Guertin, Treas.
Bernard J. Mansheim, Sr. VP/Chief Medical Officer
Ronald M. Chaffin, Sr. VP/CEO-Coventry Health Care of Delaware
Davina C. Lane, Pres./CEO-HealthCare USA of Missouri
Janet M. Stallmeyer, Sr. VP/CEO-Coventry Health Care of Kansas
John H. Austin, Chmn.

Phone: 301-581-0600 Fax: 301-493-0752
Toll-Free:
Address: 6705 Rockledge Dr., Ste. 900, Bethesda, MD 20817 US

GROWTH PLANS/SPECIAL FEATURES:
Coventry Health Care, Inc., formerly Coventry Corporation, is a managed health care company operating under the names Coventry Health Care, Coventry Health and Life, Carelink Health Plans, Group Health Plan, HealthAmerica, HealthAssurance, HealthCare USA, Southern Health and WellPath. The firm provides a full range of managed care products and services, including health maintenance organization (HMO), point-of-service (POS) and preferred provider organization (PPO) products. Coventry also administers self-insured plans for large employer groups and recently began offering defined contribution health plans. Coventry's HMO products provide comprehensive health care benefits to members, including ambulatory and inpatient physician services, hospitalization, pharmacy, dental, optical, mental health and ancillary diagnostic and therapeutic services. Aside from providing HMO products, the firm's health plans offer management services to large employers who self-insure their employees. Under related contracts, employers who fund their own health plans receive the benefit of provider pricing arrangements from the health plan. Such plans also provide a variety of administrative services such as claims processing, utilization review and quality assurance for employers. Coventry has begun implementing web-based services to manage the electronic submission and processing of eligibility determination, authorization submission and status, claims submission and status and reporting. The company recently completed the acquisition of PersonalCare Health Management and has entered into a definitive agreement to acquire Altius Health Plans, which together increase Coventry's membership by almost 240,000. In October 2004, Coventry Health Care agreed to purchase First Health Group for $1.8 billion in cash and stock.

Coventry offers its employees medical, dental and vision plans, as well as tuition assistance and sponsored educational programs.

FINANCIALS:
Sales and profits are in thousands of dollars—add 000 to get the full amount. Year 2004 note: Complete fiscal 2004 results were not available for all companies at press time. For this company, year 2004 is for 9 months.

2004 Sales: $3,927,789 (9 months)	2004 Profits: $245,351 (9 months)	Stock Ticker: CVH
2003 Sales: $4,535,143	2003 Profits: $250,145	Employees: 4,203
2002 Sales: $3,576,900	2002 Profits: $145,600	Fiscal Year Ends: 12/31
2001 Sales: $3,147,200	2001 Profits: $84,400	
2000 Sales: $2,604,910	2000 Profits: $61,340	

SALARIES/BENEFITS:
| Pension Plan: | ESOP Stock Plan: | Profit Sharing: | Top Exec. Salary: $900,000 | Bonus: $2,100,000 |
| Savings Plan: Y | Stock Purch. Plan: Y | | Second Exec. Salary: $600,000 | Bonus: $1,000,000 |

OTHER THOUGHTS:
Apparent Top Female Officers: 2
Hot Spot for Advancement for Women/Minorities:

LOCATIONS: ("Y" = Yes)
| West: | Southwest: Y | Midwest: Y | Southeast: Y | Northeast: Y | International: |

CR BARD INC

www.crbard.com

Industry Group Code: 339113 **Ranks within this company's industry group:** Sales: 19 Profits: 13

Insurance/HMO/PPO:	Drugs:	Equipment/Supplies:		Hospitals/Clinics:		Services:		Health Care:	
Insurance:	Manufacturer:	Manufacturer:	Y	Acute Care:		Diagnostics:		Home Health:	
Managed Care:	Distributor:	Distributor:		Sub-Acute Care:		Labs/Testing:		Long-Term Care:	
Utilization Mgmt.:	Specialty Pharm.:	Leasing/Finance:		Outpatient Surgery:		Staffing:		Physical Therapy:	
Payment Proc.:	Vitamins/Nutri.:	Information Sys.:		Phys. Rehab. Center:		Waste Disposal:		Phys. Practice Mgmt.:	
	Clinical Trials:			Psychiatric Clinics:		Specialty Services:	Y		

TYPES OF BUSINESS:
Equipment-Urological Catheters
Diagnostic and Interventional Products
Minimally Invasive Vascular Products
Surgical Specialty Products
Supply Chain and Business Services

BRANDS/DIVISIONS/AFFILIATES:
Bard Access Systems
Bard Devices, Inc.
Bard Medical Systems
PerFix
Composix
HydroFlex
Uryxr
Genyx Medical, Inc.

CONTACTS:
Note: Officers with more than one job title may be intentionally listed here more than once.
Timothy M. Ring, CEO
John H. Weiland, Pres.
John H. Weiland, COO
Todd C. Schermerhorn, Sr. VP/CFO
Bronwen K. Kelly, VP-Human Resources
Vincent J. Gurnari, Jr., VP-IT
Nadia J. Bernstein, General Counsel
Joseph A. Cherry, VP-Oper.
Robert L. Mellen, VP-Strategic Planning & Bus. Dev.
Eric J. Shick, VP-Investor Rel.
Scott T. Lowry, VP/Treas.
Amy S. Paul, Group VP
Timothy M. Ring, Group VP
Christopher D. Gasner, VP-Regulatory Sciences
Brian R. Barry, VP-Regulatory & Clinical Affairs
Timothy M. Ring, Chmn.

Phone: 908-277-8000   **Fax:** 908-277-8240
Toll-Free: 800-367-2273
Address: 730 Central Ave., Murray Hill, NJ 07974 US

GROWTH PLANS/SPECIAL FEATURES:
C.R. Bard, Inc. designs, manufactures, packages, distributes and sells medical, surgical and diagnostic devices. The company commands a strong market share in vascular, urological, oncological and surgical diagnostic and interventional products. C.R. Bard's line of minimally invasive vascular products includes peripheral angioplasty stents, catheters, guidewires, introducers and accessories, vena cava filters and biopsy devices; electrophysiology products including cardiac mapping and electrophysiology laboratory systems and diagnostic and temporary pacing electrode catheters; fabrics and meshes; and implantable blood vessel replacements. Its surgical specialty products include meshes for vessel and hernia repair; irrigation devices for orthopaedic, laparoscopic and gynecological procedures; and products for topical hemostasis. These products include the PerFix plug, Composix sheet, HydroFlex Multi-Application Irrigation Pump System, Avitene and Avifoam. The company also offers account management, supply chain and business enhancement services. C.R. Bard markets its products, through 22 subsidiaries and a joint venture, in 92 countries outside the United States. Its principal markets are Japan, Canada, the United Kingdom and continental Europe. During 2003, the company acquired the assets of Genyx Medical, Inc., a privately held medical device company that develops, manufactures and markets Uryxr, a proprietary injectable bulking agent for the treatment of stress urinary incontinence. In October 2004, Bard sold portions of its endoscopic technologies division to Conmed Corporation.

C.R. Bard offers employment with an emphasis on engineering and research. The company provides its employees with medical, vision, prescription drug and dental insurance.

FINANCIALS:
Sales and profits are in thousands of dollars—add 000 to get the full amount. Year 2004 note: Complete fiscal 2004 results were not available for all companies at press time. For this company, year 2004 is for 9 months.

2004 Sales: $1,232,000 (9 months)   2004 Profits: $130,600 (9 months)
2003 Sales: $1,433,100   2003 Profits: $233,000
2002 Sales: $1,273,800   2002 Profits: $155,000
2001 Sales: $1,181,300   2001 Profits: $143,200
2000 Sales: $1,098,800   2000 Profits: $106,900

Stock Ticker: BCR
Employees: 8,300
Fiscal Year Ends: 12/31

SALARIES/BENEFITS:
Pension Plan: Y   ESOP Stock Plan: Profit Sharing: Top Exec. Salary: $653,079   Bonus: $1,307,660
Savings Plan: Y   Stock Purch. Plan: Second Exec. Salary: $668,750   Bonus: $871,773

OTHER THOUGHTS:
Apparent Top Female Officers: 3
Hot Spot for Advancement for Women/Minorities: Y

LOCATIONS: ("Y" = Yes)

West	Southwest	Midwest	Southeast	Northeast	International
Y	Y	Y	Y	Y	Y

CRITICARE SYSTEMS INC

www.csiusa.com

Industry Group Code: 339113   Ranks within this company's industry group: Sales: 127   Profits: 111

Insurance/HMO/PPO:	Drugs:	Equipment/Supplies:		Hospitals/Clinics:	Services:	Health Care:
Insurance: Managed Care: Utilization Mgmt.: Payment Proc.:	Manufacturer: Distributor: Specialty Pharm.: Vitamins/Nutri.: Clinical Trials:	Manufacturer: Distributor: Leasing/Finance: Information Sys.:	Y	Acute Care: Sub-Acute Care: Outpatient Surgery: Phys. Rehab. Center: Psychiatric Clinics:	Diagnostics: Labs/Testing: Staffing: Waste Disposal: Specialty Services:	Home Health: Long-Term Care: Physical Therapy: Phys. Practice Mgmt.:

TYPES OF BUSINESS:
Equipment-Vital Sign Monitors
Patient Monitoring Systems
Noninvasive Sensors

BRANDS/DIVISIONS/AFFILIATES:
VitalView

CONTACTS:
Note: Officers with more than one job title may be intentionally listed here more than once.

Emil H. Soika, CEO
Emil H. Soika, Pres.
Deborah A. Zane, VP-Mktg.
Reinhart B. Van Deuren, General Counsel
Deborah A. Zane, VP-Bus. Dev.
Joel D. Knudson, VP-Finance/Corp. Sec.
Stephen D. Okland, VP-Domestic Sales
Joseph P. Lester, VP/General Mgr.
Drew M. Diaz, VP-Worldwide Sales
Michael T. Larson, VP-Quality Control & Assurance
Higgins D. Bailey, Chmn.

Phone: 262-798-8282	Fax: 262-798-8290
Toll-Free:	
Address: 20925 Crossroads Cir., Ste. 100, Waukesha, WI 53186-4054 US	

GROWTH PLANS/SPECIAL FEATURES:

Criticare Systems, Inc. designs, manufactures and markets cost-effective patient monitoring systems and noninvasive sensors for hospitals and alternate health care facilities throughout the world. The company has established product and technological leadership in pulse oximetry, vital signs monitoring, gas and agent analysis and central station and wireless monitoring systems. Its monitoring equipment improves patient safety by delivering accurate, comprehensive and instantaneous patient information to the clinician. Its products also help hospitals to contain costs by substituting cost-effective reusable pulse oximetry sensors for disposable sensors, controlling the use of expensive anesthetics and increasing personnel productivity. Its the VitalView telemetry system allows one nurse to monitor up to eight patients simultaneously from a convenient central location, therefore allowing hospitals to move out of the intensive care unit (ICU) those patients that require continuous monitoring but do not need all of the ICU's extensive and costly personnel and equipment resources. Criticare recently received FDA approval to market of its new arrhythmia detection and alarm software, which provides real-time analysis of ECG traces and has an integrated alarm system.

FINANCIALS:
Sales and profits are in thousands of dollars—add 000 to get the full amount. Year 2004 note: Complete fiscal 2004 results were not available for all companies at press time. For this company, year 2004 is for 12 months.

2004 Sales: $28,591 (12 months)	2004 Profits: $-2,100 (12 months)	
2003 Sales: $28,600	2003 Profits: $- 900	Stock Ticker: CMD
2002 Sales: $26,200	2002 Profits: $-1,400	Employees: 87
2001 Sales: $27,700	2001 Profits: $- 200	Fiscal Year Ends: 6/30
2000 Sales: $27,154	2000 Profits: $- 186	

SALARIES/BENEFITS:
Pension Plan:	ESOP Stock Plan:	Profit Sharing:	Top Exec. Salary: $225,000	Bonus: $25,000
Savings Plan: Y	Stock Purch. Plan:		Second Exec. Salary: $269,205	Bonus: $67,252

OTHER THOUGHTS:
Apparent Top Female Officers: 1
Hot Spot for Advancement for Women/Minorities:

LOCATIONS: ("Y" = Yes)
West:	Southwest:	Midwest:	Southeast:	Northeast:	International:
		Y			

CRYOLIFE INC

www.cryolife.com

Industry Group Code: 621511 Ranks within this company's industry group: Sales: 10 Profits: 10

Insurance/HMO/PPO:	Drugs:	Equipment/Supplies:		Hospitals/Clinics:	Services:	Health Care:
Insurance:	Manufacturer:	Manufacturer:	Y	Acute Care:	Diagnostics:	Home Health:
Managed Care:	Distributor:	Distributor:		Sub-Acute Care:	Labs/Testing:	Long-Term Care:
Utilization Mgmt.:	Specialty Pharm.:	Leasing/Finance:		Outpatient Surgery:	Staffing:	Physical Therapy:
Payment Proc.:	Vitamins/Nutri.:	Information Sys.:		Phys. Rehab. Center:	Waste Disposal:	Phys. Practice Mgmt.:
	Clinical Trials:			Psychiatric Clinics:	Specialty Services: Y	

TYPES OF BUSINESS:
Services-Tissue Preservation
Surgical Adhesives
Heart Valves
Biomedical Research

BRANDS/DIVISIONS/AFFILIATES:
BioGlue
SynerGraft
CryoLife International, Inc.
CryoLife Europa, Ltd.
AuraZyme Pharmaceuticals, Inc.
Activation Control Technology (ACT)
BioFoam

CONTACTS:
Note: Officers with more than one job title may be intentionally listed here more than once.

Steven G. Anderson, CEO
Steven G. Anderson, Pres.
D. Ashley Lee, Exec. VP/COO
D. Ashley Lee, CFO
Sidney B. Ashmore, VP-Mktg.
Kirby S. Black, Sr. VP-Research & Dev.
Albert E. Heacox, Sr. VP-Laboratory Oper.
Joseph Schepers, VP-Corp. Comm.
D. Ashley Lee, Treas.
David M. Fronk, VP-Clinical Research
Thomas J. Lynch, VP-Regulatory Affairs & Quality Assurance
Suzanne K. Gabbert, Corp. Sec.
Gerald B. Seery, Pres., CryoLife Europa
Steven G. Anderson, Chmn.

Phone: 770-419-3355 Fax: 770-426-0031
Toll-Free: 800-438-8285
Address: 1655 Roberts Blvd. NW, Ste. 142, Kennesaw, GA 30144 US

GROWTH PLANS/SPECIAL FEATURES:

CryoLife, Inc. is the leader in the preservation of human tissues for cardiovascular and vascular transplant applications. Additionally, the company develops and commercializes implantable medical devices, including BioGlue surgical adhesive, glutaraldehyde-fixed stentless porcine heart valves and tissue-engineered SynerGraft porcine heart valves and bovine vascular grafts. The company maintains two separate facilities: one in Atlanta, Georgia, which consists of laboratories, warehouse space and offices, and another facility in Fareham in the United Kingdom. Through CryoLife International, Inc. and CryoLife Europa, Ltd., the company offers its products and services in 42 countries around the world. CryoLife uses its expertise in biochemistry, cell biology, immunology and protein chemistry and its understanding of the needs of the cardiovascular, vascular and orthopedic surgery medical specialties to continue the expansion of its core preservation business and to develop or acquire complementary implantable products and technologies for these surgical specialties. The firm formed AuraZyme Pharmaceuticals, Inc. in 2001 to foster the commercial development of its Activation Control Technology (ACT), allowing CryoLife to focus on its core business practices. ACT is a reversible linker technology that has potential uses in the areas of cancer therapy, blood clot dissolving and other drug delivery applications. The company was recently granted $1 million in government funding to develop BioFoam, a protein hydrogel adhesive designed to rapidly arrest bleeding of large vessel injuries and seal the wound, a technology with potentially life-saving applications for soldiers in combat.

CryoLife offers its employees medical, drug and dental coverage, as well as tuition reimbursement.

FINANCIALS:
Sales and profits are in thousands of dollars—add 000 to get the full amount. Year 2004 note: Complete fiscal 2004 results were not available for all companies at press time. For this company, year 2004 is for 9 months.

2004 Sales: $46,518 (9 months)   2004 Profits: $-16,386 (9 months)
2003 Sales: $59,532   2003 Profits: $-32,294
2002 Sales: $77,800   2002 Profits: $-27,800
2001 Sales: $87,700   2001 Profits: $9,200
2000 Sales: $77,100   2000 Profits: $7,800

Stock Ticker: CRY
Employees: 326
Fiscal Year Ends: 12/31

SALARIES/BENEFITS:
Pension Plan: ESOP Stock Plan: Profit Sharing: Top Exec. Salary: $600,000   Bonus: $300,000
Savings Plan: Y   Stock Purch. Plan: Y   Second Exec. Salary: $261,333   Bonus: $60,000

OTHER THOUGHTS:
Apparent Top Female Officers: 1
Hot Spot for Advancement for Women/Minorities:

LOCATIONS: ("Y" = Yes)

West:	Southwest:	Midwest:	Southeast:	Northeast:	International:
			Y		Y

CTI MOLECULAR IMAGING

www.ctimi.com

Industry Group Code: 339113   Ranks within this company's industry group: Sales: 49   Profits: 57

Insurance/HMO/PPO:	Drugs:		Equipment/Supplies:		Hospitals/Clinics:	Services:	Health Care:
Insurance:	Manufacturer:	Y	Manufacturer:	Y	Acute Care:	Diagnostics:	Home Health:
Managed Care:	Distributor:	Y	Distributor:		Sub-Acute Care:	Labs/Testing:	Long-Term Care:
Utilization Mgmt.:	Specialty Pharm.:		Leasing/Finance:		Outpatient Surgery:	Staffing:	Physical Therapy:
Payment Proc.:	Vitamins/Nutri.:		Information Sys.:	Y	Phys. Rehab. Center:	Waste Disposal:	Phys. Practice Mgmt.:
	Clinical Trials:				Psychiatric Clinics:	Specialty Services:	

TYPES OF BUSINESS:
Positron Emission Tomography Imaging Equipment
Radiopharmaceuticals
Imaging Software

BRANDS/DIVISIONS/AFFILIATES:
LSO
PETNET Pharmaceuticals, Inc.
Mirada Solutions, Ltd.
PETNET Solutions
Imaging Choice Consortium
Concorde Microsystem, Inc.
CTI Molecular Technologies, Inc.
LSO HI-REZ Reveal PET/CT

CONTACTS:
Note: Officers with more than one job title may be intentionally listed here more than once.

Ronald Nutt, CEO
Ronald Nutt, Pres.
Cliffreda W. Gilreath, Sr. VP/COO
David N. Gill, Sr. VP/CFO
Joe Sardano, Sr. VP-Sales & Mktg.
Michael A. Lawless, Sr. Dir.-Investor Rel.
Michael A. Lawless, Sr. Dir.-Finance
Mark Andreaco, Sr. VP-PETNET Pharmaceuticals, Inc.
Christian P. Behrenbruch, Pres., Mirada Solutions, Ltd.
Terry D. Douglass, Chmn.

Phone: 865-218-2000   Fax: 865-218-3000
Toll-Free: 800-841-7226
Address: 810 Innovation Dr., Knoxville, TN 37932-2571 US

GROWTH PLANS/SPECIAL FEATURES:
CTI Molecular Imaging, Inc. is a leading provider of positron emission tomography (PET) imaging equipment and services. PET enables early detection of cancer, cardiac disease and neurological disorders by providing physicians with information about the body's biochemical processes and location of disease at the molecular level. The firm provides a complete line of PET scanners, cyclotrons, molecular biomarkers, detector materials and support services. It also sells LSO, its proprietary detector material. LSO reduces the duration of a PET scan by at least 50%. In addition, the company is developing new proprietary molecular probes to monitor biological processes that current probes do not track. The firm's PETNET Solutions subsidiary manufactures radiopharmaceuticals and distributes them through approximately 30 locations across the U.S. Subsidiary Mirada Solutions Ltd. is a leading developer of software and analytical tools for medical imaging workstations, OEM imaging platforms and pharmaceutical applications. The company's clients include hospitals, universities and imaging and cancer treatment centers. In recent news, PETNET formed a product consortium, the Imaging Choice Consortium (ICC), with three other companies in the radiology and radiopharmaceutical business: Bracco Diagnostics, Inc., E-Z-EM, Inc. and Berlex, a U.S. affiliate of Schering AG. ICC will combine the four companies' wide array of marketed products in the areas of MRI, x-ray, computed tomography and radiopharmacy, which includes PET, into one purchasing portfolio. The company agreed to acquire Concorde Microsystems, Inc., a leading provider of small animal PET systems for imaging laboratory animals used in medical research. CTI also launched a new research and development subsidiary, CTI Molecular Technologies, Inc. It also released LSO HI-REZ Reveal PET/CT, a high-resolution PET/CT system.

FINANCIALS:
Sales and profits are in thousands of dollars—add 000 to get the full amount. Year 2004 note: Complete fiscal 2004 results were not available for all companies at press time. For this company, year 2004 is for 9 months.

2004 Sales: $272,174 (9 months)	2004 Profits: $9,228 (9 months)	Stock Ticker: CTMI
2003 Sales: $362,289	2003 Profits: $20,563	Employees: 915
2002 Sales: $258,395	2002 Profits: $-3,419	Fiscal Year Ends: 9/30
2001 Sales: $	2001 Profits: $	
2000 Sales: $	2000 Profits: $	

SALARIES/BENEFITS:
Pension Plan: ESOP Stock Plan: Profit Sharing: Top Exec. Salary: $275,000   Bonus: $107,250
Savings Plan: Stock Purch. Plan: Second Exec. Salary: $269,958 Bonus: $187,500

OTHER THOUGHTS:
Apparent Top Female Officers:
Hot Spot for Advancement for Women/Minorities:

LOCATIONS: ("Y" = Yes)
West:	Southwest:	Midwest:	Southeast:	Northeast:	International:
			Y		Y

CURATIVE HEALTH SERVICES INC

www.curative.com

Industry Group Code: 621490   Ranks within this company's industry group: Sales: 7   Profits: 8

Insurance/HMO/PPO:	Drugs:		Equipment/Supplies:		Hospitals/Clinics:	Services:		Health Care:	
Insurance:	Manufacturer:		Manufacturer:		Acute Care:	Diagnostics:		Home Health:	
Managed Care:	Distributor:	Y	Distributor:	Y	Sub-Acute Care:	Labs/Testing:		Long-Term Care:	
Utilization Mgmt.:	Specialty Pharm.:	Y	Leasing/Finance:		Outpatient Surgery:	Staffing:		Physical Therapy:	
Payment Proc.:	Vitamins/Nutri.:		Information Sys.:		Phys. Rehab. Center:	Waste Disposal:		Phys. Practice Mgmt.:	
	Clinical Trials:				Psychiatric Clinics:	Specialty Services:	Y		

TYPES OF BUSINESS:
Clinics-Chronic Wound Care
Specialty Pharmacy Services
Direct-to-Patient Distribution Services
Online Pharmacy

BRANDS/DIVISIONS/AFFILIATES:
eBioCare
Apex
Critical Care Systems

CONTACTS:
Note: Officers with more than one job title may be intentionally listed here more than once.

Paul F. McConnell, CEO
Paul F. McConnell, Pres.
John C. Prior, COO
Thomas Axmacher, CFO
Michelle LeDell, Sr. VP-Human Resources
Anne S. Bruce, Sr. VP/CIO
Nancy Lanis, Exec. VP/General Counsel
Jason R. Escamilla, Sr. VP-Bus. Dev.
Roy McKinley, Sr. VP-Wound Care Mgmt.
Joseph L. Feshbach, Chmn.

Phone: 631-232-7000   **Fax:** 631-232-9322
Toll-Free: 800-966-5656
Address: 150 Motor Pkwy., Hauppauge, NY 11788 US

GROWTH PLANS/SPECIAL FEATURES:
Curative Health Services, Inc. provides health care products, services and support to patients with chronic medical conditions. Its specialty health care division is a leader in the treatment of chronic wounds resulting from diabetes, venous insufficiency, immobility and other causes. The company operates 86 chronic wound care clinics nationwide. Curative's specialty pharmacy services unit provides pharmacy products and services to patients with chronic and critical diseases. The company purchases pharmaceutical products from suppliers and contracts with insurance companies to distribute drugs directly to patients, provide educational materials and offer other support services. Curative also operates eBioCare, a specialty online pharmacy, and Apex, a company that caters to the needs of hemophiliacs. In recent news, Curative acquired Critical Care Systems, a national provider of specialty infusion pharmaceuticals and comprehensive clinical services. After the acquisition, the firm opened two new Critical Care Systems branch locations, one in Kansas and the other in South Carolina. These locations will provide products, clinical services and disease management support to patients suffering from hemophilia, chronic or severe infections, gastrointestinal illnesses, immune system disorders and cancer.

Curative offers its employees a benefits plan that includes car allowances and stock options.

FINANCIALS:
Sales and profits are in thousands of dollars—add 000 to get the full amount. Year 2004 note: Complete fiscal 2004 results were not available for all companies at press time. For this company, year 2004 is for 9 months.

2004 Sales: $198,740 (9 months)   2004 Profits: $-2,065   (9 months)
2003 Sales: $214,741   2003 Profits: $13,075
2002 Sales: $139,200   2002 Profits: $14,600
2001 Sales: $81,600   2001 Profits: $-22,200
2000 Sales: $77,691   2000 Profits: $-128

Stock Ticker: CURE
Employees: 371
Fiscal Year Ends: 12/31

SALARIES/BENEFITS:
Pension Plan: ESOP Stock Plan: Profit Sharing: Top Exec. Salary: $423,942   Bonus: $333,333
Savings Plan: Y   Stock Purch. Plan: Second Exec. Salary: $274,656   Bonus: $122,850

OTHER THOUGHTS:
Apparent Top Female Officers: 3
Hot Spot for Advancement for Women/Minorities: Y

LOCATIONS: ("Y" = Yes)
West:	Southwest:	Midwest:	Southeast:	Northeast:	International:
Y	Y	Y	Y	Y	

CVS CORPORATION

www.cvs.com

Industry Group Code: 446110 Ranks within this company's industry group: Sales: 2 Profits: 2

Insurance/HMO/PPO:	Drugs:	Equipment/Supplies:	Hospitals/Clinics:	Services:	Health Care:
Insurance:	Manufacturer:	Manufacturer:	Acute Care:	Diagnostics:	Home Health:
Managed Care:	Distributor:	Distributor:	Sub-Acute Care:	Labs/Testing:	Long-Term Care:
Utilization Mgmt.:	Specialty Pharm.: Y	Leasing/Finance:	Outpatient Surgery:	Staffing:	Physical Therapy:
Payment Proc.: Y	Vitamins/Nutri.:	Information Sys.: Y	Phys. Rehab. Center:	Waste Disposal:	Phys. Practice Mgmt.:
	Clinical Trials:		Psychiatric Clinics:	Specialty Services:	

TYPES OF BUSINESS:
Drug Stores
Mail-Order Pharmacy
Pharmacy Benefits Management
Online Pharmacy Services
Claims Processing

BRANDS/DIVISIONS/AFFILIATES:
Eckerd
cvs.com
PharmaCare Management Services
CVS ProCare
CVS Realty Co.

CONTACTS: Note: Officers with more than one job title may be intentionally listed here more than once.
Thomas M. Ryan, CEO
Thomas M. Ryan, Pres.
David B. Rickard, Exec. VP/CFO
Chris W. Bodine, Exec. VP-Mktg.
V. Michael Ferdinandi, Sr. VP-Human Resources
Chris W. Bodine, Exec. VP-Merch.
David B. Rickard, Chief Admin. Officer
Douglas A. Sgarro, Chief Legal Officer
Douglas A. Sgarro, Exec. VP-Strategy
V. Michael Ferdinandi, Sr. VP-Corp. Comm.
Larry D. Solberg, Sr. VP-Finance/Controller
Douglas A. Sgarro, Pres., CVS Realty Co.
Larry J. Merlo, Exec. VP-Stores
Greg S. Weishar, Pres./CEO-PharmaCare Management Services
Thomas M. Ryan, Chmn.

Phone: 401-765-1500 Fax: 401-766-2917
Toll-Free: 888-607-4287
Address: One CVS Dr., Woonsocket, RI 02895 US

GROWTH PLANS/SPECIAL FEATURES:
CVS Corporation is a leader in the U.S. chain drug store industry. Its retail pharmacy business includes over 4,100 retail drug stores in 27 states and the District of Columbia. CVS pharmacy stores sell prescription drugs and a wide assortment of general merchandise, including over-the-counter drugs, greeting cards, film and photo-finishing services, beauty products and cosmetics, seasonal merchandise and convenience foods. Stores typically include a drive-thru pharmacy. The firm's Internet pharmacy business includes a mail-order facility and a complete online retail pharmacy, operating as cvs.com. PharmaCare Management Services, CVS's pharmacy benefit management and specialty pharmacy subsidiary, provides a full range of services to managed care organizations, insurance companies, corporate health plans, unions, government agencies and other funded benefit plans. Its services include plan design and administration, formulary management, mail-order pharmacy services, claims processing and generic substitution. PharmaCare also operates 47 CVS ProCare specialty pharmacies in 19 states that support individuals requiring complex and expensive drug therapies to treat conditions such as organ transplants, HIV/AIDS, infertility, multiple sclerosis and certain cancers. The firm has continued to expand its operations with the opening of stores in several new U.S. markets, including Phoenix, Arizona; Las Vegas, Nevada; Chicago, Illinois; and Dallas, Houston and Fort Worth, Texas. In recent news, CVS purchased 1,260 Eckerd drugstores for $2.15 billion in cash. This makes CVS the largest drug store chain in North America, with more than 5,000 stores.

Full-time pharmacists enjoy benefits including comprehensive medical insurance, prescription coverage, medical and personal leave, life insurance, adoption assistance, education assistance, a performance-based incentive plan and merchandise discounts.

FINANCIALS: Sales and profits are in thousands of dollars—add 000 to get the full amount. Year 2004 note: Complete fiscal 2004 results were not available for all companies at press time. For this company, year 2004 is for 9 months.

2004 Sales: $21,671,100 (9 months) 2004 Profits: $663,700 (9 months)
2003 Sales: $26,588,000 2003 Profits: $847,300
2002 Sales: $24,182,000 2002 Profits: $717,000
2001 Sales: $22,241,000 2001 Profits: $413,000
2000 Sales: $20,087,500 2000 Profits: $746,000

Stock Ticker: CVS
Employees: 110,000
Fiscal Year Ends: 12/31

SALARIES/BENEFITS:
Pension Plan: ESOP Stock Plan: Y Profit Sharing: Top Exec. Salary: $1,000,000 Bonus: $3,500,000
Savings Plan: Y Stock Purch. Plan: Y Second Exec. Salary: $617,500 Bonus: $1,400,000

OTHER THOUGHTS:
Apparent Top Female Officers:
Hot Spot for Advancement for Women/Minorities:

LOCATIONS: ("Y" = Yes)

West:	Southwest:	Midwest:	Southeast:	Northeast:	International:
Y	Y	Y	Y	Y	

Note: Financial information, benefits and other data can change quickly and may vary from those stated here.

CYBERONICS INC

www.cyberonics.com

Industry Group Code: 339113 **Ranks within this company's industry group:** Sales: 90 Profits: 85

Insurance/HMO/PPO:	Drugs:	Equipment/Supplies:	Hospitals/Clinics:	Services:	Health Care:
Insurance:	Manufacturer:	Manufacturer: Y	Acute Care:	Diagnostics:	Home Health:
Managed Care:	Distributor:	Distributor:	Sub-Acute Care:	Labs/Testing:	Long-Term Care:
Utilization Mgmt.:	Specialty Pharm.:	Leasing/Finance:	Outpatient Surgery:	Staffing:	Physical Therapy:
Payment Proc.:	Vitamins/Nutri.:	Information Sys.:	Phys. Rehab. Center:	Waste Disposal:	Phys. Practice Mgmt.:
	Clinical Trials:		Psychiatric Clinics:	Specialty Services:	

TYPES OF BUSINESS:
Equipment-Epilepsy Therapy
Vagus Nerve Stimulation Devices

BRANDS/DIVISIONS/AFFILIATES:
Vagus Nerve Stimulation Therapy System

CONTACTS:
Note: Officers with more than one job title may be intentionally listed here more than once.

Robert P. Cummins, CEO
Robert P. Cummins, Pres.
Pamela B. Westbrook, CFO
Michael A. Cheney, VP-Mktg.
George E. Parker, III, VP-Human Resources
Shawn P. Lunney, VP-Eng.
Pamela B. Westbrook, VP-Admin.
David S. Wise, VP/General Counsel
Randal L. Simpson, VP-Oper.
Shawn P. Lunney, VP-Market Dev.
Pamela B. Westbrook, VP-Finance
W. Steven Jennings, VP-Sales
Alan D. Totah, VP-Regulatory Affairs & Quality
Richard L. Rudolph, Chief Medical Officer/VP-Clinical Affairs
Robert P. Cummins, Chmn.

Phone: 281-228-7200 **Fax:** 281-218-9332
Toll-Free: 800-332-1375
Address: 100 Cyberonics Blvd., Ste. 600, Houston, TX 77058 US

GROWTH PLANS/SPECIAL FEATURES:

Cyberonics, Inc. is the designer, developer, manufacturer and marketer of the Vagus Nerve Stimulation (VNS) Therapy System, an implantable medical device for the treatment of epilepsy and other debilitating chronic disorders. The VNS system is the only FDA-approved medical device for the treatment of epilepsy, departing from the traditional drug and surgery methods, both of which expose epileptics to significant risks or drastic side effects. It delivers an electrical signal through an implantable lead to the left cervical vagus nerve in the patient's neck on a chronic, intermittent basis. Stimulation may also be initiated by the patient or caregiver with a hand-held magnet. Treatment groups using the VNS system reported a mean seizure reduction of approximately 24% to 28% during the three-month acute phase of the studies. Additionally, many patients, including some who reported no change or an increase in seizure frequency, reported a reduction in seizure severity. Other studies suggest that efficacy is maintained and, for many patients, improves over time when the VNS Therapy System is used with drugs as part of a patient's optimized long-term treatment regimen. Cyberonics is also conducting clinical studies of this system for the treatment of depression in patients who have not responded to other treatments and has small pilot studies underway for the treatment of Alzheimer's disease and anxiety.

Benefits at Cyberonics include medical, dental, vision and life insurance, education assistance and an employee assistance program.

FINANCIALS:
Sales and profits are in thousands of dollars—add 000 to get the full amount. Year 2004 note: Complete fiscal 2004 results were not available for all companies at press time. For this company, year 2004 is for 12 months.

2004 Sales: $110,721 (12 months)	2004 Profits: $6,759 (12 months)	**Stock Ticker:** CYBX
2003 Sales: $104,500	2003 Profits: $5,200	**Employees:** 478
2002 Sales: $70,100	2002 Profits: $-26,100	**Fiscal Year Ends:** 4/30
2001 Sales: $43,400	2001 Profits: $-24,700	
2000 Sales: $47,888	2000 Profits: $-3,053	

SALARIES/BENEFITS:

Pension Plan:	ESOP Stock Plan:	Profit Sharing:	Top Exec. Salary: $410,257	Bonus: $244,918
Savings Plan: Y	Stock Purch. Plan: Y		Second Exec. Salary: $311,538	Bonus: $87,331

OTHER THOUGHTS:
Apparent Top Female Officers: 1
Hot Spot for Advancement for Women/Minorities:

LOCATIONS: ("Y" = Yes)

West:	Southwest:	Midwest:	Southeast:	Northeast:	International:
	Y				Y

D & K HEALTHCARE RESOURCES INC
www.dkwd.com

Industry Group Code: 422210   Ranks within this company's industry group: Sales: 4   Profits: 4

Insurance/HMO/PPO:	Drugs:		Equipment/Supplies:		Hospitals/Clinics:	Services:		Health Care:	
Insurance:	Manufacturer:		Manufacturer:		Acute Care:	Diagnostics:		Home Health:	
Managed Care:	Distributor:	Y	Distributor:		Sub-Acute Care:	Labs/Testing:		Long-Term Care:	
Utilization Mgmt.:	Specialty Pharm.:		Leasing/Finance:		Outpatient Surgery:	Staffing:		Physical Therapy:	
Payment Proc.:	Vitamins/Nutri.:		Information Sys.:	Y	Phys. Rehab. Center:	Waste Disposal:		Phys. Practice Mgmt.:	
	Clinical Trials:				Psychiatric Clinics:	Specialty Services:	Y		

TYPES OF BUSINESS:
Distribution-Drugs
Group Purchasing Program
Information Systems & Services

BRANDS/DIVISIONS/AFFILIATES:
Pharmaceutical Buyers, Inc.
Tykon, Inc.

CONTACTS:
Note: Officers with more than one job title may be intentionally listed here more than once.

J. Hord Armstrong, III, CEO
Martin D. Wilson, Pres.
Martin D. Wilson, COO
Thomas S. Hilton, Sr. VP/CFO
P. Denise Wiesemann, VP-Mktg.
Michael J. Kurtz, Dir.-Human Resources
Brian G. Landry, CIO
Richard Keffer, VP/General Counsel
Brian G. Landry, Sr. VP-Oper.
James D. Largent, Corp. VP-Bus. Dev.
J. Richard Gist, VP/Controller
Edward G. Petrella, Sr. VP-Sales & Bus. Dev.
Mark H. Ehrhardt, VP-Info. Services
Charles M. Levy, VP-Financial Services
Rick A. Jeter, VP-Distribution Services
J. Hord Armstrong, III, Chmn.
Mark H. Sitz, VP-Purchasing

Phone: 314-727-3485   Fax: 314-727-5759
Toll-Free:
Address: 8235 Forsyth Blvd., St. Louis, MO 63105 US

GROWTH PLANS/SPECIAL FEATURES:
D&K Healthcare Resources, Inc. is a leading national and regional pharmaceutical distributor. The company supplies pharmaceuticals, over-the-counter products, health and beauty aids and related items to independent, regional and national pharmacies, hospitals and pharmacy benefit companies in 27 states, primarily in the midwestern and southern portions of the U.S. The firm has a more flexible organization than large national wholesalers, allowing it to respond rapidly to change and customize its systems to customers' requirements. In addition, the company has a growing array of information systems products and services, including Tykon, Inc.'s proprietary order entry and confirmation system. D&K has virtually 100% electronic communications with customers and suppliers, providing its customers with customized price information and allowing its warehouses to ship orders within 24 hours. The company also has a 70% ownership in Pharmaceutical Buyers, Inc. (PBI), one of the nation's leading alternate-site group purchasing organizations. In response to the increasing number of health care procedures that are taking place outside of hospitals, PBI has shifted its focus to include the vast spectrum of providers servicing alternate-site patients, delivering optimal patient care to network independent providers, payers, manufacturers, wholesalers and distributors. In October 2004, D&K completed its acquisition of the remaining 30% of PBI, making it a wholly-owned subsidiary.

FINANCIALS:
Sales and profits are in thousands of dollars—add 000 to get the full amount. Year 2004 note: Complete fiscal 2004 results were not available for all companies at press time. For this company, year 2004 is for 12 months.

2004 Sales: $2,541,190 (12 months)	2004 Profits: $10,214 (12 months)	
2003 Sales: $2,223,400	2003 Profits: $9,686	Stock Ticker: DKHR
2002 Sales: $2,453,700	2002 Profits: $21,100	Employees: 784
2001 Sales: $1,646,000	2001 Profits: $9,100	Fiscal Year Ends: 6/30
2000 Sales: $1,458,047	2000 Profits: $8,199	

SALARIES/BENEFITS:
Pension Plan: ESOP Stock Plan: Profit Sharing: Top Exec. Salary: $650,000   Bonus: $326,625
Savings Plan: Y   Stock Purch. Plan: Second Exec. Salary: $550,000   Bonus: $248,738

OTHER THOUGHTS:
Apparent Top Female Officers: 1
Hot Spot for Advancement for Women/Minorities:

LOCATIONS: ("Y" = Yes)
West:	Southwest:	Midwest:	Southeast:	Northeast:	International:
Y	Y	Y	Y		

Plunkett's Health Care Industry Almanac 2005   339

DADE BEHRING HOLDINGS INC   www.dadebehring.com

Industry Group Code: 339113   Ranks within this company's industry group: Sales: 18   Profits: 34

Insurance/HMO/PPO:	Drugs:	Equipment/Supplies:		Hospitals/Clinics:	Services:	Health Care:
Insurance:	Manufacturer:	Manufacturer:	Y	Acute Care:	Diagnostics:	Home Health:
Managed Care:	Distributor:	Distributor:		Sub-Acute Care:	Labs/Testing:	Long-Term Care:
Utilization Mgmt.:	Specialty Pharm.:	Leasing/Finance:		Outpatient Surgery:	Staffing:	Physical Therapy:
Payment Proc.:	Vitamins/Nutri.:	Information Sys.:		Phys. Rehab. Center:	Waste Disposal:	Phys. Practice Mgmt.:
	Clinical Trials:			Psychiatric Clinics:	Specialty Services:	

TYPES OF BUSINESS:
Equipment/Supplies-Diagnostic & Testing Instruments
Clinical Chemistry Instrument Systems
Immunochemistry Instrument Systems
Automated Microbiology Instrument Systems
Hemostasis Instrument Systems
Cardiac Diagnostic Systems

BRANDS/DIVISIONS/AFFILIATES:
BN II
BN Prospec
TurbiTime System
Syva
MicroScan
BNA
BN100

CONTACTS: Note: Officers with more than one job title may be intentionally listed here more than once.
James Reid-Anderson, CEO
James Reid-Anderson, Pres.
John M. Duffey, Sr. VP/CFO
Kathy Kennedy, Sr. VP-Human Resources
David G. Edelstein, CIO
Mark Wolsey-Paige, Sr. VP-Tech.
Louise Pearson, VP/General Counsel
Mark Wolsey-Paige, Sr. VP-Strategy
Hiroshi Uchida, Pres.-Global Oper.
Donal M. Quinn, Pres.-Global Customer Mgmt.
James Reid-Anderson, Chmn.

Phone: 847-267-5300   Fax: 847-267-1066
Toll-Free:
Address: 1717 Deerfield Rd., Deerfield, IL 60015-0778 US

GROWTH PLANS/SPECIAL FEATURES:
Dade Behring Holdings, Inc. manufactures in vitro diagnostics (IVD) products for clinical laboratories worldwide. The company focuses primarily on the central lab segment of the IVD market, manufacturing and marketing a broad offering of IVD products and services, which include medical diagnostic instruments (12% of sales), reagents and consumables (84% of sales) and maintenance services (4% of sales). Dade Behring has a strong position in each of its core product markets: chemistry, hemostasis, microbiology and infectious disease diagnostics. The company has a leading share in the cardiac test market and was the first to introduce a widely adopted testing system for the cardiac proteins Troponin I, CK-MB and Myoglobin. The firm is also the market leader in the worldwide nephelometric plasma protein market, offering five dedicated plasma protein instruments: the BN II instrument, targeted at large, high-volume hospital and commercial laboratories; the BNA, BN100 and BN Prospec instruments, sold to small to medium-size labs; and the TurbiTime System, a manual instrument sold to small hospitals and private labs. In addition, Dade Behring manufactures drug abuse testing products under the Syva brand name and serves the microbiology market with its MicroScan products. The company is functionally organized into three segments: global customer management (GCM) North America, GCM international and global operations. GCM North America and GCM international are the firm's sales and service organizations. The global operations segment primarily includes all manufacturing and research and development activities, which occur in the United States and Germany. In recent news, Dade Behring entered into an excusive agreement with the University of Frankfurt and Innovectis, which will provide the company with worldwide rights to the inventions created through the university's research of cardiovascular disease markers.

FINANCIALS: Sales and profits are in thousands of dollars—add 000 to get the full amount. Year 2004 note: Complete fiscal 2004 results were not available for all companies at press time. For this company, year 2004 is for 9 months.

2004 Sales: $1,139,800 (9 months)   2004 Profits: $55,900   (9 months)
2003 Sales: $1,436,400   2003 Profits: $48,100   Stock Ticker: DADE
2002 Sales: $1,281,500   2002 Profits: $-48,600   Employees: 6,000
2001 Sales: $1,235,000   2001 Profits: $ Fiscal Year Ends: 12/31
2000 Sales: $1,184,000   2000 Profits: $

SALARIES/BENEFITS:
Pension Plan: Y   ESOP Stock Plan: Profit Sharing: Top Exec. Salary: $794,215   Bonus: $1,629,342
Savings Plan: Y   Stock Purch. Plan: Second Exec. Salary: $475,940   Bonus: $690,249

OTHER THOUGHTS:
Apparent Top Female Officers: 2
Hot Spot for Advancement for Women/Minorities:

LOCATIONS: ("Y" = Yes)
West:	Southwest:	Midwest:	Southeast:	Northeast:	International:
Y		Y	Y	Y	Y

Note: Financial information, benefits and other data can change quickly and may vary from those stated here.

DATASCOPE CORP

www.datascope.com

Industry Group Code: 339113   Ranks within this company's industry group: Sales: 54   Profits: 52

Insurance/HMO/PPO:	Drugs:	Equipment/Supplies:		Hospitals/Clinics:	Services:	Health Care:
Insurance:	Manufacturer:	Manufacturer:	Y	Acute Care:	Diagnostics:	Home Health:
Managed Care:	Distributor:	Distributor:		Sub-Acute Care:	Labs/Testing:	Long-Term Care:
Utilization Mgmt.:	Specialty Pharm.:	Leasing/Finance:		Outpatient Surgery:	Staffing:	Physical Therapy:
Payment Proc.:	Vitamins/Nutri.:	Information Sys.:		Phys. Rehab. Center:	Waste Disposal:	Phys. Practice Mgmt.:
	Clinical Trials:			Psychiatric Clinics:	Specialty Services:	

TYPES OF BUSINESS:
Equipment-Intra-Aortic Pumps & Catheters
Cardiac Assist Products
Patient Monitoring Systems
Collagen Products
Vascular Products

BRANDS/DIVISIONS/AFFILIATES:
VasoSeal
InterVascular, Inc.
Panorama Patient Monitoring Network

CONTACTS: Note: Officers with more than one job title may be intentionally listed here more than once.
Lawrence Saper, CEO
Murray Pitkowsky, Sr. VP/CFO
James Cooper, VP-Human Resources
S. Arieh Zak, Corp. Counsel
Hank Scaramelli, VP-Oper.
Murray Pitkowsky, Treas.
Nicholas E. Barker, VP-Corp. Design
S. Arieh Zak, VP-Regulatory Affairs
Terrence J. Gunning, VP/Pres.-Cardiac Assist
Lawrence Saper, Chmn.

Phone: 201-391-8100	Fax: 201-307-5400
Toll-Free:	
Address: 14 Phillips Pkwy., Montvale, NJ 07645 US	

GROWTH PLANS/SPECIAL FEATURES:
Datascope Corp. is a diversified medical device company that manufactures and markets proprietary products for clinical health care markets in interventional cardiology and radiology, cardiovascular and vascular surgery, anesthesiology, emergency medicine and critical care. Cardiac assist, patient monitoring, interventional and InterVascular products constitute the company's four main product lines. Cardiac assist products include intra-aortic balloon pump and catheter technologies. The intra-aortic balloon system is used principally to treat cardiac shock, acute heart failure and irregular heart rhythms. Patient monitoring systems encompass a broad line of physiological monitors designed to provide for patient safety and management of patient care. Datascope's monitors are capable of continuous and simultaneous measurement of many different vital signs and are utilized in operating rooms, clinical care units, post-anesthesia care units and recovery rooms, intensive care units, labor and delivery rooms as well as magnetic resonance imaging (MRI) units. The company's VasoSeal wound closure product revolutionized the technology used to seal arterial puncture wounds to stop bleeding after catheterization processes and is the first vascular sealing device to be approved in the U.S. Datascope's InterVascular subsidiary markets and sells a proprietary line of knitted and woven polyester vascular grafts, patches and interventional products for reconstructive vascular and cardiovascular surgery. All of the company's products are sold through direct sales representatives in the U.S. and a combination of direct sales representatives and independent distributors in international markets. In recent news, Datascope launched the Panorama Patient Monitoring Network, a line of patient monitoring products that allow hospitals to share patient information via one network.

The firm offers a comprehensive medical and insurance program as well as tuition assistance, an employee referral program, in-house training, credit union membership and a business-casual dress code.

FINANCIALS: Sales and profits are in thousands of dollars—add 000 to get the full amount. Year 2004 note: Complete fiscal 2004 results were not available for all companies at press time. For this company, year 2004 is for 12 months.

2004 Sales: $343,300 (12 months)	2004 Profits: $23,908 (12 months)	
2003 Sales: $328,300	2003 Profits: $23,300	Stock Ticker: DSCP
2002 Sales: $317,400	2002 Profits: $13,900	Employees: 1,320
2001 Sales: $312,800	2001 Profits: $34,200	Fiscal Year Ends: 6/30
2000 Sales: $298,800	2000 Profits: $33,100	

SALARIES/BENEFITS:
Pension Plan: Y	ESOP Stock Plan:	Profit Sharing:	Top Exec. Salary: $1,000,000	Bonus: $500,000
Savings Plan: Y	Stock Purch. Plan: Y		Second Exec. Salary: $238,750	Bonus: $42,000

OTHER THOUGHTS:
Apparent Top Female Officers:
Hot Spot for Advancement for Women/Minorities:

LOCATIONS: ("Y" = Yes)
West:	Southwest:	Midwest:	Southeast:	Northeast:	International:
Y	Y	Y	Y	Y	Y

DAVITA INC

www.davita.com

Industry Group Code: 621490 Ranks within this company's industry group: Sales: 3 Profits: 2

Insurance/HMO/PPO:	Drugs:	Equipment/Supplies:	Hospitals/Clinics:		Services:		Health Care:	
Insurance:	Manufacturer:	Manufacturer:	Acute Care:		Diagnostics:		Home Health:	
Managed Care:	Distributor:	Distributor:	Sub-Acute Care:	Y	Labs/Testing:	Y	Long-Term Care:	
Utilization Mgmt.:	Specialty Pharm.:	Leasing/Finance:	Outpatient Surgery:		Staffing:		Physical Therapy:	
Payment Proc.:	Vitamins/Nutri.:	Information Sys.:	Phys. Rehab. Center:		Waste Disposal:		Phys. Practice Mgmt.:	
	Clinical Trials:		Psychiatric Clinics:		Specialty Services:	Y		

TYPES OF BUSINESS:
Clinics-Dialysis
Clinical Research

BRANDS/DIVISIONS/AFFILIATES:
Total Renal Care Holdings, Inc.
DaVita Clinical Research, Inc.
Total Renal Research, Inc.
Physicians Dialysis, Inc.

CONTACTS:
Note: Officers with more than one job title may be intentionally listed here more than once.

Kent J. Thiry, CEO
Joseph C. Mello, COO
Denise K. Fletcher, Sr. VP/CFO
LeAnne Zumwalt, VP-Investor Rel.
Gary W. Beil, Controller
Lori S. Richardson-Pelliccioni, VP/Chief Compliance Officer/Acting General Counsel
Charlie McAllister, Chief Medical Officer
Tom Kelly, Exec. VP
Kent J. Thiry, Chmn.

Phone: 310-536-2400	Fax: 310-536-2675
Toll-Free: 800-310-4872	
Address: 601 Hawaii St., El Segundo, CA 90245 US	

GROWTH PLANS/SPECIAL FEATURES:

DaVita, Inc., formerly known as Total Renal Care Holdings, is the second-largest provider of dialysis services in the United States for patients suffering from chronic kidney failure. The company treats approximately 52,000 patients through a network of over 611 outpatient facilities in 35 states and the District of Columbia. In addition, DaVita provides acute dialysis services at over 330 hospitals. The company's dialysis services include hemodialysis, peritoneal dialysis, acute dialysis and pre-end stage renal disease (ESRD) education. The firm offers ancillary services including ESRD laboratory and ESRD clinical research programs. DaVita also operates DaVita Clinical Research, formerly Total Renal Research, Inc., which conducts Phase I and II studies and manages a network of trial sites involved in Phase II-IV clinical trials. The company has focused in recent years on a multiyear turnaround to improve its financial and operational structure. As part of that shift, DaVita completed the sale of its international operations, settled a securities class action lawsuit, improved cash flow, stabilized core operations and completed the name change from Total Renal Care. The company plans to continue expanding capacity at some centers and opening or acquiring additional centers in the near future, as well as investing in new systems and processes. Recently, DaVita acquired 21 dialysis programs/centers in California, Michigan, Texas, Ohio, Nebraska, Kentucky, Louisiana, Georgia, North Carolina, West Virginia and Maryland, serving over 1,370 patients. It also acquired Physicians Dialysis, Inc., which operates 24 dialysis centers serving approximately 1,700 patients, for $150 million in cash.

Both full- and part-time employees qualify for benefits including flexible scheduling, profit sharing, educational opportunities and a comprehensive health care package. In addition, DaVita provides $1,000 vacation rewards for employees with no unplanned absences, a college scholarship fund for children of employees, loan assistance and continued education opportunities for RNs and financial aid for employees during times of crises.

FINANCIALS:
Sales and profits are in thousands of dollars—add 000 to get the full amount. Year 2004 note: Complete fiscal 2004 results were not available for all companies at press time. For this company, year 2004 is for 9 months.

2004 Sales: $1,682,592 (9 months)	2004 Profits: $165,652 (9 months)	**Stock Ticker:** DVA
2003 Sales: $2,016,418	2003 Profits: $175,791	Employees: 13,800
2002 Sales: $1,854,600	2002 Profits: $157,300	Fiscal Year Ends: 12/31
2001 Sales: $1,650,800	2001 Profits: $137,300	
2000 Sales: $1,486,302	2000 Profits: $13,485	

SALARIES/BENEFITS:

Pension Plan:	ESOP Stock Plan:	Profit Sharing: Y	Top Exec. Salary: $640,385	Bonus: $840,000
Savings Plan: Y	Stock Purch. Plan: Y		Second Exec. Salary: $383,616	Bonus: $339,000

OTHER THOUGHTS:
Apparent Top Female Officers: 3
Hot Spot for Advancement for Women/Minorities: Y

LOCATIONS: ("Y" = Yes)

West:	Southwest:	Midwest:	Southeast:	Northeast:	International:
Y	Y	Y	Y	Y	

DELTA DENTAL PLANS ASSOCIATION

www.deltadental.com

Industry Group Code: 524114A **Ranks within this company's industry group:** Sales: Profits:

Insurance/HMO/PPO:	Drugs:	Equipment/Supplies:	Hospitals/Clinics:	Services:	Health Care:
Insurance: Y	Manufacturer:	Manufacturer:	Acute Care:	Diagnostics:	Home Health:
Managed Care: Y	Distributor:	Distributor:	Sub-Acute Care:	Labs/Testing:	Long-Term Care:
Utilization Mgmt.:	Specialty Pharm.:	Leasing/Finance:	Outpatient Surgery:	Staffing:	Physical Therapy:
Payment Proc.:	Vitamins/Nutri.:	Information Sys.:	Phys. Rehab. Center:	Waste Disposal:	Phys. Practice Mgmt.:
	Clinical Trials:		Psychiatric Clinics:	Specialty Services: Y	

TYPES OF BUSINESS:
HMO/PPO
Dental Insurance & Dental Care

BRANDS/DIVISIONS/AFFILIATES:
DeltaUSA
DeltaPremier USA
DeltaPreferred Option USA
DeltaCare USA
DeltaSelect USA/TRICARE

CONTACTS:
Note: Officers with more than one job title may be intentionally listed here more than once.
Kim Volk, CEO
Kim Volk, Pres.
Tom Dolatowski, VP-Mktg.
Karron Callaghan, VP-Tech.
Janis Oshensky, Dir.-Product & Network Dev., DeltaUSA
Stefany Soutor, Corp. Administrator
Susan Morris, VP-Corp. Comm. & Public Policy
Lucia Clark, Dir.-Education & Meeting Planning

Phone: 630-574-6001 **Fax:** 630-574-6999
Toll-Free:
Address: 1515 W. 22nd St., Ste. 1200, Oak Brook, IL 60523 US

GROWTH PLANS/SPECIAL FEATURES:
Delta Dental Plans Association (DDPA), a nonprofit organization, is the nation's largest dental benefits system and dental service corporation. The firm serves more than one-quarter of the U.S. population, nearly 45 million people, enrolled in 76,000 employer groups. Its nationwide network of 39 independent affiliates operates in all 50 states, the District of Columbia and Puerto Rico. The company administers both large and small employer groups locally or nationally through DeltaUSA. It processes nearly 62 million dental claims per year. DeltaPremier USA, DDPA's traditional fee-for-service program, offers a provider network that encompasses more than 110,000 providers and 145,000 office locations. It is the largest network in the country. DeltaPreferred Option USA, the firm's preferred provider option, has a national network of more than 50,000 dentists practicing in over 71,000 locations. DeltaCare USA, the company's dental health maintenance organization, consists of a network of more than 8,000 contracted dentists practicing in over 13,000 office locations. DeltaSelect USA/TRICARE is the firm's national program for group-voluntary customers, including the TRICARE program, which covers the nation's non-active military personnel and their dependents.

FINANCIALS:
Sales and profits are in thousands of dollars—add 000 to get the full amount. Year 2004 note: Complete fiscal 2004 results were not available for all companies at press time. For this company, year 2004 is for   months.

2004 Sales: $ (months)   2004 Profits: $ (months)
2003 Sales: $ 2003 Profits: $
2002 Sales: $ 2002 Profits: $
2001 Sales: $ 2001 Profits: $
2000 Sales: $ 2000 Profits: $

Stock Ticker: Nonprofit
Employees:
Fiscal Year Ends: 12/31

SALARIES/BENEFITS:
Pension Plan: ESOP Stock Plan: Profit Sharing: Top Exec. Salary: $ Bonus: $
Savings Plan: Stock Purch. Plan: Second Exec. Salary: $ Bonus: $

OTHER THOUGHTS:
Apparent Top Female Officers: 6
Hot Spot for Advancement for Women/Minorities: Y

LOCATIONS: ("Y" = Yes)
West:	Southwest:	Midwest:	Southeast:	Northeast:	International:
Y	Y	Y	Y	Y	Y

DENTAL BENEFITS PROVIDERS

www.dbp.com

Industry Group Code: 524114A   Ranks within this company's industry group: Sales: Profits:

Insurance/HMO/PPO:	Drugs:	Equipment/Supplies:	Hospitals/Clinics:	Services:	Health Care:
Insurance:	Manufacturer: Y	Manufacturer:	Acute Care:	Diagnostics:	Home Health:
Managed Care:	Distributor:	Distributor:	Sub-Acute Care:	Labs/Testing:	Long-Term Care:
Utilization Mgmt.:	Specialty Pharm.:	Leasing/Finance:	Outpatient Surgery:	Staffing:	Physical Therapy:
Payment Proc.:	Vitamins/Nutri.:	Information Sys.:	Phys. Rehab. Center:	Waste Disposal:	Phys. Practice Mgmt.:
	Clinical Trials:		Psychiatric Clinics:	Specialty Services:	

TYPES OF BUSINESS:
Dental Benefits

GROWTH PLANS/SPECIAL FEATURES:
Dental Benefits Providers, Inc. (DBP), a subsidiary of UnitedHealth Group, is one of the largest dental benefit companies in the U.S. It has more than 4 million members and dentist networks in 48 states, the District of Columbia, Puerto Rico and the Virgin Islands. The company subcontracts dental health maintenance organization plans (DHMOs), PPOs, POS plans, indemnity plans, preventive plans, Medicaid/Child Health Plus Plans and Medicare plans, as well as claims and administrative services to HMOs, unions, insurance companies, municipalities and large corporations.

BRANDS/DIVISIONS/AFFILIATES:
UnitedHealth Group

CONTACTS:
Note: Officers with more than one job title may be intentionally listed here more than once.

David Hall, CEO
Kevin Ruth, Pres.
Kevin Ruth, COO
Mete Sahin, CFO

Phone: 240-632-8000   **Fax:** 240-632-8100
Toll-Free: 800-445-9090
Address: 3 Irvington Center, 800 King Farm Blvd., Ste. 600, Bethesda, MD 20850 US

FINANCIALS:
Sales and profits are in thousands of dollars—add 000 to get the full amount. Year 2004 note: Complete fiscal 2004 results were not available for all companies at press time. For this company, year 2004 is for months.

2004 Sales: $ (months)   2004 Profits: $ (months)
2003 Sales: $ 2003 Profits: $
2002 Sales: $ 2002 Profits: $
2001 Sales: $ 2001 Profits: $
2000 Sales: $ 2000 Profits: $

Stock Ticker: Subsidiary
Employees:
Fiscal Year Ends: 12/31

SALARIES/BENEFITS:
Pension Plan: ESOP Stock Plan: Profit Sharing: Top Exec. Salary: $ Bonus: $
Savings Plan: Stock Purch. Plan: Second Exec. Salary: $ Bonus: $

OTHER THOUGHTS:
Apparent Top Female Officers:
Hot Spot for Advancement for Women/Minorities:

LOCATIONS: ("Y" = Yes)

West:	Southwest:	Midwest:	Southeast:	Northeast:	International:
Y	Y	Y	Y	Y	Y

DENTSPLY INTERNATIONAL INC

www.dentsply.com

Industry Group Code: 339113   Ranks within this company's industry group: Sales: 17   Profits: 15

Insurance/HMO/PPO:	Drugs:	Equipment/Supplies:		Hospitals/Clinics:	Services:	Health Care:
Insurance:	Manufacturer:	Manufacturer:	Y	Acute Care:	Diagnostics:	Home Health:
Managed Care:	Distributor:	Distributor:	Y	Sub-Acute Care:	Labs/Testing:	Long-Term Care:
Utilization Mgmt.:	Specialty Pharm.:	Leasing/Finance:		Outpatient Surgery:	Staffing:	Physical Therapy:
Payment Proc.:	Vitamins/Nutri.:	Information Sys.:		Phys. Rehab. Center:	Waste Disposal:	Phys. Practice Mgmt.:
	Clinical Trials:			Psychiatric Clinics:	Specialty Services:	

TYPES OF BUSINESS:
Supplies-Dental Consumable & Laboratory Products
Dental Practice Software
Crown & Bridge Materials
Dental Sealants
Dental Implants
Dental X-Ray Systems
Dental Cutting Instruments
Ultrasonic Scalers

BRANDS/DIVISIONS/AFFILIATES:
Oraqix

CONTACTS:
Note: Officers with more than one job title may be intentionally listed here more than once.

Gerald K. Kunkle, Jr., CEO
Thomas L. Whiting, Pres.
Thomas L. Whiting, COO
Bret W. Wise, Sr. VP/CFO
Rachel P. McKinney, Corp. VP-Human Resources
Steven R. Jefferies, VP-Advanced Tech.
Brian M. Addison, VP/General Counsel
George R. Rhodes, VP-Corp. Comm. & Professional Rel.
William E. Reardon, Corp. Treas.
Timothy S. Warady, Corp. Controller
Christopher T. Clark, Sr. VP
J. Henrik Roos, Sr. VP
William R. Jellison, Sr. VP
John C. Miles, II, Chmn.

Phone: 717-845-7511   **Fax:** 717-849-4762
Toll-Free: 800-877-0200
Address: 221 W. Philadelphia St., P.O. Box 872, York, PA 17405 US

GROWTH PLANS/SPECIAL FEATURES:

DENTSPLY International, Inc., through its many subsidiaries, designs, develops, manufactures and markets a broad range of products for the dental market. The company is one of the world's leading manufacturers and distributors of dental consumables, dental laboratory products and dental specialty products, with facilities in 22 nations and operations in over 120 countries. The firm also operates a clinical education web site that provides access to information about the newest materials, concepts and techniques in dentistry, and it is a member of the ADA Continuing Education Recognition Program, which is designed to facilitate license renewal requirements for dentists, hygienists and dental assistants. Its dental consumables segment provides dentists with anesthetics, prophylaxis paste, dental sealants, impression materials, restorative materials, tooth whiteners and topical fluoride. This segment also produces small equipment products including high- and low-speed handpieces, intraoral curing light systems and ultrasonic scalers and polishers. DENTSPLY's laboratory products are used in the preparation of dental appliances and consist of dental prosthetics including artificial teeth, precious metal dental alloys, dental ceramics and crown and bridge materials. Small equipment in this category includes computer-aided machining ceramics systems and porcelain furnaces. Finally, specialty products include endodontic instruments and materials, implants and orthodontic appliances and accessories. DENTSPLY announced recently that its Oraqix needle-free local anesthetic had been approved for release in the U.S. and is now distributed through an agreement with Johnson & Johnson.

DENTSPLY International offers its employees flexible medical, dental, disability and life insurance, educational assistance and paid holidays. Specialized training programs are available in certain job categories.

FINANCIALS:
Sales and profits are in thousands of dollars—add 000 to get the full amount. Year 2004 note: Complete fiscal 2004 results were not available for all companies at press time. For this company, year 2004 is for 9 months.

2004 Sales: $1,231,298 (9 months)	2004 Profits: $184,558 (9 months)	**Stock Ticker:** XRAY
2003 Sales: $1,570,925	2003 Profits: $174,183	Employees: 7,600
2002 Sales: $1,513,700	2002 Profits: $148,000	Fiscal Year Ends: 12/31
2001 Sales: $1,129,100	2001 Profits: $121,500	
2000 Sales: $889,800	2000 Profits: $101,100	

SALARIES/BENEFITS:
Pension Plan:	ESOP Stock Plan: Y	Profit Sharing:	Top Exec. Salary: $740,000	Bonus: $606,200
Savings Plan: Y	Stock Purch. Plan:		Second Exec. Salary: $512,000	Bonus: $340,800

OTHER THOUGHTS:
Apparent Top Female Officers: 1
Hot Spot for Advancement for Women/Minorities:

LOCATIONS: ("Y" = Yes)
West:	Southwest:	Midwest:	Southeast:	Northeast:	International:
Y	Y	Y	Y	Y	Y

DEPUY INC

www.depuy.com

Industry Group Code: 339113 **Ranks within this company's industry group:** Sales: Profits:

Insurance/HMO/PPO:	Drugs:	Equipment/Supplies:		Hospitals/Clinics:	Services:	Health Care:
Insurance:	Manufacturer:	Manufacturer:	Y	Acute Care:	Diagnostics:	Home Health:
Managed Care:	Distributor:	Distributor:	Y	Sub-Acute Care:	Labs/Testing:	Long-Term Care:
Utilization Mgmt.:	Specialty Pharm.:	Leasing/Finance:		Outpatient Surgery:	Staffing:	Physical Therapy:
Payment Proc.:	Vitamins/Nutri.:	Information Sys.:		Phys. Rehab. Center:	Waste Disposal:	Phys. Practice Mgmt.:
	Clinical Trials:			Psychiatric Clinics:	Specialty Services:	

TYPES OF BUSINESS:
Equipment/Supplies-Orthopedic Devices
Fixative Products

BRANDS/DIVISIONS/AFFILIATES:
Johnson & Johnson
DePuy Trauma & Extremities
DePuy Spine, Inc.
DePuy International
Codman and Shurtleff, Inc.
DePuy Orthopaedics

CONTACTS:
Note: Officers with more than one job title may be intentionally listed here more than once.
Kevin K. Sidow, Worldwide Pres.
Diogo Moreira-Rato, U.S. Pres.-Orthopedics, Trauma & Extremities
Michael J. Dormer, Chmn.

Phone: 574-267-8143 **Fax:** 574-267-7196
Toll-Free: 800-473-3789
Address: 700 Orthopaedic Dr., Warsaw, IN 46581 US

GROWTH PLANS/SPECIAL FEATURES:
DePuy, Inc., a subsidiary of Johnson & Johnson, is a leading designer, manufacturer and distributor of orthopedic devices and supplies. Its products are used primarily by orthopedic medical specialists and, in the case of the company's spinal implants, spinal specialists and neurosurgeons. The products are used in both surgical and non-surgical therapies to treat patients with musculoskeletal conditions resulting from degenerative diseases, deformities, trauma and sports-related injuries. The company operates through five subsidiaries. DePuy Orthopaedics develops products for hip and extremity implants, knee implants, environmental protection products and other surgical equipment. Codman and Shurtleff, Inc. enables treatment of central nervous system disorders through its hydrocephalic shunt valve systems, neuro endoscopes and spinal fixation implant products, distributing over 7,000 different products. DePuy Trauma & Extremities produces orthopedic trauma products and joint reconstructive products for shoulder, ankle, elbow, wrist and finger joints. Subsidiary DePuy Spine, Inc. develops, manufactures and markets implants and technologies for the treatment of cervical, thoracic, lumbar and sacral spinal pathologies. Its many products include the world's first artificial disc, various spinal systems, bone graft replacements and a bone growth stimulator. DePuy International, based in England, represents the company's interests abroad. DePuy also operates several web sites providing educational information on joint replacement, hydrocephalus, back and neck pain, arthritis and other medical conditions.

FINANCIALS:
Sales and profits are in thousands of dollars—add 000 to get the full amount. Year 2004 note: Complete fiscal 2004 results were not available for all companies at press time. For this company, year 2004 is for   months.

2004 Sales: $ (months)
2003 Sales: $
2002 Sales: $
2001 Sales: $
2000 Sales: $

2004 Profits: $ (months)
2003 Profits: $
2002 Profits: $
2001 Profits: $
2000 Profits: $

Stock Ticker: Subsidiary
Employees:
Fiscal Year Ends: 12/31

SALARIES/BENEFITS:
Pension Plan:	ESOP Stock Plan:	Profit Sharing:	Top Exec. Salary: $	Bonus: $
Savings Plan:	Stock Purch. Plan:		Second Exec. Salary: $	Bonus: $

OTHER THOUGHTS:
Apparent Top Female Officers:
Hot Spot for Advancement for Women/Minorities:

LOCATIONS: ("Y" = Yes)
West:	Southwest:	Midwest:	Southeast:	Northeast:	International:
Y	Y	Y	Y	Y	Y

DETROIT MEDICAL CENTER

www.dmc.org

Industry Group Code: 622110 Ranks within this company's industry group: Sales: 35 Profits:

Insurance/HMO/PPO:	Drugs:	Equipment/Supplies:	Hospitals/Clinics:		Services:		Health Care:	
Insurance: Managed Care: Utilization Mgmt.: Payment Proc.:	Manufacturer: Distributor: Specialty Pharm.: Vitamins/Nutri.: Clinical Trials:	Manufacturer: Distributor: Leasing/Finance: Information Sys.:	Acute Care: Sub-Acute Care: Outpatient Surgery: Phys. Rehab. Center: Psychiatric Clinics:	Y Y Y Y	Diagnostics: Labs/Testing: Staffing: Waste Disposal: Specialty Services:		Home Health: Long-Term Care: Physical Therapy: Phys. Practice Mgmt.:	Y Y Y

TYPES OF BUSINESS:
Hospitals
Clinical Research

BRANDS/DIVISIONS/AFFILIATES:
Wayne State University School of Medicine
Kresge Eye Institute
Barbara Ann Karmanos Cancer Institute
Sinai-Grace Hospital
Rehabilitation Institute of Michigan
Hutzel Hospital
Huron Valley-Sinai Hospital
Harper University Hospital

GROWTH PLANS/SPECIAL FEATURES:
Detroit Medical Center (DMC), established as a not-for-profit organization in 1985, is the largest health care provider in southeast Michigan, with two nursing centers, more than 100 outpatient facilities and seven hospitals: Children's Hospital of Michigan, Detroit Receiving Hospital, Harper University Hospital, Huron Valley-Sinai Hospital, Hutzel Hospital, the Rehabilitation Institute of Michigan and Sinai-Grace Hospital. The system has a combined 2,000 licensed beds and roughly 3,000 affiliated physicians. DMC also manages the Barbara Ann Karmanos Cancer Institute, one of the nation's leading cancer treatment facilities, and the Kresge Eye Institute, both located in Detroit. DMC also serves as the teaching and clinical research site for Wayne State University's School of Medicine, the nation's fourth-largest medical school.

CONTACTS:
Note: Officers with more than one job title may be intentionally listed here more than once.
Michael E. Duggan, CEO
Michael E. Duggan, Pres.
David Ellis, Corp. Dir.-Planning & Future Studies
Chuck O'Brien, Chmn.

Phone: 313-578-2000 Fax: 313-578-3225
Toll-Free: 888-362-2500
Address: 3900 John R. St., Detroit, MI 48201 US

FINANCIALS:
Sales and profits are in thousands of dollars—add 000 to get the full amount. Year 2004 note: Complete fiscal 2004 results were not available for all companies at press time. For this company, year 2004 is for months.

2004 Sales: $ (months)   2004 Profits: $ (months)
2003 Sales: $1,600,000   2003 Profits: $
2002 Sales: $1,600,000   2002 Profits: $
2001 Sales: $ 2001 Profits: $
2000 Sales: $ 2000 Profits: $

Stock Ticker: Nonprofit
Employees: 14,311
Fiscal Year Ends:

SALARIES/BENEFITS:
Pension Plan: ESOP Stock Plan: Profit Sharing: Top Exec. Salary: $ Bonus: $
Savings Plan: Stock Purch. Plan: Second Exec. Salary: $ Bonus: $

OTHER THOUGHTS:
Apparent Top Female Officers:
Hot Spot for Advancement for Women/Minorities:

LOCATIONS: ("Y" = Yes)

West:	Southwest:	Midwest:	Southeast:	Northeast:	International:
		Y			

DIAGNOSTIC PRODUCTS CORPORATION
www.dpcweb.com

Industry Group Code: 339113   Ranks within this company's industry group: Sales: 47   Profits: 27

Insurance/HMO/PPO:	Drugs:	Equipment/Supplies:		Hospitals/Clinics:	Services:	Health Care:
Insurance:	Manufacturer:	Manufacturer:	Y	Acute Care:	Diagnostics:	Home Health:
Managed Care:	Distributor:	Distributor:		Sub-Acute Care:	Labs/Testing:	Long-Term Care:
Utilization Mgmt.:	Specialty Pharm.:	Leasing/Finance:		Outpatient Surgery:	Staffing:	Physical Therapy:
Payment Proc.:	Vitamins/Nutri.:	Information Sys.:	Y	Phys. Rehab. Center:	Waste Disposal:	Phys. Practice Mgmt.:
	Clinical Trials:			Psychiatric Clinics:	Specialty Services:	

TYPES OF BUSINESS:
Supplies-Immunodiagnostic Kits
Nonisotopic Diagnostic Tests
Immunoassay Analyzers

BRANDS/DIVISIONS/AFFILIATES:
IMMULITE
IMMULITE 1000
IMMULITE 2000
IMMULITE Turbo
Sample Management System

CONTACTS:
Note: Officers with more than one job title may be intentionally listed here more than once.

Michael Ziering, CEO
James L. Brill, CFO
Nicholas Arnold, VP-Mktg. & Sales
Said El Shami, Sr. VP-R&D
Sidney A. Aroesty, Sr. VP-Oper.
James L. Brill, VP-Finance
Ira Ziering, VP-Bus. and Legal
Marilyn Ziering, Sr. VP
Michael Ziering, Chmn.

Phone: 310-645-8200	Fax: 310-645-9999
Toll-Free: 800-372-1782	
Address: 5700 W. 96th St., Los Angeles, CA 90045-5597 US	

GROWTH PLANS/SPECIAL FEATURES:

Diagnostic Products Corp. (DPC) manufactures and distributes medical immunodiagnostic test kits and related instrumentation based on technology derived from immunology and molecular biology. The tests are used to diagnose and manage a wide variety of medical conditions, such as allergies, anemia, cancer, diabetes, infectious disease and substance abuse. The tests can also be used for veterinary applications. The company has two principal immunoassay platforms. IMMULITE 2000 addresses the needs of high-volume laboratories, while IMMULITE serves lower-volume facilities and niche markets. The original IMMULITE system was first introduced in 1993. Computer-driven, it uses a patented solid-phase wash technology and chemiluminescent detection method, which together are capable of measurements at exceptionally low concentrations. The system is totally automated with respect to sample and reagent handling, incubation, washing and substrate addition. DPC's IMMULITE has the capacity for walk-away processing of up to 120 samples per hour, on a random access basis, meaning that it can perform any test, or combination of tests, on any patient sample at any time. The current top of the line, IMMULITE 2000, is an upgraded version of the original IMMULITE, capable of 200 tests per hour, as well as additional storage and enhanced interface (for transferring data to a computer). The firm also offers IMMULITE 1000, which has a menu of nearly 100 assays, and IMMULITE Turbo, which provides test results in 15 minutes. In addition, DPC is preparing to launch its newest product, the Sample Management System (SMS), which will allow a platform of 220 samples at a time and a universal robotic interface that can be linked to almost any of the workcell/automated systems available.

The company offers its employees medical, disability and life insurance, education assistance, flexible spending accounts and credit union membership.

FINANCIALS:
Sales and profits are in thousands of dollars—add 000 to get the full amount. Year 2004 note: Complete fiscal 2004 results were not available for all companies at press time. For this company, year 2004 is for 9 months.

2004 Sales: $325,514 (9 months)	2004 Profits: $50,593 (9 months)	
2003 Sales: $381,386	2003 Profits: $61,795	Stock Ticker: DP
2002 Sales: $324,100	2002 Profits: $47,300	Employees: 2,235
2001 Sales: $283,400	2001 Profits: $39,000	Fiscal Year Ends: 12/31
2000 Sales: $247,867	2000 Profits: $28,250	

SALARIES/BENEFITS:
| Pension Plan: Y | ESOP Stock Plan: | Profit Sharing: Y | Top Exec. Salary: $530,000 | Bonus: $80,000 |
| Savings Plan: Y | Stock Purch. Plan: | | Second Exec. Salary: $357,000 | Bonus: $22,500 |

OTHER THOUGHTS:
Apparent Top Female Officers: 1
Hot Spot for Advancement for Women/Minorities:

LOCATIONS: ("Y" = Yes)
West:	Southwest:	Midwest:	Southeast:	Northeast:	International:
Y				Y	Y

DIGENE CORPORATION

www.digene.com

Industry Group Code: 339113   **Ranks within this company's industry group:** Sales: 105   Profits: 118

Insurance/HMO/PPO:	Drugs:	Equipment/Supplies:		Hospitals/Clinics:	Services:	Health Care:
Insurance: Managed Care: Utilization Mgmt.: Payment Proc.:	Manufacturer: Distributor: Specialty Pharm.: Vitamins/Nutri.: Clinical Trials:	Manufacturer: Distributor: Leasing/Finance: Information Sys.:	Y Y	Acute Care: Sub-Acute Care: Outpatient Surgery: Phys. Rehab. Center: Psychiatric Clinics:	Diagnostics: Labs/Testing: Staffing: Waste Disposal: Specialty Services:	Home Health: Long-Term Care: Physical Therapy: Phys. Practice Mgmt.:

TYPES OF BUSINESS:
Supplies-DNA/RNA Tests
Genomics Research

BRANDS/DIVISIONS/AFFILIATES:
Hybrid Capture Gene Analysis System
DNAwithPap
Rapid Capture System
Hybrid Capture 2

CONTACTS:
Note: Officers with more than one job title may be intentionally listed here more than once.
Evan Jones, CEO
Charles M. Fleischman, Pres.
Charles M. Fleischman, COO
Charles M. Fleischman, CFO
Robert M. Lilley, Sr. VP-Global Sales and Mktg.
Larry Welman, VP-Human Resources
Attila T. Lorincz, Sr. VP-Research & Dev.
Joseph P. Slattery, Sr. VP-Info. Systems
Allison Cullen, VP-Product Dev.
Jay Payne, VP-Eng.
Belinda O. Patrick, Sr. VP-Mfg. Oper.
Donna M. Seyfried, VP-Bus. Dev.
Pamela Rasmussen, VP-Corp. Comm.
Joseph P. Slattery, Sr. VP-Finance
Susan M. Keese, VP-Global Product Oper.
Linda Alexander, VP-Women's Health
Douglas White, VP-North American Mktg.
Evan Jones, Chmn.

Phone: 301-944-7000   **Fax:** 301-944-7121
Toll-Free: 800-344-3631
Address: 1201 Clopper Rd., Gaithersburg, MD 20878 US

GROWTH PLANS/SPECIAL FEATURES:

Digene Corp. develops, manufactures and markets its proprietary DNA and RNA testing systems for the screening, monitoring and diagnosis of human diseases. The company uses its patented Hybrid Capture Gene Analysis System to focus on women's cancer and infectious diseases. The firm's lead product is the only FDA-approved test for human papillomavirus (HPV), the cause of more than 99% of cervical cancer cases. Digene is currently working to establish its HPV test as the standard for cervical cancer screening. Clinical studies have indicated that the test can detect cervical disease in more than 95% of the cases where it is present. Combined with the Pap smear, the test can detect virtually all instances of cervical cancer. Digene also developed its Hybrid Capture technology to include DNA tests for the detection of chlamydia, gonorrhea and other sexually transmitted infections. In addition, the firm operates in genomics research with the goal of applying its technology platform to develop gene expression DNA microarray products and services, expand its clinical testing services for use in the pharmaceutical market and correlate proprietary gene-based information with clinical diseases. The company markets its products through a direct sales force in the U.S. and through distributors in other countries. In recent years, the FDA approved Digene's DNAwithPap test, which is used to adjunctively screen women ages 30 and older to assess the presence or absence of high-risk HPV types. The FDA has also approved Digene's Rapid Capture System application that speeds up the processing of the DNAwithPap test. In other news, the Medical Services Advisory Committee of Australia recently recognized the usefulness of Digene's Hybrid Capure 2 technology in assessing the success of cervical cancer treatment.

Digene offers its employees a health care plan; dental, vision and prescription drug coverage; life insurance; short- and long-term disability insurance; and tuition reimbursement. The company also offers computer discounts and an on-site fitness center.

FINANCIALS:
Sales and profits are in thousands of dollars—add 000 to get the full amount. Year 2004 note: Complete fiscal 2004 results were not available for all companies at press time. For this company, year 2004 is for 12 months.

2004 Sales: $90,160 (12 months)	2004 Profits: $21,542 (12 months)	**Stock Ticker:** DIGE
2003 Sales: $63,100	2003 Profits: $-4,300	**Employees:** 359
2002 Sales: $48,800	2002 Profits: $-9,400	**Fiscal Year Ends:** 6/30
2001 Sales: $34,200	2001 Profits: $-6,500	
2000 Sales: $23,000	2000 Profits: $-6,800	

SALARIES/BENEFITS:
Pension Plan: ESOP Stock Plan: Profit Sharing: Top Exec. Salary: $322,708   Bonus: $165,000
Savings Plan: Y   Stock Purch. Plan: Second Exec. Salary: $322,708   Bonus: $150,975

OTHER THOUGHTS:
Apparent Top Female Officers: 6
Hot Spot for Advancement for Women/Minorities: Y

LOCATIONS: ("Y" = Yes)

West:	Southwest:	Midwest:	Southeast:	Northeast:	International:
				Y	Y

Note: Financial information, benefits and other data can change quickly and may vary from those stated here.

DJ ORTHOPEDICS INC

www.djortho.com

Industry Group Code: 339113 **Ranks within this company's industry group:** Sales: 64 Profits: 68

Insurance/HMO/PPO:	Drugs:	Equipment/Supplies:		Hospitals/Clinics:		Services:		Health Care:	
Insurance:	Manufacturer:	Manufacturer:	Y	Acute Care:		Diagnostics:		Home Health:	
Managed Care:	Distributor:	Distributor:	Y	Sub-Acute Care:		Labs/Testing:		Long-Term Care:	
Utilization Mgmt.:	Specialty Pharm.:	Leasing/Finance:		Outpatient Surgery:		Staffing:		Physical Therapy:	
Payment Proc.:	Vitamins/Nutri.:	Information Sys.:		Phys. Rehab. Center:		Waste Disposal:		Phys. Practice Mgmt.:	
	Clinical Trials:			Psychiatric Clinics:		Specialty Services:			

TYPES OF BUSINESS:
Orthopedic Device Manufacturing
Bone Growth Stimulators

BRANDS/DIVISIONS/AFFILIATES:
DonJoy
Regentek
KD Innovation

CONTACTS:
Note: Officers with more than one job title may be intentionally listed here more than once.

Leslie H. Cross, CEO
Leslie H. Cross, Pres.
Vickie L. Capps, CFO
Louis Ruggiero, Sr. VP-Mktg. & Sales
Don M. Roberts, VP/General Counsel
Luke T. Faulstick, Sr. VP-Oper.
Michael R. McBrayer, Sr. VP-Bus. Dev.
Vickie L. Capps, Sr. VP-Finance
Michael R. McBrayer, Sr. VP-Professional Rel.
Jack R. Blair, Chmn.

Phone: 760-727-1280	Fax: 760-734-3595
Toll-Free: 800-336-5690	
Address: 2985 Scott St., Vista, CA 92081 US	

GROWTH PLANS/SPECIAL FEATURES:

DJ Orthopedics, Inc. is a global orthopedic sports medicine company specializing in the design, manufacture and marketing of surgical and non-surgical products and services that repair, regenerate and rehabilitate soft tissue and bone; help protect against injury; and treat osteoarthritis of the knee. Its broad range of over 600 products, many of which are based on proprietary technologies, include rigid knee braces, soft goods and specialty and other complementary orthopedic products. DJ Orthopedics' DonJoy line of rigid knee braces includes ligament braces, which provide support for knee ligament instabilities; post-operative braces, which provide both knee immobilization and a protected range of motion; and osteoarthritic braces, which provide relief of knee pain due to osteoarthritis. The firm's soft goods products, most of which are constructed from fabric or neoprene materials, provide support and/or heat retention and compression of the knee, ankle, back and upper extremities, including the shoulder, elbow, neck and wrist. Its portfolio of specialty and other complementary orthopedic products includes a continuous cold therapy system to assist in the reduction of pain and swelling and a pain management delivery system that employs ambulatory infusion pumps for the delivery of local anesthetic to the surgical site. In addition, DJ Orthopedics offers a line of bone and soft tissue regeneration products through its recently acquired subsidiary, Regentek (formerly OrthoLogic). In recent news, the company acquired KD Innovation A/S, one of its third-party distributors in Scandinavia. The acquisition will allow the firm to directly distribute its products in Denmark, Finland, Norway and Sweden

DJ Orthopedics offers its employees HMO or PPO health and dental insurance plans, vision coverage, a fitness room, tuition reimbursement and credit union membership.

FINANCIALS:
Sales and profits are in thousands of dollars—add 000 to get the full amount. Year 2004 note: Complete fiscal 2004 results were not available for all companies at press time. For this company, year 2004 is for 9 months.

2004 Sales: $187,898 (9 months)	2004 Profits: $8,715 (9 months)	**Stock Ticker:** DJO
2003 Sales: $197,939	2003 Profits: $12,071	Employees: 1,300
2002 Sales: $182,600	2002 Profits: $-15,200	Fiscal Year Ends: 12/31
2001 Sales: $169,200	2001 Profits: $56,500	
2000 Sales: $143,600	2000 Profits: $5,200	

SALARIES/BENEFITS:

Pension Plan:	ESOP Stock Plan:	Profit Sharing:	Top Exec. Salary: $322,505	Bonus: $203,027
Savings Plan: Y	Stock Purch. Plan:		Second Exec. Salary: $252,024	Bonus: $134,114

OTHER THOUGHTS:
Apparent Top Female Officers: 1
Hot Spot for Advancement for Women/Minorities:

LOCATIONS: ("Y" = Yes)

West:	Southwest:	Midwest:	Southeast:	Northeast:	International:
Y					Y

DRUGMAX INC

www.drugmax.com

Industry Group Code: 422210   Ranks within this company's industry group: Sales: 5   Profits: 6

Insurance/HMO/PPO:	Drugs:	Equipment/Supplies:	Hospitals/Clinics:	Services:	Health Care:
Insurance: Managed Care: Utilization Mgmt.: Payment Proc.:	Manufacturer: Distributor: Y Specialty Pharm.: Y Vitamins/Nutri.: Clinical Trials:	Manufacturer: Distributor: Leasing/Finance: Information Sys.:	Acute Care: Sub-Acute Care: Outpatient Surgery: Phys. Rehab. Center: Psychiatric Clinics:	Diagnostics: Labs/Testing: Staffing: Waste Disposal: Specialty Services:	Home Health: Long-Term Care: Physical Therapy: Phys. Practice Mgmt.:

TYPES OF BUSINESS:
Wholesale Distribution of Drug Products
Online Trade Exchange

BRANDS/DIVISIONS/AFFILIATES:
drugmax.com
Valley Drug Company
drugmaxtrading.com
pharmacymax.com
Familymeds Group, Inc.

CONTACTS: Note: Officers with more than one job title may be intentionally listed here more than once.
Jugal K. Taneja, CEO
William L. LaGamba, Pres.
William L. LaGamba, COO
Ronald J. Patrick, VP/CFO
Ronald J. Patrick, Treas.
William L. LaGamba, Corp. Sec.
Jugal K. Taneja, Chmn.

Phone: 727-533-0431   Fax: 727-531-1280
Toll-Free: 888-550-4312
Address: 25400 US Hwy. 19 N., Ste. 137, Clearwater, FL 33763 US

GROWTH PLANS/SPECIAL FEATURES:
DrugMax, Inc. is primarily a full-line, wholesale distributor of pharmaceuticals, over-the-counter products, health and beauty care products and nutritional supplements. The company brings retailers, manufacturers, wholesalers and end users into a single, efficient marketplace for buying and selling as well as industry news. It maintains distribution centers in Pennsylvania, Ohio and Louisiana. DrugMax serves over 9,000 members and offers over 20,000 products spanning a broad range of categories, including batteries, brand-name and generic pharmaceuticals, diabetic products, dietary supplements, herbals, over-the-counter, pet health and short-dated items. The company purchases products from approximately 400 vendors, such as Pfizer, Eli Lilly, Merck and others. The firm's electronic commerce marketplace uses Internet technology that eliminates territorial and regional borders. In addition, DrugMax provides a community environment for news, information and online forums. The company also pioneered an online trade exchange, drugmaxtrading.com, which offers one of the first business-to-business online trade exchanges for pharmaceuticals, over-the-counter products, health and beauty care products and nutritional supplements dedicated exclusively to manufacturers, distributors, wholesalers and retailers in the pharmaceutical and over-the-counter product markets. In March 2004, DrugMax announced a merger with Familymeds Group, Inc., a specialty pharmacy group operating 82 pharmacies in 14 states. The company's VetMall and Desktop subsidiaries are no longer in operation.

FINANCIALS: Sales and profits are in thousands of dollars—add 000 to get the full amount. Year 2004 note: Complete fiscal 2004 results were not available for all companies at press time. For this company, year 2004 is for 12 months.

2004 Sales: $213,789 (12 months)   2004 Profits: $-7,039   (12 months)
2003 Sales: $291,800   2003 Profits: $-13,200
2002 Sales: $271,300   2002 Profits: $2,000
2001 Sales: $177,700   2001 Profits: $-7,800
2000 Sales: $21,100   2000 Profits: $-2,000

Stock Ticker: DMAX
Employees: 80
Fiscal Year Ends: 3/31

SALARIES/BENEFITS:
Pension Plan: ESOP Stock Plan: Profit Sharing: Top Exec. Salary: $160,413   Bonus: $5,500
Savings Plan: Stock Purch. Plan: Second Exec. Salary: $137,000   Bonus: $5,000

OTHER THOUGHTS:
Apparent Top Female Officers:
Hot Spot for Advancement for Women/Minorities:

LOCATIONS: ("Y" = Yes)
West:	Southwest:	Midwest:	Southeast:	Northeast:	International:
		Y	Y	Y	

DUANE READE INC

www.duanereade.com

Industry Group Code: 446110   Ranks within this company's industry group: Sales: 5   Profits: 4

Insurance/HMO/PPO	Drugs:	Equipment/Supplies:	Hospitals/Clinics:	Services:	Health Care:
Insurance:	Manufacturer:	Manufacturer:	Acute Care:	Diagnostics:	Home Health:
Managed Care:	Distributor:	Distributor:	Sub-Acute Care:	Labs/Testing:	Long-Term Care:
Utilization Mgmt.:	Specialty Pharm.: Y	Leasing/Finance:	Outpatient Surgery:	Staffing:	Physical Therapy:
Payment Proc.:	Vitamins/Nutri.:	Information Sys.:	Phys. Rehab. Center:	Waste Disposal:	Phys. Practice Mgmt.:
	Clinical Trials:		Psychiatric Clinics:	Specialty Services:	

TYPES OF BUSINESS:
Drug Stores

BRANDS/DIVISIONS/AFFILIATES:
Rock Bottom
Value Drug
Oak Hill Capital Partners

CONTACTS:
Note: Officers with more than one job title may be intentionally listed here more than once.

Anthony J. Cuti, CEO
Anthony J. Cuti, Pres.
John K. Henry, Sr. VP/CFO
Gary Charboneau, Sr. VP-Sales & Mktg.
James M. Rizzo, VP-Human Resources
Joseph S. Lacko, VP-MIS
Timothy R. Labeau, Sr. VP-Merch.
Michelle Bergman, General Counsel
Jerry M. Ray, Sr. VP-Store & Pharmacy Oper.
Cara O'Brien, Investor Rel.
Don Yuhaz, VP-Distribution
Anthony M. Goldrick, VP-Finance
Chris Lane, VP-Pharmacy Oper.
Mike Knievel, VP-Asset Protection
Anthony J. Cuti, Chmn.

Phone: 212-273-5700   **Fax:** 212-244-6527
Toll-Free:
Address: 440 9th Ave., New York, NY 10001 US

GROWTH PLANS/SPECIAL FEATURES:
Named after the two streets where its first store was located, Duane Reade is the largest retail drug store chain in New York City. The market leader in the Manhattan area, the company operates approximately 247 drug stores in commercial and residential neighborhoods throughout New York, with 87 in New York's outer boroughs and densely populated suburbs. The purchase of the Rock Bottom and Value Drug chains strengthened Duane Reade's presence in Manhattan, making it the most recognized drug store chain in metropolitan New York. The company's stores are small and tightly packed. Products and services offered include prescription and over-the-counter medications, vitamins, food and beverages, health aids, beauty products, greeting cards and photo processing. Duane Reade's extensive network of conveniently located pharmacies, strong local market position, pricing policies and reputation for high-quality health care products and services provide it with a competitive advantage in attracting pharmacy business from individual customers as well as managed care organizations, insurance companies and employers. The company's pharmacies employ computer systems that link all Duane Reade stores and enable them to provide customers with a broad range of services. The firm's pharmacy computer network profiles customer medical and other relevant information, supplies customers with information concerning their drug purchases for income tax and insurance purposes and prepares prescription labels and receipts. The firm has consolidated its distribution infrastructure into one mammoth 500,000-square-foot center in Queens, New York. Duane Reade plans to continue expansion with as many as 50 new stores planned in 2005, furthering entry into markets other than Manhattan. In August 2004, Duane Reade was acquired by the private equity firm Oak Hill Capital Partners for approximately $700 million.

FINANCIALS:
Sales and profits are in thousands of dollars—add 000 to get the full amount. Year 2004 note: Complete fiscal 2004 results were not available for all companies at press time. For this company, year 2004 is for 6 months.

2004 Sales: $714,756 (6 months)   2004 Profits: $4,324 (6 months)
2003 Sales: $1,383,828   2003 Profits: $5,074
2002 Sales: $1,274,500   2002 Profits: $15,600
2001 Sales: $1,143,600   2001 Profits: $24,700
2000 Sales: $1,000,068   2000 Profits: $22,676

Stock Ticker: DRD
Employees: 6,100
Fiscal Year Ends: 12/31

SALARIES/BENEFITS:
Pension Plan:	ESOP Stock Plan:	Profit Sharing:	Top Exec. Salary: $750,000	Bonus: $1,500,000
Savings Plan: Y	Stock Purch. Plan:		Second Exec. Salary: $330,000	Bonus: $396,000

OTHER THOUGHTS:
Apparent Top Female Officers: 2
Hot Spot for Advancement for Women/Minorities:

LOCATIONS: ("Y" = Yes)
West:	Southwest:	Midwest:	Southeast:	Northeast:	International:
				Y	

DYNACQ HEALTHCARE INC

www.dynacq.com

Industry Group Code: 621490　　Ranks within this company's industry group: Sales: 14　Profits: 6

Insurance/HMO/PPO:	Drugs:	Equipment/Supplies:	Hospitals/Clinics:		Services:		Health Care:	
Insurance:	Manufacturer:	Manufacturer:	Acute Care:	Y	Diagnostics:		Home Health:	
Managed Care:	Distributor:	Distributor:	Sub-Acute Care:		Labs/Testing:		Long-Term Care:	
Utilization Mgmt.:	Specialty Pharm.:	Leasing/Finance:	Outpatient Surgery:	Y	Staffing:		Physical Therapy:	
Payment Proc.:	Vitamins/Nutri.:	Information Sys.:	Phys. Rehab. Center:		Waste Disposal:		Phys. Practice Mgmt.:	Y
	Clinical Trials:		Psychiatric Clinics:		Specialty Services:	Y		

TYPES OF BUSINESS:
Emergency & Inpatient Surgery Facilities
Outpatient Surgery Facilities
Acute Care Hospital

BRANDS/DIVISIONS/AFFILIATES:
Dynacq International, Inc.
Vista Medical Center Hospital
Vista Fertility Institute

CONTACTS: Note: Officers with more than one job title may be intentionally listed here more than once.
Chiu Moon Chan, CEO
Chiu Moon Chan, Pres.
Philip S. Chan, VP/CFO
Tammy Danberg-Farney, Exec. VP/General Counsel
Richard D. Valentine, VP-Oper.
James N. Baxter, Exec. VP-Investor Rel.
Philip S. Chan, Treas.
Christina L. Gutel-Williams, Sr. Staff Attorney-Reimbursement
Chiu Moon Chan, Chmn.

Phone: 713-378-2000	Fax: 713-673-6432
Toll-Free:	
Address: 10304 Interstate 10 E., Ste. 369, Pasadena, TX 77029 US	

GROWTH PLANS/SPECIAL FEATURES:
Dynacq Healthcare, Inc., formerly Dynacq International, Inc., is a hospital holding company that, through its subsidiaries, develops and manages general acute hospitals providing specialized general surgeries. The firm does not operate any of its hospitals or medical facilities, but has management contracts with various subsidiaries and affiliates. These facilities include a central surgical campus in Pasadena, Texas, which is home to Vista Medical Center Hospital; a surgery center in Houston; a surgical hospital in Dallas; and one in Baton Rouge, Louisiana. Each includes operating rooms, pre- and post-operative space, intensive care units, nursing units and modern diagnostic facilities, and is designed to handle complex orthopedic and general surgeries, such as spine and bariatric surgeries. The Houston facility also houses the Vista Fertility Institute, which provides invitro fertilization services to couples. In addition to these, Dynacq plans to construct new hospitals in the Woodlands, Texas and Shanghai, China. In October 2004, the subsidiary that operates the Baton Rouge facility filed for bankruptcy protection, continuing to operate as a debtor in possession.

FINANCIALS:
Sales and profits are in thousands of dollars—add 000 to get the full amount. Year 2004 note: Complete fiscal 2004 results were not available for all companies at press time. For this company, year 2004 is for 9 months.

2004 Sales: $47,921 (9 months)	2004 Profits: $1,070 (9 months)	
2003 Sales: $90,000	2003 Profits: $21,000	Stock Ticker: DYII
2002 Sales: $64,900	2002 Profits: $15,400	Employees: 338
2001 Sales: $43,800	2001 Profits: $11,100	Fiscal Year Ends: 8/31
2000 Sales: $26,000	2000 Profits: $5,900	

SALARIES/BENEFITS:
Pension Plan:	ESOP Stock Plan:	Profit Sharing:	Top Exec. Salary: $180,000	Bonus: $50,000
Savings Plan: Y	Stock Purch. Plan:		Second Exec. Salary: $180,000	Bonus: $11,000

OTHER THOUGHTS:
Apparent Top Female Officers: 2
Hot Spot for Advancement for Women/Minorities:

LOCATIONS: ("Y" = Yes)
West:	Southwest:	Midwest:	Southeast:	Northeast:	International:
	Y		Y		Y

Plunkett's Health Care Industry Almanac 2005 — 353

ECLIPSYS CORPORATION

www.eclipsys.com

Industry Group Code: 511200 **Ranks within this company's industry group:** Sales: 5 Profits: 12

Insurance/HMO/PPO:	Drugs:	Equipment/Supplies:	Hospitals/Clinics:	Services:	Health Care:
Insurance:	Manufacturer:	Manufacturer:	Acute Care:	Diagnostics:	Home Health:
Managed Care:	Distributor:	Distributor:	Sub-Acute Care:	Labs/Testing:	Long-Term Care:
Utilization Mgmt.:	Specialty Pharm.:	Leasing/Finance:	Outpatient Surgery:	Staffing:	Physical Therapy:
Payment Proc.:	Vitamins/Nutri.:	Information Sys.: Y	Phys. Rehab. Center:	Waste Disposal:	Phys. Practice Mgmt.:
	Clinical Trials:		Psychiatric Clinics:	Specialty Services: Y	

TYPES OF BUSINESS:
Computer Software
Health Care IT Products and Services

BRANDS/DIVISIONS/AFFILIATES:
SunriseXA
Sunrise Clinical Manager
Sunrise Access Manager
Sunrise Patient Financial Manager
Sunrise Decision Support Manager
Sunrise Record Manager
eWebIT

CONTACTS: Note: Officers with more than one job title may be intentionally listed here more than once.
Paul L. Ruflin, CEO
Paul L. Ruflin, Pres.
John Patton, COO
Robert J. Colletti, Sr. VP/CFO
John Cooper, Exec. VP-Sales & Mktg.
Steven Kinderman, Sr. VP-Human Resources
Richard P. Mansour, Chief Medical Officer
John Gomez, Sr. VP/Chief Tech. Officer
Hans Boerma, VP-Product Solutions
Brent A. Friedman, VP/General Counsel
Michael B. Kaufman, Exec. VP-Corp. Dev.
John Depierro, Exec. VP
Russ J. Rudish, Exec. VP-Services
Mike Etue, Sr. VP-Implementation & Customer Support
Frank Stearns, Sr. VP-Consulting Services
Eugene V. Fife, Chmn.

Phone: 561-322-4321   **Fax:** 561-322-4320
Toll-Free:
Address: 1750 Clint Moore Rd., Boca Raton, FL 33487 US

GROWTH PLANS/SPECIAL FEATURES:
Eclipsys Corporation is a health care information technology company that develops and licenses its proprietary software to hospitals. The company's applications, which are installed in over 1,500 hospitals, are available for implementation on-site or through its remote hosting service. In addition, Eclipsys offers complementary services to its customers, including implementation, integration, support, maintenance and training. The company's flagship is the SunriseXA line of products, which includes Sunrise Clinical Manager, Sunrise Access Manager, Sunrise Patient Financial Manager, Sunrise Decision Support Manager, Sunrise Record Manager and eWebIT. This software allows hospitals to automate many of the key clinical, administrative and financial functions that they require, letting them admit patients, maintain patient records, create invoices for billing, control inventories, effect cost accounting, schedule doctor's visits and understand the profitability of specific medical procedures. It also enables physicians and nurses to check on a patient's condition, order tests, review test results, monitor a patient's medications and provide alerts to changes in a patient's condition.

The company offers its employees medical, dental, disability and life insurance.

FINANCIALS: Sales and profits are in thousands of dollars—add 000 to get the full amount. Year 2004 note: Complete fiscal 2004 results were not available for all companies at press time. For this company, year 2004 is for 9 months.

2004 Sales: $221,842 (9 months)   2004 Profits: $-29,674 (9 months)
2003 Sales: $254,679   2003 Profits: $-55,964
2002 Sales: $218,068   2002 Profits: $-29,763
2001 Sales: $239,676   2001 Profits: $4,408
2000 Sales: $ 2000 Profits: $

Stock Ticker: ECLP
Employees: 1,877
Fiscal Year Ends: 12/31

SALARIES/BENEFITS:
Pension Plan: ESOP Stock Plan: Profit Sharing: Top Exec. Salary: $750,000   Bonus: $75,000
Savings Plan: Y   Stock Purch. Plan: Second Exec. Salary: $375,000   Bonus: $25,000

OTHER THOUGHTS:
Apparent Top Female Officers:
Hot Spot for Advancement for Women/Minorities:

LOCATIONS: ("Y" = Yes)

West:	Southwest:	Midwest:	Southeast:	Northeast:	International:
Y	Y	Y	Y	Y	Y

Note: Financial information, benefits and other data can change quickly and may vary from those stated here.

EDWARDS LIFESCIENCES CORP
www.edwards.com

Industry Group Code: 339113 Ranks within this company's industry group: Sales: 31 Profits: 21

Insurance/HMO/PPO:	Drugs:	Equipment/Supplies:	Hospitals/Clinics:	Services:	Health Care:
Insurance:	Manufacturer:	Manufacturer: Y	Acute Care:	Diagnostics:	Home Health:
Managed Care:	Distributor:	Distributor:	Sub-Acute Care:	Labs/Testing:	Long-Term Care:
Utilization Mgmt.:	Specialty Pharm.:	Leasing/Finance:	Outpatient Surgery:	Staffing:	Physical Therapy:
Payment Proc.:	Vitamins/Nutri.:	Information Sys.:	Phys. Rehab. Center:	Waste Disposal:	Phys. Practice Mgmt.:
	Clinical Trials:		Psychiatric Clinics:	Specialty Services:	

TYPES OF BUSINESS:
Supplies-Cardiovascular Disease Related
Cardiac Surgery Products
Critical Care Products
Vascular Products

BRANDS/DIVISIONS/AFFILIATES:
Carpentier-Edwards
Cosgrove-Edwards
Swan-Ganz
Lifepath AAA
Fogarty
XenoLogiX
Advanced Venous Access
AVA 3Xi

CONTACTS: Note: Officers with more than one job title may be intentionally listed here more than once.
Michael A. Mussallem, CEO
Corinne H. Lyle, Corp. VP/CFO
Stuart L. Foster, Corp. VP-Tech. & Discovery
Corinne H. Lyle, Treas.
Anita Bessler, Corp. VP-Global Franchise Mgmt.
Michael A. Mussallem, Chmn.
Andre-Michel Ballester, Corp. VP-Europe & Intercontinental

Phone: 949-250-2500 Fax: 949-250-2525
Toll-Free:
Address: One Edwards Way, Irvine, CA 92614 US

GROWTH PLANS/SPECIAL FEATURES:
Edwards Lifesciences is an international leader in providing products and services for patients with cardiovascular disease. The firm designs products for four main cardiovascular diseases: heart valve disease, coronary artery disease, peripheral vascular disease and congestive heart failure. Its products and technologies are categorized into four main areas: cardiac surgery, critical care, vascular and perfusion. Products in the cardiac surgery category include tissue heart valves and repair products manufactured under several private labels, including Carpentier-Edwards and Cosgrove-Edwards. The company's critical care line of products includes hemodynamic monitoring devices, which are used for measuring heart pressure and output during surgery, under the Swan-Ganz brand name. Edwards additionally markets a range of products required to perform hemofiltration, such as access catheters, filters and solutions. The critical care line also consists of central venous catheters, including the firm's Advanced Venous Access, AVA HF and AVA 3Xi devices. Vascular products include balloon-tipped, catheter-based products, surgical clips and inserts. Edwards developed the Lifepath AAA endovascular graft system to treat potentially life-threatening abdominal aortic aneurysms. The company has sold its U.S. perfusion services operation to Fresenuis Medical Care A.G., although it still maintains a small perfusion services operation in Europe. The firm's products and services are supplied throughout the world via direct sales and distributor relationships with several companies, including Baxter International. In recent news, the company announced the acquisition of technology and intellectual property from ev3, Inc., mainly a percutaneous mitral valve repair program, for $15 million.

The company offers its employees medical, dental, life and vision insurance; health care reimbursement plans; dependent care reimbursement plans; and employee assistance programs. Benefits vary by country location.

FINANCIALS: Sales and profits are in thousands of dollars—add 000 to get the full amount. Year 2004 note: Complete fiscal 2004 results were not available for all companies at press time. For this company, year 2004 is for 9 months.

2004 Sales: $694,400 (9 months)   2004 Profits: $-24,200 (9 months)
2003 Sales: $860,500   2003 Profits: $79,000   Stock Ticker: EW
2002 Sales: $704,000   2002 Profits: $55,700   Employees: 5,000
2001 Sales: $692,000   2001 Profits: $-11,000   Fiscal Year Ends: 12/31
2000 Sales: $804,000   2000 Profits: $-272,000

SALARIES/BENEFITS:
Pension Plan: ESOP Stock Plan: Profit Sharing: Top Exec. Salary: $664,615   Bonus: $356,440
Savings Plan: Y   Stock Purch. Plan: Y   Second Exec. Salary: $360,962   Bonus: $122,360

OTHER THOUGHTS:
Apparent Top Female Officers: 2
Hot Spot for Advancement for Women/Minorities:

LOCATIONS: ("Y" = Yes)
West:	Southwest:	Midwest:	Southeast:	Northeast:	International:
Y			Y		Y

Plunkett's Health Care Industry Almanac 2005   355

ELAN CORP PLC   www.elan.com

Industry Group Code: 325412   Ranks within this company's industry group: Sales: 30   Profits: 41

Insurance/HMO/PPO:	Drugs:		Equipment/Supplies:	Hospitals/Clinics:	Services:	Health Care:
Insurance:	Manufacturer:	Y	Manufacturer:	Acute Care:	Diagnostics:	Home Health:
Managed Care:	Distributor:		Distributor:	Sub-Acute Care:	Labs/Testing:	Long-Term Care:
Utilization Mgmt.:	Specialty Pharm.:		Leasing/Finance:	Outpatient Surgery:	Staffing:	Physical Therapy:
Payment Proc.:	Vitamins/Nutri.:		Information Sys.:	Phys. Rehab. Center:	Waste Disposal:	Phys. Practice Mgmt.:
	Clinical Trials:			Psychiatric Clinics:	Specialty Services:	

TYPES OF BUSINESS:
Drugs-Neurology
Acute Care Drugs
Pain Management Drugs
Autoimmune Disease Drugs
Drug Delivery Technologies

BRANDS/DIVISIONS/AFFILIATES:
Antegren
Zonegran
Prialt

CONTACTS: Note: Officers with more than one job title may be intentionally listed here more than once.
Kelly Martin, CEO
Kelly Martin, Pres.
Shane Cooke, Exec. VP/CFO
Lars Ekman, Exec. VP/Pres.-R&D
Jean Duvall, Exec. VP/General Counsel
Paul Breen, VP-Oper.
Arthur Falk, VP-Corp. Compliance
Jack Laflin, Exec. VP-Global Core Services
William Daniel, Corp. Sec.
Garo Armen, Chmn.

Phone: 353-1-709-4000   Fax: 353-662-4949
Toll-Free: 866-347-3185
Address: Lincoln House, Lincoln Place, Dublin, D2 Ireland

GROWTH PLANS/SPECIAL FEATURES:
Elan Corporation, a leading global specialty pharmaceutical company, focuses on the discovery, development and marketing of therapeutic products and services in neurology, acute care and pain management. The firm also develops and commercializes products through the its extensive range of proprietary drug delivery technologies. The Irish company conducts its worldwide business through subsidiaries incorporated in Ireland, the United States, the United Kingdom and other countries. Elan is focusing its research and development on Alzheimer's disease, Parkinson's disease, multiple sclerosis, pain management and autoimmune diseases. The company uses its proprietary technologies and multidisciplinary expertise to develop, market and license drug delivery products to its pharmaceutical clients. It has developed three novel therapeutic approaches in its breakthrough research program in Alzheimer's disease: immunotherapy and beta and gamma secretase inhibitors. In collaboration with Biogen, Inc., Elan has under development certain neurologic, autoimmune and pain products including a humanized monoclonal antibody, Antegren (natalizumab), for use in multiple sclerosis and Crohn's disease. Its core pipeline is comprised of four products: Antegren, Prialt (for severe chronic pain), Zonegran (anti-epileptic for migraine and mania) and ELN-154088 (for pain). Elan recently announced an agreement with Eisai Co., Ltd. for the purchase of Elan's interests in Zonegran (zonisamide) in North America and Europe. In addition, Biogen Idec and Elan intend to submit an application for approval of Antegren as a treatment for multiple sclerosis to the European Agency for the Evaluation of Medicinal Products in the summer of 2004.
Elan offers employees a total compensation package competitive with similar biotechnology and pharmaceutical companies. Benefits include medical care, life insurance, annual paid leave and educational assistance. Details vary by country.

FINANCIALS:
Sales and profits are in thousands of dollars—add 000 to get the full amount. Year 2004 note: Complete fiscal 2004 results were not available for all companies at press time. For this company, year 2004 is for 3 months.

2004 Sales: $159,000   (3 months)   2004 Profits: $-67,100   (3 months)
2003 Sales: $746,000   2003 Profits: $-529,400   Stock Ticker: Foreign
2002 Sales: $1,470,100   2002 Profits: $-2,394,800   Employees: 4,377
2001 Sales: $1,512,900   2001 Profits: $-887,200   Fiscal Year Ends: 12/31
2000 Sales: $1,302,000   2000 Profits: $-294,500

SALARIES/BENEFITS:
Pension Plan: Y   ESOP Stock Plan: Profit Sharing: Top Exec. Salary: $520,000   Bonus: $640,000
Savings Plan: Y   Stock Purch. Plan: Y   Second Exec. Salary: $395,000   Bonus: $500,000

OTHER THOUGHTS:
Apparent Top Female Officers: 1
Hot Spot for Advancement for Women/Minorities:

LOCATIONS: ("Y" = Yes)
West:	Southwest:	Midwest:	Southeast:	Northeast:	International:
Y	Y	Y	Y	Y	Y

Note: Financial information, benefits and other data can change quickly and may vary from those stated here.

ELI LILLY & CO

www.lilly.com

Industry Group Code: 325412 **Ranks within this company's industry group:** Sales: 11 Profits: 8

Insurance/HMO/PPO:	Drugs:		Equipment/Supplies:		Hospitals/Clinics:	Services:		Health Care:
Insurance:	Manufacturer:	Y	Manufacturer:	Y	Acute Care:	Diagnostics:		Home Health:
Managed Care:	Distributor:		Distributor:		Sub-Acute Care:	Labs/Testing:		Long-Term Care:
Utilization Mgmt.: Y	Specialty Pharm.:		Leasing/Finance:		Outpatient Surgery:	Staffing:		Physical Therapy:
Payment Proc.: Y	Vitamins/Nutri.:	Y	Information Sys.:	Y	Phys. Rehab. Center:	Waste Disposal:		Phys. Practice Mgmt.:
	Clinical Trials:	Y			Psychiatric Clinics:	Specialty Services:	Y	

TYPES OF BUSINESS:
Drugs-Manufacturing
Computer-Based Prescription Drug Claims Processing
Pharmacy Benefit Design
Administration & Management Services
Disease Management Services
Animal Health Products
Vitamins
Medical Communication Networks

BRANDS/DIVISIONS/AFFILIATES:
PCS Health Systems
Integrated Medical Systems, Inc.
Prozac
InnoCentive, LLC

CONTACTS:
Note: Officers with more than one job title may be intentionally listed here more than once.

Sidney Taurel, CEO
Sidney Taurel, Pres.
Charles E. Golden, Exec. VP/CFO
Alfonso Zulueta, VP-Mktg. & Sales
Steven Paul, Exec. VP-Science & Tech.
W. Roy Dunbar, CIO
Scott Canute, VP-Mfg.
Robert A. Armitage, General Counsel
John Lechleiter, VP-Pharmaceutical Oper.
Alpheus Bingham, VP-Lilly Research Strategy
Anne Nobles, VP-Corp. Affairs
Alan Brier, VP-Medical/Chief Medical Officer
Bryce Carmine, Pres., Primary Care Products
Lori Queisser, VP/Chief Compliance Officer
Elizabeth Klimes, Pres., Specialty Care Products
Sidney Taurel, Chmn.

Phone: 317-276-2000   **Fax:** 317-277-6579
Toll-Free: 800-545-5979
Address: Lilly Corporate Center, Drop Code 1112, Indianapolis, IN 46285-0001 US

GROWTH PLANS/SPECIAL FEATURES:
Eli Lilly and Company develops, manufactures and sells pharmaceutical products. Through PCS Health Systems, the company provides prescription benefit management services in the U.S., employing more than 35,000 people worldwide. The company markets its medicines in 140 countries, with additional major research and development facilities in nine countries. Eli Lilly, which conducts clinical trials in more than 30 countries, has annual research and development expenses of over $2 billion. The firm also owns Integrated Medical Systems, Inc., which develops and operates physician-focused medical communication networks. Eli Lily's Prozac is the most widely prescribed, branded antidepressant worldwide. The company's products include central nervous system agents, anti-infectives, endocrine products, an anti-ulcer agent, oncolytic agents, cardiovascular therapy products, sedatives and vitamins. Eli Lilly's separate e-business venture, InnoCentive, LLC, uses the Internet to create and enhance open-source scientific research and development. During 2002, CEO Sidney Taurel chose to accept an annual salary of $1.00 as a reflection of his confidence in and commitment to the company. Had Mr. Taurel not taken this action, his base salary would have been $1,391,100 for 2002. Also, Eli Lilly recently announced it will donate $6 million to the Oklahoma Medical Research Foundation (OMRF). OMRF will use the gift to create a pair of endowed faculty chairs, the Eli Lilly Chairs in Biomedical Research. The company has been named as one of Fortune's 100 Best Companies to Work for in America and was named to Working Mother magazine's list of the 100 best companies for working mothers in the United States for the eighth consecutive year.

Eli Lilly offers its employees health insurance, domestic partner benefits and an employee assistance program, as well as one week of vacation when they get married and up to 10 weeks of paid maternity leave. The firm also offers an on-site fitness center, flexible hours or telecommuting, parenting and dependant care leaves, adoption assistance and tuition reimbursement.

FINANCIALS:
Sales and profits are in thousands of dollars—add 000 to get the full amount. Year 2004 note: Complete fiscal 2004 results were not available for all companies at press time. For this company, year 2004 is for 9 months.

2004 Sales: $10,213,600 (9 months)   2004 Profits: $1,812,500 (9 months)
2003 Sales: $12,582,500   2003 Profits: $2,560,800
2002 Sales: $11,078,000   2002 Profits: $2,708,000
2001 Sales: $11,542,000   2001 Profits: $2,780,000
2000 Sales: $10,862,200   2000 Profits: $3,057,800

Stock Ticker: LLY
Employees: 46,100
Fiscal Year Ends: 12/31

SALARIES/BENEFITS:
Pension Plan: Y   ESOP Stock Plan: Profit Sharing: Top Exec. Salary: $1,432,860   Bonus: $1,193,595
Savings Plan: Y   Stock Purch. Plan: Second Exec. Salary: $858,510   Bonus: $490,118

OTHER THOUGHTS:
Apparent Top Female Officers: 3
Hot Spot for Advancement for Women/Minorities: Y

LOCATIONS: ("Y" = Yes)
West:	Southwest:	Midwest:	Southeast:	Northeast:	International:
Y	Y	Y	Y	Y	Y

Note: Financial information, benefits and other data can change quickly and may vary from those stated here.

EMERGENCY FILTRATION PRODUCTS INC

www.emergencyfiltration.com

Industry Group Code: 339113   Ranks within this company's industry group: Sales: 135   Profits: 109

Insurance/HMO/PPO:	Drugs:	Equipment/Supplies:	Hospitals/Clinics:	Services:	Health Care:
Insurance: Managed Care: Utilization Mgmt.: Payment Proc.:	Manufacturer: Distributor: Specialty Pharm.: Vitamins/Nutri.: Clinical Trials:	Manufacturer: Distributor: Leasing/Finance: Information Sys.: Y	Acute Care: Sub-Acute Care: Outpatient Surgery: Phys. Rehab. Center: Psychiatric Clinics:	Diagnostics: Labs/Testing: Staffing: Waste Disposal: Specialty Services:	Home Health: Long-Term Care: Physical Therapy: Phys. Practice Mgmt.:

TYPES OF BUSINESS:
Medical Equipment
Filtration Products

BRANDS/DIVISIONS/AFFILIATES:
Nanomask
RespAide
Superstat

CONTACTS:
Note: Officers with more than one job title may be intentionally listed here more than once.

Sherman Lazrus, Interim CEO
Douglas K. Beplate, Pres.
Steve M. Hanni, CFO
Peter Clark, Treas.

Phone: 702-558-5164   Fax: 702-567-1893
Toll-Free:
Address: 175 Cassia Way, Ste. A115, Henderson, NV 89014-6643 US

GROWTH PLANS/SPECIAL FEATURES:
Emergency Filtration is a specialty filter products company that has developed a state-of-the-art air filtration technology for removing infectious bacteria and viruses in air flow systems. The company's RespAide dual-filtered vapor isolation valve (VIV) technology is currently being marketed in CPR isolation masks to protect emergency response personnel against infectious diseases during mouth-to-mouth resuscitation. The same filter used in the RespAide product is ideal for reducing the risk of exposure to viruses and bacteria and equipment contamination during the use of bag valve mask (BVM) resuscitation devices. The company also markets Superstat, a product that provides rapid, safe, effective surgical clotting of the blood for surgery, trauma and burn wound management. Another configuration of the firm's technology is a personal environmental mask designed to address concerns of biological contamination in a workplace or other environment. The mask possesses a disposable filter and an enhanced matrix of charged nanoparticles designed to protect the user from possible inhalation of biological contaminants. Emergency Filtration has introduced two new configurations of its technology, a one-way and a two-way breathing circuit filter for applications where ambient air flow must pass evenly in both directions while still protecting equipment and hoses. The filters are used inline with circuitry, hoses and anesthesia, ventilation and respiratory equipment. The use of the filter serves to remove viruses and bacteria from the airflow, control the moisture delivered to the patient and keep equipment contaminant-free. The company has also designed a self-contained device that delivers medicine in aerosol form and a bag with built-in $CO(2)$ monitoring capabilities. In recent news, Emergency Filtration announced the mass marketing of its Nanomask personal filtration system, which is effective against SARS, to China and Taiwan.

FINANCIALS:
Sales and profits are in thousands of dollars—add 000 to get the full amount. Year 2004 note: Complete fiscal 2004 results were not available for all companies at press time. For this company, year 2004 is for 6 months.

2004 Sales: $ 325 (6 months)   2004 Profits: $- 515   (6 months)
2003 Sales: $ 764   2003 Profits: $- 706
2002 Sales: $ 260   2002 Profits: $-1,141
2001 Sales: $ 461   2001 Profits: $-1,123
2000 Sales: $ 2000 Profits: $

Stock Ticker: EMFP
Employees: 4
Fiscal Year Ends: 12/31

SALARIES/BENEFITS:
Pension Plan: ESOP Stock Plan: Profit Sharing: Top Exec. Salary: $96,000   Bonus: $111,000
Savings Plan: Stock Purch. Plan: Second Exec. Salary: $96,000   Bonus: $34,300

OTHER THOUGHTS:
Apparent Top Female Officers:
Hot Spot for Advancement for Women/Minorities:

LOCATIONS: ("Y" = Yes)
West:	Southwest:	Midwest:	Southeast:	Northeast:	International:
Y					Y

EMERGING VISION INC

www.sterlingoptical.com

Industry Group Code: 446130   Ranks within this company's industry group: Sales: 3   Profits: 1

Insurance/HMO/PPO:	Drugs:	Equipment/Supplies:	Hospitals/Clinics:	Services:	Health Care:
Insurance:	Manufacturer:	Manufacturer: Y	Acute Care:	Diagnostics:	Home Health:
Managed Care: Y	Distributor:	Distributor:	Sub-Acute Care:	Labs/Testing:	Long-Term Care:
Utilization Mgmt.:	Specialty Pharm.:	Leasing/Finance:	Outpatient Surgery:	Staffing:	Physical Therapy:
Payment Proc.:	Vitamins/Nutri.:	Information Sys.:	Phys. Rehab. Center:	Waste Disposal:	Phys. Practice Mgmt.:
	Clinical Trials:		Psychiatric Clinics:	Specialty Services: Y	

TYPES OF BUSINESS:
Eyeglasses & Related Products, Retail
Franchise Operations
Group Vision Plan

BRANDS/DIVISIONS/AFFILIATES:
Sterling Optical
Sterling Vision
Site For Sore Eyes
VisionCare of California, Inc.
Duling Optical
Singer Specs
Insight Managed Vision Care

CONTACTS:
Note: Officers with more than one job title may be intentionally listed here more than once.

Christopher G. Payan, Co-COO
Christopher G. Payan, CFO
Samuel Z. Herskowitz, Chief Mktg. Officer
Myles Lewis, Co-COO/Sr. VP-Bus. Dev.
Nicholas Shashati, Pres., VisionCare of California, Inc.
Christopher G. Payan, Corp. Sec.
Samuel Z. Herskowitz, Co-COO
Alan Cohen, Chmn.

Phone: 516-390-2100   Fax: 516-390-2190
Toll-Free:
Address: 100 Quentin Roosevelt Blvd., Ste. 508, Garden City, NY 11530 US

GROWTH PLANS/SPECIAL FEATURES:
Emerging Vision, Inc., formerly Sterling Vision, is one of the largest chains of retail optical stores and the fastest-growing optical franchise in the industry. The company and its franchises develop and operate retail optical stores principally under such trade names as Sterling Optical, Site for Sore Eyes, Duling Optical and Singer Specs. The firm also operates VisionCare of California, Inc. (VCC), a specialized health care maintenance organization. VCC employs licensed optometrists who render services in offices located immediately adjacent to, or within, most Sterling stores located in California. Currently, there are over 172 stores in operation in 20 states, the District of Columbia, Canada and the U.S. Virgin Islands. Most Sterling stores offer eye care products and services such as prescription and non-prescription eyeglasses, eyeglass frames, ophthalmic lenses, contact lenses, sunglasses and a broad range of ancillary items. Emerging Vision also fills prescriptions from its own or affiliated optometrists, as well as from unaffiliated optometrists and ophthalmologists. Most Sterling stores have an inventory of ophthalmic and contact lenses, as well as on-site lab equipment for cutting and edging ophthalmic lenses to fit into eyeglass frames. In many cases, the stores offer same-day service. The company also offers four simple vision tests online to help customers identify possible vision problems that they can then discuss with an eye care professional. Emerging Vision also owns and manages an exclusive group vision plan, Insight Managed Vision Care. Under the plan, the company contracts with payors that offer eye care benefits to their covered participants and offers discounted prices to members of the plan.

FINANCIALS:
Sales and profits are in thousands of dollars—add 000 to get the full amount. Year 2004 note: Complete fiscal 2004 results were not available for all companies at press time. For this company, year 2004 is for 6 months.

2004 Sales: $7,387 (6 months)   2004 Profits: $683 (6 months)
2003 Sales: $13,980   2003 Profits: $-2,967
2002 Sales: $17,400   2002 Profits: $-4,600
2001 Sales: $20,600   2001 Profits: $-3,800
2000 Sales: $23,058   2000 Profits: $-38,992

Stock Ticker: ISEE
Employees: 132
Fiscal Year Ends: 12/31

SALARIES/BENEFITS:
Pension Plan: ESOP Stock Plan: Profit Sharing: Top Exec. Salary: $175,000   Bonus: $26,000
Savings Plan: Stock Purch. Plan: Second Exec. Salary: $156,000   Bonus: $26,000

OTHER THOUGHTS:
Apparent Top Female Officers:
Hot Spot for Advancement for Women/Minorities:

LOCATIONS: ("Y" = Yes)
West:	Southwest:	Midwest:	Southeast:	Northeast:	International:
Y	Y	Y	Y	Y	Y

EMERITUS CORP

www.emeritus.com

Industry Group Code: 623110 **Ranks within this company's industry group:** Sales: 10 Profits: 9

Insurance/HMO/PPO:	Drugs:	Equipment/Supplies:	Hospitals/Clinics:	Services:	Health Care:
Insurance: Managed Care: Utilization Mgmt.: Payment Proc.:	Manufacturer: Distributor: Specialty Pharm.: Vitamins/Nutri.: Clinical Trials:	Manufacturer: Distributor: Leasing/Finance: Information Sys.:	Acute Care: Sub-Acute Care: Outpatient Surgery: Phys. Rehab. Center: Psychiatric Clinics:	Diagnostics: Labs/Testing: Staffing: Waste Disposal: Specialty Services:	Home Health: Long-Term Care: Y Physical Therapy: Phys. Practice Mgmt.:

TYPES OF BUSINESS:
Long-Term Health Care
Assisted Living Communities

BRANDS/DIVISIONS/AFFILIATES:

CONTACTS:
Note: Officers with more than one job title may be intentionally listed here more than once.

Daniel R. Baty, CEO
Kellie Murray, Dir.-Human Resources
Frank A. Ruffo, VP-Admin.
Gary S. Becker, Sr. VP-Oper.
Martin D. Roffe, VP-Financial Planning
Raymond R. Brandstorm, VP-Finance
Russell G. Kubik, VP-Oper., Central Div.
Suzette McCanless, VP-Oper., Eastern Div.
Peter K. Kang, VP-Oper., Western Div.
Susan Scherr, VP-Signature Services
Daniel R. Baty, Chmn.

Phone: 206-298-2909 **Fax:** 206-301-4500
Toll-Free: 800-429-4828
Address: 3131 Elliott Ave., Ste. 500, Seattle, WA 98121 US

GROWTH PLANS/SPECIAL FEATURES:

Emeritus Corp. is a leading provider of retirement and assisted living services for senior citizens worldwide, with an interest in 180 communities located across 33 states, totaling approximately 14,845 units with a total capacity for 18,208 residents. These communities offer an alternative to residential housing for senior citizens who need help with the activities of daily living. Emeritus residents are typically unable to live independently but do not require the intensive care provided in skilled nursing facilities. Under the company's approach, seniors reside in a private or semi-private residential unit for a monthly fee based on each resident's individual service needs. The firm believes its residential assisted living communities allow seniors to maintain a more independent lifestyle than is possible in the institutional environment of skilled nursing facilities, while still receiving assistance with activities of daily living they would not otherwise receive at independent living facilities. Emeritus offers three tiers of service to its occupants. All residents receive the basic level, which includes restaurant-style meals, a full-time activity program, scheduled transportation to off-site activities and appointments, laundry service and 24-hour emergency response. Enhanced living services apply to those individuals who need more frequent or intensive assistance or increased care or supervision, including daily assistance with bathing, dressing and grooming, medication management, dining assistance/special diets, assistance with reminders and redirection, diabetic management, respiratory care, grooming assistance, behavior management and individualized treatment depending on need. The special care program is for Alzheimer's and related dementia patients and is designed to meet the specialized medical, psychological and social needs of those residents affected by such conditions.

FINANCIALS:
Sales and profits are in thousands of dollars—add 000 to get the full amount. Year 2004 note: Complete fiscal 2004 results were not available for all companies at press time. For this company, year 2004 is for 6 months.

2004 Sales: $145,253 (6 months)	2004 Profits: $-2,625 (6 months)	**Stock Ticker:** ESC
2003 Sales: $206,657	2003 Profits: $-3,825	**Employees:** 7,500
2002 Sales: $153,100	2002 Profits: $-6,200	**Fiscal Year Ends:** 12/31
2001 Sales: $140,600	2001 Profits: $-4,200	
2000 Sales: $125,200	2000 Profits: $-21,900	

SALARIES/BENEFITS:
Pension Plan: ESOP Stock Plan: Profit Sharing: Top Exec. Salary: $197,783 Bonus: $65,000
Savings Plan: Y Stock Purch. Plan: Y Second Exec. Salary: $194,750 Bonus: $65,000

OTHER THOUGHTS:
Apparent Top Female Officers: 3
Hot Spot for Advancement for Women/Minorities: Y

LOCATIONS: ("Y" = Yes)

West:	Southwest:	Midwest:	Southeast:	Northeast:	International:
Y	Y	Y	Y	Y	

EMPI INC

www.empi.com

Industry Group Code: 339113 **Ranks within this company's industry group:** Sales: 71 Profits: 64

Insurance/HMO/PPO:	Drugs:	Equipment/Supplies:		Hospitals/Clinics:		Services:	Health Care:
Insurance:	Manufacturer:	Manufacturer:	Y	Acute Care:		Diagnostics:	Home Health:
Managed Care:	Distributor:	Distributor:	Y	Sub-Acute Care:		Labs/Testing:	Long-Term Care:
Utilization Mgmt.:	Specialty Pharm.:	Leasing/Finance:		Outpatient Surgery:		Staffing:	Physical Therapy:
Payment Proc.:	Vitamins/Nutri.:	Information Sys.:		Phys. Rehab. Center:		Waste Disposal:	Phys. Practice Mgmt.:
	Clinical Trials:			Psychiatric Clinics:		Specialty Services:	

TYPES OF BUSINESS:
Medical Device Manufacturing
Pain Management Products
Tissue Rehabilitation Products
Incontinence Products
Clinic Supplies

BRANDS/DIVISIONS/AFFILIATES:
Encore Medical Corporation
Epix VT
Dupel Iontophoresis System
Saunders/Pronex Traction Devices
300 PV
Advance Dynamic ROM
Innosense Minnova

CONTACTS:
Note: Officers with more than one job title may be intentionally listed here more than once.
H. Philip Vierling, CEO
H. Philip Vierling, Pres.
Patrick D. Spangler, Exec. VP/CFO
Joseph E. Laptewicz, Jr., Chmn.

Phone: 651-415-9000   **Fax:** 651-415-7447
Toll-Free: 888-328-3536
Address: 599 Cardigan Rd., St. Paul, MN 55126-4099 US

GROWTH PLANS/SPECIAL FEATURES:
Empi, Inc. is a leading medical device company that develops, manufactures, markets and distributes a range of products for pain management, tissue rehabilitation and incontinence, as well as clinic supplies. The firm's pain management products include Epix VT, a non-invasive, non-addictive pain control system that works through transcutaneous electrical nerve stimulation; the Dupel Iontophoresis System, a non-invasive drug delivery system that uses electricity to administer medicine through the skin; and Saunders/Pronex Traction Devices, providing cervical and lumbar traction for effective spine pain management. The company's tissue rehabilitation products include 300 PV, a neuromuscular electrical stimulation portable multifunction device that helps slow or prevent disuse atrophy, re-educate muscles and control pain; Advance Dynamic ROM, a stretching device that provides low-load prolonged stretches to increase joint range of motion through both extension and flexion models for the knee, elbow, wrist, ankle dorsiflexion, forearm supination and below-knee amputation; and Innosense Minnova, a pelvic floor stimulation device that helps treat urinary incontinence through biofeedback and strengthening. In addition, Empi markets clinic supplies, such as electrodes, lead wires, batteries and electrotherapy skin care products. The firm sells its products to more than 13,000 clinics nationwide and markets its products throughout Asia, Canada and Europe. In October 2004, Encore Medical Corporation, which designs, manufactures and sells joint treatment and replacement products, acquired Empi.

FINANCIALS:
Sales and profits are in thousands of dollars—add 000 to get the full amount. Year 2004 note: Complete fiscal 2004 results were not available for all companies at press time. For this company, year 2004 is for months.

2004 Sales: $ (months)
2003 Sales: $150,300
2002 Sales: $136,900
2001 Sales: $
2000 Sales: $

2004 Profits: $ (months)
2003 Profits: $13,300
2002 Profits: $18,900
2001 Profits: $
2000 Profits: $

Stock Ticker: Private
Employees: 780
Fiscal Year Ends: 12/31

SALARIES/BENEFITS:
Pension Plan:	ESOP Stock Plan:	Profit Sharing:	Top Exec. Salary: $	Bonus: $
Savings Plan:	Stock Purch. Plan:		Second Exec. Salary: $	Bonus: $

OTHER THOUGHTS:
Apparent Top Female Officers:
Hot Spot for Advancement for Women/Minorities:

LOCATIONS: ("Y" = Yes)
West:	Southwest:	Midwest:	Southeast:	Northeast:	International:
		Y			

ENCORE MEDICAL CORPORATION

www.encoremed.com

Industry Group Code: 339113 **Ranks within this company's industry group:** Sales: 86 Profits: 115

Insurance/HMO/PPO:	Drugs:	Equipment/Supplies:		Hospitals/Clinics:	Services:	Health Care:
Insurance:	Manufacturer:	Manufacturer:	Y	Acute Care:	Diagnostics:	Home Health:
Managed Care:	Distributor:	Distributor:	Y	Sub-Acute Care:	Labs/Testing:	Long-Term Care:
Utilization Mgmt.:	Specialty Pharm.:	Leasing/Finance:		Outpatient Surgery:	Staffing:	Physical Therapy:
Payment Proc.:	Vitamins/Nutri.:	Information Sys.:		Phys. Rehab. Center:	Waste Disposal:	Phys. Practice Mgmt.:
	Clinical Trials:			Psychiatric Clinics:	Specialty Services:	

TYPES OF BUSINESS:
Supplies-Joint & Bone Damage
Reconstructive Total Joint Implants
Specialty Trauma Products
Spinal Implants
Orthopedic Supply Distribution
Rehabilitation Products

BRANDS/DIVISIONS/AFFILIATES:
Chattanooga Group
Empi, Inc.

CONTACTS:
Note: Officers with more than one job title may be intentionally listed here more than once.
Kenneth W. Davidson, CEO
Paul Chapman, Pres.
Paul Chapman, COO
William W. Burke, Exec. VP/CFO
Craig L. Smith, Chief Scientific Officer
Harry L. Zimmerman, Exec. VP/General Counsel
Jack F. Cahill, Exec. VP/Pres.-Surgical Div.
Scott A. Klosterman, Exec. VP-Chattanooga Group
Kenneth W. Davidson, Chmn.

Phone: 512-832-9500 **Fax:** 512-834-6300
Toll-Free:
Address: 9800 Metric Blvd., Austin, TX 78758 US

GROWTH PLANS/SPECIAL FEATURES:
Encore Medical Corporation designs, manufactures, markets and distributes orthopedic devices, sports medicine equipment and other related products for the orthopedic industry worldwide. Encore's products are used to treat patients with musculoskeletal conditions resulting from degenerative diseases, deformities, traumatic events and participation in sporting events. These products serve the needs of physical therapists, chiropractors and sports medicine professionals. The company is divided into three operating segments: the surgical division, the soft goods division and the Chattanooga Group. The surgical division manufactures hard goods for surgical implantation and reconstruction, including hip, knee and shoulder implants, trauma products and spinal implants. Encore's soft goods division offers goods and devices used to assist in the repair and rehabilitation of soft tissue and bone, to protect patients from injury and to aid patients in their recovery from orthopedic trauma and surgery. The Chattanooga Group manufactures rehabilitation products for patient care and electrotherapy, as well as physical therapy tables, traction and chiropractic devices. The company places a strong emphasis on research and development for its surgical implant product pipeline, which has led to the approval of over 100 patents. Encore recently received pre-market clearance from the FDA for several clinical physical therapy laser devices, which it plans to introduce under the Chattanooga brand in early 2005. These devices will be indicated for topical heating for local blood circulation; minor muscle and joint aches, pains and stiffness; muscle spasm; arthritic pain and stiffness; and muscle relaxation. In October 2004, the company completed its acquisition of Empi, Inc., a manufacturer of orthopedic products.

FINANCIALS:
Sales and profits are in thousands of dollars—add 000 to get the full amount. Year 2004 note: Complete fiscal 2004 results were not available for all companies at press time. For this company, year 2004 is for 6 months.

2004 Sales: $60,340 (6 months)   2004 Profits: $3,212   (6 months)
2003 Sales: $108,059   2003 Profits: $-2,517
2002 Sales: $95,500   2002 Profits: $ 6
2001 Sales: $42,700   2001 Profits: $ 500
2000 Sales: $30,113   2000 Profits: $-3,263

Stock Ticker: ENMC
Employees: 450
Fiscal Year Ends: 12/31

SALARIES/BENEFITS:
Pension Plan: ESOP Stock Plan: Profit Sharing: Top Exec. Salary: $311,500   Bonus: $320,000
Savings Plan: Stock Purch. Plan: Second Exec. Salary: $225,385   Bonus: $170,000

OTHER THOUGHTS:
Apparent Top Female Officers:
Hot Spot for Advancement for Women/Minorities:

LOCATIONS: ("Y" = Yes)
West:	Southwest:	Midwest:	Southeast:	Northeast:	International:
	Y		Y		

ENDO PHARMACEUTICALS HOLDINGS INC

www.endo.com

Industry Group Code: 325412 Ranks within this company's industry group: Sales: 36 Profits: 30

Insurance/HMO/PPO:	Drugs:		Equipment/Supplies:	Hospitals/Clinics:	Services:	Health Care:	
Insurance: Managed Care: Utilization Mgmt.: Payment Proc.:	Manufacturer: Distributor: Specialty Pharm.: Vitamins/Nutri.: Clinical Trials:	Y	Manufacturer: Distributor: Leasing/Finance: Information Sys.:	Acute Care: Sub-Acute Care: Outpatient Surgery: Phys. Rehab. Center: Psychiatric Clinics:	Diagnostics: Labs/Testing: Staffing: Waste Disposal: Specialty Services:	Home Health: Long-Term Care: Physical Therapy: Phys. Practice Mgmt.:	

TYPES OF BUSINESS:
Drugs-Pain Management

BRANDS/DIVISIONS/AFFILIATES:
Endo Pharmaceuticals, Inc.
Lidoderm
Percocet
Zydone
Percodan

CONTACTS:
Note: Officers with more than one job title may be intentionally listed here more than once.

Carol A. Ammon, CEO
Peter A. Lankau, Pres.
Peter A. Lankau, COO
Jeffrey R. Black, Exec. VP/CFO
David Bass, VP-Human Resources
David A. Lee, VP-R&D
Caroline B. Manogue, General Counsel
Mariann T. MacDonald, Exec. VP-Oper.
Jeffrey R. Black, Treas.
Carol A. Ammon, Chmn.

Phone: 610-558-9800 Fax: 610-558-8979
Toll-Free:
Address: 100 Painters Dr., Chadds Ford, PA 19317 US

GROWTH PLANS/SPECIAL FEATURES:

Endo Pharmaceuticals Holdings, Inc. is a fully integrated specialty pharmaceutical company with market leadership in pain management. The company discovers, produces and markets pharmaceutical products, principally for the treatment of pain, under both generic and brand names. The branded products, Percodan, Zydone, Lidoderm and Percocet, are sold to health care professionals throughout the U.S. Percocet and Zydone are used to treat moderate to severe pain, Lidoderm is used to treat postherpetic neuralgia and Percodan is used to treat severe pain. The company offers a generic version of Sinemet (carbidopa/levodopa) for the treatment of the symptoms of idiopathic Parkinson's disease. Endo focuses on generic products that are challenging to bring to market due to complex formulation, regulatory or legal problems or barriers in raw material sourcing. Recently, Endo Pharmaceuticals signed a licensing agreement with Vernalis to market Froval, an acute migraine treatment for adults. In addition, the company has come to an agreement with the U.S. FDA over its design of clinical trials for oxymorphone extended-release tablets. The trials are expected to provide the additional clarification and information requested by the FDA to finalize the drug's NDA.

The firm offers employees medical, dental and prescription coverage, life insurance, AD&D, long- and short-term disability, a dependent care spending account, a medical spending account and an educational assistance program.

FINANCIALS:
Sales and profits are in thousands of dollars—add 000 to get the full amount. Year 2004 note: Complete fiscal 2004 results were not available for all companies at press time. For this company, year 2004 is for 9 months.

2004 Sales: $457,806 (9 months)	2004 Profits: $114,099 (9 months)	Stock Ticker: ENDP
2003 Sales: $595,608	2003 Profits: $69,790	Employees: 492
2002 Sales: $399,000	2002 Profits: $30,800	Fiscal Year Ends: 12/31
2001 Sales: $252,000	2001 Profits: $-36,500	
2000 Sales: $197,429	2000 Profits: $-156,840	

SALARIES/BENEFITS:
Pension Plan:	ESOP Stock Plan:	Profit Sharing:	Top Exec. Salary: $480,000	Bonus: $420,000
Savings Plan: Y	Stock Purch. Plan: Y		Second Exec. Salary: $368,333	Bonus: $346,500

OTHER THOUGHTS:
Apparent Top Female Officers: 3
Hot Spot for Advancement for Women/Minorities: Y

LOCATIONS: ("Y" = Yes)
West:	Southwest:	Midwest:	Southeast:	Northeast: Y	International:

ENVIRONMENTAL TECTONICS CORP

www.etcusa.com

Industry Group Code: 339113 Ranks within this company's industry group: Sales: 116 Profits: 96

Insurance/HMO/PPO:	Drugs:	Equipment/Supplies:		Hospitals/Clinics:		Services:		Health Care:	
Insurance:	Manufacturer:	Manufacturer:	Y	Acute Care:		Diagnostics:		Home Health:	
Managed Care:	Distributor:	Distributor:		Sub-Acute Care:		Labs/Testing:		Long-Term Care:	
Utilization Mgmt.:	Specialty Pharm.:	Leasing/Finance:		Outpatient Surgery:		Staffing:		Physical Therapy:	
Payment Proc.:	Vitamins/Nutri.:	Information Sys.:	Y	Phys. Rehab. Center:		Waste Disposal:		Phys. Practice Mgmt.:	
	Clinical Trials:			Psychiatric Clinics:		Specialty Services:			

TYPES OF BUSINESS:
Medical Equipment & Supplies Manufacturing
Flight Simulators
Decompression Chambers
Hyperbaric Chambers
Human Centrifuges
Amusement Ride Simulators
Steam & Gas Sterilizers
Environmental Simulation Systems

BRANDS/DIVISIONS/AFFILIATES:
Space Traveler

GROWTH PLANS/SPECIAL FEATURES:
Environmental Tectonics Corp. (ETC) designs, manufactures and sells software-driven products used to create and monitor the physiological effects of motion on humans and equipment or to control, modify, simulate and measure environmental conditions. Its product line includes aircrew training systems, entertainment products, medical sterilizers, environmental and hyperbaric chambers and other products that involve similar manufacturing techniques and engineering technologies. ETC operates in two primary business segments: aircrew training systems and the industrial group. The aircrew training division manufactures devices used for medical research, advanced flight training and the indoctrination and testing of military and commercial pilots. Its products include night vision trainers, water survival training equipment, flight simulators and real-time interactive training programs. This segment also produces real-time interactive training programs for various disaster situations and entertainment products such as motion-based simulation rides. ETC's industrial group manufactures steam and gas sterilizers for various industrial and pharmaceutical applications, environmental systems, sampling and analysis systems, test equipment and a hyperbaric line that includes monoplace and multiplace chambers for high-altitude training, decompression and wound care applications. Predicting commercial spaceflight in the near future, the company plans to offer Space Traveler training solutions for physiological issues associated with space travel.

CONTACTS: Note: Officers with more than one job title may be intentionally listed here more than once.
William F. Mitchell, CEO
William F. Mitchell, Pres.
Duane D. Deaner, CFO
Husnu Onus, VP-Int'l Mktg. & Sales
Robert B. Henstenburg, Chief Eng.-High-Performance Composites
Dick Leland, VP-Aircrew Training Systems
William F. Mitchell, Chmn.

Phone: 215-355-9100   Fax: 215-357-4000
Toll-Free:
Address: 125 James Way, Southampton, PA 18966 US

FINANCIALS: Sales and profits are in thousands of dollars—add 000 to get the full amount. Year 2004 note: Complete fiscal 2004 results were not available for all companies at press time. For this company, year 2004 is for 12 months.

2004 Sales: $25,995 (12 months)   2004 Profits: $-793 (12 months)
2003 Sales: $43,100   2003 Profits: $2,500
2002 Sales: $32,500   2002 Profits: $1,700
2001 Sales: $32,500   2001 Profits: $2,000
2000 Sales: $34,900   2000 Profits: $2,800

Stock Ticker: ETC
Employees: 241
Fiscal Year Ends: 2/28

SALARIES/BENEFITS:
Pension Plan: ESOP Stock Plan: Profit Sharing: Top Exec. Salary: $225,000   Bonus: $10,051
Savings Plan: Y   Stock Purch. Plan: Second Exec. Salary: $ Bonus: $

OTHER THOUGHTS:
Apparent Top Female Officers:
Hot Spot for Advancement for Women/Minorities:

LOCATIONS: ("Y" = Yes)
West:	Southwest:	Midwest:	Southeast:	Northeast:	International:
		Y		Y	Y

EON LABS INC

www.eonlabs.com

Industry Group Code: 325412 **Ranks within this company's industry group:** Sales: 42 Profits: 29

Insurance/HMO/PPO:	Drugs:	Equipment/Supplies:	Hospitals/Clinics:	Services:	Health Care:
Insurance:	Manufacturer: Y	Manufacturer:	Acute Care:	Diagnostics:	Home Health:
Managed Care:	Distributor:	Distributor:	Sub-Acute Care:	Labs/Testing:	Long-Term Care:
Utilization Mgmt.:	Specialty Pharm.:	Leasing/Finance:	Outpatient Surgery:	Staffing:	Physical Therapy:
Payment Proc.:	Vitamins/Nutri.:	Information Sys.:	Phys. Rehab. Center:	Waste Disposal:	Phys. Practice Mgmt.:
	Clinical Trials:		Psychiatric Clinics:	Specialty Services:	

TYPES OF BUSINESS:
Drugs-Generic

BRANDS/DIVISIONS/AFFILIATES:
Metformin
Bupropion
Fluoxetine
Sucralfate
Midodrine
Ciprofloxacin

CONTACTS:
Note: Officers with more than one job title may be intentionally listed here more than once.

Bernhard Hampl, CEO
Bernhard Hampl, Pres.
William F. Holt, CFO
Frank J. Della Fera, VP-Mktg. & Sales
Nitin V. Sheth, VP-R&D
Rathnam Kumar, VP-Mfg.
Jeffery S. Bauer, VP-Bus. Dev.
William F. Holt, VP-Finance/Treas./Corp. Sec.
Pranab K. Bhattacharyya, VP-Quality Mgmt.
Sadie M. Ciganek, VP-Regulatory Affairs
William B. Eversgerd, VP-Plant Facilities
Leon Shargel, VP-Biopharmaceutics

Phone: 212-728-8116 **Fax:** 718-949-3120
Toll-Free: 800-526-0225
Address: 227-15 N. Conduit Ave., Laurelton, NY 11413 US

GROWTH PLANS/SPECIAL FEATURES:
Eon Labs, Inc. is a generic pharmaceutical company that develops, licenses, manufactures, sells and distributes a broad range of prescription pharmaceutical products primarily in the United States. The firm focuses on drugs in a range of solid oral dosage forms, using both immediate and sustained-release delivery, in tablet, multiple-layer tablet, film-coated tablet and capsule forms. Its diverse product line includes approximately 117 products representing various dosage strengths of 55 drugs. These products include Bupropion, a generic form of Wellbutrin; Fluoxetine, a generic form of Prozac; Metformin, a generic form of Glucophage; and Sucralfate, a generic form of Carafate. Eon Labs obtains new generic pharmaceutical products through internal product development and from strategic licensing or co-development arrangements with Hexal AG and other companies. The firm stresses timely execution of the product development process as it strives to be the first to market with a generic product. Being first to market on a number of products has given Eon Labs favorable market share for those products. Recently, the company received final approval for Midodrine tablets, the generic equivalent of ProAmatine, and for Ciprofloxacin, the generic equivalent of Cipro.

The company offers its employee medical and dental coverage and tuition reimbursement.

FINANCIALS:
Sales and profits are in thousands of dollars—add 000 to get the full amount. Year 2004 note: Complete fiscal 2004 results were not available for all companies at press time. For this company, year 2004 is for 9 months.

2004 Sales: $320,969 (9 months)   2004 Profits: $89,194 (9 months)
2003 Sales: $329,538   2003 Profits: $70,135
2002 Sales: $244,269   2002 Profits: $43,263
2001 Sales: $165,443   2001 Profits: $15,791
2000 Sales: $ 2000 Profits: $

Stock Ticker: ELAB
Employees: 153
Fiscal Year Ends: 12/31

SALARIES/BENEFITS:
Pension Plan: ESOP Stock Plan: Profit Sharing: Top Exec. Salary: $313,343   Bonus: $1,250,000
Savings Plan: Y   Stock Purch. Plan: Second Exec. Salary: $200,930   Bonus: $200,000

OTHER THOUGHTS:
Apparent Top Female Officers: 1
Hot Spot for Advancement for Women/Minorities:

LOCATIONS: ("Y" = Yes)

West:	Southwest:	Midwest:	Southeast:	Northeast:	International:
				Y	

Plunkett's Health Care Industry Almanac 2005 365

EPIC SYSTEMS CORPORATION
www.epicsys.com

Industry Group Code: 511200   Ranks within this company's industry group: Sales: 14   Profits:

Insurance/HMO/PPO:	Drugs:	Equipment/Supplies:	Hospitals/Clinics:	Services:	Health Care:
Insurance:	Manufacturer:	Manufacturer:	Acute Care:	Diagnostics:	Home Health:
Managed Care:	Distributor:	Distributor:	Sub-Acute Care:	Labs/Testing:	Long-Term Care:
Utilization Mgmt.:	Specialty Pharm.:	Leasing/Finance:	Outpatient Surgery:	Staffing:	Physical Therapy:
Payment Proc.:	Vitamins/Nutri.:	Information Sys.: Y	Phys. Rehab. Center:	Waste Disposal:	Phys. Practice Mgmt.:
	Clinical Trials:		Psychiatric Clinics:	Specialty Services: Y	

TYPES OF BUSINESS:
Computer Software
Support Services

BRANDS/DIVISIONS/AFFILIATES:
EpicCare
SuccessWorks
EKG Enabler
Spirometer Enabler

CONTACTS: Note: Officers with more than one job title may be intentionally listed here more than once.
Judith R. Faulkner, CEO
Carl D. Dvorak, COO
Robert M. Fahrenbach, CFO
Brad Eichhorst, VP-Clinical Informatics
Tim Escher, VP-Tech.
Stephen J. Dickman, Chief Admin. Officer
Ken Hansen, VP/General Counsel
David W. Hall, VP
Patricia Thompson, VP-Industry Practice Program
Daniel S. Bormann, Chief Security Officer

Phone: 608-271-9000   Fax: 608-271-7237
Toll-Free:
Address: 5301 Tokay Blvd., Madison, WI 53711 US

GROWTH PLANS/SPECIAL FEATURES:
Epic Systems Corp. is a developer of integrated inpatient, ambulatory and payor systems. All Epic software applications are designed to share a single database so that each viewer can access all available patient data through a single interface from anywhere in the organization. The firm's products include programs that share medical records between affiliates, hospital and professional billing, data repository management, nursing documentation, ambulatory clinical systems, inpatient pharmacy systems, operating room management, ICU/acute care support and radiology information systems. Most systems have software that allows access to data using handheld and portable technology. The company's technology is chosen for speed and ease of access. Epic can deploy its systems with full-client workstations, thin-client devices, wireless laptops, handheld devices, the Internet, remote access servers and virtual private networks. It uses the Bridges Interface Development Toolkit to create a variety of message formats, providing data mapping capabilities and flexible data formatting. The firm's EpicCare system supports off-the-shelf speech recognitions tools, such as IBM ViaVoice, while its EKG and Spirometer Enabler modules allow the system to capture and display EKGs and spirometer readings. EpicCare also allows data capture from monitoring devices such as ventilators, infusion pumps and acute care physiological monitors. SuccessWorks is the company's collection of client-centered services, including training, tailoring of applications to the client's situation, access to hardware and network specialists who plan and implement the client's system and access to the firm's community library exchange, an online collection of application tools and pre-made content that allows clients to share care templates, custom forms, enterprise report formats and documentation shortcuts.

Epic offers its employees a comprehensive insurance plan, flexible spending accounts, a casual dress policy and bonuses for certification in the firm's software applications.

FINANCIALS: Sales and profits are in thousands of dollars—add 000 to get the full amount. Year 2004 note: Complete fiscal 2004 results were not available for all companies at press time. For this company, year 2004 is for months.

2004 Sales: $ (months)   2004 Profits: $ (months)
2003 Sales: $15,300   2003 Profits: $
2002 Sales: $ 2002 Profits: $
2001 Sales: $ 2001 Profits: $
2000 Sales: $ 2000 Profits: $

Stock Ticker: Private
Employees: 36
Fiscal Year Ends: 12/31

SALARIES/BENEFITS:
Pension Plan: ESOP Stock Plan: Profit Sharing: Top Exec. Salary: $ Bonus: $
Savings Plan: Y   Stock Purch. Plan: Second Exec. Salary: $ Bonus: $

OTHER THOUGHTS:
Apparent Top Female Officers: 2
Hot Spot for Advancement for Women/Minorities:

LOCATIONS: ("Y" = Yes)
| West: | Southwest: | Midwest: Y | Southeast: | Northeast: | International: |

Note: Financial information, benefits and other data can change quickly and may vary from those stated here.

ERESEARCH TECHNOLOGY INC

www.ert.com

Industry Group Code: 511200   Ranks within this company's industry group: Sales: 8   Profits: 4

Insurance/HMO/PPO:	Drugs:	Equipment/Supplies:	Hospitals/Clinics:	Services:		Health Care:	
Insurance:	Manufacturer:	Manufacturer:	Acute Care:	Diagnostics:	Y	Home Health:	
Managed Care:	Distributor:	Distributor:	Sub-Acute Care:	Labs/Testing:		Long-Term Care:	
Utilization Mgmt.:	Specialty Pharm.:	Leasing/Finance:	Outpatient Surgery:	Staffing:		Physical Therapy:	
Payment Proc.:	Vitamins/Nutri.:	Information Sys.:	Y	Phys. Rehab. Center:	Waste Disposal:		Phys. Practice Mgmt.:	
	Clinical Trials:		Psychiatric Clinics:	Specialty Services:	Y		

TYPES OF BUSINESS:
Software-Clinical Trials
Technology Consulting Services
Cardiac Safety Services

BRANDS/DIVISIONS/AFFILIATES:
EXPeRT
eResearch Network
eData Entry
Enterprise EDC
eResearch Community

CONTACTS: Note: Officers with more than one job title may be intentionally listed here more than once.
Joseph A. Esposito, CEO
Joseph A. Esposito, Pres.
Bruce Johnson, Sr. VP/CFO
Scott Grisanti, Chief Mktg. Officer
Joel Morganroth, Chief Scientist
Vincent Renz, Chief Tech. Officer
Thomas P. Devine, Sr. VP/Chief Dev. Officer
Anna Marie Pagliaccetti, VP/General Counsel
Scott Grisanti, Sr. VP-Bus. Dev.
Robert S. Brown, Sr. VP-Outsourcing Partnerships
Jeffrey S. Litwin, Sr. VP/Chief Medical Officer
Anna Marie Pagliaccetti, Corp. Sec.
Vincent Renz, Sr. VP-Tech. & Consulting
Joel Morganroth, Chmn.

Phone: 215-972-0420   Fax: 215-972-0414
Toll-Free:
Address: 30 S. 17th St., Philadelphia, PA 19103-4001 US

GROWTH PLANS/SPECIAL FEATURES:
eResearch Technology, Inc. (ERT) provides technology and services that improve the accuracy, timeliness and efficiency of trial set-up, data collection and interpretation and new drug, biologic and device application submission. The company provides centralized cardiac safety services and clinical research technology and services, which include the development, marketing and support of clinical research technology. Clinical trial sponsors and clinical research organizations use the cardiac safety services during clinical trials. ERT's clinical research technology and services include the licensing of its proprietary software products and the provision of maintenance and consulting services supporting its proprietary software products. The eResearch Network (eResNet) technology provides an integrated end-to-end clinical research platform that includes trials, data and safety management modules. The eResearch Community is a central command and control web portal that provides real-time information related to monitoring clinical trial activities, data quality and safety. The EXPeRT Cardiac Safety Intelligent Data Management System provides cardiac safety data collection, interpretation and distribution of electrocardiographic (ECG) data and images. Recently, ERT agreed to service the University of Rochester with access to its Enterprise EDC platform and web portal for access to real-time data.

FINANCIALS: Sales and profits are in thousands of dollars—add 000 to get the full amount. Year 2004 note: Complete fiscal 2004 results were not available for all companies at press time. For this company, year 2004 is for 9 months.

2004 Sales: $45,823 (9 months)   2004 Profits: $9,097   (9 months)
2003 Sales: $66,842   2003 Profits: $14,463
2002 Sales: $41,500   2002 Profits: $6,200
2001 Sales: $28,000   2001 Profits: $-3,800
2000 Sales: $28,100   2000 Profits: $100

Stock Ticker: ERES
Employees: 284
Fiscal Year Ends: 12/31

SALARIES/BENEFITS:
Pension Plan: ESOP Stock Plan: Profit Sharing: Top Exec. Salary: $300,000   Bonus: $404,846
Savings Plan: Y   Stock Purch. Plan: Second Exec. Salary: $200,000   Bonus: $161,939

OTHER THOUGHTS:
Apparent Top Female Officers: 1
Hot Spot for Advancement for Women/Minorities:

LOCATIONS: ("Y" = Yes)

West:	Southwest:	Midwest:	Southeast:	Northeast:	International:
				Y	Y

ESSILOR INTERNATIONAL SA

www.essilor.com

Industry Group Code: 339113 Ranks within this company's industry group: Sales: 9 Profits: 12

Insurance/HMO/PPO:	Drugs:	Equipment/Supplies:		Hospitals/Clinics:	Services:	Health Care:
Insurance:	Manufacturer:	Manufacturer:	Y	Acute Care:	Diagnostics:	Home Health:
Managed Care:	Distributor:	Distributor:	Y	Sub-Acute Care:	Labs/Testing:	Long-Term Care:
Utilization Mgmt.:	Specialty Pharm.:	Leasing/Finance:		Outpatient Surgery:	Staffing:	Physical Therapy:
Payment Proc.:	Vitamins/Nutri.:	Information Sys.:		Phys. Rehab. Center:	Waste Disposal:	Phys. Practice Mgmt.:
	Clinical Trials:			Psychiatric Clinics:	Specialty Services:	

TYPES OF BUSINESS:
Supplies-Ophthalmic Products
Corrective Lenses

BRANDS/DIVISIONS/AFFILIATES:
Essilor of America, Inc.
Select Optical
Opal-Lite
Tri Supreme
LTL
City Optical
Crizal Alize
Varilux Ipseo

CONTACTS: Note: Officers with more than one job title may be intentionally listed here more than once.
Xavier Fontanet, CEO
Philippe Alfroid, COO
Fabienne Lecorvaisier, CFO
Thierry Robin, VP-Strategic Mktg.
Henri Vidal, VP-Human Resources
Jean-Luc Schuppiser, VP-Research & Dev.
Didier Lambert, VP-Info. Systems
Carol Xueref, VP-Legal Affairs
Claude Brignon, VP-Oper.
Carol Xueref, VP-Group Dev.
Hubert Sagnieres, Pres., Essilor of America, Inc.
Bertrand de Lime, Exec. VP-Europe
Patrick Cherrier, VP-Asia
Olivier Mathieux, VP-Latin America
Xavier Fontanet, Chmn.

Phone: 33-1-49-77-42-24   **Fax:** 33-1-49-77-44-20
Toll-Free:
Address: 147, rue de Paris, Charenton-le-Pont, 94227 France

GROWTH PLANS/SPECIAL FEATURES:
Essilor International S.A. is a leading global designer, manufacturer and distributor of ophthalmic/optical products and supplies, especially corrective lenses. Its products treat common sight problems, including myopia (nearsightedness), hyperopia (farsightedness), astigmatism and presbyopia. The company's brands include Varilux Panamic, its fifth generation of progressive lenses; Airwear polycarbonate lenses, which block UVA and UVB rays; and Transitions variable-tint lenses. The firm supplies its products through a global network of 173 prescription laboratories and 18 production plants. In recent news, Essilor of America, Inc., the firm's wholly-owned U.S. subsidiary, acquired three prescription laboratories: Select Optical, Opal-Lite, Inc. and Tri Supreme, one of the 10 largest prescription laboratories in the U.S. The company also acquired LTL, a major distributor of finished lenses in Europe and in the ophthalmic lens market in Italy. In addition, it acquired a 50% stake in City Optical, an Australian prescription laboratory. Essilor's newest products include the Crizal Alize anti-reflective treatment, the Varilux Ellipse small-frame progressive lenses and the Varilux Ipseo line of personalized progressive lenses.

FINANCIALS:
Sales and profits are in thousands of dollars—add 000 to get the full amount. Year 2004 note: Complete fiscal 2004 results were not available for all companies at press time. For this company, year 2004 is for months.

2004 Sales: $ (months)   2004 Profits: $ (months)
2003 Sales: $2,656,500   2003 Profits: $251,500
2002 Sales: $2,241,100   2002 Profits: $191,100
2001 Sales: $ 2001 Profits: $
2000 Sales: $ 2000 Profits: $

Stock Ticker: Foreign
Employees: 23,607
Fiscal Year Ends: 12/31

SALARIES/BENEFITS:
| Pension Plan: | ESOP Stock Plan: | Profit Sharing: | Top Exec. Salary: $ | Bonus: $ |
| Savings Plan: | Stock Purch. Plan: | | Second Exec. Salary: $ | Bonus: $ |

OTHER THOUGHTS:
Apparent Top Female Officers: 1
Hot Spot for Advancement for Women/Minorities:

LOCATIONS: ("Y" = Yes)
West:	Southwest:	Midwest:	Southeast:	Northeast:	International:
Y	Y	Y	Y	Y	Y

ns
ETHICON INC

www.ethiconinc.com

Industry Group Code: 339113 Ranks within this company's industry group: Sales: Profits:

Insurance/HMO/PPO:	Drugs:	Equipment/Supplies:		Hospitals/Clinics:		Services:		Health Care:	
Insurance:	Manufacturer:	Manufacturer:	Y	Acute Care:		Diagnostics:		Home Health:	
Managed Care:	Distributor:	Distributor:	Y	Sub-Acute Care:		Labs/Testing:		Long-Term Care:	
Utilization Mgmt.:	Specialty Pharm.:	Leasing/Finance:		Outpatient Surgery:		Staffing:		Physical Therapy:	
Payment Proc.:	Vitamins/Nutri.:	Information Sys.:		Phys. Rehab. Center:		Waste Disposal:		Phys. Practice Mgmt.:	
	Clinical Trials:			Psychiatric Clinics:		Specialty Services:			

TYPES OF BUSINESS:
Sutures, Surgical Mesh, Needles & Skin Adhesives
Wound Management Products
Burn & Skin Care Products
Women's Health Surgical Products
Cardiovascular Surgery Products

BRANDS/DIVISIONS/AFFILIATES:
Johnson & Johnson
GYNECARE
CARDIOVATIONS
Johnson & Johnson Wound Management
ETHICON Products
HARMONIC SCALPEL
PREVACARE
Heartpoint, Inc.

CONTACTS:
Note: Officers with more than one job title may be intentionally listed here more than once.
Robert Coradini, Worldwide Pres., CARDIOVATIONS
Rodrigo Bianchi, Worldwide Pres., ETHICON Products
Dan Wildman, Worldwide Pres., Johnson & Johnson Wound Mgmt.
Barbara Schwartz, Worldwide Pres., GYNECARE

Phone: 908-218-0707	Fax: 908-218-2471
Toll-Free: 800-255-2500	
Address: Rte. 22, Box 151, Somerville, NJ 08876 US	

GROWTH PLANS/SPECIAL FEATURES:
ETHICON, Inc., a Johnson & Johnson subsidiary, markets wound management, women's health and cardiovascular surgery products in 52 countries around the world. The company has four business units: GYNECARE, its women's health business unit; CARDIOVATIONS, which manufactures surgical devices for the treatment of cardiovascular diseases; Johnson & Johnson Wound Management (WM), which sells burn and skin care products; and ETHICON Products (EP), one of the leading manufacturers of wound closure and cardiovascular surgery products. GYNECARE currently offers GYNECARE THERMACHOICHE Uterine Balloon Therapy, a less invasive surgical device to treat excessive menstrual bleeding; GYNECARE TVT Tension-free Support for Incontinence; the GYNECARE VERSAPOINT Bipolar Electrosurgery System, which treats uterine fibroids and polyps; and the GYNECARE INTERCEED (TC7) Absorbable Adhesion Barrier, which treats surgical adhesions. CARDIOVATIONS products include the CLEARGLIDE Endoscopic Vein Harvesting System; the Watchband Incision for Endoscopic Radial Artery Harvesting; the HARMONIC SCALPEL, which uses ultrasonic energy to harvest radial arteries; the FLEXSITE heart stabilizer; MYOLIFT, which eliminates the need to place patients on cardiopulmonary bypass for coronary artery surgery; and the PORT ACCESS valve repair surgery product line. WM's key brands are TIELLE Hydropolymer Adhesive dressings; FIBRACOL Collagen Wound Dressings for the management of pressure ulcers, diabetic foot ulcers and venous leg ulcers; INTEGRA Dermal Generation Template for the regeneration of burned skin; and the PREVACARE line of skin care products for damaged or compromised skin. In addition, it sells traditional wound care products, such as sponges, bandages, dressings, transparent films and tapes, as well as hemostasis products, which are used by surgeons to control mild to moderate bleeding. EP's products include PROCEED Surgical Mesh, MultiPass Needles, PROLENE polypropylene sutures and DERMABOND ProPen Topical Skin Adhseive. Recently, Johnson & Johnson agreed to acquire Heartpoint, Inc., a leading manufacturer of less invasive cardiac surgery products, which will operate as part of ETHICON.

FINANCIALS:
Sales and profits are in thousands of dollars—add 000 to get the full amount. Year 2004 note: Complete fiscal 2004 results were not available for all companies at press time. For this company, year 2004 is for months.

2004 Sales: $ (months) 2004 Profits: $ (months)
2003 Sales: $ 2003 Profits: $
2002 Sales: $ 2002 Profits: $
2001 Sales: $ 2001 Profits: $
2000 Sales: $ 2000 Profits: $

Stock Ticker: Subsidiary
Employees:
Fiscal Year Ends: 12/31

SALARIES/BENEFITS:
Pension Plan: ESOP Stock Plan: Profit Sharing: Top Exec. Salary: $ Bonus: $
Savings Plan: Stock Purch. Plan: Second Exec. Salary: $ Bonus: $

OTHER THOUGHTS:
Apparent Top Female Officers: 1
Hot Spot for Advancement for Women/Minorities:

LOCATIONS: ("Y" = Yes)
West:	Southwest:	Midwest:	Southeast:	Northeast:	International:
	Y		Y	Y	

Note: Financial information, benefits and other data can change quickly and may vary from those stated here.

EXACTECH INC

www.exac.com

Industry Group Code: 339113   **Ranks within this company's industry group:** Sales: 104   Profits: 80

Insurance/HMO/PPO:	Drugs:	Equipment/Supplies:		Hospitals/Clinics:	Services:	Health Care:
Insurance: Managed Care: Utilization Mgmt.: Payment Proc.:	Manufacturer: Distributor: Specialty Pharm.: Vitamins/Nutri.: Clinical Trials:	Manufacturer: Distributor: Leasing/Finance: Information Sys.:	Y	Acute Care: Sub-Acute Care: Outpatient Surgery: Phys. Rehab. Center: Psychiatric Clinics:	Diagnostics: Labs/Testing: Staffing: Waste Disposal: Specialty Services:	Home Health: Long-Term Care: Physical Therapy: Phys. Practice Mgmt.:

TYPES OF BUSINESS:
Equipment-Joint Replacement
Orthopedic Implant Devices
Surgical Instruments
Biologic Products

BRANDS/DIVISIONS/AFFILIATES:
AcuMatch
AcuDriver Automated Osteotome System
Optetrak
Opteform
Cemex
Link S.T.A.R.
Optefil
M-Series

CONTACTS:
Note: Officers with more than one job title may be intentionally listed here more than once.
William Petty, CEO
William Petty, Pres.
Joel C. Phillips, CFO
David W. Petty, Exec. VP-Mktg. & Sales
Betty Petty, VP-Human Resources
Gary J. Miller, Exec. VP-Research & Dev.
Betty Petty, VP-Admin.
Joel C. Phillips, Treas.
Betty Petty, Corp. Sec.
William Petty, Chmn.

Phone: 352-377-1140   **Fax:** 352-378-2617
Toll-Free: 800-392-2832
Address: 2320 NW 66th Ct., Gainsville, FL 32653 US

GROWTH PLANS/SPECIAL FEATURES:
Exactech, Inc. develops, manufactures, markets and sells orthopedic implant devices and related surgical instrumentation and materials and distributes biologic materials to hospitals and physicians in the U.S. and internationally. The company's orthopedic implant products are used to replace joints that have deteriorated as a result of injury or diseases such as arthritis. These products include Optetrak, a total primary knee replacement system, and the AcuMatch integrated hip system with M-Series modular femoral stem, L-Series femoral stem, C-Series cemented femoral stem and P-Series press fit femoral stem. Biologic allograft materials, such as Exactech's Opteform and Optefil, are used by surgeons when indicated to repair bone defects and provide an interface to stimulate new bone growth. The company also offers Cemex, a bone cement system, and the AcuDriver Automated Osteotome System, an air-driven impact hand piece used by surgeons during joint implant revision procedures to remove failed prostheses and bone cement. Additionally, Exactech's Link S.T.A.R. ankle, which provides an alternative to fusion that maintains motion and pain relief in some arthritic patients, is currently being distributed under an FDA Investigational Device Exemption.

FINANCIALS:
Sales and profits are in thousands of dollars—add 000 to get the full amount. Year 2004 note: Complete fiscal 2004 results were not available for all companies at press time. For this company, year 2004 is for 9 months.

2004 Sales: $60,855 (9 months)	2004 Profits: $5,447 (9 months)	
2003 Sales: $71,255	2003 Profits: $6,501	**Stock Ticker:** EXAC
2002 Sales: $59,300	2002 Profits: $5,300	Employees: 154
2001 Sales: $46,600	2001 Profits: $3,500	Fiscal Year Ends: 12/31
2000 Sales: $41,900	2000 Profits: $4,200	

SALARIES/BENEFITS:
Pension Plan:	ESOP Stock Plan:	Profit Sharing:	Top Exec. Salary: $294,731	Bonus: $55,910
Savings Plan: Y	Stock Purch. Plan:		Second Exec. Salary: $205,657	Bonus: $30,064

OTHER THOUGHTS:
Apparent Top Female Officers: 1
Hot Spot for Advancement for Women/Minorities:

LOCATIONS: ("Y" = Yes)
West:	Southwest:	Midwest:	Southeast:	Northeast:	International:
			Y	Y	

EXCEL TECHNOLOGY INC

www.exceltechinc.com

Industry Group Code: 339113 **Ranks within this company's industry group:** Sales: 82 Profits: 70

Insurance/HMO/PPO:	Drugs:	Equipment/Supplies:	Hospitals/Clinics:	Services:	Health Care:
Insurance:	Manufacturer:	Manufacturer: Y	Acute Care:	Diagnostics:	Home Health:
Managed Care:	Distributor:	Distributor:	Sub-Acute Care:	Labs/Testing:	Long-Term Care:
Utilization Mgmt.:	Specialty Pharm.:	Leasing/Finance:	Outpatient Surgery:	Staffing:	Physical Therapy:
Payment Proc.:	Vitamins/Nutri.:	Information Sys.:	Phys. Rehab. Center:	Waste Disposal:	Phys. Practice Mgmt.:
	Clinical Trials:		Psychiatric Clinics:	Specialty Services:	

TYPES OF BUSINESS:
Equipment-Electro-Optical Components & Laser Systems
Optical Scanning Equipment
Photomask Repair Systems
Scientific & Industrial Lasers

BRANDS/DIVISIONS/AFFILIATES:
Control Systemation, Inc.
Baublys
Control Laser
Synrad
Cambridge Technology
Quantronix
Photo Research
Continuum

CONTACTS:
Note: Officers with more than one job title may be intentionally listed here more than once.
Antoine Dominic, CEO
Antoine Dominic, Pres.
Antoine Dominic, COO
Antoine Dominic, CFO
Francis A. Dominic, Pres., Photo Research, Inc.
J. Donald Hill, Chmn.

Phone: 631-784-6175	Fax: 631-784-6195
Toll-Free:	
Address: 41 Research Way, East Setauket, NY 11733 US	

GROWTH PLANS/SPECIAL FEATURES:
Excel Technology, Inc. designs, develops, manufactures and markets laser systems and electro-optical components for industry, science and medicine. The company's many subsidiaries include Control Systemation, Inc., which focuses on turn-key laser-based micro-machining systems and part-handling workstations for factory automation. In recent years, Excel consolidated the product lines and development efforts of subsidiaries Baublys and Control Laser to eliminate duplicative products and efforts, to increase efficiency and to create a unified market presence for the firm's marking operations. Current products and applications include Baublys-Control Laser marking and engraving systems, Synrad carbon dioxide lasers, Cambridge scanners, Quantronix photomask repair systems and scientific and industrial solid-state lasers, TOC optical products and Photo Research light and color measurement products. Excel's Cambridge Technology subsidiary manufactures high-speed mirror-positioning components used to direct laser energy, servicing a growing number of laser-based medical applications. These include digital radiography, skin resurfacing and eye treatment. The firm also sells spare parts and related consumable materials used primarily in semiconductor, industrial and scientific systems. Through its subsidiary Continuum, Excel develops, manufactures and markets pulsed lasers and related accessories for the scientific and commercial marketplaces. Excel Technology Japan Holdings Co., Ltd., the firm's Japanese subsidiary, focuses on distributing the products of Quantronix, Baublys-Control Laser, Control Systemation and Continuum.

FINANCIALS:
Sales and profits are in thousands of dollars—add 000 to get the full amount. Year 2004 note: Complete fiscal 2004 results were not available for all companies at press time. For this company, year 2004 is for 9 months.

2004 Sales: $105,355 (9 months)	2004 Profits: $12,246 (9 months)	
2003 Sales: $122,681	2003 Profits: $11,318	**Stock Ticker:** XLTC
2002 Sales: $94,500	2002 Profits: $8,500	Employees: 619
2001 Sales: $88,500	2001 Profits: $5,900	Fiscal Year Ends: 12/31
2000 Sales: $107,700	2000 Profits: $15,600	

SALARIES/BENEFITS:
Pension Plan:	ESOP Stock Plan:	Profit Sharing:	Top Exec. Salary: $425,000	Bonus: $885,500
Savings Plan: Y	Stock Purch. Plan: Y		Second Exec. Salary: $305,769	Bonus: $50,000

OTHER THOUGHTS:
Apparent Top Female Officers:
Hot Spot for Advancement for Women/Minorities:

LOCATIONS: ("Y" = Yes)
West: Y	Southwest:	Midwest:	Southeast: Y	Northeast: Y	International: Y

EXPRESS SCRIPTS INC
www.express-scripts.com

Industry Group Code: 522320A Ranks within this company's industry group: Sales: 3 Profits: 2

Insurance/HMO/PPO:	Drugs:		Equipment/Supplies:	Hospitals/Clinics:	Services:		Health Care:
Insurance:	Manufacturer:		Manufacturer:	Acute Care:	Diagnostics:		Home Health:
Managed Care:	Distributor:		Distributor:	Sub-Acute Care:	Labs/Testing:		Long-Term Care:
Utilization Mgmt.: Y	Specialty Pharm.:	Y	Leasing/Finance:	Outpatient Surgery:	Staffing:		Physical Therapy:
Payment Proc.: Y	Vitamins/Nutri.:		Information Sys.:	Phys. Rehab. Center:	Waste Disposal:		Phys. Practice Mgmt.:
	Clinical Trials:			Psychiatric Clinics:	Specialty Services:	Y	

TYPES OF BUSINESS:
Pharmacy Benefits Management
Mail & Internet Pharmacies
Formulary Management
Integrated Drug & Medical Data Analysis
Market Research Programs
Medical Information Management
Workers' Compensation Programs
Informed-Decision Counseling

BRANDS/DIVISIONS/AFFILIATES:
CuraScript

CONTACTS:
Note: Officers with more than one job title may be intentionally listed here more than once.
Barrett A. Toan, CEO
George Paz, Pres.
David A. Lowenberg, COO
Edward J. Stiften, Sr. VP/CFO
Barrett A. Toan, Chmn.

Phone: 314-770-1666 **Fax:** 314-702-7037
Toll-Free:
Address: 13900 Riverport Dr., Maryland Heights, MO 63043 US

GROWTH PLANS/SPECIAL FEATURES:
Express Scripts, Inc. is one of the nation's largest independent pharmacy benefit managers, providing pharmacy service and pharmacy benefit plan design consultation for more than 16,000 clients including HMOs, unions and government health care plans. The company's core services include pharmacy network management, mail and Internet pharmacies, formulary management, targeted clinical programs, integrated drug and medical data analysis, market research programs, medical information management, workers' compensation programs and informed-decision counseling. Express Scripts provides progressive health care management by leveraging expertise in pharmacy benefit management (PBM) in order to positively impact clients' total health care benefits. The firm combines pharmacy and medical claims data to develop new strategies for decreasing total health care spending and improving health outcomes. The PBM business provides managed prescription drug services to 50 million members in the United States and Canada. Health Management Services, a subsidiary, provides comprehensive demand and disease management support services through a 24-hour call center staffed by registered nurses and pharmacists. Through pharmacy network management, Express Scripts contracts with retail pharmacies to provide prescription drugs to members of the pharmacy benefit plans it manages. Express Scripts also provides a number of Internet-based services, including disease tracking, consumer prescription drug information and electronic claim processing. In recent news, Express Scripts acquired CuraScript, one of the largest pharmacy companies.

FINANCIALS:
Sales and profits are in thousands of dollars—add 000 to get the full amount. Year 2004 note: Complete fiscal 2004 results were not available for all companies at press time. For this company, year 2004 is for 9 months.

2004 Sales: $11,175,010 (9 months)	2004 Profits: $197,300 (9 months)	**Stock Ticker:** ESRX
2003 Sales: $13,294,517	2003 Profits: $249,600	**Employees:** 8,575
2002 Sales: $12,261,000	2002 Profits: $203,000	**Fiscal Year Ends:** 12/31
2001 Sales: $9,329,000	2001 Profits: $125,000	
2000 Sales: $6,786,900	2000 Profits: $-9,100	

SALARIES/BENEFITS:
Pension Plan:	ESOP Stock Plan:	Profit Sharing:	Top Exec. Salary: $750,000	Bonus: $637,500
Savings Plan: Y	Stock Purch. Plan: Y		Second Exec. Salary: $486,331	Bonus: $471,308

OTHER THOUGHTS:
Apparent Top Female Officers:
Hot Spot for Advancement for Women/Minorities:

LOCATIONS: ("Y" = Yes)
West:	Southwest:	Midwest:	Southeast:	Northeast:	International:
Y	Y	Y	Y	Y	Y

EXTENDICARE INC

www.extendicare.com

Industry Group Code: 623110 Ranks within this company's industry group: Sales: 5 Profits: 4

Insurance/HMO/PPO:	Drugs:	Equipment/Supplies:	Hospitals/Clinics:	Services:	Health Care:
Insurance:	Manufacturer:	Manufacturer:	Acute Care:	Diagnostics:	Home Health:
Managed Care:	Distributor:	Distributor:	Sub-Acute Care: Y	Labs/Testing:	Long-Term Care: Y
Utilization Mgmt.:	Specialty Pharm.:	Leasing/Finance:	Outpatient Surgery:	Staffing:	Physical Therapy:
Payment Proc.:	Vitamins/Nutri.:	Information Sys.:	Phys. Rehab. Center: Y	Waste Disposal:	Phys. Practice Mgmt.:
	Clinical Trials:		Psychiatric Clinics:	Specialty Services:	

TYPES OF BUSINESS:
Long-Term Care
Assisted Living Facilities
Sub-Acute Care
Rehabilitative Services

BRANDS/DIVISIONS/AFFILIATES:
Extendicare Health Services, Inc.
Assisted Living Concepts, Inc.

GROWTH PLANS/SPECIAL FEATURES:
Extendicare, Inc. is one of the largest operators of long-term care and assisted living facilities in North America. The company owns and operates approximately 273 locations in the U.S. and Canada with a capacity of about 27,700 residents. In the U.S., the firm provides medical specialty services, such as sub-acute care and rehabilitative therapy services, while in Canada it provides home health care services. In recent news, Extendicare Health Services, Inc., a wholly-owned subsidiary of the company, agreed to acquire Assisted Living Concepts, Inc., which has 177 assisted living facilities, composed of 122 owned properties and 55 leased facilities representing 6,838 units, located in 14 states.

CONTACTS:
Note: Officers with more than one job title may be intentionally listed here more than once.

Mel Rhinelander, CEO
Mel Rhinelander, Pres.
Richard L. Bertrand, Sr. VP/CFO
Christina L. McKey, VP-Human Resources
R. Gordon Spear, VP-Admin.
Len G. Koroneos, VP-Bus. Dev./Privacy Officer
Christopher Barnes, Mgr.-Investor Rel.
Elaine E. Everson, VP/Controller
Mark W. Durishan, VP
Jillian E. Fountain, Corp. Sec.
Paul Tuttle, VP-Eastern Oper.
Paul Rushforth, VP-Western Oper.
David J. Hennigar, Chmn.

Phone: 905-470-4000 **Fax:** 905-470-5588
Toll-Free:
Address: 3000 Steeles Ave. E., Markham, Ontario L3R 9W2 Canada

FINANCIALS:
Sales and profits are in thousands of dollars—add 000 to get the full amount. Year 2004 note: Complete fiscal 2004 results were not available for all companies at press time. For this company, year 2004 is for 6 months.

2004 Sales: $661,500 (6 months)   2004 Profits: $35,300 (6 months)
2003 Sales: $1,338,800   2003 Profits: $47,100
2002 Sales: $1,115,600   2002 Profits: $12,000
2001 Sales: $ 2001 Profits: $
2000 Sales: $ 2000 Profits: $

Stock Ticker: Foreign
Employees: 35,800
Fiscal Year Ends: 12/31

SALARIES/BENEFITS:
Pension Plan: ESOP Stock Plan: Profit Sharing: Top Exec. Salary: $ Bonus: $
Savings Plan: Stock Purch. Plan: Second Exec. Salary: $ Bonus: $

OTHER THOUGHTS:
Apparent Top Female Officers: 3
Hot Spot for Advancement for Women/Minorities: Y

LOCATIONS: ("Y" = Yes)

West:	Southwest:	Midwest:	Southeast:	Northeast:	International:
Y	Y	Y	Y	Y	Y

E-Z-EM INC

www.ezem.com

Industry Group Code: 325413 Ranks within this company's industry group: Sales: 1 Profits: 2

Insurance/HMO/PPO:	Drugs:	Equipment/Supplies:	Hospitals/Clinics:	Services:	Health Care:
Insurance:	Manufacturer: Y	Manufacturer: Y	Acute Care:	Diagnostics:	Home Health:
Managed Care:	Distributor:	Distributor:	Sub-Acute Care:	Labs/Testing:	Long-Term Care:
Utilization Mgmt.:	Specialty Pharm.:	Leasing/Finance:	Outpatient Surgery:	Staffing:	Physical Therapy:
Payment Proc.:	Vitamins/Nutri.:	Information Sys.:	Phys. Rehab. Center:	Waste Disposal:	Phys. Practice Mgmt.:
	Clinical Trials:		Psychiatric Clinics:	Specialty Services:	

TYPES OF BUSINESS:
Equipment-Diagnostic Imaging
Therapeutic Devices
Contrast Systems
Diagnostic Radiology Devices
Custom Pharmaceuticals
Gastrointestinal Products
Immunoassay Tests
X-Ray Protection Equipment

BRANDS/DIVISIONS/AFFILIATES:
AngioDynamics, Inc.
CT Smoothies
Readi-CAT
Varibar dysphagia line
Endovascular Laser Venous System
Dura-Flow Chronic Dialysis catheter

CONTACTS:
Note: Officers with more than one job title may be intentionally listed here more than once.

Anthony A. Lombardo, CEO
Anthony A. Lombardo, Pres.
Dennis J. Curtin, CFO
Joseph J. Palma, Sr. VP-Global Sales
Sandra D. Baron, VP-Global Human Resources
Jeffrey S. Peacock, Sr. VP-Global Scientific & Tech. Oper.
Jeffrey S. Peacock, Sr. VP-Global Scientific & Tech. Oper.
Craig A. Burk, VP-Mfg.
Peter J. Graham, General Counsel
Brad S. Schreck, Sr. VP-Global Mktg.
Arthur L. Zimmet, Sr. VP-Special Projects
Robert M. Bloomfield, VP-Market Research
Eamonn P. Hobbs, Sr. VP-AngioDynamics
Howard S. Stern, Chmn.

Phone: 516-333-8230 Fax: 516-333-8278
Toll-Free: 800-544-4624
Address: 717 Main St., Westbury, NY 11590 US

GROWTH PLANS/SPECIAL FEATURES:

E-Z-EM, Inc. is primarily engaged in developing, manufacturing and marketing diagnostic products used by physicians during image-assisted procedures to detect anatomic abnormalities and diseases. Its products and services are designed for use in the radiology, gastroenterology, speech pathology and virtual colonoscopy industries. The company's lead products include CT Smoothies, Readi-CAT contrast products, Varibar dysphagia line and CT injector systems. Through wholly-owned subsidiary AngioDynamics, Inc., the company also manufactures and markets a variety of therapeutic and diagnostic products used to diagnose and treat vascular disease, including the Endovascular Laser Venous System and the Dura-Flow Chronic Dialysis catheter. E-Z-EM provides contract manufacturing in the areas of diagnostic contrast media, pharmaceuticals, cosmetics and defense decontaminants. It has three laboratories specializing in liquids, powders and immunodiagnostic tests for GI disease, and an engineering department that specializes in FDA Class 2 Medical Device development, manufacturing and regulation.

The company offers its employees a comprehensive health plan, along with discounts at optical retail stores, employee training, development programs, tuition reimbursement and business-casual attire.

FINANCIALS:
Sales and profits are in thousands of dollars—add 000 to get the full amount. Year 2004 note: Complete fiscal 2004 results were not available for all companies at press time. For this company, year 2004 is for 12 months.

2004 Sales: $148,771 (12 months)   2004 Profits: $6,726 (12 months)
2003 Sales: $133,200   2003 Profits: $2,700
2002 Sales: $122,100   2002 Profits: $600
2001 Sales: $113,300   2001 Profits: $3,300
2000 Sales: $112,100   2000 Profits: $6,000

Stock Ticker: EZM
Employees: 759
Fiscal Year Ends: 5/31

SALARIES/BENEFITS:
Pension Plan: ESOP Stock Plan: Profit Sharing: Y   Top Exec. Salary: $320,000   Bonus: $96,600
Savings Plan: Y   Stock Purch. Plan: Y   Second Exec. Salary: $240,000   Bonus: $46,560

OTHER THOUGHTS:
Apparent Top Female Officers: 1
Hot Spot for Advancement for Women/Minorities:

LOCATIONS: ("Y" = Yes)
West:	Southwest:	Midwest:	Southeast:	Northeast: Y	International: Y

FAIRVIEW HEALTH SERVICES

www.fairview.org

Industry Group Code: 622110 **Ranks within this company's industry group:** Sales: Profits:

Insurance/HMO/PPO:	Drugs:	Equipment/Supplies:	Hospitals/Clinics:		Services:		Health Care:	
Insurance:	Manufacturer:	Manufacturer:	Acute Care:	Y	Diagnostics:		Home Health:	Y
Managed Care:	Distributor:	Distributor:	Sub-Acute Care:	Y	Labs/Testing:		Long-Term Care:	Y
Utilization Mgmt.:	Specialty Pharm.:	Leasing/Finance:	Outpatient Surgery:	Y	Staffing:		Physical Therapy:	
Payment Proc.:	Vitamins/Nutri.:	Information Sys.:	Phys. Rehab. Center:	Y	Waste Disposal:		Phys. Practice Mgmt.:	
	Clinical Trials:		Psychiatric Clinics:		Specialty Services:	Y		

TYPES OF BUSINESS:
Hospitals
Specialty Clinics
Home Care
Hospice Services
Children's Services
Book Publishing

BRANDS/DIVISIONS/AFFILIATES:
Ebenezer
Minnesota Heart and Vascular Center
Brain Tumor Center of Minnesota
Fairview Hand Center
Institute for Athletic Medicine
Fairview Foundation
Fairview Press
Fairview-University Medical Center

CONTACTS:
Note: Officers with more than one job title may be intentionally listed here more than once.
David Page, CEO
David Page, Pres.
William Maxwell, Exec. VP/COO
James Fox, Sr. VP/CFO
Paul Torgerson, Sr. VP/Chief Admin. Officer
Paul Torgerson, General Counsel
Rodney Burwell, Chmn.

Phone: 612-672-6141 **Fax:** 612-672-7186
Toll-Free:
Address: 2450 Riverside Ave., Minneapolis, MN 55454 US

GROWTH PLANS/SPECIAL FEATURES:
Fairview Health Services is one of the top integrated health networks in the Midwest, serving the Twin Cities area and suburbs, the Minnesota Valley and the Red Wing, Northland, Lakes and Range areas of Minnesota. The system includes seven hospitals with 2,567 licensed beds, including six community hospitals, an academic teaching hospital, comprehensive children's services, more than 50 primary care and specialty clinics and home care and hospice services. Fairview also provides 20 senior housing facilities through Ebenezer and is home to the Minnesota Heart and Vascular Center, the Brain Tumor Center of Minnesota, Fairview Hand Center and 24 Institute for Athletic Medicine locations. The Fairview Foundation is the group's funding entity for special projects, programs, allocations and endowments, supporting patient care, medical staff education needs and publication of books through Fairview Press. Fairview-University Medical Center recently added a TomoTherapy cancer treatment system and Gamma Knife radiosurgery system, enhancing its neuroscience and radiation therapy services. The center has also recently been honored by United Resource Networks for its transplant services.

FINANCIALS:
Sales and profits are in thousands of dollars—add 000 to get the full amount. Year 2004 note: Complete fiscal 2004 results were not available for all companies at press time. For this company, year 2004 is for months.

2004 Sales: $ (months)   2004 Profits: $ (months)
2003 Sales: $ 2003 Profits: $
2002 Sales: $1,623,300   2002 Profits: $
2001 Sales: $ 2001 Profits: $
2000 Sales: $ 2000 Profits: $

Stock Ticker: Nonprofit
Employees:
Fiscal Year Ends: 12/31

SALARIES/BENEFITS:
Pension Plan: Y   ESOP Stock Plan: Profit Sharing: Top Exec. Salary: $ Bonus: $
Savings Plan: Y   Stock Purch. Plan: Second Exec. Salary: $ Bonus: $

OTHER THOUGHTS:
Apparent Top Female Officers:
Hot Spot for Advancement for Women/Minorities:

LOCATIONS: ("Y" = Yes)
West:	Southwest:	Midwest:	Southeast:	Northeast:	International:
		Y			

FIRST CHOICE HEALTH NETWORK INC

www.fchn.com

Industry Group Code: 524114   Ranks within this company's industry group: Sales: Profits:

Insurance/HMO/PPO:	Drugs:	Equipment/Supplies:	Hospitals/Clinics:	Services:	Health Care:
Insurance:	Manufacturer:	Manufacturer:	Acute Care:	Diagnostics:	Home Health:
Managed Care:	Distributor:	Distributor:	Sub-Acute Care:	Labs/Testing:	Long-Term Care:
Utilization Mgmt.: Y	Specialty Pharm.:	Leasing/Finance:	Outpatient Surgery:	Staffing:	Physical Therapy:
Payment Proc.:	Vitamins/Nutri.:	Information Sys.:	Phys. Rehab. Center:	Waste Disposal:	Phys. Practice Mgmt.:
	Clinical Trials:		Psychiatric Clinics:	Specialty Services:	

TYPES OF BUSINESS:
PPO
Utilization Management

BRANDS/DIVISIONS/AFFILIATES:

CONTACTS:
Note: Officers with more than one job title may be intentionally listed here more than once.
Gary R. Gannaway, CEO
Gary R. Gannaway, Pres.
Kenneth Hamm, Exec. VP/CFO
Ross D. Heyl, VP/Chief Mktg. Officer
Ze'ev Young, VP/Chief Medical Officer

Phone: 206-292-8255   Fax:
Toll-Free: 800-783-7312
Address: 600 University St., Ste 1400, Seattle, WA 98101 US

GROWTH PLANS/SPECIAL FEATURES:
First Choice Health Network, Inc. (FCHN) is a physician- and hospital-owned company offering a preferred provider organization (PPO) and health benefits management services to large self-funded plan sponsors. The company's principal business is the development and operation of a preferred provider network of hospitals, physicians and ancillary service providers, which currently consists of approximately 21,700 professional providers and 110 hospitals. The network serves approximately 1.1 million employees and dependents through contracts with 125 payors including insurers, third-party administrators, union trusts and employers. FCHN's network is located primarily in Washington, with additional health care providers located in Alaska, Idaho and Montana. It also contracts with self-insured employers, indemnity insurers, health maintenance organizations, union trusts and third-party administrators to provide subscribers with access to the PPO, for which it receives a fee. Additionally, hospitals participating in the PPO pay the network an administrative fee. FCHN's health benefits management business segment offers benefits management and administration services to self-funded employers and insurance carriers. Services include flexible spending account and health reimbursement account administration, COBRA benefits administration and medical management services.

FINANCIALS:
Sales and profits are in thousands of dollars—add 000 to get the full amount. Year 2004 note: Complete fiscal 2004 results were not available for all companies at press time. For this company, year 2004 is for months.

2004 Sales: $ (months)	2004 Profits: $ (months)	Stock Ticker: Private
2003 Sales: $	2003 Profits: $	Employees: 146
2002 Sales: $93,034	2002 Profits: $1,924	Fiscal Year Ends: 12/31
2001 Sales: $122,625	2001 Profits: $-1,407	
2000 Sales: $139,144	2000 Profits: $-1,350	

SALARIES/BENEFITS:
Pension Plan:	ESOP Stock Plan:	Profit Sharing:	Top Exec. Salary: $304,452	Bonus: $145,411
Savings Plan: Y	Stock Purch. Plan:		Second Exec. Salary: $238,989	Bonus: $123,408

OTHER THOUGHTS:
Apparent Top Female Officers:
Hot Spot for Advancement for Women/Minorities:

LOCATIONS: ("Y" = Yes)
West:	Southwest:	Midwest:	Southeast:	Northeast:	International:
Y					

FIRST CONSULTING GROUP INC

www.fcg.com

Industry Group Code: 541512   Ranks within this company's industry group: Sales: 1 Profits: 2

Insurance/HMO/PPO:	Drugs:	Equipment/Supplies:	Hospitals/Clinics:	Services:	Health Care:
Insurance:	Manufacturer:	Manufacturer:	Acute Care:	Diagnostics:	Home Health:
Managed Care:	Distributor:	Distributor:	Sub-Acute Care:	Labs/Testing:	Long-Term Care:
Utilization Mgmt.:	Specialty Pharm.:	Leasing/Finance:	Outpatient Surgery:	Staffing: Y	Physical Therapy:
Payment Proc.:	Vitamins/Nutri.:	Information Sys.: Y	Phys. Rehab. Center:	Waste Disposal:	Phys. Practice Mgmt.:
	Clinical Trials:		Psychiatric Clinics:	Specialty Services: Y	

TYPES OF BUSINESS:
Integration Services
Drug Development Consulting
Data Warehousing
Call Center Management
Application Integration
Information Technology Consulting
Systems Development and Implementation
Outsourcing Services

BRANDS/DIVISIONS/AFFILIATES:
FCG Management Services, LLC

CONTACTS:
Note: Officers with more than one job title may be intentionally listed here more than once.
Luther J. Nussbaum, CEO
Steven Heck, Pres.
Walter J. McBride, Exec. VP/CFO
Michael A. Zuercher, General Counsel
Bill Van Nostrand, Exec. VP-Life Sciences Bus. Unit
Mary Franz, Exec. VP-Consulting & Systems Integration
Guy L. Scalzi, Sr. VP-Outsourcing Services Bus. Unit
Barbara Hoehn, VP-Gov't Bus. Unit
Luther J. Nussbaum, Chmn.

Phone: 562-624-5200   Fax: 562-432-5774
Toll-Free: 800-345-0957
Address: 111 W. Ocean Blvd., 4th Fl., Long Beach, CA 90802 US

GROWTH PLANS/SPECIAL FEATURES:
First Consulting Group, Inc. (FCG) provides information-based consulting, integration and outsourcing services primarily to health-related industries in North America and Europe. Services are designed to increase efficiency of clients' operations through reduced cost, improved customer services, enhanced quality of patient care and more rapid introduction of new pharmaceutical compounds. The company applies industry knowledge and skills combined with advanced technologies, including the Internet, to make improvements in health care delivery, financing and administration, maintenance and research and development. FCG provides services primarily to health care delivery organizations, health plans, government health care organizations and pharmaceutical and life sciences organizations. Clients have included Fortune 500 companies, 17 of the top 20 managed care firms and two of the largest government health care IDNs. The firm assembles multi-disciplinary teams that provide comprehensive services. These professionals are supported by internal research and a centralized information system that provides real-time access to current industry information and project methodologies, experiences, models and tools. In recent news, FCG signed an agreement with Ardent Health Services to assist in improving the availability and reliability of information technology within Ardent's member hospitals.

FCG offers its employees medical, dental, disability and life insurance, discretionary performance rewards, recruiting referral fees, a matching gift program and tuition reimbursement.

FINANCIALS:
Sales and profits are in thousands of dollars—add 000 to get the full amount. Year 2004 note: Complete fiscal 2004 results were not available for all companies at press time. For this company, year 2004 is for 9 months.

2004 Sales: $212,894 (9 months)   2004 Profits: $1,662 (9 months)
2003 Sales: $287,739   2003 Profits: $-16,953
2002 Sales: $282,700   2002 Profits: $2,000
2001 Sales: $266,900   2001 Profits: $-6,900
2000 Sales: $248,885   2000 Profits: $-13,874

Stock Ticker: FCGI
Employees: 2,066
Fiscal Year Ends: 12/31

SALARIES/BENEFITS:
Pension Plan: ESOP Stock Plan: Profit Sharing: Top Exec. Salary: $475,000   Bonus: $23,750
Savings Plan: Y   Stock Purch. Plan: Y   Second Exec. Salary: $445,000   Bonus: $20,025

OTHER THOUGHTS:
Apparent Top Female Officers: 2
Hot Spot for Advancement for Women/Minorities:

LOCATIONS: ("Y" = Yes)

West:	Southwest:	Midwest:	Southeast:	Northeast:	International:
Y	Y	Y	Y	Y	Y

FIRST HEALTH GROUP CORP

www.firsthealth.com

Industry Group Code: 524114   Ranks within this company's industry group: Sales: 48   Profits: 23

Insurance/HMO/PPO:		Drugs:		Equipment/Supplies:		Hospitals/Clinics:		Services:		Health Care:	
Insurance:	Y	Manufacturer:		Manufacturer:		Acute Care:		Diagnostics:		Home Health:	
Managed Care:	Y	Distributor:		Distributor:		Sub-Acute Care:		Labs/Testing:		Long-Term Care:	
Utilization Mgmt.:	Y	Specialty Pharm.:		Leasing/Finance:		Outpatient Surgery:		Staffing:		Physical Therapy:	
Payment Proc.:	Y	Vitamins/Nutri.:		Information Sys.:	Y	Phys. Rehab. Center:		Waste Disposal:		Phys. Practice Mgmt.:	
		Clinical Trials:				Psychiatric Clinics:		Specialty Services:	Y		

TYPES OF BUSINESS:
PPO
Insurance Underwriting
Claims Administration
Pharmacy Benefit Management
Utilization Review Services
Workers' Compensation Services
Managed Care Services
IT Services

BRANDS/DIVISIONS/AFFILIATES:
First Health Network
Coventry Health Care, Inc.

CONTACTS:
Note: Officers with more than one job title may be intentionally listed here more than once.
Edward L. Wristen, CEO
Edward L. Wristen, Pres.
William R. McManaman, Sr. VP/CFO
Scott P. Smith, Chief Medical Officer
Ronald S. Boeving, CIO/VP-Info. Systems
Susan T. Smith, VP/General Counsel
Susan Oberling, Sr. VP-Oper.
David R. Studenmund, VP-Strategic Planning
Joseph E. Whitters, VP-Finance
Mary Baranowski, Sr. VP-Care Delivery Systems
Susan M. Fleming, Sr. VP-Product Mgmt. & External Affairs
A. Lee Dickerson, Exec. VP-Provider Networks & Bill Review Admin.
Karyn R. Glogowski, Sr. VP-Group Health & Account Mgmt.
James C. Smith, Chmn.

Phone: 630-737-7900   Fax:
Toll-Free:
Address: 3200 Highland Ave., Downers Grove, IL 60515 US

GROWTH PLANS/SPECIAL FEATURES:
First Health Group Corp. is one of the nation's premier full-service national health benefits companies, referred to as a preferred provider organization (PPO). Its First Health Network has approximately 4,300 participating hospitals and 450,000 outpatient care providers. The company specializes in providing large, national employers with a fully integrated single source for their group health programs. Its offerings include clinical programs such as case management, disease management and return-to-work programs; administrative products such as bill review, first report of injury and front end processing; pharmacy benefit management; fiscal agent services; and group health insurance products. These are supported by an IT infrastructure that includes proprietary integrated applications, centralized data, 24-hour customer service and member, provider, client and consultant web sites. First Health serves federal employees, self-insured corporations, third-party administrators, worker's compensation payors, small and mid-sized group health insurers and state Medicaid programs. In October 2004, Coventry Health Care, Inc. agreed to purchase First Health Group for $1.8 billion in cash and stock.

FINANCIALS:
Sales and profits are in thousands of dollars—add 000 to get the full amount. Year 2004 note: Complete fiscal 2004 results were not available for all companies at press time. For this company, year 2004 is for 9 months.

2004 Sales: $657,300 (9 months)   2004 Profits: $86,500 (9 months)
2003 Sales: $890,926   2003 Profits: $152,734
2002 Sales: $760,000   2002 Profits: $132,900
2001 Sales: $593,100   2001 Profits: $102,900
2000 Sales: $506,741   2000 Profits: $82,619

Stock Ticker: FHCC
Employees: 6,000
Fiscal Year Ends: 12/31

SALARIES/BENEFITS:
Pension Plan: ESOP Stock Plan: Profit Sharing: Top Exec. Salary: $798,663   Bonus: $440,005
Savings Plan: Y Stock Purch. Plan: Y   Second Exec. Salary: $705,388 Bonus: $114,412

OTHER THOUGHTS:
Apparent Top Female Officers: 5
Hot Spot for Advancement for Women/Minorities: Y

LOCATIONS: ("Y" = Yes)

West:	Southwest:	Midwest:	Southeast:	Northeast:	International:
Y	Y	Y	Y	Y	

Note: Financial information, benefits and other data can change quickly and may vary from those stated here.

FISCHER IMAGING CORP

www.fischerimaging.com

Industry Group Code: 339113   Ranks within this company's industry group: Sales: 114   Profits: 128

Insurance/HMO/PPO:	Drugs:	Equipment/Supplies:	Hospitals/Clinics:	Services:	Health Care:
Insurance:	Manufacturer:	Manufacturer: Y	Acute Care:	Diagnostics:	Home Health:
Managed Care:	Distributor:	Distributor:	Sub-Acute Care:	Labs/Testing:	Long-Term Care:
Utilization Mgmt.:	Specialty Pharm.:	Leasing/Finance:	Outpatient Surgery:	Staffing:	Physical Therapy:
Payment Proc.:	Vitamins/Nutri.:	Information Sys.:	Phys. Rehab. Center:	Waste Disposal:	Phys. Practice Mgmt.:
	Clinical Trials:		Psychiatric Clinics:	Specialty Services:	

TYPES OF BUSINESS:
Equipment-X-Ray Imaging Systems
Needle Biopsy Platforms
Digital Mammography Systems

BRANDS/DIVISIONS/AFFILIATES:
MammoTest
SenoScan

CONTACTS: Note: Officers with more than one job title may be intentionally listed here more than once.
Harris Ravine, CEO
Harris Ravine, Pres.
David Kirwan, CFO
Bob Hoffman, VP-North American Sales
Laurie Clyne, VP-Human Resources
Roman Janer, Chief Tech. Officer
Steve Moseley, Exec. VP-Bus. Dev.
David Kirwan, Sr. VP-Finance
Janine Broda, VP-Mktg. & Strategic Alliances
Peter Cardle, VP-EMEA
Tom Gibson, VP-National Service
Gary Turner, VP-Quality & Regulatory Affairs
Gail Schoettler, Chmn.

Phone: 303-254-2525   Fax: 303-254-2502
Toll-Free:
Address: 12300 N. Grant St., Denver, CO 80241 US

GROWTH PLANS/SPECIAL FEATURES:

Fischer Imaging Corp. develops, manufactures and markets medical imaging systems for the detection, diagnosis and treatment of breast cancer. Fischer serves the breast care needs of women around the world and has installed systems in over 1,500 clinics, hospitals and imaging centers in the U.S. and Europe. The company's main products are the SenoScan digital mammography system and the MammoTest stereotactic breast biopsy machine. SenoScan's advantages over conventional x-ray film mammography systems stem from the ability to acquire high-resolution images at reduced radiation doses, to manipulate the digital image, to transmit the images to facilitate remote diagnosis and to store the images in a cost-effective digital archive. MammoTest allows for a breast biopsy procedure that is less invasive and expensive than surgical biopsy and can be performed under local anesthetic on an outpatient basis. Fischer's radiology, electrophysiology and surgery division produces a line of film and digital general x-ray imaging systems and a number of specialized x-ray systems used in electrophysiology procedures. Current research and development efforts are focused on providing new imaging technology for breast cancer screening and treatment, particularly the development of computer-aided detection software for use with SenoScan.

Employee benefits at Fischer include medical, dental, long-term disability and basic life insurance, as well as tuition reimbursement, an employee assistance program, credit union membership and relocation assistance.

FINANCIALS:
Sales and profits are in thousands of dollars—add 000 to get the full amount. Year 2004 note: Complete fiscal 2004 results were not available for all companies at press time. For this company, year 2004 is for 6 months.

2004 Sales: $31,785 (6 months)   2004 Profits: $-1,323   (6 months)
2003 Sales: $46,200   2003 Profits: $-14,400
2002 Sales: $45,000   2002 Profits: $10,000
2001 Sales: $41,900   2001 Profits: $-800
2000 Sales: $54,100   2000 Profits: $200

Stock Ticker: FIMG
Employees: 232
Fiscal Year Ends: 12/31

SALARIES/BENEFITS:
Pension Plan: ESOP Stock Plan: Profit Sharing: Top Exec. Salary: $236,172   Bonus: $91,100
Savings Plan: Y Stock Purch. Plan: Second Exec. Salary: $204,217 Bonus: $139,390

OTHER THOUGHTS:
Apparent Top Female Officers: 3
Hot Spot for Advancement for Women/Minorities: Y

LOCATIONS: ("Y" = Yes)
West	Southwest	Midwest	Southeast	Northeast	International
Y					Y

ative
FISHER SCIENTIFIC INTERNATIONAL INC   www.fisherscientific.com

Industry Group Code: 421450   Ranks within this company's industry group: Sales: 2   Profits: 3

Insurance/HMO/PPO:	Drugs:		Equipment/Supplies:		Hospitals/Clinics:	Services:		Health Care:	
Insurance:	Manufacturer:	Y	Manufacturer:	Y	Acute Care:	Diagnostics:		Home Health:	
Managed Care:	Distributor:	Y	Distributor:	Y	Sub-Acute Care:	Labs/Testing:		Long-Term Care:	
Utilization Mgmt.:	Specialty Pharm.:		Leasing/Finance:		Outpatient Surgery:	Staffing:		Physical Therapy:	
Payment Proc.:	Vitamins/Nutri.:		Information Sys.:		Phys. Rehab. Center:	Waste Disposal:		Phys. Practice Mgmt.:	
	Clinical Trials:				Psychiatric Clinics:	Specialty Services:	Y		

TYPES OF BUSINESS:
Equipment/Supplies Distributor
Contract Manufacturing
Equipment Calibration and Repair
Clinical Trial Services
Laboratory Workstations
Clinical Consumables
Diagnostic Reagents
Custom Chemical Synthesis

BRANDS/DIVISIONS/AFFILIATES:
Fisher Research
Fisher Science Education
Fisher HealthCare
Medical Analysis Systems, Inc.
Fisher Hamilton
Fisher Clinical Services, Inc.
Dharmacon, Inc.
Apogent Technologies, Inc.

CONTACTS:
Note: Officers with more than one job title may be intentionally listed here more than once.

Paul M. Montrone, CEO
David T. Della Penta, Pres.
David T. Della Penta, COO
Kevin P. Clark, VP/CFO
Todd M. DuChene, VP/General Counsel
Gia L. Oei, Media Rel. Contact
Carolyn J. Miller, Investor Rel. Contact
Gregory J. Heinlein, Treas.
Patrick J. Balthrop, Pres., Fisher HealthCare
Todd M. DuChene, Corp. Sec.
Paul M. Montrone, Chmn.

Phone: 603-926-5911   **Fax:** 603-926-0222
Toll-Free: 800-395-5442
Address: One Liberty Ln., Hampton, NH 03842 US

GROWTH PLANS/SPECIAL FEATURES:
Fisher Scientific International, Inc. is a world leader in servicing the needs of the scientific community. The company provides more than 600,000 products and services to research, health care, industrial, educational and government customers in 145 countries. The firm's products and services enable scientific discovery and clinical laboratory testing for more than 350,000 customers. Fisher strives to serve as a one-stop source for the scientific and laboratory needs of its customers. Products include scientific instruments and equipment, clinical consumables, diagnostic reagents, safety and clean room supplies, laboratory equipment and workstations. Over 80% of the firm's revenue comes from the sales of consumable products. Services include pharmaceutical services for Phase III and Phase IV clinical trials, laboratory instrument calibration and repair, contract manufacturing and custom chemical synthesis. The domestic distribution segment manufactures, sells and distributes products to three primary customer markets: scientific research (pharmaceutical, biotechnology, industrial customers and colleges and universities), clinical laboratory (group purchasing organizations, reference laboratories and independent hospital and physician office laboratories) and industrial safety (industrial companies, public safety organizations and controlled environments). The international distribution segment consists of distribution businesses located in Europe, Canada, Asia and Latin America that sell and distribute products primarily to the scientific research market. The laboratory workstations segment engages in the manufacture and sale of laboratory furniture and fume hoods to the scientific research laboratory market and the manufacture and sale of consoles and enclosures to the technology, communications and financial markets. In recent news, the company announced that it will acquire for $2.7 billion and merge with Apogent Technologies, Inc., a global provider of laboratory and life science products. Fisher Scientific also acquired Dharmacon, Inc., a leader in RNA interference technology.

Fisher Scientific provides a competitive bonus package and the opportunity to work in a variety of fields at locations in various countries around the world.

FINANCIALS:
Sales and profits are in thousands of dollars—add 000 to get the full amount. Year 2004 note: Complete fiscal 2004 results were not available for all companies at press time. For this company, year 2004 is for 9 months.

2004 Sales: $3,331,600 (9 months)	2004 Profits: $90,100 (9 months)	**Stock Ticker:** FSH
2003 Sales: $3,564,400	2003 Profits: $78,400	Employees: 10,200
2002 Sales: $3,238,400	2002 Profits: $50,600	Fiscal Year Ends: 12/31
2001 Sales: $2,880,000	2001 Profits: $16,400	
2000 Sales: $2,622,300	2000 Profits: $22,700	

SALARIES/BENEFITS:
Pension Plan:	ESOP Stock Plan:	Profit Sharing: Y	Top Exec. Salary: $815,000	Bonus: $1,100,000
Savings Plan: Y	Stock Purch. Plan:		Second Exec. Salary: $300,000	Bonus: $810,000

OTHER THOUGHTS:
Apparent Top Female Officers: 2
Hot Spot for Advancement for Women/Minorities:

LOCATIONS: ("Y" = Yes)
West:	Southwest:	Midwest:	Southeast:	Northeast:	International:
Y	Y	Y	Y	Y	Y

FOREST LABORATORIES INC

www.frx.com

Industry Group Code: 325412 **Ranks within this company's industry group:** Sales: 21 Profits: 15

Insurance/HMO/PPO:	Drugs:		Equipment/Supplies:	Hospitals/Clinics:	Services:	Health Care:
Insurance:	Manufacturer:	Y	Manufacturer:	Acute Care:	Diagnostics:	Home Health:
Managed Care:	Distributor:	Y	Distributor:	Sub-Acute Care:	Labs/Testing:	Long-Term Care:
Utilization Mgmt.:	Specialty Pharm.:		Leasing/Finance:	Outpatient Surgery:	Staffing:	Physical Therapy:
Payment Proc.:	Vitamins/Nutri.:		Information Sys.:	Phys. Rehab. Center:	Waste Disposal:	Phys. Practice Mgmt.:
	Clinical Trials:			Psychiatric Clinics:	Specialty Services:	

TYPES OF BUSINESS:
Drugs-Manufacturing
Over-the-Counter Pharmaceuticals
Generic Pharmaceuticals
Antidepressants
Asthma Medications

BRANDS/DIVISIONS/AFFILIATES:
Lexapro
Namenda
Celexa
Benicar
Tiazac
Aerobid
AeroChamber Plus
Infasurf

CONTACTS:
Note: Officers with more than one job title may be intentionally listed here more than once.
Howard Solomon, CEO
Kenneth E. Goodman, Pres.
Kenneth E. Goodman, COO
John E. Eggers, CFO
Elaine Hochberg, Sr. VP-Mktg.
Bernard J. McGovern, VP-Human Resources
Lawrence S. Olanoff, Exec. VP-Scientific Affairs
Richard Overton, VP-Oper. & Facilities
Mary E. Prehn, VP-Licensing & Corp. Dev.
Charles E. Triano, VP-Investor Rel.
John E. Eggers, VP-Finance
Terrill J. Howell, VP-Oper., Forest Pharmaceuticals
Howard Solomon, Chmn.

Phone: 212-421-7850   **Fax:** 212-750-9152
Toll-Free: 800-947-5227
Address: 909 3rd Ave., New York, NY 10022 US

GROWTH PLANS/SPECIAL FEATURES:
Forest Laboratories, Inc. develops, manufactures and sells branded and generic prescription and over-the-counter pharmaceuticals that are used to treat a wide range of illnesses. The company's Lexapro and Celexa products are used to treat central nervous system disorders like major depressive disorder, generalized anxiety disorder and depression. Forest offers the first and only medication approved for use with moderate and severe Alzheimer's disease, Namenda. Benicar and Tiazac both treat cardiovascular disease. The company also offers medications to treat asthma and an inhalent delivery system called AeroChamber Plus. Armour Thyroid, Levothroid and Thyroloar all treat conditions of the endocrine system. Recently, Forest agreed to develop and market PAION's desmotesplase, a blood-clot-dissolving agent under development for the treatment of acute ischemic stroke.

Forest offers its employees medical, dental and vision insurance, plus financial assistance for adoption and fertility treatments.

FINANCIALS:
Sales and profits are in thousands of dollars—add 000 to get the full amount. Year 2004 note: Complete fiscal 2004 results were not available for all companies at press time. For this company, year 2004 is for 12 months.

2004 Sales: $2,650,432 (12 months)   2004 Profits: $735,874 (12 months)
2003 Sales: $2,206,700   2003 Profits: $622,000
2002 Sales: $1,566,600   2002 Profits: $338,000
2001 Sales: $1,205,200   2001 Profits: $215,100
2000 Sales: $899,300   2000 Profits: $112,688

Stock Ticker: FRX
Employees: 4,967
Fiscal Year Ends: 3/31

SALARIES/BENEFITS:
Pension Plan: ESOP Stock Plan: Profit Sharing: Top Exec. Salary: $991,250   Bonus: $550,000
Savings Plan: Y   Stock Purch. Plan: Y   Second Exec. Salary: $669,250   Bonus: $350,000

OTHER THOUGHTS:
Apparent Top Female Officers: 2
Hot Spot for Advancement for Women/Minorities:

LOCATIONS: ("Y" = Yes)
West:	Southwest:	Midwest:	Southeast:	Northeast:	International:
		Y		Y	Y

Note: Financial information, benefits and other data can change quickly and may vary from those stated here.

FRESENIUS AG

www.fresenius-ag.com

Industry Group Code: 621490 **Ranks within this company's industry group:** Sales: 1 Profits: 3

Insurance/HMO/PPO:	Drugs:		Equipment/Supplies:		Hospitals/Clinics:		Services:		Health Care:	
Insurance:	Manufacturer:	Y	Manufacturer:	Y	Acute Care:		Diagnostics:		Home Health:	
Managed Care:	Distributor:	Y	Distributor:	Y	Sub-Acute Care:	Y	Labs/Testing:		Long-Term Care:	
Utilization Mgmt.:	Specialty Pharm.:		Leasing/Finance:		Outpatient Surgery:		Staffing:		Physical Therapy:	
Payment Proc.:	Vitamins/Nutri.:		Information Sys.:		Phys. Rehab. Center:		Waste Disposal:		Phys. Practice Mgmt.:	
	Clinical Trials:				Psychiatric Clinics:		Specialty Services:	Y		

TYPES OF BUSINESS:
Dialysis Products & Services
Nutrition, Infusion Therapy & Transfusion Technology Products
Ambulatory Care Services
Management & Consulting Services
Biopharmaceuticals
Information Technology Services

BRANDS/DIVISIONS/AFFILIATES:
Fresenius Health Care Group
Fresenius Medical Care AG
Fresenius Kabi
Fresenius ProServe
Fresenius Biotech
Fresenius Netcare
Wittgensteiner Kliniken-WKA
Fresenius Biotech

CONTACTS:
Note: Officers with more than one job title may be intentionally listed here more than once.
Ulf M. Schneider, Chmn.-Mgmt. Board
Stephan Sturm, CFO
Stephan Sturm, Dir.-Labor Rel.
Dieter Schenk, Lawyer/Tax Consultant
Joachim Weith, Sr. VP-Corp. Comm. & Gov't Affairs
Rainer Baule, CEO-Fresenius Kabi
Rainer Hohmann, CEO-Fresenius ProServe
Ben Lipps, CEO-Fresenius Medical Care
Gerd Krick, Chmn.

Phone: 49-6172-608-0   **Fax:** 49-6172-608-2488
Toll-Free:
Address: Else-Kroner-Strasse 1, Bas Homburg, 61346 Germany

GROWTH PLANS/SPECIAL FEATURES:
Fresenius AG is an international health care group offering products and services for dialysis, hospitals and the ambulatory medical care of patients. The firm has operation sin 100 countries. The company operates the Fresenius Health Care Group (FHCG), which has three core segments: Fresenius Medical Care AG (FMC), Fresenius Kabi and Fresenius ProServe. FMC is a leading manufacturer of chronic kidney failure products, such as hemodialysis machines, dialyzers and related disposable products. It also owns and operates 1,595 dialysis clinics worldwide. Kabi provides parenteral nutrition products, which supply nutrients to the body while avoiding the gastro-intestinal tract; enteral nutrition products, which artificially feed via the intestinal tract; infusion therapy products, including electrolyte and glucose solutions, blood replacement solutions and medical products, such as rinsing solutions, and drugs and anesthetics for injection or infusion; transfusion technology products, including cell separators, blood bag systems, blood filters and products for the blood bank; and ambulatory care services. ProServe operates through several subsidiaries, including Wittgensteiner Kliniken-WKA, hospitals activHealth, hospitalia care, hospitalia international, Pharmaplan and VAMED. It offers management services to hospitals and other health care facilities, including project development, consulting and staff training. In addition, the firm operates through two other FHCG subsidiaries: Fresenius Biotech, which develops and markets biopharmaceuticals in the fields of oncology, immunology and regenerative medicine; and Fresenius Netcare, which offers services in the field of information technology both inside and outside of the company. In recent news, Fresenius agreed to sell its hospitalia care subsidiary, which operates and manages 23 nursing care facilities in Germany with more than 2,600 beds.

FINANCIALS:
Sales and profits are in thousands of dollars—add 000 to get the full amount. Year 2004 note: Complete fiscal 2004 results were not available for all companies at press time. For this company, year 2004 is for months.

2004 Sales: $ (months)	2004 Profits: $ (months)	**Stock Ticker:** Foreign
2003 Sales: $8,866,700	2003 Profits: $144,300	**Employees:** 65,243
2002 Sales: $7,868,100	2002 Profits: $140,400	**Fiscal Year Ends:** 12/31
2001 Sales: $	2001 Profits: $	
2000 Sales: $	2000 Profits: $	

SALARIES/BENEFITS:
| Pension Plan: | ESOP Stock Plan: | Profit Sharing: | Top Exec. Salary: $ | Bonus: $ |
| Savings Plan: | Stock Purch. Plan: | | Second Exec. Salary: $ | Bonus: $ |

OTHER THOUGHTS:
Apparent Top Female Officers:
Hot Spot for Advancement for Women/Minorities:

LOCATIONS: ("Y" = Yes)
West:	Southwest:	Midwest:	Southeast:	Northeast:	International:
Y	Y			Y	Y

FUJISAWA PHARMACEUTICALS COMPANY LTD

www.fujisawa.co.jp

Industry Group Code: 325412   Ranks within this company's industry group: Sales: 19   Profits: 21

Insurance/HMO/PPO:	Drugs:	Equipment/Supplies:	Hospitals/Clinics:	Services:	Health Care:
Insurance:	Manufacturer: Y	Manufacturer:	Acute Care:	Diagnostics:	Home Health:
Managed Care:	Distributor:	Distributor:	Sub-Acute Care:	Labs/Testing:	Long-Term Care:
Utilization Mgmt.:	Specialty Pharm.:	Leasing/Finance:	Outpatient Surgery:	Staffing:	Physical Therapy:
Payment Proc.:	Vitamins/Nutri.:	Information Sys.:	Phys. Rehab. Center:	Waste Disposal:	Phys. Practice Mgmt.:
	Clinical Trials:		Psychiatric Clinics:	Specialty Services: Y	

TYPES OF BUSINESS:

Drugs, Manufacturing
Immunological Pharmaceuticals
Chemicals
Over-the-Counter Products
Medical Systems and Home Care Devices
Reagents
Genomic Research

BRANDS/DIVISIONS/AFFILIATES:

Fujisawa Healthcare, Inc.
Fujisawa GmbH
Prograf
Protopic
Astellas Pharma, Inc.
Zepharma, Inc.
Yamanouchi Pharmaceutical Company

CONTACTS: Note: Officers with more than one job title may be intentionally listed here more than once.

Hatsuo Aoki, CEO
Hatsuo Aoki, Pres.
Osamu Nagai, Corp. VP/CFO
Takeshi Shimomura, Corp. Exec. VP-Sales & Mktg.
Toshio Goto, Corp. VP-Global Research
Hitoshi Ohta, Corp. VP-Global Mfg.
Koichi Sejima, Corp. Exec. VP/Chief Admin. Officer
Masafumi Nogimori, Corp. Sr. VP-Global Strategy
Tadahiko Inoue, Corp. VP-General Affairs
Hideo Fukumoto, Corp. VP/CEO-Fujisawa Healthcare, Inc.
Masaji Ohe, Corp. VP-OTC & Consumer Products
Masao Shimizu, Corp. VP-Global Dev.
Akira Fujiyama, Chmn.

Phone: 81-6-6202-1141	Fax: 81-6-6206-7926
Toll-Free:	
Address: 4-7, Doshomachi 3-chome, Chuo-ku, Osaka, 541-8514 Japan	

GROWTH PLANS/SPECIAL FEATURES:

Fujisawa Pharmaceuticals Company, Ltd. is a global biopharmaceutical company based in Japan, with operations in Europe and North America, as well as in Taiwan, Hong Kong, China and South Korea. Roughly 90% of company revenues relate to sales of pharmaceuticals, led by Prograf (tacrolimus), which is used as an immunosuppressant in conjunction with organ transplantation. Other Fujisawa products target needs in cardiology and dermatology, including Protopic, the firest topical immunomodulator for the treatment of atopic dermatitis. Approximately half of company sales are derived overseas, led by U.S. division Fujisawa Healthcare, Inc. and the company's German-based European headquarters, Fujisawa GmbH. Other Fujisawa businesses include manufacturing and distribution of over-the-counter (OTC) products in Japan, as well as the domestic supply of medical systems and home care devices and the production of chemicals ranging from industrial compounds to food additives. Within its medical supply and systems division, Fujisawa serves the biotechnology industry by providing access to more than 7,000 reagents used in immunology and genetic research. In addition to ongoing in-house genomic research, Fujisawa is engaged in a collaborative effort with Quark Biotech, Inc. focused on the discovery of new medicines for the treatment of stroke. In early 2004, Fujisawa entered into an agreement to be acquired by Yamanouchi Pharmaceutical Co. for a reported price of $7.6 billion in a stock-for-stock transaction. The resulting company, to be launched in August 2005, will be called Astellas Pharma, Inc., with Yamanouchi chief executive Toichi Takenaka assuming executive control and Fujisawa head Hatsuo Aoki becoming board chairman. The new company should rank as Japan's second-largest drug company (behind Takeda Chemical Industries, Ltd.) and as the 17th-largest drug company in the world. Fujisawa and Yamanouchi have already started the integration process, relaunching their respective OTC businesses in a new joint venture named Zepharma, Inc.

FINANCIALS: Sales and profits are in thousands of dollars—add 000 to get the full amount. Year 2004 note: Complete fiscal 2004 results were not available for all companies at press time. For this company, year 2004 is for 12 months.

2004 Sales: $3,742,900 (12 months)   2004 Profits: $392,500   (12 months)
2003 Sales: $3,188,300   2003 Profits: $238,900
2002 Sales: $2,573,500   2002 Profits: $197,200
2001 Sales: $2,355,100   2001 Profits: $162,500
2000 Sales: $ 2000 Profits: $

Stock Ticker: Foreign
Employees: 8,000
Fiscal Year Ends: 3/31

SALARIES/BENEFITS:

Pension Plan:	ESOP Stock Plan:	Profit Sharing:	Top Exec. Salary: $	Bonus: $
Savings Plan:	Stock Purch. Plan:		Second Exec. Salary: $	Bonus: $

OTHER THOUGHTS:

Apparent Top Female Officers:
Hot Spot for Advancement for Women/Minorities:

LOCATIONS: ("Y" = Yes)

West:	Southwest:	Midwest:	Southeast:	Northeast:	International:
		Y			Y

# GAMBRO AB

www.gambro.com

Industry Group Code: 621490　Ranks within this company's industry group: Sales: 2　Profits: 1

Insurance/HMO/PPO:	Drugs:	Equipment/Supplies:		Hospitals/Clinics:	Services:		Health Care:	
Insurance: Managed Care: Utilization Mgmt.: Payment Proc.:	Manufacturer: Distributor: Specialty Pharm.: Vitamins/Nutri.: Clinical Trials:	Manufacturer: Distributor: Leasing/Finance: Information Sys.:	Y	Acute Care: Sub-Acute Care: Outpatient Surgery: Phys. Rehab. Center: Psychiatric Clinics:	Diagnostics: Labs/Testing: Staffing: Waste Disposal: Specialty Services:	Y	Home Health: Long-Term Care: Physical Therapy: Phys. Practice Mgmt.:	

TYPES OF BUSINESS:
Dialysis Products & Services
Dialysis Clinics
Cell Therapy & Apheresis Technologies
Blood Component Collection & Purification Technologies
Liver Failure Products & Services
Sterile Solutions

BRANDS/DIVISIONS/AFFILIATES:
Gambro, Inc.
Gambro Healthcare, Inc.
Gambro Healthcare Laboratory Services, Inc.
Gambro BCT
Gambro Renal Products
Hospal
Teraklin AG
Navigant Biotechnologies, Inc.

CONTACTS: Note: Officers with more than one job title may be intentionally listed here more than once.
Soren Mellstig, CEO
Soren Mellstig, Pres.
Lars Granlof, Sr. VP/CFO
Lars Fahlen, Sr. VP-Corp. Human Resources
Maris Harmanis, Sr. VP/Head-Corp. Research
Ingmar Magnusson, General Counsel
Asa Hedin, Head-Strategic Dev.
Karin Avasalu, VP-Corp. Comm.
Pia Irell, VP-Investor Rel.
Pia Irell, VP-Corp. Finance
Larry C. Buckelew, Pres./CEO-Gambro Healthcare U.S.
Jon Risfelt, Pres., Gambro Renal Products
David B. Perez, Pres., Gambro BCT, Inc.
Kevin Smith, Pres., Gambro, Inc.
Claes Dahlback, Chmn.
Bo-Inge Hansson, Head-Gambro Healthcare Int'l

Phone: 46-8-613-65-00	Fax: 46-8-611-28-30
Toll-Free:	
Address: Jakobsgatan 6, Stockholm, SE-103 91 Sweden	

GROWTH PLANS/SPECIAL FEATURES:
Gambro AB is a global medical technology and health care company that manufactures dialysis products, operates kidney dialysis clinics and develops and supplies blood bank technology worldwide. The firm operates through three businesses: Gambro Healthcare (GH), Gambro Renal Products (GRP) and Gambro BCT (blood component technology). GH is a leading provider of dialysis services worldwide. It includes two organizational segments: Gambro Healthcare U.S., which operates 565 clinics in the U.S., and Gambro Healthcare International, which operates 146 clinics outside of the U.S. GRP is a leading developer, manufacturer and supplier of hemodialysis, peritoneal dialysis and acute dialysis products and equipment, including dialysis machines, dialyzers, blood lines, sterile solutions and liquid and dry concentrates. It provides products and services under the Gambro and Hospal brand names and has production facilities in 12 countries and sales organizations in 28 countries. Gambro BCT provides technology, products and systems to blood centers and hospital blood banks worldwide. It is a global leader in cell therapy and apheresis (the separation of blood into its components, i.e. red blood cells, white blood cells, blood platelets and plasma), as well as in the development of blood component collection and purification technologies. The company's wholly-owned subsidiary Gambro, Inc. operates through two subsidiaries: Gambro Healthcare, Inc. and Gambro Healthcare Laboratory Services, Inc. In recent news, Gambro expanded into the emerging acute liver failure market through the acquisition of Teraklin AG. The company launched Prismaflex, a new system for the treatment of acute renal failure and fluid management. The firm's wholly-owned subsidiary Navigant Biotechnologies, Inc. announced positive clinical trial results demonstrating the recovery and survival of platelets treated with its Mirasol Pathogen Technology for the removal of blood-born pathogens. Gambro BCT agreed to acquire the assets of Ivex Pharmaceuticals, Ltd., which develops and manufactures sterile solutions for the pharmaceutical and medical device industry.

FINANCIALS: Sales and profits are in thousands of dollars—add 000 to get the full amount. Year 2004 note: Complete fiscal 2004 results were not available for all companies at press time. For this company, year 2004 is for months.

2004 Sales: $ (months)
2003 Sales: $3,606,400
2002 Sales: $3,151,700
2001 Sales: $
2000 Sales: $

2004 Profits: $ (months)
2003 Profits: $196,200
2002 Profits: $70,000
2001 Profits: $
2000 Profits: $

Stock Ticker: Foreign
Employees: 21,273
Fiscal Year Ends: 12/31

SALARIES/BENEFITS:
Pension Plan:	ESOP Stock Plan:	Profit Sharing:	Top Exec. Salary: $	Bonus: $
Savings Plan:	Stock Purch. Plan:		Second Exec. Salary: $	Bonus: $

OTHER THOUGHTS:
Apparent Top Female Officers: 3
Hot Spot for Advancement for Women/Minorities: Y

LOCATIONS: ("Y" = Yes)
West: Y	Southwest:	Midwest:	Southeast:	Northeast:	International: Y

GE COMMERCIAL FINANCE
www.gecommercialfinance.com

Industry Group Code: 522220A   Ranks within this company's industry group: Sales: 1   Profits:

Insurance/HMO/PPO:	Drugs:	Equipment/Supplies:	Hospitals/Clinics:	Services:	Health Care:
Insurance:	Manufacturer:	Manufacturer:	Acute Care:	Diagnostics:	Home Health:
Managed Care:	Distributor:	Distributor:	Sub-Acute Care:	Labs/Testing:	Long-Term Care:
Utilization Mgmt.:	Specialty Pharm.:	Leasing/Finance: Y	Outpatient Surgery:	Staffing:	Physical Therapy:
Payment Proc.:	Vitamins/Nutri.:	Information Sys.:	Phys. Rehab. Center:	Waste Disposal:	Phys. Practice Mgmt.:
	Clinical Trials:		Psychiatric Clinics:	Specialty Services: Y	

TYPES OF BUSINESS:
Lending-Commercial
Commercial Equipment Leasing
Finance Program Development
Real Estate Finance
Health Care Finance
Fleet Management
Specialty Financing

BRANDS/DIVISIONS/AFFILIATES:
General Electric Co.
GE Corporate Financial Services
GE Vendor Financial Services
GE Commercial Equipment Financing
GE Aviation Services
GE European Equipment Finance
GE Real Estate
GE Healthcare Financial Services

CONTACTS:
Note: Officers with more than one job title may be intentionally listed here more than once.
Michael A. Neal, CEO
Michael A. Neal, Pres.
Marissa Moretti, Media Rel. Contact
Paul T. Bossidy, Pres./CEO-GE Commercial Equipment Financing
Michael A. Gaudino, Pres./CEO-GE Corporate Financial Services
Rick Wolfert, Pres./CEO-GE Healthcare Financial Services
Kathryn V. Marinello, Pres./CEO-GE Fleet Services
Roman Oryschuk, Pres./CEO-GE European Equipment Finance

Phone: 203-357-4000	Fax:
Toll-Free:	
Address: 260 Long Ridge Rd., Stamford, CT 06927 US	

GROWTH PLANS/SPECIAL FEATURES:
GE Commercial Finance, a result of the June 2003 reorganization of GE Capital, provides both small and large businesses across the globe with a wide variety of financial services and products. The company offers financing programs, loans, operating leases and other services. In addition, it supplies specialized loans and financing leases for major capital assets such as aircraft fleets, industrial facilities and equipment, as well as loans to and investments in public and private entities in diverse industries. The firm is divided into eight smaller businesses. GE Aviation Services serves customers in more than 60 nations, providing funding for more than 1,200 owned aircraft and managing nearly 300 others. Commercial equipment financing is provided for a wide variety of equipment, facility and office needs, ranging from $50,000 to $50 million per transaction. GE Corporate Financial Services provides financing solutions primarily for non-investment-grade companies, including revolving credit facilities, term debt, asset securitization, trade finance, factoring, debtor-in-possession facilities and plan-of-reorganization facilities, as well as preferred and common equity. GE Energy Financial Services is a global leader in energy investing and financing that provides a wide range of financial products and services to companies throughout the energy industry. GE European Equipment Finance makes equipment leasing, business financing and other associated services available to European businesses of varying size. GE Fleet Services is one of the largest fleet management companies in the world with more than 1.4 million cars and trucks under lease and service management globally. GE Healthcare Financial Services is a specialty finance entity dealing only with the health care industry's unique requirements. GE Real Estate offers intermediate to long-term mortgage financing, restructuring and acquisition capital and niche equity investments. GE Vendor Financial Services develops and provides financial solutions and services to equipment manufacturers, distributors, dealers and their end users.

FINANCIALS:
Sales and profits are in thousands of dollars—add 000 to get the full amount. Year 2004 note: Complete fiscal 2004 results were not available for all companies at press time. For this company, year 2004 is for months.

2004 Sales: $ (months)   2004 Profits: $ (months)
2003 Sales: $18,869,000   2003 Profits: $
2002 Sales: $16,040,000   2002 Profits: $3,185,000
2001 Sales: $13,880,000   2001 Profits: $2,724,000
2000 Sales: $11,982,000   2000 Profits: $2,294,000

Stock Ticker: Subsidiary
Employees:
Fiscal Year Ends: 12/31

SALARIES/BENEFITS:
Pension Plan: ESOP Stock Plan: Profit Sharing: Top Exec. Salary: $ Bonus: $
Savings Plan: Stock Purch. Plan: Second Exec. Salary: $ Bonus: $

OTHER THOUGHTS:
Apparent Top Female Officers: 2
Hot Spot for Advancement for Women/Minorities:

LOCATIONS: ("Y" = Yes)
West:	Southwest:	Midwest:	Southeast:	Northeast:	International:
Y	Y	Y	Y	Y	Y

GE HEALTHCARE

www.gehealthcare.com

Industry Group Code: 339113 Ranks within this company's industry group: Sales: 2 Profits:

Insurance/HMO/PPO:	Drugs:	Equipment/Supplies:		Hospitals/Clinics:	Services:		Health Care:
Insurance:	Manufacturer:	Manufacturer:	Y	Acute Care:	Diagnostics:		Home Health:
Managed Care:	Distributor:	Distributor:		Sub-Acute Care:	Labs/Testing:		Long-Term Care:
Utilization Mgmt.:	Specialty Pharm.:	Leasing/Finance:		Outpatient Surgery:	Staffing:		Physical Therapy:
Payment Proc.:	Vitamins/Nutri.:	Information Sys.:	Y	Phys. Rehab. Center:	Waste Disposal:		Phys. Practice Mgmt.:
	Clinical Trials:			Psychiatric Clinics:	Specialty Services:	Y	

TYPES OF BUSINESS:
Equipment-X-Ray & Ultrasound Bone Densitometers
Magnetic Resonance Imaging Systems
Patient Monitoring Systems
Clinical Information Systems
Information Technology
Surgery & Vascular Imaging
Nuclear Medicine
Clinical & Business Services

BRANDS/DIVISIONS/AFFILIATES:
GE Electric Co.
GE Healthcare Bio-Sciences
GE Healthcare Technologies
GE Healthcare Information Technologies
Centricity
Giraffe OmniBed
Innova
InstaTrak

CONTACTS:
Note: Officers with more than one job title may be intentionally listed here more than once.
William Castell, CEO
William Castell, Pres.
Mark Vachon, Exec. VP/CFO
Jean-Mitchel Cossery, Exec. VP-Strategic Mktg.
John Lynch, Exec. VP-Human Resources
Stuart Scott, CIO
William R. Clarke, Chief Tech. Officer/Chief Medical Officer
Peter Y. Solmssen, Exec. VP/General Counsel
Michael A. Jones, Exec. VP-Bus. Dev.
Pam Wickham, Exec. VP-Global Comm.
Steve Bolze, Exec. VP-Integration
Michael Stevens, Exec. VP/Staff Exec.
Peter Loescher, Pres./CEO-GE Healthcare Bio-Sciences
Joseph M. Hogan, Pres./CEO-GE Healthcare Technologies

Phone: 44-1494-544-000 Fax:
Toll-Free:
Address: Pollards Wood, Nightingales Ln., Chalfont St. Giles, HP8 4SP UK

GROWTH PLANS/SPECIAL FEATURES:
GE Healthcare, a subsidiary of GE, is a global leader in medical imaging and information technologies, patient monitoring systems and health care services. Some of the company's well-known products include Centricity, a suite of applications designed to provide real-time patient information at the point of care; Giraffe OmniBed and Incubators for critically ill and premature infants; Innova 3100, a digital imaging system for visualizing the heart and fine vessels; InstaTrak, which creates an anatomical roadmap and real-time visualization of surgical instrumentation to guide surgeons during life-critical procedures; Lightspeed RT, the first multi-slice CT system with special applications for more precise cancer care; Myoview, an advanced cardiac imaging agent; MegaBace, a DNA analysis system used to sequence the first chromosome completely mapped during the Human Genome Project; Optison, a second-generation ultrasound medical diagnostic product; and Voluson 730 EXPERT, an ultrasound system that allows physicians to perform volume scanning in real time, creating a 4-D image. GE Healthcare operates through two subsidiaries: GE Healthcare Bio-Sciences (BS) and GE Healthcare Technologies (HT), formerly GE Medical Systems. BS provides medical diagnostics, drug discovery and protein separation systems. Its diagnostic imaging agents are used during medical scanning procedures to highlight organs, tissues and cells inside the human body and for early detection, diagnosis and management of diseases. BS's chromatography and filtration purification systems are applied to research and drug development programs to yield more targeted and effective therapies, while its drug discovery systems provide cellular and protein analysis, DNA sequencing, gene expression and genetic variation. HT manufactures diagnostic imaging equipment, such as computer-based x-ray and fluoroscopic imaging systems. Its subsidiary, GE Healthcare Information Technologies (formerly GE Medical Systems Information Technologies), provides information technology products for the health care industry.

GE Healthcare provides general benefits to employees, as well as advanced training programs in sales, finance, human resources, information technology, operations, design engineering and quality control/Six Sigma.

FINANCIALS:
Sales and profits are in thousands of dollars—add 000 to get the full amount. Year 2004 note: Complete fiscal 2004 results were not available for all companies at press time. For this company, year 2004 is for months.

2004 Sales: $ (months) 2004 Profits: $ (months)
2003 Sales: $10,200,000 2003 Profits: $
2002 Sales: $ 2002 Profits: $
2001 Sales: $ 2001 Profits: $
2000 Sales: $ 2000 Profits: $

Stock Ticker: Subsidiary
Employees: 42,500
Fiscal Year Ends: 12/31

SALARIES/BENEFITS:
Pension Plan: Y ESOP Stock Plan: Profit Sharing: Top Exec. Salary: $ Bonus: $
Savings Plan: Y Stock Purch. Plan: Second Exec. Salary: $ Bonus: $

OTHER THOUGHTS:
Apparent Top Female Officers: 1
Hot Spot for Advancement for Women/Minorities:

LOCATIONS: ("Y" = Yes)

West:	Southwest:	Midwest:	Southeast:	Northeast:	International:
		Y			Y

Note: Financial information, benefits and other data can change quickly and may vary from those stated here.

GENENTECH INC

www.gene.com

Industry Group Code: 325412 **Ranks within this company's industry group:** Sales: 20 Profits: 17

Insurance/HMO/PPO:	Drugs:		Equipment/Supplies:	Hospitals/Clinics:	Services:	Health Care:
Insurance:	Manufacturer:	Y	Manufacturer:	Acute Care:	Diagnostics:	Home Health:
Managed Care:	Distributor:		Distributor:	Sub-Acute Care:	Labs/Testing:	Long-Term Care:
Utilization Mgmt.:	Specialty Pharm.:		Leasing/Finance:	Outpatient Surgery:	Staffing:	Physical Therapy:
Payment Proc.:	Vitamins/Nutri.:		Information Sys.:	Phys. Rehab. Center:	Waste Disposal:	Phys. Practice Mgmt.:
	Clinical Trials:			Psychiatric Clinics:	Specialty Services:	

TYPES OF BUSINESS:
Drugs-Biotechnology
Genetically Engineered Drugs
Cardiovascular and Oncology Research

BRANDS/DIVISIONS/AFFILIATES:
Avastin
TNKase
Herceptin
Rituxan
Activase
Pulmozyme
Nutropin Depot
Xolair

CONTACTS:
Note: Officers with more than one job title may be intentionally listed here more than once.
Arthur D. Levinson, CEO
Arthur D. Levinson, Pres.
Myrtle S. Potter, COO
David Ebersman, Exec. VP/CFO
Richard H. Scheller, Sr. VP-Research
Stephen G. Juelsgaard, General Counsel
Myrtle S. Potter, Exec. VP-Commercial Oper.
Susan Desmond-Hellmann, Exec. VP-Dev.
Susan Desmond-Hellmann, Exec. VP-Product Oper.
Susan Desmond-Hellmann, Chief Medical Officer
Stephen G. Juelsgaard, Exec. VP/Corp. Sec.
Arthur D. Levinson, Chmn.

Phone: 650-225-1000 **Fax:** 650-225-6000
Toll-Free:
Address: One DNA Way, South San Francisco, CA 94080-4990 US

GROWTH PLANS/SPECIAL FEATURES:
Genentech, Inc. launched the biotechnology industry by making medicines from splicing genes into fast-growing bacteria that produced theraputic proteins. Using molecular biology, the firm creates drugs that combat diseases on a molecular level. Genentech uses cutting edge technologies such as computer visualization of molecules, micro arrays and sensitive assaying techniques to discover, develop, manufacture and market human pharmaceuticals for significant unmet medical needs. The company's products consist of a variety of cardio-centric medications, as well as cancer, GHD and cystic fibrosis treatments. Biotechnology products offered by Genentech include Herceptin, which is used in treatments of certain metastatic breast cancers; Nutropin, a sustained-release formulation of growth hormone for the treatment of growth hormone deficiency (GHD) in children; TNKase single-bolus thrombolytic agent for the treatment of acute myocardial infarction; and Pulmozyme Inhalation Solution for the treatment of cystic fibrosis. The company also produces the Rituxan antibody, which it markets together with IDEC Pharmaceuticals, for the treatment of patients with relapsed or refractory low-grade or follicular, CD20-positive B-cell non-Hodgkin's lymphoma. Through its long-standing Patient Assistance Program, Genentech assures that everyone who needs these important medicines can get them. The firm also supports the continuing improvement of patient care through its post-marketing studies, which collect data on the health progress of patients who use Genentech medicines nationwide. Scientists of the company publish around 250 scientific papers per year and are highly regarded as among the most prolific in the scientific industry. The firm's scientists focus mainly in the areas of cardiovascular disease and cancer, the number one and number two fatal diseases in the U.S. In recent news, the company announced its launch of Avastin. Avastin is an antibody developed to inhibit angiogenesis (the formation of new blood vessels) as a treatment for solid-tumor cancers.

Company perks include on-campus bicycles, an on-site hair salon and free espresso. Genentech is also consistently voted by Fortune magazine as one of the top 100 Best Companies To Work For.

FINANCIALS:
Sales and profits are in thousands of dollars—add 000 to get the full amount. Year 2004 note: Complete fiscal 2004 results were not available for all companies at press time. For this company, year 2004 is for 9 months.

2004 Sales: $2,682,577 (9 months)   2004 Profits: $578,321 (9 months)
2003 Sales: $2,799,400   2003 Profits: $562,527
2002 Sales: $2,252,300   2002 Profits: $63,800
2001 Sales: $2,081,700   2001 Profits: $150,300
2000 Sales: $1,736,400   2000 Profits: $-74,200

Stock Ticker: DNA
Employees: 6,226
Fiscal Year Ends: 12/31

SALARIES/BENEFITS:
Pension Plan: ESOP Stock Plan: Profit Sharing: Top Exec. Salary: $860,000   Bonus: $1,204,000
Savings Plan: Y   Stock Purch. Plan: Y   Second Exec. Salary: $562,400   Bonus: $575,000

OTHER THOUGHTS:
Apparent Top Female Officers: 2
Hot Spot for Advancement for Women/Minorities:

LOCATIONS: ("Y" = Yes)
West	Southwest	Midwest	Southeast	Northeast	International
Y					Y

Note: Financial information, benefits and other data can change quickly and may vary from those stated here.

GENERAL NUTRITION COMPANIES INC

www.gnc.com

Industry Group Code: 446191 Ranks within this company's industry group: Sales: 1 Profits:

Insurance/HMO/PPO:	Drugs:	Equipment/Supplies:	Hospitals/Clinics:	Services:	Health Care:
Insurance:	Manufacturer:	Manufacturer:	Acute Care:	Diagnostics:	Home Health:
Managed Care:	Distributor:	Distributor:	Sub-Acute Care:	Labs/Testing:	Long-Term Care:
Utilization Mgmt.:	Specialty Pharm.:	Leasing/Finance:	Outpatient Surgery:	Staffing:	Physical Therapy:
Payment Proc.:	Vitamins/Nutri.: Y	Information Sys.:	Phys. Rehab. Center:	Waste Disposal:	Phys. Practice Mgmt.:
	Clinical Trials:		Psychiatric Clinics:	Specialty Services:	

TYPES OF BUSINESS:
Nutritional Supplements, Retail
Fitness Equipment
Online Sales

BRANDS/DIVISIONS/AFFILIATES:
GNC Corporation
www.gncgear.com
PharmAssure
GNC Live Well
Mega Men
Total Lean
Preventive Nutrition
50 Gram Slam

CONTACTS:
Note: Officers with more than one job title may be intentionally listed here more than once.

Louis Mancini, CEO
Louis Mancini, Pres.
Joseph Fortunato, Exec. VP/COO
David R. Heilman, Exec. VP/CFO
Margaret Alison Peet, Dir.-Nat'l Sales
Eileen Scott, Sr. VP-Human Resources
Margaret Alison Peet, Sr. VP-Scientific Affairs
Michael Locke, Sr. VP-Mfg.
James M. Sander, Sr. VP-Law/Chief Legal Officer
Curtis J. Larrimer, Sr. VP-Finance
Tom Dowd, Sr. VP-Stores
J.J. Sorrenti, Sr. VP/General Mgr.-Franchising
Reginald N. Steele, Sr. VP-Int'l Franchising
Robert J. DiNicola, Chmn.
Lee Karayusuf, Sr. VP-Distribution & Transportation

Phone: 412-288-4600 Fax: 412-288-4764
Toll-Free:
Address: 300 6th Ave., Pittsburgh, PA 15222 US

GROWTH PLANS/SPECIAL FEATURES:
General Nutrition Companies, Inc. (GNC) is the largest specialty retailer of nutritional supplements in the United States. The firm was a subsidiary of Dutch firm Royal Numico for some time. However, Royal Numico agreed to sell GNC to Apollo Management, a U.S. private equity firm, in late 2003, for $750 million. The company operates more than 5,600 retail outlets throughout the United States and in foreign markets, including Puerto Rico, Canada and Mexico. The company's new GNC Live Well store format offers a full range of supplements and expanded product lines, such as aromatherapy, bath and spa and a broad selection of self-care-related products. The company has a Gold Card membership program through which subscribers receive a 20% discount on GNC products during the first seven days of every month, including fitness gear purchased from GNC's www.gncgear.com web site. The firm has developed a strategic alliance with Rite Aid Corporation, whereby Rite Aid will open 1,500 GNC areas within its retail drug stores nationwide over a three-year period. GNC will also manufacture Rite Aid private-label products. In addition, the companies have introduced a vitamin and supplement line under the PharmAssure brand name. GNC also entered into a partnership with Drugstore.com, giving it the exclusive online rights to sell GNC-brand products, as well as the PharmAssure brand of vitamins and nutritional supplements. The firm's products are sold under proprietary brands including Mega Men, Pro Performance, Total Lean and Preventive Nutrition and under nationally recognized third-party brands including Muscletech, EAS and Atkins. The company operates two manufacturing facilities in South Carolina and three distribution centers in Pennsylvania, South Carolina and Arizona. In recent news, GNC introduced the 50 Gram Slam, a new ready-to-drink protein shake that contains 50 grams of protein from milk and whey protein concentrates.

FINANCIALS:
Sales and profits are in thousands of dollars—add 000 to get the full amount. Year 2004 note: Complete fiscal 2004 results were not available for all companies at press time. For this company, year 2004 is for months.

2004 Sales: $ (months)   2004 Profits: $ (months)
2003 Sales: $1,429,500   2003 Profits: $
2002 Sales: $1,500,900   2002 Profits: $
2001 Sales: $1,428,000   2001 Profits: $
2000 Sales: $1,399,000   2000 Profits: $

Stock Ticker: Subsidiary
Employees: 14,251
Fiscal Year Ends: 12/31

SALARIES/BENEFITS:
Pension Plan: ESOP Stock Plan: Profit Sharing: Top Exec. Salary: $ Bonus: $
Savings Plan: Stock Purch. Plan: Second Exec. Salary: $ Bonus: $

OTHER THOUGHTS:
Apparent Top Female Officers: 3
Hot Spot for Advancement for Women/Minorities: Y

LOCATIONS: ("Y" = Yes)
West:	Southwest:	Midwest:	Southeast:	Northeast:	International:
Y	Y	Y	Y	Y	Y

GENTIVA HEALTH SERVICES INC

www.gentiva.com

Industry Group Code: 621610   Ranks within this company's industry group: Sales: 2   Profits: 3

Insurance/HMO/PPO:	Drugs:	Equipment/Supplies:	Hospitals/Clinics:		Services:		Health Care:	
Insurance:	Manufacturer:	Manufacturer:	Acute Care:		Diagnostics:		Home Health:	Y
Managed Care:	Distributor:	Distributor:	Sub-Acute Care:		Labs/Testing:		Long-Term Care:	
Utilization Mgmt.:	Specialty Pharm.:	Leasing/Finance:	Outpatient Surgery:		Staffing:	Y	Physical Therapy:	Y
Payment Proc.:	Vitamins/Nutri.:	Information Sys.:	Phys. Rehab. Center:	Y	Waste Disposal:		Phys. Practice Mgmt.:	
	Clinical Trials:		Psychiatric Clinics:		Specialty Services:	Y		

TYPES OF BUSINESS:
Home Health Care
Disease Management
Skilled Nursing Services
Physical & Occupational Therapy
Health Care Consulting
Infusion Therapy
Rehabilitation Services

BRANDS/DIVISIONS/AFFILIATES:
CareCentrix
Gentiva Orthopedic Services
Rehab Without Walls
Gentiva Business Services

CONTACTS: Note: Officers with more than one job title may be intentionally listed here more than once.
Ron Malone, CEO
Al Perry, Pres.
Al Perry, COO
John Potapchuk, Sr. VP/CFO
Mary Morrisey-Gabriel, Sr. VP-Sales
Nicholas Florio, VP-Human Resources
Brian Jones, VP/CIO
Stephen Paige, VP/General Counsel
Bob Creamer, Sr. VP-Nursing Oper.
Chris Anderson, VP-Audit Services & Quality Assurance
Chris Anderson, Chief Compliance Officer
Murray Mease, VP-CareCentrix
Susan Sender, VP/Chief Nursing Exec.
Ron Malone, Chmn.

Phone: 631-501-7000   Fax: 631-501-7148
Toll-Free:
Address: 3 Huntington Quadrangle, 2S, Melville, NY 11747 US

GROWTH PLANS/SPECIAL FEATURES:
Gentiva Health Services, Inc. is a leading provider of home health care services through more than 350 locations. The firm delivers a wide range of services, principally through its Gentiva Health Services and CareCentrix brands. The company operates licensed and Medicare-certified nursing agencies located in 35 states, substantially all of which are currently accredited by the Joint Commission on Accreditation of Healthcare Organizations (JCAHO). These agencies provide various combinations of skilled nursing and therapy services, paraprofessional nursing services and homemaker services to pediatric, adult and elder patients. The CareCentrix operation provides an array of administrative services and coordinates the delivery of home nursing services, acute and chronic infusion therapies, durable medical equipment and respiratory products and services for managed care organizations and health plans. Other divisions of the company include Gentiva Orthopedic Services, which provides specialty care for patients recovering from bone and joint replacement surgery; Rehab Without Walls, a rehabilitation service that is specially suited to patients with spinal or brain injuries and diseases; and Gentiva Business Services, which provides software, billing management, training and consulting services to other health agencies.

The company offers its employees competitive benefits packages that usually include full health coverage.

FINANCIALS:
Sales and profits are in thousands of dollars—add 000 to get the full amount. Year 2004 note: Complete fiscal 2004 results were not available for all companies at press time. For this company, year 2004 is for 9 months.

2004 Sales: $620,223 (9 months)	2004 Profits: $19,594 (9 months)	Stock Ticker: GTIV
2003 Sales: $814,029	2003 Profits: $56,766	Employees: 15,100
2002 Sales: $768,500	2002 Profits: $-49,000	Fiscal Year Ends: 12/31
2001 Sales: $1,377,700	2001 Profits: $21,000	
2000 Sales: $1,506,600	2000 Profits: $-104,200	

SALARIES/BENEFITS:
Pension Plan: ESOP Stock Plan: Profit Sharing: Top Exec. Salary: $471,539   Bonus: $500,000
Savings Plan: Y   Stock Purch. Plan: Second Exec. Salary: $274,308   Bonus: $175,000

OTHER THOUGHTS:
Apparent Top Female Officers: 2
Hot Spot for Advancement for Women/Minorities:

LOCATIONS: ("Y" = Yes)
West:	Southwest:	Midwest:	Southeast:	Northeast:	International:
Y	Y	Y	Y	Y	

GENZYME CORP

www.genzyme.com

Industry Group Code: 325412 Ranks within this company's industry group: Sales: 24 Profits: 36

Insurance/HMO/PPO:	Drugs:	Equipment/Supplies:	Hospitals/Clinics:	Services:	Health Care:
Insurance:	Manufacturer: Y	Manufacturer: Y	Acute Care:	Diagnostics:	Home Health:
Managed Care:	Distributor:	Distributor:	Sub-Acute Care:	Labs/Testing:	Long-Term Care:
Utilization Mgmt.:	Specialty Pharm.:	Leasing/Finance:	Outpatient Surgery:	Staffing:	Physical Therapy:
Payment Proc.:	Vitamins/Nutri.:	Information Sys.:	Phys. Rehab. Center:	Waste Disposal:	Phys. Practice Mgmt.:
	Clinical Trials: Y		Psychiatric Clinics:	Specialty Services:	

TYPES OF BUSINESS:
Drugs
Genetic Disease Treatments
Surgical Products
Diagnostic Products
Genetic Testing Services
Oncology Products
Biomaterials
Drug Materials

BRANDS/DIVISIONS/AFFILIATES:
Genzyme Biosurgery
Genzyme Molecular Oncology
Alfigen, Inc.
ILEX Oncology, Inc.
Fabrazyme
Renagel
Cerezyme
Aldurazyme

CONTACTS:
Note: Officers with more than one job title may be intentionally listed here more than once.

Henri A. Termeer, CEO
Henri A. Termeer, Pres.
Michael S. Wyzga, Exec. VP/CFO/Chief Acc. Officer
Zoltan Csimma, Sr. VP-Human Resources
Alan E. Smith, Sr. VP-Research/Chief Scientific Officer
Thomas J. DesRosier, Sr. VP/General Counsel/Chief Patent Counsel
Mark Bamforth, Sr. VP-Corp. Oper. & Pharmaceuticals
Richard H. Douglas, Sr. VP-Corp. Dev.
Elliott D. Hillback, Jr., Sr. VP-Corp. Affairs
Evan M. Lebson, VP/Treas.
Mara G. Aspinall, Pres., Genetics
Donald E. Pogorzelski, Pres., Diagnostic Products
David Meeker, Pres., LSD Therapeutics
Ann Merrifield, Pres., Genzyme Biosurgery
Henri A. Termeer, Chmn.
Sandford D. Smith, Sr. VP-Int'l Group

Phone: 617-252-7500 **Fax:** 617-252-7600
Toll-Free:
Address: 500 Kendall St., Cambridge, MA 02142 US

GROWTH PLANS/SPECIAL FEATURES:

Genzyme Corporation develops, manufactures and markets innovative products and services for major unmet medical needs, such as rare genetic disorders, renal disease, osteoarthritis and organ transplant. The company operates worldwide in 26 countries, primarily in North America and Europe. The firm conducts operations through two wholly-owned subsidiaries, Genzyme Biosurgery and Genzyme Molecular Oncology, as well as the company's main operating unit, Genzyme General, which operates through several business units, including diagnostics, genetics, pharmaceuticals and advanced biomaterials. Genzyme Biosurgery develops and markets a portfolio of devices, advanced biomaterials and biotherapeutics primarily for the orthopedic, general surgery and severe burn treatment markets. Genzyme Molecular Oncology is developing a new generation of cancer products, focusing primarily on cancer vaccines and angiogenesis inhibitors. Genzyme General primarily develops and markets drugs and services for the treatment of genetic disorders and their chronic debilitating diseases. This division's major products include Cerezyme, its predecessor Ceredase and Fabrazyme (for the treatment of Gaucher's disease); Renagel, which reduces phosphorus levels in hemodialysis patients; and Aldurazyme for the treatment of mucopolysaccharidosis, a rare but often fatal genetic disease. The diagnostics unit offers a line of products for the diagnostics industry and clinical laboratories, in three key product areas: clinical chemistry, rapid tests and point-of-care diagnostics. The genetics unit is a leading nationwide provider of high-quality genetic testing and genetic counseling services for physicians and their patients. The pharmaceuticals division develops and manufactures specialty pharmaceuticals and drug materials and provides products and services in the lipid, peptide, amino acid derivatives and drug delivery markets. The advanced biomaterials unit develops sodium hyaluronate products using three proprietary technology platforms: surface modification, drug delivery and drug conjugation. Recently, Genzyme's genetics unit acquired IMPATH, Inc.'s physician services business unit, Alfigen, Inc. The firm also acquired ILEX Oncology, Inc.

FINANCIALS:
Sales and profits are in thousands of dollars—add 000 to get the full amount. Year 2004 note: Complete fiscal 2004 results were not available for all companies at press time. For this company, year 2004 is for 9 months.

2004 Sales: $1,610,068 (9 months)   2004 Profits: $243,869 (9 months)
2003 Sales: $1,713,900   2003 Profits: $-67,600
2002 Sales: $1,329,500   2002 Profits: $-13,100
2001 Sales: $1,223,600   2001 Profits: $-112,100
2000 Sales: $752,483   2000 Profits: $85,956

Stock Ticker: GENZ
Employees: 5,625
Fiscal Year Ends: 12/31

SALARIES/BENEFITS:
Pension Plan: ESOP Stock Plan: Profit Sharing: Top Exec. Salary: $1,237,745   Bonus: $1,596,692
Savings Plan: Y Stock Purch. Plan: Y   Second Exec. Salary: $600,000 Bonus: $417,000

OTHER THOUGHTS:
Apparent Top Female Officers: 2
Hot Spot for Advancement for Women/Minorities:

LOCATIONS: ("Y" = Yes)
West:	Southwest:	Midwest:	Southeast:	Northeast:	International:
Y	Y	Y	Y	Y	Y

Note: Financial information, benefits and other data can change quickly and may vary from those stated here.

GISH BIOMEDICAL INC

www.gishbiomedical.com

Industry Group Code: 339113   Ranks within this company's industry group: Sales: Profits:

Insurance/HMO/PPO:	Drugs:	Equipment/Supplies:		Hospitals/Clinics:	Services:	Health Care:
Insurance:	Manufacturer:	Manufacturer:	Y	Acute Care:	Diagnostics:	Home Health:
Managed Care:	Distributor:	Distributor:		Sub-Acute Care:	Labs/Testing:	Long-Term Care:
Utilization Mgmt.:	Specialty Pharm.:	Leasing/Finance:		Outpatient Surgery:	Staffing:	Physical Therapy:
Payment Proc.:	Vitamins/Nutri.:	Information Sys.:		Phys. Rehab. Center:	Waste Disposal:	Phys. Practice Mgmt.:
	Clinical Trials:			Psychiatric Clinics:	Specialty Services:	

TYPES OF BUSINESS:
Equipment-Cardiac & Orthopedic Surgical Products
Disposable Surgical Devices

BRANDS/DIVISIONS/AFFILIATES:
CardioTech International, Inc.
StatSat
Orthofuser
Vision
Hemed
CAPVRF44
Gish Biocompatible Surfaces Coating

CONTACTS:
Note: Officers with more than one job title may be intentionally listed here more than once.

Leslie M. Taeger, CFO
Michael Szycher, Pres./CEO-CardioTech

Phone: 800-938-0531   Fax: 949-635-6296
Toll-Free: 866-221-9911
Address: 22942 Arroyo Vista, Rancho Santa Margarita, CA 92688 US

GROWTH PLANS/SPECIAL FEATURES:
Gish Biomedical, Inc., a subsidiary of CardioTech International, Inc., designs, produces and markets innovative specialty surgical devices for various applications, including cardiovascular surgery, orthopedics and oncology. All of the company's products are single-use disposable products or have a disposable component. Gish's primary markets include products for use in open-heart and other cardiac surgeries, myocardial management, infusion therapy and post-operative blood salvage. Products include custom cardiovascular tubing systems, arterial filters, cardiotomy reservoirs, Vision oxygenators, CAPVRF44 venous reservoirs, cardioplegia delivery systems, StatSat oxygen saturation monitors, Hemed critical care central venous access catheters and ports and the Orthofuser product for orthopedic procedures. In 2004, Gish received FDA clearance for its Gish Biocompatible Surfaces Coating, a heparin-based coating that inhibits blood coagulation, decreases risk of systemic inflammatory response syndrome, provides stable antithrombotic activity and reduces thrombus formation, platelet adhesion, blood loss and hemolysis. This coating will be used to cover the surfaces of the company's disposable products.

FINANCIALS:
Sales and profits are in thousands of dollars—add 000 to get the full amount. Year 2004 note: Complete fiscal 2004 results were not available for all companies at press time. For this company, year 2004 is for months.

2004 Sales: $ (months)   2004 Profits: $ (months)
2003 Sales: $ 2003 Profits: $
2002 Sales: $ 2002 Profits: $
2001 Sales: $18,000   2001 Profits: $-2,900
2000 Sales: $17,700   2000 Profits: $-2,800

Stock Ticker: Subsidiary
Employees: 161
Fiscal Year Ends: 3/31

SALARIES/BENEFITS:
Pension Plan: ESOP Stock Plan: Profit Sharing: Top Exec. Salary: $180,000   Bonus: $28,650
Savings Plan: Y   Stock Purch. Plan: Second Exec. Salary: $118,750   Bonus: $

OTHER THOUGHTS:
Apparent Top Female Officers:
Hot Spot for Advancement for Women/Minorities:

LOCATIONS: ("Y" = Yes)
West:	Southwest:	Midwest:	Southeast:	Northeast:	International:
Y					

GLAXOSMITHKLINE PLC

www.gsk.com

Industry Group Code: 325412 **Ranks within this company's industry group:** Sales: 9 Profits: 13

Insurance/HMO/PPO:	Drugs:		Equipment/Supplies:	Hospitals/Clinics:	Services:	Health Care:
Insurance:	Manufacturer:	Y	Manufacturer:	Acute Care:	Diagnostics:	Home Health:
Managed Care:	Distributor:	Y	Distributor:	Sub-Acute Care:	Labs/Testing:	Long-Term Care:
Utilization Mgmt.:	Specialty Pharm.:		Leasing/Finance:	Outpatient Surgery:	Staffing:	Physical Therapy:
Payment Proc.:	Vitamins/Nutri.:		Information Sys.:	Phys. Rehab. Center:	Waste Disposal:	Phys. Practice Mgmt.:
	Clinical Trials:	Y		Psychiatric Clinics:	Specialty Services:	

TYPES OF BUSINESS:
Drugs-Prescription
Asthma Drugs
Respiratory Drugs
Antibiotics
Antivirals
Dermatological
Neurologicals
Oral Care Products

BRANDS/DIVISIONS/AFFILIATES:
Lanoxin
Flovent
Paxil
Augmentin
Zantac
Relafen
Tums
Citrucel

CONTACTS: Note: Officers with more than one job title may be intentionally listed here more than once.
Jean-Pierre Garnier, CEO
Robert Ingram, COO
John Coombe, CFO
Daniel Phelan, Sr. VP-Human Resources
Tachi Yamada, Pres., R&D
Ford Calhoun, CIO
David Pulman, Pres.-Global Mfg. and Supply
Rupert Bondy, Sr. VP/General Counsel
David Stout, Pres.-Pharmaceutical Oper.
Jennie Younger, Sr. VP-Corp. Comm. & Partnerships
Marc Dunoyer, Pres., Pharmaceuticals, Japan
Chris Viehbacher, Pres., Pharmaceuticals, US
John Ziegler, Pres., Consumer Health Care
Andrew Witty, Pres., Pharmaceuticals, Europe
Christopher Gent, Chmn.
Russell Greig, Pres.-Pharmaceuticals, Int'l

Phone: 44-20-8047-5000 **Fax:** 44-20-8047-7807
Toll-Free: 888-825-5249
Address: 980 Great West Rd., Brentford, Middlesex TW8 9GS UK

GROWTH PLANS/SPECIAL FEATURES:

GlaxoSmithKline (GSK) is a leading research-based pharmaceutical company. GSK was formed from the merger of Glaxo Wellcome and SmithKline Beecham, and its subsidiaries constitute a major global drug and health products company engaged in the creation, discovery, development, manufacture and marketing of pharmaceutical and consumer health-related products. GSK's headquarters are located in Middlesex, England, with operation headquarters in Philadelphia, Pennsylvania and Triangle Park, North Carolina, in addition to operating companies in approximately 102 countries. The firm's major markets are the U.S., Japan, the U.K., Germany and Italy. GSK operates in two industry segments: pharmaceuticals (prescription drugs and vaccines) and consumer health care (over-the-counter medicines, oral care and nutritional health care). Pharmaceutical products include treatments for central nervous system disorders, such as Paxil for depression and anxiety and Lamictal for epilepsy; respiratory treatments, such as Flovent for asthma and Ventolin for bronchitis; anti-bacterials such as Augmentin and Amoxil; anti-virals such as Valtrex for genital herpes and Zeffix for hepatitis B; gastro-intestinal treatments such as Zantac for ulcer, reflux and dyspepsia; cardiovascular treatments such as Lanoxin for congestive heart failure; and arthritis treatments such as Relafen for osteoarthritis. Consumer health care products include over-the-counter medicines such as Tums, Citrucel and Nicorette; oral care products such as Aquafresh and Polident; and nutritional health care products. GSK R&D operates at 24 sites in seven countries with a leading position in genomics/genetics and new drug discovery technologies and an annual budget of about $4 billion. Recently, the Nanotechnology Institute (NTI) signed GSK as a corporate member, reflecting NTI's efforts to commercialize the basic research done at NTI, and this partnership matches GSK's efforts to identify technologies that enable new product and research methodologies.

U.S. employees of GlaxoSmithKline are offered a competitive benefits package including health care and other insurance, an employee assistance program, dependent care resources and corporate discounts.

FINANCIALS:
Sales and profits are in thousands of dollars—add 000 to get the full amount. Year 2004 note: Complete fiscal 2004 results were not available for all companies at press time. For this company, year 2004 is for 6 months.

2004 Sales: $18,315,000 (6 months)	2004 Profits: $4,252,000 (6 months)	**Stock Ticker:** Foreign
2003 Sales: $17,251,000	2003 Profits: $1,949,000	Employees: 100,000
2002 Sales: $31,819,000	2002 Profits: $5,903,000	Fiscal Year Ends: 12/31
2001 Sales: $29,858,600	2001 Profits: $-158,800	
2000 Sales: $26,346,500	2000 Profits: $-7,537,200	

SALARIES/BENEFITS:
Pension Plan: Y	ESOP Stock Plan: Y	Profit Sharing: Y	Top Exec. Salary: $1,084,544	Bonus: $1,758,240
Savings Plan: Y	Stock Purch. Plan:		Second Exec. Salary: $580,160	Bonus: $864,320

OTHER THOUGHTS:
Apparent Top Female Officers: 1
Hot Spot for Advancement for Women/Minorities:

LOCATIONS: ("Y" = Yes)
West:	Southwest:	Midwest:	Southeast:	Northeast:	International:
Y	Y	Y	Y	Y	Y

GROUP HEALTH COOPERATIVE OF PUGET SOUND   www.ghc.org

Industry Group Code: 524114   Ranks within this company's industry group: Sales: 34   Profits: 22

Insurance/HMO/PPO:	Drugs:	Equipment/Supplies:	Hospitals/Clinics:		Services:		Health Care:	
Insurance:	Manufacturer:	Manufacturer:	Acute Care:	Y	Diagnostics:		Home Health:	
Managed Care: Y	Distributor:	Distributor:	Sub-Acute Care:	Y	Labs/Testing:		Long-Term Care:	Y
Utilization Mgmt.:	Specialty Pharm.: Y	Leasing/Finance:	Outpatient Surgery:		Staffing:		Physical Therapy:	
Payment Proc.:	Vitamins/Nutri.:	Information Sys.:	Phys. Rehab. Center:		Waste Disposal:		Phys. Practice Mgmt.:	
	Clinical Trials:		Psychiatric Clinics:		Specialty Services:			

TYPES OF BUSINESS:
Hospitals
HMO, PPO & Point-of-Service Plans
Clinics & Long-Term Facilities
Medical Research
Pharmacies

BRANDS/DIVISIONS/AFFILIATES:
Group Health Options, Inc.
Group Health Permanente
Group Heatlh Center for Health Studies
Group Health Community Foundation

CONTACTS:
Note: Officers with more than one job title may be intentionally listed here more than once.
Scott Armstrong, CEO
Scott Armstrong, Pres.
Jim Truess, Exec. VP/CFO
Maureen McLaughlin, Exec. VP/Chief Mktg. Officer
Larry Yok, Dir.-Human Resources
Rick Woods, VP/General Counsel
Theresa Boyle, Exec. Dir.-Strategy & Planning
Pam MacEwan, VP-Public Affairs & Governance
Hugh Straley, Medical Dir.
Jack Dutzar, Medical Dir.-Community Networks & Clinical Support
Stephen Tarnoff, Medical Dir.-Integrated Group Practice
Peter Adler, Exec. VP-Integrated Group Practice
Grant Hendrickson, Chmn.

Phone: 206-448-5600   **Fax:** 206-448-4010
Toll-Free: 888-901-4636
Address: 521 Wall St., Seattle, WA 98121-539 US

GROWTH PLANS/SPECIAL FEATURES:
Group Health Cooperative of Puget Sound (GHCPS) is a consumer-governed, not-for-profit health care system that provides both medical coverage and care. It is owned by and serves nearly 540,000 members in all 20 counties in Washington and two counties in northern Idaho. The company's members participate in HMO, PPO or point-of-service health plans. Its facilities include behavioral health clinics, breast centers, hearing and sight centers, medical centers, nursing homes, urgent care centers, hospitals, specialty care units, emergency rooms and pharmacies. The firm's family of organizations includes Group Health Options, Inc., a wholly-owned subsidiary that offers coordinated-care plans for both groups and individuals, a Medicare plan and a plan for residents who qualify for Health Options (Medicaid), Basic Health and the State Children's Health Insurance Plan; Group Health Permanente, a multi-specialty medical group whose doctors and other clinicians provide care at company-operated medical facilities; Group Health Center for Health Studies, a research center that conducts epidemiologic, health services and clinical research; and Group Health Community Foundation, a charitable foundation. GHCPS's affiliates include Kaiser Permanente, which works with the company in areas such as marketing to regional and national customers, sharing best clinical practices and providing full-service member reciprocity. In addition, the firm has an alliance to share medical centers and hospitals with Virginia Mason Medical Center and the Everett Clinic.

FINANCIALS:
Sales and profits are in thousands of dollars—add 000 to get the full amount. Year 2004 note: Complete fiscal 2004 results were not available for all companies at press time. For this company, year 2004 is for months.

2004 Sales: $ (months)	2004 Profits: $ (months)	**Stock Ticker:** Nonprofit
2003 Sales: $1,966,100	2003 Profits: $155,700	Employees: 9,708
2002 Sales: $1,760,000	2002 Profits: $	Fiscal Year Ends: 12/31
2001 Sales: $	2001 Profits: $	
2000 Sales: $	2000 Profits: $	

SALARIES/BENEFITS:
Pension Plan:	ESOP Stock Plan:	Profit Sharing:	Top Exec. Salary: $	Bonus: $
Savings Plan:	Stock Purch. Plan:		Second Exec. Salary: $	Bonus: $

OTHER THOUGHTS:
Apparent Top Female Officers: 3
Hot Spot for Advancement for Women/Minorities: Y

LOCATIONS: ("Y" = Yes)
West:	Southwest:	Midwest:	Southeast:	Northeast:	International:
Y					

GROUP HEALTH INCORPORATED

www.ghi.com

Industry Group Code: 524114 **Ranks within this company's industry group:** Sales: 31 Profits: 41

Insurance/HMO/PPO:	Drugs:	Equipment/Supplies:	Hospitals/Clinics:	Services:	Health Care:
Insurance:	Manufacturer: Y	Manufacturer:	Acute Care:	Diagnostics:	Home Health:
Managed Care: Y	Distributor:	Distributor:	Sub-Acute Care:	Labs/Testing:	Long-Term Care:
Utilization Mgmt.:	Specialty Pharm.:	Leasing/Finance:	Outpatient Surgery:	Staffing:	Physical Therapy:
Payment Proc.:	Vitamins/Nutri.:	Information Sys.:	Phys. Rehab. Center:	Waste Disposal:	Phys. Practice Mgmt.:
	Clinical Trials:		Psychiatric Clinics:	Specialty Services:	

TYPES OF BUSINESS:
HMO
Health Insurance

BRANDS/DIVISIONS/AFFILIATES:
GHI HMO

GROWTH PLANS/SPECIAL FEATURES:
Group Health Incorporated (GHI) is a not-for-profit organization that offers health insurance and related services to approximately 2.5 million members in the state of New York. Founded in 1937, GHI provides affordable health care to a broad segment of the population. The company and its subsidiary, GHI HMO, offer a range of flexible plans including medical, dental, vision, hospital, prescription drug and managed mental health coverage options, in addition to administrative-services-only plans. Offerings include plans for small groups, with two to 50 employees; plans for large groups, with more than 50 employees; and individual and family plans for people without a group. The firm has locations in New York City, Albany, Buffalo, Lake Katrine and Syracuse, New York. GHI recently introduced a new diabetes management initiative for qualified diabetic members.

CONTACTS:
Note: Officers with more than one job title may be intentionally listed here more than once.

Frank J. Branchini, CEO
Frank J. Branchini, Pres.
Donna Lynne, Exec. VP/COO
David Henderson, Chief Mktg. Officer
Mariann Drohan, VP-Human Resources
Robert Allen, VP-IT & Tech. Services
William Guerci, Sr. VP-Admin.
Jeffrey Chansler, Sr. VP/General Counsel
Thomas Dwyer, Sr. VP-Oper.
Martin Adelstein, VP-Labor & Bus. Dev.
Ilene Margolin, Sr. VP-Corp. Affairs
William Guerci, Sr. VP-Finance/Corp. Treas.
William Mastro, Sr. VP/Corp. Sec.
Marilyn DeQuatro, Sr. VP-Service
Steven Kessler, Sr. VP-Actuarial & Underwriting
Aran Ron, Medical Dir.
James F. Gill, Chmn.

Phone: 212-615-0000 **Fax:** 212-563-8561
Toll-Free:
Address: 441 9th Ave., New York, NY 10001-1681 US

FINANCIALS:
Sales and profits are in thousands of dollars—add 000 to get the full amount. Year 2004 note: Complete fiscal 2004 results were not available for all companies at press time. For this company, year 2004 is for months.

2004 Sales: $ (months)
2003 Sales: $2,157,500
2002 Sales: $
2001 Sales: $
2000 Sales: $

2004 Profits: $ (months)
2003 Profits: $5,600
2002 Profits: $
2001 Profits: $
2000 Profits: $

Stock Ticker: Nonprofit
Employees: 2,400
Fiscal Year Ends: 12/31

SALARIES/BENEFITS:
Pension Plan: ESOP Stock Plan: Profit Sharing: Top Exec. Salary: $ Bonus: $
Savings Plan: Stock Purch. Plan: Second Exec. Salary: $ Bonus: $

OTHER THOUGHTS:
Apparent Top Female Officers: 4
Hot Spot for Advancement for Women/Minorities: Y

LOCATIONS: ("Y" = Yes)
West:	Southwest:	Midwest:	Southeast:	Northeast:	International:
				Y	

Note: Financial information, benefits and other data can change quickly and may vary from those stated here.

GSI LUMONICS INC

www.gsilumonics.com

Industry Group Code: 339113 **Ranks within this company's industry group:** Sales: 65 Profits: 113

Insurance/HMO/PPO:	Drugs:	Equipment/Supplies:	Hospitals/Clinics:	Services:	Health Care:
Insurance:	Manufacturer:	Manufacturer: Y	Acute Care:	Diagnostics:	Home Health:
Managed Care:	Distributor:	Distributor:	Sub-Acute Care:	Labs/Testing:	Long-Term Care:
Utilization Mgmt.:	Specialty Pharm.:	Leasing/Finance:	Outpatient Surgery:	Staffing:	Physical Therapy:
Payment Proc.:	Vitamins/Nutri.:	Information Sys.:	Phys. Rehab. Center:	Waste Disposal:	Phys. Practice Mgmt.:
	Clinical Trials:		Psychiatric Clinics:	Specialty Services:	

TYPES OF BUSINESS:
Equipment-Laser Systems
Motion Control Components

BRANDS/DIVISIONS/AFFILIATES:

CONTACTS:
Note: Officers with more than one job title may be intentionally listed here more than once.
Charles D. Winston, CEO
Charles D. Winston, Pres.
Thomas R. Swain, CFO
Linda Palmer, VP-Human Resources
Kurt A. Pelsue, VP-Tech./Chief Tech. Officer
Eileen Casal, General Counsel
Felix I. Stukalin, VP-Bus. Dev.
Linda Palmer, VP-Corp. Comm.
Thomas R. Swain, VP-Finance

Phone: 978-439-5511 **Fax:**
Toll-Free:
Address: 39 Manning Rd., Billerica, MA 01821 US

GROWTH PLANS/SPECIAL FEATURES:
GSI Lumonics, Inc. designs, develops, manufactures and markets components, lasers and laser-based advanced manufacturing systems as enabling tools for a wide range of applications in the medical, automotive, semiconductor, electronics, light industrial and aerospace industries. With operations in nine countries, the firm sells to original equipment manufacturers (OEMs) worldwide. The company's component products include optical scanners and subsystems used by OEMs for materials processing, test and measurement, alignment, inspection, imaging, and rapid prototyping, a well as medical applications in dermatology and ophthalmology. Components are also used in film imaging subsystems for CAT scans and magnetic resonance imaging systems. GSI Lumonics' lasers are primarily used in materials processing applications in light automotive, electronics, aerospace, medical and light industrial markets. Laser systems are also used in applications such as laser repair to improve yields in the production of dynamic random access memory chips, permanent marking systems for silicon wafers and individual dies for traceability and quality control, circuit processing systems for linear and mixed signal devices, as well as for certain passive electronic components and printed circuit board manufacturing systems for via hole drilling, solder paste inspection and component placement inspection.

The firm offers employees PPO and HMO health coverage, life insurance, tuition reimbursement, paid memberships to professional organizations, an employee referral program and membership in a credit union.

FINANCIALS:
Sales and profits are in thousands of dollars—add 000 to get the full amount. Year 2004 note: Complete fiscal 2004 results were not available for all companies at press time. For this company, year 2004 is for 9 months.

2004 Sales: $250,061 (9 months)	2004 Profits: $32,876 (9 months)	**Stock Ticker:** GSLI
2003 Sales: $185,561	2003 Profits: $-2,170	Employees: 1,067
2002 Sales: $159,100	2002 Profits: $-27,700	Fiscal Year Ends: 12/31
2001 Sales: $247,900	2001 Profits: $-14,700	
2000 Sales: $373,900	2000 Profits: $45,400	

SALARIES/BENEFITS:
Pension Plan:	ESOP Stock Plan:	Profit Sharing:	Top Exec. Salary: $400,000	Bonus: $239,540
Savings Plan: Y	Stock Purch. Plan: Y		Second Exec. Salary: $209,720	Bonus: $216,960

OTHER THOUGHTS:
Apparent Top Female Officers: 2
Hot Spot for Advancement for Women/Minorities:

LOCATIONS: ("Y" = Yes)
West:	Southwest:	Midwest:	Southeast:	Northeast:	International:
Y		Y		Y	Y

GTC BIOTHERAPEUTICS INC

www.gtc-bio.com

Industry Group Code: 325414　　Ranks within this company's industry group: Sales: 4　Profits: 3

Insurance/HMO/PPO:	Drugs:	Equipment/Supplies:	Hospitals/Clinics:	Services:	Health Care:
Insurance: Managed Care: Utilization Mgmt.: Payment Proc.:	Manufacturer: Y Distributor: Specialty Pharm.: Vitamins/Nutri.: Clinical Trials:	Manufacturer: Distributor: Leasing/Finance: Information Sys.:	Acute Care: Sub-Acute Care: Outpatient Surgery: Phys. Rehab. Center: Psychiatric Clinics:	Diagnostics: Labs/Testing: Staffing: Waste Disposal: Specialty Services:	Home Health: Long-Term Care: Physical Therapy: Phys. Practice Mgmt.:

TYPES OF BUSINESS:
Drugs-Anticoagulants
Recombinant Proteins
Transgenic Animals

BRANDS/DIVISIONS/AFFILIATES:
Genzyme Transgenics Corp.
Remicade
Antegren

CONTACTS:
Note: Officers with more than one job title may be intentionally listed here more than once.
Geoffrey F. Cox, CEO
Geoffrey F. Cox, Pres.
John B. Green, CFO
Harry M. Meade, Sr. VP-Research & Dev.
Daniel S. Woloshen, General Counsel
Gregory Liposky, Sr. VP-Oper.
Paul Horan, Sr. VP-Corp. Dev.
Thomas E. Newberry, VP-Corp. Comm.
Thomas E. Newberry, VP-Investor Rel.
John B. Green, Sr. VP-Finance/Treas.
Carol A. Ziomek, VP-Dev.
Suzanne Groet, VP-Therapeutic Protein Dev.
Richard A. Scotland, VP-Regulatory Affairs
Geoffrey F. Cox, Chmn.

Phone: 508-620-9700　　**Fax:** 508-370-3797
Toll-Free:
Address: 175 Crossing Blvd., Ste. 410, Framingham, MA 01702-9322 US

GROWTH PLANS/SPECIAL FEATURES:
GTC Biotherapeutics, Inc. (GTC), formerly Genzyme Transgenics Corp., applies transgenic technology to develop recombinant proteins for therapeutic uses. The company uses transgenic animals that express specific recombinant proteins in their milk. Its technology platform includes the ability to generate animals and provide for animal husbandry, breeding and milking, as well as the ability to purify the milk to a clarified intermediate bulk material that may undergo manufacturing to obtain a clinical grade product. The firm generates transgenic animals through microinjection and nuclear transfer, and it expects to rely primarily on nuclear transfer techniques in new program development work. GTC uses goats in most of its commercial development programs due to relatively short gestation times and relatively high milk production volume of the animals. The company's products include Remicade, a monoclonal antibody marketed for rheumatoid arthritis, and Antegren, for neurological disorders. GTC has development partnerships with companies including Abbott Labs, Bristol-Myers Squibb, Centocor, Elan Pharmaceuticals, Progenics and ImmunoGen. In May 2004, GTC, along with Mayo Clinic, began developing an agonistic antibody to CD137 as a potential therapeutic for solid tumors.

GTC offers its employees dental insurance, tuition reimbursement and fitness club membership rebates.

FINANCIALS:
Sales and profits are in thousands of dollars—add 000 to get the full amount. Year 2004 note: Complete fiscal 2004 results were not available for all companies at press time. For this company, year 2004 is for 9 months.

2004 Sales: $3,429 (9 months)　　2004 Profits: $-21,985 (9 months)
2003 Sales: $9,764　　2003 Profits: $-29,537
2002 Sales: $10,400　　2002 Profits: $-24,300
2001 Sales: $13,700　　2001 Profits: $-16,600
2000 Sales: $16,200　　2000 Profits: $-14,100

Stock Ticker: GTCB
Employees: 159
Fiscal Year Ends: 12/31

SALARIES/BENEFITS:
Pension Plan:　　ESOP Stock Plan:　　Profit Sharing:　　Top Exec. Salary: $420,056　　Bonus: $110,000
Savings Plan: Y　　Stock Purch. Plan: Y　　　　　　　　Second Exec. Salary: $271,543　　Bonus: $25,421

OTHER THOUGHTS:
Apparent Top Female Officers: 2
Hot Spot for Advancement for Women/Minorities:

LOCATIONS: ("Y" = Yes)
West:	Southwest:	Midwest:	Southeast:	Northeast:	International:
				Y	

Note: Financial information, benefits and other data can change quickly and may vary from those stated here.

GUIDANT CORP

www.guidant.com

Industry Group Code: 339113 Ranks within this company's industry group: Sales: 6 Profits: 9

Insurance/HMO/PPO:	Drugs:	Equipment/Supplies:		Hospitals/Clinics:	Services:	Health Care:
Insurance:	Manufacturer:	Manufacturer:	Y	Acute Care:	Diagnostics:	Home Health:
Managed Care:	Distributor:	Distributor:		Sub-Acute Care:	Labs/Testing:	Long-Term Care:
Utilization Mgmt.:	Specialty Pharm.:	Leasing/Finance:		Outpatient Surgery:	Staffing:	Physical Therapy:
Payment Proc.:	Vitamins/Nutri.:	Information Sys.:		Phys. Rehab. Center:	Waste Disposal:	Phys. Practice Mgmt.:
	Clinical Trials:			Psychiatric Clinics:	Specialty Services:	

TYPES OF BUSINESS:

Equipment-Cardiovascular Therapeutic Devices
Implantable Cardiovascular Devices
Vascular Intervention Products
Pacemakers
Catheters & Stents

BRANDS/DIVISIONS/AFFILIATES:

VITALITY
CROSSAIL
OPENSAIL
MULTI-LINK
VASOVIEW

CONTACTS: Note: Officers with more than one job title may be intentionally listed here more than once.

Ronald W. Dollens, CEO
Ronald W. Dollens, Pres.
Guido J. Neels, COO
Keith E. Brauer, VP/CFO
Mark C. Bartell, Pres.-U.S. Sales Oper.
Roger Marchetti, VP-Human Resources
William F. McConnell, Jr., VP/CIO
Beverly H. Lorell, VP/Chief Medical & Tech. Officer
Bernard E. Kury, VP/General Counsel
Keith E. Brauer, VP-Finance
Ronald K. Lattanze, Pres.-Japan
Beverly Huss, Pres.-Endovascular Solutions
Maria Degois-Sainz, Pres.-Cardiac Surgery
Dana G. Mead, Jr., Pres.-Vascular Intervention
James M. Cornelius, Chmn.
Ronald N. Spaulding, Pres.-Europe, Middle East, Africa & Canada

Phone: 317-971-2000 Fax: 317-971-2040
Toll-Free:
Address: 111 Monument Cir., 29th Fl., Indianapolis, IN 46204 US

GROWTH PLANS/SPECIAL FEATURES:

Guidant Corporation designs, develops, manufactures and markets a broad range of products for use in cardiac rhythm management, vascular intervention and cardiac surgery. The company offers a number of stents, angioplasty systems, cardiac surgery systems and implantable devices that can monitor the heart and deliver electricity to treat coronary abnormalities such as tachycardia, bradycardia and heart failure. The company's VITALITY implantable cardioverter defibrillator (ICD) system combines complete ventricular and atrial therapies in the world's smallest (30 cubic centimeters) and thinnest (11 millimeters) dual-chamber ICD. The firm also manufactures a number of pacemakers that feature blended sensor technology designed to measure patient workload through respiration and motion, providing rate response based on the patient's activity. Guidant's CROSSAIL and OPENSAIL dilation catheters and MULTI-LINK stents are used in angioplasty procedures, reducing the need for more invasive treatments. The company produces surgical devices that allow physicians to perform a coronary artery bypass while a patient's heart remains beating, as well as biliary stent systems, coronary dilation catheters, coronary guide wires and postoperative atrial fibrillation management devices. In October 2004, the FDA approved the company's VASOVIEW endoscopic vessel harvesting system, which facilitates the removal of leg or arm arteries for use in bypass surgeries. Also in 2004, Guidant acquired the remaining stake in a company that is developing bioabsorbable drug eluting stents.

Guidant offers its employees tuition reimbursement, dental and vision insurance and matching gifts to charity. The company's offices in Santa Clara, Temecula and St. Paul feature on-site fitness centers, and employees at other locations receive reimbursement for a portion of their health club membership fees.

FINANCIALS: Sales and profits are in thousands of dollars—add 000 to get the full amount. Year 2004 note: Complete fiscal 2004 results were not available for all companies at press time. For this company, year 2004 is for 9 months.

2004 Sales: $2,797,400 (9 months) 2004 Profits: $419,500 (9 months)
2003 Sales: $3,698,000 2003 Profits: $330,300
2002 Sales: $3,239,600 2002 Profits: $611,800
2001 Sales: $2,707,600 2001 Profits: $484,000
2000 Sales: $2,548,700 2000 Profits: $374,300

Stock Ticker: GDT
Employees: 12,000
Fiscal Year Ends: 12/31

SALARIES/BENEFITS:

Pension Plan: Y ESOP Stock Plan: Y Profit Sharing: Top Exec. Salary: $700,008 Bonus: $437,500
Savings Plan: Y Stock Purch. Plan: Y Second Exec. Salary: $427,212 Bonus: $187,500

OTHER THOUGHTS:

Apparent Top Female Officers: 3
Hot Spot for Advancement for Women/Minorities: Y

LOCATIONS: ("Y" = Yes)

West:	Southwest:	Midwest:	Southeast:	Northeast:	International:
Y	Y	Y			Y

GYRUS GROUP

www.gyrusplc.com

Industry Group Code: 339113   Ranks within this company's industry group: Sales: 76 Profits: 72

Insurance/HMO/PPO:	Drugs:	Equipment/Supplies:		Hospitals/Clinics:		Services:	Health Care:
Insurance:	Manufacturer:	Manufacturer:	Y	Acute Care:		Diagnostics:	Home Health:
Managed Care:	Distributor:	Distributor:	Y	Sub-Acute Care:		Labs/Testing:	Long-Term Care:
Utilization Mgmt.:	Specialty Pharm.:	Leasing/Finance:		Outpatient Surgery:		Staffing:	Physical Therapy:
Payment Proc.:	Vitamins/Nutri.:	Information Sys.:		Phys. Rehab. Center:		Waste Disposal:	Phys. Practice Mgmt.:
	Clinical Trials:			Psychiatric Clinics:		Specialty Services:	

TYPES OF BUSINESS:
Supplies-Surgical Instruments
Ear, Nose and Throat Products
Urologic and Gynecologic Products

BRANDS/DIVISIONS/AFFILIATES:
RetroX
Gyrus North America Sales, Inc.
Gyrus International, Ltd.
PlasmaKinetic

CONTACTS: Note: Officers with more than one job title may be intentionally listed here more than once.
Roy Davis, Group COO
Simon Shaw, CFO
Colin Goble, Group Tech. Dir.
Mark Goble, Dir.-Strategic Dev.
Jon Moore, Managing Dir.-Gyrus Medical, Ltd.
Thomas Murphy, Pres.-Surgical Div.
Jerry Dowdy, Pres.-ENT Div.
Michael Geraghty, Pres., Gyrus North America Sales, Inc.
Brian Steer, Exec. Chmn.
Davic Ball, Managing Dir.-Int'l

Phone: 44-29-2077-6300   Fax: 44-29-2077-6301
Toll-Free:
Address: Fortran Rd., St. Mellons, Cardiff CF3 0LT UK

GROWTH PLANS/SPECIAL FEATURES:
Gyrus Group plc is a medical technology company that develops and manufactures products that reduce trauma and complications during open and endoscopic surgical procedures. The company's products are based on its PlasmaKinetic technology, which uses radio frequencies to cut, vaporize and coagulate tissue or seal blood vessels. Gyrus operates through three global business divisions: ear, nose and throat (ENT), surgical and partnered technologies (PT). The ENT division provides surgical instruments, packing materials, scopes and implants for otology, rhinology, and head, neck, throat and upper airway surgery. The otology unit also licenses its RetroX hearing enhancement system to treat high-frequency hearing loss. The surgical segment offers a range of surgical instruments for general surgery, as well as a line of specialty products for gynecological and urological surguery. The PT division develops, licenses and commercializes Gyrus technology outside of its core areas by out-licensing to a number of marketing partners, including Johnson & Johnson (Depuy Mitek, Ethicon Endo-Surgery and Gynecare), Bard and Guidant. In addition, the firm directly sells its products through two organizations: Gyrus North America Sales, Inc. and Gyrus International, Ltd. The firm's main customers include ear, nose and throat (ENT) surgeons, gynecologists and urologists. Through strategic relationships, the company also sells to the arthroscopic, cardiac, gastrointestinal and hysteroscopic markets.

FINANCIALS: Sales and profits are in thousands of dollars—add 000 to get the full amount. Year 2004 note: Complete fiscal 2004 results were not available for all companies at press time. For this company, year 2004 is for months.

2004 Sales: $ (months)   2004 Profits: $ (months)
2003 Sales: $138,900   2003 Profits: $10,600   Stock Ticker: Foreign
2002 Sales: $120,300   2002 Profits: $3,300   Employees: 641
2001 Sales: $ 2001 Profits: $ Fiscal Year Ends: 12/31
2000 Sales: $ 2000 Profits: $

SALARIES/BENEFITS:
Pension Plan: ESOP Stock Plan: Profit Sharing: Top Exec. Salary: $ Bonus: $
Savings Plan: Stock Purch. Plan: Second Exec. Salary: $ Bonus: $

OTHER THOUGHTS:
Apparent Top Female Officers:
Hot Spot for Advancement for Women/Minorities:

LOCATIONS: ("Y" = Yes)

West:	Southwest:	Midwest:	Southeast:	Northeast:	International:
		Y	Y		Y

Note: Financial information, benefits and other data can change quickly and may vary from those stated here.

HAEMONETICS CORPORATION

www.haemonetics.com

Industry Group Code: 339113 Ranks within this company's industry group: Sales: 51 Profits: 45

Insurance/HMO/PPO:	Drugs:	Equipment/Supplies:	Hospitals/Clinics:	Services:	Health Care:
Insurance:	Manufacturer:	Manufacturer: Y	Acute Care:	Diagnostics:	Home Health:
Managed Care:	Distributor:	Distributor:	Sub-Acute Care:	Labs/Testing:	Long-Term Care:
Utilization Mgmt.:	Specialty Pharm.:	Leasing/Finance:	Outpatient Surgery:	Staffing:	Physical Therapy:
Payment Proc.:	Vitamins/Nutri.:	Information Sys.:	Phys. Rehab. Center:	Waste Disposal:	Phys. Practice Mgmt.:
	Clinical Trials:		Psychiatric Clinics:	Specialty Services:	

TYPES OF BUSINESS:
Equipment-Blood-Recovery Systems
Surgical Blood Salvage Equipment
Blood Component Therapy Equipment
Automated Blood Collection Equipment

BRANDS/DIVISIONS/AFFILIATES:
Cell Saver
ACP
OrthoPAT
Bloodless Surgery Station
SmartSuction
SmartCell

CONTACTS:
Note: Officers with more than one job title may be intentionally listed here more than once.

Brad Nutter, CEO
Brad Nutter, Pres.
Ronald Ryan, CFO
Lisa Lopez, General Counsel
Robert Ebbeling, VP-Oper.
Lisa Lopez, VP-Investor Rel.
Ronald Ryan, VP-Finance
Brian Concannon, Pres.-Patient Div.
Peter Allen, Pres.-Donor Div.
Yutaka Sakurada, Pres.-Japan/Asia
Mark Popovsky, VP/Corp. Medical Dir.
Ronald A. Matricaria, Chmn.
Ulrich Eckert, Pres.-Europe

Phone: 781-848-7100 Fax:
Toll-Free: 800-225-5242
Address: 400 Wood Rd., Braintree, MA 02184 US

GROWTH PLANS/SPECIAL FEATURES:

Haemonetics Corporation is a global medical devices company that manufactures automated systems for the collection, processing and surgical salvage of blood. Haemonetics markets its products to hospitals, commercial plasma fractionators and national health organizations in over 50 countries. The company's blood donor products automate the collection of blood parts, such as plasma, platelets and red blood cells, allowing donors to give larger volumes of desired blood cells. Its ACP-brand system automates the process of freezing, thawing and washing red blood cells in a closed system, allowing for 14-day storage of thawed cells. It is used by the U.S. Military to freeze red blood cells for up to 10 years. Haemonetics' surgical patient products are blood salvage systems used during and after surgery to collect a patient's blood for reinfusion. These include the Cell Saver for high-blood-loss surgeries and the OrthoPAT for slower-blood-loss procedures, typically orthopedic surgeries. All of the firm's equipment is designed to regulate blood processing while ensuring patient and donor safety. It incorporates various processes and devices such as centrifugal drives, ultrasonic sensors, pneumatics, various electromechanical assemblies and optical systems using combinations of light emitting diodes, lensing arrays, fiber optics and charge coupled devices in conjunction with the system's microprocessor. A revolutionary component of the firm's equipment was its introduction of disposable parts, which, in conjunction with specialized programming, maximizes donor-patient safety. Haemonetics recently received regulatory clearance to market two blood sampling systems that facilitate the collection of small samples for bacterial screening, further increasing blood safety. In August 2004, the company announced that it would acquire the Bloodless Surgery Station product line from Harvest Technologies Corporation. This technology consists of the SmartSuction, the SmartCell and an autotransfusion blood bag with integral transfusion filter.

U.S. workers are offered on-site child care and a cafeteria, tuition reimbursement, a referral bonus program, service awards and a wellness program.

FINANCIALS:
Sales and profits are in thousands of dollars—add 000 to get the full amount. Year 2004 note: Complete fiscal 2004 results were not available for all companies at press time. For this company, year 2004 is for 12 months.

2004 Sales: $364,229 (12 months)
2003 Sales: $337,000
2002 Sales: $320,000
2001 Sales: $293,900
2000 Sales: $280,600

2004 Profits: $29,320 (12 months)
2003 Profits: $28,400
2002 Profits: $30,000
2001 Profits: $7,200
2000 Profits: $15,400

Stock Ticker: HAE
Employees: 1,438
Fiscal Year Ends: 3/31

SALARIES/BENEFITS:
Pension Plan: ESOP Stock Plan: Profit Sharing: Top Exec. Salary: $500,000   Bonus: $225,000
Savings Plan: Y   Stock Purch. Plan: Y   Second Exec. Salary: $306,014 Bonus: $129,600

OTHER THOUGHTS:
Apparent Top Female Officers: 1
Hot Spot for Advancement for Women/Minorities:

LOCATIONS: ("Y" = Yes)
West:	Southwest:	Midwest:	Southeast:	Northeast:	International:
			Y	Y	Y

Note: Financial information, benefits and other data can change quickly and may vary from those stated here.

HANGER ORTHOPEDIC GROUP INC

www.hanger.com

Industry Group Code: 621340　Ranks within this company's industry group: Sales: 1　Profits: 1

Insurance/HMO/PPO:	Drugs:	Equipment/Supplies:		Hospitals/Clinics:		Services:		Health Care:	
Insurance:	Manufacturer:	Manufacturer:	Y	Acute Care:		Diagnostics:		Home Health:	
Managed Care:	Distributor:	Distributor:	Y	Sub-Acute Care:		Labs/Testing:		Long-Term Care:	
Utilization Mgmt.:	Specialty Pharm.:	Leasing/Finance:		Outpatient Surgery:		Staffing:		Physical Therapy:	
Payment Proc.:	Vitamins/Nutri.:	Information Sys.:		Phys. Rehab. Center:	Y	Waste Disposal:		Phys. Practice Mgmt.:	
	Clinical Trials:			Psychiatric Clinics:		Specialty Services:			

TYPES OF BUSINESS:
Hospitals/Clinics-Physical Rehab Centers
Orthotic/Prosthetic Patient Care Centers
Orthotic/Prosthetic Devices & Components, Distribution

BRANDS/DIVISIONS/AFFILIATES:
Southern Prosthetic Supply, Inc.
Hanger Prosthetics & Orthotics, Inc.
Innovative Neurotronics, Inc.
Linkia
Insignia
Brace Shop Prosthetic Orthotic Centers, Inc. (The)
Rehab Designs of America Corporation

CONTACTS:
Note: Officers with more than one job title may be intentionally listed here more than once.

Ivan R. Sabel, CEO
Thomas F. Kirk, Pres.
Thomas F. Kirk, COO
George E. McHenry, Exec. VP/CFO
Michael F. Murphy, VP-Mktg.
Brian A. Wheeler, VP-Human Resources
Edward L. Mitzel, VP/CIO
Michael F. Murphy, VP-Bus. Dev.
Jason P. Owen, Treas.
Richmond L. Taylor, Pres./COO-Hanger Prosthetics & Orthotics, Inc.
Glenn M. Lohrmann, VP/Controller/Corp. Sec.
Ronald N. May, Pres., Southern Prosthetic Supply, Inc.
Ivan R. Sabel, Chmn.

Phone: 301-986-0701	Fax: 301-986-0702
Toll-Free: 800-466-7638	
Address: 2 Bethesda Metro Center, Ste. 1300, Bethesda, MD 20814 US	

GROWTH PLANS/SPECIAL FEATURES:
Hanger Orthopedic Group, Inc. is one of the leading providers of orthotic and prosthetic (O/P) patient care. The company operates through two businesses: Southern Prosthetic Supply, Inc. (SPS), the world's largest distributor of O/P devices; and Hanger Prosthetics & Orthotics, Inc. (HP&O), the nation's largest O/P patient care company. Through SPS, the company is a leading distributor of branded and private-label O/P devices and components in the U.S., all of which are manufactured by third parties. In addition, Hanger designs, fabricates, fits and maintains a wide range of standard and custom-made orthotics, including spinal, knee and sports-medicine braces, which provide external support to patients suffering from musculoskeletal disorders, as well as prosthetics, including custom-made artificial limbs for patients who are without limbs as a result of traumatic injuries, vascular diseases, diabetes, cancer or congenital disorders. Insignia, the company's newest proprietary technology, provides an alternative to traditional plaster casting methods by using 3D motion-tracking laser scanners and proprietary CAD software to provide a faster, cleaner and less invasive image capture experience. Through HP&O, the firm operates the largest O/P patient care network in the U.S., with 614 O/P patient care centers in 44 states and the District of Columbia, employing 1,016 certified practitioners. In recent news, Hanger formed two new wholly-owned subsidiaries: Innovative Neurotronics, Inc., which will specialize in the development and commercialization of devices that use electrical stimulation to improve the functionality of an impaired extremity; and Linkia, the first managed care organization dedicated solely to serving the O/P market. In addition, the firm acquired The Brace Shop Prosthetic Orthotic Centers, Inc., which has four full-time and two part-time offices in the northeast. It also acquired Rehab Designs of America Corporation, with 19 patient centers in Missouri, Kansas, Wisconsin, Colorado and Texas.

Hanger offers employees medical, dental and life insurance, as well as relocation assistance.

FINANCIALS:
Sales and profits are in thousands of dollars—add 000 to get the full amount. Year 2004 note: Complete fiscal 2004 results were not available for all companies at press time. For this company, year 2004 is for 9 months.

2004 Sales: $422,867　(9 months)	2004 Profits: $-27,346　(9 months)	
2003 Sales: $547,903	2003 Profits: $16,239	**Stock Ticker: HGR**
2002 Sales: $525,500	2002 Profits: $23,600	Employees: 3,007
2001 Sales: $508,100	2001 Profits: $-8,900	Fiscal Year Ends: 12/31
2000 Sales: $486,000	2000 Profits: $-14,000	

SALARIES/BENEFITS:
Pension Plan:	ESOP Stock Plan:	Profit Sharing:	Top Exec. Salary: $495,000	Bonus: $124,480
Savings Plan: Y	Stock Purch. Plan:		Second Exec. Salary: $450,000	Bonus: $113,164

OTHER THOUGHTS:
Apparent Top Female Officers:
Hot Spot for Advancement for Women/Minorities:

LOCATIONS: ("Y" = Yes)
West:	Southwest:	Midwest:	Southeast:	Northeast:	International:
Y	Y	Y	Y	Y	Y

HARBORSIDE HEALTHCARE CORP

www.hbrside.com

Industry Group Code: 623110   Ranks within this company's industry group: Sales: Profits:

Insurance/HMO/PPO:	Drugs:	Equipment/Supplies:	Hospitals/Clinics:		Services:		Health Care:	
Insurance:	Manufacturer:	Manufacturer:	Acute Care:		Diagnostics:		Home Health:	
Managed Care:	Distributor:	Distributor:	Sub-Acute Care:	Y	Labs/Testing:		Long-Term Care:	Y
Utilization Mgmt.:	Specialty Pharm.:	Leasing/Finance:	Outpatient Surgery:		Staffing:	Y	Physical Therapy:	Y
Payment Proc.:	Vitamins/Nutri.:	Information Sys.:	Phys. Rehab. Center:	Y	Waste Disposal:		Phys. Practice Mgmt.:	
	Clinical Trials:		Psychiatric Clinics:		Specialty Services:			

TYPES OF BUSINESS:
Long-Term Health Care/Nursing Homes
Sub-Acute Care Facilities
Rehabilitation Services
Temporary Staffing Services

BRANDS/DIVISIONS/AFFILIATES:
Theracor
Sowerby Health Centers
Associated Healthcare
ReadyNurse

CONTACTS: Note: Officers with more than one job title may be intentionally listed here more than once.
Stephen L. Guillard, CEO
Damian N. Dell'Anno, Pres.
Damian N. Dell'Anno, COO
William H. Stephan, Sr. VP/CFO
Michael J. Reed, Sr. VP-Mktg. & Sales
Robert Haggerty, Sr. VP-Human Resources
John Guida, Sr. VP/CIO
Susan Gwyn, Sr. VP-Ancillary Services
Bruce J. Beardsley, Sr. VP-Acquisitions
Susan Coppola, Sr. VP-Clinical Services
Stephen L. Guillard, Chmn.

Phone: 617-646-5400   Fax: 617-646-5454
Toll-Free:
Address: One Beacon St., Ste. 1100, Boston, MA 02108 US

GROWTH PLANS/SPECIAL FEATURES:

Harborside Healthcare Corporation provides high-quality long-term care, sub-acute care and other specialty medical services in the mid-Atlantic, Midwest and New England. The company operates 45 facilities in Maryland, New Jersey, Connecticut, Massachusetts, New Hampshire, Rhode Island, Indiana and Ohio. The firm provides traditional skilled nursing care; a wide range of sub-acute care programs such as orthopedic, CVA/stroke, cardiac, pulmonary and wound care; as well as distinct programs for the provision of care to Alzheimer's and hospice patients. In addition, Harborside provides rehabilitation therapy services both at company-operated and non-affiliated facilities. Each facility offers a number of individualized therapeutic practices designed to enhance the quality of life of its patients. Entertainment events, musical productions, trips, arts and crafts and volunteer and other programs encourage community interaction. Harborside also provides support services, including dietary services, social services, housekeeping and laundry services, pharmaceutical and medical supplies and routine rehabilitation therapy. Subsidiary ReadyNurse provides temporary registered nurses (RNs), licensed practical nurses (LPNs) and certified nursing aides (CNAs) to the company's facilities as well as a variety of other clinical settings.

The company offers its workforce medical and dental coverage, employee meals, a prescription drug plan and continuing education.

FINANCIALS: Sales and profits are in thousands of dollars—add 000 to get the full amount. Year 2004 note: Complete fiscal 2004 results were not available for all companies at press time. For this company, year 2004 is for months.

2004 Sales: $ (months)	2004 Profits: $ (months)	
2003 Sales: $	2003 Profits: $	Stock Ticker: Private
2002 Sales: $400,224	2002 Profits: $-5,659	Employees: 8,000
2001 Sales: $346,738	2001 Profits: $-16,902	Fiscal Year Ends: 12/31
2000 Sales: $322,672	2000 Profits: $-36,706	

SALARIES/BENEFITS:

Pension Plan:	ESOP Stock Plan:	Profit Sharing:	Top Exec. Salary: $397,523	Bonus: $86,250
Savings Plan: Y	Stock Purch. Plan:		Second Exec. Salary: $281,259	Bonus: $45,000

OTHER THOUGHTS:
Apparent Top Female Officers: 2
Hot Spot for Advancement for Women/Minorities:

LOCATIONS: ("Y" = Yes)

West:	Southwest:	Midwest:	Southeast:	Northeast:	International:
		Y		Y	

HARVARD PILGRIM HEALTH CARE INC   www.harvardpilgrim.org

Industry Group Code: 524114   Ranks within this company's industry group: Sales: 32   Profits: 35

Insurance/HMO/PPO:		Drugs:		Equipment/Supplies:		Hospitals/Clinics:		Services:		Health Care:	
Insurance:		Manufacturer:		Manufacturer:		Acute Care:		Diagnostics:		Home Health:	
Managed Care:	Y	Distributor:		Distributor:		Sub-Acute Care:		Labs/Testing:		Long-Term Care:	
Utilization Mgmt.:		Specialty Pharm.:		Leasing/Finance:		Outpatient Surgery:		Staffing:		Physical Therapy:	
Payment Proc.:		Vitamins/Nutri.:		Information Sys.:		Phys. Rehab. Center:		Waste Disposal:		Phys. Practice Mgmt.:	
		Clinical Trials:				Psychiatric Clinics:		Specialty Services:			

TYPES OF BUSINESS:
HMO/PPO
Indemnity Insurance

BRANDS/DIVISIONS/AFFILIATES:
Harvard Pilgrim Health Care of New England
HPHC Insurance Company
First Seniority
Medicare Enhance
HPHConnect

CONTACTS: Note: Officers with more than one job title may be intentionally listed here more than once.
Charles D. Baker, Jr., CEO
Charles D. Baker, Jr., Pres.
Bruce M. Bullen, COO
Joseph C. Capezza, CFO
Vincent Capozzi, Sr. VP-Sales & Mktg.
Deborah A. Hicks, VP-Human Resources
Deborah A. Norton, Sr. VP/CIO
William F. Frado, Jr., Sr. VP/General Counsel
Beth-Ann Roberts, VP-Northern New England Oper.
David Cochran, Sr. VP-Strategic Dev.
Alan G. Raymond, Sr. VP-Comm. & Mktg.
Marie Montgomery, VP-Corp. Acct./Controller
Roberta Herman, Sr. VP/Chief Medical Officer
Leanne Berge, Sr. VP-Network Services & Oper.
David Segal, Sr. VP-Customer Service & Oper.
Vicki Coates, VP-Oper. Integration & Product Admin.
Charles D. Baker, Chmn.

Phone: 617-745-1000   **Fax:** 617-509-7590
Toll-Free: 888-888-4742
Address: 93 Worcester St., Wellesley, MA 02481 US

GROWTH PLANS/SPECIAL FEATURES:
Harvard Pilgrim Health Care, Inc. is a not-for-profit health plan with approximately 800,000 members and a network of more than 22,000 doctors and 130 hospitals. The firm provides health coverage in Massachusetts and Maine, as well as in Vermont and New Hampshire through its Harvard Pilgrim Health Care of New England (NE) subsidiary. In addition, the firm is the parent company of HPHC Insurance Company, an indemnity insurance company in Massachusetts and New Hampshire. The firm offers a variety of plan choices, including HMOs, PPOs and a point-of-service plans. The company also enrolls Medicare beneficiaries through its First Seniority and Medicare Enhance programs, as well as offering its HPHConnect web site for online benefits administration. In recent news, Harvard Pilgrim formed a strategic business and marketing alliance with UnitedHealth Group that combines the company's network of doctors and hospitals with UnitedHealth's national network. It also offers a simplified administration and care management portfolio in a single integrated package. In addition, NE partnered with New Hampshire Public Risk Management Exchange (also known as Primex3) to create a health insurance program for local government in the southern area of New Hampshire.

FINANCIALS: Sales and profits are in thousands of dollars—add 000 to get the full amount. Year 2004 note: Complete fiscal 2004 results were not available for all companies at press time. For this company, year 2004 is for months.

2004 Sales: $ (months)   2004 Profits: $ (months)
2003 Sales: $2,100,000   2003 Profits: $44,200   **Stock Ticker:** Nonprofit
2002 Sales: $ 2002 Profits: $ Employees: 1,400
2001 Sales: $ 2001 Profits: $ Fiscal Year Ends: 12/31
2000 Sales: $ 2000 Profits: $

SALARIES/BENEFITS:
Pension Plan: ESOP Stock Plan: Profit Sharing: Top Exec. Salary: $ Bonus: $
Savings Plan: Stock Purch. Plan: Second Exec. Salary: $ Bonus: $

OTHER THOUGHTS:
Apparent Top Female Officers: 7
Hot Spot for Advancement for Women/Minorities: Y

LOCATIONS: ("Y" = Yes)
West:	Southwest:	Midwest:	Southeast:	Northeast:	International:
				Y	

HCA INC

www.hcahealthcare.com

Industry Group Code: 622110 Ranks within this company's industry group: Sales: 2 Profits: 1

Insurance/HMO/PPO:	Drugs:	Equipment/Supplies:	Hospitals/Clinics:		Services:		Health Care:	
Insurance:	Manufacturer:	Manufacturer:	Acute Care:	Y	Diagnostics:		Home Health:	
Managed Care:	Distributor:	Distributor:	Sub-Acute Care:	Y	Labs/Testing:		Long-Term Care:	
Utilization Mgmt.:	Specialty Pharm.:	Leasing/Finance:	Outpatient Surgery:	Y	Staffing:		Physical Therapy:	
Payment Proc.:	Vitamins/Nutri.:	Information Sys.:	Phys. Rehab. Center:	Y	Waste Disposal:		Phys. Practice Mgmt.:	
	Clinical Trials:		Psychiatric Clinics:		Specialty Services:			

TYPES OF BUSINESS:
Hospitals-General
Outpatient Surgery Centers
Sub-Acute Care
Psychiatric Hospitals
Rehabilitation Services

BRANDS/DIVISIONS/AFFILIATES:

CONTACTS:
Note: Officers with more than one job title may be intentionally listed here more than once.

Jack O. Bovender, Jr., CEO
Richard M. Bracken, Pres.
Richard M. Bracken, COO
R. Milton Johnson, Exec. VP/CFO
John M. Steele, Sr. VP-Human Resources
Noel B. Williams, CIO
A. Bruce Moore, Jr., Sr. VP-Admin.
Robert A. Waterman, Sr. VP/General Counsel
A. Bruce Moore, Jr., Sr. VP-Oper.
V. Carl George, VP-Dev.
David G. Anderson, Sr. VP-Finance/Treas.
Charles R. Evans, Pres.-Eastern Group
Victor L. Campbell, Sr. VP
Rosalyn S. Elton, Sr. VP-Oper. Finance
Alan R. Yuspeh, Sr. VP-Ethics, Compliance & Corp. Responsibility
Jack O. Bovender, Jr., Chmn.
James A. Fitzgerald, Jr., Sr. VP-Supply Chain Oper.

Phone: 615-344-9551 **Fax:** 615-344-2266
Toll-Free:
Address: One Park Plaza, Nashville, TN 37203 US

GROWTH PLANS/SPECIAL FEATURES:

HCA, Inc., formerly known as HCA Healthcare Co., owns and operates approximately 191 hospitals and more than 80 outpatient surgery centers in 23 states, the U.K. and Switzerland, with a total of 43,441 licensed beds. Of the hospitals, 176 are general, acute care hospitals, seven are psychiatric hospitals, one is a rehabilitation center and seven are hospitals acquired in joint ventures. The company's acute care hospitals provide a full range of services, including intensive care, cardiac care, diagnostic and emergency services, radiology, respiratory therapy, cardiology and physical therapy. The psychiatric hospitals provide therapeutic programs including child, adolescent and adult psychiatric care and adult and adolescent alcohol and drug abuse treatment and counseling. In the mid-1990s, the firm underwent significant downsizing and restructuring and almost a complete turnover of senior management in response to a widespread government investigation into its business practices. More recently, the company has established a comprehensive ethics and compliance program and has begun to expand again. In recent news, the board of directors extended an offer to repurchase up to 61 million shares of its outstanding stock.

FINANCIALS:
Sales and profits are in thousands of dollars—add 000 to get the full amount. Year 2004 note: Complete fiscal 2004 results were not available for all companies at press time. For this company, year 2004 is for 9 months.

2004 Sales: $17,562,000 (9 months)	2004 Profits: $770,000 (9 months)	**Stock Ticker:** HCA
2003 Sales: $21,808,000	2003 Profits: $1,332,000	Employees: 242,000
2002 Sales: $19,729,000	2002 Profits: $833,000	Fiscal Year Ends: 12/31
2001 Sales: $17,953,000	2001 Profits: $886,000	
2000 Sales: $16,670,000	2000 Profits: $219,000	

SALARIES/BENEFITS:
Pension Plan: Y   ESOP Stock Plan: Profit Sharing: Top Exec. Salary: $1,191,102   Bonus: $
Savings Plan: Y   Stock Purch. Plan: Y   Second Exec. Salary: $831,604   Bonus: $

OTHER THOUGHTS:
Apparent Top Female Officers: 2
Hot Spot for Advancement for Women/Minorities:

LOCATIONS: ("Y" = Yes)
West:	Southwest:	Midwest:	Southeast:	Northeast:	International:
Y	Y	Y	Y	Y	Y

HEALTH CARE SERVICE CORPORATION

www.hcsc.net

Industry Group Code: 524114 Ranks within this company's industry group: Sales: 12 Profits: 6

Insurance/HMO/PPO:	Drugs:	Equipment/Supplies:	Hospitals/Clinics:	Services:	Health Care:
Insurance: Y	Manufacturer:	Manufacturer:	Acute Care:	Diagnostics:	Home Health:
Managed Care: Y	Distributor:	Distributor:	Sub-Acute Care:	Labs/Testing:	Long-Term Care:
Utilization Mgmt.:	Specialty Pharm.:	Leasing/Finance:	Outpatient Surgery:	Staffing:	Physical Therapy:
Payment Proc.: Y	Vitamins/Nutri.:	Information Sys.:	Phys. Rehab. Center:	Waste Disposal:	Phys. Practice Mgmt.:
	Clinical Trials:		Psychiatric Clinics:	Specialty Services: Y	

TYPES OF BUSINESS:
Insurance
HMO, PPO, POS & Traditional Indemnity
Medicare Supplemental Health
Life Insurance
Dental Insurance
Electronic Claims & Information Network
Workers' Compensation
Retirement Services

BRANDS/DIVISIONS/AFFILIATES:
Blue Cross and Blue Shield of Illinois
Blue Cross and Blue Shield of Texas
Blue Cross and Blue Shield of New Mexico
Preferred Financial Group
Fort Dearborn Life Insurance Company
Medical Life Insurance Company
Dental Network of America, Inc.
Health Information Network, Inc. (The)

CONTACTS:
Note: Officers with more than one job title may be intentionally listed here more than once.

Raymond R. McCaskey, CEO
Raymond R. McCaskey, Pres.
Sherman M. Wolff, Exec. VP/COO
Denise A. Bujack, Sr. VP/CFO
Patrick F. O'Connor, Sr. VP/Chief Human Resources Officer
Patrick E. Moroney, Sr. VP/CIO
Hugo Tagli, Jr., Sr. VP/Chief Legal Officer
Larry J. Newsom, Sr. VP/CEO-Subsidiary Oper.
Robert Kieckhefer, VP-Public Affairs
Patricia A. Hemingway Hall, Pres.-Texas Div.
Gail K. Boudreaux, Pres.-Illinois Div.
Elizabeth A. Watrin, Pres.-New Mexico Div.
Ray A. Angeli, Sr. VP-Subscriber Services
Milton Carroll, Chmn.

Phone: 312-653-6000 Fax: 312-819-1220
Toll-Free:
Address: 300 E. Randolph St., Chicago, IL 60601-5099 US

GROWTH PLANS/SPECIAL FEATURES:
Health Care Service Corporation (HCSC) is a licensee of the Blue Cross and Blue Shield Association. It provides PPOs, HMOs, POS plans, traditional indemnity and Medicare supplemental health plans to approximately 9.5 million members through Blue Cross and Blue Shield of Illinois (BCBSI), Blue Cross and Blue Shield of Texas (BCBST) and Blue Cross and Blue Shield of New Mexico (BCBSNM). Through its non-Blue Cross and Blue Shield subsidiaries, the company offers prescription drug plans, Medicare supplement insurance, dental and vision coverage, life and disability insurance, workers' compensation, retirement services and medical financial services. One such subsidiary, Preferred Financial Group, is made up of HSCS's various life insurance subsidiaries: Fort Dearborn Life Insurance Company of Illinois (FDL), Medical Life Insurance Company in Ohio (MLI) and Colorado Bankers Life Insurance Company. Another subsidiary, Dental Network of America, Inc., functions as a third-party administrator for all company dental programs and is registered in every state except Florida. It also offers a dental discount card program. The Health Information Network, Inc., a wholly-owned subsidiary, is an electronic claims and information network that acts as a clearinghouse for physicians, hospitals and other providers to file patient claims and other transactions electronically with their billing agents. Hallmark Services Corporation, another wholly-owned subsidiary, provides administration and claim adjudication services for individual policies to the direct markets divisions of BCBSI and BCBST. Recently, FDL and MLI agreed to merge. FDL also agreed to acquire Combined Services, a general insurance agency owned by Blue Cross and Blue Shield of Vermont, which operates extensive broker distribution networks in Connecticut, Maine, Massachusetts, New Hampshire, Rhode Island and Vermont. In addition, FDL acquired Omaha Life Insurance Company from Blue Cross and Blue Shield of Nebraska.

FINANCIALS:
Sales and profits are in thousands of dollars—add 000 to get the full amount. Year 2004 note: Complete fiscal 2004 results were not available for all companies at press time. For this company, year 2004 is for months.

2004 Sales: $ (months)
2003 Sales: $8,190,400
2002 Sales: $7,312,300
2001 Sales: $
2000 Sales: $

2004 Profits: $ (months)
2003 Profits: $624,600
2002 Profits: $245,900
2001 Profits: $
2000 Profits: $

Stock Ticker: Private
Employees: 13,000
Fiscal Year Ends: 12/31

SALARIES/BENEFITS:
Pension Plan: ESOP Stock Plan: Profit Sharing: Top Exec. Salary: $ Bonus: $
Savings Plan: Stock Purch. Plan: Second Exec. Salary: $ Bonus: $

OTHER THOUGHTS:
Apparent Top Female Officers: 4
Hot Spot for Advancement for Women/Minorities: Y

LOCATIONS: ("Y" = Yes)
West:	Southwest:	Midwest:	Southeast:	Northeast:	International:
Y	Y	Y		Y	

HEALTH FITNESS CORP

www.hfit.com

Industry Group Code: 713940 **Ranks within this company's industry group:** Sales: 1 Profits: 1

Insurance/HMO/PPO:	Drugs:	Equipment/Supplies:	Hospitals/Clinics:	Services:	Health Care:
Insurance:	Manufacturer:	Manufacturer:	Acute Care:	Diagnostics:	Home Health:
Managed Care:	Distributor:	Distributor:	Sub-Acute Care:	Labs/Testing:	Long-Term Care:
Utilization Mgmt.:	Specialty Pharm.:	Leasing/Finance:	Outpatient Surgery:	Staffing:	Physical Therapy: Y
Payment Proc.:	Vitamins/Nutri.:	Information Sys.:	Phys. Rehab. Center:	Waste Disposal:	Phys. Practice Mgmt.:
	Clinical Trials:		Psychiatric Clinics:	Specialty Services: Y	

TYPES OF BUSINESS:
Corporate & Hospital-Based Fitness Centers
Consulting Services
Fitness Center Management
Fitness Center Design
Wellness Programs
Health & Fitness Assessment
On-Site Physical Therapy Services

BRANDS/DIVISIONS/AFFILIATES:
HFC Assessment Services
HFC Wellness Programs
HFC Fitness Programs
HFC Treatment Services

CONTACTS:
Note: Officers with more than one job title may be intentionally listed here more than once.

Jerry V. Noyce, CEO
Jerry V. Noyce, Pres.
Wesley W. Winnekins, CFO
Katherine Hamlin, VP-Mktg. & Strategic Dev.
Jeanne C. Crawford, VP-Human Resources
James A. Narum, Sr. VP-Corp. Bus. Dev.
Wesley W. Winnekins, Treas.
David T. Hurt, VP-Acct. Services
Ralph Colao, VP-Consulting & Best Practices
Geri Martin, VP-Mktg.
Mike Seethaler, VP-New Bus. Dev.
John C. Penn, Chmn.

Phone: 612-831-6830 **Fax:** 952-897-5173
Toll-Free: 800-639-7913
Address: 3600 American Blvd. W., Ste. 560, Bloomington, MN 55431 US

GROWTH PLANS/SPECIAL FEATURES:

Health Fitness Corp. (HFC) and its subsidiaries provide fitness and wellness management services and programs to corporations, hospitals, communities and universities in the U.S. and Canada. The firm also provides injury prevention programs and on-site physical therapy services. Currently, HFC is under contract to manage 393 sites, including 223 corporate fitness centers, 47 corporate wellness programs, 12 occupational health programs, 15 hospital-, community- or university-based fitness centers and 96 corporate sites that do not have full-time staff. The company provides a full range of development, management, marketing and consulting services, including demographic analysis, space planning, interior design, floor plan design, selection and sourcing of fitness equipment, fitness program design and occupational health consulting services. HFC also manages the operations of established fitness centers, including staff selection and implementation of programs. Programs offered include HFC Assessment Services, a full range of tools to assess the health and well-being of individuals, including screenings and education; HFC Wellness Programs, a menu of lifestyle programs addressing the specific needs of a company's workforce, including weight loss and stress management; HFC Fitness Programs, customized exercise-based programs including personal training and specialty group classes; and HFC Treatment Services, on-site services designed to prevent, manage and treat musculo-skeletal disorders in the work environment.

The company offers employees health and dental coverage, baby care and an employee assistance program. In addition, HFC has introduced an eTraining center, wherein associate employees pick up the latest information and instructional material for learning about safety, member retention, quality customer service and practices.

FINANCIALS:
Sales and profits are in thousands of dollars—add 000 to get the full amount. Year 2004 note: Complete fiscal 2004 results were not available for all companies at press time. For this company, year 2004 is for 9 months.

2004 Sales: $38,950 (9 months)	2004 Profits: $1,337 (9 months)	**Stock Ticker:** HFIT
2003 Sales: $31,478	2003 Profits: $ 632	Employees: 2,965
2002 Sales: $27,900	2002 Profits: $3,000	Fiscal Year Ends: 12/31
2001 Sales: $25,900	2001 Profits: $1,800	
2000 Sales: $26,200	2000 Profits: $ 900	

SALARIES/BENEFITS:
Pension Plan: ESOP Stock Plan: Profit Sharing: Top Exec. Salary: $238,050   Bonus: $20,230
Savings Plan: Y   Stock Purch. Plan: Y   Second Exec. Salary: $131,159   Bonus: $10,000

OTHER THOUGHTS:
Apparent Top Female Officers: 3
Hot Spot for Advancement for Women/Minorities: Y

LOCATIONS: ("Y" = Yes)

West:	Southwest:	Midwest:	Southeast:	Northeast:	International:
Y	Y	Y	Y	Y	Y

Note: Financial information, benefits and other data can change quickly and may vary from those stated here.

HEALTH GRADES INC

www.healthgrades.com

Industry Group Code: 514199 Ranks within this company's industry group: Sales: 1 Profits: 1

Insurance/HMO/PPO:	Drugs:	Equipment/Supplies:	Hospitals/Clinics:	Services:	Health Care:
Insurance:	Manufacturer:	Manufacturer:	Acute Care:	Diagnostics:	Home Health:
Managed Care:	Distributor:	Distributor:	Sub-Acute Care:	Labs/Testing:	Long-Term Care:
Utilization Mgmt.:	Specialty Pharm.:	Leasing/Finance:	Outpatient Surgery:	Staffing:	Physical Therapy:
Payment Proc.:	Vitamins/Nutri.:	Information Sys.:	Phys. Rehab. Center:	Waste Disposal:	Phys. Practice Mgmt.:
	Clinical Trials:		Psychiatric Clinics:	Specialty Services: Y	

TYPES OF BUSINESS:
Online Health Information
Health Providers Ratings Data
Consulting Services

BRANDS/DIVISIONS/AFFILIATES:

CONTACTS:
Note: Officers with more than one job title may be intentionally listed here more than once.

Kerry R. Hicks, CEO
Kerry R. Hicks, Pres.
G. Allen Dodge, CFO
Michael D. Phillips, Sr. VP-Provider Sales
David G. Hicks, Exec. VP-IT
John R. Morrow, Sr. VP-Strategic Dev.
G. Allen Dodge, Sr. VP-Finance
Sarah P. Loughran, Exec. VP-Provider Services
Peter A. Fatianow, Sr. VP-Corp. Services

Phone: 303-716-0041 **Fax:** 303-716-1298
Toll-Free:
Address: 44 Union Blvd., Ste. 600, Lakewood, CO 80228 US

GROWTH PLANS/SPECIAL FEATURES:
Health Grades, Inc. (HGI) is a health care ratings and consulting company that provides consumers with the means to assess and compare the quality or qualifications of health care providers including hospitals, nursing homes, home health agencies, hospice programs and fertility clinics. It currently provides ratings or profile information on over 4,700 hospitals, 620,000 physicians in over 120 specialties and 16,000 nursing homes. This information is available on the firm's web site free of charge to consumers, employers and health plans, with more detailed reports available for a fee. For hospitals with high ratings, HGI offers the opportunity to license its ratings and trademarks and provides assistance in marketing programs. The company also offers consulting services to hospitals that either want to build a reputation based on quality of care or are working to identify areas to improve quality. HGI has an ongoing collaboration with the Leapfrog Group to analyze and report the findings of hospital patient safety surveys. Leapfrog's survey assesses the extent to which hospitals strive to implement patient safety practices and rewards for advances in safety.

FINANCIALS:
Sales and profits are in thousands of dollars—add 000 to get the full amount. Year 2004 note: Complete fiscal 2004 results were not available for all companies at press time. For this company, year 2004 is for 6 months.

2004 Sales: $6,718 (6 months)	2004 Profits: $824 (6 months)	**Stock Ticker:** HGRD
2003 Sales: $8,805	2003 Profits: $-1,284	**Employees:** 56
2002 Sales: $5,300	2002 Profits: $-1,700	**Fiscal Year Ends:** 12/31
2001 Sales: $3,600	2001 Profits: $-7,400	
2000 Sales: $5,800	2000 Profits: $-7,500	

SALARIES/BENEFITS:
Pension Plan:	ESOP Stock Plan:	Profit Sharing:	Top Exec. Salary: $285,499	Bonus: $220,205
Savings Plan: Y	Stock Purch. Plan:		Second Exec. Salary: $254,735	Bonus: $91,227

OTHER THOUGHTS:
Apparent Top Female Officers: 1
Hot Spot for Advancement for Women/Minorities:

LOCATIONS: ("Y" = Yes)
West:	Southwest:	Midwest:	Southeast:	Northeast:	International:
Y					

HEALTH INSURANCE PLAN OF GREATER NEW YORK

www.hipusa.com

Industry Group Code: 524114   Ranks within this company's industry group: Sales: 25   Profits: 11

Insurance/HMO/PPO:	Drugs:	Equipment/Supplies:	Hospitals/Clinics:	Services:	Health Care:
Insurance:	Manufacturer:	Manufacturer:	Acute Care:	Diagnostics:	Home Health:
Managed Care: Y	Distributor:	Distributor:	Sub-Acute Care:	Labs/Testing:	Long-Term Care:
Utilization Mgmt.:	Specialty Pharm.:	Leasing/Finance:	Outpatient Surgery:	Staffing:	Physical Therapy:
Payment Proc.:	Vitamins/Nutri.:	Information Sys.:	Phys. Rehab. Center:	Waste Disposal:	Phys. Practice Mgmt.:
	Clinical Trials:		Psychiatric Clinics:	Specialty Services:	

Insurance: Y (Managed Care: Y)

TYPES OF BUSINESS:
HMO

BRANDS/DIVISIONS/AFFILIATES:
ConnectiCare Holding Company
Vytra Health Plans
HIP Integrative Wellness

CONTACTS:
Note: Officers with more than one job title may be intentionally listed here more than once.

Anthony L. Watson, CEO
Daniel T. McGowan, Pres.
Daniel T. McGowan, COO
Michael D. Fullwood, Exec. VP/CFO
Larry G. Posner, Sr. VP-Mktg. & Sales
Fred Blickman, Sr. VP-Human Resources
Pedro Villalba, Sr. VP-IT
Pedro Villalba, Chief Tech. Officer
Michael D. Fullwood, General Counsel/Corp. Sec.
David S. Abernethy, Exec. VP-Oper.
Arthur J. Byrd, VP-Investor Rel.
Domini F. D'Adamo, Sr. VP-Finance/Corp. Controller
Arthur H. Barnes, Sr. VP-External Affairs & Corp. Contributions
Ronald I. Platt, Exec. VP-Medical Affairs/Chief Medical Officer
Anthony L. Watson, Chmn.

Phone: 212-630-5000   Fax:
Toll-Free: 800-447-8255
Address: 55 Water St., New York, NY 10041-8190 US

GROWTH PLANS/SPECIAL FEATURES:

Health Insurance Plan of Greater New York (HIP) provides health insurance products to a membership of more than 1 million, spread throughout New York City, Long Island and Westchester County. It is the largest HMO in New York City and has been a leader in utilizing the Internet to provide not only reduced costs but improved customer service. For example, HIP was the first health insurance company in the nation to translate its web site into Chinese and Korean in addition to Spanish, as well as being rated the number-one insurance company in the country for the innovative use of technology by Information Week Magazine. HIP maintains a network of approximately 22,000 physicians and provides care through a number of top New York City area hospitals, including Beth Israel Medical Center, St. Luke's-Roosevelt Hospital Center, Montefiore Medical Center, Lenox Hill Hospital and St. Barnabas Hospital. In addition to HIP's comprehensive heath insurance options, the company provides programs and discounts for alternative medicine such as acupuncture, massage therapy and nutritional counseling, mental health services and chemical dependency treatment, pharmacy services, dental plans and women's wellness programs. HIP Integrative Wellness is an initiative supporting the belief that the best patient care will be attentive to the patient's spiritual, emotional and mental states as well as the physical. The company recently acquired Vytra Health Plans of Long Island, putting HIP's membership over 1 million. Another recent acquisition is ConnectiCare Holding Company, a managed health care company with approximately 270,000 members in Connecticut and Massachusetts. Subject to regulatory approval, stock from ConnectiCare's current owners, The Carlyle Group and Liberty Partners, will be transferred to HIP, though ConnectiCare will maintain its headquarters and offices independently in Connecticut and will retain all its current management.

FINANCIALS:
Sales and profits are in thousands of dollars—add 000 to get the full amount. Year 2004 note: Complete fiscal 2004 results were not available for all companies at press time. For this company, year 2004 is for months.

2004 Sales: $ (months)	2004 Profits: $ (months)
2003 Sales: $3,369,900	2003 Profits: $274,800
2002 Sales: $2,901,700	2002 Profits: $178,400
2001 Sales: $	2001 Profits: $
2000 Sales: $	2000 Profits: $

Stock Ticker: Nonprofit
Employees: 2,000
Fiscal Year Ends: 12/31

SALARIES/BENEFITS:
Pension Plan: ESOP Stock Plan: Profit Sharing: Top Exec. Salary: $ Bonus: $
Savings Plan: Stock Purch. Plan: Second Exec. Salary: $ Bonus: $

OTHER THOUGHTS:
Apparent Top Female Officers:
Hot Spot for Advancement for Women/Minorities:

LOCATIONS: ("Y" = Yes)
West:	Southwest:	Midwest:	Southeast:	Northeast:	International:
				Y	

HEALTH MANAGEMENT ASSOCIATES INC   www.hma-corp.com

Industry Group Code: 622110   Ranks within this company's industry group: Sales: 24   Profits: 6

Insurance/HMO/PPO:	Drugs:	Equipment/Supplies:	Hospitals/Clinics:		Services:	Health Care:
Insurance: Managed Care: Utilization Mgmt.: Payment Proc.:	Manufacturer: Distributor: Specialty Pharm.: Vitamins/Nutri.: Clinical Trials:	Manufacturer: Distributor: Leasing/Finance: Information Sys.:	Acute Care: Sub-Acute Care: Outpatient Surgery: Phys. Rehab. Center: Psychiatric Clinics:	Y	Diagnostics: Labs/Testing: Staffing: Waste Disposal: Specialty Services:	Home Health: Long-Term Care: Physical Therapy: Phys. Practice Mgmt.:

TYPES OF BUSINESS:
Hospitals-General
Psychiatric Hospitals

GROWTH PLANS/SPECIAL FEATURES:
Health Management Associates, Inc. operates a network of acute care hospitals in the rural southeastern and southwestern United States. The company currently operates 41 general acute care hospitals, with a total of 5,769 licensed beds, and two psychiatric hospitals, with a total of 134 licensed beds. The firm is rapidly growing through acquisitions. In evaluating potential acquisitions, Health Management Associates requires a hospital's market service area to exhibit a demographic need for the facility and to have an established physician base that can be augmented by the company's ability to attract additional physicians to the community. Many hospitals acquired by the firm are unprofitable at the time of acquisition. Recent additions include the acquisition of Chester County Hospital, an 82-bed hospital in Chester, South Carolina, and the building of the 100-bed Collier Regional Medical Center. The operations of Health Management Associates' psychiatric hospitals focus mainly on child and adolescent residential treatment programs. Some of the company's hospitals provide services to retired and certain other military personnel and their families, pursuant to the Civilian Health and Medical Program of Uniformed Services (CHAMPUS). The firm has been named to the Forbes Platinum 400 for the best large companies in America for the third consecutive year. In recent news, Health Management Associates exchanged the 76-bed Williamson Memorial Hospital, located in Williamson, West Virginia, with LifePoint Hospitals, Inc. for nearly all of the assets of Bartow Memorial Hospital.

BRANDS/DIVISIONS/AFFILIATES:
East Pointe Hospital
Lee County Community Hospital
Charlie Hospital
Medical Center of Southeastern Oklahoma
Charlotte Regional Medical Center
Davis Medical Center
Walton Medical Center
Yakima Medical Center

CONTACTS:
Note: Officers with more than one job title may be intentionally listed here more than once.
Joseph V. Vumbacco, CEO
Joseph V. Vumbacco, Pres.
Robert E. Farnham, Sr. VP/CFO
Timothy R. Parry, VP/General Counsel
Peter M. Lawson, Exec. VP-Oper.
John C. Merriwether, VP-Financial Rel.
Jon P. Vollmer, Exec. VP-Hospital Oper.
Timothy R. Parry, Corp. Sec.
William J. Schoen, Chmn.

Phone: 239-598-3131   Fax: 239-598-2705
Toll-Free: 800-829-8432
Address: 5811 Pelican Bay Blvd., Ste. 500, Naples, FL 34108-2710 US

FINANCIALS:
Sales and profits are in thousands of dollars—add 000 to get the full amount. Year 2004 note: Complete fiscal 2004 results were not available for all companies at press time. For this company, year 2004 is for 9 months.

2004 Sales: $1,903,018 (9 months)   2004 Profits: $213,642 (9 months)
2003 Sales: $2,560,600   2003 Profits: $283,400
2002 Sales: $2,262,600   2002 Profits: $246,400
2001 Sales: $1,879,800   2001 Profits: $195,000
2000 Sales: $1,577,800   2000 Profits: $167,700

Stock Ticker: HMA
Employees: 24,000
Fiscal Year Ends: 9/30

SALARIES/BENEFITS:
Pension Plan: ESOP Stock Plan: Profit Sharing: Top Exec. Salary: $650,000   Bonus: $812,500
Savings Plan: Y   Stock Purch. Plan: Second Exec. Salary: $300,000   Bonus: $157,500

OTHER THOUGHTS:
Apparent Top Female Officers:
Hot Spot for Advancement for Women/Minorities:

LOCATIONS: ("Y" = Yes)

West:	Southwest:	Midwest:	Southeast:	Northeast:	International:
Y	Y	Y	Y	Y	

HEALTH MANAGEMENT SYSTEMS INC

www.hmsy.com

Industry Group Code: 522320 Ranks within this company's industry group: Sales: 1 Profits: 1

Insurance/HMO/PPO:	Drugs:	Equipment/Supplies:	Hospitals/Clinics:	Services:	Health Care:
Insurance:	Manufacturer:	Manufacturer:	Acute Care:	Diagnostics:	Home Health:
Managed Care:	Distributor:	Distributor:	Sub-Acute Care:	Labs/Testing:	Long-Term Care:
Utilization Mgmt.: Y	Specialty Pharm.:	Leasing/Finance:	Outpatient Surgery:	Staffing:	Physical Therapy:
Payment Proc.: Y	Vitamins/Nutri.:	Information Sys.: Y	Phys. Rehab. Center:	Waste Disposal:	Phys. Practice Mgmt.:
	Clinical Trials:		Psychiatric Clinics:	Specialty Services: Y	

TYPES OF BUSINESS:
Data Processing-Health Care
Information Management Services
Outsourcing Services
Bills/Claims Management

BRANDS/DIVISIONS/AFFILIATES:
HMS Holdings Corp.

CONTACTS:
Note: Officers with more than one job title may be intentionally listed here more than once.

William F. Miller, CEO
William C. Lucia, Pres.
Thomas Archbold, Interim CFO
Joseph Joy, VP/CIO
Michael Hostetler, VP-Product Dev.
Stephen Vaccaro, Sr. VP-Oper.
Chuck Anderson, VP-Corp. Dev.
Donna Price, Sr. VP-Client Rel.
Helene Garrick, Dir.-Compliance & Quality Assurance
Carl Borgatti, VP-Contract Oper.
Thomas A. Baggett, Jr., VP-Overpayment Recovery Services

Phone: 212-685-4545 Fax: 212-889-8776
Toll-Free: 888-467-0184
Address: 401 Park Ave. S., New York, NY 10016 US

GROWTH PLANS/SPECIAL FEATURES:
Health Management Systems, Inc., a wholly-owned subsidiary of HMS Holdings Corp., provides information-based revenue enhancement services to health care providers and payers. The company's services benefit clients by increasing revenue, accelerating cash flow and reducing operating and administrative costs. The firm is organized into two business units: the provider services division and the payer services division. The provider services division offers hospitals and other health care providers a comprehensive array of technology-based revenue cycle services. These services include identifying third-party resources, submitting timely and accurate bills to third-party payers and patients, recovering and properly accounting for the amounts due and securing the appropriate cost-based reimbursement from entitlement programs. Clients may use one or more of the services or outsource the entirety of their business office operations to Health Management Systems. The payer services division offers a broad range of services to state Medicaid and other government agencies that administer health care entitlement programs. The firm's services are designed to identify and recover amounts that should have been the responsibility of a third party or that were paid inappropriately. The company has contracts in 30 states to detect Medicaid fraud. In recent news, the company announced that it has recovered over $2 billion to date.

The company offers its employees comprehensive health care coverage and tuition reimbursement.

FINANCIALS:
Sales and profits are in thousands of dollars—add 000 to get the full amount. Year 2004 note: Complete fiscal 2004 results were not available for all companies at press time. For this company, year 2004 is for 9 months.

2004 Sales: $50,638 (9 months)   2004 Profits: $750 (9 months)
2003 Sales: $74,400   2003 Profits: $2,300
2002 Sales: $32,300   2002 Profits: $935
2001 Sales: $58,700   2001 Profits: $-19,500
2000 Sales: $8,200   2000 Profits: $-900

Stock Ticker: Subsidiary
Employees: 493
Fiscal Year Ends: 12/31

SALARIES/BENEFITS:
Pension Plan: ESOP Stock Plan: Profit Sharing: Top Exec. Salary: $400,000   Bonus: $200,000
Savings Plan: Y Stock Purch. Plan: Second Exec. Salary: $225,000 Bonus: $132,500

OTHER THOUGHTS:
Apparent Top Female Officers: 2
Hot Spot for Advancement for Women/Minorities:

LOCATIONS: ("Y" = Yes)
West:	Southwest:	Midwest:	Southeast:	Northeast:	International:
Y	Y	Y	Y	Y	

HEALTH NET INC

www.healthnet.com

Industry Group Code: 524114   **Ranks within this company's industry group:** Sales: 11   Profits: 14

Insurance/HMO/PPO:		Drugs:	Equipment/Supplies:	Hospitals/Clinics:	Services:		Health Care:	
Insurance:	Y	Manufacturer:	Manufacturer:	Acute Care:	Diagnostics:		Home Health:	
Managed Care:	Y	Distributor:	Distributor:	Sub-Acute Care:	Labs/Testing:		Long-Term Care:	
Utilization Mgmt.:	Y	Specialty Pharm.:	Leasing/Finance:	Outpatient Surgery:	Staffing:		Physical Therapy:	
Payment Proc.:		Vitamins/Nutri.:	Information Sys.:	Phys. Rehab. Center:	Waste Disposal:		Phys. Practice Mgmt.:	
		Clinical Trials:		Psychiatric Clinics:	Specialty Services:	Y		

TYPES OF BUSINESS:
HMO/PPO
Utilization Management
Health Care Services Management
Administrative Services
Health Insurance Underwriting
Life Insurance Underwriting

BRANDS/DIVISIONS/AFFILIATES:
Rosetta Stone
Decision Power
Hospital Comparison Report
Evidence Based Medicine

CONTACTS:
Note: Officers with more than one job title may be intentionally listed here more than once.

Jay M. Gellert, CEO
Jay M. Gellert, Pres.
Anthony Piszel, Exec. VP/CFO
Jay L. Silverstein, Sr. VP/Chief Mktg. Officer
B. Curtis Westen, Sr. VP/General Counsel
Marvin P. Rich, Exec. VP-Oper.
David W. Olson, Sr. VP-Corp. Comm.
Karin D. Mayhew, Sr. VP-Organization Effectiveness
Jonathan H. Scheff, Sr. VP/Chief Medical Officer
Christopher P. Wing, Exec. VP-Reg. Health Plans & Specialty Companies
Jeffrey M. Folick, Exec. VP-Reg. Health Plans & Specialty Companies
Roger F. Greaves, Chmn.

Phone: 818-676-6000   **Fax:** 818-676-8591
Toll-Free: 800-291-6911
Address: 21650 Oxnard St., Woodland Hills, CA 91367 US

GROWTH PLANS/SPECIAL FEATURES:
Health Net, Inc. is one of the largest publicly traded managed health care companies in the U.S. The company's HMO, insured PPO and government contract subsidiaries provide health benefits to more than 7.3 million individuals in 27 states through group, individual, Medicare, Medicaid and TRICARE programs. Health Net also offers managed health care products for behavioral health and prescription drugs, and it owns health and life insurance companies licensed to sell exclusive provider organization, PPO, POS and indemnity products, as well as life and accidental death and disability insurance, in 36 states and the District of Columbia. Health plan services are provided to the firm's commercial and individual members in Arizona, California, Oregon, Connecticut, New Jersey and New York, and include primary and specialty physician care, hospital care, pharmacy services, behavioral health and ancillary diagnostic and therapeutic services. Health Net's HMO includes nearly 45,000 primary care physicians and 100,000 specialist physicians. Moreover, the company provides managed health care product coordination for multi-region employers and administrative services for medical groups and self-funded benefits programs. The firm also receives contracts from federal government programs such as TRICARE to perform administrative and management services. Health Net's new Rosetta Stone initiative provides information to consumers so that they can make better informed decisions about their health care. It incorporates Decision Power, which provides members with electronic and telephonic interactive modes of acquiring information about health care issues; a Hospital Comparison Report, which allows them to compare hospital clinical and cost performance for a variety of common procedures; and Evidence Based Medicine, which provides data on evidence-based standards of care.

FINANCIALS:
Sales and profits are in thousands of dollars—add 000 to get the full amount. Year 2004 note: Complete fiscal 2004 results were not available for all companies at press time. For this company, year 2004 is for 9 months.

2004 Sales: $8,778,800 (9 months)   2004 Profits: $128,233   (9 months)
2003 Sales: $10,959,000   2003 Profits: $234,000
2002 Sales: $10,149,000   2002 Profits: $229,000
2001 Sales: $9,980,000   2001 Profits: $86,000
2000 Sales: $9,076,600   2000 Profits: $163,623

Stock Ticker: HNT
Employees: 9,053
Fiscal Year Ends: 12/31

SALARIES/BENEFITS:
Pension Plan: ESOP Stock Plan: Profit Sharing: Top Exec. Salary: $891,731   Bonus: $800,000
Savings Plan: Y   Stock Purch. Plan: Second Exec. Salary: $520,865   Bonus: $700,000

OTHER THOUGHTS:
Apparent Top Female Officers: 1
Hot Spot for Advancement for Women/Minorities:

LOCATIONS: ("Y" = Yes)
West:	Southwest:	Midwest:	Southeast:	Northeast:	International:
Y	Y			Y	

HEALTHAXIS INC

www.healthaxis.com

Industry Group Code: 511200 Ranks within this company's industry group: Sales: 13 Profits: 9

Insurance/HMO/PPO:	Drugs:	Equipment/Supplies:	Hospitals/Clinics:	Services:	Health Care:
Insurance: Managed Care: Utilization Mgmt.: Payment Proc.:	Manufacturer: Distributor: Specialty Pharm.: Vitamins/Nutri.: Clinical Trials:	Manufacturer: Distributor: Leasing/Finance: Information Sys.: Y	Acute Care: Sub-Acute Care: Outpatient Surgery: Phys. Rehab. Center: Psychiatric Clinics:	Diagnostics: Labs/Testing: Staffing: Waste Disposal: Specialty Services: Y	Home Health: Long-Term Care: Physical Therapy: Phys. Practice Mgmt.:

TYPES OF BUSINESS:
Software-Health Care Administration
Benefit Administration Systems
Web-Enabled Administration Systems
Imaging Services
Outsourcing Services

BRANDS/DIVISIONS/AFFILIATES:

CONTACTS:
Note: Officers with more than one job title may be intentionally listed here more than once.

James W. McLane, CEO
John M. Carradine, Pres.
John M. Carradine, COO
John M. Carradine, CFO
Emry Sisson, Exec. VP-IT
Brent Webb, Sr. VP/General Counsel
Mark H. Airhart, Sr. VP-Oper.
Jimmy D. Taylor, VP-Finance
James W. McLane, Chmn.

Phone: 972-443-5000 Fax: 972-556-0572
Toll-Free: 800-519-0679
Address: 5215 N. O'Connor Blvd., Ste. 800, Irving, TX 75039 US

GROWTH PLANS/SPECIAL FEATURES:
Healthaxis, Inc. provides configurable Internet-based connectivity and application solutions for health benefit distribution and administration. Its software products and related services assist health insurance payers, third-party administrators, intermediaries and employers to provide enhanced services to members, employees and providers. Healthaxis's operations are divided into four business units: application solutions, web technology, imaging services and outsourcing. The application solutions group provides comprehensive benefit administration systems for enrollment, group and individual billing and premium collection and reconciliation. The web technology group provides Internet platforms enrollment, sale, distribution and post-sale administration of insurance policies, including health, vision and dental insurance. The imaging services group provides automated capture, imaging, storage and retrieval of electronic claims, attachments and related correspondence. The outsourcing group provides system technology support services to the firm's largest client, UICI.

FINANCIALS:
Sales and profits are in thousands of dollars—add 000 to get the full amount. Year 2004 note: Complete fiscal 2004 results were not available for all companies at press time. For this company, year 2004 is for 6 months.

2004 Sales: $8,143 (6 months)   2004 Profits: $-3,555 (6 months)
2003 Sales: $20,851   2003 Profits: $-4,264
2002 Sales: $19,800   2002 Profits: $-8,600
2001 Sales: $43,800   2001 Profits: $-310,600
2000 Sales: $42,800   2000 Profits: $-35,000

Stock Ticker: HAXS
Employees: 237
Fiscal Year Ends: 12/31

SALARIES/BENEFITS:
Pension Plan: ESOP Stock Plan: Profit Sharing: Top Exec. Salary: $251,150   Bonus: $
Savings Plan: Y   Stock Purch. Plan: Second Exec. Salary: $298,000   Bonus: $35,000

OTHER THOUGHTS:
Apparent Top Female Officers:
Hot Spot for Advancement for Women/Minorities:

LOCATIONS: ("Y" = Yes)
West:	Southwest:	Midwest:	Southeast:	Northeast:	International:
	Y				

HEALTHNOW NEW YORK

www.healthnowny.com

Industry Group Code: 524114 Ranks within this company's industry group: Sales: 36 Profits: 31

Insurance/HMO/PPO:	Drugs:	Equipment/Supplies:	Hospitals/Clinics:	Services:	Health Care:
Insurance: Y	Manufacturer:	Manufacturer:	Acute Care:	Diagnostics:	Home Health:
Managed Care: Y	Distributor:	Distributor:	Sub-Acute Care:	Labs/Testing:	Long-Term Care:
Utilization Mgmt.:	Specialty Pharm.:	Leasing/Finance:	Outpatient Surgery:	Staffing:	Physical Therapy:
Payment Proc.:	Vitamins/Nutri.:	Information Sys.:	Phys. Rehab. Center:	Waste Disposal:	Phys. Practice Mgmt.:
	Clinical Trials:		Psychiatric Clinics:	Specialty Services:	

TYPES OF BUSINESS:
Insurance
HMO, PPO, POS & Traditional Indemnity Plans

GROWTH PLANS/SPECIAL FEATURES:
HealthNow New York, Inc. provides health insurance and related services to more than 900,000 members in New York State. It operates through two subsidiaries: BlueCross BlueShield of Western New York (BCBS) and BlueShield of Northeastern New York (BSNN). Both subsidiaries provide health insurance products and related services, include PPO, HMO, POS and traditional indemnity plans under the Community Blue, Traditional Blue and HealthNow brands. In addition, the firm provides Medicare and Medicaid services through its upstate Medicare division and durable medical equipment regional carrier (DMERC).

BRANDS/DIVISIONS/AFFILIATES:
BlueCross BlueShield of Western New York
BlueShield of Northeastern New York
Community Blue
Traditional Blue
HealthNow

CONTACTS:
Note: Officers with more than one job title may be intentionally listed here more than once.

Alphonso O'Neil-White, CEO
Alphonson O'Neil-White, Pres.
James A. Cardone, Exec. VP/CFO/Treas.
Nora K. McGuire, Sr. VP-Mktg.
Ralph Volpe, VP-Human Resources
Gary J. Kerl, Sr. VP/CIO
Ralph Volpe, VP-Admin. Services
Nora K. McGuire, Sr. VP-Bus. Dev.
Laura Perry, Media Contact
George L. Busch, VP-Finance
Brian O'Grady, Acting COO-BlueShield of Northeastern New York
Cheryl A. Howe, Exec. VP-Health Services & Mktg. Mgmt.
Renee R. Fleming, VP-Corp. Pharmacy Services
William T. Wickis, Sr. VP-Customer Services & Claim Oper.
Joseph J. Castiglia, Chmn.

Phone: 716-887-6900 Fax: 716-887-8981
Toll-Free: 888-249-2583
Address: 1901 Main St., Buffalo, NY 14240-0080 US

FINANCIALS:
Sales and profits are in thousands of dollars—add 000 to get the full amount. Year 2004 note: Complete fiscal 2004 results were not available for all companies at press time. For this company, year 2004 is for months.

2004 Sales: $ (months)   2004 Profits: $ (months)
2003 Sales: $1,775,600   2003 Profits: $55,200
2002 Sales: $ 2002 Profits: $
2001 Sales: $ 2001 Profits: $
2000 Sales: $ 2000 Profits: $

Stock Ticker: Nonprofit
Employees: 2,000
Fiscal Year Ends:

SALARIES/BENEFITS:
Pension Plan: ESOP Stock Plan: Profit Sharing: Top Exec. Salary: $ Bonus: $
Savings Plan: Stock Purch. Plan: Second Exec. Salary: $ Bonus: $

OTHER THOUGHTS:
Apparent Top Female Officers: 4
Hot Spot for Advancement for Women/Minorities: Y

LOCATIONS: ("Y" = Yes)
| West: | Southwest: | Midwest: | Southeast: | Northeast: Y | International: |

HEALTHSOUTH CORP

www.healthsouth.com

Industry Group Code: 621490 **Ranks within this company's industry group:** Sales: Profits:

Insurance/HMO/PPO:	Drugs:	Equipment/Supplies:	Hospitals/Clinics:		Services:		Health Care:	
Insurance:	Manufacturer:	Manufacturer:	Acute Care:		Diagnostics:	Y	Home Health:	
Managed Care:	Distributor:	Distributor:	Sub-Acute Care:		Labs/Testing:		Long-Term Care:	
Utilization Mgmt.:	Specialty Pharm.:	Leasing/Finance:	Outpatient Surgery:	Y	Staffing:		Physical Therapy:	
Payment Proc.:	Vitamins/Nutri.:	Information Sys.:	Phys. Rehab. Center:	Y	Waste Disposal:		Phys. Practice Mgmt.:	
	Clinical Trials:		Psychiatric Clinics:		Specialty Services:	Y		

TYPES OF BUSINESS:
Rehabilitative Health Care
Diagnostic Centers
Outpatient Surgery Services
Worksite Services
Acute Care Hospitals

BRANDS/DIVISIONS/AFFILIATES:

CONTACTS:
Note: Officers with more than one job title may be intentionally listed here more than once.

Jay Grinney, CEO
Jay Grinney, Pres.
Mike Snow, COO
John Workman, CFO
Gregory L. Doody, General Counsel
Karen G. Davis, Pres./COO-Diagnostic Div.
Mark Tarr, Pres.-Inpatient Div.

Phone: 205-967-7116 **Fax:** 205-969-4719
Toll-Free:
Address: One HealthSouth Pkwy., Birmingham, AL 35243 US

GROWTH PLANS/SPECIAL FEATURES:

Healthsouth Corporation is the nation's largest provider of outpatient surgery, outpatient diagnostic and rehabilitative health care services through a national network of rehabilitation facilities, outpatient surgery centers, diagnostic centers and occupational medical facilities. The firm's outpatient surgery centers perform procedures including orthopedic, ophthalmologic, gynecologic and podiatric procedures. Healthsouth's outpatient rehabilitation centers provide common sports medicine treatments such as stretching, strengthening, conditioning and muscle re-education. They also provide orthopedic programs for people recovering from stroke, amputation, brain injury, spinal cord injury and arthritis. The firm provides worksite services including occupational medicine, return-to-work consultation, ergonomic jobsite analysis, workstation modification, physical therapy and fitness and health enhancement programs. Healthsouth recently opened a new 20-bed long-term acute care hospital in Winnfield, Louisiana and is planning the opening of a 40-bed acute care hospital for January 2005. In March 2003, the company was investigated for massive financial fraud, including consistently over-reporting earnings for as much as $1.4 billion. This investigation led to the dismissal of the firm's CEO and president as well as multiple executives and members of the board of directors. In response to pressure from its ongoing financial problems, Healthsouth is undertaking extensive restructuring, including layoffs, debt management and the sale of some of its properties.

FINANCIALS:
Sales and profits are in thousands of dollars—add 000 to get the full amount. Year 2004 note: Complete fiscal 2004 results were not available for all companies at press time. For this company, year 2004 is for months.

2004 Sales: $ (months)   2004 Profits: $ (months)
2003 Sales: $ 2003 Profits: $
2002 Sales: $4,310,800   2002 Profits: $-270,100
2001 Sales: $4,380,500   2001 Profits: $202,400
2000 Sales: $4,195,100   2000 Profits: $278,500

Stock Ticker: HLSH.PK
Employees: 51,000
Fiscal Year Ends: 12/31

SALARIES/BENEFITS:
Pension Plan:	ESOP Stock Plan:	Profit Sharing:	Top Exec. Salary: $3,961,169	Bonus: $6,500,000
Savings Plan:	Stock Purch. Plan:		Second Exec. Salary: $502,115	Bonus: $1,500,000

OTHER THOUGHTS:
Apparent Top Female Officers: 1
Hot Spot for Advancement for Women/Minorities:

LOCATIONS: ("Y" = Yes)
West:	Southwest:	Midwest:	Southeast:	Northeast:	International:
Y	Y	Y	Y	Y	Y

HEALTHSTREAM INC

www.healthstream.com

Industry Group Code: 611410 Ranks within this company's industry group: Sales: 1 Profits: 1

Insurance/HMO/PPO:	Drugs:	Equipment/Supplies:	Hospitals/Clinics:	Services:	Health Care:
Insurance:	Manufacturer:	Manufacturer:	Acute Care:	Diagnostics:	Home Health:
Managed Care:	Distributor:	Distributor:	Sub-Acute Care:	Labs/Testing:	Long-Term Care:
Utilization Mgmt.:	Specialty Pharm.:	Leasing/Finance:	Outpatient Surgery:	Staffing:	Physical Therapy:
Payment Proc.:	Vitamins/Nutri.:	Information Sys.: Y	Phys. Rehab. Center:	Waste Disposal:	Phys. Practice Mgmt.:
	Clinical Trials:		Psychiatric Clinics:	Specialty Services: Y	

TYPES OF BUSINESS:
Educational and Training Content
Health Care e-Learning Solutions

BRANDS/DIVISIONS/AFFILIATES:
Education Design, Inc.
Healthcare Learning Center
de'MEDICI Systems
SynQuest Technologies
Emergency Medical Internetwork
Multimedia Marketing, Inc.
Quick Study, Inc.

CONTACTS:
Note: Officers with more than one job title may be intentionally listed here more than once.
Robert A. Frist, Jr., CEO
Arthur E. Newman, Sr. VP/CFO
Scott Portis, VP-Tech.
Robert H. Laird, VP/General Counsel
Michael Pote, Sr. VP
Fred Perner, Sr. VP
Robert D. Wiemer, VP
Robert H. Laird, Corp. Sec.

Phone: 615-301-3100 **Fax:** 615-301-3200
Toll-Free: 800-933-9293
Address: 209 10th Ave. S., Ste. 450, Nashville, TN 37203 US

GROWTH PLANS/SPECIAL FEATURES:

HealthStream, Inc. provides Internet-based training and services for the health care industry. The firm provides services throughout the U.S. and Canada, focusing primarily on health care organizations and pharmaceutical and medical device companies. Within its health care organization business unit (HCO), HealthStream focuses on expanding its web-based application service provider (ASP), e-learning and installed learning management products, long-term care and outpatient facilities. Within its pharmaceutical and medical device company business unit (PMD), the company focuses on providing services such as live and online educational and training activities aimed at health care professionals, as well as online training for medical industry sales representatives. HealthStream's Healthcare Learning Center (HLC) product provides organizations with the firm's training and continuing education services over the Internet. Training material is hosted on a central data center that allows end users to access services online, eliminating the need for on-site installations. HLC also provides tools that enable administrators to configure and modify materials, track completion and predict training expenses. The service is subscription-based. HealthStream has provided training to major health care institutions and firms. The company's acquisition of Education Design, Inc. expanded its product offerings in the PMD unit. Its other acquisitions include de'MEDICI Systems, SynQuest Technologies, Emergency Medical Internetwork (EMINet), Multimedia Marketing and Quick Study, Inc. HealthStream's customers include HCA Health, Inc., Merck & Co. and Medtronic, Inc. In recent news, Henry Ford Health System chose HealthStream's HLC to deliver online training to its 16,000 employees under a three-year contract.

FINANCIALS:
Sales and profits are in thousands of dollars—add 000 to get the full amount. Year 2004 note: Complete fiscal 2004 results were not available for all companies at press time. For this company, year 2004 is for 6 months.

2004 Sales: $9,599 (6 months) 2004 Profits: $-947 (6 months)
2003 Sales: $18,195 2003 Profits: $-3,412
2002 Sales: $15,800 2002 Profits: $-16,600
2001 Sales: $13,500 2001 Profits: $-19,600
2000 Sales: $9,652 2000 Profits: $-20,285

Stock Ticker: HSTM
Employees: 143
Fiscal Year Ends: 12/31

SALARIES/BENEFITS:
Pension Plan: ESOP Stock Plan: Profit Sharing: Top Exec. Salary: $96,250 Bonus: $10,000
Savings Plan: Y Stock Purch. Plan: Second Exec. Salary: $157,500 Bonus: $23,154

OTHER THOUGHTS:
Apparent Top Female Officers:
Hot Spot for Advancement for Women/Minorities:

LOCATIONS: ("Y" = Yes)
West:	Southwest:	Midwest:	Southeast:	Northeast:	International:
Y			Y		Y

HEALTHTRONICS INC

www.healthtronics.com

Industry Group Code: 621490 Ranks within this company's industry group: Sales: 11 Profits: 13

Insurance/HMO/PPO:	Drugs:	Equipment/Supplies:		Hospitals/Clinics:		Services:		Health Care:	
Insurance:	Manufacturer:	Manufacturer:	Y	Acute Care:		Diagnostics:		Home Health:	
Managed Care:	Distributor:	Distributor:		Sub-Acute Care:		Labs/Testing:		Long-Term Care:	
Utilization Mgmt.:	Specialty Pharm.:	Leasing/Finance:		Outpatient Surgery:		Staffing:	Y	Physical Therapy:	
Payment Proc.:	Vitamins/Nutri.:	Information Sys.:		Phys. Rehab. Center:		Waste Disposal:		Phys. Practice Mgmt.:	Y
	Clinical Trials:			Psychiatric Clinics:		Specialty Services:	Y		

TYPES OF BUSINESS:
Lithotripsy Services
Medical Trailer Manufacturing & Services
Orthopedics Practice Management
Urologic Staffing

BRANDS/DIVISIONS/AFFILIATES:
AK Specialty Vehicles
Calumet Coach Company
Smit Mobile Equipment Company
Frontline Communications Corp.
HealthTronics Surgical Services, Inc.
Prime Medical Services, Inc.

CONTACTS:
Note: Officers with more than one job title may be intentionally listed here more than once.
Brad A. Hummel, CEO
Brad A. Hummel, Pres.
John Q. Barnidge, CFO
Klaas F. Vlietstra, Interim Pres.-Mfg.
James S.B. Whittenburg, General Counsel
James S.B. Whittenburg, Sr. VP-Dev.
Richard A. Rusk, VP/Controller
Joseph M. Jenkins, Pres.-Urology
James S.B. Whittenburg, Corp. Sec.

Phone: 512-328-2892 Fax: 512-328-8510
Toll-Free: 888-252-6575
Address: 1301 Capital of Texas Hwy., Ste. 200B, Austin, TX 78746 US

GROWTH PLANS/SPECIAL FEATURES:
HealthTronics, Inc., formed by the November 2004 merger of Prime Medical Services, Inc. and HealthTronics Surgical Services, Inc., is a health care service provider in three business segments: urological services and products; orthopedic services and products; and specialty vehicles. HealthTronics' urological unit focuses on lithotripsy systems, which serve a network of 3,000 physicians in 47 states. Lithotripsy is the treatment of kidney stones using shockwaves to break up the stones and allow them to pass painlessly from the body. The treatment procedure is non-invasive and requires only a short recovery period, usually a matter of hours. The company's lithotripsy services include scheduling, staffing, training, quality assurance, maintenance, regulatory compliance and contracting with hospitals and surgery centers. In the orthopedics sector, HealthTronics offers turnkey operations management, which includes billing, collections, scheduling and reporting. The unit also offers an equipment maintenance program. The firm was the first health care company to debut the Extracorporeal Shock Wave system, a non-invasive procedure that uses shockwaves to treat musculoskeletal injuries. Subsidiary AK Specialty Vehicles provides manufacturing services, installation, refurbishment and repair of trailers and coaches for mobile medical services providers. This specialty vehicle segment was expanded by the acquisition of the assets of Calumet Coach Company, Frontline Communications Corporation and Smit Mobile Medical Equipment Company, which allowed the manufacture of vehicles and installation of equipment for a broad array of diagnostic and communications equipment. In addition to lithotripsy, the vehicles are equipped for medical services such as magnetic resonance imaging (MRI), cardiac catheterization, CT scanners and positron emission tomography, as well as non-medical devices for communications and broadcasting applications.

FINANCIALS:
Sales and profits are in thousands of dollars—add 000 to get the full amount. Year 2004 note: Complete fiscal 2004 results were not available for all companies at press time. For this company, year 2004 is for 9 months.

2004 Sales: $137,163 (9 months) 2004 Profits: $4,745 (9 months)
2003 Sales: $160,393 2003 Profits: $6,223
2002 Sales: $169,900 2002 Profits: $800
2001 Sales: $154,900 2001 Profits: $-14,500
2000 Sales: $130,700 2000 Profits: $10,700

Stock Ticker: HTRN
Employees: 1,050
Fiscal Year Ends: 12/31

SALARIES/BENEFITS:
Pension Plan: ESOP Stock Plan: Profit Sharing: Top Exec. Salary: $400,000 Bonus: $325,000
Savings Plan: Stock Purch. Plan: Second Exec. Salary: $230,000 Bonus: $50,000

OTHER THOUGHTS:
Apparent Top Female Officers:
Hot Spot for Advancement for Women/Minorities:

LOCATIONS: ("Y" = Yes)
West:	Southwest:	Midwest:	Southeast:	Northeast:	International:
	Y		Y	Y	

# HEARUSA INC

www.hearx.com

Industry Group Code: 621490 Ranks within this company's industry group: Sales: 16 Profits: 17

Insurance/HMO/PPO:	Drugs:	Equipment/Supplies:	Hospitals/Clinics:	Services:	Health Care:
Insurance:	Manufacturer:	Manufacturer:	Acute Care:	Diagnostics:	Home Health:
Managed Care:	Distributor:	Distributor:	Sub-Acute Care:	Labs/Testing:	Long-Term Care:
Utilization Mgmt.:	Specialty Pharm.:	Leasing/Finance:	Outpatient Surgery:	Staffing:	Physical Therapy:
Payment Proc.:	Vitamins/Nutri.:	Information Sys.:	Phys. Rehab. Center:	Waste Disposal:	Phys. Practice Mgmt.:
	Clinical Trials:		Psychiatric Clinics:	Specialty Services: Y	

TYPES OF BUSINESS:
Hearing Care Centers
Hearing Benefits Management

BRANDS/DIVISIONS/AFFILIATES:
HEARx

CONTACTS: Note: Officers with more than one job title may be intentionally listed here more than once.
Stephen J. Hansbrough, CEO
Stephen J. Hansbrough, Pres.
Kenneth Schofield, COO
Gino Chouinard, Exec. VP/CFO
Donna L. Taylor, Sr. VP-Sales
Robert C. Packard, VP-Human Resources
Nancy Bacigalupi, VP-Admin.
Donna L. Taylor, Sr. VP-Oper.
Candace P. Brough, Sr. VP-Corp. Comm.
Denise Pottlitzer, VP-Acc.
Cynthia M. Beyer, Sr. VP-Professional Services
Paul A. Brown, Chmn.

Phone: 561-478-8770 Fax: 888-888-0009
Toll-Free: 800-323-3277
Address: 1250 Northpoint Pkwy., West Palm Beach, FL 33407 US

GROWTH PLANS/SPECIAL FEATURES:
HearUSA, Inc. owns or manages a network of 157 HearUSA and HEARx hearing care centers that provide a full range of audiological products and services for the hearing impaired. The company serves customers in Florida, New York, New Jersey, Massachusetts, Ohio, Michigan, Wisconsin, Minnesota, Missouri, Washington, California and Ontario, Canada. The firm services over 170 benefit programs for hearing care with various health maintenance organizations, preferred provider organizations, insurers, benefit administrators and health care providers. Each HearUSA or HEARx center is staffed by a licensed audiologist or hearing instrument specialist, and most are conveniently located in shopping or medical centers. The centers offer a complete range of quality hearing aids, with emphasis on digital technology. Though they are currently operating under multiple names, the company's goal is to have all centers similar in design, exterior marking and signage.

Employment benefits at HearUSA include medical benefits and ongoing education programs.

FINANCIALS: Sales and profits are in thousands of dollars—add 000 to get the full amount. Year 2004 note: Complete fiscal 2004 results were not available for all companies at press time. For this company, year 2004 is for 9 months.

2004 Sales: $52,325 (9 months)   2004 Profits: $-2,266 (9 months)
2003 Sales: $70,545   2003 Profits: $-1,109
2002 Sales: $59,600   2002 Profits: $-6,900
2001 Sales: $48,800   2001 Profits: $-8,600
2000 Sales: $56,409   2000 Profits: $-3,317

Stock Ticker: EAR
Employees: 505
Fiscal Year Ends: 12/31

SALARIES/BENEFITS:
Pension Plan: ESOP Stock Plan: Profit Sharing: Top Exec. Salary: $250,000   Bonus: $125,000
Savings Plan: Y   Stock Purch. Plan: Second Exec. Salary: $240,000   Bonus: $112,500

OTHER THOUGHTS:
Apparent Top Female Officers: 5
Hot Spot for Advancement for Women/Minorities: Y

LOCATIONS: ("Y" = Yes)
West	Southwest	Midwest	Southeast	Northeast	International
Y		Y	Y	Y	Y

HEMACARE CORPORATION

www.hemacare.com

Industry Group Code: 621991 Ranks within this company's industry group: Sales: 2 Profits: 2

Insurance/HMO/PPO:	Drugs:	Equipment/Supplies:	Hospitals/Clinics:	Services:	Health Care:
Insurance:	Manufacturer:	Manufacturer:	Acute Care:	Diagnostics:	Home Health:
Managed Care:	Distributor:	Distributor:	Sub-Acute Care:	Labs/Testing: Y	Long-Term Care:
Utilization Mgmt.:	Specialty Pharm.:	Leasing/Finance:	Outpatient Surgery:	Staffing:	Physical Therapy:
Payment Proc.:	Vitamins/Nutri.:	Information Sys.:	Phys. Rehab. Center:	Waste Disposal:	Phys. Practice Mgmt.:
	Clinical Trials:		Psychiatric Clinics:	Specialty Services: Y	

TYPES OF BUSINESS:
Management-Blood Collection Centers and Blood Banks
Blood Products

BRANDS/DIVISIONS/AFFILIATES:
Coral Blood Services, Inc.

CONTACTS:
Note: Officers with more than one job title may be intentionally listed here more than once.
Judi Irving, CEO
Judi Irving, Pres.
Dana Belisle, COO
Robert S. Chilton, Exec. VP/CFO
Robert L. Johnson, Sr. VP/General Counsel
Linda Mondor, Dir.-Oper., Northeast Region
Dana Belisle, Pres., Coral Blood Services
David Ciavarella, Medical Dir.-Coral Blood Services
Jacquelyn Hedlund, Medical Dir.-Coral Blood Services
Nurit Degani, Dir.-Therapeutic Services, West Coast
Julian Steffenhagen, Chmn.

Phone: 818-226-1968 Fax: 818-251-5300
Toll-Free: 877-310-0717
Address: 21101 Oxnard St., Woodland Hills, CA 91367 US

GROWTH PLANS/SPECIAL FEATURES:
HemaCare Corporation and its wholly-owned subsidiary, Coral Blood Services, Inc., collect, process and distribute blood services and products to hospitals and medical centers. The company divides its business into two categories: blood products and blood services. The blood products segment provides hospitals with significant portions of their blood supply needs. HemaCare's blood products operations specialize in the collection and distribution of apheresis platelets, focusing on single-donor platelets. The firm's blood services operations provide hospitals with specialty-trained nurses and specialized equipment on a mobile basis. Other services include stem cell collection and an assortment of therapeutic treatments, which are provided to patients with a variety of disorders. Additionally, the company has entered into blood management programs (BMPs) with many of its hospital customers. In BMP arrangements, HemaCare provides its products and services, as well as donor testing, community blood drives and specialized collections, under multi-year contractual agreements. HemaCare believes its BMPs benefit hospitals in several ways, including greater reliability than local blood centers, overall reduction in blood procurement costs and access to experienced nurses and physicians. The firm plans to expand its blood collections and blood management programs to new hospital customers.

The company offers its employees medical, dental and life insurance; employee assistance plans; tuition reimbursement; and credit union membership.

FINANCIALS:
Sales and profits are in thousands of dollars—add 000 to get the full amount. Year 2004 note: Complete fiscal 2004 results were not available for all companies at press time. For this company, year 2004 is for 6 months.

2004 Sales: $13,657 (6 months) 2004 Profits: $734 (6 months)
2003 Sales: $27,488 2003 Profits: $-4,679
2002 Sales: $27,817 2002 Profits: $-591
2001 Sales: $25,200 2001 Profits: $300
2000 Sales: $21,500 2000 Profits: $600

Stock Ticker: HEMA
Employees: 270
Fiscal Year Ends: 12/31

SALARIES/BENEFITS:
Pension Plan: ESOP Stock Plan: Profit Sharing: Top Exec. Salary: $200,000 Bonus: $65,000
Savings Plan: Y Stock Purch. Plan: Second Exec. Salary: $151,900 Bonus: $80,000

OTHER THOUGHTS:
Apparent Top Female Officers: 4
Hot Spot for Advancement for Women/Minorities: Y

LOCATIONS: ("Y" = Yes)
West:	Southwest:	Midwest:	Southeast:	Northeast:	International:
Y	Y	Y	Y	Y	

HENRY FORD HEALTH SYSTEMS

www.henryfordhealth.org

Industry Group Code: 622110 **Ranks within this company's industry group:** Sales: 23 Profits:

Insurance/HMO/PPO:	Drugs:	Equipment/Supplies:	Hospitals/Clinics:	Services:	Health Care:
Insurance:	Manufacturer:	Manufacturer: Y	Acute Care: Y	Diagnostics:	Home Health: Y
Managed Care: Y	Distributor:	Distributor: Y	Sub-Acute Care: Y	Labs/Testing:	Long-Term Care: Y
Utilization Mgmt.:	Specialty Pharm.:	Leasing/Finance:	Outpatient Surgery:	Staffing:	Physical Therapy:
Payment Proc.:	Vitamins/Nutri.:	Information Sys.:	Phys. Rehab. Center:	Waste Disposal:	Phys. Practice Mgmt.:
	Clinical Trials:		Psychiatric Clinics:	Specialty Services:	

TYPES OF BUSINESS:
Hospitals-General
Nursing Homes
Home Health Care
Medical Equipment
Insurance
Psychiatric Services

BRANDS/DIVISIONS/AFFILIATES:
Health Alliance Plan of Michigan
Henry Ford Heart and Vascular Institute
Kingsworth Hospital
Henry Ford Wyandotte Hospital
Henry Ford Hospital

GROWTH PLANS/SPECIAL FEATURES:
The Henry Ford Health System, founded in 1915 by automobile manufacturer Henry Ford, is a collection of hospitals and other health care facilities in southeastern Michigan. The health system includes three hospitals: the Henry Ford Hospital, the Henry Ford Wyandotte Hospital and the Kingsworth Hospital, which treats psychiatric disorders. The Henry Ford Heart and Vascular Institute offers prevention, treatment, transplantation and rehabilitation for high-risk patients. The firm also manages nursing homes, hospice needs, home health care, a medical equipment supplier and a health insurance provider called Health Alliance Plan of Michigan, which has more than 560,000 policy holders.

CONTACTS:
Note: Officers with more than one job title may be intentionally listed here more than once.
Nancy M. Schlichting, CEO
Nancy M. Schlichting, Pres.
James M. Connelly, CFO

Phone: 313-876-8700 **Fax:** 313-876-9243
Toll-Free: 800-653-6568
Address: One Ford Pl., Detroit, MI 48202-3450 US

FINANCIALS:
Sales and profits are in thousands of dollars—add 000 to get the full amount. Year 2004 note: Complete fiscal 2004 results were not available for all companies at press time. For this company, year 2004 is for months.

2004 Sales: $ (months)   2004 Profits: $ (months)
2003 Sales: $2,600,000   2003 Profits: $
2002 Sales: $2,400,000   2002 Profits: $
2001 Sales: $ 2001 Profits: $
2000 Sales: $ 2000 Profits: $

Stock Ticker: Nonprofit
Employees: 12,700
Fiscal Year Ends: 12/31

SALARIES/BENEFITS:
Pension Plan: ESOP Stock Plan: Profit Sharing: Top Exec. Salary: $ Bonus: $
Savings Plan: Stock Purch. Plan: Second Exec. Salary: $ Bonus: $

OTHER THOUGHTS:
Apparent Top Female Officers: 1
Hot Spot for Advancement for Women/Minorities:

LOCATIONS: ("Y" = Yes)
West:	Southwest:	Midwest:	Southeast:	Northeast:	International:
		Y			

Note: Financial information, benefits and other data can change quickly and may vary from those stated here.

HENRY SCHEIN INC

www.henryschein.com

Industry Group Code: 421450   Ranks within this company's industry group: Sales: 3   Profits: 1

Insurance/HMO/PPO:	Drugs:	Equipment/Supplies:	Hospitals/Clinics:	Services:	Health Care:
Insurance: Managed Care: Utilization Mgmt.: Payment Proc.:	Manufacturer: Distributor: Specialty Pharm.: Vitamins/Nutri.: Clinical Trials:	Manufacturer: Distributor: Y Leasing/Finance: Information Sys.:	Acute Care: Sub-Acute Care: Outpatient Surgery: Phys. Rehab. Center: Psychiatric Clinics:	Diagnostics: Labs/Testing: Staffing: Waste Disposal: Specialty Services:	Home Health: Long-Term Care: Physical Therapy: Phys. Practice Mgmt.:

TYPES OF BUSINESS:
Health Care Products Distribution
Dental Supplies Distribution
Veterinary Products Distribution
Electronic Catalogs

BRANDS/DIVISIONS/AFFILIATES:
Dentrix Dental Systems, Inc.
Micro Bio-Medics, Inc.
Schein Empire Dental Chair
Smith Holden, Inc.
Spherecom Dental Supply, Inc.
Sullivan Dental Products
ORALCDx
Hager Dental GmbH

CONTACTS:
Note: Officers with more than one job title may be intentionally listed here more than once.

Stanley M. Bergman, CEO
Stanley M. Bergman, Pres.
Steven Paladino, Exec. VP/CFO
Leonard A. David, VP-Human Resources
Gerald A. Benjamin, Exec. VP/Chief Admin. Officer
Leonard A. David, Special Counsel
Mark E. Mlotek, Sr. VP-Corp. Bus. Dev.
James P. Breslawski, Exec. VP/Pres.-U.S. Dental
Michael Racioppi, Pres.-Medical Group
Stanley M. Bergman, Chmn.
Michael Zack, Sr. VP-Int'l Group

Phone: 631-843-5500   Fax: 631-843-5658
Toll-Free:
Address: 135 Duryea Rd., Melville, NY 11747 US

GROWTH PLANS/SPECIAL FEATURES:
Henry Schein, Inc. is a leading distributor of health care products to office-based practitioners in the North American and European markets. The company markets its products and services to over 450,000 customers, primarily dental practices and dental laboratories. Other customers include physician practices, veterinary clinics and institutions. The firm offers a broad selection of more than 90,000 branded and Henry Schein private-brand products. These include surgical, dental, pharmaceutical, vitamin, veterinary, medical equipment and diagnostic testing products. The company employs an integrated sales and marketing approach, merging direct marketing programs with 700 telemarketing representatives and 1,350 field sales consultants. Henry Schein currently distributes over 22 million pieces of direct marketing material to approximately 650,000 office-based health care practitioners. The firm is divided into four primary business segments: dental, medical, international and technology and value-added services. The segments operate through a centralized and automated distribution network that supplies customers in more than 125 countries worldwide. The company is a pioneer in developing electronic catalogs and ordering systems for its health care professional customers. The firm has provided a PC-based ordering option since the mid-1980s. Henry Schein's web site provides an array of value-added features including instant customer registration, easy shopping and ordering and improved customer service and supply procurement capabilities. In recent news, the company signed an agreement to acquire the dental distribution operations of Hager Dental GmbH in Germany.
Henry Schein offers employees business-casual dress, a company cafeteria, referral bonuses, service awards, an employee assistance program, insurance plans and tuition reimbursement.

FINANCIALS:
Sales and profits are in thousands of dollars—add 000 to get the full amount. Year 2004 note: Complete fiscal 2004 results were not available for all companies at press time. For this company, year 2004 is for 9 months.

2004 Sales: $2,865,946 (9 months)   2004 Profits: $98,633 (9 months)
2003 Sales: $3,353,805   2003 Profits: $137,501   **Stock Ticker:** HSIC
2002 Sales: $2,825,000   2002 Profits: $118,000   Employees: 7,900
2001 Sales: $2,558,200   2001 Profits: $87,400   Fiscal Year Ends: 12/31
2000 Sales: $2,381,700   2000 Profits: $56,700

SALARIES/BENEFITS:
Pension Plan: ESOP Stock Plan: Profit Sharing: Top Exec. Salary: $800,000   Bonus: $1,250,000
Savings Plan: Y   Stock Purch. Plan: Second Exec. Salary: $383,000   Bonus: $18,874

OTHER THOUGHTS:
Apparent Top Female Officers:
Hot Spot for Advancement for Women/Minorities:

LOCATIONS: ("Y" = Yes)
West:	Southwest:	Midwest:	Southeast:	Northeast:	International:
Y	Y	Y	Y	Y	Y

Plunkett's Health Care Industry Almanac 2005   419

HIGHMARK INC
www.highmark.com

Industry Group Code: 524114   Ranks within this company's industry group: Sales: 13   Profits: 27

Insurance/HMO/PPO:	Drugs:	Equipment/Supplies:	Hospitals/Clinics:	Services:	Health Care:
Insurance:	Manufacturer:	Manufacturer:	Acute Care:	Diagnostics:	Home Health:
Managed Care: Y	Distributor:	Distributor:	Sub-Acute Care:	Labs/Testing:	Long-Term Care:
Utilization Mgmt.:	Specialty Pharm.:	Leasing/Finance:	Outpatient Surgery:	Staffing:	Physical Therapy:
Payment Proc.:	Vitamins/Nutri.:	Information Sys.:	Phys. Rehab. Center:	Waste Disposal:	Phys. Practice Mgmt.:
	Clinical Trials:		Psychiatric Clinics:	Specialty Services:	

TYPES OF BUSINESS:
Insurance
Administrative Services

BRANDS/DIVISIONS/AFFILIATES:
Western Pennsylvania Caring Foundation
Insurer Physicians Services Organization, Inc.
HGSAdministrators
Veritus Medicare Services
Highmark Life and Casualty Group (The)
Davis Vision
United Concordia
Mountain State Blue Cross Blue Shield

CONTACTS: Note: Officers with more than one job title may be intentionally listed here more than once.
Kenneth R. Melani, CEO
Kenneth R. Melani, Pres.
Robert C. Gray, CFO
S. Tyrone Alexander, VP-Human Resources
S. Tyrone Alexander, VP-Admin.
Gary R. Truitt, General Counsel
Robert C. Gray, Exec. VP-Finance
J. Robert Baum, Vice-Chmn.
James M. Klingensmith, Exec. VP-Health Services
David M. O'Brien, Exec. VP-Gov't Services
Michael A. Romano, Sr. VP-Corp. Compliance
John N. Shaffer, Chmn.

Phone: 412-544-7000   Fax:
Toll-Free:
Address: 5th Ave. Pl., 120 5th Ave., Pittsburg, PA 15222-3099 US

GROWTH PLANS/SPECIAL FEATURES:
Highmark, an independent licensee of the Blue Cross Blue Shield Association, is one of the largest health insurers in the United States and provides health insurance to 23 million customers primarily in Pennsylvania. Insurance plans include medical, dental, vision, indemnity and casualty insurance. The firm was created in 1996 by the consolidation of Pennsylvania Blue Shield, now called Highmark Blue Shield, and a Blue Cross plan in western Pennsylvania, now called Highmark Blue Cross Blue Shield. Subsidiaries offering the Blue Cross Blue Shield plans include Mountain State Blue Cross Blue Shield, Keystone Health Plan West and HealthGuard. Other subsidiaries, such as GateWay Health Plan, United Concordia, Clarity Vision, Davis Vision, the Highmark Life and Casualty Group and Veritus Medicare Services, sell independently owned insurance plans. Other subsidiaries include HGSAdministrators, which provides professional assistance to insurers, and Insurer Physicians Services Organization, Inc., which develops joint ventures with private practice physicians. Through the Western Pennsylvania Caring Foundation, Highmark offers free health care coverage to children whose parents exceed the financial requirements for public aid but still cannot afford private insurance.

FINANCIALS: Sales and profits are in thousands of dollars—add 000 to get the full amount. Year 2004 note: Complete fiscal 2004 results were not available for all companies at press time. For this company, year 2004 is for months.

2004 Sales: $ (months)   2004 Profits: $ (months)
2003 Sales: $8,104,800   2003 Profits: $75,700   Stock Ticker: Nonprofit
2002 Sales: $7,400,000   2002 Profits: $-83,400   Employees: 11,000
2001 Sales: $ 2001 Profits: $ Fiscal Year Ends: 12/31
2000 Sales: $ 2000 Profits: $

SALARIES/BENEFITS:
Pension Plan: ESOP Stock Plan: Profit Sharing: Top Exec. Salary: $ Bonus: $
Savings Plan: Stock Purch. Plan: Second Exec. Salary: $ Bonus: $

OTHER THOUGHTS:
Apparent Top Female Officers:
Hot Spot for Advancement for Women/Minorities:

LOCATIONS: ("Y" = Yes)
West:	Southwest:	Midwest:	Southeast:	Northeast:	International:
				Y	

Note: Financial information, benefits and other data can change quickly and may vary from those stated here.

HILLENBRAND INDUSTRIES

www.hillenbrand.com

Industry Group Code: 339113 **Ranks within this company's industry group:** Sales: 12 Profits: 16

Insurance/HMO/PPO:		Drugs:		Equipment/Supplies:		Hospitals/Clinics:		Services:		Health Care:	
Insurance:		Manufacturer:	Y	Manufacturer:	Y	Acute Care:		Diagnostics:		Home Health:	
Managed Care:		Distributor:		Distributor:		Sub-Acute Care:		Labs/Testing:		Long-Term Care:	
Utilization Mgmt.:		Specialty Pharm.:		Leasing/Finance:	Y	Outpatient Surgery:		Staffing:		Physical Therapy:	
Payment Proc.:		Vitamins/Nutri.:		Information Sys.:		Phys. Rehab. Center:		Waste Disposal:		Phys. Practice Mgmt.:	
		Clinical Trials:				Psychiatric Clinics:		Specialty Services:	Y		

TYPES OF BUSINESS:
Equipment-Hospital Beds & Related Products
Funeral Planning Financial Services
Burial Caskets & Related Products
Life Insurance Products
Specialized Therapy Products

BRANDS/DIVISIONS/AFFILIATES:
Batesville Casket Company
Forethought Financial Services
Forethought Federal Savings Bank
Forethought Life Insurance Company
Forethought Group, Inc. (The)
Arkansas National Life Insurance Company
Hill-Rom, Inc.
Basic Care

CONTACTS:
Note: Officers with more than one job title may be intentionally listed here more than once.
Frederick W. Rockwood, CEO
Frederick W. Rockwood, Pres.
Scott K. Sorensen, VP/CFO
Bruce Bonnevier, VP-Human Resources
Patrick D. de Maynadier, VP/General Counsel
Catherine Greany, VP-Corp. Dev.
Wendy Wilson, VP-Investor Rel.
Mark R. Lanning, VP/Treas.
Kimberly K. Dennis, VP-Shared Services
Stephen W. McMillen, VP-Exec. Leadership Dev.
Kenneth A. Camp, VP/Pres., Batesville Casket Company
Ray J. Hillenbrand, Chmn.

Phone: 812-934-7000 **Fax:** 812-934-7371
Toll-Free:
Address: 700 State Rte. 46 E., Batesville, IN 47006-8835 US

GROWTH PLANS/SPECIAL FEATURES:
Hillenbrand Industries, Inc. is a holding company for three major operating companies serving the funeral services and health care industries. The funeral services group consists of two companies, Batesville Casket Company and Forethought Financial Services. Batesville is among the world's leading casket makers and also sells cremation urns as well as related support services. It serves funeral directors operating licensed funeral homes in North America and certain export markets. Forethought provides funeral planning financial products and marketing services in the U.S. Its customers are licensed funeral homes, funeral professionals, licensed agents and other death care providers. Forethought also manages Forethought Federal Savings Bank, which gives individuals the opportunity to save for their own funeral arrangements. In addition, the subsidiary manages Forethought Life Insurance Co., the Forethought Group, Inc. and Arkansas National Life Insurance Company. The health care group consists of Hill-Rom, Inc., a manufacturer of equipment for the health care market and a provider of specialized rental therapy products designed to assist with the problems of patient immobility. It serves acute, ambulatory and long-term health care facilities and home care patients worldwide. In addition to its domestic operations, Hill-Rom operates hospital bed, therapy bed and patient room manufacturing facilities in France. These products are sold and leased directly to hospitals and nursing homes throughout Europe. In recent news, Hill-Rom launched a new bed, the Basic Care, for hospitals in Latin America, Asia and the Middle East.

FINANCIALS:
Sales and profits are in thousands of dollars—add 000 to get the full amount. Year 2004 note: Complete fiscal 2004 results were not available for all companies at press time. For this company, year 2004 is for 9 months.

2004 Sales: $1,355,000 (9 months)	2004 Profits: $48,000 (9 months)	**Stock Ticker:** HB
2003 Sales: $2,042,000	2003 Profits: $138,000	Employees: 9,900
2002 Sales: $1,757,000	2002 Profits: $-10,000	Fiscal Year Ends: 9/30
2001 Sales: $2,107,000	2001 Profits: $170,000	
2000 Sales: $2,096,000	2000 Profits: $154,000	

SALARIES/BENEFITS:
Pension Plan: Y	ESOP Stock Plan:	Profit Sharing:	Top Exec. Salary: $996,354	Bonus: $1,882,188
Savings Plan: Y	Stock Purch. Plan:		Second Exec. Salary: $427,882	Bonus: $769,811

OTHER THOUGHTS:
Apparent Top Female Officers: 3
Hot Spot for Advancement for Women/Minorities: Y

LOCATIONS: ("Y" = Yes)
West:	Southwest:	Midwest:	Southeast:	Northeast:	International:
		Y	Y	Y	Y

HILL-ROM COMPANY INC

www.hill-rom.com

Industry Group Code: 339113 Ranks within this company's industry group: Sales: 24 Profits:

Insurance/HMO/PPO:	Drugs:	Equipment/Supplies:		Hospitals/Clinics:		Services:	Health Care:
Insurance:	Manufacturer:	Manufacturer:	Y	Acute Care:	Y	Diagnostics:	Home Health:
Managed Care:	Distributor:	Distributor:	Y	Sub-Acute Care:		Labs/Testing:	Long-Term Care:
Utilization Mgmt.:	Specialty Pharm.:	Leasing/Finance:		Outpatient Surgery:		Staffing:	Physical Therapy:
Payment Proc.:	Vitamins/Nutri.:	Information Sys.:		Phys. Rehab. Center:		Waste Disposal:	Phys. Practice Mgmt.:
	Clinical Trials:			Psychiatric Clinics:		Specialty Services:	

TYPES OF BUSINESS:
Equipment-Hospital Beds & Related Products
Communication Systems
Stretchers

BRANDS/DIVISIONS/AFFILIATES:
Hillenbrand Industries
TotalCare
Advanta
AvantGuard
CareAssist
TranStar
Flexicair Eclipse
Silkair

CONTACTS:
Note: Officers with more than one job title may be intentionally listed here more than once.
R. Ernest Wasser, CEO
R. Ernest Wasser, Pres.
Mike Murren, CFO

Phone: 812-934-7777   Fax: 812-934-8189
Toll-Free:
Address: 1069 State Rd. 46 E., Batesville, IN 47006 US

GROWTH PLANS/SPECIAL FEATURES:
Hill-Rom Company, a subsidiary of Hillenbrand Industries, sells, rents and services hospital products including hospital beds; non-invasive therapeutic surfaces and devices; stretchers and other transport systems; furniture; communication and locating systems; and operating room accessories. The firm primarily focuses on a line of electrically adjustable hospital beds that can be adjusted to varied orthopedic and therapeutic contours and positions. Hospital bed models include the TotalCare Sp02RT bed, a pulmonary bed that delivers rotation, percussion, and vibration; the TotalCare bed, a bed designed for acute patients with little to no mobility; the Advanta, AvantGuard and CareAssist beds, designed for a variety of medical and surgical applications; and the Affinity III bed, specifically designed for the maternity department. The firm also provides therapy products for acute care, home care and long-term care. Hill-Rom also manufactures a full line of stretchers under the TranStar name. Other products include nurse call systems, fetal monitoring information systems, siderail communications, surgical table accessories, bedside cabinets, tables and mattresses. The company's architectural products include customized, prefabricated modules that are either wall-mounted or on freestanding columns and allow medical equipment such as gases, communication accessories and electrical services to be kept safely in patient rooms. Other wound and pulmonary care technology include low-airloss therapy, such as the Flexicair Eclipse mattress, a portable rental mattress replacement for the acute care environment; the Silkair mattress, a low-airloss overlay product for home care; and the V-Cue mattress, a rotational mattress. Hill-Rom therapy systems are provided to hospitals, long-term care facilities and homes through more than 200 service centers located in the United States, Canada and Western Europe. In recent news, the company's newest product, the Basic Care Bed, has been made available for use by hospitals in Latin America, Asia and the Middle East.

Hill-Rom's employee benefits vary by country and may include health and life insurance, paid vacation and tuition assistance.

FINANCIALS:
Sales and profits are in thousands of dollars—add 000 to get the full amount. Year 2004 note: Complete fiscal 2004 results were not available for all companies at press time. For this company, year 2004 is for months.

2004 Sales: $ (months)   2004 Profits: $ (months)
2003 Sales: $1,067,000   2003 Profits: $
2002 Sales: $883,000   2002 Profits: $
2001 Sales: $ 2001 Profits: $
2000 Sales: $ 2000 Profits: $

Stock Ticker: Subsidiary
Employees:
Fiscal Year Ends: 9/30

SALARIES/BENEFITS:
Pension Plan: Y   ESOP Stock Plan: Profit Sharing: Top Exec. Salary: $ Bonus: $
Savings Plan: Stock Purch. Plan: Second Exec. Salary: $ Bonus: $

OTHER THOUGHTS:
Apparent Top Female Officers:
Hot Spot for Advancement for Women/Minorities:

LOCATIONS: ("Y" = Yes)
West	Southwest	Midwest	Southeast	Northeast	International
		Y		Y	Y

HOLOGIC INC

www.hologic.com

Industry Group Code: 339113   Ranks within this company's industry group: Sales: 62   Profits: 93

Insurance/HMO/PPO:	Drugs:	Equipment/Supplies:		Hospitals/Clinics:	Services:	Health Care:
Insurance: Managed Care: Utilization Mgmt.: Payment Proc.:	Manufacturer: Distributor: Specialty Pharm.: Vitamins/Nutri.: Clinical Trials:	Manufacturer: Distributor: Leasing/Finance: Information Sys.:	Y	Acute Care: Sub-Acute Care: Outpatient Surgery: Phys. Rehab. Center: Psychiatric Clinics:	Diagnostics: Labs/Testing: Staffing: Waste Disposal: Specialty Services:	Home Health: Long-Term Care: Physical Therapy: Phys. Practice Mgmt.:

TYPES OF BUSINESS:
Equipment-X-Ray Bone Densitometers
Mammography Systems
Radiography Systems

BRANDS/DIVISIONS/AFFILIATES:
LORAD
QDR
Sahara
Selenia
Flouroscan

GROWTH PLANS/SPECIAL FEATURES:
Hologic, Inc. is a leading developer, manufacturer and marketer of diagnostic and medical imaging systems primarily serving the health care needs of women. Its core women's health care business units are focused on bone densitometry, mammography, breast biopsy and direct-to-digital x-ray radiography. The company's QDR x-ray bone densitometry product line and Sahara portable ultrasound bone analyzer aid in early detection of osteoporosis. Its LORAD division produces the Selenia line of mammography systems, which is a premier brand in its market. In addition, Hologic develops, manufactures and supplies other x-ray-based imaging systems, such as general-purpose direct-to-digital x-ray equipment and Flouroscan mini C-arm imaging products. Customers include hospitals, imaging clinics, private practices and major pharmaceutical companies that use its products in conducting clinical trials.

CONTACTS: Note: Officers with more than one job title may be intentionally listed here more than once.
John W. Cumming, CEO
John W. Cumming, Pres.
Robert Cascella, COO
John Pekarsky, Sr. VP-Sales & Strategic Accounts
Jay A. Stein, Chief Tech. Officer
Glenn P. Muir, Exec. VP-Admin.
Glenn P. Muir, Exec. VP-Finance/Treas.
Peter Soltani, VP-Direct Radiography Corp.
John W. Cumming, Chmn.

Phone: 781-999-7300   Fax:
Toll-Free: 800-343-9729
Address: 35 Crosby Dr., Bedford, MA 01730 US

FINANCIALS:
Sales and profits are in thousands of dollars—add 000 to get the full amount. Year 2004 note: Complete fiscal 2004 results were not available for all companies at press time. For this company, year 2004 is for 9 months.

2004 Sales: $164,756 (9 months)   2004 Profits: $6,954 (9 months)
2003 Sales: $204,035   2003 Profits: $2,882
2002 Sales: $190,200   2002 Profits: $200
2001 Sales: $178,500   2001 Profits: $-20,900
2000 Sales: $93,700   2000 Profits: $-18,600

Stock Ticker: HOLX
Employees: 722
Fiscal Year Ends: 9/30

SALARIES/BENEFITS:
Pension Plan: ESOP Stock Plan: Profit Sharing: Top Exec. Salary: $390,952   Bonus: $358,995
Savings Plan: Y   Stock Purch. Plan: Second Exec. Salary: $245,258   Bonus: $60,000

OTHER THOUGHTS:
Apparent Top Female Officers:
Hot Spot for Advancement for Women/Minorities:

LOCATIONS: ("Y" = Yes)
West:	Southwest:	Midwest:	Southeast:	Northeast:	International:
				Y	Y

HOOPER HOLMES INC

www.hooperholmes.com

Industry Group Code: 621511 Ranks within this company's industry group: Sales: 5 Profits: 4

Insurance/HMO/PPO:	Drugs:	Equipment/Supplies:	Hospitals/Clinics:	Services:		Health Care:	
Insurance:	Manufacturer:	Manufacturer:	Acute Care:	Diagnostics:		Home Health:	
Managed Care:	Distributor:	Distributor:	Sub-Acute Care:	Labs/Testing:	Y	Long-Term Care:	
Utilization Mgmt.:	Specialty Pharm.:	Leasing/Finance:	Outpatient Surgery:	Staffing:		Physical Therapy:	
Payment Proc.:	Vitamins/Nutri.:	Information Sys.:	Y	Phys. Rehab. Center:	Waste Disposal:		Phys. Practice Mgmt.:
	Clinical Trials:		Psychiatric Clinics:	Specialty Services:	Y		

TYPES OF BUSINESS:
Services-Testing (Health & Life Insurance Prospects)
Health Information Underwriting Services
Home Medical Examinations
Outsourced Information Services
Electronic Case Management

BRANDS/DIVISIONS/AFFILIATES:
Heritage Labs
Portamedic
Portamedic Select
Michigan Evaluation Group
Infolink
Fax And Scan Today (FAST)
Heritage Labs

CONTACTS:
Note: Officers with more than one job title may be intentionally listed here more than once.

James M. McNamee, CEO
James M. McNamee, Pres.
Fred Lash, Sr. VP/CFO
David J. Goldberg, Sr. VP/Chief Mktg. Officer
Robert W. Jewett, Sr. VP/General Counsel
Fred Lash, Treas.
Joseph A. Marone, Jr., VP/Controller
Raymond A. Sinclair, Sr. VP
Alexander Warren, Sr. VP-Health Info.
James M. McNamee, Chmn.

Phone: 908-766-5000 **Fax:** 908-953-6304
Toll-Free:
Address: 170 Mt. Airy Rd., Basking Ridge, NJ 07920 US

GROWTH PLANS/SPECIAL FEATURES:
Hooper Holmes, Inc. is a leading provider of risk assessment services to the life and health insurance industry and medical evaluation and claims management services to the automobile insurance and workers' compensation industries. It provides medical examinations, frequently conducted in the patient's home by paramedicals; personal health interviews; record collection; and laboratory testing, which help life insurance companies evaluate the risks associated with underwriting policies. The company's Portamedic health division conducts paramedical and medical exams in an insurance applicant's home or office and offers comprehensive coverage to its customers. Its Fax And Scan Today (FAST) service indexes and images underwriting documents and makes them available on the company's web site or through a securely encrypted file transfer protocol site. The Portamedic Select unit is geared toward alternative distribution of life and health insurance, as well as electronic case management. Under the Infolink name, Hooper Holmes offers personal health interviews and medical record collection, including attending physician statements. The firm also owns a 55% interest in Heritage Labs, a laboratory that provides testing services for both Hooper Holmes' customers and third-party health information service providers. Hooper Holmes' diversified business unit provides independent medical examinations and peer reviews to the automobile no-fault insurance market and workers' compensation in New York, Pennsylvania and New Jersey. The company operates a network of over 275 branch and contract affiliate offices nationwide and in the U.K., with an army of registered nurses, licensed practical nurses, physicians, phlebotomists and medical and EKG technicians. In 2004, the firm completed its acquisition of the Michigan Evaluation Group, which provides the insurance, legal and business community direct access to accredited and board-certified physicians for the purpose of conducting independent medical examinations.

FINANCIALS:
Sales and profits are in thousands of dollars—add 000 to get the full amount. Year 2004 note: Complete fiscal 2004 results were not available for all companies at press time. For this company, year 2004 is for 9 months.

2004 Sales: $245,281 (9 months)   2004 Profits: $8,800 (9 months)
2003 Sales: $300,182   2003 Profits: $15,847
2002 Sales: $260,300   2002 Profits: $14,300
2001 Sales: $245,200   2001 Profits: $15,200
2000 Sales: $275,000   2000 Profits: $21,000

Stock Ticker: HH
Employees: 2,570
Fiscal Year Ends: 12/31

SALARIES/BENEFITS:
| Pension Plan: | ESOP Stock Plan: | Profit Sharing: | Top Exec. Salary: $700,000 | Bonus: $100,000 |
| Savings Plan: | Stock Purch. Plan: | | Second Exec. Salary: $230,000 | Bonus: $20,000 |

OTHER THOUGHTS:
Apparent Top Female Officers:
Hot Spot for Advancement for Women/Minorities:

LOCATIONS: ("Y" = Yes)
West:	Southwest:	Midwest:	Southeast:	Northeast:	International:
Y	Y	Y	Y	Y	Y

— 424 —

HORIZON BLUE CROSS BLUE SHIELD OF NEW JERSEY
www.horizon-bcbsnj.com

Industry Group Code: 524114   Ranks within this company's industry group: Sales: 22   Profits: 21

Insurance/HMO/PPO:	Drugs:	Equipment/Supplies:	Hospitals/Clinics:	Services:	Health Care:
Insurance: Y	Manufacturer:	Manufacturer:	Acute Care:	Diagnostics:	Home Health:
Managed Care: Y	Distributor:	Distributor:	Sub-Acute Care:	Labs/Testing:	Long-Term Care:
Utilization Mgmt.: Y	Specialty Pharm.:	Leasing/Finance:	Outpatient Surgery:	Staffing:	Physical Therapy:
Payment Proc.:	Vitamins/Nutri.:	Information Sys.:	Phys. Rehab. Center:	Waste Disposal:	Phys. Practice Mgmt.:
	Clinical Trials:		Psychiatric Clinics:	Specialty Services:	

TYPES OF BUSINESS:
Insurance
HMO, PPO, POS & Traditional Indemnity Plans
Medical Savings Accounts & Open Access Plans
Dental & Behavioral Health Insurance
Medicaid & Medicare
Casualty & Life Insurance
Utilization Management
Workers' Compensation

BRANDS/DIVISIONS/AFFILIATES:
Blue Cross Blue Shield
Horizon HMO
Magellan Behavioral Health
Horizon Healthcare Dental, Inc.
Horizon Casualty Services, Inc.
Horizon Healthcare Insurance Company of New York
Horizon Healthcare Insurance Agency, Inc.
Horizon NJ Health

CONTACTS:
Note: Officers with more than one job title may be intentionally listed here more than once.

William J. Marino, CEO
William J. Marino, Pres.
Robert J. Pures, CFO
Lawrence B. Altman, VP-Corp. Mktg.
Carole C. Soldo, VP-Human Resources
Charles C. Emery, Jr., Sr. VP-Info. Systems/CIO
Robert J. Pures, Sr. VP-Admin.
John W. Campbel, Sr. VP/General Counsel/Corp. Sec.
Lawrence B. Altman, VP-Corp. Comm.
Robert J. Pures, Treas.
Christy W. Bell, Sr. VP-Health Care Mgmt.
Carol A. Banks, VP-State Health Benefits Plan
Donna M. Celestini, VP-Health Care Services
Richard G. Popiel, VP-Health Affairs/Chief Medical Officer

Phone: 973-466-4000   Fax: 973-466-4317
Toll-Free: 800-355-2583
Address: 3 Penn Plaza E., Newark, NJ 07101 US

GROWTH PLANS/SPECIAL FEATURES:
Horizon Blue Cross Blue Shield of New Jersey (HBCBSNJ) is the only licensed Blue Cross Blue Shield plan in New Jersey. It is also one of New Jersey's leading health insurance providers, serving nearly 2 million members throughout north, south and central New Jersey. The firm's insurance plans include traditional indemnity, Horizon HMO, Horizon PPO, Horizon POS, Horizon MSA (a medical savings account) and Horizon Direct Access (an open access plan). The company also offers dental, Medicare supplment and behavioral health insurance, as well as workers' compensation. Magellan Behavioral Health provides utilization reviews and management services to HBCBDNJ customers receiving mental health and substance abuse treatment. In addition, HBCBSNJ provides services through two affiliates: Horizon Healthcare Dental, Inc., which provides managed dental plans for individuals and groups; and Horizon Casualty Services, Inc., which provides workers' compensation managed care and claims administration services, as well as auto injury management services. The firm also operates through several subsidiaries that are not Blue Cross and Blue Shield licensed companies. Horizon Healthcare Insurance Company of New York provides managed care and traditional health plans in New York State, a growing regional market for the company. Horizon Healthcare Insurance Agency, Inc. offers group life and employee benefit coverage, including accidental death and dismemberment, dependent life, premium conversions, weekly income, long-term disability, flexible spending accounts and group term life insurance. Horizon NJ Health, New Jersey's largest managed health care organization, serves the publicly insured Medicaid and NJ FamilyCare populations.

FINANCIALS:
Sales and profits are in thousands of dollars—add 000 to get the full amount. Year 2004 note: Complete fiscal 2004 results were not available for all companies at press time. For this company, year 2004 is for months.

2004 Sales: $ (months)   2004 Profits: $ (months)
2003 Sales: $5,082,400   2003 Profits: $171,100
2002 Sales: $4,097,500   2002 Profits: $114,100
2001 Sales: $ 2001 Profits: $
2000 Sales: $ 2000 Profits: $

Stock Ticker: Nonprofit
Employees: 4,600
Fiscal Year Ends: 12/31

SALARIES/BENEFITS:
Pension Plan: ESOP Stock Plan: Profit Sharing: Top Exec. Salary: $ Bonus: $
Savings Plan: Stock Purch. Plan: Second Exec. Salary: $ Bonus: $

OTHER THOUGHTS:
Apparent Top Female Officers: 4
Hot Spot for Advancement for Women/Minorities: Y

LOCATIONS: ("Y" = Yes)
West:	Southwest:	Midwest:	Southeast:	Northeast:	International:
				Y	

HORIZON HEALTH CORPORATION

www.horz.com

Industry Group Code: 621490 Ranks within this company's industry group: Sales: 9 Profits: 10

Insurance/HMO/PPO:	Drugs:	Equipment/Supplies:	Hospitals/Clinics:	Services:	Health Care:
Insurance: Managed Care: Utilization Mgmt.: Y Payment Proc.:	Manufacturer: Distributor: Specialty Pharm.: Vitamins/Nutri.: Clinical Trials:	Manufacturer: Distributor: Leasing/Finance: Information Sys.: Y	Acute Care: Sub-Acute Care: Outpatient Surgery: Phys. Rehab. Center: Y Psychiatric Clinics:	Diagnostics: Labs/Testing: Staffing: Y Waste Disposal: Specialty Services: Y	Home Health: Long-Term Care: Physical Therapy: Y Phys. Practice Mgmt.:

TYPES OF BUSINESS:
Mental Health and Physical Rehabilitation Programs
Psychiatric Health Databases
Specialty Mental Health Services
Employee Assistance Plans
Outsourcing and Staffing Services

BRANDS/DIVISIONS/AFFILIATES:
Horizon Mental Health Management, Inc.
Mental Health Outcomes, Inc.
Horizon Behavioral Services, Inc.
Specialty Rehab Management, Inc.
ProCare One Nurses, LLC
CQI+TM Outcomes Measurement Systems
PsychScope
Employee Assistance Programs International, Inc.

CONTACTS:
Note: Officers with more than one job title may be intentionally listed here more than once.

James K. Newman, CEO
James K. Newman, Pres.
David S. Tingue, Sr. VP-Mktg.
Frank C. Meyercord, Sr. VP/General Counsel
Frank J. Baumann, Sr. VP-Oper.
Donald W. Thayer, Sr. VP-Acquisitions & Dev.
James K. Newman, Chmn.

Phone: 972-420-8200 Fax: 972-420-8252
Toll-Free: 800-931-4646
Address: 1500 Waters Ridge Dr., Lewisville, TX 75057-6011 US

GROWTH PLANS/SPECIAL FEATURES:
Horizon Health Corp. is a provider of employee assistance plans (EAPs) and behavioral health services to business and managed care organizations, as well as a leading contract manager of psychiatric and physical rehabilitation clinical programs offered by general acute care hospitals in the United States. The firm was the first psychiatric contract manager to implement geriatric psychiatry, outpatient, partial hospitalization and home health services through subsidiary Horizon Mental Health Management, Inc. Mental Health Outcomes, Inc., a psychiatric subsidiary, focuses on the design and management of psychiatric outcomes measurement systems. It also supports pharmaceutical research by providing the nation's most comprehensive psychiatric databases, such as CQI+TM Outcome Measurement Systems and PsychScope. Horizon Behavioral Services, Inc. (HBS), a leader in the EAP business, provides employers with administration and management of behavioral health, substance abuse and work life services for employees. Members of HBS have full access to licensed counselors, mental health and substance abuse treatment facilities and consultation services. Another subsidiary, Specialty Rehab Management, Inc., provides physical medicine and rehabilitation services to general hospitals. The company specializes in helping individuals who are disabled due to a chronic disease, major trauma and/or premature birth and congenital defects.

Horizon Health offers employees medical, dental and pharmacy coverage, as well as life and disability insurance. It also offers a flexible benefit plan with tax deduction features for health and dependent care expenses.

FINANCIALS:
Sales and profits are in thousands of dollars—add 000 to get the full amount. Year 2004 note: Complete fiscal 2004 results were not available for all companies at press time. For this company, year 2004 is for 9 months.

2004 Sales: $128,941 (9 months)   2004 Profits: $7,980 (9 months)
2003 Sales: $166,300   2003 Profits: $9,600
2002 Sales: $143,700   2002 Profits: $8,900
2001 Sales: $127,700   2001 Profits: $6,800
2000 Sales: $133,700   2000 Profits: $7,100

Stock Ticker: HORC
Employees: 1,876
Fiscal Year Ends: 8/31

SALARIES/BENEFITS:
Pension Plan: ESOP Stock Plan: Profit Sharing: Top Exec. Salary: $288,446 Bonus: $251,417
Savings Plan: Y Stock Purch. Plan: Second Exec. Salary: $240,000 Bonus: $167,165

OTHER THOUGHTS:
Apparent Top Female Officers:
Hot Spot for Advancement for Women/Minorities:

LOCATIONS: ("Y" = Yes)
West:	Southwest:	Midwest:	Southeast:	Northeast:	International:
Y	Y	Y	Y	Y	

HOSPIRA INC

www.hospira.com

Industry Group Code: 325414 **Ranks within this company's industry group:** Sales: 1 Profits:

Insurance/HMO/PPO:	Drugs:	Equipment/Supplies:	Hospitals/Clinics:	Services:	Health Care:
Insurance:	Manufacturer: Y	Manufacturer:	Acute Care:	Diagnostics:	Home Health:
Managed Care:	Distributor:	Distributor:	Sub-Acute Care:	Labs/Testing:	Long-Term Care:
Utilization Mgmt.:	Specialty Pharm.:	Leasing/Finance:	Outpatient Surgery:	Staffing:	Physical Therapy:
Payment Proc.:	Vitamins/Nutri.:	Information Sys.: Y	Phys. Rehab. Center:	Waste Disposal:	Phys. Practice Mgmt.:
	Clinical Trials:		Psychiatric Clinics:	Specialty Services:	

TYPES OF BUSINESS:
Drugs, Manufacturing
Hospital Products
Medication Delivery Systems
Anesthetics
Injectables
Diagnostic Imaging Agents
Drug Library Software
Monitoring Systems

BRANDS/DIVISIONS/AFFILIATES:
Abbott Laboratories
One 2 One

CONTACTS:
Note: Officers with more than one job title may be intentionally listed here more than once.
Christopher B. Begley, CEO
Terrence C. Kearney, CFO
Edward A. Ogunro, Sr. VP-Research & Dev.
Brian J. Smith, Sr. VP/General Counsel
John Arnott, Sr. VP-Global Commercial Oper.
Terrence C. Kearney, Sr. VP-Finance
David A. Jones, Chmn.

Phone: 224-212-2000 **Fax:**
Toll-Free:
Address: 275 N. Field Dr., Lake Forest, IL 60045 US

GROWTH PLANS/SPECIAL FEATURES:
Hospira, Inc. was established in 2003 by Abbott Laboratories in order to facilitate the company's planned spin-off of a new, separate company specializing in the manufacture and sale of hospital products, including injectable pharmaceuticals and medication delivery systems. Operating independently since May 2004, Hospira oversees most of Abbott's former hospital products division and select operations formerly managed by Abbott's international segment. Hospira's pharmaceutical offerings include anesthetics, acute care injectables and diagnostic imaging agents, as well as prefilled syringes and premixed intravenous delivery systems for quick administration. The company also markets invasive monitoring systems, like angiography kits and cardiac catheters; medical infusion systems, including patient-controlled drug pumps for pain management; and drug library software for customized installation in various hospital and clinical settings. Hospira's One 2 One unit is a leading provider of contract manufacturing services, partnering with pharmaceutical and biotechnology companies on all aspects of formulation development, filling and finishing of injectables, as well as providing access to a range of delivery systems and related products including stoppers, I.V. administration sets and latex, rubber and vinyl items. Hospira recently announced that it would acquire a 100,000-square-foot manufacturing facility in North Carolina and related equipment from Fresenius Kabi in order to keep pace with industry demand for pharmaceutical injectables, intravenous drugs and expanded contract pharmaceutical manufacturing.

FINANCIALS:
Sales and profits are in thousands of dollars—add 000 to get the full amount. Year 2004 note: Complete fiscal 2004 results were not available for all companies at press time. For this company, year 2004 is for 9 months.

2004 Sales: $1,810,749 (9 months)	2004 Profits: $252,076 (9 months)	**Stock Ticker:** HSP
2003 Sales: $2,500,000	2003 Profits: $	**Employees:** 14,000
2002 Sales: $	2002 Profits: $	**Fiscal Year Ends:** 12/31
2001 Sales: $	2001 Profits: $	
2000 Sales: $	2000 Profits: $	

SALARIES/BENEFITS:
Pension Plan:	ESOP Stock Plan:	Profit Sharing:	Top Exec. Salary: $	Bonus: $
Savings Plan:	Stock Purch. Plan:		Second Exec. Salary: $	Bonus: $

OTHER THOUGHTS:
Apparent Top Female Officers:
Hot Spot for Advancement for Women/Minorities:

LOCATIONS: ("Y" = Yes)
West:	Southwest:	Midwest:	Southeast:	Northeast:	International:
Y	Y	Y	Y	Y	Y

HUMAN GENOME SCIENCES INC

www.hgsi.com

Industry Group Code: 541710   Ranks within this company's industry group: Sales: 12   Profits: 12

Insurance/HMO/PPO:	Drugs:	Equipment/Supplies:	Hospitals/Clinics:	Services:	Health Care:
Insurance: Managed Care: Utilization Mgmt.: Payment Proc.:	Manufacturer: Distributor: Specialty Pharm.: Vitamins/Nutri.: Clinical Trials: Y	Manufacturer: Distributor: Leasing/Finance: Information Sys.:	Acute Care: Sub-Acute Care: Outpatient Surgery: Phys. Rehab. Center: Psychiatric Clinics:	Diagnostics: Labs/Testing: Staffing: Waste Disposal: Specialty Services:	Home Health: Long-Term Care: Physical Therapy: Phys. Practice Mgmt.:

TYPES OF BUSINESS:
Research and Development-Genetics and Biotechnology
Human Gene and Microbe Database
Protein-Based Drug Development

BRANDS/DIVISIONS/AFFILIATES:
LymphoStat-B
Albuferon

CONTACTS: Note: Officers with more than one job title may be intentionally listed here more than once.
William A. Haseltine, CEO
Craig A. Rosen, Pres.
Craig A. Rosen, COO
Steven C. Mayer, Exec. VP/CFO
Jeanne M. Riley, VP-Strategic Mktg.
Susan B. McKay, Sr. VP-Human Resources
Craig A. Rosen, Pres.-R&D
Michael R. Fannon, VP/CIO
David C. Stump, Sr. VP-Drug Dev.
James H. Davis, General Counsel/Corp. Sec.
Perry Karsen, Sr. VP-Bus. Dev.
Argeris N. Karabelas,

Phone: 301-309-8504   Fax: 301-309-8512
Toll-Free:
Address: 14200 Shady Grove Rd., Rockville, MD 20850 US

GROWTH PLANS/SPECIAL FEATURES:
Human Genome Sciences, Inc. possesses one of the largest databases of human genes and microbes in the world. Initially focused on genetic research, the firm has successfully become a drug development company engaged in the research and development of proprietary pharmaceutical and diagnostic products. In March 2004, the company announced that it would further restrict its focus, dropping several of its drugs under development to focus on the five most promising projects. These projects include LymphoStat-B for the treatment of systemic lupus erythematosus and rheumatoid arthritis, currently in Phase II trials; a long-acting alpha interferon for the treatment of hepatitis C; anti-TRAIL Receptor 1 and TRAIL Receptor 2 monoclonal antibodies for the treatment of cancer, currently in Phase I trials; Albuferon for the treatment of chronic hepatitis C, now in Phase II trials; and an anti-CCR5 monoclonal antibody for the treatment of HIV/AIDS, for which the company plans to file an Investigational New Drug (NDA) during 2004. At the same time, Human Genome Sciences announced the reduction of its workforce by about 20% and the installation of a new CEO by the end of 2004, as founder Haseltine retires.

The firm encourages employees to enhance their professional development by providing tuition reimbursement programs, encouraging attendance at professional conferences and sponsoring skill-building seminars.

FINANCIALS:
Sales and profits are in thousands of dollars—add 000 to get the full amount. Year 2004 note: Complete fiscal 2004 results were not available for all companies at press time. For this company, year 2004 is for 9 months.

2004 Sales: $3,004 (9 months)   2004 Profits: $-176,192 (9 months)
2003 Sales: $8,168   2003 Profits: $-185,324
2002 Sales: $3,600   2002 Profits: $-219,700
2001 Sales: $12,800   2001 Profits: $-117,200
2000 Sales: $22,100   2000 Profits: $-243,800

Stock Ticker: HGSI
Employees: 1,100
Fiscal Year Ends: 12/31

SALARIES/BENEFITS:
Pension Plan: ESOP Stock Plan: Profit Sharing: Top Exec. Salary: $5,000,000   Bonus: $200,850
Savings Plan: Y   Stock Purch. Plan: Y   Second Exec. Salary: $390,000   Bonus: $200,850

OTHER THOUGHTS:
Apparent Top Female Officers: 2
Hot Spot for Advancement for Women/Minorities:

LOCATIONS: ("Y" = Yes)
West:	Southwest:	Midwest:	Southeast:	Northeast:	International:
				Y	

HUMANA INC

www.humana.com

Industry Group Code: 524114   **Ranks within this company's industry group:** Sales: 8   Profits: 16

Insurance/HMO/PPO:	Drugs:	Equipment/Supplies:	Hospitals/Clinics:	Services:	Health Care:
Insurance:	Manufacturer:	Manufacturer:	Acute Care:	Diagnostics:	Home Health:
Managed Care: Y	Distributor:	Distributor:	Sub-Acute Care:	Labs/Testing:	Long-Term Care:
Utilization Mgmt.:	Specialty Pharm.:	Leasing/Finance:	Outpatient Surgery:	Staffing:	Physical Therapy:
Payment Proc.:	Vitamins/Nutri.:	Information Sys.:	Phys. Rehab. Center:	Waste Disposal:	Phys. Practice Mgmt.:
	Clinical Trials:		Psychiatric Clinics:	Specialty Services:	

TYPES OF BUSINESS:
HMO
Mental Health Plans
Workers' Compensation
Dental Plans
Group Life Plans
Wellness Programs

BRANDS/DIVISIONS/AFFILIATES:
HumanaOne

CONTACTS:
Note: Officers with more than one job title may be intentionally listed here more than once.

Michael B. McCallister, CEO
Michael B. McCallister, Pres.
James H. Bloem, Sr. VP/CFO
Steven O. Moya, Sr. VP/Chief Mktg. Officer
Bonnie C. Hathcock, Sr. VP/Chief Human Resources Officer
Bruce J. Goodman, Sr. VP/Chief Service & Info. Officer
Arthur P. Hipwell, Sr. VP/General Counsel
Thomas J. Liston, Sr. VP-Strategy & Corp. Dev.
Steven E. McCulley, VP/Controller
Jonathan T. Lord, Chief Clinical Strategy & Innovation Officer
Heidi S. Margulis, Sr. VP-Gov't Rel.
R. Eugene Shields, Sr. VP-Gov't Programs
James E. Murray, COO-Market & Bus. Segment Oper.
David A. Jones, Chmn.

Phone: 502-580-1000   **Fax:** 502-580-3677
Toll-Free: 800-486-2620
Address: 500 W. Main St., Louisville, KY 40202 US

GROWTH PLANS/SPECIAL FEATURES:

Humana, Inc. is one of the nation's largest health benefits companies, offering coordinated health insurance coverage and related services for employer groups, government-sponsored programs and individuals. The company serves approximately 8.5 million members, primarily in the South and Midwest. Its services are marketed mostly through health maintenance organizations (HMOs) and preferred provider organizations (PPOs) that promote or require the use of contracted providers. To meet that end, Humana contracts with over 463,000 physicians, hospitals, dentists and other providers, in one of the largest networks in the U.S. The company also offers a wide variety of services to employers, such as workers' compensation, dental plans, group life plans and an administrative-services-only plan. Humana provides health benefits and related services to companies ranging from fewer than 10 to over 10,000 employees. More than 120,000 small businesses with an average size of nine employees rely on the company for medical coverage. In addition, the company's HumanaOne product is available directly to individuals. Humana also markets products to government segment members and beneficiaries, including Medicaid contracts and supplemental plans for those covered by Medicare. Its TRICARE program provides health insurance coverage to the dependents of active-duty military personnel and to retired military personnel and their dependents.

Humana offers its employees a broad array of benefits including medical and dental plans, disability, fitness centers, tuition reimbursement, scholarship programs for children of employees and adoption assistance.

FINANCIALS:
Sales and profits are in thousands of dollars—add 000 to get the full amount. Year 2004 note: Complete fiscal 2004 results were not available for all companies at press time. For this company, year 2004 is for 9 months.

2004 Sales: $9,894,700 (9 months)   2004 Profits: $232,886 (9 months)
2003 Sales: $12,226,311   2003 Profits: $228,934
2002 Sales: $11,175,000   2002 Profits: $143,000
2001 Sales: $10,076,000   2001 Profits: $117,000
2000 Sales: $10,514,000   2000 Profits: $90,000

Stock Ticker: HUM
Employees: 13,700
Fiscal Year Ends: 12/31

SALARIES/BENEFITS:
Pension Plan:	ESOP Stock Plan:	Profit Sharing:	Top Exec. Salary: $713,923	Bonus: $1,070,885
Savings Plan: Y	Stock Purch. Plan:		Second Exec. Salary: $476,630	Bonus: $571,956

OTHER THOUGHTS:
Apparent Top Female Officers: 2
Hot Spot for Advancement for Women/Minorities:

LOCATIONS: ("Y" = Yes)
West:	Southwest:	Midwest:	Southeast:	Northeast:	International:
Y	Y	Y	Y	Y	

HUNTLEIGH TECHNOLOGIES PLC

www.huntleigh-technology.com

Industry Group Code: 339113   Ranks within this company's industry group: Sales: 52   Profits: 46

Insurance/HMO/PPO:	Drugs:	Equipment/Supplies:	Hospitals/Clinics:	Services:	Health Care:
Insurance:	Manufacturer:	Manufacturer: Y	Acute Care:	Diagnostics:	Home Health:
Managed Care:	Distributor:	Distributor: Y	Sub-Acute Care:	Labs/Testing:	Long-Term Care:
Utilization Mgmt.:	Specialty Pharm.:	Leasing/Finance:	Outpatient Surgery:	Staffing:	Physical Therapy:
Payment Proc.:	Vitamins/Nutri.:	Information Sys.:	Phys. Rehab. Center:	Waste Disposal:	Phys. Practice Mgmt.:
	Clinical Trials:		Psychiatric Clinics:	Specialty Services:	

TYPES OF BUSINESS:
Medical Equipment Manufacturing, Sales and Rental
Patient Positioning and Transportation Equipment
Pressure Area Care Management Products
Pneumatic Compression Devices
Ultrasonic Diagnostic Equipment

BRANDS/DIVISIONS/AFFILIATES:
Nimbus Logic 200

CONTACTS:
Note: Officers with more than one job title may be intentionally listed here more than once.
David Schild, CEO
Craig Smith, CFO
Stephen Cook, Chief Tech. Officer
Geoff Cox, Group Managing Dir.
Robert Angel, CEO-Huntleigh Healthcare, Inc.
Richard Newbery, Corp. Sec.
Julian Schild, Chmn.

Phone: 44-1582-413104   Fax: 44-1582 402589
Toll-Free:
Address: 310-312 Dallow Rd., Luton, Bedfordshire LU1 1TD UK

GROWTH PLANS/SPECIAL FEATURES:
Huntleigh Technology plc, based in the United Kingdom, manufactures, sells and rents medical equipment and instruments internationally. The firm offers products in four sectors: patient positioning and transportation; pressure area care management; intermittent pneumatic compression devices; and ultrasonic diagnostic equipment. Patient positioning and transportation systems include electric and manual medical and surgical beds; maternity beds and cribs; and other furniture for hospitals. Pressure area care management products are mattress replacement systems for the prevention and treatment of pressure ulcers, including the Nimbus Logic 200. Intermittent pneumatic compression devices are designed for the prevention of deep vein thrombosis, venous leg ulcers, edema and inflammatory arthritis on joints and limbs. Ultrasonic diagnostic equipment is used in vascular assessment, vital sign readings, obstetrics and veterinary practices. The firm distributes products to over 120 countries, with manufacturing sites in the U.K., U.S., Australia and South Africa.

FINANCIALS:
Sales and profits are in thousands of dollars—add 000 to get the full amount. Year 2004 note: Complete fiscal 2004 results were not available for all companies at press time. For this company, year 2004 is for months.

2004 Sales: $ (months)   2004 Profits: $ (months)
2003 Sales: $332,800   2003 Profits: $27,500
2002 Sales: $283,000   2002 Profits: $23,800
2001 Sales: $ 2001 Profits: $
2000 Sales: $ 2000 Profits: $

Stock Ticker: Foreign
Employees: 2,330
Fiscal Year Ends: 12/31

SALARIES/BENEFITS:
Pension Plan: ESOP Stock Plan: Profit Sharing: Top Exec. Salary: $ Bonus: $
Savings Plan: Stock Purch. Plan: Second Exec. Salary: $ Bonus: $

OTHER THOUGHTS:
Apparent Top Female Officers:
Hot Spot for Advancement for Women/Minorities:

LOCATIONS: ("Y" = Yes)
West:	Southwest:	Midwest:	Southeast:	Northeast:	International:
				Y	Y

I FLOW CORPORATION

www.i-flowcorp.com

Industry Group Code: 339113 **Ranks within this company's industry group:** Sales: 113 Profits: 100

Insurance/HMO/PPO:	Drugs:	Equipment/Supplies:	Hospitals/Clinics:	Services:	Health Care:
Insurance:	Manufacturer:	Manufacturer: Y	Acute Care:	Diagnostics:	Home Health:
Managed Care:	Distributor:	Distributor:	Sub-Acute Care:	Labs/Testing:	Long-Term Care:
Utilization Mgmt.:	Specialty Pharm.:	Leasing/Finance: Y	Outpatient Surgery:	Staffing:	Physical Therapy:
Payment Proc.:	Vitamins/Nutri.:	Information Sys.:	Phys. Rehab. Center:	Waste Disposal:	Phys. Practice Mgmt.:
	Clinical Trials:		Psychiatric Clinics:	Specialty Services:	

TYPES OF BUSINESS:
Medical Equipment-Mobile Infusion Systems
Anesthesia Kits
Rental Infusion Equipment

BRANDS/DIVISIONS/AFFILIATES:
InfuSystem, Inc.
Block Medical de Mexico, S.A. de C.V.
askyoursurgeon.com
ON-Q Post-Operative Pain Relief System

CONTACTS:
Note: Officers with more than one job title may be intentionally listed here more than once.
Donald M. Earhart, CEO
Donald M. Earhart, Pres.
James J. Dal Porto, Exec. VP/COO
James R. Talevich, CFO
James R. Talevich, Treas.
Donald M. Earhart, Chmn.

Phone: 949-206-2700   **Fax:** 949-206-2600
Toll-Free: 800-448-3569
Address: 20202 Windrow Dr., Lake Forest, CA 92630 US

GROWTH PLANS/SPECIAL FEATURES:
I-Flow designs, develops and markets technically advanced, low-cost ambulatory drug delivery systems. Its products are used both in hospitals and alternate site settings, including freestanding surgery centers and physicians' offices. The firm's family of products is focused on three primary market segments: regional anesthesia, intravenous (IV) infusion therapy and oncology infusion services. I-Flow currently manufactures a line of compact, portable infusion pumps, catheters, needles and pain kits that administer medication directly to the wound site as well as administer local anesthetics, chemotherapies, antibiotics, diagnostic agents, nutritional supplements and other medications. Subsidiary InfuSystem, Inc. provides infusion pumps for rent on a month-to-month basis to the cancer infusion therapy market. I-Flow also owns a subsidiary in Mexico, Block Medical de Mexico, which manufactures a substantial portion of the company's products. I-Flow's askyoursurgeon.com web site educates consumers about their post-surgical pain treatment options and highlights the company's ON-Q family of products. The ON-Q family provides regionally administered medication through catheters providing continuous post-operative wound site pain management through nerve blocks or direct application at the surgical incision sites. Recently, I-Flow sold its Spinal Specialties subsidiary, a designer and manufacturer of custom spinal, epidermal and nerve block infusion kits, to Integra LifeSciences Holdings Corporation for approximately $6 million.

FINANCIALS:
Sales and profits are in thousands of dollars—add 000 to get the full amount. Year 2004 note: Complete fiscal 2004 results were not available for all companies at press time. For this company, year 2004 is for 9 months.

2004 Sales: $50,024 (9 months)	2004 Profits: $-4,774 (9 months)	**Stock Ticker:** IFLO
2003 Sales: $47,043	2003 Profits: $457	Employees: 520
2002 Sales: $38,100	2002 Profits: $-3,100	Fiscal Year Ends: 12/31
2001 Sales: $33,300	2001 Profits: $1,300	
2000 Sales: $32,000	2000 Profits: $1,600	

SALARIES/BENEFITS:
Pension Plan:	ESOP Stock Plan:	Profit Sharing:	Top Exec. Salary: $355,626	Bonus: $300,000
Savings Plan: Y	Stock Purch. Plan:		Second Exec. Salary: $231,570	Bonus: $255,000

OTHER THOUGHTS:
Apparent Top Female Officers:
Hot Spot for Advancement for Women/Minorities:

LOCATIONS: ("Y" = Yes)
West:	Southwest:	Midwest:	Southeast:	Northeast:	International:
Y		Y			Y

ICU MEDICAL INC

www.icumed.com

Industry Group Code: 339113   Ranks within this company's industry group: Sales: 87   Profits: 54

Insurance/HMO/PPO:	Drugs:	Equipment/Supplies:		Hospitals/Clinics:	Services:	Health Care:
Insurance:	Manufacturer:	Manufacturer:	Y	Acute Care:	Diagnostics:	Home Health:
Managed Care:	Distributor:	Distributor:		Sub-Acute Care:	Labs/Testing:	Long-Term Care:
Utilization Mgmt.:	Specialty Pharm.:	Leasing/Finance:		Outpatient Surgery:	Staffing:	Physical Therapy:
Payment Proc.:	Vitamins/Nutri.:	Information Sys.:		Phys. Rehab. Center:	Waste Disposal:	Phys. Practice Mgmt.:
	Clinical Trials:			Psychiatric Clinics:	Specialty Services:	

TYPES OF BUSINESS:
Equipment-Intravenous Connection Devices
Custom IV Systems

BRANDS/DIVISIONS/AFFILIATES:
CLAVE
CLC2000
1o2 Valve
Bio-Plexus, Inc.
Punctur-Guard

CONTACTS:
Note: Officers with more than one job title may be intentionally listed here more than once.

George Lopez, CEO
George Lopez, Pres.
Francis J. O'Brien, CFO
Alison D. Burcar, VP-Mktg.
James Reitz, Dir.-Human Resources
Steven C. Riggs, VP-Oper.
Richard A. Costello, VP-Sales

Phone: 949-366-2183   Fax: 949-366-8368
Toll-Free: 800-824-7890
Address: 951 Calle Amanecer, San Clemente, CA 92673 US

GROWTH PLANS/SPECIAL FEATURES:
ICU Medical is a leader in the development, manufacture and sale of disposable medical connection systems for use in intravenous (IV) therapy applications. Its devices are designed to protect health care workers and their patients from exposure to infectious diseases such as hepatitis B and C and HIV through accidental needlesticks. The firm is also a leader in the production of custom IV systems and low-cost generic IV systems. The company's main product, the CLAVE, is an innovative one-piece, needleless IV connection device that accounts for approximately 59% of the company's revenue (exclusive of CLAVEs incorporated into custom IV systems). The CLAVE allows protected, secure and sterile IV connections without needles and without failure-prone mechanical valves used in other IV connection systems. It was designed to eliminate needles from certain applications in acute care hospitals, home health care, ambulatory surgical centers, nursing homes, convalescent facilities, physicians' offices, medical clinics and emergency centers. Principal products introduced in recent years are the CLC2000, the 1o2 Valve and, with the acquisition of Bio-Plexus, Inc., the Punctur-Guard line of blood collection needles, which reduce the risk of needlesticks by allowing the practitioner to blunt the needle while it is still in the vein. A key element in ICU's strategy to expand its custom IV system business has been the development and implementation of proprietary software for custom product design, customer orders and order tracking, combined with an innovative system to coordinate the manufacture of components in the U.S., assembly of components into sets in Mexico and Italy and distribution of finished products. Currently, ICU sells substantially all of its products to IV product manufacturers and independent distributors. Its largest customer is Abbott Laboratories, which accounts for 67% of the company's revenues.

FINANCIALS:
Sales and profits are in thousands of dollars—add 000 to get the full amount. Year 2004 note: Complete fiscal 2004 results were not available for all companies at press time. For this company, year 2004 is for 9 months.

2004 Sales: $60,366 (9 months)	2004 Profits: $6,514 (9 months)	Stock Ticker: ICUI
2003 Sales: $107,354	2003 Profits: $22,297	Employees: 574
2002 Sales: $87,800	2002 Profits: $19,700	Fiscal Year Ends: 12/31
2001 Sales: $69,100	2001 Profits: $15,400	
2000 Sales: $56,200	2000 Profits: $11,800	

SALARIES/BENEFITS:
Pension Plan:	ESOP Stock Plan:	Profit Sharing:	Top Exec. Salary: $340,000	Bonus: $187,000
Savings Plan: Y	Stock Purch. Plan: Y		Second Exec. Salary: $222,000	Bonus: $27,750

OTHER THOUGHTS:
Apparent Top Female Officers: 1
Hot Spot for Advancement for Women/Minorities:

LOCATIONS: ("Y" = Yes)
West:	Southwest:	Midwest:	Southeast:	Northeast:	International:
Y				Y	Y

IDEXX LABORATORIES INC

www.idexx.com

Industry Group Code: 339113   Ranks within this company's industry group: Sales: 41   Profits: 30

Insurance/HMO/PPO:	Drugs:		Equipment/Supplies:		Hospitals/Clinics:	Services:		Health Care:	
Insurance:	Manufacturer:		Manufacturer:		Acute Care:	Diagnostics:	Y	Home Health:	
Managed Care:	Distributor:		Distributor:		Sub-Acute Care:	Labs/Testing:	Y	Long-Term Care:	
Utilization Mgmt.:	Specialty Pharm.:	Y	Leasing/Finance:		Outpatient Surgery:	Staffing:		Physical Therapy:	
Payment Proc.:	Vitamins/Nutri.:		Information Sys.:	Y	Phys. Rehab. Center:	Waste Disposal:		Phys. Practice Mgmt.:	
	Clinical Trials:				Psychiatric Clinics:	Specialty Services:	Y		

TYPES OF BUSINESS:
Veterinary Laboratory Testing & Consulting
Point-of-Care Diagnostic Products
Veterinary Pharmaceuticals
Information Management Software
Contaminant Test Products

BRANDS/DIVISIONS/AFFILIATES:
Colilert-18
SNAP
Parallux
Colisure
SURPASS
HerdCheck

CONTACTS: Note: Officers with more than one job title may be intentionally listed here more than once.
Jonathan W. Ayers, CEO
Jonathan W. Ayers, Pres.
Merilee Raines, VP/CFO
William C. Wallen, Sr. VP/Chief Scientific Officer
S. Sam Fratoni, VP/CIO
Conan R. Deady, VP/General Counsel & Sec.
Laurel E. LaBauve, VP-Worldwide Oper.
Merilee Raines, Treas.
Quentin J. Tonelli, VP/General Mgr.-Production Animal Services
Robert S. Hulsy, VP/Pres., IDEXX Reference Laboratories
Jonathan W. Ayers, Chmn.

Phone: 207-856-0300   Fax: 207-856-0346
Toll-Free: 800-548-6733
Address: One IDEXX Dr., Westbrook, ME 04092-2041 US

GROWTH PLANS/SPECIAL FEATURES:
IDEXX Laboratories, Inc. is a worldwide leader in providing diagnostic, detection and information products for various industries. The company's primary business focus is on pet health. Its companion animal and equine veterinary offerings include in-clinic diagnostic tests and instrumentation, laboratory services, pharmaceuticals and veterinary practice information management software. The firm also operates in three other business areas. It provides assay kits, software and instrumentation for accurate assessment of infectious disease in production animals, such as cattle, swine and poultry, as well as diagnostics for the detection of microbiological contamination in drinking water and for the screening of antibiotic residues in milk. It provides a broad range of single-use, hand-held test kits that allow quick, accurate and convenient testing for a variety of companion animal diseases and health conditions. The principal single-use tests, sold under the SNAP name, include a feline combination test, the SNAP Combo FIV antibody/FeLV antigen test, which enables veterinarians to test simultaneously for feline leukemia virus and feline immunodeficiency virus; a canine combination test, the SNAP 3Dx, which tests simultaneously for Lyme disease, Ehrlichia canis and heartworm; and a canine heartworm-only test. The company currently offers commercial veterinary laboratory and consulting services in the U.S. through facilities located in Arizona, California, Colorado, Illinois, Maryland, Massachusetts, New Jersey, Oregon and Texas. IDEXX also sells products that detect microbial contaminants in water and antibiotic residues in milk. Its Colilert-18 and Colisure tests simultaneously detect total coliforms and E. coli in water. The company's two principal products for use in testing for antibiotic residue in milk are the SNAP Beta-lactam test and the Parallux system. Recently, IDEXX received FDA approval for its topical equine anti-inflammatory SURPASS. It also received USDA approval for IDEXX HerdCheck, a rapid test for mad cow disease.

IDEXX provides performance bonuses, a tuition assistance program, an employee referral program and personal growth leave.

FINANCIALS: Sales and profits are in thousands of dollars—add 000 to get the full amount. Year 2004 note: Complete fiscal 2004 results were not available for all companies at press time. For this company, year 2004 is for 9 months.

2004 Sales: $404,907 (9 months)   2004 Profits: $61,397 (9 months)
2003 Sales: $475,992   2003 Profits: $57,090
2002 Sales: $412,700   2002 Profits: $45,400
2001 Sales: $386,100   2001 Profits: $37,600
2000 Sales: $367,400   2000 Profits: $36,600

Stock Ticker: IDXX
Employees: 2,473
Fiscal Year Ends: 12/31

SALARIES/BENEFITS:
Pension Plan: ESOP Stock Plan: Profit Sharing: Top Exec. Salary: $520,000   Bonus: $546,000
Savings Plan: Y   Stock Purch. Plan: Y   Second Exec. Salary: $268,000   Bonus: $196,980

OTHER THOUGHTS:
Apparent Top Female Officers: 2
Hot Spot for Advancement for Women/Minorities:

LOCATIONS: ("Y" = Yes)
West:	Southwest:	Midwest:	Southeast:	Northeast:	International:
Y	Y	Y	Y	Y	Y

IDX SYSTEMS CORP

www.idx.com

Industry Group Code: 511200   Ranks within this company's industry group: Sales: 3   Profits: 2

Insurance/HMO/PPO:	Drugs:	Equipment/Supplies:	Hospitals/Clinics:	Services:	Health Care:
Insurance:	Manufacturer:	Manufacturer:	Acute Care:	Diagnostics:	Home Health:
Managed Care:	Distributor:	Distributor:	Sub-Acute Care:	Labs/Testing:	Long-Term Care:
Utilization Mgmt.:	Specialty Pharm.:	Leasing/Finance:	Outpatient Surgery:	Staffing:	Physical Therapy:
Payment Proc.:	Vitamins/Nutri.:	Information Sys.: Y	Phys. Rehab. Center:	Waste Disposal:	Phys. Practice Mgmt.:
	Clinical Trials:		Psychiatric Clinics:	Specialty Services: Y	

TYPES OF BUSINESS:
Computer Software-Health Care
Practice Management Software
e-Commerce Services
Clinical Documentation
Transcription Services

BRANDS/DIVISIONS/AFFILIATES:
Flowcast
IDXtend for the Web
Carecast
Groupcast
Imagecast
EDiX Corp.

CONTACTS:
Note: Officers with more than one job title may be intentionally listed here more than once.

James H. Crook, Jr., CEO
Thomas W. Butts, Pres.
Thomas W. Butts, COO
John A. Kane, CFO
Robert F. Galin, Sr. VP-Sales
Cynthia B. Limoges, VP-Human Resources
Michael J. Whalen, CIO/VP-Info. Systems Support & Planning
John A. Kane, Sr. VP-Admin
Robert W. Baker, Jr., Sr. VP/General Counsel/Corp. Sec.
Margo C. Happer, VP-Corp. Comm.
Margo C. Happer, VP-Investor Rel.
John A. Kane, Sr. VP-Finance/Treas.
Richard E. Tarrant, Chmn.

Phone: 802-862-1022   Fax: 802-862-6848
Toll-Free:
Address: 40 IDX Dr., Burlington, VT 05402-1070 US

GROWTH PLANS/SPECIAL FEATURES:

IDX Systems is a leading provider of software, services and technologies for health care organizations. The company's Flowcast division markets business performance solutions for large group practices, academic medical centers and hospitals. Flowcast solutions, marketed under the name IDXtend for the Web, include products for patient access, financial management, decision support, document management and connectivity. The Carecast system division represents the next generation of electronic clinical information solutions, delivering sub-second response time and 99.9% up-time reliability to support clinical environments. The system enables rapid access to patient records across the care continuum, from admission to discharge, including pharmacy and ambulatory care. It integrates orders, results, pharmacy and clinical documentation with administrative and financial processes for scheduling, registration, admitting, charging and billing. The Groupcast practice management division provides solutions for patient management, financial management, administrative efficiency and decision support for medical group practices, management service organizations and other billing organizations that service the health care marketplace. Groupcast solutions help clients streamline patient flow and business processes such as patient interactive web services, scheduling, referral management, eligibility, demographic management, collections, document imaging and decision support tools. Relational reporting using Microsoft SQL Server turns data into meaningful information for decision makers. The Imagecast radiology information system automates and manages a radiology department's clinical, demographic, administrative, billing, scheduling and image management information. The company recently sold its EDiX Corp. subsidiary, which offered Internet-based services for patients and physicians and e-commerce services for efficient health care delivery, to Spheris, a medical transcription company, for approximately $64 million.

IDX offers its employees a child care resource center; medical, dental and vision insurance; an employee assistance program; short- and long-term disability; and tuition assistance. New hires start with three weeks of vacation.

FINANCIALS:
Sales and profits are in thousands of dollars—add 000 to get the full amount. Year 2004 note: Complete fiscal 2004 results were not available for all companies at press time. For this company, year 2004 is for 9 months.

2004 Sales: $369,016 (9 months)   2004 Profits: $19,432 (9 months)
2003 Sales: $400,000   2003 Profits: $58,400
2002 Sales: $348,000   2002 Profits: $10,000
2001 Sales: $379,900   2001 Profits: $-8,600
2000 Sales: $341,893   2000 Profits: $-35,968

Stock Ticker: IDXC
Employees: 2,048
Fiscal Year Ends: 12/31

SALARIES/BENEFITS:
Pension Plan: ESOP Stock Plan: Profit Sharing: Top Exec. Salary: $500,000   Bonus: $113,200
Savings Plan: Y   Stock Purch. Plan: Y   Second Exec. Salary: $290,000   Bonus: $217,500

OTHER THOUGHTS:
Apparent Top Female Officers: 2
Hot Spot for Advancement for Women/Minorities:

LOCATIONS: ("Y" = Yes)
West:	Southwest:	Midwest:	Southeast:	Northeast:	International:
Y	Y	Y	Y	Y	

Note: Financial information, benefits and other data can change quickly and may vary from those stated here.

IMMUCOR INC

www.immucor.com

Industry Group Code: 339113 Ranks within this company's industry group: Sales: 93 Profits: 62

Insurance/HMO/PPO:	Drugs:	Equipment/Supplies:	Hospitals/Clinics:	Services:	Health Care:
Insurance:	Manufacturer:	Manufacturer: Y	Acute Care:	Diagnostics:	Home Health:
Managed Care:	Distributor:	Distributor: Y	Sub-Acute Care:	Labs/Testing:	Long-Term Care:
Utilization Mgmt.:	Specialty Pharm.:	Leasing/Finance:	Outpatient Surgery:	Staffing:	Physical Therapy:
Payment Proc.:	Vitamins/Nutri.:	Information Sys.:	Phys. Rehab. Center:	Waste Disposal:	Phys. Practice Mgmt.:
	Clinical Trials:		Psychiatric Clinics:	Specialty Services:	

TYPES OF BUSINESS:
Equipment-Blood Testing
Automated Blood Bank Instruments
Blood Reagents

BRANDS/DIVISIONS/AFFILIATES:
ABS2000
ROSYS Plato
DIAS Plus
Galileo
I-TRAC Plus
BioTek
Capture
ReACT

CONTACTS: Note: Officers with more than one job title may be intentionally listed here more than once.
Edward L. Gallup, CEO
Gioacchino De Chirico, Pres.
Steven C. Ramsey, CFO
Michael C. Poynter, VP-Sales
Ralph A. Eatz, Sr. VP/Chief Scientific Officer
Gioacchino DeChirico, Pres., Immucor Italia
Didier L. Lanson, Dir.-European Oper.
Bill Weiss, Dir.-U.S. Sales
Marilyn Moulds, VP-Reference & Education Services
Edward L. Gallup, Chmn.

Phone: 770-441-2051 Fax: 770-441-3807
Toll-Free: 800-829-2553
Address: 3130 Gateway Dr., Norcross, GA 30091-5625 US

GROWTH PLANS/SPECIAL FEATURES:
Immucor, Inc. develops, manufactures and sells a line of reagents and automated systems used primarily by hospitals, clinical laboratories and blood banks for tests that detect and identify properties of the cell and serum components of human blood prior to a blood transfusion. The company's blood bank systems include ABS2000, ROSYS Plato, DIAS Plus, Multireader Plus and I-TRAC Plus. Immucor has an ongoing agreement with Bio-Tek, a subsidiary of Lionheart Technologies, for the development of an automated blood bank analyzer, the ABS2000. The firm also distributes laboratory equipment designed to automate certain blood testing procedures and to be used in conjunction with its Capture and ReACT products. In addition, Immucor has received FDA approval for its proprietary solid-phase blood testing system, which is easier to interpret than the subjective results sometimes obtained from existing agglutination technology. Immucor's latest automated walk-away instrument for the hospital blood bank transfusion laboratory is the Galileo, which recently received clearance for distribution from the Japanese and Canadian health ministries. The product is still awaiting FDA approval.

FINANCIALS: Sales and profits are in thousands of dollars—add 000 to get the full amount. Year 2004 note: Complete fiscal 2004 results were not available for all companies at press time. For this company, year 2004 is for 12 months.

2004 Sales: $112,558 (12 months)	2004 Profits: $12,538 (12 months)	Stock Ticker: BLUD
2003 Sales: $98,300	2003 Profits: $14,400	Employees: 531
2002 Sales: $84,100	2002 Profits: $8,800	Fiscal Year Ends: 5/31
2001 Sales: $69,400	2001 Profits: $-8,000	
2000 Sales: $76,500	2000 Profits: $2,800	

SALARIES/BENEFITS:
Pension Plan:	ESOP Stock Plan:	Profit Sharing:	Top Exec. Salary: $329,500	Bonus: $40,391
Savings Plan: Y	Stock Purch. Plan:		Second Exec. Salary: $309,650	Bonus: $25,399

OTHER THOUGHTS:
Apparent Top Female Officers: 1
Hot Spot for Advancement for Women/Minorities:

LOCATIONS: ("Y" = Yes)
West:	Southwest: Y	Midwest:	Southeast: Y	Northeast:	International: Y

ic
IMPATH INC

www.impath.com

Industry Group Code: 541690 Ranks within this company's industry group: Sales: Profits:

Insurance/HMO/PPO:	Drugs:	Equipment/Supplies:	Hospitals/Clinics:	Services:		Health Care:
Insurance:	Manufacturer:	Manufacturer:	Acute Care:	Diagnostics:	Y	Home Health:
Managed Care:	Distributor:	Distributor:	Sub-Acute Care:	Labs/Testing:		Long-Term Care:
Utilization Mgmt.:	Specialty Pharm.:	Leasing/Finance:	Outpatient Surgery:	Staffing:		Physical Therapy:
Payment Proc.:	Vitamins/Nutri.:	Information Sys.: Y	Phys. Rehab. Center:	Waste Disposal:		Phys. Practice Mgmt.:
	Clinical Trials:		Psychiatric Clinics:	Specialty Services:	Y	

TYPES OF BUSINESS:
Consulting-Patient-Specific Information
Cancer Treatment Data
Information Services

BRANDS/DIVISIONS/AFFILIATES:
Genzyme Genetics

CONTACTS: Note: Officers with more than one job title may be intentionally listed here more than once.
Carter H. Eckert, CEO
Iris D. Daniels, VP-Corp. Comm.
Iris D. Daniels, VP-Investor Rel.
Carter H. Eckert, Chmn.

Phone: 212-698-0300 Fax: 212-258-2137
Toll-Free: 800-447-5816
Address: 521 W. 57th St., 6th Fl., New York, NY 10019 US

GROWTH PLANS/SPECIAL FEATURES:
IMPATH, Inc., a subsidiary of Genzyme Genetics, facilitiates the clinical application of advanced technologies in community hospitals in order to enable clinicians to make better treatment decisions for cancer patients. The company works exclusively on cancer analysis, combining advanced technologies and medical expertise to provide patient-specific diagnostic, prognostic and treatment information to physicians treating the disiaease. IMPATH operates in three divisions. The physician services division, which accounts for approximately 81% of revenues, provides patient-specific cancer diagnostic and prognostic information, with particular expertise in difficult-to-diagnose tumors, prognostic profiles in breast cancer and other cancers as well as lymphoma and leukemia analyses. The predictive oncology division provides integrated services and information resources for genomics, biopharmaceutical, diagnostic products and pharmaceutical companies in the development and commercialization of targeted gene- and protein-based therapies. The information services division licenses tumor registry software to hospitals that treat cancer patients. As an increased understanding of the molecular basis of cancer leads to new evaluation methods and therapeutic tools, IMPATH expects that the information it provides will become increasingly significant in optimizing the management of all phases of cancer, including cancer predisposition, diagnosis, prognosis, treatment determination and patient follow-up. In March 2004, IMPATH entered into a multi-year provider participation agreement with Humana, Inc., wherein it will provide Humana members with its full suite of cancer diagnostic and prognostic services. Genzyme acquired the company in May 2004.

FINANCIALS: Sales and profits are in thousands of dollars—add 000 to get the full amount. Year 2004 note: Complete fiscal 2004 results were not available for all companies at press time. For this company, year 2004 is for months.

2004 Sales: $ (months) 2004 Profits: $ (months)
2003 Sales: $ 2003 Profits: $
2002 Sales: $188,100 2002 Profits: $10,500
2001 Sales: $189,600 2001 Profits: $11,000
2000 Sales: $138,200 2000 Profits: $13,000

Stock Ticker: Subsidiary
Employees: 1,219
Fiscal Year Ends: 12/31

SALARIES/BENEFITS:
Pension Plan: ESOP Stock Plan: Profit Sharing: Top Exec. Salary: $365,000   Bonus: $294,500
Savings Plan: Y   Stock Purch. Plan: Second Exec. Salary: $325,000   Bonus: $152,000

OTHER THOUGHTS:
Apparent Top Female Officers: 1
Hot Spot for Advancement for Women/Minorities:

LOCATIONS: ("Y" = Yes)
West:	Southwest:	Midwest:	Southeast:	Northeast:	International:
Y	Y			Y	

IMS HEALTH INC

www.imshealth.com

Industry Group Code: 511200 **Ranks within this company's industry group:** Sales: 1 Profits: 1

Insurance/HMO/PPO:	Drugs:	Equipment/Supplies:	Hospitals/Clinics:	Services:	Health Care:
Insurance:	Manufacturer:	Manufacturer:	Acute Care:	Diagnostics:	Home Health:
Managed Care:	Distributor: Y	Distributor:	Sub-Acute Care:	Labs/Testing:	Long-Term Care:
Utilization Mgmt.:	Specialty Pharm.:	Leasing/Finance:	Outpatient Surgery:	Staffing:	Physical Therapy:
Payment Proc.:	Vitamins/Nutri.:	Information Sys.: Y	Phys. Rehab. Center:	Waste Disposal:	Phys. Practice Mgmt.:
	Clinical Trials:		Psychiatric Clinics:	Specialty Services: Y	

TYPES OF BUSINESS:
Software-Sales Management & Market Research
Pharmaceutical Sales Tracking
Health Care Databases
Consulting Services
Physician Profiling
Industry Audits

BRANDS/DIVISIONS/AFFILIATES:
United Research China Shanghai
IMS Inpatient Therapy Profiler
IMS Knowledge Link 2

CONTACTS:
Note: Officers with more than one job title may be intentionally listed here more than once.

David M. Thomas, CEO
David R. Carlucci, Pres.
David R. Carlucci, COO
Nancy E. Cooper, Sr.VP/CFO
Robert H. Steinfeld, Sr. VP/General Counsel & Corp. Sec.
Murray L. Aitken, Sr. VP-Corp. Strategy
Caroline Lappetito, Dir.-U.S. Public Rel.
William J. Nelligan, Pres., IMS Asia Pacific
Tatsuyuki Saeki, Pres.,-IMS Japan
Bruce F. Boggs, Pres., IMS Americas
Gilles V.J. Pajot, Exec. VP/Pres.-IMS European Region
David M. Thomas, Chmn.

Phone: 203-319-4700   **Fax:** 203-319-4701
Toll-Free:
Address: 1499 Post Rd., Fairfield, CT 06430 US

GROWTH PLANS/SPECIAL FEATURES:
IMS Health, Inc. is one of the world's leading providers of information solutions to the pharmaceutical and health care industries. Key services offered by the company include market research for prescription and over-the-counter pharmaceutical products, sales management information to optimize sales force productivity and consulting services to assist in decision-making. Due to the company's international presence, with more than 100 offices worldwide, half of its sales come from outside the U.S. IMS Health provides syndicated pharmaceutical, medical, hospital, promotional and prescription audits in 45 countries. In addition, the company performs sales territory reports, prescription tracking reports and doctor profiling services. Customers of the firm include major pharmaceutical manufacturers, biotechnology firms, financial analysts, government and regulatory agencies, researchers and educators. IMS Health utilizes powerful database management tools in processing over one billion medical transactions a month. The firm captures data on 75% of prescription sales worldwide and 90% of U.S. prescription sales. It tracks more than one million products from more than 3,000 active drug manufacturers. The company then takes its accumulated data and turns it industry into trends, perspectives and forecasts. In recent news, IMS Health acquired United Research China Shanghai, which offers comprehensive coverage of China's over-the-counter market, as well as consumer health consulting services. The company entered into an exclusive co-marketing agreement with Premier Healthcare Informatics for IMS Inpatient Therapy Profiler, a new information service designed to provide better insights into hospital drug and medical device utilization and disease treatment. The firm announced an agreement with the World Health Organization Collaborating Centre for international drug monitoring for its drug dictionary. IMS launched IMS Knowledge Link 2, an enhanced version of its premier web-based information resource for its customers.

FINANCIALS:
Sales and profits are in thousands of dollars—add 000 to get the full amount. Year 2004 note: Complete fiscal 2004 results were not available for all companies at press time. For this company, year 2004 is for 9 months.

2004 Sales: $1,125,330 (9 months)   2004 Profits: $211,831 (9 months)
2003 Sales: $1,381,800   2003 Profits: $639,000
2002 Sales: $1,428,100   2002 Profits: $266,100
2001 Sales: $1,332,900   2001 Profits: $185,400
2000 Sales: $1,424,400   2000 Profits: $120,800

Stock Ticker: RX
Employees: 6,000
Fiscal Year Ends: 12/31

SALARIES/BENEFITS:
Pension Plan: Y   ESOP Stock Plan: Profit Sharing: Top Exec. Salary: $787,500   Bonus: $984,375
Savings Plan: Y   Stock Purch. Plan: Second Exec. Salary: $550,000   Bonus: $660,000

OTHER THOUGHTS:
Apparent Top Female Officers: 2
Hot Spot for Advancement for Women/Minorities:

LOCATIONS: ("Y" = Yes)
West:	Southwest:	Midwest:	Southeast:	Northeast:	International:
Y				Y	Y

Note: Financial information, benefits and other data can change quickly and may vary from those stated here.

INAMED CORP

www.inamedcorp.com

Industry Group Code: 339113 **Ranks within this company's industry group:** Sales: 53 Profits: 32

Insurance/HMO/PPO:	Drugs:	Equipment/Supplies:	Hospitals/Clinics:	Services:	Health Care:
Insurance: Managed Care: Utilization Mgmt.: Payment Proc.:	Manufacturer: Distributor: Specialty Pharm.: Vitamins/Nutri.: Clinical Trials:	Manufacturer: Y Distributor: Leasing/Finance: Information Sys.:	Acute Care: Sub-Acute Care: Outpatient Surgery: Phys. Rehab. Center: Psychiatric Clinics:	Diagnostics: Labs/Testing: Staffing: Waste Disposal: Specialty Services:	Home Health: Long-Term Care: Physical Therapy: Phys. Practice Mgmt.:

TYPES OF BUSINESS:
Supplies-Prostheses
Breast Implants
Tissue Expanders
Facial Implants
Obesity Products

BRANDS/DIVISIONS/AFFILIATES:
INAMED Aesthetics
INAMED Health
INAMED International
Hylaform Plus

CONTACTS:
Note: Officers with more than one job title may be intentionally listed here more than once.
Nicholas L. Teti, CEO
Nicholas L. Teti, Pres.
Vicente Trelles, Exec. VP/COO
Declan Daly, Exec. VP/CFO
Patricia Cooper, VP-Human Resources
Joseph A. Newcomb, Exec. VP/General Counsel
Robert S. Vaters, Exec. VP-Strategy & Corp. Dev.
Hani M. Zeini, Exec. VP-Aesthetics
Ronald J. Ehmsen, VP-Clinical & Regulatory Affairs
Joseph A. Newcomb, Corp. Sec.
Nicholas L. Teti, Chmn.

Phone: 805-692-5400 **Fax:** 805-692-5432
Toll-Free:
Address: 5540 Ekwill St., Ste. D, Santa Barbara, CA 93111-2919 US

GROWTH PLANS/SPECIAL FEATURES:
Inamed Corporation is a global surgical and medical device company engaged in the development, manufacturing and marketing of products for the plastic and reconstructive surgery, aesthetic medicine and obesity markets. The company operates through two primary subsidiaries, INAMED Aesthetics and INAMED Health. INAMED Aesthetics offers a line of breast implants for augmentation and reconstruction surgeries following mastectomies as well as collagen-based facial implants to correct facial wrinkles and improve lip definition. INAMED Health develops and markets medical devices to treat obesity using minimally invasive surgery. INAMED International extends the company's sales, marketing and manufacturing presence to locations in Canada, Germany, France, Spain, Italy, Ireland, the U.K., Costa Rica, Japan and Australia. In recent news, Inamed announced that the FDA is considering reintroducing silicon breast implants in the U.S. Inamed is one of the largest produces of silicon breast implants for the export market. The FDA also recently approved Hylaform Plus, a product developed and marketed in partnership with Genzyme Corporation for the correction of moderate to severe facial wrinkles and folds. The product won Allure Magazine's 2004 Best of Beauty Breakthrough Award.

FINANCIALS:
Sales and profits are in thousands of dollars—add 000 to get the full amount. Year 2004 note: Complete fiscal 2004 results were not available for all companies at press time. For this company, year 2004 is for 9 months.

2004 Sales: $280,600 (9 months)	2004 Profits: $44,200 (9 months)	**Stock Ticker:** IMDC
2003 Sales: $332,600	2003 Profits: $53,000	Employees: 1,200
2002 Sales: $275,700	2002 Profits: $32,900	Fiscal Year Ends: 12/31
2001 Sales: $238,100	2001 Profits: $21,000	
2000 Sales: $240,100	2000 Profits: $37,000	

SALARIES/BENEFITS:
Pension Plan: Y	ESOP Stock Plan:	Profit Sharing:	Top Exec. Salary: $452,698	Bonus: $625,100
Savings Plan: Y	Stock Purch. Plan: Y		Second Exec. Salary: $296,068	Bonus: $315,000

OTHER THOUGHTS:
Apparent Top Female Officers: 1
Hot Spot for Advancement for Women/Minorities:

LOCATIONS: ("Y" = Yes)
West:	Southwest:	Midwest:	Southeast:	Northeast:	International:
Y					Y

INCYTE CORP

www.incyte.com

Industry Group Code: 541710   Ranks within this company's industry group: Sales: 10   Profits: 11

Insurance/HMO/PPO:	Drugs:	Equipment/Supplies:	Hospitals/Clinics:	Services:	Health Care:
Insurance:	Manufacturer:	Manufacturer:	Acute Care:	Diagnostics:	Home Health:
Managed Care:	Distributor:	Distributor:	Sub-Acute Care:	Labs/Testing:	Long-Term Care:
Utilization Mgmt.:	Specialty Pharm.:	Leasing/Finance:	Outpatient Surgery:	Staffing:	Physical Therapy:
Payment Proc.:	Vitamins/Nutri.:	Information Sys.: Y	Phys. Rehab. Center:	Waste Disposal:	Phys. Practice Mgmt.:
	Clinical Trials:		Psychiatric Clinics:	Specialty Services: Y	

TYPES OF BUSINESS:
Research-Genetic Information (Drug Discovery)
Genomic Databases
Gene Expression Services

GROWTH PLANS/SPECIAL FEATURES:
Incyte Corp., formerly Incyte Genomics, was historically involved with marketing and selling access to its proprietary genomic information databases, the BioKnowledge Library (BKL). The company underwent a restructuring in early 2004, and though it will still offer customers access to BKL, Incyte is now focused on drug discovery and development. The firm intends to use its intellectual property and genomic information to become a leader in therapeutic small-molecule, secreted protein and antibody discoveries for use against HIV, cancer, inflammation and metabolic diseases like diabetes and obesity. The firm's lead product candidate, in-licensed from Pharmasset, Ltd., is Reverset, a reverse transcription inhibitor that is currently in Phase II clinical trials for use against HIV.

BRANDS/DIVISIONS/AFFILIATES:
Incyte Genomics
BioKnowledge Library
Reverset

CONTACTS:
Note: Officers with more than one job title may be intentionally listed here more than once.
Paul A. Friedman, CEO
Paul A. Friedman, Pres.
David C. Hastings, CFO/Exec. VP
Paula J. Swain, Exec. VP-Human Resources
Patricia A. Schreck, Exec. VP/General Counsel
Jim Merryweather, Exec. VP-Bus. Dev.
Pamela M. Murphy, VP-Corp. Comm.
Pamela M. Murphy, VP-Investor Rel.
John A. Keller, Exec. VP/Chief Bus. Officer
Brian W. Metcalf, Exec. VP/Chief Drug Discovery Scientist
Richard U. DeSchutter, Chmn.

Phone: 302-498-6700   Fax: 302-425-2750
Toll-Free:
Address: Rte 141 & Henry Clay Rd., Bldg. E336, Wilmington, DE 19880 US

FINANCIALS:
Sales and profits are in thousands of dollars—add 000 to get the full amount. Year 2004 note: Complete fiscal 2004 results were not available for all companies at press time. For this company, year 2004 is for 9 months.

2004 Sales: $15,198 (9 months)   2004 Profits: $-127,291 (9 months)
2003 Sales: $47,092   2003 Profits: $-166,463
2002 Sales: $101,612   2002 Profits: $-136,885
2001 Sales: $219,300   2001 Profits: $-183,200
2000 Sales: $194,200   2000 Profits: $-29,700

Stock Ticker: INCY
Employees: 454
Fiscal Year Ends: 12/31

SALARIES/BENEFITS:
Pension Plan: ESOP Stock Plan: Profit Sharing: Top Exec. Salary: $642,308   Bonus: $276,250
Savings Plan: Stock Purch. Plan: Second Exec. Salary: $473,649   Bonus: $217,000

OTHER THOUGHTS:
Apparent Top Female Officers: 3
Hot Spot for Advancement for Women/Minorities: Y

LOCATIONS: ("Y" = Yes)
West:	Southwest:	Midwest:	Southeast:	Northeast:	International:
				Y	

INSTITUT STRAUMANN AG

www.straumann.com

Industry Group Code: 339113 **Ranks within this company's industry group:** Sales: 58 Profits: 26

Insurance/HMO/PPO:	Drugs:		Equipment/Supplies:		Hospitals/Clinics:	Services:	Health Care:	
Insurance:	Manufacturer:	Y	Manufacturer:	Y	Acute Care:	Diagnostics:	Home Health:	
Managed Care:	Distributor:		Distributor:		Sub-Acute Care:	Labs/Testing:	Long-Term Care:	
Utilization Mgmt.:	Specialty Pharm.:		Leasing/Finance:		Outpatient Surgery:	Staffing:	Physical Therapy:	
Payment Proc.:	Vitamins/Nutri.:		Information Sys.:		Phys. Rehab. Center:	Waste Disposal:	Phys. Practice Mgmt.:	
	Clinical Trials:				Psychiatric Clinics:	Specialty Services:		

TYPES OF BUSINESS:
Dental Implants
Dental Tissue Regeneration
Dental Drugs, Manufacturing

BRANDS/DIVISIONS/AFFILIATES:
Straumann Dental Implant System
Emdogain
Biora AB
SynOcta
TE

CONTACTS:
Note: Officers with more than one job title may be intentionally listed here more than once.

Gilbert Achermann, CEO
Martin Gartsch, CFO
Thomas Jaberg, Head-Mktg. Support Div.
Dieter Lipp, Head-Oper. Div.
Markus Koller, Head-Implants Div.
Sandro Matter, Head-Biologics Div.
Rudolf Maag, Chmn.

Phone: 41-61-965-11-11 **Fax:** 41-61-965-11-06
Toll-Free:
Address: Hauptstrasse 26d, Waldenburg, CH-4437 Switzerland

GROWTH PLANS/SPECIAL FEATURES:

Institut Straumann AG is the world's second-largest producer of dental implants and a major provider of dental tissue regeneration products. Based in Switzerland, Straumann maintains subsidiaries and distributors in countries throughout the world, with its most important markets being Germany and the United States. The company is organized into two segments, the implants division and the biologics division. The implants division produces a range of products for the Straumann Dental Implant System, which include implants, prosthetic components and instruments. Brand names include the TE implant and the SynOcta prosthetic product lines. The biologics division focuses on biotechnology for the reconstruction of dental bone and soft tissue. The company acquired Biora AB, the developer of Enamel Matrix Derivative (EMD) protein, as a major stepping stone in the expansion of its biologics activities. Its Emdogain gel for the treatment of periodontitis has firmly positioned the company in the market for periodontal tissue regeneration. In 2004 and 2005 respectively, Straumann plans to launch a bone substitute material and a new type of membrane used to cover bone tissue and protect bone defects during tissue regeneration. In recent news, the company broke ground in Andover, Massachusetts for a new combined U.S. headquarters, training and production center with an anticipated completion date in mid-2005.

FINANCIALS:
Sales and profits are in thousands of dollars—add 000 to get the full amount. Year 2004 note: Complete fiscal 2004 results were not available for all companies at press time. For this company, year 2004 is for months.

2004 Sales: $ (months)
2003 Sales: $269,400
2002 Sales: $215,350
2001 Sales: $
2000 Sales: $

2004 Profits: $ (months)
2003 Profits: $62,900
2002 Profits: $43,860
2001 Profits: $
2000 Profits: $

Stock Ticker: Foreign
Employees: 903
Fiscal Year Ends: 12/31

SALARIES/BENEFITS:
| Pension Plan: | ESOP Stock Plan: | Profit Sharing: | Top Exec. Salary: $ | Bonus: $ |
| Savings Plan: | Stock Purch. Plan: | | Second Exec. Salary: $ | Bonus: $ |

OTHER THOUGHTS:
Apparent Top Female Officers:
Hot Spot for Advancement for Women/Minorities:

LOCATIONS: ("Y" = Yes)
West:	Southwest:	Midwest:	Southeast:	Northeast:	International:
Y				Y	Y

Note: Financial information, benefits and other data can change quickly and may vary from those stated here.

INSTRUMENTARIUM CORPORATION
www.instrumentarium.com

Industry Group Code: 339113   Ranks within this company's industry group: Sales: Profits:

Insurance/HMO/PPO:	Drugs:	Equipment/Supplies:		Hospitals/Clinics:	Services:		Health Care:	
Insurance:	Manufacturer:	Manufacturer:	Y	Acute Care:	Diagnostics:		Home Health:	
Managed Care:	Distributor:	Distributor:		Sub-Acute Care:	Labs/Testing:		Long-Term Care:	
Utilization Mgmt.:	Specialty Pharm.:	Leasing/Finance:		Outpatient Surgery:	Staffing:		Physical Therapy:	
Payment Proc.:	Vitamins/Nutri.:	Information Sys.:	Y	Phys. Rehab. Center:	Waste Disposal:		Phys. Practice Mgmt.:	
	Clinical Trials:			Psychiatric Clinics:	Specialty Services:	Y		

TYPES OF BUSINESS:
Equipment-Patient Monitoring Devices
Anesthesia Systems
Clinical Information Systems
Consulting and Integration Services
Diagnostic Imaging Equipment
Infant Care Equipment

BRANDS/DIVISIONS/AFFILIATES:
GE Medical Systems
Spacelabs Medical, Inc.
Deio
Soredex
Medko
Datex-Ohmeda
Ultraview
Ohmeda Medical

CONTACTS:
Note: Officers with more than one job title may be intentionally listed here more than once.
Olli Rikkala, CEO
Olli Rikkala, Pres.
Peter Tchernych, VP-Project Sales
Ritva Sotamaa, General Counsel
Juhani Lassila, VP-Investor Rel.
Juhani Lassila, VP-Finance/Treas.

Phone: 358-10-394-11   Fax: 359-9-146-4172
Toll-Free:
Address: Kuortaneenkatu 2, Helsinki, 00031 Finland

GROWTH PLANS/SPECIAL FEATURES:
Instrumentarium Corporation, a subsidiary of GE Medical Systems, is a global leader in medical technology. The company operates through two segments: anesthesia and critical care, and medical equipment. The anesthesia and critical care segment, which accounts for 80% of sales, includes subsidiaries Datex-Ohmeda, Spacelabs Medical, Deio and Instrumed. Datex-Ohmeda supplies systems and solutions for operating rooms and critical care areas of the hospital, including anesthesia systems, equipment and services, patient monitors, ventilators and workstations, such as the System 5 Integrated Anesthesia Workstation. Spacelabs Medical oversees critical care patient monitoring, anesthesia delivery, diagnostic cardiology and clinical information systems and provides patient monitors and clinical information systems. Among its products are the Ultraview Anesthesia Delivery System and the Ultraview Web Source. Deio provides clinical information management solutions. Instrumed provides installation, information system integration, training and technical support to customers in Finland. The company's medical equipment segment includes Soredex, Ohmeda Medical and Medko Medical. The medical equipment division develops, manufactures and markets diagnostic x-ray, mammography, dental and surgical imaging equipment. Soredex also provides diagnostic imaging equipment and manufactures dental imaging products. Ohmeda Medical manufactures infant care equipment such as infant incubators, warmers, jaundice management systems and vital signs monitors. Medko Medical provides customers with consulting, planning, delivery, installation, training and warranty services. General Electric acquired Instrumentarium through GE Finland in January 2004.

FINANCIALS:
Sales and profits are in thousands of dollars—add 000 to get the full amount. Year 2004 note: Complete fiscal 2004 results were not available for all companies at press time. For this company, year 2004 is for   months.

2004 Sales: $ (months)	2004 Profits: $ (months)	
2003 Sales: $	2003 Profits: $	Stock Ticker: Foreign
2002 Sales: $1,183,400	2002 Profits: $163,600	Employees: 1,177
2001 Sales: $242,100	2001 Profits: $-2,100	Fiscal Year Ends: 12/31
2000 Sales: $249,000	2000 Profits: $-4,700	

SALARIES/BENEFITS:
Pension Plan: Y   ESOP Stock Plan: Profit Sharing: Top Exec. Salary: $440,000   Bonus: $
Savings Plan: Y   Stock Purch. Plan: Second Exec. Salary: $200,000   Bonus: $

OTHER THOUGHTS:
Apparent Top Female Officers: 1
Hot Spot for Advancement for Women/Minorities:

LOCATIONS: ("Y" = Yes)
West:	Southwest:	Midwest:	Southeast:	Northeast:	International:
		Y			Y

INTEGRA LIFESCIENCES HOLDINGS CORP   www.integra-ls.com

Industry Group Code: 339113   Ranks within this company's industry group: Sales: 70   Profits: 48

Insurance/HMO/PPO:	Drugs:	Equipment/Supplies:	Hospitals/Clinics:	Services:	Health Care:
Insurance:	Manufacturer: Y	Manufacturer: Y	Acute Care:	Diagnostics:	Home Health:
Managed Care:	Distributor:	Distributor:	Sub-Acute Care:	Labs/Testing:	Long-Term Care:
Utilization Mgmt.:	Specialty Pharm.:	Leasing/Finance:	Outpatient Surgery:	Staffing:	Physical Therapy:
Payment Proc.:	Vitamins/Nutri.:	Information Sys.:	Phys. Rehab. Center:	Waste Disposal:	Phys. Practice Mgmt.:
	Clinical Trials:		Psychiatric Clinics:	Specialty Services:	

TYPES OF BUSINESS:
Drugs-Human Tissue
Skin Replacement Products
Absorbable Medical Products
Tissue Regeneration Technology
Neurosurgery Products

BRANDS/DIVISIONS/AFFILIATES:
Integra NeuroSciences
Integra Plastic and Reconstructive Surgery
JARIT Surgical Instruments, Inc.
DuraGen Dural Graft Matrix
NeuraGen Nerve Guide
INTEGRA Dermal Regeneration Template
INTEGRA Bilayer Matrix Wound Dressing
BUDDE Halo Retractor System

CONTACTS: Note: Officers with more than one job title may be intentionally listed here more than once.
Stuart M. Essig, CEO
Stuart M. Essig, Pres.
Gerard S. Carlozzi, Exec. VP/COO
Deborah A. Leonetti, Sr. VP-Global Mktg.
Wilma J. Davis, VP-Human Resources
Randy Gottlieb, VP/CIO
Donald R. Nociolo, Sr. VP-Mfg. Oper.
John B. Henneman, III, Exec. VP/Chief Admin. Officer
Richard D. Gorelick, VP/General Counsel
David B. Holtz, Sr. VP-Finance/Treas.
Simon J. Archibald, VP-Clinical Affairs
Judith E. O'Grady, Sr. VP-Quality, Regulatory and Clinical Affairs
Leigh DeFilippis, VP/Corp. Controller
Robert D. Paltridge, Sr. VP-Global Sales
Richard E. Caruso, Chmn.

Phone: 609-936-2239   Fax: 609-799-3297
Toll-Free: 800-654-0500
Address: 311 Enterprise Dr., Plainsboro, NJ 08536 US

GROWTH PLANS/SPECIAL FEATURES:
Integra Lifesciences Holdings Corporation develops, manufactures and markets medical devices, implants and biomaterials for use in neurotrauma, neurosurgery, plastic and reconstructive surgery and general surgery. The company's product lines include traditional medical devices, such as monitoring and drainage systems, surgical instruments and fixation systems, as well as innovative tissue repair products, such as the DuraGen Dural Graft Matrix, the NeuraGen Nerve Guide, the INTEGRA Dermal Regeneration Template and the INTEGRA Bilayer Matrix Wound Dressing, which incorporate Integra's proprietary absorbable implant technology. Products focus on injuries involving the brain, cranium, spine and central nervous system and the repair and reconstruction of soft tissue. They are marketed and sold through subsidiaries Integra NeuroSciences and Integra Plastic and Reconstructive Surgery, through a distributor network managed by subsidiary JARIT Surgical Instruments, Inc. and through strategic alliances. Through acquisitions and internal growth, the firm has rapidly grown into a leading provider of products used in the diagnosis, monitoring and treatment of chronic diseases and acute injuries. The company has completed over 15 acquisitions since 1999, the latest of which include obtaining the MAYFIELD Cranial Stabilization and Positioning Systems and the BUDDE Halo Retractor System from Schaerer Mayfield USA, Inc., as well as acquiring Berchtold Medizin-Elektronik GmbH, a German manufacturer and marketer of surgical products.

FINANCIALS:
Sales and profits are in thousands of dollars—add 000 to get the full amount. Year 2004 note: Complete fiscal 2004 results were not available for all companies at press time. For this company, year 2004 is for 9 months.

2004 Sales: $168,014 (9 months)   2004 Profits: $7,358 (9 months)
2003 Sales: $166,695   2003 Profits: $26,861
2002 Sales: $112,600   2002 Profits: $35,300
2001 Sales: $87,700   2001 Profits: $26,200
2000 Sales: $71,600   2000 Profits: $-11,400

Stock Ticker: IART
Employees: 880
Fiscal Year Ends: 12/31

SALARIES/BENEFITS:
Pension Plan: Y   ESOP Stock Plan: Profit Sharing: Top Exec. Salary: $402,821   Bonus: $
Savings Plan: Y   Stock Purch. Plan: Y   Second Exec. Salary: $297,132 Bonus: $

OTHER THOUGHTS:
Apparent Top Female Officers: 4
Hot Spot for Advancement for Women/Minorities: Y

LOCATIONS: ("Y" = Yes)

West:	Southwest:	Midwest:	Southeast:	Northeast:	International:
Y				Y	Y

Note: Financial information, benefits and other data can change quickly and may vary from those stated here.

INTEGRAMED AMERICA INC

www.integramed.com

Industry Group Code: 621111   Ranks within this company's industry group: Sales: 9   Profits: 7

Insurance/HMO/PPO:	Drugs:		Equipment/Supplies:		Hospitals/Clinics:		Services:		Health Care:	
Insurance: Managed Care: Utilization Mgmt.: Payment Proc.:	Manufacturer: Distributor: Specialty Pharm.: Vitamins/Nutri.: Clinical Trials:	Y	Manufacturer: Distributor: Leasing/Finance: Information Sys.:	Y Y	Acute Care: Sub-Acute Care: Outpatient Surgery: Phys. Rehab. Center: Psychiatric Clinics:		Diagnostics: Labs/Testing: Staffing: Waste Disposal: Specialty Services:	Y	Home Health: Long-Term Care: Physical Therapy: Phys. Practice Mgmt.:	Y

TYPES OF BUSINESS:
Physician Practice Management-Reproductive Services
Fertility-Related Pharmaceutical Distribution
Treatment Financing Programs

BRANDS/DIVISIONS/AFFILIATES:
FertilityWeb
IntegraMed Pharmaceutical Services, Inc.
IntegraMed Financial Services
FertilityMarKit
ARTWorks Practice Management Information System
FertilityPartners
ARTWorks Clinical Information System
Ivpcare, Inc.

CONTACTS: Note: Officers with more than one job title may be intentionally listed here more than once.
Gerardo Canet, CEO
Jay Higham, Pres.
Jay Higham, COO
John W. Hlywak, Jr., Sr. VP/CFO
Jay Higham, Sr. VP-Mktg. & Dev.
Lisa Marin, VP-Human Resources
Peter Cucchiara, VP-Info. Systems
Lisa Marin, VP-Admin.
Claude E. White, VP/General Counsel
Kevin Conroy, VP/Treas.
Pamela Schumann, VP-Consumer Services
Gerardo Canet, Chmn.

Phone: 914-253-8000   Fax: 914-253-8008
Toll-Free: 800-458-0044
Address: 2 Manhattanville Rd., 3rd Fl., Purchase, NY 10577 US

GROWTH PLANS/SPECIAL FEATURES:
IntegraMed America, Inc. offers products and services to patients and providers in the fertility industry. The company provides services to a network of 25 reproductive science centers including fertility clinics, embryologic laboratories and clinical research sites, which are all leaders in conventional fertility and assisted reproductive technology (ART) services. Its discrete service packages include FertilityWeb, a web site development, hosting and marketing service; FertilityPurchase, a group purchasing program; FertilityMarKit marketing and sales programs; ARTWorks Clinical Information System; ARTWorks Practice Management Information System; and FertilityPartners, its turnkey fertility center operation. FertilityPartners entails administrative services such as accounting, human resources and purchasing of supplies; servicing and financing patient accounts receivable; marketing and sales; and integrated information systems. In addition, the firm distributes pharmaceutical products and services directly to patients through subsidiary IntegraMed Pharmaceutical Services, Inc., which, through a partnership with Ivpcare, Inc., has access to programs such as CycleTrack and Education Matters. CycleTrack allows the firm to limit drug distribution to only the amount required by each individual patient, minimizing the cost to third-party payers and patients. Education Matters is a comprehensive patient education program that offers videos and written materials devoted to educating patients on the proper handling and administration of complex fertility products. Through IntegraMed Financial Services, the firm also provides patients with treatment financing programs, allowing them to select the option that best suits their financial situations from a full range of payment choices.

FINANCIALS: Sales and profits are in thousands of dollars—add 000 to get the full amount. Year 2004 note: Complete fiscal 2004 results were not available for all companies at press time. For this company, year 2004 is for 6 months.

2004 Sales: $52,287 (6 months)   2004 Profits: $507 (6 months)
2003 Sales: $93,690   2003 Profits: $1,044
2002 Sales: $88,200   2002 Profits: $1,100
2001 Sales: $74,800   2001 Profits: $6,500
2000 Sales: $57,900   2000 Profits: $1,900

Stock Ticker: INMD
Employees: 700
Fiscal Year Ends: 12/31

SALARIES/BENEFITS:
Pension Plan: ESOP Stock Plan: Profit Sharing: Top Exec. Salary: $275,000   Bonus: $24,750
Savings Plan: Stock Purch. Plan: Second Exec. Salary: $206,000   Bonus: $16,480

OTHER THOUGHTS:
Apparent Top Female Officers: 2
Hot Spot for Advancement for Women/Minorities:

LOCATIONS: ("Y" = Yes)
West:	Southwest:	Midwest:	Southeast:	Northeast:	International:
Y	Y	Y	Y	Y	

ns
INTERMAGNETICS GENERAL CORP

www.igc.com

Industry Group Code: 335929 Ranks within this company's industry group: Sales: 1 Profits: 1

Insurance/HMO/PPO:	Drugs:	Equipment/Supplies:		Hospitals/Clinics:	Services:	Health Care:
Insurance:	Manufacturer:	Manufacturer:	Y	Acute Care:	Diagnostics:	Home Health:
Managed Care:	Distributor:	Distributor:	Y	Sub-Acute Care:	Labs/Testing:	Long-Term Care:
Utilization Mgmt.:	Specialty Pharm.:	Leasing/Finance:		Outpatient Surgery:	Staffing:	Physical Therapy:
Payment Proc.:	Vitamins/Nutri.:	Information Sys.:		Phys. Rehab. Center:	Waste Disposal:	Phys. Practice Mgmt.:
	Clinical Trials:			Psychiatric Clinics:	Specialty Services:	

TYPES OF BUSINESS:
Superconducting Magnets, Wire & Cable Manufacturing
Magnetic Resonance Imaging Systems
Radio-Frequency Coils
Cryogenic Applications
Superconductivity Technology

BRANDS/DIVISIONS/AFFILIATES:
IGC-Medical Advances, Inc.
IGC-Polycold Systems, Inc.
SuperPower, Inc.
MRI Devices Corp.
Matrix Fault Current Limiter

CONTACTS:
Note: Officers with more than one job title may be intentionally listed here more than once.

Glenn H. Epstein, CEO
Glenn H. Epstein, Pres.
Michael K. Burke, Exec. VP/CFO
Kevin Lake, VP-Human Resources
Katherine M. Sheehan, General Counsel
Thomas O'Brien, Exec. VP-Corp. Dev.
Leo Blecher, Sector Pres.-MRI
Philip J. Pellegrino, Sector Pres.-Energy Tech.
David E. Thielman, VP/Mgr.-Invivo
Glenn H. Epstein, Chmn.

Phone: 518-782-1122   **Fax:** 518-786-8216
Toll-Free:
Address: 450 Old Niskayuna Rd., Latham, NY 12210-0461 US

GROWTH PLANS/SPECIAL FEATURES:
Intermagnetics General Corp. has a 30-year history as a leading global developer and manufacturer of superconducting materials, radio-frequency coils, magnets and devices utilizing low- and high-temperature superconductors and cryogenic refrigeration systems. The firm sells its products primarily in the magnetic resonance imaging (MRI), analytical instrumentation and industrial processing markets. Intermagnetics is also investing in the development of high-temperature superconducting materials and products for the energy technology market, specifically transmission and distribution of electric power. The company operates through three products segments: MRI, instrumentation and energy technology. The MRI segment principally provides products to the diagnostic imaging market. Its magnet business group develops, manufactures and sells low-temperature superconducting magnets. The segment also manufactures radio-frequency coils through IGC-Medical Advances, Inc. The instrumentation segment provides cryogenic refrigeration equipment used primarily in ultra-high-vacuum applications, industrial coatings, analytical instrumentation and semiconductor processing and testing through subsidiary IGC-Polycold Systems, Inc. Through subsidiary SuperPower, Inc., the energy technology segment is developing second-generation high-temperature superconducting materials and devices designed to enhance capacity, reliability and quality of electrical power transmission and distribution. In 2002, the company completed two major divestitures, selling IGC-Advanced Superconductor and IGC-APD Cryogenics, Inc. In recent news, Intermagnetics expanded its strategic supply agreement with Philips Medical Systems to include magnets for Philips' Enterprise MRI systems. In May 2004, the company acquired MRI Devices Corp. for $100 million. In August of the same year, SuperPower, in partnership with the Department of Energy and the Electric Power Research Institute, successfully tested the Matrix Fault Current Limiter, designed to protect utility transmission grids from damaging power surges.

Intermagnetics offers employees health and dental insurance, a fitness reimbursement program, tuition reimbursement, credit union membership and flexible spending accounts.

FINANCIALS:
Sales and profits are in thousands of dollars—add 000 to get the full amount. Year 2004 note: Complete fiscal 2004 results were not available for all companies at press time. For this company, year 2004 is for 12 months.

2004 Sales: $164,447 (12 months)   2004 Profits: $14,860 (12 months)
2003 Sales: $147,400   2003 Profits: $14,900
2002 Sales: $153,300   2002 Profits: $20,600
2001 Sales: $138,200   2001 Profits: $11,100
2000 Sales: $112,800   2000 Profits: $6,500

Stock Ticker: IMGC
Employees: 1,038
Fiscal Year Ends: 5/31

SALARIES/BENEFITS:
| Pension Plan: | ESOP Stock Plan: | Profit Sharing: | Top Exec. Salary: $485,264 | Bonus: $360,000 |
| Savings Plan: Y | Stock Purch. Plan: | | Second Exec. Salary: $247,536 | Bonus: $93,413 |

OTHER THOUGHTS:
Apparent Top Female Officers: 1
Hot Spot for Advancement for Women/Minorities:

LOCATIONS: ("Y" = Yes)
West:	Southwest:	Midwest:	Southeast:	Northeast:	International:
Y		Y		Y	

INTERMOUNTAIN HEALTH CARE

www.ihc.com

Industry Group Code: 622110 **Ranks within this company's industry group:** Sales: 17 Profits: 3

Insurance/HMO/PPO:	Drugs:	Equipment/Supplies:	Hospitals/Clinics:	Services:	Health Care:
Insurance: Y	Manufacturer:	Manufacturer:	Acute Care: Y	Diagnostics:	Home Health: Y
Managed Care:	Distributor:	Distributor: Y	Sub-Acute Care: Y	Labs/Testing:	Long-Term Care:
Utilization Mgmt.:	Specialty Pharm.: Y	Leasing/Finance:	Outpatient Surgery: Y	Staffing:	Physical Therapy:
Payment Proc.:	Vitamins/Nutri.:	Information Sys.:	Phys. Rehab. Center: Y	Waste Disposal:	Phys. Practice Mgmt.:
	Clinical Trials:		Psychiatric Clinics:	Specialty Services: Y	

TYPES OF BUSINESS:
Hospitals-General
Surgical Centers
Pharmacies
Counseling Services
Rehabilitation Centers
Emergency Air Transport
Home Care
Health Insurance

BRANDS/DIVISIONS/AFFILIATES:
IHC Physician Group
IHC HomeCare
IHC Health Plans
IHC/AmeriNet

CONTACTS:
Note: Officers with more than one job title may be intentionally listed here more than once.
William H. Nelson, CEO
William H. Nelson, Pres.
Charles W. Sorenson, Jr., COO
Everett Goodwin, CFO
Kent H. Murdock, Vice-Chmn.
Linda C. Leckman, CEO-IHC Physician Div.
Brent E. Wallace, Chmn.-IHC Physician Div.
Gregory P. Steven, Medical Dir.
Merrill Gappmayer, Chmn.

Phone: 801-442-2000 **Fax:** 801-442-3327
Toll-Free:
Address: 36 S. State St., Salt Lake City, UT 84111 US

GROWTH PLANS/SPECIAL FEATURES:

Intermountain Health Care, Inc. (IHC) is a nonprofit health care provider for Utah and Idaho. The firm operates 20 hospitals, health care agencies, 14 surgical centers and a minor emergency pediatric clinic. IHC also runs an emergency air transport system, a collection of physician clinics, pharmacies, counseling and dialysis and rehabilitation centers. The IHC Physician Group has 400 full-time clinical and general practice doctors as well as over 600 doctors working with the firm's subsidiaries. The firm also runs a variety of subsidiaries for additional patient assistance. IHC HomeCare offers home nursing, a hospice center, pharmacy delivery and medical equipment and supplies for the elderly and infirmed. IHC Health Plans supplies medical, prescription and dental insurance to corporate and individual clients. Joint venture IHC/AmeriNet is a group purchasing organization.

IHC offers medical, life and dental insurance along with flexible spending accounts, on-site exercise facilities, tuition reimbursement and classes through the IHC University, child care and eldercare centers, adoption benefits, a credit union and discounted home and auto insurance.

FINANCIALS:
Sales and profits are in thousands of dollars—add 000 to get the full amount. Year 2004 note: Complete fiscal 2004 results were not available for all companies at press time. For this company, year 2004 is for months.

2004 Sales: $ (months)	2004 Profits: $ (months)	**Stock Ticker:** Nonprofit
2003 Sales: $3,266,700	2003 Profits: $893,200	Employees:
2002 Sales: $2,847,300	2002 Profits: $	Fiscal Year Ends: 12/31
2001 Sales: $	2001 Profits: $	
2000 Sales: $	2000 Profits: $	

SALARIES/BENEFITS:
Pension Plan: Y   ESOP Stock Plan: Profit Sharing: Top Exec. Salary: $ Bonus: $
Savings Plan: Y   Stock Purch. Plan: Second Exec. Salary: $ Bonus: $

OTHER THOUGHTS:
Apparent Top Female Officers: 1
Hot Spot for Advancement for Women/Minorities:

LOCATIONS: ("Y" = Yes)
West	Southwest	Midwest	Southeast	Northeast	International
Y					

INTERPORE CROSS INTERNATIONAL   www.interpore.com

Industry Group Code: 325414   Ranks within this company's industry group: Sales: 2   Profits: 2

Insurance/HMO/PPO:	Drugs:	Equipment/Supplies:		Hospitals/Clinics:		Services:		Health Care:	
Insurance:	Manufacturer:	Manufacturer:	Y	Acute Care:		Diagnostics:		Home Health:	
Managed Care:	Distributor:	Distributor:		Sub-Acute Care:		Labs/Testing:		Long-Term Care:	
Utilization Mgmt.:	Specialty Pharm.:	Leasing/Finance:		Outpatient Surgery:		Staffing:		Physical Therapy:	
Payment Proc.:	Vitamins/Nutri.:	Information Sys.:		Phys. Rehab. Center:		Waste Disposal:		Phys. Practice Mgmt.:	
	Clinical Trials:			Psychiatric Clinics:		Specialty Services:			

TYPES OF BUSINESS:
Synthetically Produced Bone Repair Material
Soft Tissue Repair Products
Minimally Invasive Surgery Products

GROWTH PLANS/SPECIAL FEATURES:

Interpore Cross International, a member of EBI Medical, Inc., a subsidiary of Biomet, is a biomaterials company that specializes in developing, manufacturing and marketing medical devices for bone and soft tissue repair, especially for spinal surgery. It manufactured the first synthetically produced bone repair material approved in the U.S. for orthopedic, oral and maxillofacial applications. The company's synthetic bone graft products are derived from marine coral using a process that converts coral skeleton into hydroxyapatite, a biocompatible implant material. The company's spinal implant product offerings include the SYNERGY Spinal System, the C-TEK Anterior Cervical Plate system, the Telescopic Plate Spacer and the GEO Structure vertebral body replacement device. Its orthobiologic offerings include Pro Osteon synthetic bone graft products; BonePlast Bone Void Filler, an absorbable temporary bone grafter; and Autologous Growth Factors-related products. The firm's American Osteomedix Corp. subsidiary develops and markets a category of minimally invasive surgery products including the CDO System and the LP System, designed to assist physicians in the delivery of biocompatible materials into bone through small incisions.

BRANDS/DIVISIONS/AFFILIATES:
Pro Osteon Implant 500
American Osteomedix Corp.
SYNERGY Spinal System
C-TEK Anterior Cervical Plate
GEO Structure
EBI Medical, Inc.
Biomet
BonePlast Bone Void Filler

CONTACTS: Note: Officers with more than one job title may be intentionally listed here more than once.
David C. Mercer, CEO
Joseph A. Mussey, Pres.
Joseph A. Mussey, COO
Richard L. Harrison, CFO
M. Ross Simmonds, Sr. VP-Sales & Distribution
Edwin C. Shors, VP-Research
Edwin C. Shors, VP-New Tech.
Philip A. Mellinger, VP-Product Dev.
R. Park Carmon, VP-Oper.
Richard L. Harrison, Sr. VP-Finance
Richard L. Harrison, Corp. Sec.
David C. Mercer, Chmn.

Phone: 949-453-3200   Fax: 949-453-3225
Toll-Free:
Address: 181 Technology Dr., Irvine, CA 92618-2402 US

FINANCIALS:
Sales and profits are in thousands of dollars—add 000 to get the full amount. Year 2004 note: Complete fiscal 2004 results were not available for all companies at press time. For this company, year 2004 is for months.

2004 Sales: $ (months)   2004 Profits: $ (months)
2003 Sales: $70,718   2003 Profits: $14,934
2002 Sales: $58,900   2002 Profits: $4,100
2001 Sales: $51,300   2001 Profits: $4,300
2000 Sales: $44,300   2000 Profits: $4,100

Stock Ticker: Subsidiary
Employees: 213
Fiscal Year Ends: 12/31

SALARIES/BENEFITS:
Pension Plan: ESOP Stock Plan: Profit Sharing: Top Exec. Salary: $272,500   Bonus: $32,688
Savings Plan: Stock Purch. Plan: Y   Second Exec. Salary: $272,500   Bonus: $24,375

OTHER THOUGHTS:
Apparent Top Female Officers:
Hot Spot for Advancement for Women/Minorities:

LOCATIONS: ("Y" = Yes)

West:	Southwest:	Midwest:	Southeast:	Northeast:	International:
Y			Y	Y	

Note: Financial information, benefits and other data can change quickly and may vary from those stated here.

INTUITIVE SURGICAL INC

www.intuitivesurgical.com

Industry Group Code: 339113   Ranks within this company's industry group: Sales: 96   Profits: 124

Insurance/HMO/PPO:	Drugs:	Equipment/Supplies:	Hospitals/Clinics:	Services:	Health Care:
Insurance:	Manufacturer:	Manufacturer: Y	Acute Care:	Diagnostics:	Home Health:
Managed Care:	Distributor:	Distributor:	Sub-Acute Care:	Labs/Testing:	Long-Term Care:
Utilization Mgmt.:	Specialty Pharm.:	Leasing/Finance:	Outpatient Surgery:	Staffing:	Physical Therapy:
Payment Proc.:	Vitamins/Nutri.:	Information Sys.:	Phys. Rehab. Center:	Waste Disposal:	Phys. Practice Mgmt.:
	Clinical Trials:		Psychiatric Clinics:	Specialty Services:	

TYPES OF BUSINESS:
Endoscopic Surgery Products
Operative Surgical Robots

BRANDS/DIVISIONS/AFFILIATES:
da Vinci Surgical System
EndoWrist
Computer Motion, Inc.
SOCRATES
InSite
ZEUS
HERMES
AESOP

CONTACTS: Note: Officers with more than one job title may be intentionally listed here more than once.
Lonnie M. Smith, CEO
Lonnie M. Smith, Pres.
Susan K. Barnes, Sr. VP/CFO
Eric C. Miller, Sr. VP-Mktg.
Augusto V. Castello, VP-Mfg.
Frank D. Nguyen, VP/General Counsel
Gary S. Guthart, Sr. VP-Product Oper.
Aleks Cukic, VP-Bus. Dev. & Strategic Planning
Benjamin Gong, VP-Finance
Louis J. Mazzarese, VP-Quality, Clinical & Regulatory Affairs
Jerry McNamara, Sr. VP-Worldwide Sales

Phone: 408-523-2100   Fax: 408-523-1390
Toll-Free: 888-868-4647
Address: 950 Kifer Rd., Sunnyvale, CA 94086 US

GROWTH PLANS/SPECIAL FEATURES:
Intuitive Surgical, Inc. is a leading manufacturer of operative surgical robotics. The firm designs and manufactures the da Vinci Surgical System, which consists of a surgeon's console, a patient-side cart, a high-performance vision system and Intuitive's proprietary wristed instruments. The system provides the surgeon with the intuitive control, range of motion, fine tissue manipulation capability and 3-D visualization characteristics of open surgery, while simultaneously allowing the surgeon to work through the small ports of minimally invasive surgery (MIS). The da Vinci Surgical System can be used to control Intuitive's endoscopic instruments including rigid endoscopes, blunt and sharp endoscopic dissectors, scissors, scalpels, forceps/pickups, needle holders, endoscopic retractors, stabilizers, electrocautery and accessories during a wide range of surgical procedures. Surgeons operate while seated comfortably at a console viewing a bright and sharp 3-D image of the surgical field. This immersive visualization, the InSite vision system, results in surgeons no longer feeling disconnected from the surgical field and the instruments, as they do when using an endoscope in MIS. Intuitive also manufactures a variety of EndoWrist instruments, each of which incorporates a wrist joint for natural dexterity with tips customized for various surgical procedures. Through subsidiary Computer Motion, Inc., the company has access to the ZEUS, HERMES, AESOP and SOCRATES robotic and telecommunicative surgery systems. It has discontinued pursuing further regulatory approvals or promoting these products, though it continues to support systems already installed at customer sites.

The company offers employees health, dental and life insurance, as well as a medical expense reimbursement plan and an employee assistance program.

FINANCIALS: Sales and profits are in thousands of dollars—add 000 to get the full amount. Year 2004 note: Complete fiscal 2004 results were not available for all companies at press time. For this company, year 2004 is for 9 months.

2004 Sales: $93,609 (9 months)   2004 Profits: $11,796 (9 months)
2003 Sales: $91,675   2003 Profits: $-9,623
2002 Sales: $72,000   2002 Profits: $-18,400
2001 Sales: $51,700   2001 Profits: $-16,700
2000 Sales: $26,600   2000 Profits: $-18,500

Stock Ticker: ISRG
Employees: 325
Fiscal Year Ends: 12/31

SALARIES/BENEFITS:
Pension Plan: ESOP Stock Plan: Profit Sharing: Top Exec. Salary: $358,000   Bonus: $178,125
Savings Plan: Y   Stock Purch. Plan: Y   Second Exec. Salary: $230,000   Bonus: $80,000

OTHER THOUGHTS:
Apparent Top Female Officers: 1
Hot Spot for Advancement for Women/Minorities:

LOCATIONS: ("Y" = Yes)
West:	Southwest:	Midwest:	Southeast:	Northeast:	International:
Y					Y

/ Plunkett's Health Care Industry Almanac 2005

INVACARE CORP

www.invacare.com

Industry Group Code: 339113   Ranks within this company's industry group: Sales: 22   Profits: 23

Insurance/HMO/PPO:	Drugs:	Equipment/Supplies:		Hospitals/Clinics:	Services:	Health Care:
Insurance:	Manufacturer:	Manufacturer:	Y	Acute Care:	Diagnostics:	Home Health:
Managed Care:	Distributor:	Distributor:	Y	Sub-Acute Care:	Labs/Testing:	Long-Term Care:
Utilization Mgmt.:	Specialty Pharm.:	Leasing/Finance:		Outpatient Surgery:	Staffing:	Physical Therapy:
Payment Proc.:	Vitamins/Nutri.:	Information Sys.:		Phys. Rehab. Center:	Waste Disposal:	Phys. Practice Mgmt.:
	Clinical Trials:			Psychiatric Clinics:	Specialty Services:	

TYPES OF BUSINESS:
Supplies-Wheelchairs
Home Health Care Equipment
Home Respiratory Products
Medical Supplies

BRANDS/DIVISIONS/AFFILIATES:
Highly Maneuverable Vehicle
Pronto Heavy Duty Power Wheelchair
Home Care Bed
WP Domus GmbH

CONTACTS: Note: Officers with more than one job title may be intentionally listed here more than once.
A. Malachi Mixon, III, CEO
Gerald B. Blouch, Pres.
Gerald B. Blouch, COO
Gregory C. Thompson, Sr. VP/CFO
Louis F.J. Slangen, Sr. VP-Sales & Mktg.
Joe Usaj, Sr. VP-Human Resources
Russ Lenahan, VP-IT
Joseph B. Richey, II, Pres.-Tech.
Neal J. Curran, VP-Eng. & Product Dev.
Joseph B. Richey, II, Sr. VP-Electronics & Design Eng.
Bridget A. Miller, VP/General Counsel
Stephen D. Neese, VP-Customer Oper.
Louis F.J. Slangen, Sr. VP-Global Market Dev.
Stephen D. Neese, VP-e-Bus.
Bill Corcoran, VP-Financial Services
Judy Kovacs, VP/Mgr.-Invacare Service & Parts
John Ledek, VP-Respiratory Products
Matt Mullarkey, VP/Mgr.-Home Medical Equipment
Michael A. Perry, VP-Invacare Supply Group
A. Malachi Mixon, III, Chmn.
Kenneth A. Sparrow, Pres.-Int'l
W. Darrel Lowery, VP-North American Logistics

Phone: 440-329-6000   Fax:
Toll-Free:
Address: One Invacare Way, P.O. Box 4028, Elyria, OH 44036 US

GROWTH PLANS/SPECIAL FEATURES:
Invacare Corp. is a leading manufacturer and distributor of health care products for the non-acute care environment, including the home health care and retail care markets. The firm sells its products to over 25,000 home health care and retail locations in the U.S., Australia, Canada, Europe and New Zealand. The company's product line includes power and manual wheelchairs, motorized scooters, home care beds, mattress overlays, home respiratory products, bathing equipment and patient aids. In addition, the firm is a manufacturer and distributor of beds and furnishings for non-acute care markets and numerous lines of branded medical supplies including ostomy, incontinence, diabetic, wound care and other home products. The company also manufactures, markets and distributes many accessory products, including spare parts, wheelchair cushions, arm rests, wheels and respiratory parts. New product development has been given a strong emphasis as part of Invacare's strategy to gain market share and maintain competitive advantage. As a result, the company introduced 40 new products in 2003, including the Highly Maneuverable Vehicle, the Pronto Heavy Duty Power Wheelchair and the Home Care Bed, a more durable, easy-to-clean bed. In September 2004, Invacare completed its acquisition of WP Domus GmbH, a designer and manufacturer of power add-on products, bath lifts and walking aids, among other products.

FINANCIALS:
Sales and profits are in thousands of dollars—add 000 to get the full amount. Year 2004 note: Complete fiscal 2004 results were not available for all companies at press time. For this company, year 2004 is for 9 months.

2004 Sales: $1,010,138 (9 months)   2004 Profits: $54,753 (9 months)
2003 Sales: $1,247,176   2003 Profits: $71,409
2002 Sales: $1,089,161   2002 Profits: $64,770
2001 Sales: $1,053,600   2001 Profits: $35,200
2000 Sales: $1,013,200   2000 Profits: $59,900

Stock Ticker: IVC
Employees: 5,300
Fiscal Year Ends: 12/31

SALARIES/BENEFITS:
Pension Plan: ESOP Stock Plan: Profit Sharing: Top Exec. Salary: $948,000   Bonus: $948,000
Savings Plan: Y   Stock Purch. Plan: Second Exec. Salary: $585,833   Bonus: $557,650

OTHER THOUGHTS:
Apparent Top Female Officers: 2
Hot Spot for Advancement for Women/Minorities:

LOCATIONS: ("Y" = Yes)
West:	Southwest:	Midwest:	Southeast:	Northeast:	International:
Y	Y	Y	Y	Y	Y

Note: Financial information, benefits and other data can change quickly and may vary from those stated here.

INVERNESS MEDICAL INNOVATIONS INC
www.invernessmedical.com

Industry Group Code: 339113   Ranks within this company's industry group: Sales: 56   Profits: 67

Insurance/HMO/PPO:	Drugs:		Equipment/Supplies:		Hospitals/Clinics:	Services:	Health Care:
Insurance:	Manufacturer:		Manufacturer:	Y	Acute Care:	Diagnostics:	Home Health:
Managed Care:	Distributor:		Distributor:	Y	Sub-Acute Care:	Labs/Testing:	Long-Term Care:
Utilization Mgmt.:	Specialty Pharm.:		Leasing/Finance:		Outpatient Surgery:	Staffing:	Physical Therapy:
Payment Proc.:	Vitamins/Nutri.:	Y	Information Sys.:		Phys. Rehab. Center:	Waste Disposal:	Phys. Practice Mgmt.:
	Clinical Trials:				Psychiatric Clinics:	Specialty Services:	

TYPES OF BUSINESS:
Supplies-Over-the-Counter Health Care Products
Self-Test Diagnostic Products
Vitamins & Nutritional Supplements
Professional Diagnostic Products

BRANDS/DIVISIONS/AFFILIATES:
Clearblue
Fact Plus
Accu-Clear
Persona
SmartCare
Wampole
Clearview
DoubleCheck

CONTACTS:
Note: Officers with more than one job title may be intentionally listed here more than once.

Ron Zwanziger, CEO
Ron Zwanziger, Pres.
Anthony J. Bernardo, VP/COO
Christopher J. Lindop, CFO
John Yonkin, VP-U.S. Mktg. & Sales
Jerry McAleer, VP-Research & Dev.
Paul T. Hempel, General Counsel
Doug Shaffer, VP-U.S. Oper.
Duane L. James, Treas./VP-Finance
David Toohey, VP-Professional Diagnostics
David Scott, Chief Scientific Officer
John B. Wilkens, VP-Consumer Diagnostics
Ron Zwanziger, Chmn.

Phone: 781-647-3900	Fax: 781-647-3939
Toll-Free:	
Address: 51 Sawyer Rd., Ste. 200, Waltham, MA 02453 US	

GROWTH PLANS/SPECIAL FEATURES:
Inverness Medical Innovations, Inc. (IMI) develops, manufactures and markets consumer health care products, including self-test diagnostic products for the women's health market, as well as vitamins and nutritional supplements. To a lesser extent, the firm also manufactures and markets diagnostic products for use by medical professionals. Its consumer diagnostic products target the worldwide over-the-counter pregnancy and fertility/ovulation test market, providing a safe, easy and effective method for women to manage their reproductive health without the expense, inconvenience and delay associated with physician visits or laboratory testing. Products include the Clearblue and Fact Plus lines of pregnancy tests, Accu-Clear pregnancy and fertility/ovulation prediction products and Persona, a hand-held menstrual cycle monitoring device that is sold in Germany and the U.K. as a contraceptive device. IMI's professional diagnostic products are sold under the Wampole, SureStep, Signify, TestPack and Clearview labels, and include rapid membrane tests for pregnancy, drug abuse, mononucleosis, strep throat, lyme disease, chlamydia, H.pylori and rubella; ELISA tests for infectious and sexually transmitted diseases; IFA and microbiology assays for over 20 viral, bacterial and autoimmune diseases; and a line of serology diagnostic products for mononucleosis, rheumatoid arthritis, C-reactive protein, syphilis, rubella and streptococcal infections. In addition, its DoubleCheck and ImmunoGold HIV and hepatitis platforms are low-cost rapid tests sold outside of the U.S. IMI also markets a variety of vitamins and nutritional supplements, including Stresstabs, a B-complex vitamin with added antioxidants; Ferro-Sequels, a time-release iron supplement; Protegra, an antioxidant vitamin and mineral supplement; Posture-D, a calcium supplement; SoyCare, a soy supplement for menopause; ALLBEE, a line of B-complex vitamins; and Z-BEC, a zinc supplement with B-complex vitamins and added antioxidants. These are often sold under the SmartCare program, which assists consumers in matching their health concerns to the appropriate supplement.

FINANCIALS:
Sales and profits are in thousands of dollars—add 000 to get the full amount. Year 2004 note: Complete fiscal 2004 results were not available for all companies at press time. For this company, year 2004 is for 9 months.

2004 Sales: $276,933 (9 months)	2004 Profits: $-8,516 (9 months)	
2003 Sales: $296,712	2003 Profits: $12,269	Stock Ticker: IMA
2002 Sales: $207,900	2002 Profits: $-31,100	Employees: 1,435
2001 Sales: $49,400	2001 Profits: $-24,700	Fiscal Year Ends: 12/31
2000 Sales: $51,100	2000 Profits: $2,200	

SALARIES/BENEFITS:
Pension Plan: Y	ESOP Stock Plan:	Profit Sharing:	Top Exec. Salary: $295,553	Bonus: $550,000
Savings Plan: Y	Stock Purch. Plan:		Second Exec. Salary: $234,439	Bonus: $200,000

OTHER THOUGHTS:
Apparent Top Female Officers:
Hot Spot for Advancement for Women/Minorities:

LOCATIONS: ("Y" = Yes)
West:	Southwest:	Midwest:	Southeast:	Northeast:	International:
Y				Y	Y

IRIDEX CORP

www.iridex.com

Industry Group Code: 339113 Ranks within this company's industry group: Sales: 124 Profits: 102

Insurance/HMO/PPO:	Drugs:	Equipment/Supplies:		Hospitals/Clinics:	Services:	Health Care:
Insurance:	Manufacturer:	Manufacturer:	Y	Acute Care:	Diagnostics:	Home Health:
Managed Care:	Distributor:	Distributor:	Y	Sub-Acute Care:	Labs/Testing:	Long-Term Care:
Utilization Mgmt.:	Specialty Pharm.:	Leasing/Finance:		Outpatient Surgery:	Staffing:	Physical Therapy:
Payment Proc.:	Vitamins/Nutri.:	Information Sys.:		Phys. Rehab. Center:	Waste Disposal:	Phys. Practice Mgmt.:
	Clinical Trials:			Psychiatric Clinics:	Specialty Services:	

TYPES OF BUSINESS:
Equipment-Diversified Laser Systems
Ophthalmological & Dermatological Laser Systems

GROWTH PLANS/SPECIAL FEATURES:
IRIDEX Corporation manufactures semiconductor-based laser systems for use in ophthalmology and dermatology. The company's family of OcuLight laser systems is used in hospitals, clinics and doctors' offices to treat serious eye disorders, including age-related macular degeneration, glaucoma and diabetic retinopathy, which are the three leading causes of irreversible blindness. Its DioLite 523 and Apex 800 dermatology systems treat skin conditions such as vascular and pigmented lesions and remove unwanted hair. Each system includes a console, which generates the laser energy, and a number of interchangeable peripheral delivery devices, including disposable delivery devices, for use in specific clinical applications. This allows customers to purchase a basic console system and add additional delivery devices as their needs expand or as the company develops new applications. IRIDEX markets its products through a direct sales force in the U.S. and a network of 66 distributors that sells to 107 countries around the world. Recently, the company received FDA clearance for its solid-state IRIS Medical IQ 810 infrared diode laser photocoagulator for the treatment of retinal disorders and glaucoma, and for its VariLite dual-wavelength laser to be used on 19 dermatology indications, including vascular, pigmented and cutaneous lesions, leg veins, hair removal and moderate inflammatory acne vulgaris.

BRANDS/DIVISIONS/AFFILIATES:
IRIS Medical IQ 810
OcuLight
DioLite 532
Apex 800
VariLite

CONTACTS:
Note: Officers with more than one job title may be intentionally listed here more than once.
Theodore A. Boutacoff, CEO
Theodore A. Boutacoff, Pres.
Larry Tannenbaum, CFO
Eduardo Arias, Sr. VP-Int'l Sales
Larry Tannenbaum, Sr. VP-Admin.
Timothy Powers, VP-Oper.
Eduardo Arias, Sr. VP-Bus. Dev.
Larry Tannenbaum, Sr. VP-Finance
James L. Donovan, VP-Corp. Bus. Dev.
Donald L. Hammond, Chmn.

Phone: 650-940-4700 **Fax:** 650-940-4710
Toll-Free: 800-338-9087
Address: 1212 Terra Bella Ave., Mountain View, CA 94043-1824 US

FINANCIALS:
Sales and profits are in thousands of dollars—add 000 to get the full amount. Year 2004 note: Complete fiscal 2004 results were not available for all companies at press time. For this company, year 2004 is for 6 months.

2004 Sales: $15,501 (6 months)   2004 Profits: $ 116   (6 months)
2003 Sales: $31,699   2003 Profits: $ 371
2002 Sales: $30,600   2002 Profits: $ 200
2001 Sales: $27,300   2001 Profits: $-1,300
2000 Sales: $33,400   2000 Profits: $2,400

Stock Ticker: IRIX
Employees: 108
Fiscal Year Ends: 12/31

SALARIES/BENEFITS:
Pension Plan: ESOP Stock Plan: Profit Sharing: Top Exec. Salary: $240,000   Bonus: $
Savings Plan: Y   Stock Purch. Plan: Y   Second Exec. Salary: $167,400   Bonus: $

OTHER THOUGHTS:
Apparent Top Female Officers:
Hot Spot for Advancement for Women/Minorities:

LOCATIONS: ("Y" = Yes)
West:	Southwest:	Midwest:	Southeast:	Northeast:	International:
Y					

IRIS INTERNATIONAL INC

www.proiris.com

Industry Group Code: 339113   Ranks within this company's industry group: Sales: 125   Profits: 108

Insurance/HMO/PPO:	Drugs:	Equipment/Supplies:		Hospitals/Clinics:	Services:		Health Care:	
Insurance:	Manufacturer:	Manufacturer:	Y	Acute Care:	Diagnostics:		Home Health:	
Managed Care:	Distributor:	Distributor:		Sub-Acute Care:	Labs/Testing:		Long-Term Care:	
Utilization Mgmt.:	Specialty Pharm.:	Leasing/Finance:		Outpatient Surgery:	Staffing:		Physical Therapy:	
Payment Proc.:	Vitamins/Nutri.:	Information Sys.:	Y	Phys. Rehab. Center:	Waste Disposal:		Phys. Practice Mgmt.:	
	Clinical Trials:			Psychiatric Clinics:	Specialty Services:	Y		

TYPES OF BUSINESS:
Equipment-Body Fluid Analysis
Automated Urinalysis Workstations
Digital Imaging Software, Research & Development

BRANDS/DIVISIONS/AFFILIATES:
International Remote Imaging Systems, Inc.
Automated Intelligent Microscopy
StatSpin, Inc.
Advanced Digital Imaging Research, LLC
iQ200 Automated Urine Microscopy Analyzer

CONTACTS: Note: Officers with more than one job title may be intentionally listed here more than once.
Cesar M. Garcia, CEO
Cesar M. Garcia, Pres.
Cesar M. Garcia, COO
Martin G. Paravato, VP/CFO
Allen W. Nemeth, VP-U.S. Sales
John Yi, VP-Oper.
Robert O'Malley, VP-Global Mktg., Planning & Svcs.
Robert A. Mello, VP/Pres., StatSpin
Richard H. Williams, Chmn.
Bernardo M. Alfano, VP-Int'l Sales & Tech. Svcs.

Phone: 818-709-1244   Fax: 818-700-9661
Toll-Free: 800-776-4747
Address: 9172 Eton Ave., Chatsworth, CA 91311-5874 US

GROWTH PLANS/SPECIAL FEATURES:
IRIS International, Inc., formerly International Remote Imaging Systems, Inc., manufactures and markets automated urinalysis imaging systems and medical devices used in hospitals and clinical reference laboratories worldwide. The company is a leader in the automated urinalysis workstation market. All of its imaging systems use patented and proprietary Automated Intelligent Microscopy (AIM) technology for automated specimen presentation, allowing its products to classify and present images of microscopic particles in easy-to-view displays. IRIS's StatSpin subsidiary manufactures and markets products for blood analysis, including a variety of benchtop centrifuges, small instruments and supplies for the laboratory market. These products are used primarily for cytology, hematology and urinalysis. It also operates Advanced Digital Imaging Research, LLC (ADIR), which specializes in the research and development of digital imaging software and algorithm development, thus assisting in the advancement of proprietary imaging technology. It also conducts government-sponsored research and development in medical imaging and software, as well as contract research for corporate clients. The company's recently launched iQ200 Automated Urine Microscopy Analyzer uses image flow cytometry and IRIS' patented AIM technology to reduce cost and time spent on manual microscopic analysis. The iQ200 has numerous benefits over competing products, including increased accuracy, fully automated walk-away urinalysis and user-defined reflexive testing. In recent news, IRIS signed a five-year purchasing agreement with the U.S. Department of Veterans Affairs (VA) that will put the firm's technology in 10 VA health care centers. The company also received a $2-million grant from the U.S. government to develop 3-D face recognition technology for use in security screening.

FINANCIALS: Sales and profits are in thousands of dollars—add 000 to get the full amount. Year 2004 note: Complete fiscal 2004 results were not available for all companies at press time. For this company, year 2004 is for 9 months.

2004 Sales: $31,464 (9 months)   2004 Profits: $ 967   (9 months)
2003 Sales: $31,345   2003 Profits: $1,448   Stock Ticker: IRIS
2002 Sales: $28,200   2002 Profits: $ 900   Employees: 156
2001 Sales: $28,600   2001 Profits: $1,500   Fiscal Year Ends: 12/31
2000 Sales: $28,600   2000 Profits: $2,300

SALARIES/BENEFITS:
Pension Plan: ESOP Stock Plan: Profit Sharing: Top Exec. Salary: $272,800   Bonus: $50,000
Savings Plan: Y   Stock Purch. Plan: Y   Second Exec. Salary: $246,492   Bonus: $100,000

OTHER THOUGHTS:
Apparent Top Female Officers:
Hot Spot for Advancement for Women/Minorities:

LOCATIONS: ("Y" = Yes)
West:	Southwest:	Midwest:	Southeast:	Northeast:	International:
Y	Y			Y	Y

Note: Financial information, benefits and other data can change quickly and may vary from those stated here.

I-STAT CORP

www.i-stat.com

Industry Group Code: 339113   Ranks within this company's industry group: Sales: Profits:

Insurance/HMO/PPO:	Drugs:	Equipment/Supplies:		Hospitals/Clinics:	Services:	Health Care:
Insurance:	Manufacturer:	Manufacturer:	Y	Acute Care:	Diagnostics:	Home Health:
Managed Care:	Distributor:	Distributor:	Y	Sub-Acute Care:	Labs/Testing:	Long-Term Care:
Utilization Mgmt.:	Specialty Pharm.:	Leasing/Finance:		Outpatient Surgery:	Staffing:	Physical Therapy:
Payment Proc.:	Vitamins/Nutri.:	Information Sys.:		Phys. Rehab. Center:	Waste Disposal:	Phys. Practice Mgmt.:
	Clinical Trials:			Psychiatric Clinics:	Specialty Services:	

TYPES OF BUSINESS:
Supplies-Handheld Blood Test Products
Diagnostic Products

BRANDS/DIVISIONS/AFFILIATES:
i-STAT System
i-STAT Canada, Ltd.
Heska Corp.
Abbott Laboratories

GROWTH PLANS/SPECIAL FEATURES:
i-STAT Corp., a subsidiary of Abbott Laboratories, develops, manufactures and markets medical diagnostic products for blood analysis that provide health care professionals with immediate and accurate information at the point of patient care. Its current products, marketed under the i-STAT System brand, consist of a portable, handheld analyzer and a variety of single-use disposable cartridges. Each cartridge simultaneously performs different combinations of commonly ordered blood tests in approximately two minutes. The i-STAT System provides accurate and reliable blood tests faster and easier than most other advanced clinical laboratory equipment of its kind. The firm markets its products overseas to hospitals in Japan, Europe, Canada, South America, Mexico, Latin America, South Africa, Hong Kong, China and other countries in Asia.

The firm's employee benefits program includes medical, dental, life and disability insurance.

CONTACTS:
Note: Officers with more than one job title may be intentionally listed here more than once.

Lorin J. Randall, CFO
Noah J. Kroloff, VP-Int'l Sales & Mktg.
Michael P. Zelin, Exec. VP/Chief Tech. Officer
Noah J. Kroloff, VP-Corp. Dev.
Lorin J. Randall, Treas.

Phone: 609-443-9300   **Fax:** 609-443-9310
Toll-Free:
Address: 104 Windsor Center Dr., East Windsor, NJ 08520 US

FINANCIALS:
Sales and profits are in thousands of dollars—add 000 to get the full amount. Year 2004 note: Complete fiscal 2004 results were not available for all companies at press time. For this company, year 2004 is for   months.

2004 Sales: $ (months)	2004 Profits: $ (months)	**Stock Ticker:** Subsidiary
2003 Sales: $	2003 Profits: $	Employees: 706
2002 Sales: $59,900	2002 Profits: $-62,800	Fiscal Year Ends: 12/31
2001 Sales: $58,800	2001 Profits: $-23,200	
2000 Sales: $55,000	2000 Profits: $-7,500	

SALARIES/BENEFITS:
Pension Plan:	ESOP Stock Plan:	Profit Sharing:	Top Exec. Salary: $403,000	Bonus:	$80,197
Savings Plan: Y	Stock Purch. Plan:		Second Exec. Salary: $285,000	Bonus:	$70,894

OTHER THOUGHTS:
Apparent Top Female Officers:
Hot Spot for Advancement for Women/Minorities:

LOCATIONS: ("Y" = Yes)

West:	Southwest:	Midwest:	Southeast:	Northeast:	International:
				Y	Y

JEFFERSON HEALTH SYSTEM INC

www.jeffersonhealth.org

Industry Group Code: 622110 Ranks within this company's industry group: Sales: 28 Profits:

Insurance/HMO/PPO:	Drugs:	Equipment/Supplies:	Hospitals/Clinics:		Services:		Health Care:	
Insurance:	Manufacturer:	Manufacturer:	Acute Care:	Y	Diagnostics:		Home Health:	
Managed Care:	Distributor:	Distributor:	Sub-Acute Care:	Y	Labs/Testing:		Long-Term Care:	Y
Utilization Mgmt.:	Specialty Pharm.:	Leasing/Finance:	Outpatient Surgery:	Y	Staffing:		Physical Therapy:	Y
Payment Proc.:	Vitamins/Nutri.:	Information Sys.:	Phys. Rehab. Center:	Y	Waste Disposal:		Phys. Practice Mgmt.:	
	Clinical Trials:		Psychiatric Clinics:		Specialty Services:			

TYPES OF BUSINESS:
Hospitals
Sub-Acute Care
Behavioral Health Services
Ambulatory Care Centers
Rehabilitation Services
Long-Term Care
Teaching Hospitals

BRANDS/DIVISIONS/AFFILIATES:
Albert Einstein Healthcare Network
Frankford Hospitals
Magee Rehabilitation
Main Line Health
Thomas Jefferson University Hospitals
Jefferson HealthCARE
Jefferson Radiation Oncology
Regional Spinal Cord Injury Centers

CONTACTS:
Note: Officers with more than one job title may be intentionally listed here more than once.

Joseph T. Sebastianelli, CEO
Joseph T. Sebastianelli, Pres.
Kirk E. Gorman, CFO
David F. Simon, Sr. VP/General Counsel
Diane Salter, VP-Insurance

Phone: 610-255-6200	Fax:
Toll-Free:	
Address: 259 N. Radnor-Chester Rd., Ste. 290, Radnor, PA 19087 US	

GROWTH PLANS/SPECIAL FEATURES:
Jefferson Health System, Inc. (JHS) is a nonprofit group consisting of five member health care organizations in the greater Philadelphia area. The Albert Einstein Healthcare Network operates six major facilities and many outpatient centers, including a tertiary care teaching hospital, a behavioral health center, two general care centers, a nationally recognized rehabilitation facility, a sub-acute care center and a long-term care residence for seniors. Frankford Hospitals' system includes three hospital campuses in Philadelphia and Bucks County, three ambulatory care sites and several primary care satellites and specialty practices. Magee Rehabilitation's hospital is one of 16 federally designated model Regional Spinal Cord Injury Centers and is home to the nation's first brain injury rehabilitation program to be accredited by the Commission on the Accreditation of Rehabilitation Facilities. The hospital provides inpatient and outpatient services for people with spinal cord injuries, brain injuries, strokes, orthopedic injuries and amputations, as well as general rehabilitation and ventilator services. Main Line Health, one of the founding members of JHS, operates four hospitals and a number of health centers in the suburbs of Philadelphia. Its clinical specialties include behavioral health, pediatrics, geriatrics, women's health and cancer, cardiac, pulmonary, orthopedic and stroke care. The other founding member, Thomas Jefferson University Hospitals, operates two Philadelphia teaching hospitals as well as Jefferson HealthCARE in Voorhees, New Jersey and Jefferson Radiation Oncology sites throughout the Delaware Valley.

FINANCIALS:
Sales and profits are in thousands of dollars—add 000 to get the full amount. Year 2004 note: Complete fiscal 2004 results were not available for all companies at press time. For this company, year 2004 is for months.

2004 Sales: $ (months)	2004 Profits: $ (months)	**Stock Ticker: Nonprofit**
2003 Sales: $2,499,900	2003 Profits: $	Employees: 27,000
2002 Sales: $	2002 Profits: $	Fiscal Year Ends: 6/30
2001 Sales: $	2001 Profits: $	
2000 Sales: $	2000 Profits: $	

SALARIES/BENEFITS:
Pension Plan:	ESOP Stock Plan:	Profit Sharing:	Top Exec. Salary: $	Bonus: $
Savings Plan:	Stock Purch. Plan:		Second Exec. Salary: $	Bonus: $

OTHER THOUGHTS:
Apparent Top Female Officers: 1
Hot Spot for Advancement for Women/Minorities:

LOCATIONS: ("Y" = Yes)
West:	Southwest:	Midwest:	Southeast:	Northeast: Y	International:

Note: Financial information, benefits and other data can change quickly and may vary from those stated here.

JENNY CRAIG INC

www.jennycraig.com

Industry Group Code: 446190   Ranks within this company's industry group: Sales: 2   Profits:

Insurance/HMO/PPO:	Drugs:	Equipment/Supplies:	Hospitals/Clinics:	Services:	Health Care:
Insurance:	Manufacturer:	Manufacturer:	Acute Care:	Diagnostics:	Home Health:
Managed Care:	Distributor:	Distributor:	Sub-Acute Care:	Labs/Testing:	Long-Term Care:
Utilization Mgmt.:	Specialty Pharm.:	Leasing/Finance:	Outpatient Surgery:	Staffing:	Physical Therapy:
Payment Proc.:	Vitamins/Nutri.:	Information Sys.:	Phys. Rehab. Center:	Waste Disposal:	Phys. Practice Mgmt.:
	Clinical Trials:		Psychiatric Clinics:	Specialty Services: Y	

TYPES OF BUSINESS:
Weight Management Centers
Packaged Food
Video Production
Franchising

BRANDS/DIVISIONS/AFFILIATES:
ACI Capital Co., Inc.
DB Capital Partners, Inc.

CONTACTS:
Note: Officers with more than one job title may be intentionally listed here more than once.

James P. Evans, CEO
Patricia A. Larchet, Pres.
Patricia A. Larchet, COO
Cynthia P. Kellogg, CFO
Scott Parket, VP-Mktg.
Roberta C. Baade, VP-Human Resources
Bob Fried, VP/CIO
Lewis Shender, VP/General Counsel
Norma Hubble, VP-Oper.
Kent R. Coykendall, VP-Strategic Planning and Bus. Dev.
Cynthia P. Kellogg, Treas.
Alan V. Dobies, VP-Corp. Services
Doug Fisher, VP-Franchise/Jenny Direct Oper.
Kent Q. Kreh, Chmn.

Phone: 760-696-4000   **Fax:** 760-696-4607
Toll-Free: 800-597-5366
Address: 5770 Fleet St., Carlsbad, CA 92008 US

GROWTH PLANS/SPECIAL FEATURES:
Jenny Craig, Inc. is one of the largest weight management companies in the world. The firm has approximately 648 owned and franchised locations throughout the U.S., Canada, Australia, New Zealand, Puerto Rico and Guam. Jenny Craig offers clients who wish to lose weight personalized diet programs with the help of one-on-one consultations with weight loss counselors. Once a weight goal is achieved, Jenny Craig offers weight maintenance programs with services such as consultations and menu planning. In addition, the company manufactures and sells over 70 packaged food products including freeze-dried and frozen entrees, packaged nutrition bars, popcorn and other assorted meals and snacks. Moreover, the company publishes reduced-fat/calorie cookbooks and exercise audio and videotapes. Jenny Craig is owned by ACI Capital Co., Inc. and DB Capital Partners, Inc. In 2004, the company opened new centers in New York, New York, with four additional openings planned for Des Moines, Iowa; Iowa City, Iowa; Oklahoma City, Oklahoma; and Edmonton, Alberta in Canada.

Jenny Craig employees receive basic life insurance, disability insurance, an employee assistance program and company discounts. Optional benefits include group health insurance, supplemental life insurance and health care and dependent care flexible spending accounts.

FINANCIALS:
Sales and profits are in thousands of dollars—add 000 to get the full amount. Year 2004 note: Complete fiscal 2004 results were not available for all companies at press time. For this company, year 2004 is for months.

2004 Sales: $ (months)   2004 Profits: $ (months)
2003 Sales: $280,000   2003 Profits: $
2002 Sales: $300,000   2002 Profits: $
2001 Sales: $283,600   2001 Profits: $-19,300
2000 Sales: $ 2000 Profits: $

Stock Ticker: Private
Employees: 3,000
Fiscal Year Ends: 6/30

SALARIES/BENEFITS:
Pension Plan: ESOP Stock Plan: Profit Sharing: Top Exec. Salary: $ Bonus: $
Savings Plan: Y   Stock Purch. Plan: Second Exec. Salary: $ Bonus: $

OTHER THOUGHTS:
Apparent Top Female Officers: 4
Hot Spot for Advancement for Women/Minorities: Y

LOCATIONS: ("Y" = Yes)

West:	Southwest:	Midwest:	Southeast:	Northeast:	International:
Y	Y	Y	Y	Y	Y

JOHNS HOPKINS MEDICINE

www.hopkinsmedicine.org

Industry Group Code: 622110   Ranks within this company's industry group: Sales: 36   Profits:

Insurance/HMO/PPO:	Drugs:	Equipment/Supplies:	Hospitals/Clinics:		Services:		Health Care:	
Insurance:	Manufacturer:	Manufacturer:	Acute Care:	Y	Diagnostics:		Home Health:	Y
Managed Care:	Distributor:	Distributor:	Sub-Acute Care:	Y	Labs/Testing:		Long-Term Care:	
Utilization Mgmt.:	Specialty Pharm.:	Leasing/Finance:	Outpatient Surgery:		Staffing:		Physical Therapy:	
Payment Proc.:	Vitamins/Nutri.:	Information Sys.:	Phys. Rehab. Center:	Y	Waste Disposal:		Phys. Practice Mgmt.:	Y
	Clinical Trials:		Psychiatric Clinics:		Specialty Services:	Y		

TYPES OF BUSINESS:
Medical Care
Medical Research
Medical School
Home Care Services
Physician Network Management

BRANDS/DIVISIONS/AFFILIATES:
Johns Hopkins University School of Medicine
Johns Hopkins Health System
Johns Hopkins Hospital and Outpatient Center
Johns Hopkins Bayview Medical Center
Johns Hopkins HealthCare

CONTACTS:
Note: Officers with more than one job title may be intentionally listed here more than once.

Edward D. Miller, CEO
Richard A. Grossi, VP/CFO
Chi V. Dang, Vice Dean-Research
Stephanie Reel, VP-Info. Services
Steven J. Thompson, Vice Dean-Admin.
Joanne E. Pollak, VP/General Counsel
Toby A. Gordon, VP-Strategic Planning & Market Research
Elaine Freeman, VP-Corp. Comm.
William R. Brody, Pres., Johns Hopkins University
Ronald R. Peterson, Pres., Johns Hopkins Hospital & Health System
Judy Reitz, VP-Quality Improvement
Joseph R. Coppola, VP-Corp. Security
Lenox D. Baker, Jr., Chmn.

Phone: 410-955-5000   Fax: 410-955-4452
Toll-Free:
Address: 720 Rutland Ave., Baltimore, MD 21205 US

GROWTH PLANS/SPECIAL FEATURES:
Johns Hopkins Medicine is a nonprofit organization that includes Johns Hopkins University School of Medicine and the Johns Hopkins Health System. The medical school, ranked number two in the U.S., consists of 32 academic departments from anesthesiology to urology. Its nursing program has also been honored with magnet status by the American Nurses Credentialing Center. The school opened its first international division in Singapore in 1999, where 12 full-time faculty members lead training and research on endemic Southeast Asian diseases. Johns Hopkins Health System provides comprehensive health care services, operating primarily through its three Maryland hospitals. The Johns Hopkins Hospital and Outpatient Center has been rated the best hospital in the nation for over a decade, treating patients from around the world. Johns Hopkins Bayview Medical Center is a teaching hospital housing a neonatal intensive care unit, sleep disorders center, area-wide trauma center, regional burn center and a nationally regarded geriatrics center on its 130-acre campus. The organization also offers a home care group that provides visits by nurses, physical, occupational and speech therapists, home health aides and social workers; a network of physicians providing community-based health care; three facilities at which faculty physicians practice; and programs to assists patients and families from foreign countries or other U.S. cities with physician appointments, lodging, transportation, interpreter services, financial arrangements, day care centers and sightseeing. Johns Hopkins HealthCare serves medical professionals and payers by providing eligibility database management, member-physician services, claims adjudication, care management, patient outreach programs, decision support matrices, client-focused product development and physician/facility network development and management.

FINANCIALS:
Sales and profits are in thousands of dollars—add 000 to get the full amount. Year 2004 note: Complete fiscal 2004 results were not available for all companies at press time. For this company, year 2004 is for months.

2004 Sales: $ (months)
2003 Sales: $1,600,000
2002 Sales: $925,800
2001 Sales: $
2000 Sales: $

2004 Profits: $ (months)
2003 Profits: $
2002 Profits: $
2001 Profits: $
2000 Profits: $

Stock Ticker: Nonprofit
Employees: 25,000
Fiscal Year Ends: 6/30

SALARIES/BENEFITS:
Pension Plan: ESOP Stock Plan: Profit Sharing: Top Exec. Salary: $ Bonus: $
Savings Plan: Stock Purch. Plan: Second Exec. Salary: $ Bonus: $

OTHER THOUGHTS:
Apparent Top Female Officers: 4
Hot Spot for Advancement for Women/Minorities: Y

LOCATIONS: ("Y" = Yes)
West:	Southwest:	Midwest:	Southeast:	Northeast:	International:
				Y	Y

JOHNSON & JOHNSON

www.jnj.com

Industry Group Code: 325412 Ranks within this company's industry group: Sales: 2 Profits: 1

Insurance/HMO/PPO:	Drugs:		Equipment/Supplies:		Hospitals/Clinics:	Services:	Health Care:
Insurance:	Manufacturer:	Y	Manufacturer:	Y	Acute Care:	Diagnostics:	Home Health:
Managed Care:	Distributor:	Y	Distributor:	Y	Sub-Acute Care:	Labs/Testing:	Long-Term Care:
Utilization Mgmt.:	Specialty Pharm.:		Leasing/Finance:		Outpatient Surgery:	Staffing:	Physical Therapy:
Payment Proc.:	Vitamins/Nutri.:		Information Sys.:		Phys. Rehab. Center:	Waste Disposal:	Phys. Practice Mgmt.:
	Clinical Trials:				Psychiatric Clinics:	Specialty Services:	

TYPES OF BUSINESS:
Drugs-Personal Health Care and Hygiene Products Manufacturer
Sterilization Products
Surgical Products
Pharmaceuticals
Skin Care Products
Self Diagnostic Products
Drug Research and Development
Medical Equipment

BRANDS/DIVISIONS/AFFILIATES:
Risperdal
Mylanta
Band-Aid
Tylenol
Monistat

CONTACTS: Note: Officers with more than one job title may be intentionally listed here more than once.
William C. Weldon, CEO
James T. Lenehan, Pres.
Robert J. Darretta, CFO
Nicholas J. Valeriani, VP-Human Resources
Theodore J. Torphy, VP-Science & Tech.
JoAnn H. Heisen, CIO
Russell Deyo, VP-Admin.
Roger S. Fine, General Counsel
David P. Holveck, VP-Corp. Dev.
John A. Papa, Treas.
Colleen A. Goggins, Worldwide Chmn.-Consumer & Personal Care
Christine A. Poon, Worldwide Chmn. Medicine & Nutritionals
Per A. Peterson, Chmn.-Research & Dev., Pharmaceuticals Group
J. Andrea Alstrup, VP-Advertising
William C. Weldon, Chmn.

Phone: 732-524-0400 **Fax:** 732-524-3300
Toll-Free: 800-328-9033
Address: One Johnson & Johnson Plaza, New Brunswick, NJ 08933 US

GROWTH PLANS/SPECIAL FEATURES:
Johnson & Johnson, founded in 1886, is one of the world's largest, most comprehensive and well known manufacturers of health care products. The company has more than 200 companies in 54 countries and markets its products in almost every country in the world. Johnson & Johnson's worldwide operations are divided into three segments: consumer, pharmaceutical and medical devices and diagnostics. The company's principal consumer goods are personal care and hygiene products, including nonprescription drug, adult skin and hair care, baby care, oral care, first aid and sanitary protection products. Major brands in this segment include Mylanta, Band-Aid, Tylenol, Aveeno and Monistat. The pharmaceutical segment covers a wide spectrum of health fields, including antifungal, anti-infective, cardiovascular, dermatology, hematology, immunology, pain management, psychotropic and women's health. Among Johnson & Johnson's pharmaceutical products are Risperdal, an antipsychotic used to treat schizophrenia, and Remicade for the treatment of Crohn's Disease and rheumatoid arthritis. In the medical devices and diagnostics segment, Johnson & Johnson makes a number of professional products including suture and mechanical wound closure products, surgical instruments, disposable contact lenses, joint replacement products, intravenous catheters and medical equipment. Johnson & Johnson's medical device units develop, market and sell more medical devices than any other company in the world and its Vision Care, Inc. unit is the world leader in contact lenses. Johnson & Johnson is pursuing nanotech applications in the biomedical fields primarily through research and funding agreements with other biotech companies including Cordis and Affymetrix.

Johnson & Johnson offers employees medical and dental coverage with reimbursement accounts, life and disability insurance, comprehensive heath and wellness programs and flexible vacation schedules. Some locations offer on-site child care centers and Nurture Space programs where new mothers get counseling on how to return to work while breastfeeding.

FINANCIALS:
Sales and profits are in thousands of dollars—add 000 to get the full amount. Year 2004 note: Complete fiscal 2004 results were not available for all companies at press time. For this company, year 2004 is for 9 months.

2004 Sales: $30,608,000 (9 months) 2004 Profits: $5,352,000 (9 months)
2003 Sales: $41,862,000 2003 Profits: $7,197,000
2002 Sales: $36,298,000 2002 Profits: $6,597,000
2001 Sales: $33,004,000 2001 Profits: $5,668,000
2000 Sales: $30,129,000 2000 Profits: $5,023,000

Stock Ticker: JNJ
Employees: 110,600
Fiscal Year Ends: 12/31

SALARIES/BENEFITS:
Pension Plan: Y ESOP Stock Plan: Profit Sharing: Top Exec. Salary: $1,266,154 Bonus: $1,950,000
Savings Plan: Y Stock Purch. Plan: Second Exec. Salary: $1,037,308 Bonus: $860,000

OTHER THOUGHTS:
Apparent Top Female Officers: 3
Hot Spot for Advancement for Women/Minorities: Y

LOCATIONS: ("Y" = Yes)
West:	Southwest:	Midwest:	Southeast:	Northeast:	International:
Y	Y	Y	Y	Y	Y

Note: Financial information, benefits and other data can change quickly and may vary from those stated here.

ns
KAISER PERMANENTE

www.kaiserpermanente.org

Industry Group Code: 622110 Ranks within this company's industry group: Sales: 1 Profits: 2

Insurance/HMO/PPO:	Drugs:	Equipment/Supplies:	Hospitals/Clinics:		Services:		Health Care:	
Insurance: Managed Care: Y Utilization Mgmt.: Payment Proc.:	Manufacturer: Distributor: Specialty Pharm.: Vitamins/Nutri.: Clinical Trials:	Manufacturer: Distributor: Leasing/Finance: Information Sys.:	Acute Care: Sub-Acute Care: Outpatient Surgery: Phys. Rehab. Center: Psychiatric Clinics:	Y Y Y	Diagnostics: Labs/Testing: Staffing: Waste Disposal: Specialty Services:		Home Health: Long-Term Care: Physical Therapy: Phys. Practice Mgmt.:	Y

TYPES OF BUSINESS:
Hospitals/Clinics-General & Specialty Hospitals
HMO/PPO
Outpatient Facilities

BRANDS/DIVISIONS/AFFILIATES:
Kaiser Foundation Health Plans
Kaiser Foundation Hospitals
Permanente Medical Groups

CONTACTS:
Note: Officers with more than one job title may be intentionally listed here more than once.

George C. Halvorson, CEO
Robert E. Briggs, Sr. VP/CFO
Laurence G. O'Neil, Sr. VP-Human Resources
Robert M. Crane, Sr. VP-Research & Policy Dev.
J. Clifford Dodd, Sr. VP/CIO
Arthur M. Southam, Sr. VP-Product & Market Mgmt.
J. Clifford Dodd, Sr. VP/Chief Admin. Officer
Leslie A. Margolin, Sr. VP-Health Plan & Hospital Oper.
Bernard J. Tyson, Sr. VP-Comm. & External Rel.
Francis J. Crosson, Exec. Dir.-The Permanente Federation
Raymond J. Baxter, Sr. VP-Community Benefits
Louise L. Liang, Sr. VP-Quality & Clinical Systems Support
Steven Zatkin, Sr. VP-Gov't Rel.
George C. Halvorson, Chmn.

Phone: 510-271-5800 Fax: 510-267-7524
Toll-Free:
Address: One Kaiser Plaza, Ste. 2600, Oakland, CA 94612-3673 US

GROWTH PLANS/SPECIAL FEATURES:
Kaiser Permanente is a private, not-for-profit health care organization dedicated to providing integrated health care coverage. The company operates in nine states and Washington, D.C., serving a total of 8.2 million members, with about 6 million of those in California. Kaiser is separated into three operating divisions: Kaiser Foundation Health Plans, which contracts with individuals and groups to provide medical coverage; Kaiser Foundation Hospitals, which operates community hospitals and outpatient facilities in several states; and Permanente Medical Groups, which is the company's network of physicians who provide health care to its members. In total, the company operates through 30 medical centers, including hospitals and outpatient facilities, 431 medical offices and 11,000 physicians. In addition, Kaiser Foundation Hospitals fund medical and health-related research. The company recently received approval for the construction of a new hospital in Antioch, California. The new facility, a 600,000-square-foot building, will contain office space, 150 beds and six operating rooms; it is due for completion in 2007.

Kaiser Permanente offers health coverage for its employees, their spouses, domestic partners and children, as well as paid time off and life/disability insurance.

FINANCIALS:
Sales and profits are in thousands of dollars—add 000 to get the full amount. Year 2004 note: Complete fiscal 2004 results were not available for all companies at press time. For this company, year 2004 is for months.

2004 Sales: $ (months)   2004 Profits: $ (months)
2003 Sales: $25,300,000   2003 Profits: $996,000
2002 Sales: $22,500,000   2002 Profits: $
2001 Sales: $ 2001 Profits: $
2000 Sales: $ 2000 Profits: $

Stock Ticker: Nonprofit
Employees: 147,000
Fiscal Year Ends: 12/31

SALARIES/BENEFITS:
Pension Plan: Y   ESOP Stock Plan: Profit Sharing: Top Exec. Salary: $ Bonus: $
Savings Plan: Y   Stock Purch. Plan: Second Exec. Salary: $ Bonus: $

OTHER THOUGHTS:
Apparent Top Female Officers: 2
Hot Spot for Advancement for Women/Minorities:

LOCATIONS: ("Y" = Yes)
West:	Southwest:	Midwest:	Southeast:	Northeast:	International:
Y		Y	Y	Y	

Note: Financial information, benefits and other data can change quickly and may vary from those stated here.

KENDLE INTERNATIONAL INC

www.kendle.com

Industry Group Code: 541710 Ranks within this company's industry group: Sales: 6 Profits: 6

Insurance/HMO/PPO:	Drugs:	Equipment/Supplies:	Hospitals/Clinics:	Services:		Health Care:	
Insurance:	Manufacturer:	Manufacturer:	Acute Care:	Diagnostics:		Home Health:	
Managed Care:	Distributor:	Distributor:	Sub-Acute Care:	Labs/Testing:	Y	Long-Term Care:	
Utilization Mgmt.:	Specialty Pharm.:	Leasing/Finance:	Outpatient Surgery:	Staffing:		Physical Therapy:	
Payment Proc.:	Vitamins/Nutri.:	Information Sys.: Y	Phys. Rehab. Center:	Waste Disposal:		Phys. Practice Mgmt.:	
	Clinical Trials: Y		Psychiatric Clinics:	Specialty Services:	Y		

TYPES OF BUSINESS:
Research & Development-Clinical Trials
Statistical Analysis
Technical Writing
Consulting Services
e-Learning
Clinical Trial Software
Clinical Data Management

BRANDS/DIVISIONS/AFFILIATES:
eKendleCollege
TriAlert
TrialWare
TrialWeb
TrialBase
TrialView
TriaLine

CONTACTS: Note: Officers with more than one job title may be intentionally listed here more than once.
Candace K. Kendle, CEO
Christopher C. Bergen, Pres.
Christopher C. Bergen, COO
Karl Brenkert, III, CFO/Sr. VP
Thomas Stilgenbauer, Exec. VP/Chief Mktg. Officer
Anthony L. Forcellini, Sr. VP-Oper.
Karl Brenkert, III, Treas.
Keith A. Cheesman, Dir.-Admin.
Malcolm Summers, Dir.-European Regulatory Consulting
Melanie A. Bruno, VP-Global Regulatory Affairs
Candace K. Kendle, Chmn.

Phone: 513-381-5550 Fax: 513-381-5870
Toll-Free: 800-733-1572
Address: 1200 Carew Tower, 441 Vine St., Cincinnati, OH 45202 US

GROWTH PLANS/SPECIAL FEATURES:
Kendle International, Inc. is a contract research organization that provides drug research and development services in the pharmaceutical and biotechnology industries. Its services include clinical trial management, clinical data management, statistical analysis, technical writing and regulatory consulting and representation. Kendle runs a state-of-the-art clinical pharmacology unit in The Netherlands, where it offers services for drugs undergoing Phase I and IIA clinical trials. Through its health care communications division, the firm provides organizational, meeting management and publication services to various professional associations and pharmaceutical companies. The firm's proprietary software, TrialWare, processes clinical trial data through automated workflow and parallel processing in a standard format. The TrialWare product line includes a database management system, TrialBase; an interactive voice response patient randomization system, TriaLine; an online case report forms review system, TrialView; and a coding enhancement feature, TriAlert. The company also operates eKendleCollege, an online e-learning division that runs seminars and training programs, focusing on the organization of clinical trials. Kendle has been working to expand its overseas operations with strategic acquisitions of foreign contract research organizations. In June 2004 Kendle opened new offices in Bucharest, Romania and in Sofia, Bulgaria. The company has also recently updated TrialView to provide planimetry capabilities. The new function helps biopharmaceutical companies to measure body areas and volume during the conduct of clinical trials.
Kendle offers its employees stock options, flexible work schedules, business-casual dress and continuing education through its corporate university and tuition reimbursement program, as well as the option to telecommute. Additionally, senior personnel are eligible for a management bonus. Full- or part-time associates who work at least 24 hours a week are eligible for benefits.

FINANCIALS: Sales and profits are in thousands of dollars—add 000 to get the full amount. Year 2004 note: Complete fiscal 2004 results were not available for all companies at press time. For this company, year 2004 is for 9 months.

2004 Sales: $156,697 (9 months) 2004 Profits: $1,484 (9 months)
2003 Sales: $209,657 2003 Profits: $-1,690
2002 Sales: $214,000 2002 Profits: $-54,800
2001 Sales: $154,300 2001 Profits: $4,200
2000 Sales: $120,500 2000 Profits: $-2,100

Stock Ticker: KNDL
Employees: 1,680
Fiscal Year Ends: 12/31

SALARIES/BENEFITS:
Pension Plan: ESOP Stock Plan: Profit Sharing: Y Top Exec. Salary: $290,338 Bonus: $33,518
Savings Plan: Y Stock Purch. Plan: Y Second Exec. Salary: $251,815 Bonus: $22,669

OTHER THOUGHTS:
Apparent Top Female Officers: 2
Hot Spot for Advancement for Women/Minorities:

LOCATIONS: ("Y" = Yes)
West:	Southwest:	Midwest:	Southeast:	Northeast:	International:
Y		Y		Y	Y

KIMBERLY CLARK CORP

www.kimberly-clark.com

Industry Group Code: 322000 Ranks within this company's industry group: Sales: 1 Profits: 1

Insurance/HMO/PPO:	Drugs:	Equipment/Supplies:	Hospitals/Clinics:	Services:	Health Care:
Insurance:	Manufacturer:	Manufacturer: Y	Acute Care:	Diagnostics:	Home Health:
Managed Care:	Distributor:	Distributor:	Sub-Acute Care:	Labs/Testing:	Long-Term Care:
Utilization Mgmt.:	Specialty Pharm.:	Leasing/Finance:	Outpatient Surgery:	Staffing:	Physical Therapy:
Payment Proc.:	Vitamins/Nutri.:	Information Sys.:	Phys. Rehab. Center:	Waste Disposal:	Phys. Practice Mgmt.:
	Clinical Trials:		Psychiatric Clinics:	Specialty Services:	

TYPES OF BUSINESS:
Personal Paper Products Manufacturer
Facial & Bathroom Tissue
Disposable Diapers
Health Care Products
Printing Products

BRANDS/DIVISIONS/AFFILIATES:
Kleenex
Scott
Huggies
Kotex
Depend
Pull-Ups
Safeskin
Wypall

CONTACTS: Note: Officers with more than one job title may be intentionally listed here more than once.
Thomas J. Falk, CEO
Mark A. Buthman, Sr. VP/CFO
Lizanne C. Gottung, Sr. VP-Human Resources
Cheryl A. Perkins, Sr. VP/Chief Tech. Officer
Ronald D. Mc Cray, Sr. VP-Law & Gov't Affairs
Robert E. Abernathy, Group Pres.-Dev. & Emerging Markets
Steven R. Kalmanson, Group Pres.-North Atlantic Personal Care
W. Dudley Lehman, Group Pres.-Business-to-Business
Robert P. van der Merwe, Group Pres.-North Atlantic Consumer Tissue
Thomas J. Falk, Chmn.

Phone: 972-281-1200 Fax: 972-281-1490
Toll-Free:
Address: 351 Phelps Dr., Irving, TX 75038 US

GROWTH PLANS/SPECIAL FEATURES:
Kimberly-Clark is a leading global manufacturer of consumer tissue, personal care and business-to-business products. The consumer tissue segment manufactures and markets facial and bathroom tissue, paper towels and napkins for household use, wet wipes and related products. Products in this segment are sold under the Kleenex, Scott, Cottonelle, Viva, Andrex, Scottex, Page, Huggies and other brand names. The newest product in this segment is Kleenex's Anti-Viral tissue, designed to kill 99.9% of cold and flu viruses in the tissue within 15 minutes. The firm's personal care segment manufactures and markets disposable diapers, training and youth pants, swimpants, feminine and incontinence care products and other related products. These products are sold under a variety of well-known brand names, including Huggies, Pull-Ups, Little Swimmers, GoodNites, Kotex, Lightdays, Depend and Poise. Kimberly-Clark's business-to-business segment manufactures and markets facial and bathroom tissue, paper towels, wipes and napkins for away-from-home use; health care products such as surgical gowns, drapes, infection control products, sterilization wraps, disposable face masks and exam gloves, respiratory products and other disposable medical products; printing, premium business and correspondence papers; specialty and technical papers; and other products. Products in this segment are sold under the Kimberly-Clark, Kleenex, Scott, Kimwipes, WypAll, Surpass, Safeskin, Tecnol, Ballard and other brand names. In July 2004, the company announced plans to spin-off its paper business into a $655-million-a-year company.

Kimberly-Clark offers its employees tuition reimbursement and medical and dental insurance.

FINANCIALS: Sales and profits are in thousands of dollars—add 000 to get the full amount. Year 2004 note: Complete fiscal 2004 results were not available for all companies at press time. For this company, year 2004 is for 9 months.

2004 Sales: $1,144,100 (9 months)   2004 Profits: $1,354,900 (9 months)
2003 Sales: $14,348,000   2003 Profits: $1,694,200
2002 Sales: $13,566,000   2002 Profits: $1,675,000
2001 Sales: $14,524,000   2001 Profits: $1,610,000
2000 Sales: $13,982,000   2000 Profits: $1,800,600

Stock Ticker: KMB
Employees: 62,000
Fiscal Year Ends: 12/31

SALARIES/BENEFITS:
Pension Plan: Y ESOP Stock Plan: Profit Sharing: Top Exec. Salary: $987,500 Bonus: $840,000
Savings Plan: Y Stock Purch. Plan: Second Exec. Salary: $520,000 Bonus: $346,710

OTHER THOUGHTS:
Apparent Top Female Officers: 2
Hot Spot for Advancement for Women/Minorities:

LOCATIONS: ("Y" = Yes)
West:	Southwest:	Midwest:	Southeast:	Northeast:	International:
Y	Y	Y	Y	Y	Y

Note: Financial information, benefits and other data can change quickly and may vary from those stated here.

KINDRED HEALTHCARE INC

www.kindredhealthcare.com

Industry Group Code: 623110   Ranks within this company's industry group: Sales: 1   Profits: 13

Insurance/HMO/PPO:	Drugs:	Equipment/Supplies:	Hospitals/Clinics:		Services:		Health Care:	
Insurance: Managed Care: Utilization Mgmt.: Payment Proc.:	Manufacturer: Distributor: Specialty Pharm.: Y Vitamins/Nutri.: Clinical Trials:	Manufacturer: Distributor: Leasing/Finance: Information Sys.:	Acute Care: Sub-Acute Care: Outpatient Surgery: Phys. Rehab. Center: Psychiatric Clinics:	Y Y	Diagnostics: Labs/Testing: Staffing: Waste Disposal: Specialty Services:		Home Health: Long-Term Care: Physical Therapy: Phys. Practice Mgmt.:	Y Y

TYPES OF BUSINESS:
Nursing Homes
Acute Care Hospitals
Rehabilitation Therapy
Specialty Pharmacies

BRANDS/DIVISIONS/AFFILIATES:
Peoplefirst Rehabilitation

CONTACTS:
Note: Officers with more than one job title may be intentionally listed here more than once.
Paul J. Diaz, CEO
Paul J. Diaz, Pres.
Richard A. Lechleiter, Sr. VP/CFO
Richard E. Chapman, Sr. VP/CIO
Richard E. Chapman, Chief Admin. Officer
M. Suzanne Riedman, Sr. VP/General Counsel
Susan E. Moss, VP-Corp. Comm.
Frank J. Battafarano, Pres.-Hospital Div.
Lane M. Bowen, Pres.-Health Services Div.
William M. Altman, VP-Compliance & Gov't Programs
Mark A. McCullough, Pres.-Pharmacy Div.
Edward L. Kuntz, Chmn.

Phone: 502-596-7300   **Fax:** 502-596-4170
Toll-Free:
Address: 680 S. 4th St., Louisville, KY 40202 US

GROWTH PLANS/SPECIAL FEATURES:
Kindred Healthcare, Inc. provides long-term health care services primarily through the operation of nursing centers and hospitals. The firm is organized into three operating divisions. The health services division provides long-term care services through 255 nursing centers, with nearly 33,000 licensed beds in 30 states, and a physical, occupational and speech rehabilitation therapy business operating under the name Peoplefirst Rehabilitation. A number of these nursing centers offer specialized programs for residents suffering from Alzheimer's disease and dementia, in addition to standard long-term care, pharmacy, medical, clinical, dietary, social and recreational services. Kindred's hospital division provides long-term acute care services to medically complex patients by operating 66 hospitals, with over 5,200 licensed beds in 23 states. This is the largest network of long-term acute care hospitals in the U.S. based on revenues, treating patients who suffer from multiple organ system failures, neurological disorders, head injuries, brain stem and spinal cord trauma, cerebral vascular accidents, chemical brain injuries, central nervous system disorders, developmental anomalies and cardiopulmonary disorders. The company's pharmacy division provides services to nursing centers and specialized care centers, operating 30 institutional pharmacies in 19 states that serve approximately 61,400 patients. This division serves over 680 facilities, including skilled nursing facilities, assisted living facilities and psychiatric hospitals. A major portion of Kindred's revenue comes from Medicare and Medicaid reimbursements.

FINANCIALS:
Sales and profits are in thousands of dollars—add 000 to get the full amount. Year 2004 note: Complete fiscal 2004 results were not available for all companies at press time. For this company, year 2004 is for 9 months.

2004 Sales: $2,643,783 (9 months)   2004 Profits: $51,177   (9 months)
2003 Sales: $3,284,019   2003 Profits: $-75,336
2002 Sales: $3,357,800   2002 Profits: $34,700
2001 Sales: $3,081,400   2001 Profits: $523,600
2000 Sales: $2,888,500   2000 Profits: $-64,751

Stock Ticker: KIND
Employees: 50,900
Fiscal Year Ends: 12/31

SALARIES/BENEFITS:
Pension Plan: ESOP Stock Plan: Profit Sharing: Top Exec. Salary: $844,200   Bonus: $1,587,560
Savings Plan: Y   Stock Purch. Plan: Second Exec. Salary: $618,000   Bonus: $1,142,585

OTHER THOUGHTS:
Apparent Top Female Officers: 2
Hot Spot for Advancement for Women/Minorities:

LOCATIONS: ("Y" = Yes)

West	Southwest	Midwest	Southeast	Northeast	International
Y	Y	Y	Y	Y	

KINETIC CONCEPTS INC

www.kci1.com

Industry Group Code: 339113 **Ranks within this company's industry group:** Sales: 32 Profits: 28

Insurance/HMO/PPO:	Drugs:	Equipment/Supplies:		Hospitals/Clinics:	Services:	Health Care:
Insurance:	Manufacturer:	Manufacturer:	Y	Acute Care:	Diagnostics:	Home Health:
Managed Care:	Distributor:	Distributor:	Y	Sub-Acute Care:	Labs/Testing:	Long-Term Care:
Utilization Mgmt.:	Specialty Pharm.:	Leasing/Finance:		Outpatient Surgery:	Staffing:	Physical Therapy:
Payment Proc.:	Vitamins/Nutri.:	Information Sys.:		Phys. Rehab. Center:	Waste Disposal:	Phys. Practice Mgmt.:
	Clinical Trials:			Psychiatric Clinics:	Specialty Services:	

TYPES OF BUSINESS:
Equipment-Specialized Mattresses & Beds
Kinetic Therapy Products
Therapeutic Support Surfaces
Wound Closure Devices
Circulatory Devices

BRANDS/DIVISIONS/AFFILIATES:
Roto Rest Delta
FirstStep
KinAir
AtmosAir
V.A.C. System
TheraPulse
TriaDyne
PediDyne

CONTACTS:
Note: Officers with more than one job title may be intentionally listed here more than once.

Dennert O. Ware, CEO
Dennert O. Ware, Pres.
Martin J. Landon, VP/CFO
R. James Cravens, VP-Human Resources
Daniel C. Wadsworth, Jr., VP-Global Research & Dev.
Michael J. Burke, VP-Mfg.
Dennis E. Noll, Sr. VP/General Counsel
G. Frederick Rush, VP-Corp. Dev.
Martin J. Landon, VP-Finance
Christopher M. Fashek, Pres.-USA
Michael J. Burke, VP-Quality
Steven J. Hartpence, VP-Bus. Systems
Robert Jaunich, II, Chmn.
Jorg W. Menten, Pres.-Int'l

Phone: 210-524-9000 **Fax:** 210-255-6998
Toll-Free: 888-275-4524
Address: 8023 Vantage Dr., San Antonio, TX 78230 US

GROWTH PLANS/SPECIAL FEATURES:
Kinetic Concepts, Inc. (KCI) is a global medical technology company that designs, manufactures, markets and services proprietary products that can improve clinical outcomes by accelerating the healing process or preventing complications. The company's medical systems and therapeutic surfaces are used in four major clinical applications. Its five wound healing and tissue repair systems incorporate Vacuum Assisted Closure (V.A.C.) technology, consisting of the therapy unit, a foam dressing, an occlusive drape, a tube system connecting the dressing to the therapy unit and a canister. This negative pressure therapy is used on serious trauma wounds, failed surgical closures, amputations, burns covering a large portion of the body, serious pressure ulcers and other difficult wounds. For treatment of complications of immobility KCI offers the TriaDyne, Roto Rest Delta and PediDyne therapy systems, which rotate the patient by up to 62 degrees on either side, using kinetic therapy to promote pulmonary health. The company's therapeutic surfaces for wound treatment and prevention treat pressure sores, burns, ulcers, skin grafts and other skin conditions. They also help prevent the formation of pressure sores in certain immobile individuals by reducing friction between skin and bed and by using surfaces supported by air, foam, silicon beads or viscous fluid. These include the KinAir and FluidAir beds, FirstStep and TriCell overlays and AtmosAir seating surfaces. The TheraPulse framed beds and DynaPulse overlay also provide treatment through a continuous pulsating action which improves capillary and lymphatic circulation in patients suffering from severe pressure sores, burns, skin grafts or flaps, swelling or circulatory problems. Finally, the company produces bariatric support surfaces and aids for obese patients, including the BariAir Therapy System, which can serve as both a bed and an examination table.

FINANCIALS:
Sales and profits are in thousands of dollars—add 000 to get the full amount. Year 2004 note: Complete fiscal 2004 results were not available for all companies at press time. For this company, year 2004 is for 6 months.

2004 Sales: $461,819 (6 months)	2004 Profits: $29,493 (6 months)	**Stock Ticker:** KCI
2003 Sales: $763,800	2003 Profits: $60,200	**Employees:** 2,820
2002 Sales: $579,000	2002 Profits: $106,400	**Fiscal Year Ends:** 12/31
2001 Sales: $455,947	2001 Profits: $23,901	
2000 Sales: $352,032	2000 Profits: $9,129	

SALARIES/BENEFITS:
Pension Plan:	ESOP Stock Plan:	Profit Sharing:	Top Exec. Salary: $525,359	Bonus: $393,000
Savings Plan:	Stock Purch. Plan:		Second Exec. Salary: $266,595	Bonus: $152,306

OTHER THOUGHTS:
Apparent Top Female Officers:
Hot Spot for Advancement for Women/Minorities:

LOCATIONS: ("Y" = Yes)
West:	Southwest:	Midwest:	Southeast:	Northeast:	International:
	Y				Y

KYPHON INC

www.kyphon.com

Industry Group Code: 339113 Ranks within this company's industry group: Sales: 79 Profits: 47

Insurance/HMO/PPO:	Drugs:	Equipment/Supplies:		Hospitals/Clinics:	Services:	Health Care:
Insurance:	Manufacturer:	Manufacturer:	Y	Acute Care:	Diagnostics:	Home Health:
Managed Care:	Distributor:	Distributor:		Sub-Acute Care:	Labs/Testing:	Long-Term Care:
Utilization Mgmt.:	Specialty Pharm.:	Leasing/Finance:		Outpatient Surgery:	Staffing:	Physical Therapy:
Payment Proc.:	Vitamins/Nutri.:	Information Sys.:		Phys. Rehab. Center:	Waste Disposal:	Phys. Practice Mgmt.:
	Clinical Trials:			Psychiatric Clinics:	Specialty Services:	

TYPES OF BUSINESS:
Surgical Equipment-Spinal

BRANDS/DIVISIONS/AFFILIATES:
KyphX
KyphOs
KyphX HV-R
Sanatis GmbH

CONTACTS:
Note: Officers with more than one job title may be intentionally listed here more than once.

Richard W. Mott, CEO
Richard W. Mott, Pres.
Arthur T. Taylor, VP/CFO
Julie D. Tracy, VP-Mktg.
Stephen C. Hams, VP-Human Resources
Karen D. Talmadge, Exec. VP/Chief Science Officer
David M. Shaw, General Counsel/VP-Legal Affairs
Elizabeth A. Rothwell, VP-Oper. & Quality
Cindy M. Domescus, VP-Clinical Research & Regulatory Affairs
Mary K. Hailey, VP-Reimbursement
Avram A. Edidin, VP-Research & Dev.
Anthony J. Recupero, VP-Sales

Phone: 408-548-6500 Fax: 408-548-6501
Toll-Free:
Address: 1221 Crossman Ave., Sunnyvale, CA 94089 US

GROWTH PLANS/SPECIAL FEATURES:
Kyphon, Inc. develops medical devices to restore spinal anatomy using minimally invasive technology. Its devices are used primarily by surgeons who repair compression fractures of the spine caused by osteoporosis and cancer. The firm's commercial products, including its KyphX instruments, utilize its proprietary balloon technology. Instruments include bone access systems, inflatable bone tamps, inflation syringes, bone filler devices, bone biopsy devices and curettes. Surgeons use these instruments to help repair compression fractures during minimally invasive spine surgeries. Most alternative spine fracture treatments are either highly invasive or are pain management therapies. As of December 2003, Kyphon had trained more than 3,900 physicians in the U.S., Europe and Asia Pacific in the use of its KyphX instruments, and these physicians had used these instruments in over 60,000 spine surgeries. The company believes the use of KyphX instruments leads to significant patient benefits, including the ability to reverse the collapse of the bone caused by the spine fracture. Reversal of collapsed spine can reduce spine deformity, thereby increasing mobility and improving respiratory function in patients. In February 2003, Kyphon acquired Sanatis GmbH, a developer and manufacturer of orthopedic biomaterials, which can resorb or remodel into bone in traumatic fracture patients when used instead of more traditional bone filler materials. The company has obtained authorization to sell its first product from this acquisition, KyphOs calcium phosphate cement, in Europe. Kyphon recently launched KyphX HV-R bone cement, the first product on the market specifically indicated for treating spinal fractures caused by osteoporosis.

FINANCIALS:
Sales and profits are in thousands of dollars—add 000 to get the full amount. Year 2004 note: Complete fiscal 2004 results were not available for all companies at press time. For this company, year 2004 is for 9 months.

2004 Sales: $150,989 (9 months)   2004 Profits: $15,648 (9 months)
2003 Sales: $131,028   2003 Profits: $27,323
2002 Sales: $76,316   2002 Profits: $-15,338
2001 Sales: $ 2001 Profits: $
2000 Sales: $ 2000 Profits: $

Stock Ticker: KYPH
Employees: 441
Fiscal Year Ends: 12/31

SALARIES/BENEFITS:
| Pension Plan: | ESOP Stock Plan: | Profit Sharing: | Top Exec. Salary: $317,500 | Bonus: $54,634 |
| Savings Plan: | Stock Purch. Plan: | | Second Exec. Salary: $226,000 | Bonus: $53,750 |

OTHER THOUGHTS:
Apparent Top Female Officers: 5
Hot Spot for Advancement for Women/Minorities: Y

LOCATIONS: ("Y" = Yes)
West:	Southwest:	Midwest:	Southeast:	Northeast:	International:
Y					Y

LABONE INC

www.labone.com

Industry Group Code: 621511 Ranks within this company's industry group: Sales: 4 Profits: 3

Insurance/HMO/PPO:	Drugs:	Equipment/Supplies:	Hospitals/Clinics:	Services:	Health Care:
Insurance: Managed Care: Utilization Mgmt.: Payment Proc.:	Manufacturer: Distributor: Specialty Pharm.: Vitamins/Nutri.: Clinical Trials:	Manufacturer: Distributor: Leasing/Finance: Information Sys.:	Acute Care: Sub-Acute Care: Outpatient Surgery: Phys. Rehab. Center: Psychiatric Clinics:	Diagnostics: Labs/Testing: Y Staffing: Waste Disposal: Specialty Services: Y	Home Health: Long-Term Care: Physical Therapy: Phys. Practice Mgmt.:

TYPES OF BUSINESS:
Services-Testing (Life, Disability & Medical Insurance Prospects)
Risk Assessment Services
Health Care Laboratory Testing
Substance Abuse Testing

BRANDS/DIVISIONS/AFFILIATES:
Northwest Toxicology
ExamOne

CONTACTS: Note: Officers with more than one job title may be intentionally listed here more than once.
W. Thomas Grant, II, CEO
W. Thomas Grant, II, Pres.
Michael J. Asselta, Exec. VP/COO
John W. McCarty, CFO
Philip A. Spencer, Exec. VP-Health Care Mktg.
Dan McCabe, VP-Shared IT Services
Michael G. Dorman, Chief Tech. Officer
Joseph C. Benage, Exec. VP/General Counsel
Craig R. Meegan, VP/Controller
Troy L. Hartman, Exec. VP/Pres., ExamOne
James J. Mussatto, Exec. VP-Health Care & Substance Abuse Testing
Joseph C. Benage, Corp. Sec.
Gregg R. Sadler, Exec. VP/Pres.-Insurance Services
W. Thomas Grant, II, Chmn.

Phone: 913-888-1770 Fax: 913-888-0771
Toll-Free:
Address: 10101 Renner Blvd., Lenexa, KS 66219 US

GROWTH PLANS/SPECIAL FEATURES:
LabOne, Inc., provides risk assessment services for the insurance industry, laboratory testing services for the health care industry and substance abuse testing services for employers and third-party administrators. The firm's risk assessment division provides underwriting and claims support services including tele-underwriting, specimen collection and paramedical examinations, laboratory testing, telephone inspections, motor vehicle reports and medical information retrieval to the insurance industry. Laboratory tests performed by the company are specifically designed to assist an insurance company in objectively evaluating the mortality and morbidity risks posed by policy applicants. The majority of the testing is performed on specimens of individual life insurance policy applicants but also includes specimens of individuals applying for individual and group medical and disability policies. The clinical division includes laboratory testing services for the health care industry as an aid in the diagnosis and treatment of patients. The most frequently requested tests include blood chemistry analyses, urinalyses, blood cell counts, Pap smears and infectious disease tests. LabOne operates a highly automated and centralized laboratory, which the company believes has significant economic advantages over other conventional laboratory competitors. The firm markets its clinical testing services to managed care companies, insurance companies, self-insured groups and physicians. The clinical division also includes substance abuse testing services provided to employers who adhere to drug screening guidelines. The company's rapid turnaround times and multiple testing options help clients reduce downtime for affected employees and meet mandated drug screening guidelines. In recent news, LabOne announced the acquisition of the assets of the drug testing division, Northwest Toxicology, of NWT, Inc.

LabOne provides employees with a choice of health plans, dental coverage, life insurance, tuition reimbursement and training and seminar opportunities. The company also offers a wide range of services including an apartment search service, child care referral, dry cleaning, mail services, massages, film development, windshield repair, YMCA membership and an on-site ATM, basketball court, cafeteria, store, fitness center and travel agent.

FINANCIALS: Sales and profits are in thousands of dollars—add 000 to get the full amount. Year 2004 note: Complete fiscal 2004 results were not available for all companies at press time. For this company, year 2004 is for 9 months.

2004 Sales: $348,146 (9 months)   2004 Profits: $18,781 (9 months)
2003 Sales: $346,020   2003 Profits: $20,732
2002 Sales: $298,100   2002 Profits: $14,800
2001 Sales: $233,900   2001 Profits: $-1,000
2000 Sales: $169,200   2000 Profits: $- 500

Stock Ticker: LABS
Employees: 3,000
Fiscal Year Ends: 12/31

SALARIES/BENEFITS:
Pension Plan: Y   ESOP Stock Plan: Profit Sharing: Top Exec. Salary: $325,000   Bonus: $320,125
Savings Plan: Y   Stock Purch. Plan: Second Exec. Salary: $225,000 Bonus: $166,219

OTHER THOUGHTS:
Apparent Top Female Officers:
Hot Spot for Advancement for Women/Minorities:

LOCATIONS: ("Y" = Yes)
West:	Southwest:	Midwest:	Southeast:	Northeast:	International:
		Y			Y

Note: Financial information, benefits and other data can change quickly and may vary from those stated here.

LABORATORY CORP OF AMERICA HOLDINGS   www.labcorp.com

Industry Group Code: 621511   Ranks within this company's industry group: Sales: 2   Profits: 2

Insurance/HMO/PPO:	Drugs:	Equipment/Supplies:	Hospitals/Clinics:	Services:		Health Care:
Insurance:	Manufacturer:	Manufacturer:	Acute Care:	Diagnostics:		Home Health:
Managed Care:	Distributor:	Distributor:	Sub-Acute Care:	Labs/Testing:	Y	Long-Term Care:
Utilization Mgmt.:	Specialty Pharm.:	Leasing/Finance:	Outpatient Surgery:	Staffing:		Physical Therapy:
Payment Proc.:	Vitamins/Nutri.:	Information Sys.:	Phys. Rehab. Center:	Waste Disposal:		Phys. Practice Mgmt.:
	Clinical Trials:		Psychiatric Clinics:	Specialty Services:		

TYPES OF BUSINESS:
Clinical Laboratory Testing
Diagnostics
Urinalyses
Blood Cell Counts
Blood Chemistry Analysis
HIV Tests
Pap Smears
Specialty & Niche Tests

BRANDS/DIVISIONS/AFFILIATES:
DIANON Systems, Inc.
Dynacare, Inc.

CONTACTS: Note: Officers with more than one job title may be intentionally listed here more than once.
Thomas P. Mac Mahon, CEO
Thomas P. Mac Mahon, Pres.
Richard L. Novak, Exec. VP/COO
Wesley R. Elingburg, Exec. VP/CFO
William B. Haas, Exec. VP-Sales & Mktg.
Myla P. Lai-Goldman, Exec. VP/Chief Scientific Officer
David P. King, Exec. VP-Strategic Planning & Corp. Dev.
Bradford T. Smith, Exec. VP-Corp. Affairs
Wesley R. Elingburg, Treas.
Myla P. Lai-Goldman, Medical Dir.
Bradford T. Smith, Chief Legal Officer
Thomas P. Mac Mahon, Chmn.

Phone: 336-229-1127   Fax:
Toll-Free:
Address: 358 S. Main St., Burlington, NC 27215 US

GROWTH PLANS/SPECIAL FEATURES:
Laboratory Corporation of America Holdings (LabCorp) is the second-largest independent clinical laboratory company in the U.S., offering more than 4,400 different health-related laboratory tests to the medical industry. The tests are primarily used in routine screening, patient diagnosis and the monitoring and treatment of disease. The company operates a nationwide network of 31 primary testing facilities and over 1,100 service centers, consisting of branches, patient service centers and STAT labs, which can perform routine tests quickly and report results to the physician immediately. The most common tests performed by the firm include blood chemistry analysis, urinalyses, blood cell counts, Pap smears, HIV tests, microbiology cultures and substance abuse tests. The firm generally performs and reports routine tests within 24 hours, utilizing a variety of sophisticated and computer-enhanced laboratory testing equipment. The company processes an average of approximately 340,000 patient specimens per day, serving clients in all 50 states, the District of Columbia, Puerto Rico and Canada. LabCorp also performs specialty and niche testing including infectious disease and allergy testing and a number of diagnostic genetics testing services and forensic identity tests. The company provides clinical laboratory testing for pharmaceutical companies conducting clinical research trials on new drugs. The expansion of its specialty and niche testing business is currently a primary growth strategy for the company. LabCorp continually seeks new and improved technologies to enhance its testing services and increase the broad range of tests it offers. The company has grown significantly in recent years, primarily through the acquisitions of Dynacare, Inc., a provider of clinical laboratory testing services in the U.S. and Canada; and DIANON Systems, Inc., a leading national provider of anatomic pathology and genetic testing services.

FINANCIALS:
Sales and profits are in thousands of dollars—add 000 to get the full amount. Year 2004 note: Complete fiscal 2004 results were not available for all companies at press time. For this company, year 2004 is for 9 months.

2004 Sales: $2,318,300 (9 months)	2004 Profits: $278,200 (9 months)	Stock Ticker: LH
2003 Sales: $2,939,400	2003 Profits: $321,000	Employees: 23,000
2002 Sales: $2,507,700	2002 Profits: $254,600	Fiscal Year Ends: 12/31
2001 Sales: $2,199,800	2001 Profits: $179,500	
2000 Sales: $1,919,300	2000 Profits: $112,100	

SALARIES/BENEFITS:
Pension Plan: Y   ESOP Stock Plan: Profit Sharing: Top Exec. Salary: $845,625   Bonus: $1,297,910
Savings Plan: Stock Purch. Plan: Second Exec. Salary: $469,040   Bonus: $571,709

OTHER THOUGHTS:
Apparent Top Female Officers: 1
Hot Spot for Advancement for Women/Minorities:

LOCATIONS: ("Y" = Yes)
West:	Southwest:	Midwest:	Southeast:	Northeast:	International:
Y	Y	Y	Y	Y	Y

Plunkett's Health Care Industry Almanac 2005

LAKELAND INDUSTRIES INC
www.lakeland.com

Industry Group Code: 339113 Ranks within this company's industry group: Sales: 101 Profits: 94

Insurance/HMO/PPO:	Drugs:	Equipment/Supplies:		Hospitals/Clinics:	Services:	Health Care:
Insurance:	Manufacturer:	Manufacturer:	Y	Acute Care:	Diagnostics:	Home Health:
Managed Care:	Distributor:	Distributor:		Sub-Acute Care:	Labs/Testing:	Long-Term Care:
Utilization Mgmt.:	Specialty Pharm.:	Leasing/Finance:		Outpatient Surgery:	Staffing:	Physical Therapy:
Payment Proc.:	Vitamins/Nutri.:	Information Sys.:		Phys. Rehab. Center:	Waste Disposal:	Phys. Practice Mgmt.:
	Clinical Trials:			Psychiatric Clinics:	Specialty Services:	

TYPES OF BUSINESS:
Safety Clothing
Reusable Industrial and Medical Apparel
Protective Systems and Body Suits
Specialty Safety Gloves

BRANDS/DIVISIONS/AFFILIATES:
Lakeland Protective Wear, Inc.

CONTACTS:
Note: Officers with more than one job title may be intentionally listed here more than once.

Christopher J. Ryan, CEO
Christopher J. Ryan, Pres.
James M. McCormick, CFO
Harvey Pride, Jr., VP-Mfg.
Christopher J. Ryan, General Counsel
James M. McCormick, Treas.
Christopher J. Ryan, Corp. Sec.
Raymond J. Smith, Chmn.

Phone: 631-981-9700   **Fax:** 631-981-9751
Toll-Free: 800-645-9291
Address: 711-2 Koehler Ave., Ronkonkorna, NY 11779-7410 US

GROWTH PLANS/SPECIAL FEATURES:

Lakeland Industries, Inc. manufactures and sells a comprehensive line of safety garments and accessories for the industrial safety and protective clothing industries in the United States. The company's major product areas include disposable and limited-use protective industrial garments; specialty safety and industrial work gloves; reusable woven industrial and medical apparel; fire- and heat-protective clothing; and protective systems and body suits for use by toxic waste clean-up teams, hazardous material clean-up teams and first responders to acts of terrorism. The firm's garments protect the wearer from contaminants or irritants, such as chemicals, pesticides, fertilizers, paint, grease and dust, and from limited exposure to hazardous waste and toxic chemicals including acids, asbestos, lead and hydro-carbons (PCBs). Lakeland's products are also used to prevent human contamination of manufacturing processes in clean-room environments. Lakeland's disposable clothing products protect a wearer's hands and arms from lacerations, heat and chemical irritants without sacrificing manual dexterity or comfort. Health care workers at hospitals, clinics and emergency rescue sites use Lakeland products to protect themselves from viruses, bacteria and contagious diseases such as AIDS and hepatitis. Finally, the firm's products protect wearers from highly concentrated and powerful chemical and biological toxins such as toxic wastes at Super Fund sites, accidental toxic chemical spills or biological discharges, the handling of chemical or biological warfare weapons and the cleaning and maintenance of chemical, petro-chemical and nuclear facilities. Lakeland buys most of its raw materials for manufacturing from DuPont, including Kevlar and Tyvek. Recently, due to increased demand by first responders for its chemical and fire gear, the company's seasonal selling pattern has shifted. Based on the size and timing of governmental orders, which depend upon disbursals that do not follow ordinary seasonal sales patterns, the company anticipates unusual fluctuations in working capital requirements.

About 78% of the company's employees work in its international facilities in Burlington, Ontario; Celaya, Mexico; and AnQui City, China. All employees in Mexico and China belong to labor unions.

FINANCIALS:
Sales and profits are in thousands of dollars—add 000 to get the full amount. Year 2004 note: Complete fiscal 2004 results were not available for all companies at press time. For this company, year 2004 is for 12 months.

2004 Sales: $89,717 (12 months)   2004 Profits: $3,638 (12 months)
2003 Sales: $77,800   2003 Profits: $2,600
2002 Sales: $76,400   2002 Profits: $2,000
2001 Sales: $76,100   2001 Profits: $1,100
2000 Sales: $58,600   2000 Profits: $1,700

Stock Ticker: LAKE
Employees: 1,292
Fiscal Year Ends: 1/31

SALARIES/BENEFITS:
Pension Plan: Y   ESOP Stock Plan: Profit Sharing: Top Exec. Salary: $262,500   Bonus: $82,500
Savings Plan: Y   Stock Purch. Plan: Second Exec. Salary: $215,000   Bonus: $40,300

OTHER THOUGHTS:
Apparent Top Female Officers:
Hot Spot for Advancement for Women/Minorities:

LOCATIONS: ("Y" = Yes)
West:	Southwest:	Midwest:	Southeast:	Northeast:	International:
			Y	Y	Y

Note: Financial information, benefits and other data can change quickly and may vary from those stated here.

LASERSCOPE

www.laserscope.com

Industry Group Code: 339113   Ranks within this company's industry group: Sales: 109   Profits: 95

Insurance/HMO/PPO:	Drugs:	Equipment/Supplies:		Hospitals/Clinics:	Services:	Health Care:
Insurance: Managed Care: Utilization Mgmt.: Payment Proc.:	Manufacturer: Distributor: Specialty Pharm.: Vitamins/Nutri.: Clinical Trials:	Manufacturer: Distributor: Leasing/Finance: Information Sys.:	Y	Acute Care: Sub-Acute Care: Outpatient Surgery: Phys. Rehab. Center: Psychiatric Clinics:	Diagnostics: Labs/Testing: Staffing: Waste Disposal: Specialty Services:	Home Health: Long-Term Care: Physical Therapy: Phys. Practice Mgmt.:

TYPES OF BUSINESS:
Equipment-Medical Laser Systems
Energy Delivery Devices

BRANDS/DIVISIONS/AFFILIATES:
KTP/532
Niagara
Lyra
Lyra XP
Wavelight
NWL
GreenLight
800 Series

CONTACTS:
Note: Officers with more than one job title may be intentionally listed here more than once.

Eric M. Reuter, CEO
Eric M. Reuter, Pres.
Dennis LaLumandiere, CFO
William Kelley, VP-Int'l Sales
Marsha Harris, Human Resources
Ken Arnold, VP-Research & Dev.
Kerrick Securda, VP-Bus. Dev.
Dennis LaLumandiere, VP-Finance
Van A. Frazier, VP-Regulatory, Quality & Clinical
Bob Mathews, Exec. VP-Oper. & Service
Robert Mann, VP-North American Sales & Mktg.
Robert J. Pressley, Chmn.

Phone: 408-943-0636   Fax: 408-943-9630
Toll-Free: 800-356-7600
Address: 3070 Orchard Dr., San Jose, CA 95134-2011 US

GROWTH PLANS/SPECIAL FEATURES:

Laserscope designs, manufactures, sells and services an advanced line of medical laser systems and related energy devices for the medical office, outpatient surgical center and hospital markets. The company is a pioneer in the development and commercialization of lasers and advanced fiber-optic devices for a wide variety of applications. Laserscope's product portfolio consists of more than 350 products, including KTP/532, CO2, Nd:YAG, Er:YAG and Dye medical laser systems and related energy delivery devices. The firm's primary medical markets are aesthetic surgery and urology. Secondary markets include ear, nose and throat surgery, dermatology, general surgery, gynecology, photodynamic therapy and other surgical specialties. The company's Niagara laser system is a KTP single-wavelength laser used for photo vaporization of the prostate, a procedure to treat benign prostatic hyperplasia. The Lyra and Lyra XP laser systems are compact Nd:YAG, single-wavelength lasers used primarily for hair removal and leg vein treatments in doctors' offices. These lasers are approved by the FDA for hair removal on all skin color types and were the first lasers FDA-approved for treatment of pseudo folliculitis barbae, or ingrown hairs. The 800 Series KTP/YAG Surgical Laser System is designed for use in hospitals. It is a high-power, dual-wavelength system with applications in urology, general surgery and other surgical specialties. The KTP/532 beam surgically cuts, vaporizes and coagulates tissue with minimal disruption to adjacent areas. Cutting and vaporization are achieved hemostatically, making the system effective for endoscopic as well as open surgical procedures. In recent news, the firm received a patent for the technology and applications for its newest laser, the GreenLight PV, which offers laser treatment for men suffering from an enlarged prostate, also known as BPH.

FINANCIALS:
Sales and profits are in thousands of dollars—add 000 to get the full amount. Year 2004 note: Complete fiscal 2004 results were not available for all companies at press time. For this company, year 2004 is for 9 months.

2004 Sales: $64,340 (9 months)   2004 Profits: $9,555   (9 months)
2003 Sales: $57,427   2003 Profits: $2,517
2002 Sales: $43,100   2002 Profits: $ 300
2001 Sales: $35,100   2001 Profits: $- 800
2000 Sales: $35,400   2000 Profits: $ 200

Stock Ticker: LSCP
Employees: 195
Fiscal Year Ends: 12/31

SALARIES/BENEFITS:

Pension Plan:	ESOP Stock Plan:	Profit Sharing:	Top Exec. Salary: $280,000	Bonus: $
Savings Plan: Y	Stock Purch. Plan: Y		Second Exec. Salary: $187,000	Bonus: $

OTHER THOUGHTS:
Apparent Top Female Officers: 1
Hot Spot for Advancement for Women/Minorities:

LOCATIONS: ("Y" = Yes)

West:	Southwest:	Midwest:	Southeast:	Northeast:	International:
Y					

LCA VISION INC

www.lasikplus.com

Industry Group Code: 621490 **Ranks within this company's industry group:** Sales: 15 Profits: 12

Insurance/HMO/PPO:	Drugs:	Equipment/Supplies:	Hospitals/Clinics:		Services:		Health Care:
Insurance:	Manufacturer:	Manufacturer:	Acute Care:		Diagnostics:		Home Health:
Managed Care:	Distributor:	Distributor:	Sub-Acute Care:		Labs/Testing:		Long-Term Care:
Utilization Mgmt.:	Specialty Pharm.:	Leasing/Finance:	Outpatient Surgery:	Y	Staffing:		Physical Therapy:
Payment Proc.:	Vitamins/Nutri.:	Information Sys.:	Phys. Rehab. Center:		Waste Disposal:		Phys. Practice Mgmt.:
	Clinical Trials:		Psychiatric Clinics:		Specialty Services:		

TYPES OF BUSINESS:
Services-Laser Vision Correction Surgery Centers

BRANDS/DIVISIONS/AFFILIATES:
LasikPlus

CONTACTS:
Note: Officers with more than one job title may be intentionally listed here more than once.
Stephen N. Joffe, CEO
Kevin M. Hassey, Pres.
Alan H. Buckey, CFO
Craig P.R. Joffe, Sr. VP/General Counsel
Alan H. Buckey, Exec. VP-Finance
Craig P.R. Joffe, Corp. Sec.
Stephen N. Joffe, Chmn.

Phone: 513-792-9292   Fax: 513-792-5620
Toll-Free: 800-334-2224
Address: 7840 Montgomery Rd., Cincinnati, OH 45236 US

GROWTH PLANS/SPECIAL FEATURES:
LCA-Vision, Inc. is a leading provider and operator of laser vision correction centers for the treatment of nearsightedness, farsightedness and astigmatism. Treatments are done by using one of two methods: PRK (photo-refractive keratectomy) or LASIK (Laser-In-Situ Keratomileusis). PRK removes the epithelium of the cornea and treats it with excimer laser pulses. LASIK reshapes the cornea with an excimer laser by cutting a flap in the top of the cornea to expose the inner cornea. The corneal flap is then treated with excimer laser pulses according to the patient's prescription. The LASIK procedure now accounts for virtually all of the procedures performed by LCA, as recovery time is significantly shorter and patient discomfort is negligible. The company has a total of 40 wholly owned correction centers located in large metropolitan centers throughout the United States, with three joint ventures in Canada and one in Europe. In addition, the firm has licensed its business to Rei Corporation in Japan, which has introduced LCA technologies to additional locations in Japan. LCA has gradually transferred all of its facilities to closed-access, meaning LCA maintains full operational and financial control over its business, directly employing its own ophthalmologists and taking on full responsibility for marketing and patient acquisition. The company has also unified all its vision centers under the name LasikPlus and has begun marketing that name accordingly. LCA recently began offering the new wavefront-guided LASIK system, a groundbreaking system that allows doctors to map out the exact surface of the cornea before surgery, and thus provide personalized, more accurate modifications to the cornea, with an end result of clearer, crisper vision.

FINANCIALS:
Sales and profits are in thousands of dollars—add 000 to get the full amount. Year 2004 note: Complete fiscal 2004 results were not available for all companies at press time. For this company, year 2004 is for 9 months.

2004 Sales: $94,406 (9 months)	2004 Profits: $27,173 (9 months)	
2003 Sales: $81,423	2003 Profits: $7,269	Stock Ticker: LCAV
2002 Sales: $61,800	2002 Profits: $-3,800	Employees: 274
2001 Sales: $68,000	2001 Profits: $-23,400	Fiscal Year Ends: 12/31
2000 Sales: $63,400	2000 Profits: $-2,400	

SALARIES/BENEFITS:
Pension Plan:	ESOP Stock Plan:	Profit Sharing:	Top Exec. Salary: $300,000	Bonus: $50,000
Savings Plan: Y	Stock Purch. Plan:		Second Exec. Salary: $175,000	Bonus: $100,000

OTHER THOUGHTS:
Apparent Top Female Officers:
Hot Spot for Advancement for Women/Minorities:

LOCATIONS: ("Y" = Yes)
West:	Southwest:	Midwest:	Southeast:	Northeast:	International:
Y	Y	Y	Y	Y	Y

# LIFE CARE CENTERS OF AMERICA

www.lcca.com

Industry Group Code: 623110   Ranks within this company's industry group: Sales: Profits:

Insurance/HMO/PPO:	Drugs:	Equipment/Supplies:	Hospitals/Clinics:	Services:	Health Care:
Insurance:	Manufacturer:	Manufacturer:	Acute Care:	Diagnostics:	Home Health: Y
Managed Care:	Distributor:	Distributor:	Sub-Acute Care: Y	Labs/Testing:	Long-Term Care: Y
Utilization Mgmt.:	Specialty Pharm.:	Leasing/Finance:	Outpatient Surgery:	Staffing:	Physical Therapy: Y
Payment Proc.:	Vitamins/Nutri.:	Information Sys.:	Phys. Rehab. Center: Y	Waste Disposal:	Phys. Practice Mgmt.:
	Clinical Trials:		Psychiatric Clinics:	Specialty Services:	

TYPES OF BUSINESS:
Assisted Living Facilities
Home Care
Respite Care
Alzheimer's Care
Hospice
Rehabilitation

BRANDS/DIVISIONS/AFFILIATES:
American Lifestyles
Life Care at Home

CONTACTS: Note: Officers with more than one job title may be intentionally listed here more than once.
Don J. Giardina, Pres.
Diana Kodadek, Dir.-Sales & Hospitality
Allison Pierce, Sr. VP-People Dev.
Alison Shaw, Corp. Legal Counsel
Beecher Hunter, Exec. VP-Corp. & Comm. Rel.
Jim Bello, Dir.-Clinical Services
Forrest L. Preston, Chmn.

Phone: 423-472-9585   Fax: 423-339-8337
Toll-Free: 800-554-9585
Address: 3570 Keith St. NW, Cleveland, TN 37320 US

GROWTH PLANS/SPECIAL FEATURES:
Life Care Centers of America (LCCA) operates over 260 skilled nursing, assisted living, retirement, home care and Alzheimer's centers in 28 states. Its assisted living centers promote independence and dignity while providing help with tasks such as dressing, bathing and grooming. The staff of these facilities also assist with medications and discretely monitor patients' health. Through American Lifestyles, LCCA operates 40 additional retirement communities for more affluent seniors. These offer fine accommodations, trained chefs and minimal assistance. Most of the firm's locations also provide Alzheimer's care, respite care, subacute medical care, wound care, adult day care, hospice and rehabilitation services such as physical, occupational and speech therapy. LCCA's senior living campuses provide various types of facilities in one location, offering retirement, assisted living and nursing care depending on the changing needs of the patients. The company's Life Care at Home agencies offer health and social services for people who prefer to stay at home yet require care that cannot be provided by family members. Services range from intermittent to live-in and may include administration of medication, physical therapy, occupational therapy, speech therapy and errands such as grocery shopping. The company prides itself on being based in a Judeo-Christian ethic of treating people with compassion, dignity and respect.

FINANCIALS: Sales and profits are in thousands of dollars—add 000 to get the full amount. Year 2004 note: Complete fiscal 2004 results were not available for all companies at press time. For this company, year 2004 is for months.

2004 Sales: $ (months)   2004 Profits: $ (months)
2003 Sales: $ 2003 Profits: $
2002 Sales: $ 2002 Profits: $
2001 Sales: $ 2001 Profits: $
2000 Sales: $ 2000 Profits: $

Stock Ticker: Private
Employees:
Fiscal Year Ends: 12/31

SALARIES/BENEFITS:
Pension Plan: ESOP Stock Plan: Profit Sharing: Top Exec. Salary: $ Bonus: $
Savings Plan: Stock Purch. Plan: Second Exec. Salary: $ Bonus: $

OTHER THOUGHTS:
Apparent Top Female Officers: 3
Hot Spot for Advancement for Women/Minorities: Y

LOCATIONS: ("Y" = Yes)
West:	Southwest:	Midwest:	Southeast:	Northeast:	International:
Y	Y	Y	Y	Y	

Note: Financial information, benefits and other data can change quickly and may vary from those stated here.

LIFECELL CORPORATION

www.lifecell.com

Industry Group Code: 325414   Ranks within this company's industry group: Sales: 3   Profits: 1

Insurance/HMO/PPO:	Drugs:	Equipment/Supplies:	Hospitals/Clinics:	Services:	Health Care:
Insurance:	Manufacturer: Y	Manufacturer: Y	Acute Care:	Diagnostics:	Home Health:
Managed Care:	Distributor:	Distributor:	Sub-Acute Care:	Labs/Testing:	Long-Term Care:
Utilization Mgmt.:	Specialty Pharm.:	Leasing/Finance:	Outpatient Surgery:	Staffing:	Physical Therapy:
Payment Proc.:	Vitamins/Nutri.:	Information Sys.:	Phys. Rehab. Center:	Waste Disposal:	Phys. Practice Mgmt.:
	Clinical Trials:		Psychiatric Clinics:	Specialty Services:	

TYPES OF BUSINESS:
Drugs-Tissue Grafting
Skin Replacement Technology
Regenerative Medicine

BRANDS/DIVISIONS/AFFILIATES:
Alloderm
Cymetra
Repliform
ThromboSol
Graft Jacket
SmartPReP

CONTACTS:
Note: Officers with more than one job title may be intentionally listed here more than once.

Paul G. Thomas, CEO
Paul G. Thomas, Pres.
Steven T. Sobieski, CFO
Lisa N. Colleran, VP-Mktg.
Fred Feldman, Sr. VP-Product Dev.
Steven T. Sobieski, VP-Admin.
William E. Barnhart, Sr. VP-Oper.
Lisa N. Colleran, VP-Bus. Dev.
Steven T. Sobieski, VP-Finance
Paul G. Thomas, Chmn.

Phone: 908-947-1100   **Fax:**
Toll-Free:
Address: One Millennium Way, Branchburg, NJ 08876-3876 US

GROWTH PLANS/SPECIAL FEATURES:
LifeCell Corporation specializes in regenerative medicine, developing and manufacturing products geared toward the repair, replacement and preservation of human tissues. The company has developed and patented several proprietary technologies, including a method for producing an extracellular tissue matrix, a method for cell preservation through signal transduction and a method for freeze-drying biological cells and tissues without damage. LifeCell markets four major products based on these tissue matrix technologies: Alloderm and Cymetra for burns and plastic reconstructive surgery, Repliform for the urogynecology market (treatment of urinary incontinence) and Graft Jacket, an acellular periosteum replacement graft. Alloderm is a human tissue product that supports the regeneration of normal human soft tissue. The company also distributes cryopreserved allograft skin for use as a temporary wound dressing in the treatment of burns. LifeCell is the exclusive marketing agent for the SmartPReP Platelet Concentration System in the United States to ear, nose and throat (ENT), plastic reconstructive and general surgeons in hospitals. Additionally, the firm has a number of products currently under development, including ThromboSol, a formulation for extended storage of platelets, and technologies to enhance the storage of red blood cells for transfusion. LifeCell is currently collaborating with the University of Texas M.D. Anderson Cancer Center to evaluate ThromboSol's potential for use with patients undergoing chemotherapy and treatments for leukemia.

LifeCell offers its employees medical, dental, vision and life insurance. It also offers tuition reimbursement and a summer schedule.

FINANCIALS:
Sales and profits are in thousands of dollars—add 000 to get the full amount. Year 2004 note: Complete fiscal 2004 results were not available for all companies at press time. For this company, year 2004 is for 9 months.

2004 Sales: $44,473 (9 months)	2004 Profits: $3,042 (9 months)	
2003 Sales: $40,249	2003 Profits: $18,672	**Stock Ticker:** LIFC
2002 Sales: $34,400	2002 Profits: $1,400	Employees: 173
2001 Sales: $27,800	2001 Profits: $-2,100	Fiscal Year Ends: 12/31
2000 Sales: $22,772	2000 Profits: $-7,138	

SALARIES/BENEFITS:
Pension Plan: ESOP Stock Plan: Y   Profit Sharing: Top Exec. Salary: $330,000   Bonus: $179,520
Savings Plan: Y   Stock Purch. Plan: Second Exec. Salary: $196,900   Bonus: $67,104

OTHER THOUGHTS:
Apparent Top Female Officers: 1
Hot Spot for Advancement for Women/Minorities:

LOCATIONS: ("Y" = Yes)
West:	Southwest:	Midwest:	Southeast:	Northeast:	International:
				Y	

LIFECORE BIOMEDICAL INC
www.lifecore.com

Industry Group Code: 339113   Ranks within this company's industry group: Sales: 117   Profits: 106

Insurance/HMO/PPO:	Drugs:	Equipment/Supplies:	Hospitals/Clinics:	Services:	Health Care:
Insurance:	Manufacturer:	Manufacturer: Y	Acute Care:	Diagnostics:	Home Health:
Managed Care:	Distributor:	Distributor:	Sub-Acute Care:	Labs/Testing:	Long-Term Care:
Utilization Mgmt.:	Specialty Pharm.:	Leasing/Finance:	Outpatient Surgery:	Staffing:	Physical Therapy:
Payment Proc.:	Vitamins/Nutri.:	Information Sys.:	Phys. Rehab. Center:	Waste Disposal:	Phys. Practice Mgmt.:
	Clinical Trials:		Psychiatric Clinics:	Specialty Services:	

TYPES OF BUSINESS:
Dental Implants
Tissue Regeneration Products
Surgical Devices

BRANDS/DIVISIONS/AFFILIATES:
RENOVA Internal Hex
RESTORE
STAGE-1

CONTACTS:
Note: Officers with more than one job title may be intentionally listed here more than once.

Dennis J. Allingham, CEO
Dennis J. Allingham, Pres.
David M. Noel, CFO
Andre P. Decarie, VP-Mktg. & Sales
Larry D. Hiebert, VP-Oper.
David M. Noel, VP-Finance

Phone: 952-368-4300   **Fax:** 952-368-3411
Toll-Free:
Address: 3515 Lyman Blvd., Chaska, MN 55318 US

GROWTH PLANS/SPECIAL FEATURES:
Lifecore Biomedical, Inc. develops and manufactures dental implant systems and tissue regeneration products. The company's hyaluronan division develops products utilizing hyaluronan, a naturally occurring polysaccharide that lubricates soft tissues in the body. The division also uses hyaluronan as a component in ophthalmic, orthopedic and veterinary medical devices, including Bexco Pharma's HY-50 product, an aseptically packaged solution that is used as a veterinary orthopedic drug. The company's other customers include the Musculoskeletal Transplant Foundation and Alcon, Inc. Lifecore's oral restorative division develops and markets precision surgical and prosthetic devices for the restoration of damaged or deteriorating dentition systems and support tissues. The division offers a number of titanium-based dental implant systems, including RESTORE, STAGE-1 and the new RENOVA Internal Hex implant system. Additionally, Lifecore manufactures tissue regeneration products that restore bone and soft tissue that has deteriorated as the result of periodontal disease.

Lifecore offers its employees health, life and dental insurance, an employee assistance program and an on-site fitness center.

FINANCIALS:
Sales and profits are in thousands of dollars—add 000 to get the full amount. Year 2004 note: Complete fiscal 2004 results were not available for all companies at press time. For this company, year 2004 is for 12 months.

2004 Sales: $47,036 (12 months)	2004 Profits: $ 707 (12 months)	**Stock Ticker:** LCBM
2003 Sales: $42,400	2003 Profits: $- 400	Employees: 183
2002 Sales: $38,800	2002 Profits: $-4,700	Fiscal Year Ends: 6/30
2001 Sales: $34,100	2001 Profits: $-3,700	
2000 Sales: $32,800	2000 Profits: $-1,600	

SALARIES/BENEFITS:
Pension Plan: ESOP Stock Plan: Profit Sharing: Top Exec. Salary: $304,154   Bonus: $30,000
Savings Plan: Y   Stock Purch. Plan: Y   Second Exec. Salary: $201,907   Bonus: $19,287

OTHER THOUGHTS:
Apparent Top Female Officers:
Hot Spot for Advancement for Women/Minorities:

LOCATIONS: ("Y" = Yes)
West:	Southwest:	Midwest:	Southeast:	Northeast:	International:
		Y			Y

LIFELINE SYSTEMS INC

www.lifelinesys.com

Industry Group Code: 513390D   Ranks within this company's industry group: Sales: 1   Profits:

Insurance/HMO/PPO:	Drugs:	Equipment/Supplies:		Hospitals/Clinics:	Services:		Health Care:	
Insurance:	Manufacturer:	Manufacturer:	Y	Acute Care:	Diagnostics:		Home Health:	
Managed Care:	Distributor:	Distributor:		Sub-Acute Care:	Labs/Testing:		Long-Term Care:	
Utilization Mgmt.:	Specialty Pharm.:	Leasing/Finance:		Outpatient Surgery:	Staffing:		Physical Therapy:	
Payment Proc.:	Vitamins/Nutri.:	Information Sys.:		Phys. Rehab. Center:	Waste Disposal:		Phys. Practice Mgmt.:	
	Clinical Trials:			Psychiatric Clinics:	Specialty Services:	Y		

TYPES OF BUSINESS:
Personal Response Monitoring Systems & Services

BRANDS/DIVISIONS/AFFILIATES:
LIFELINE
PROTECT Emergency Response Systems, Inc.

CONTACTS:
Note: Officers with more than one job title may be intentionally listed here more than once.

Ronald Feinstein, CEO
Ronald Feinstein, Pres.
Mark Beucler, CFO
Donald G. Strange, Sr. VP-Sales
Ellen Berezin, VP-Human Resources
Richard M. Reich, Sr. VP/CIO
Mark Beucler, VP-Finance/Treas.
Edward Bolesky, Sr. VP-Customer Care
Leonard E. Wechsler, VP/Pres.-Canada
L. Dennis Shapiro, Chmn.

Phone: 617-679-1000   Fax:
Toll-Free:
Address: 111 Lawrence St., Framingham, MA 02139 US

GROWTH PLANS/SPECIAL FEATURES:

Lifeline Systems, Inc. provides 24-hour personal response monitoring services to its subscribers, primarily elderly individuals with medical or age-related conditions, as well as physically challenged individuals. Its principal offering, called LIFELINE, consists of a monitoring service utilizing equipment designed, assembled and marketed by the company. Subscribers to this service communicate with the company via a communicator that connects to the telephone line in the subscriber's home and a personal help button, which is worn or carried by the individual subscriber. When activated, the personal help button initiates a telephone call from the subscriber's communicator to Lifeline's central monitoring facilities. Trained employees of the company then identify the nature and extent of the subscriber's particular need and manage the situation by notifying the subscriber's friends, neighbors and/or emergency personnel, as set forth in a predetermined protocol. Most of the time, however, subscribers' calls do not require Lifeline to dispatch a responder, but instead require it to provide reassurance and support to a lonely subscriber. To provide its services, the company develops relationships with hospitals or other health care providers who establish a Lifeline program for the benefit of at-risk individuals in their coverage area or for senior living facilities in their coverage area. The firm handles over 27,000 calls per day. In recent news, Lifeline acquired PROTECT Emergency Response Systems, Inc., a supplier of wireless emergency call systems for seniors. The company intends to offer both products, allowing customers to choose which system works best for them.

Lifeline offers its employees health, dental, vision, life, business travel accident and disability coverage, in addition to tuition reimbursement, medical expense reimbursement and dependent care assistance.

FINANCIALS:
Sales and profits are in thousands of dollars—add 000 to get the full amount. Year 2004 note: Complete fiscal 2004 results were not available for all companies at press time. For this company, year 2004 is for 9 months.

2004 Sales: $95,570 (9 months)	2004 Profits: $8,015 (9 months)	Stock Ticker: LIFE
2003 Sales: $116,159	2003 Profits: $10,259	Employees: 857
2002 Sales: $105,000	2002 Profits: $8,100	Fiscal Year Ends: 12/31
2001 Sales: $96,600	2001 Profits: $6,300	
2000 Sales: $81,500	2000 Profits: $3,200	

SALARIES/BENEFITS:

Pension Plan:	ESOP Stock Plan:	Profit Sharing:	Top Exec. Salary: $335,833	Bonus: $421,600
Savings Plan: Y	Stock Purch. Plan: Y		Second Exec. Salary: $195,116	Bonus: $117,245

OTHER THOUGHTS:
Apparent Top Female Officers: 1
Hot Spot for Advancement for Women/Minorities:

LOCATIONS: ("Y" = Yes)

West:	Southwest:	Midwest:	Southeast:	Northeast:	International:
				Y	Y

LIFESCAN INC

www.lifescan.com

Industry Group Code: 339113 **Ranks within this company's industry group:** Sales: 26 Profits:

Insurance/HMO/PPO:	Drugs:	Equipment/Supplies:	Hospitals/Clinics:	Services:	Health Care:
Insurance:	Manufacturer:	Manufacturer: Y	Acute Care:	Diagnostics:	Home Health:
Managed Care:	Distributor:	Distributor:	Sub-Acute Care:	Labs/Testing:	Long-Term Care:
Utilization Mgmt.:	Specialty Pharm.:	Leasing/Finance:	Outpatient Surgery:	Staffing:	Physical Therapy:
Payment Proc.:	Vitamins/Nutri.:	Information Sys.: Y	Phys. Rehab. Center:	Waste Disposal:	Phys. Practice Mgmt.:
	Clinical Trials:		Psychiatric Clinics:	Specialty Services:	

TYPES OF BUSINESS:
Medical Testing Products
Blood Glucose Monitoring Products

BRANDS/DIVISIONS/AFFILIATES:
Johnson & Johnson
OneTouch
InDuo
OneTouch Diabetes Management Software
SureStep
Unistik
DataLink Data Management System

CONTACTS: Note: Officers with more than one job title may be intentionally listed here more than once.
Peter Luther, Pres.
Eric Compton, VP-Mktg.
Charles Renfroe, Sr. Mgr.-Professional Affairs
John Bradford, Sr. Mktg. Mgr.-OneTouch Systems
Karen McCormick, VP-Institutional & Cardiovascular Units
Eric Milledge, Chmn.

Phone: 408-263-9789 **Fax:** 408-942-6070
Toll-Free: 800-227-8862
Address: 1000 Gibraltar Dr., Milpitas, CA 95035 US

GROWTH PLANS/SPECIAL FEATURES:
LifeScan, Inc., a subsidiary of Johnson & Johnson, is a world leader in blood glucose monitoring for home and hospital use. Its OneTouch technology eliminates wiping and timing procedures, making it easier for patients to test their own blood glucose levels. These testing products require less blood than other tests, and some provide the ability to take blood from an arm rather than fingertips. They are designed to be quick and easy to use. LifeScan's InDuo is the world's first combined glucose monitoring and insulin dosing system, incorporating the ability to adjust insulin doses up or down depending on blood glucose measurements. The company also sells OneTouch test strips, lancets and Diabetes Management Software, which tracks glucose values, weight, blood pressure and cholesterol and allows patients to customize medications by name and create meal schedules and insulin regimens. Its institutional products include the SureStep testing system, Unistik lancing devices and the DataLink Data Management System, as well as an institutional version of the OneTouch system. In addition, LifeScan supports the American Diabetes Association, the Juvenile Diabetes Research Foundation, the American Association of Diabetes Educators and the landmark Diabetes Control and Complications Trial, and invests heavily in basic and applied research for new product development.

FINANCIALS:
Sales and profits are in thousands of dollars—add 000 to get the full amount. Year 2004 note: Complete fiscal 2004 results were not available for all companies at press time. For this company, year 2004 is for months.

2004 Sales: $ (months)   2004 Profits: $ (months)
2003 Sales: $1,004,000   2003 Profits: $
2002 Sales: $1,000,000   2002 Profits: $
2001 Sales: $ 2001 Profits: $
2000 Sales: $ 2000 Profits: $

Stock Ticker: Subsidiary
Employees: 2,500
Fiscal Year Ends: 12/31

SALARIES/BENEFITS:
Pension Plan: ESOP Stock Plan: Profit Sharing: Top Exec. Salary: $ Bonus: $
Savings Plan: Stock Purch. Plan: Second Exec. Salary: $ Bonus: $

OTHER THOUGHTS:
Apparent Top Female Officers: 1
Hot Spot for Advancement for Women/Minorities:

LOCATIONS: ("Y" = Yes)

West:	Southwest:	Midwest:	Southeast:	Northeast:	International:
Y					Y

LOGISTICARE INC

www.logisticare.com

Industry Group Code: 621111 Ranks within this company's industry group: Sales: 7 Profits:

Insurance/HMO/PPO:	Drugs:	Equipment/Supplies:	Hospitals/Clinics:	Services:	Health Care:
Insurance:	Manufacturer:	Manufacturer:	Acute Care:	Diagnostics:	Home Health:
Managed Care:	Distributor:	Distributor:	Sub-Acute Care:	Labs/Testing:	Long-Term Care:
Utilization Mgmt.:	Specialty Pharm.:	Leasing/Finance:	Outpatient Surgery:	Staffing:	Physical Therapy:
Payment Proc.:	Vitamins/Nutri.:	Information Sys.: Y	Phys. Rehab. Center:	Waste Disposal:	Phys. Practice Mgmt.:
	Clinical Trials:		Psychiatric Clinics:	Specialty Services: Y	

TYPES OF BUSINESS:
Medical Transportation
Outsourced Logistics Services
Logistics Software

BRANDS/DIVISIONS/AFFILIATES:
EMTrack
Medicaid NEMT

CONTACTS:
Note: Officers with more than one job title may be intentionally listed here more than once.

John L. Shermyen, CEO
Albert Cortina, COO
Steven Russell, CFO
Henry S. Gray Hardy, Exec. VP-Bus. Dev.
Ray Williams, Sr. VP-Public Affairs
Kirk J. Gonzales, VP-Bus. Implementation

Phone: 770-907-7596 Fax: 770-907-7598
Toll-Free: 800-486-7647
Address: 1640 Phoenix Blvd., Ste. 200, Atlanta, GA 30349 US

GROWTH PLANS/SPECIAL FEATURES:
LogistiCare, Inc., founded in 1994, is a provider of outsourced transportation management services to insurance companies, managed care organizations and government health agencies, with expertise in the area of non-emergency medical transportation (NEMT). It is the only company in the U.S. that uses software purpose-built for its industry. The firm has developed integrated software that manages data and costs associated with transportation, including scheduling, routing, billing verification and quality assurance reporting functions. The company provides its services on a contract or fee-for-service basis. It processes transportation requests and dispatches drivers through its network of carriers, using its proprietary EMTrack software. LogistiCare operates five network operations centers, located in Connecticut, Georgia, Florida, Virginia and Maryland, as well as a number of business office locations across the U.S. In recent news, LogistiCare plans to take over management of the Medicaid NEMT program in eight Colorado counties.

FINANCIALS:
Sales and profits are in thousands of dollars—add 000 to get the full amount. Year 2004 note: Complete fiscal 2004 results were not available for all companies at press time. For this company, year 2004 is for months.

2004 Sales: $ (months)   2004 Profits: $ (months)
2003 Sales: $180,000   2003 Profits: $ Stock Ticker: Private
2002 Sales: $100,000   2002 Profits: $ Employees: 600
2001 Sales: $91,000   2001 Profits: $ Fiscal Year Ends: 12/31
2000 Sales: $ 2000 Profits: $

SALARIES/BENEFITS:
Pension Plan: ESOP Stock Plan: Profit Sharing: Top Exec. Salary: $ Bonus: $
Savings Plan: Stock Purch. Plan: Second Exec. Salary: $ Bonus: $

OTHER THOUGHTS:
Apparent Top Female Officers:
Hot Spot for Advancement for Women/Minorities:

LOCATIONS: ("Y" = Yes)

West:	Southwest:	Midwest:	Southeast:	Northeast:	International:
Y	Y	Y	Y	Y	

LONGS DRUG STORES CORPORATION

www.longs.com

Industry Group Code: 446110 Ranks within this company's industry group: Sales: 4 Profits: 3

Insurance/HMO/PPO:	Drugs:	Equipment/Supplies:	Hospitals/Clinics:	Services:	Health Care:
Insurance:	Manufacturer:	Manufacturer:	Acute Care:	Diagnostics:	Home Health:
Managed Care:	Distributor:	Distributor:	Sub-Acute Care:	Labs/Testing:	Long-Term Care:
Utilization Mgmt.: Y	Specialty Pharm.: Y	Leasing/Finance:	Outpatient Surgery:	Staffing:	Physical Therapy:
Payment Proc.:	Vitamins/Nutri.:	Information Sys.:	Phys. Rehab. Center:	Waste Disposal:	Phys. Practice Mgmt.:
	Clinical Trials:		Psychiatric Clinics:	Specialty Services:	

TYPES OF BUSINESS:
Drug Stores
Mail-Service Pharmacy
Prescription Benefits Management

BRANDS/DIVISIONS/AFFILIATES:
RxAmerica
American Diversified Pharmacies, Inc.

CONTACTS: Note: Officers with more than one job title may be intentionally listed here more than once.
Warren F. Bryant, CEO
Warren F. Bryant, Pres.
Richard W. Dreiling, Exec. VP/COO
Steven McCann, Sr. VP/CFO
Todd J. Vasos, Sr. VP-Mktg.
Linda M. Watt, Sr. VP-Human Resources
Michael M. Laddon, Sr. VP/CIO
Bruce E. Schwallie, Exec. VP/Chief Merch. Officer
William J. Rainey, Sr. VP/General Counsel
Steven McCann, Treas.
Martin A. Bennett, Sr. VP-Stores
Gerald H. Saito, Sr. VP/District Mgr.-Hawaii
R. M. Long, Chmn.

Phone: 925-937-1170 Fax: 925-210-6886
Toll-Free:
Address: 141 N. Civic Dr., Walnut Creek, CA 94596 US

GROWTH PLANS/SPECIAL FEATURES:
Longs Drug Stores Corporation, founded in 1938 by brothers Joe and Tom Long, is one of the largest drug store chains in North America, with approximately 470 stores throughout California, Hawaii, Nevada, Oregon, Washington and Colorado. The company offers a wide array of quality merchandise and services, including pharmaceutical products, personal care items, photography supplies, gifts, groceries and greeting cards. The company's web site offers community health screening schedules, prescription refills and pharmacist access, coupons and education regarding a monthly health topic. The firm's focus is on displaying value-priced merchandise accompanied by friendly customer service. Longs stores also have large and varied photo and photo-processing departments that carry a variety of cameras, film and frames, in addition to providing processing services. Longs' subsidiary, RxAmerica, provides prescription benefits management and cost management services to more than 6 million customers. Another subsidiary, American Diversified Pharmacies, Inc., operates a state-of-the-art mail-service pharmacy.

Long's gives back to the community by providing health screenings, vaccinations, charity fundraising, recycling and disaster relief. The firm offers its employees a group health plan, a prescription plan, dental and vision plans and merchandise discounts.

FINANCIALS: Sales and profits are in thousands of dollars—add 000 to get the full amount. Year 2004 note: Complete fiscal 2004 results were not available for all companies at press time. For this company, year 2004 is for 12 months.

2004 Sales: $4,526,524 (12 months)   2004 Profits: $29,764   (12 months)
2003 Sales: $4,426,300   2003 Profits: $6,700   Stock Ticker: LDG
2002 Sales: $4,304,700   2002 Profits: $47,200   Employees: 22,900
2001 Sales: $4,027,100   2001 Profits: $44,900   Fiscal Year Ends: 1/31
2000 Sales: $3,672,413   2000 Profits: $68,974

SALARIES/BENEFITS:
Pension Plan: ESOP Stock Plan: Profit Sharing: Y   Top Exec. Salary: $750,000   Bonus: $143,040
Savings Plan: Y   Stock Purch. Plan: Second Exec. Salary: $360,224   Bonus: $60,843

OTHER THOUGHTS:
Apparent Top Female Officers: 1
Hot Spot for Advancement for Women/Minorities:

LOCATIONS: ("Y" = Yes)
West:	Southwest:	Midwest:	Southeast:	Northeast:	International:
Y					

LUMENIS LTD

www.lumenis.com

Industry Group Code: 339113 **Ranks within this company's industry group:** Sales: Profits:

Insurance/HMO/PPO:	Drugs:	Equipment/Supplies:		Hospitals/Clinics:	Services:	Health Care:
Insurance:	Manufacturer:	Manufacturer:	Y	Acute Care:	Diagnostics:	Home Health:
Managed Care:	Distributor:	Distributor:		Sub-Acute Care:	Labs/Testing:	Long-Term Care:
Utilization Mgmt.:	Specialty Pharm.:	Leasing/Finance:		Outpatient Surgery:	Staffing:	Physical Therapy:
Payment Proc.:	Vitamins/Nutri.:	Information Sys.:		Phys. Rehab. Center:	Waste Disposal:	Phys. Practice Mgmt.:
	Clinical Trials:			Psychiatric Clinics:	Specialty Services:	

TYPES OF BUSINESS:
Laser Surgery Products

BRANDS/DIVISIONS/AFFILIATES:
Intense Pulsed Light
LightSheer
ChillTip
UltraPulse
OpusDent

CONTACTS:
Note: Officers with more than one job title may be intentionally listed here more than once.

Avner Raz, CEO
Avner Raz, Pres.
Lauri A. Hanover, CFO
Kevin Morano, Sr. VP-Mktg.
Yossi Gal, Exec. VP-Human Resources
Igor Gradov, Global VP-Research & Dev.
Kevin Morano, Sr. VP-Bus. Dev.
Wade Hampton, Exec. VP-Americas
Hai Ben Israel, Exec. VP-Planning & Resources
Zhai Qiying, Exec. VP-Asia-Pacific Oper.
Amnon Harari, Exec. VP-European Oper.
Jacob A. Frenkel, Chmn.

Phone: 972-4-959-9000   **Fax:** 972-4-959-9050
Toll-Free:
Address: P.O. Box 240, Yokneam, 20692 Israel

GROWTH PLANS/SPECIAL FEATURES:
Lumenis, Ltd. is the world leader in laser and light-based technologies for medical and aesthetic applications. The company has more than 60,000 systems installed in doctors' offices, clinics and operating rooms in over 75 countries. Its technology revolves around gas-based, solid-state and diode-pumped lasers, which it uses to treat patients in the aesthetic, surgical, ophthalmic, dental and veterinary fields. Lumenis's cosmetic treatments include Intense Pulsed Light skin treatments, skin resurfacing, treatments for leg veins, vascular lesions, pigmented lesions, acne, psoriasis and vitiligo, cosmetic repigmentation and hair removal. The firm's LightSheer laser hair removal system with ChillTip cooling device and its UltraPulse laparoscopy technology are considered the top of their class. The company has recently developed products to treat glaucoma, age-related macular degeneration, kidney stones and benign prostatic hyperplasia. In veterinary medicine, Lumenis's laser products have been used in cat declaws, spays, neuters, amputations, dental procedures, mass removals and avian and exotic pet procedures, reducing the recovery time required for common animal surgeries. Subsidiary OpusDent develops and sells lasers to the dental community, which can be used for soft tissue and root canal procedures as well as for tooth whitening.

FINANCIALS:
Sales and profits are in thousands of dollars—add 000 to get the full amount. Year 2004 note: Complete fiscal 2004 results were not available for all companies at press time. For this company, year 2004 is for months.

2004 Sales: $ (months)   2004 Profits: $ (months)
2003 Sales: $ 2003 Profits: $
2002 Sales: $348,500   2002 Profits: $-44,100
2001 Sales: $ 2001 Profits: $
2000 Sales: $ 2000 Profits: $

Stock Ticker: Foreign
Employees:
Fiscal Year Ends: 12/31

SALARIES/BENEFITS:
Pension Plan: ESOP Stock Plan: Profit Sharing: Top Exec. Salary: $265,261   Bonus: $520,000
Savings Plan: Stock Purch. Plan: Second Exec. Salary: $264,974   Bonus: $163,928

OTHER THOUGHTS:
Apparent Top Female Officers: 1
Hot Spot for Advancement for Women/Minorities

LOCATIONS: ("Y" = Yes)

West:	Southwest:	Midwest:	Southeast:	Northeast:	International:
Y				Y	Y

LUXOTTICA GROUP SPA

www.loxottica.it

Industry Group Code: 333314 Ranks within this company's industry group: Sales: 1 Profits: 1

Insurance/HMO/PPO:	Drugs:	Equipment/Supplies:	Hospitals/Clinics:	Services:	Health Care:
Insurance: Y	Manufacturer:	Manufacturer: Y	Acute Care:	Diagnostics:	Home Health:
Managed Care:	Distributor:	Distributor:	Sub-Acute Care:	Labs/Testing:	Long-Term Care:
Utilization Mgmt.:	Specialty Pharm.:	Leasing/Finance:	Outpatient Surgery:	Staffing:	Physical Therapy:
Payment Proc.:	Vitamins/Nutri.:	Information Sys.:	Phys. Rehab. Center:	Waste Disposal:	Phys. Practice Mgmt.:
	Clinical Trials:		Psychiatric Clinics:	Specialty Services: Y	

TYPES OF BUSINESS:
Lens/Eyeglass Frame Manufacturing
Vision Plan Provider
Lens/Eyeglass Frame Retailer
Eye Care Services

BRANDS/DIVISIONS/AFFILIATES:
Beni Stabili
Cole National Corp.
Tristar Optical Co., Ltd.
Killer Loop
OPSM Group, Ltd.
LensCrafters
Collezione Rathschuler
EyeMed Vision Care, LLC

CONTACTS:
Note: Officers with more than one job title may be intentionally listed here more than once.
Roberto Chemello, Co-CEO
Enrico Cavatorta, CFO
Beatrice Niedda, Mgr.-Mktg.
Enzo Damin, Mgr.-Human Resources
Umberto Soccal, CIO
Andrea Gallina, Mgr.-Mfg.
Luciano Santel, Mgr.-Corp. Dev.
Sabina Grossi, Dir.-Investor Rel.
Alessandra Senici, Investor Rel.
Luigi Francavilla, Co-CEO
Cliff Bartow, COO-LensCrafters
Jack Dennis, CFO-LensCrafters
Leonardo Del Vecchio, Chmn.

Phone: 39-02-863341 Fax: 39-0437-63223
Toll-Free:
Address: Via Cantu, 2, Milan, 20123 Italy

GROWTH PLANS/SPECIAL FEATURES:
Luxottica Group is the world's largest manufacturer and retailer of prescription and fashion eyeglass frames and sunglasses. The firm conducts business through three production companies: Luxottica, SRL; Killer Loop Eyewear, SRL; and Tristar Optical Co., Ltd. It fully owns and operates four other eyewear-related companies: Collezione Rathschuler; Luxottica Leasing, SPA; Luxottica USA; and Luxottica Luxeumbourg, in addition to dozens of retail and wholesale subsidiaries located around the world. Company-owned brand names include Ray Ban, Vogue, Persol, Arnette, Killer Loop, Revo, Sferoflex, Luxottica and T3. Moreover, Luxottica licenses brands from Prada, Ungaro, Versace, Chanel, Ferragamo, Bulgari, Moschino, Brooks Brothers, Miu Miu and Anne Klein, among others. It distributes its products in 120 countries through 29 subsidiaries and over 100 independent distributors. Luxottica is also involved in the U.S. health care market through its EyeMed Vision Care, LLC subsidiary. EyeMed provides member clients with vision plan options, which include a network of optometrists, ophthalmologists and opticians; eye care services; and Luxottica eyeglass frames. The firm has contracts with several major employers and health groups including Wellpoint, American Express, Canon USA, Independent Health and Gannet Company, Inc. Luxottica manufactures the only prescription sunglass lens to receive the Skin Cancer Foundation's Seal of Recommendation, called FeatherWates SPF. The company announced in July 2004 that it has signed a definitive agreement to acquire competitor Cole National Group for $441 million, and it intends to purchase Beni Stabili, an Italian real estate manager, for more than $1 billion.

FINANCIALS:
Sales and profits are in thousands of dollars—add 000 to get the full amount. Year 2004 note: Complete fiscal 2004 results were not available for all companies at press time. For this company, year 2004 is for 6 months.

2004 Sales: $1,905,700 (6 months)   2004 Profits: $189,100 (6 months)
2003 Sales: $3,551,100   2003 Profits: $336,100
2002 Sales: $2,959,900   2002 Profits: $351,600
2001 Sales: $2,731,800   2001 Profits: $282,000
2000 Sales: $2,268,900   2000 Profits: $239,700

Stock Ticker: Foreign
Employees: 36,900
Fiscal Year Ends: 12/31

SALARIES/BENEFITS:
Pension Plan: ESOP Stock Plan: Profit Sharing: Top Exec. Salary: $ Bonus: $
Savings Plan: Stock Purch. Plan: Second Exec. Salary: $ Bonus: $

OTHER THOUGHTS:
Apparent Top Female Officers: 4
Hot Spot for Advancement for Women/Minorities: Y

LOCATIONS: ("Y" = Yes)
West:	Southwest:	Midwest:	Southeast:	Northeast:	International:
Y	Y	Y	Y	Y	Y

MAGELLAN HEALTH SERVICES INC   www.magellanhealth.com

Industry Group Code: 622210   **Ranks within this company's industry group:** Sales: 1   Profits: 1

Insurance/HMO/PPO:	Drugs:	Equipment/Supplies:	Hospitals/Clinics:	Services:	Health Care:
Insurance: Managed Care: Utilization Mgmt.: Y Payment Proc.:	Manufacturer: Distributor: Specialty Pharm.: Vitamins/Nutri.: Clinical Trials:	Manufacturer: Distributor: Leasing/Finance: Information Sys.:	Acute Care: Sub-Acute Care: Outpatient Surgery: Phys. Rehab. Center: Psychiatric Clinics:	Diagnostics: Labs/Testing: Staffing: Waste Disposal: Specialty Services: Y	Home Health: Long-Term Care: Physical Therapy: Phys. Practice Mgmt.:

TYPES OF BUSINESS:
Clinics-Psychiatric
Managed Behavioral Health Care Plans

BRANDS/DIVISIONS/AFFILIATES:
Magellan Behavioral Health
magellanassist.com
magellanprovider.com
LifeManagement

CONTACTS:
Note: Officers with more than one job title may be intentionally listed here more than once.

Steven Shulman, CEO
Rene Lerer, Pres.
Rene Lerer, COO
Mark S. Demilio, CFO
Caskie Lewis-Clapper, Chief Human Resources Officer
Jeff D. Emerson, CIO
Megan M. Arthur, General Counsel
Gregory Bayer, Exec. VP-Oper.
Anthony M. Kotin, Chief Mktg. & Strategy Officer
Erin S. Somers, VP-Public Rel.
Melissa Rose, VP-Investor Rel.
Christopher W. Cooney, Chief Branding & Comm. Officer
Alex Rodriguez, Chief Medical Officer
Steven J. Shulman, Chmn.

Phone: 860-507-1900   **Fax:** 410-953-5200
Toll-Free:
Address: 16 Munson Rd., Farmington, CT 06032 US

GROWTH PLANS/SPECIAL FEATURES:

Magellan Health Services, Inc provides services such as counseling, therapy and crisis intervention through its extensive network of behavioral health professionals, psychiatric hospitals, residential treatment centers and other treatment facilities. The company has ceased all direct health care services and now focuses exclusively on managed health care plans through its Magellan Behavioral Health, magellanassist.com and magellanprovider.com divisions. Magellan Behavioral Health manages mental health, substance abuse and child and family care health plans for employers, unions and public entities. The division also provides employee assistance programs, dependant care, public sector, pharmacy management and other wellness care products. The magellanasssist.com and magellanprovider.com sites provide web-based solutions and information for employers and employees enrolled in Magellan-managed health care programs. The company's LifeManagement division provides services such as referrals and information on child care, adoption, parenting skills, college selection, elder care, relocation, home repair and retirement planning, with the goal of decreasing worker absenteeism and increasing employee productivity, job satisfaction and retention. In January 2004, Magellan Health Services and its 88 subsidiaries emerged from Chapter 11 reorganization to become one of the nation's leading providers of managed behavioral health care services.

Magellan offers its employees comprehensive medical insurance, a life resources program and performance incentives.

FINANCIALS:
Sales and profits are in thousands of dollars—add 000 to get the full amount. Year 2004 note: Complete fiscal 2004 results were not available for all companies at press time. For this company, year 2004 is for 3 months.

2004 Sales: $440,200 (3 months)	2004 Profits: $13,100 (3 months)	**Stock Ticker:** MGLN
2003 Sales: $1,510,746	2003 Profits: $451,770	Employees: 4,700
2002 Sales: $1,753,100	2002 Profits: $-729,100	Fiscal Year Ends: 12/31
2001 Sales: $1,755,500	2001 Profits: $24,600	
2000 Sales: $1,640,900	2000 Profits: $-65,800	

SALARIES/BENEFITS:
Pension Plan:	ESOP Stock Plan: Y	Profit Sharing:	Top Exec. Salary: $516,667	Bonus: $470,813
Savings Plan: Y	Stock Purch. Plan: Y		Second Exec. Salary: $400,000	Bonus: $66,660

OTHER THOUGHTS:
Apparent Top Female Officers: 4
Hot Spot for Advancement for Women/Minorities: Y

LOCATIONS: ("Y" = Yes)
West:	Southwest:	Midwest:	Southeast:	Northeast:	International:
Y	Y	Y	Y	Y	

MALLINCKRODT INC

www.mallinckrodt.com

Industry Group Code: 339113 **Ranks within this company's industry group:** Sales: Profits:

Insurance/HMO/PPO:	Drugs:	Equipment/Supplies:	Hospitals/Clinics:	Services:	Health Care:
Insurance:	Manufacturer: Y	Manufacturer: Y	Acute Care:	Diagnostics:	Home Health:
Managed Care:	Distributor:	Distributor:	Sub-Acute Care:	Labs/Testing:	Long-Term Care:
Utilization Mgmt.:	Specialty Pharm.:	Leasing/Finance:	Outpatient Surgery:	Staffing:	Physical Therapy:
Payment Proc.:	Vitamins/Nutri.:	Information Sys.:	Phys. Rehab. Center:	Waste Disposal:	Phys. Practice Mgmt.:
	Clinical Trials:		Psychiatric Clinics:	Specialty Services:	

TYPES OF BUSINESS:
Drugs-Pain and Addiction
Imaging Agents and Radiopharmaceuticals
Bulk Analgesic Pharmaceuticals
Generic Pharmaceuticals
Active Pharmaceutical Ingredients
Medical Devices
Respiratory Products
Diagnostics Products

BRANDS/DIVISIONS/AFFILIATES:
Tyco Healthcare Group
Mallinckrodt Pharmaceuticals
Mallinckordt Respiratory
Mallinckordt Imaging
OptiMARK
OxiFirst
NeutroSpec
Puritan-Bennett

CONTACTS:
Note: Officers with more than one job title may be intentionally listed here more than once.
Douglas A. McKinney, CFO
Kathy Schaefer, VP/Controller
Richard J. Meelia, Pres., Tyco Healthcare Group
Michael J. Collins, Pres., Pharmaceuticals Div.
Mark Thom, Pres., Imaging and Respiratory Div.
Douglas A. McKinney, VP-Shared Services
C. Ray Holman, Chmn.

Phone: 314-654-2000 **Fax:** 314-654-5381
Toll-Free:
Address: 675 McDonnell Blvd., Hazelwood, MO 63042 US

GROWTH PLANS/SPECIAL FEATURES:
Mallinckrodt, Inc., a subsidiary of Tyco Healthcare Group, develops and manufactures a wide range of medical products and devices, primarily used by hospitals for diagnostic and treatment purposes. It is the world's leader in bulk analgesic pharmaceuticals and a leader in generic dosage pharmaceuticals. The company's imaging group produces a full line of imaging agents and radiopharmaceuticals, including ultrasound and MRI contrast agents, catheters for diagnosis and therapy and x-ray contrast media. Through its respiratory segment, the firm offers a variety of products, including anesthesia devices, medical gases, oxygen therapy and asthma management products, sleep diagnostics and therapy devices and blood analysis products. Its products are sold under the Shiley, DAR, Nellcor and Puritan-Bennett brands. Mallinckrodt's pharmaceuticals division is focused on providing pain relief and addiction therapy, with a product line that includes codeine, phosphate, morphine sulfate, naltrexone (for alcohol addiction) and methylphenidate (for attention deficit hyperactivity disorder). It also supplies raw materials or active pharmaceutical ingredients and is a leader in the manufacturing, formulation, packaging and distribution of a growing line of generic pharmaceuticals. Mallinckrodt has been working toward the development and release of new products. The company is the developer of the OxiFirst fetal oxygen monitoring system, widely hailed to be the first major breakthrough in obstetrical monitoring since the 1960s. This new technology enables obstetricians to monitor fetus oxygenation during labor and delivery. The firm's imaging division has developed OptiMARK, the first and only MRI contrast agent FDA-approved for administration by power injection. In recent news, the FDA approved NeutroSpec, a new imaging agent to help detect difficult-to-diagnose cases of appendicitis in patients five years and older with atypical symptoms. Mallinckrodt also received FDA approval to market its generic morphine sulfate extended-release tablets.

FINANCIALS:
Sales and profits are in thousands of dollars—add 000 to get the full amount. Year 2004 note: Complete fiscal 2004 results were not available for all companies at press time. For this company, year 2004 is for months.

2004 Sales: $ (months)   2004 Profits: $ (months)
2003 Sales: $ 2003 Profits: $
2002 Sales: $3,000,000   2002 Profits: $
2001 Sales: $3,000,000   2001 Profits: $
2000 Sales: $ 2000 Profits: $

Stock Ticker: Subsidiary
Employees: 11,000
Fiscal Year Ends: 9/30

SALARIES/BENEFITS:
Pension Plan: Y   ESOP Stock Plan: Profit Sharing: Top Exec. Salary: $732,840   Bonus: $4,072,400
Savings Plan: Y   Stock Purch. Plan: Second Exec. Salary: $322,793   Bonus: $1,095,600

OTHER THOUGHTS:
Apparent Top Female Officers: 1
Hot Spot for Advancement for Women/Minorities:

LOCATIONS: ("Y" = Yes)
West:	Southwest:	Midwest:	Southeast:	Northeast:	International:
Y	Y	Y	Y	Y	Y

MANOR CARE INC

www.hcr-manorcare.com

Industry Group Code: 623110   Ranks within this company's industry group: Sales: 2   Profits: 1

Insurance/HMO/PPO:	Drugs:	Equipment/Supplies:	Hospitals/Clinics:		Services:		Health Care:	
Insurance:	Manufacturer:	Manufacturer:	Acute Care:		Diagnostics:		Home Health:	Y
Managed Care:	Distributor:	Distributor:	Sub-Acute Care:	Y	Labs/Testing:		Long-Term Care:	Y
Utilization Mgmt.:	Specialty Pharm.:	Leasing/Finance:	Outpatient Surgery:		Staffing:		Physical Therapy:	
Payment Proc.:	Vitamins/Nutri.:	Information Sys.:	Phys. Rehab. Center:	Y	Waste Disposal:		Phys. Practice Mgmt.:	
	Clinical Trials:		Psychiatric Clinics:		Specialty Services:			

TYPES OF BUSINESS:
Long-Term Health Care/Nursing Homes
Home Health Care
Short-Term Care Facilities
Assisted Living Facilities
Rehabilitation Clinics

BRANDS/DIVISIONS/AFFILIATES:
HCR Manor Care
Springhouse
Heartland
HCR Manor Care Foundation
ManorCare
Arden Courts

CONTACTS:
Note: Officers with more than one job title may be intentionally listed here more than once.

Paul A. Ormond, CEO
Paul A. Ormond, Pres.
M. Keith Weikel, Sr. Exec. VP/COO
Geoffrey G. Meyers, Exec. VP/CFO
Wade B. O'Brian, Dir.-Human Resources & Labor Rel.
R. Jeffrey Bixler, VP/General Counsel
Nancy A. Edwards, VP/General Mgr.
Paul A. Ormond, Chmn.

Phone: 419-252-5500   Fax: 419-252-5596
Toll-Free:
Address: 333 N. Summit St., Toledo, OH 43604-2617 US

GROWTH PLANS/SPECIAL FEATURES:

Manor Care, Inc. develops, owns and manages skilled nursing and assisted living facilities, which provide convalescent care and services principally for residents over the age of 65. The firm does business through its operating group, HCR Manor Care. It operates more than 500 long-term care facilities, assisted living facilities, outpatient rehabilitation clinics and home health care offices throughout the United States, under the names Heartland, ManorCare, Arden Courts and Springhouse. Other services include Alzheimer's care, rehabilitative therapy, hospice care and vision services. Manor Care also runs a not-for-profit corporation called HCR Manor Care Foundation, which is focused on education and research of disorders affecting the elderly and the community services provided to them. It provides grants to community programs, research funding for geriatric diseases and grants for organizations that provide public education services. Partnerships and other ventures supply the firm with high-quality pharmaceutical products and management services to physician practices.

Employee benefits include medical, dental, prescription drug and vision coverage, as well as tuition reimbursement, access to a credit union and training programs.

FINANCIALS:
Sales and profits are in thousands of dollars—add 000 to get the full amount. Year 2004 note: Complete fiscal 2004 results were not available for all companies at press time. For this company, year 2004 is for 9 months.

2004 Sales: $2,403,291 (9 months)   2004 Profits: $120,300 (9 months)
2003 Sales: $3,029,441   2003 Profits: $119,007
2002 Sales: $2,905,400   2002 Profits: $130,600
2001 Sales: $2,694,100   2001 Profits: $68,500
2000 Sales: $2,380,600   2000 Profits: $39,100

Stock Ticker: HCR
Employees: 61,000
Fiscal Year Ends: 12/31

SALARIES/BENEFITS:
Pension Plan: Y   ESOP Stock Plan: Profit Sharing: Top Exec. Salary: $874,193   Bonus: $1,086,000
Savings Plan: Y   Stock Purch. Plan: Second Exec. Salary: $554,515   Bonus: $570,000

OTHER THOUGHTS:
Apparent Top Female Officers: 1
Hot Spot for Advancement for Women/Minorities:

LOCATIONS: ("Y" = Yes)
West:	Southwest:	Midwest:	Southeast:	Northeast:	International:
Y	Y	Y	Y	Y	

MARIAN HEALTH SYSTEMS
www.marianhealthsystem.com

Industry Group Code: 622110   Ranks within this company's industry group: Sales: 20   Profits:

Insurance/HMO/PPO:	Drugs:	Equipment/Supplies:	Hospitals/Clinics:		Services:	Health Care:	
Insurance:	Manufacturer:	Manufacturer:	Acute Care:	Y	Diagnostics:	Home Health:	Y
Managed Care:	Distributor:	Distributor:	Sub-Acute Care:	Y	Labs/Testing:	Long-Term Care:	Y
Utilization Mgmt.:	Specialty Pharm.:	Leasing/Finance:	Outpatient Surgery:		Staffing:	Physical Therapy:	
Payment Proc.:	Vitamins/Nutri.:	Information Sys.:	Phys. Rehab. Center:	Y	Waste Disposal:	Phys. Practice Mgmt.:	
	Clinical Trials:		Psychiatric Clinics:		Specialty Services:		

TYPES OF BUSINESS:
Hospitals
Senior Communities
Long-Term Care
Home Care Services
Rehabilitation Services
Cancer Care
Dialysis Centers

BRANDS/DIVISIONS/AFFILIATES:
Sisters of the Sorrowful Mother
Saint Clair's Health System
Ministry Health Care
Affinity Health System
Saint John Health System
Via Christi Health System

CONTACTS:
Note: Officers with more than one job title may be intentionally listed here more than once.
M. Therese Gottschalk, CEO
M. Therese Gottschalk, Pres.
Nicholas Desien, Pres./CEO-Ministry Health Care

Phone: 918-742-9988	Fax: 918-744-2716
Toll-Free:	
Address: P.O. Box 4753, Tulsa, OK 74159 US	

GROWTH PLANS/SPECIAL FEATURES:
Marian Health System manages four health care systems in Kansas, New Jersey, Oklahoma and Wisconsin. The system is sponsored by the Sisters of the Sorrowful Mother, a Catholic charity, and has decentralized management for each location to respond more efficiently to local needs. Marian has separated its organizations into five regional companies: the Saint Clair's Health System, Ministry Health Care, Affinity Health System, the Saint John Health System and the Via Christi Health System. The Saint Clair's Health System has four hospitals and four senior assistance communities. Health care services include women's health, maternal-child care, emergency services, pediatrics, behavioral therapy and cancer care through an affiliation with Memorial Sloan-Kettering Cancer Center. The Ministry Health Care system includes eight hospitals, two medical centers, clinics, long-term care facilities, home care agencies, dialysis centers and many other programs and services in Wisconsin and Minnesota. The Affinity Health System, located in Wisconsin, runs one hospital, two medical centers, a rehabilitation center, a nursing home called Saint Elisabeth's and a convalescent center. The Saint John Health System manages four health centers and six nursing homes and is a regional leader in radiology, cardiology, oncology, urology, wellness and physical rehabilitation. The Via Christi Health System, co-sponsored with the Sisters of St. Joseph of Wichita, has seven hospitals and medical centers and six senior living communities.

FINANCIALS:
Sales and profits are in thousands of dollars—add 000 to get the full amount. Year 2004 note: Complete fiscal 2004 results were not available for all companies at press time. For this company, year 2004 is for months.

2004 Sales: $ (months)	2004 Profits: $ (months)	
2003 Sales: $2,804,800	2003 Profits: $	Stock Ticker: Private
2002 Sales: $2,679,100	2002 Profits: $	Employees: 4,011
2001 Sales: $	2001 Profits: $	Fiscal Year Ends: 9/30
2000 Sales: $	2000 Profits: $	

SALARIES/BENEFITS:
Pension Plan:	ESOP Stock Plan:	Profit Sharing:	Top Exec. Salary: $	Bonus: $
Savings Plan:	Stock Purch. Plan:		Second Exec. Salary: $	Bonus: $

OTHER THOUGHTS:
Apparent Top Female Officers: 1
Hot Spot for Advancement for Women/Minorities:

LOCATIONS: ("Y" = Yes)
West:	Southwest:	Midwest:	Southeast:	Northeast:	International:
	Y	Y		Y	

MARINER HEALTH CARE INC

www.marinerhealth.com

Industry Group Code: 623110 Ranks within this company's industry group: Sales: 4 Profits: 11

Insurance/HMO/PPO:	Drugs:	Equipment/Supplies:	Hospitals/Clinics:		Services:	Health Care:	
Insurance:	Manufacturer:	Manufacturer:	Acute Care:	Y	Diagnostics:	Home Health:	
Managed Care:	Distributor:	Distributor:	Sub-Acute Care:	Y	Labs/Testing:	Long-Term Care:	Y
Utilization Mgmt.:	Specialty Pharm.:	Leasing/Finance:	Outpatient Surgery:		Staffing:	Physical Therapy:	Y
Payment Proc.:	Vitamins/Nutri.:	Information Sys.:	Phys. Rehab. Center:		Waste Disposal:	Phys. Practice Mgmt.:	
	Clinical Trials:		Psychiatric Clinics:		Specialty Services:		

TYPES OF BUSINESS:
Skilled Nursing Facilities
Long-Term Acute Care Hospitals

BRANDS/DIVISIONS/AFFILIATES:
National Senior Care, Inc.

CONTACTS:
Note: Officers with more than one job title may be intentionally listed here more than once.

C. Christian Winkle, CEO
C. Christian Winkle, Pres.
Michael Boxer, Exec. VP/CFO
Terry O'Malley, Sr. VP-Human Resources
Stefano M. Miele, Sr. VP/General Counsel
Boyd P. Gentry, Sr. VP/Treas.
Jennifer Kulla, Sr. VP-Clinical Services
Bruce Duner, Sr. VP/Chief Acct. Officer
David F. Polakoff, Chief Medical Officer
William C. Straub, Sr. VP-Internal Controls
Victor Lund, Chmn.

Phone: 678-443-7000 Fax: 770-393-8054
Toll-Free: 800-929-4762
Address: One Ravinia Dr., Ste. 1500, Atlanta, GA 30346 US

GROWTH PLANS/SPECIAL FEATURES:
Mariner Health Care, Inc., through its subsidiaries, is one of the largest providers of skilled nursing and long-term health care services in the U.S. The company operates 252 skilled nursing facilities and two stand-alone assisted living facilities with an aggregate of approximately 31,000 licensed beds, as well as 12 long-term acute care hospitals (LTACs) with 640 licensed beds. These facilities are located in 23 states, with concentrations in Texas, North Carolina, California, Colorado, South Carolina and Maryland. Mariner's skilled nursing facilities provide 24-hour care to patients requiring assistance with one or more activities of daily living, supported by rehabilitation services including physical, occupational and speech therapy. Many also include sub-acute or intensive medical care facilities that offer enteral therapy, intravenous therapy, specialized wound management, tracheotomy, cancer and HIV care for patients with complex medical conditions. Through its LTACs, the firm provides more intensive care than can be provided in a typical skilled nursing facility. In recent news, Mariner agreed to be acquired by National Senior Care, Inc., pending shareholder approval.

FINANCIALS:
Sales and profits are in thousands of dollars—add 000 to get the full amount. Year 2004 note: Complete fiscal 2004 results were not available for all companies at press time. For this company, year 2004 is for months.

2004 Sales: $ (months)	2004 Profits: $ (months)	Stock Ticker: MHCA
2003 Sales: $1,715,400	2003 Profits: $-12,800	Employees: 35,000
2002 Sales: $1,785,100	2002 Profits: $1,375,600	Fiscal Year Ends: 12/31
2001 Sales: $	2001 Profits: $	
2000 Sales: $	2000 Profits: $	

SALARIES/BENEFITS:
Pension Plan: ESOP Stock Plan: Profit Sharing: Top Exec. Salary: $750,000 Bonus: $455,560
Savings Plan: Y Stock Purch. Plan: Second Exec. Salary: $427,500 Bonus: $210,859

OTHER THOUGHTS:
Apparent Top Female Officers: 1
Hot Spot for Advancement for Women/Minorities:

LOCATIONS: ("Y" = Yes)
West:	Southwest:	Midwest:	Southeast:	Northeast:	International:
Y	Y	Y	Y	Y	

MARSH & McLENNAN COMPANIES INC

www.marshmac.com

Industry Group Code: 524210   Ranks within this company's industry group: Sales: 1 Profits: 1

Insurance/HMO/PPO:	Drugs:	Equipment/Supplies:	Hospitals/Clinics:	Services:	Health Care:
Insurance: Y	Manufacturer:	Manufacturer:	Acute Care:	Diagnostics:	Home Health:
Managed Care:	Distributor:	Distributor:	Sub-Acute Care:	Labs/Testing:	Long-Term Care:
Utilization Mgmt.:	Specialty Pharm.:	Leasing/Finance:	Outpatient Surgery:	Staffing:	Physical Therapy:
Payment Proc.:	Vitamins/Nutri.:	Information Sys.:	Phys. Rehab. Center:	Waste Disposal:	Phys. Practice Mgmt.:
	Clinical Trials:		Psychiatric Clinics:	Specialty Services: Y	

TYPES OF BUSINESS:
Insurance Brokerage and Management
Investment Management
Risk Management
Consulting Services
Human Resources Services
Benefits Administration
Mutual Funds
Annuities

BRANDS/DIVISIONS/AFFILIATES:
Marsh, Inc.
Putnam Investments, LLC
Mercer Consulting Group, Inc.
Seabury & Smith, Inc.
MMC Capital
Mercer Delta Consulting
Lippincott & Marguiles
National Economic Research Associates

CONTACTS:
Note: Officers with more than one job title may be intentionally listed here more than once.
Michael G. Cherkasky, CEO
Michael G. Cherkasky, Pres.
Sandra S. Wijnberg, Sr. VP/CFO
William L. Rosoff, Sr. VP/General Counsel
Francis N. Bonsignore, Sr. VP-Exec. Resources & Dev.
Lawrence J. Lasser, Pres., Putnam Investments
Ray J. Groves, Pres./CEO-Marsh, Inc.
Michael G. Cherkasky, Chmn.

Phone: 212-345-5000   Fax: 212-345-4838
Toll-Free:
Address: 1166 Ave. of the Americas, New York, NY 10036-2774 US

GROWTH PLANS/SPECIAL FEATURES:

Marsh & McLennan Companies, Inc. (MMC), the world's largest insurance brokerage firm, provides global professional services, with annual revenues exceeding $11 billion. It is the parent company of Marsh, Inc., the world's leading risk and insurance firm; Putnam Investments, a leading investment management company in the United States; and Mercer Consulting Group, a major global provider of consulting services. Marsh provides advice and transactional capabilities to clients in over 100 countries and consists of several risk and insurance units, including Seabury & Smith, which provides insurance program management services; MMC Capital, which offers insurance industry investment services internationally; and Guy Carpenter & Company, Inc., which is involved in reinsurance. Putnam Investments manages over 11 million shareholder accounts and over 300 institutional accounts. It offers mutual funds, institutional portfolios and retirement plans, including 401(k)s and IRAs, as well as annuities and life insurance. Mercer Consulting Group is one of the largest human resources and management consulting firms in the world. The unit consists of five segments: Mercer Human Resources Consulting, which provides professional advice and services; Mercer Management Consulting, involved in business strategy counseling; Mercer Delta Consulting, which offers expertise related to corporate organization; Lippincott & Marguiles, an image consulting unit; and National Economic Research Associates, which focuses on regulatory, financial and public policy. In addition, the firm now provides chemical and bio-terrorism risk assessment and management services to U.S. businesses and government units. In October 2004, MMC introduced significant reforms to its business model in response to allegations of price rigging by the New York attorney general. The reforms aim to increase transparency and will eliminate contingent compensation, the practice of receiving commissions from insurers for directing more business to them.

The company provides its employees with various education-related programs, personal insurance options and employee assistance resources.

FINANCIALS:
Sales and profits are in thousands of dollars—add 000 to get the full amount. Year 2004 note: Complete fiscal 2004 results were not available for all companies at press time. For this company, year 2004 is for 9 months.

2004 Sales: $9,215,000 (9 months)   2004 Profits: $856,000 (9 months)
2003 Sales: $11,588,000   2003 Profits: $1,540,000
2002 Sales: $10,440,000   2002 Profits: $1,365,000
2001 Sales: $9,943,000   2001 Profits: $974,000
2000 Sales: $10,157,000   2000 Profits: $1,181,000

Stock Ticker: MMC
Employees: 60,500
Fiscal Year Ends: 12/31

SALARIES/BENEFITS:
Pension Plan: Y   ESOP Stock Plan: Profit Sharing: Top Exec. Salary: $1,200,000   Bonus: $3,500,042
Savings Plan: Stock Purch. Plan: Y   Second Exec. Salary: $900,000   Bonus: $2,350,042

OTHER THOUGHTS:
Apparent Top Female Officers: 1
Hot Spot for Advancement for Women/Minorities:

LOCATIONS: ("Y" = Yes)
West:	Southwest:	Midwest:	Southeast:	Northeast:	International:
Y	Y	Y	Y	Y	Y

MATRIA HEALTHCARE INC

www.matria.com

Industry Group Code: 621610 Ranks within this company's industry group: Sales: 5 Profits: 8

Insurance/HMO/PPO:	Drugs:	Equipment/Supplies:	Hospitals/Clinics:	Services:	Health Care:
Insurance: Managed Care: Utilization Mgmt.: Payment Proc.:	Manufacturer: Distributor: Specialty Pharm.: Vitamins/Nutri.: Clinical Trials:	Manufacturer: Distributor: Y Leasing/Finance: Information Sys.:	Acute Care: Sub-Acute Care: Outpatient Surgery: Phys. Rehab. Center: Psychiatric Clinics:	Diagnostics: Labs/Testing: Staffing: Waste Disposal: Specialty Services: Y	Home Health: Y Long-Term Care: Physical Therapy: Phys. Practice Mgmt.:

TYPES OF BUSINESS:
Home Health Care-Obstetrical
Disease Management Services
Blood Sampling Product Distribution
Diabetes Supplies

BRANDS/DIVISIONS/AFFILIATES:
System 37
Term Guard
Genesis
MaternaLink
Healthdyne Technologies
Facet Technologies, Inc.
Health Enhancement
Quality Oncology, Inc.

CONTACTS:
Note: Officers with more than one job title may be intentionally listed here more than once.

Parker H. Petit, CEO
Thomas S. Hall, Pres.
Thomas S. Hall, COO
Stephen M. Mengert, CFO
Steven Janicak, VP/Chief Mktg. Officer
Robert W. Kelley, Jr., VP-Tech.
Thornton A. Kuntz, Jr., VP-Admin.
Roberta L. McCaw, General Counsel/VP-Legal
Martin L. Olson, VP-Program Dev.
Stephen M. Mengert, VP-Finance
Eugene E. Jennings, Pres., Health Enhancement
Yvonne V. Scoggins, VP-Financial Planning & Analysis
James P. Reichmann, VP-Strategic Sales
Jean A. Bisio, Sr. VP-Disease Mgmt.
Parker H. Petit, Chmn.

Phone: 770-767-4500 **Fax:** 770-767-4521
Toll-Free: 800-759-1601
Address: 1850 Parkway Pl., 12th Fl., Marietta, GA 30067 US

GROWTH PLANS/SPECIAL FEATURES:
Matria Healthcare, Inc. is a disease management company that helps control health care costs by providing cost-saving alternatives for some of the most expensive medical conditions in the nation: diabetes, pregnancy, select respiratory diseases, cardiovascular diseases, depression and cancer. The diabetes disease management program provides risk assessment, patient education, clinical interventions, compliance management and outcomes reporting. As part of the compliance management process, the company sells glucose testing supplies, insulin, insulin pumps, syringes and other prescription and non-prescription drugs used by patients with diabetes. Operating under the name Facet Technologies, Inc., Matria's diabetes segment is also a leading designer, assembler, packager and wholesale distributor of microsampling products used to obtain and test small samples of blood. The women's health segment offers disease management services designed to assist physicians in the management of maternity patients. Services include risk assessment, patient education and management, infusion therapy, gestational diabetes management and other monitoring and clinical services as prescribed by the patient's physician. The respiratory disease management business provides respiratory disease risk assessment, screening and case management services to patients throughout the U.S. The firm's cardiovascular management program combines education with health risk assessments to improve compliance with physician recommendations about medication, blood pressure, nutrition and exercise. Since depression is the leading cause of disability in the U.S., Matria has developed a system of coordinated educational efforts and health care interventions to promote employee self-care efforts. The company's Quality Oncology, Inc. subsidiary is the nation's premiere provider of cancer disease management programs. The firm has announced plans to sell its diabetes and respiratory supplies business, operated by Diabetes Self Care, Inc., and Diabetes Management Solutions, Inc. to a subsidiary of CCS Medical.

FINANCIALS:
Sales and profits are in thousands of dollars—add 000 to get the full amount. Year 2004 note: Complete fiscal 2004 results were not available for all companies at press time. For this company, year 2004 is for 9 months.

2004 Sales: $215,171 (9 months)   2004 Profits: $25,500 (9 months)
2003 Sales: $326,847   2003 Profits: $7,306
2002 Sales: $277,600   2002 Profits: $-16,300
2001 Sales: $264,000   2001 Profits: $6,700
2000 Sales: $225,800   2000 Profits: $13,700

Stock Ticker: MATR
Employees: 1,452
Fiscal Year Ends: 12/31

SALARIES/BENEFITS:
Pension Plan: ESOP Stock Plan: Profit Sharing: Top Exec. Salary: $462,701   Bonus: $58,131
Savings Plan: Y   Stock Purch. Plan: Y   Second Exec. Salary: $408,311 Bonus: $43,131

OTHER THOUGHTS:
Apparent Top Female Officers: 3
Hot Spot for Advancement for Women/Minorities: Y

LOCATIONS: ("Y" = Yes)
West:	Southwest:	Midwest:	Southeast:	Northeast:	International:
Y			Y	Y	

Note: Financial information, benefits and other data can change quickly and may vary from those stated here.

MAXYGEN INC

www.maxygen.com

Industry Group Code: 541710 **Ranks within this company's industry group:** Sales: 11 Profits: 9

Insurance/HMO/PPO:	Drugs:	Equipment/Supplies:	Hospitals/Clinics:	Services:	Health Care:
Insurance:	Manufacturer: Y	Manufacturer:	Acute Care:	Diagnostics:	Home Health:
Managed Care:	Distributor:	Distributor:	Sub-Acute Care:	Labs/Testing: Y	Long-Term Care:
Utilization Mgmt.:	Specialty Pharm.:	Leasing/Finance:	Outpatient Surgery:	Staffing:	Physical Therapy:
Payment Proc.:	Vitamins/Nutri.:	Information Sys.:	Phys. Rehab. Center:	Waste Disposal:	Phys. Practice Mgmt.:
	Clinical Trials:		Psychiatric Clinics:	Specialty Services: Y	

TYPES OF BUSINESS:
Research & Development-Molecular Evolution
Improved and Novel Pharmaceuticals

BRANDS/DIVISIONS/AFFILIATES:
MolecularBreeding
DNAShuffling
MaxyScan
Codexis, Inc.

CONTACTS:
Note: Officers with more than one job title may be intentionally listed here more than once.

Russell J. Howard, CEO
Simba Gill, Pres.
Lawrence W. Briscoe, Sr. VP/CFO
R. Paul Spence, VP-R&D
Michael Rabson, Sr. VP/General Counsel
Elliot Goldstein, VP-Clinical Dev. and Denmark Oper.
Alan Shaw, Pres./CEO-Codexis
Isaac Stein, Chmn.

Phone: 650-298-5300 **Fax:** 650-364-2715
Toll-Free:
Address: 200 Penobscot Dr., Redwood City, CA 94063 US

GROWTH PLANS/SPECIAL FEATURES:

Maxygen, Inc. works to create improved versions of human therapeutics that are more effective and safer than currently available treatments, as well as to develop novel drugs. Its proprietary MolecularBreeding directed evolution and protein modification technologies allow the company to rapidly move from product concept to IND-ready drug candidate, lowering costs associated with research and expanding the potential for discovery. Components of the process include DNAShuffling, a proprietary process for recombining genes into a library of novel DNA sequences, and MaxyScan, a series of screening capabilities for the identification of desired properties from the library. Maxygen currently has six product candidates in preclinical studies, for hepatitis C, multiple sclerosis, pulmonary fibrosis, tuberculosis, meningitis, myelosuppression, dengue and cancer. Many more potential products are in the creation or screening stages. The company also uses its technologies in the chemicals market through subsidiary Codexis, Inc. Codexis is involved in a number of collaborations, including one with Chevron Research and Technology Co. to develop novel bioprocesses for petrochemical products, specifically the conversion of methane to methanol. The firm's other subsidiary, Verdia, Inc., was purchased by DuPont in July 2004.

In addition to comprehensive medical insurance, the firm offers employee service awards, concierge service, a credit union, annual Costco memberships and health club and tuition reimbursement. The company also pays 75% of employee mass transit costs and provides on-site bike lockers.

FINANCIALS:
Sales and profits are in thousands of dollars—add 000 to get the full amount. Year 2004 note: Complete fiscal 2004 results were not available for all companies at press time. For this company, year 2004 is for 9 months.

2004 Sales: $17,424 (9 months)	2004 Profits: $-22,878 (9 months)	**Stock Ticker:** MAXY
2003 Sales: $30,528	2003 Profits: $-44,964	Employees: 271
2002 Sales: $41,800	2002 Profits: $-33,900	Fiscal Year Ends: 12/31
2001 Sales: $30,500	2001 Profits: $-45,000	
2000 Sales: $24,500	2000 Profits: $-59,600	

SALARIES/BENEFITS:
Pension Plan: ESOP Stock Plan: Y   Profit Sharing: Top Exec. Salary: $420,000   Bonus: $105,000
Savings Plan: Y   Stock Purch. Plan: Y   Second Exec. Salary: $339,900   Bonus: $84,975

OTHER THOUGHTS:
Apparent Top Female Officers:
Hot Spot for Advancement for Women/Minorities:

LOCATIONS: ("Y" = Yes)
West:	Southwest:	Midwest:	Southeast:	Northeast:	International:
Y					Y

MAYO FOUNDATION FOR MEDICAL EDUCATION AND RESEARCH
www.mayo.edu

Industry Group Code: 622110   Ranks within this company's industry group: Sales: 11   Profits: 5

Insurance/HMO/PPO:	Drugs:	Equipment/Supplies:	Hospitals/Clinics:		Services:		Health Care:	
Insurance:	Manufacturer:	Manufacturer:	Acute Care:	Y	Diagnostics:	Y	Home Health:	
Managed Care:	Distributor:	Distributor:	Sub-Acute Care:	Y	Labs/Testing:	Y	Long-Term Care:	Y
Utilization Mgmt.:	Specialty Pharm.:	Leasing/Finance:	Outpatient Surgery:	Y	Staffing:		Physical Therapy:	
Payment Proc.:	Vitamins/Nutri.:	Information Sys.:	Phys. Rehab. Center:		Waste Disposal:		Phys. Practice Mgmt.:	Y
	Clinical Trials: Y		Psychiatric Clinics:		Specialty Services:	Y		

TYPES OF BUSINESS:
Hospitals/Clinics-General & Specialty Hospitals
Health Care Education
Medical Research
Physician Practice Management

BRANDS/DIVISIONS/AFFILIATES:
Mayo Clinic
St. Marys Hospital
Rochester Medical Hospital
St. Luke's Hospital
Mayo Clinic Hospital
Mayo Health System
Mayo Clinic College of Medicine
Mayo School of Health Sciences

CONTACTS:
Note: Officers with more than one job title may be intentionally listed here more than once.
Denis A. Cortese, CEO
Denis A. Cortese, Pres.
Jeffrey W. Bolton, CFO/Chair-Dept. of Finance
David Alquist, Dir.-Medical Dev.
Robert K. Smoldt, VP/Chief Admin. Officer
Jonathan J. Oviatt, Corp. Sec./Chair-Legal Dev.
Michael J. McNamara, Chair-Dept. of Dev.
Jeffrey Korsmo, Admin.-Mayo Clinic, Rochester
Shirley Weis, Admin.-Mayo Clinic, Scottsdale
Craig A. Smoldt, Chair-Dept. of Facilities & Systems Support

Phone: 507-284-2511   Fax: 507-284-0161
Toll-Free:
Address: 200 1st St. SW, Rochester, MN 55905 US

GROWTH PLANS/SPECIAL FEATURES:

The Mayo Foundation for Medical Education and Research is a not-for-profit health care organization providing medical treatment, physician management, health care education, research and other specialized medical services through a network of clinics and hospitals in the Midwest, Arizona and Florida. The three primary clinics, which house physician group practices, are located in Rochester, Minnesota; Jacksonville, Florida; and Scottsdale, Arizona. These clinics are accompanied by hospitals in each of the three cities. St. Marys Hospital, with 1,157 beds, and Rochester Medical Hospital, with 794 beds, are both located in Rochester, Minnesota. St. Luke's Hospital in Florida has 289 beds, and Mayo Clinic Hospital in Arizona has 202 beds. Additionally, the nonprofit operates the Charter House, a retirement community in Rochester. In total, the group includes nearly 3,000 staff physicians and medical scientists, 520 clinical and research employees, 1,800 residents and students and 37,000 administrative and allied health staff, spread over all locations and facilities. The Mayo Health System is a provider network of clinics and hospitals serving 60 communities in Iowa, Minnesota and Wisconsin. The Mayo Clinic College of Medicine, operating through the foundation's clinics and hospitals, is broken into five segments: Mayo School of Graduate Medical Education, Mayo Graduate School, Mayo Medical School, Mayo School of Health Sciences and Mayo School of Continuing Medical Education.

Mayo was recently voted one of the 100 Best Companies to Work For by Fortune Magazine.

FINANCIALS:
Sales and profits are in thousands of dollars—add 000 to get the full amount. Year 2004 note: Complete fiscal 2004 results were not available for all companies at press time. For this company, year 2004 is for months.

2004 Sales: $ (months)	2004 Profits: $ (months)	**Stock Ticker: Nonprofit**
2003 Sales: $4,822,200	2003 Profits: $348,900	Employees: 42,620
2002 Sales: $4,425,100	2002 Profits: $-212,300	Fiscal Year Ends: 12/31
2001 Sales: $	2001 Profits: $	
2000 Sales: $	2000 Profits: $	

SALARIES/BENEFITS:
Pension Plan:	ESOP Stock Plan:	Profit Sharing:	Top Exec. Salary: $	Bonus: $
Savings Plan:	Stock Purch. Plan:		Second Exec. Salary: $	Bonus: $

OTHER THOUGHTS:
Apparent Top Female Officers: 1
Hot Spot for Advancement for Women/Minorities:

LOCATIONS: ("Y" = Yes)
West:	Southwest:	Midwest:	Southeast:	Northeast:	International:
	Y	Y	Y		

MCKESSON CORPORATION

www.mckesson.com

Industry Group Code: 422210 Ranks within this company's industry group: Sales: 1 Profits: 2

Insurance/HMO/PPO:	Drugs:	Equipment/Supplies:	Hospitals/Clinics:	Services:	Health Care:
Insurance: Managed Care: Utilization Mgmt.: Payment Proc.: Y	Manufacturer: Distributor: Y Specialty Pharm.: Vitamins/Nutri.: Clinical Trials:	Manufacturer: Distributor: Y Leasing/Finance: Information Sys.: Y	Acute Care: Sub-Acute Care: Outpatient Surgery: Phys. Rehab. Center: Psychiatric Clinics:	Diagnostics: Labs/Testing: Staffing: Waste Disposal: Specialty Services: Y	Home Health: Long-Term Care: Physical Therapy: Phys. Practice Mgmt.:

TYPES OF BUSINESS:
Drugs-Distributor
Pharmaceutical Supply Management
Health Care Information Technology
Logistical Services
Online Claims and Statement Processing
Outsourcing Services
Utilization Management
Disease Management

BRANDS/DIVISIONS/AFFILIATES:
McKesson HBOC, Inc.
McKesson Medical-Surgical
McKesson Pharmaceutical
McKesson Automation
McKesson Pharmacy Systems
McKesson Medication Management

CONTACTS:
Note: Officers with more than one job title may be intentionally listed here more than once.
John H. Hammergren, CEO
John H. Hammergren, Pres.
William R. Graber, CFO
Paul E. Kirincic, Sr. VP-Human Resources
Cheryl T. Smith, Sr. VP/CIO
Ivan D. Meyerson, General Counsel
Marc Owen, Sr. VP-Corp. Strategy & Bus. Dev.
Pamela Pure, Sr. VP/Pres.-Info. Solutions
Paul C. Julian, Sr. VP/Pres.-Supply Solutions
Marcia Argyris, Pres., McKesson Foundation
Graham O. King, Sr. VP-Info. Solutions
John H. Hammergren, Chmn.

Phone: 415-983-8300 Fax: 415-983-7160
Toll-Free:
Address: One Post St., San Francisco, CA 94104 US

GROWTH PLANS/SPECIAL FEATURES:

McKesson Corporation, formerly McKesson HBOC, Inc., is the world's largest pharmaceutical supply management and health care information technology company. The firm focuses primarily on delivering value-added logistical services, materials management, third-party reimbursement support, scheduling, clinical data capture and analysis, billing and cost accountability and decision support. The company provides products and services through four divisions: supply solutions (SS), information solutions (IS), medical management (MM) and corporate solutions (CS). SS provides health care facilities with supplies and services through its subdivisions, including McKesson Pharmaceutical, which supplies pharmaceuticals and health care products to pharmacies; McKesson Medical-Surgical, which offers medical-surgical supplies, equipment and related services; McKesson Automation, the leader in scaleable pharmacy automation for inpatient and outpatient pharmacies; McKesson Pharmacy Systems, which offers products and services to help pharmacies run more efficiently; and McKesson Medication Management, which provides integrated pharmacy management services. IS serves the information system needs of health care facilities. It develops, implements and supports software that integrates data and provides a full complement of network technologies, as well as outsourcing services for managing business offices and information system operations. MM's offering include nurse triage, utilization management, case management and disease management, as well as analytic, credentialing and patient education solutions. CS works with multi-business customers to develop a portfolio of solutions reducing cost, improving efficiency and providing medication safety solutions, all from a single-source provider. The firm recently acquired the assets of of M.E.D.S., Inc., a Montreal-based provider of automated medication packaging devices for the United States and Canada.

McKesson provides employees with medical, dental, vision and prescription drug benefits; an assistance program; resources for child care, legal counsel and financial planning; adoption assistance; and flexible spending accounts.

FINANCIALS:
Sales and profits are in thousands of dollars—add 000 to get the full amount. Year 2004 note: Complete fiscal 2004 results were not available for all companies at press time. For this company, year 2004 is for 12 months.

2004 Sales: $69,506,100 (12 months)   2004 Profits: $646,500 (12 months)
2003 Sales: $57,120,800   2003 Profits: $555,400
2002 Sales: $50,006,000   2002 Profits: $419,000
2001 Sales: $42,019,100   2001 Profits: $-42,100
2000 Sales: $36,687,000   2000 Profits: $729,900

Stock Ticker: MCK
Employees: 24,600
Fiscal Year Ends: 3/31

SALARIES/BENEFITS:
Pension Plan: ESOP Stock Plan: Profit Sharing: Top Exec. Salary: $995,000 Bonus: $2,250,000
Savings Plan: Stock Purch. Plan: Second Exec. Salary: $665,000 Bonus: $400,000

OTHER THOUGHTS:
Apparent Top Female Officers: 3
Hot Spot for Advancement for Women/Minorities: Y

LOCATIONS: ("Y" = Yes)
West:	Southwest:	Midwest:	Southeast:	Northeast:	International:
Y	Y	Y	Y	Y	Y

Note: Financial information, benefits and other data can change quickly and may vary from those stated here.

MDS INC

www.mdsintl.com

Industry Group Code: 339113   **Ranks within this company's industry group:** Sales: 21   Profits: 41

Insurance/HMO/PPO:	Drugs:		Equipment/Supplies:	Hospitals/Clinics:	Services:		Health Care:	
Insurance:	Manufacturer:	Y	Manufacturer:	Acute Care:	Diagnostics:		Home Health:	
Managed Care:	Distributor:		Distributor:	Sub-Acute Care:	Labs/Testing:		Long-Term Care:	
Utilization Mgmt.:	Specialty Pharm.:		Leasing/Finance:	Outpatient Surgery:	Staffing:		Physical Therapy:	
Payment Proc.:	Vitamins/Nutri.:		Information Sys.:	Phys. Rehab. Center:	Waste Disposal:		Phys. Practice Mgmt.:	
	Clinical Trials:			Psychiatric Clinics:	Specialty Services:	Y		

TYPES OF BUSINESS:
Laboratory Services
Research and Development Services
Imaging Agents
Medical and Surgical Supplies
Irradiation Systems

BRANDS/DIVISIONS/AFFILIATES:
MDS Nordion
MDS Sciex
MDS Diagnostic Services
MDS Pharma Services
Source Medical
MDS Capital Corp.
MDS Proteomics

CONTACTS: Note: Officers with more than one job title may be intentionally listed here more than once.
John A. Rogers, CEO
John A. Rogers, Pres.
Jim A.G. Garner, CFO
Mary E. Federau, Sr. VP-Talent Dev.
David Poirier, CIO
Alan D. Torrie, Exec. VP-Tech. and Global Markets
Peter E. Brent, Sr. VP/General Counsel/Corp. Sec.
Robert W. Breckon, Exec. VP-Corp. Dev.
Kerry A. Thomas, VP-Strategic e-Bus. Initiatives
Mike Nethercott, VP-Corp. Mktg. & Comm.
Sharon Mathers, VP-Investor Rel.
Jim A.G. Garner, Exec. VP-Finance
James M. Reid, Exec. VP-Organization Dynamics
John A. Morrison, Group Pres./CEO-Health Care Provider Markets
Andrew W. Boorn, Pres., MDS Sciex
Edward K. Rygiel, Exec. VP
Wilfred G. Lewitt, Chmn.

Phone: 416-675-7661   **Fax:** 416-675-0688
Toll-Free: 888-637-7222
Address: 100 International Blvd., Toronto, Ontario M9W 6J6 Canada

GROWTH PLANS/SPECIAL FEATURES:
MDS, Inc. is a global biotechnology firm operating in health, life sciences and venture capital, with operations in 24 countries around the world, including locations in North and South America, Europe, Asia and Africa. The life sciences segment includes MDS Pharma Services, MDS Sciex and MDS Nordion, providing drug discovery and development services; analytical instruments and technology solutions; and radioisotopes, radiation and related technologies. Customers include pharmaceutical and biotechnology companies, hospitals and health care professionals. MDS Nordion's cobalt-60 irradiation systems are used to sterilize over 40% of the world's disposable medical supplies, to irradiate blood for blood transfusions and to destroy harmful bacteria on produce. The firm's health segment, including MDS Diagnostic Services and Source Medical, provides access to clinical, anatomical, esoteric and genetic laboratory tests; manages laboratory organizations; and distributes health care products to hospitals, long-term care facilities and physicians. MDS also owns 47% of MDS Capital Corp., which manages funds totaling over $1 billion. MDS recently transferred its Ontario lab business to Hemosol, Inc., which will continue researching blood products under the name Hemosol Corp., and its New York and Georgia labs to Laboratory Corporation of America Holdings. Subsidiary MDS Proteomics has also undergone a restructuring in order to regain profitability.

The company offers its employees an on-site fitness center, aerobics, yoga and strength training classes, nature trails for jogging and walking and 52 acres of trees and wildlife to enjoy. MDS also sponsors organized sports, such as soccer, volleyball and hockey.

FINANCIALS:
Sales and profits are in thousands of dollars—add 000 to get the full amount. Year 2004 note: Complete fiscal 2004 results were not available for all companies at press time. For this company, year 2004 is for 9 months.

2004 Sales: $1,033,000 (9 months)   2004 Profits: $46,000 (9 months)
2003 Sales: $1,364,000   2003 Profits: $36,000
2002 Sales: $1,150,000   2002 Profits: $67,000
2001 Sales: $1,031,000   2001 Profits: $46,000
2000 Sales: $938,700   2000 Profits: $22,000

Stock Ticker: Foreign
Employees: 10,000
Fiscal Year Ends: 10/31

SALARIES/BENEFITS:
Pension Plan: Y   ESOP Stock Plan: Profit Sharing: Top Exec. Salary: $ Bonus: $
Savings Plan: Stock Purch. Plan: Y   Second Exec. Salary: $ Bonus: $

OTHER THOUGHTS:
Apparent Top Female Officers: 3
Hot Spot for Advancement for Women/Minorities: Y

LOCATIONS: ("Y" = Yes)
West:	Southwest:	Midwest:	Southeast:	Northeast:	International:
Y	Y	Y	Y	Y	Y

MEDCATH CORPORATION

www.medcath.com

Industry Group Code: 622110 Ranks within this company's industry group: Sales: 42 Profits: 19

Insurance/HMO/PPO:	Drugs:	Equipment/Supplies:	Hospitals/Clinics:		Services:		Health Care:	
Insurance: Managed Care: Utilization Mgmt.: Payment Proc.:	Manufacturer: Distributor: Specialty Pharm.: Vitamins/Nutri.: Clinical Trials:	Manufacturer: Distributor: Leasing/Finance: Information Sys.:	Acute Care: Sub-Acute Care: Outpatient Surgery: Phys. Rehab. Center: Psychiatric Clinics:	Y	Diagnostics: Labs/Testing: Staffing: Waste Disposal: Specialty Services:	Y Y Y	Home Health: Long-Term Care: Physical Therapy: Phys. Practice Mgmt.:	

TYPES OF BUSINESS:
Cardiac Care Hospitals
Management and Consulting Services
Cardiac Catheterization Labs

BRANDS/DIVISIONS/AFFILIATES:

CONTACTS: Note: Officers with more than one job title may be intentionally listed here more than once.
John T. Casey, CEO
John T. Casey, Pres.
Charles R. Slaton, Exec. VP/COO
James E. Harris, Exec. VP/CFO
Brian T. Atkinson, Sr. VP/General Counsel
Joan McCanless, Sr. VP-Risk Mgmt., Decision Support & Compliance
Thomas K. Hearn, III, Pres.-Diagnostic Div.
John T. Casey, Chmn.

Phone: 704-708-6600   Fax: 704-708-5035
Toll-Free:
Address: 10720 Sikes Pl., Ste. 300, Charlotte, NC 28277 US

GROWTH PLANS/SPECIAL FEATURES:

MedCath Corporation designs, develops, owns and operates cardiac care hospitals in partnership with cardiologists and cardiovascular surgeons. The company also provides consulting and management services tailored to cardiologists and cardiovascular surgeons and owns several cardiac catheterization labs. The firm's 13 hospitals are freestanding, licensed general acute care hospitals capable of providing a full complement of health services through an emergency department, operating rooms, catheterization laboratories, pharmacy, laboratory, radiology department, cafeteria and food service. The company also provides cardiovascular care services in diagnostic and therapeutic facilities located in seven states and through mobile cardiac catheterization laboratories. Physicians use mobile diagnostic facilities to evaluate the functioning of patients' hearts and coronary arteries and to serve areas that do not have the patient volume to support a full-time facility. MedCath has developed an innovative, standardized facility design and infrastructure specifically tailored to cardiovascular care. Patients remain in the same large, private room during their entire stay. Rooms are equipped for critical care, telemetry and post-surgical care. Hospital rooms can accommodate family members who wish to stay with the patient, and MedCath hospitals feature unlimited visiting hours. The firm intends to begin development on one to three new heart hospitals every year.

FINANCIALS: Sales and profits are in thousands of dollars—add 000 to get the full amount. Year 2004 note: Complete fiscal 2004 results were not available for all companies at press time. For this company, year 2004 is for 9 months.

2004 Sales: $510,697 (9 months)   2004 Profits: $3,088   (9 months)
2003 Sales: $542,986   2003 Profits: $-60,306
2002 Sales: $447,628   2002 Profits: $24,351
2001 Sales: $377,000   2001 Profits: $1,100
2000 Sales: $332,300   2000 Profits: $-13,600

Stock Ticker: MDTH
Employees: 4,124
Fiscal Year Ends: 9/30

SALARIES/BENEFITS:
Pension Plan:	ESOP Stock Plan:	Profit Sharing:	Top Exec. Salary: $481,629	Bonus: $450,000
Savings Plan:	Stock Purch. Plan:		Second Exec. Salary: $301,225	Bonus: $60,000

OTHER THOUGHTS:
Apparent Top Female Officers: 1
Hot Spot for Advancement for Women/Minorities:

LOCATIONS: ("Y" = Yes)
West:	Southwest:	Midwest:	Southeast:	Northeast:	International:
Y	Y	Y	Y	Y	

MEDCO HEALTH SOLUTIONS

www.medcohealth.com

Industry Group Code: 522320A   Ranks within this company's industry group: Sales: 1 Profits: 1

Insurance/HMO/PPO:	Drugs:	Equipment/Supplies:	Hospitals/Clinics:	Services:	Health Care:
Insurance:	Manufacturer:	Manufacturer:	Acute Care:	Diagnostics:	Home Health:
Managed Care:	Distributor: Y	Distributor:	Sub-Acute Care:	Labs/Testing:	Long-Term Care:
Utilization Mgmt.:	Specialty Pharm.: Y	Leasing/Finance:	Outpatient Surgery:	Staffing:	Physical Therapy:
Payment Proc.:	Vitamins/Nutri.:	Information Sys.:	Phys. Rehab. Center:	Waste Disposal:	Phys. Practice Mgmt.:
	Clinical Trials:		Psychiatric Clinics:	Specialty Services: Y	

TYPES OF BUSINESS:
Prescription Benefits Management
Home Delivery Pharmacies

BRANDS/DIVISIONS/AFFILIATES:
Merck, Corp.
Systemed, LLC
Blue Cross Blue Shield

CONTACTS:
Note: Officers with more than one job title may be intentionally listed here more than once.

David B. Snow, Jr., CEO
David B. Snow, Jr., Pres.
Kenneth O. Klepper, COO
JoAnn A. Reed, CFO
Jack A. Smith, Chief Mktg. Officer
Karin Princivalle, Sr. VP-Human Resources
David S. Machlowitz, General Counsel
JoAnn A. Reed, Sr. VP-Finance
Glenn C. Taylor, Sr. VP-Key Accounts
Robert S. Epstein, Chief Medical Officer
Arthur H. Nardin, Sr. VP-Pharmaceutical Contracting
Timothy C. Wentworth, Group Pres.-Nat'l Accounts
David B. Snow, Jr., Chmn.

Phone: 201-269-3400   Fax: 201-269-1109
Toll-Free:
Address: 100 Parsons Pond Dr., Franklin Lakes, NJ 07417 US

GROWTH PLANS/SPECIAL FEATURES:
Medco Health Solutions is the leading pharmacy benefits manager (PBM) in the United States. Formerly a subsidiary of Merck, Medco Health Solutions was spun-off as an independent company in August 2003. PBM services include the design and implementation of formularies, lists of preferred drugs from which clients can choose; claims adjudication and administration for pharmacies; discounts on certain pharmaceuticals that have been negotiated with drug manufacturers; and other management and control programs. Medco also runs a home drug delivery business through a network of nearly 60,000 retail pharmacies. The firm has client businesses in all of the major industry segments, including Blue Cross/Blue Shield plans; managed care organizations (HMOs and PPOs); insurance carriers; third-party benefit plan administrators; employers; federal, state and local government agencies; and union-sponsored benefit plans. Medco has developed its own technology platform that includes automated home delivery pharmacies, specialized call center pharmacies and Internet applications. The company's wholly-owned subsidiary, Systemed, LLC, uses the capabilities of Medco but specializes in delivering personalized services to small and mid-sized companies.

FINANCIALS:
Sales and profits are in thousands of dollars—add 000 to get the full amount. Year 2004 note: Complete fiscal 2004 results were not available for all companies at press time. For this company, year 2004 is for 9 months.

2004 Sales: $26,438,700 (9 months)	2004 Profits: $348,900 (9 months)	Stock Ticker: MHS
2003 Sales: $34,264,500	2003 Profits: $425,800	Employees: 13,650
2002 Sales: $32,958,000	2002 Profits: $362,000	Fiscal Year Ends: 12/31
2001 Sales: $29,070,600	2001 Profits: $256,600	
2000 Sales: $22,266,300	2000 Profits: $216,800	

SALARIES/BENEFITS:
Pension Plan:	ESOP Stock Plan:	Profit Sharing:	Top Exec. Salary: $600,000	Bonus: $800,000
Savings Plan: Y	Stock Purch. Plan:		Second Exec. Salary: $408,095	Bonus: $190,000

OTHER THOUGHTS:
Apparent Top Female Officers: 2
Hot Spot for Advancement for Women/Minorities:

LOCATIONS: ("Y" = Yes)
West:	Southwest:	Midwest:	Southeast:	Northeast:	International:
Y	Y	Y	Y	Y	

MEDEX HOLDINGS CORPORATION

www.medex.com

Industry Group Code: 339113   **Ranks within this company's industry group:** Sales: 60   Profits: 121

Insurance/HMO/PPO:	Drugs:	Equipment/Supplies:	Hospitals/Clinics:	Services:	Health Care:
Insurance: Managed Care: Utilization Mgmt.: Payment Proc.:	Manufacturer: Distributor: Specialty Pharm.: Vitamins/Nutri.: Clinical Trials:	Manufacturer: Y Distributor: Leasing/Finance: Information Sys.:	Acute Care: Sub-Acute Care: Outpatient Surgery: Phys. Rehab. Center: Psychiatric Clinics:	Diagnostics: Labs/Testing: Staffing: Waste Disposal: Specialty Services:	Home Health: Long-Term Care: Physical Therapy: Phys. Practice Mgmt.:

TYPES OF BUSINESS:
Medical Equipment & Supplies
Infusion Systems
Pressure Monitoring Systems
Cath Lab Packs
Respiratory Products

BRANDS/DIVISIONS/AFFILIATES:
Medex, Inc.
Springfusor Mechanical Infusion System
Medfusion 3500 Syringe Pump
PharmGuard Medication Safety Software

CONTACTS:
Note: Officers with more than one job title may be intentionally listed here more than once.
Dominick A. Arena, CEO
Dominick A. Arena, Pres.
Michael I. Dobrovic, VP/CFO
Charles J. Jamison, VP/General Counsel
Georg Landsberg, Sr. VP-European Oper.
Michael I. Dobrovic, Treas.
Timothy A. Dugan, Chmn.

Phone: 760-602-4400   **Fax:** 760-929-0147
Toll-Free: 800-848-1757
Address: 2231 Rutherford Rd., Carlsbad, CA 92008 US

GROWTH PLANS/SPECIAL FEATURES:
Medex Holdings Corporation, which conducts its operations through Medex, Inc. and its subsidiaries, is a leading global manufacturer and marketer of critical care disposable and non-disposable medical products. The company has a portfolio of critical care products with established brands used by hospitals and alternate care facilities for diagnostic and therapeutic procedures. Medex offers its customers a complete fluid and drug infusion system including infusion pumps, fluid and drug administration products and peripheral intravenous catheters (PIVCs), all of which function together to safely deliver measured doses of fluids and drugs into a patient's vascular system. The company categorizes its products into the following primary product lines: infusion systems, consisting of infusion pumps, disposables for fluid and drug administration and vascular access products; pressure monitoring systems, including disposable, semi-reusable and reusable pressure transducers used to measure blood pressures within the body; cath lab packs and accessories; and respiratory products, which include devices used for oxygen administration, anesthesia, drug delivery and humidification. The company has a global sales force of approximately 200 sales representatives and a network of distributors that reach over 5,500 hospitals and alternate care settings in more than 80 countries. In the United States, Medex has long-standing relationships with some of the largest and most prominent group purchasing organizations and integrated delivery networks, which allows its sales force to sell the company's entire portfolio of products to the appropriate call point within the hospital during a single sales call. In recent news, Pharmaceutical Buyers, Inc., a group purchasing organization with a focus on the alternative care market, awarded Medex a three-year contract.

FINANCIALS:
Sales and profits are in thousands of dollars—add 000 to get the full amount. Year 2004 note: Complete fiscal 2004 results were not available for all companies at press time. For this company, year 2004 is for months.

2004 Sales: $ (months)   2004 Profits: $ (months)
2003 Sales: $219,100   2003 Profits: $-7,400
2002 Sales: $100,800   2002 Profits: $-1,700
2001 Sales: $ 2001 Profits: $
2000 Sales: $ 2000 Profits: $

Stock Ticker: MDX
Employees: 2,080
Fiscal Year Ends: 12/31

SALARIES/BENEFITS:
Pension Plan: ESOP Stock Plan: Profit Sharing: Top Exec. Salary: $320,309   Bonus: $2,104,019
Savings Plan: Stock Purch. Plan: Second Exec. Salary: $268,092 Bonus: $1,098,724

OTHER THOUGHTS:
Apparent Top Female Officers:
Hot Spot for Advancement for Women/Minorities:

LOCATIONS: ("Y" = Yes)
West:	Southwest:	Midwest:	Southeast:	Northeast:	International:
Y		Y	Y	Y	Y

MEDICAL ACTION INDUSTRIES INC

www.medical-action.com

Industry Group Code: 339113   Ranks within this company's industry group: Sales: 89   Profits: 75

Insurance/HMO/PPO:	Drugs:	Equipment/Supplies:		Hospitals/Clinics:	Services:	Health Care:
Insurance:	Manufacturer:	Manufacturer:	Y	Acute Care:	Diagnostics:	Home Health:
Managed Care:	Distributor:	Distributor:	Y	Sub-Acute Care:	Labs/Testing:	Long-Term Care:
Utilization Mgmt.:	Specialty Pharm.:	Leasing/Finance:		Outpatient Surgery:	Staffing:	Physical Therapy:
Payment Proc.:	Vitamins/Nutri.:	Information Sys.:		Phys. Rehab. Center:	Waste Disposal:	Phys. Practice Mgmt.:
	Clinical Trials:			Psychiatric Clinics:	Specialty Services:	

TYPES OF BUSINESS:
Supplies-Laparotomy Sponges and Operating Room Towels
Disposable Surgical Products
Waste Collection Systems

BRANDS/DIVISIONS/AFFILIATES:
BioSafety
Maxxim Meadical

CONTACTS:
Note: Officers with more than one job title may be intentionally listed here more than once.
Paul D. Meringolo, CEO
Paul D. Meringolo, Pres.
Manuel B. Losada, VP-Mktg. & Sales
Philip R. Meringolo, Dir.-Info. Systems
Richard G. Satin, General Counsel
Richard G. Satin, VP-Oper.
Victor Bacchioni, Corp. Controller
Paul D. Meringolo, Chmn.
Eric Liu, Int'l Oper.

Phone: 631-231-4600   Fax: 631-231-3075
Toll-Free: 800-645-7042
Address: 800 Prime Pl., Hauppauge, NY 11788 US

GROWTH PLANS/SPECIAL FEATURES:
Medical Action Industries, Inc. develops, manufactures, markets and distributes a variety of disposable surgical products. The company markets its products primarily to acute care facilities in domestic and certain international markets and is expanding its end-user base to include physician, dental and veterinary offices. Medical Action is a leader in the manufacturing and distribution of collection systems for the containment of medical waste, minor procedure kits and trays, sterile laparotomy sponges and sterile operating room towels in the United States. To complement these products, Medical Action has developed several additional product lines, including gauze sponges, gauze fluffs, dry burn dressings and non-adherent gauze dressings. The company's products are marketed through an extensive network of independent distributors, direct sales personnel and manufacturers' representatives. Medical Action has made steady acquisitions of key business segments and has experienced increasing revenues for the past several years. It made its largest acquisition in company history in October 2002, with the acquisition of Maxxim Medical's BioSafety division. BioSafety's manufacturing facility makes specialty packaging and collection systems for the containment of infectious waste and a line of sharps containment systems.

FINANCIALS:
Sales and profits are in thousands of dollars—add 000 to get the full amount. Year 2004 note: Complete fiscal 2004 results were not available for all companies at press time. For this company, year 2004 is for 12 months.

2004 Sales: $127,601 (12 months)	2004 Profits: $9,434 (12 months)	**Stock Ticker: MDCI**
2003 Sales: $104,800	2003 Profits: $8,200	Employees: 356
2002 Sales: $82,800	2002 Profits: $6,300	Fiscal Year Ends: 3/31
2001 Sales: $75,400	2001 Profits: $4,400	
2000 Sales: $71,000	2000 Profits: $3,200	

SALARIES/BENEFITS:
Pension Plan:	ESOP Stock Plan:	Profit Sharing:	Top Exec. Salary: $450,981	Bonus: $106,000
Savings Plan: Y	Stock Purch. Plan:		Second Exec. Salary: $229,701	Bonus: $112,000

OTHER THOUGHTS:
Apparent Top Female Officers:
Hot Spot for Advancement for Women/Minorities:

LOCATIONS: ("Y" = Yes)
West:	Southwest:	Midwest:	Southeast:	Northeast:	International:
			Y	Y	

MEDICAL MUTUAL OF OHIO

www.medmutual.com

Industry Group Code: 524114 Ranks within this company's industry group: Sales: 39 Profits:

Insurance/HMO/PPO:	Drugs:	Equipment/Supplies:	Hospitals/Clinics:	Services:	Health Care:
Insurance: Y	Manufacturer:	Manufacturer:	Acute Care:	Diagnostics:	Home Health:
Managed Care: Y	Distributor:	Distributor:	Sub-Acute Care:	Labs/Testing:	Long-Term Care:
Utilization Mgmt.:	Specialty Pharm.:	Leasing/Finance:	Outpatient Surgery:	Staffing:	Physical Therapy:
Payment Proc.:	Vitamins/Nutri.:	Information Sys.:	Phys. Rehab. Center:	Waste Disposal:	Phys. Practice Mgmt.:
	Clinical Trials:		Psychiatric Clinics:	Specialty Services:	

TYPES OF BUSINESS:
Insurance
HMO/PPO

GROWTH PLANS/SPECIAL FEATURES:
Medical Mutual of Ohio (MMO), formerly Blue Cross Blue Shield of Ohio, is a not-for-profit health care company that provides health insurance to more than 3 million customers in Ohio and Pennsylvania through individual and corporate plans. The firm is no longer associated with the Blue Cross Blue Shield Association. MMO insurance programs include HMOs, PPOs, POSs, indemnity and Medicare supplemental. It also provides dental, vision, life and workers' compensation insurance. The firm was recently named a Fortune 1000 company, at number 797.

BRANDS/DIVISIONS/AFFILIATES:
Blue Cross Blue Shield of Ohio

CONTACTS:
Note: Officers with more than one job title may be intentionally listed here more than once.
Kent W. Clapp, CEO
Kent W. Clapp, Pres.
Susan Tyler, CFO
Kenneth Sidon, CIO
Don Olson, Media Rel. Mgr.
Joseph Krysh, VP-Claims & Customer Service
Kent W. Clapp, Chmn.

Phone: 216-687-7000   Fax: 216-687-6044
Toll-Free: 800-700-2583
Address: 2060 E. 9th St., Cleveland, OH 44115-1300 US

FINANCIALS:
Sales and profits are in thousands of dollars—add 000 to get the full amount. Year 2004 note: Complete fiscal 2004 results were not available for all companies at press time. For this company, year 2004 is for months.

2004 Sales: $ (months)   2004 Profits: $ (months)
2003 Sales: $1,600,000   2003 Profits: $
2002 Sales: $1,500,000   2002 Profits: $
2001 Sales: $ 2001 Profits: $
2000 Sales: $ 2000 Profits: $

Stock Ticker: Nonprofit
Employees: 2,500
Fiscal Year Ends: 12/31

SALARIES/BENEFITS:
Pension Plan: ESOP Stock Plan: Profit Sharing: Top Exec. Salary: $ Bonus: $
Savings Plan: Stock Purch. Plan: Second Exec. Salary: $ Bonus: $

OTHER THOUGHTS:
Apparent Top Female Officers: 1
Hot Spot for Advancement for Women/Minorities:

LOCATIONS: ("Y" = Yes)
West:	Southwest:	Midwest:	Southeast:	Northeast:	International:
		Y		Y	

MEDICORE INC

www.medicore.com

Industry Group Code: 339113 Ranks within this company's industry group: Sales: 123 Profits: 103

Insurance/HMO/PPO:	Drugs:	Equipment/Supplies:		Hospitals/Clinics:		Services:		Health Care:	
Insurance:	Manufacturer:	Manufacturer:	Y	Acute Care:		Diagnostics:		Home Health:	Y
Managed Care:	Distributor:	Distributor:	Y	Sub-Acute Care:		Labs/Testing:		Long-Term Care:	
Utilization Mgmt.:	Specialty Pharm.:	Leasing/Finance:		Outpatient Surgery:		Staffing:		Physical Therapy:	
Payment Proc.:	Vitamins/Nutri.:	Information Sys.:		Phys. Rehab. Center:		Waste Disposal:		Phys. Practice Mgmt.:	
	Clinical Trials:			Psychiatric Clinics:		Specialty Services:	Y		

TYPES OF BUSINESS:
Medical Supplies-Assorted
Blood Sampling Equipment
Diabetic Supplies
Kidney Dialysis Centers
Glass Tubing Products
Prepackaged Swabs & Bandages
Home Health Services

BRANDS/DIVISIONS/AFFILIATES:
Dialysis Corporation of America
Linux Global Partners, Inc.
DCA Medical Services, Inc.
Producers of Quality Medical Disposables
Lite Touch
Lady Lite

CONTACTS: Note: Officers with more than one job title may be intentionally listed here more than once.
Thomas K. Langbein, CEO
Thomas K. Langbein, Pres.
David R. Ouzts, VP-Finance/Treas.
Stephen W. Everett, Pres./CEO-Dialysis Corp. of America
Thomas K. Langbein, Chmn.

Phone: 305-558-4000 **Fax:**
Toll-Free:
Address: 2337 W. 76th, Hialeah, FL 33016 US

GROWTH PLANS/SPECIAL FEATURES:
Medicore, Inc. operates in three business segments: medical products, kidney dialysis centers and investment in technology companies. The company's medical products division manufactures and distributes medical supplies, primarily disposables, to domestic and foreign hospitals, blood banks, laboratories and retail pharmacies. These products include exam gloves, prepackaged swabs and bandages and glass tubing products for laboratories. The firm also distributes a line of blood lancets used to draw blood for testing. The lancets are distributed under the names Producers of Quality Medical Disposables, Lady Lite and Lite Touch, or under a private label if requested by the customer. Medicore's 19 outpatient dialysis facilities, operated by subsidiary Dialysis Corporation of America, are located in Pennsylvania, Maryland, New Jersey, Georgia, South Carolina, Virginia and Ohio. It also provides acute dialysis services through contractual relationships with seven hospitals and medical centers and provides home care services through subsidiary DCA Medical Services, Inc. The firm's technology investment is represented by a 14% share in Linux Global Partners, Inc. (LGP), a private speculative company attempting to develop and market a Linux desktop system. LGP also invests in developing Linux software companies.

FINANCIALS: Sales and profits are in thousands of dollars—add 000 to get the full amount. Year 2004 note: Complete fiscal 2004 results were not available for all companies at press time. For this company, year 2004 is for 6 months.

2004 Sales: $18,638 (6 months)   2004 Profits: $- 34 (6 months)
2003 Sales: $32,110   2003 Profits: $ 273
2002 Sales: $26,100   2002 Profits: $ 500
2001 Sales: $20,700   2001 Profits: $1,200
2000 Sales: $10,800   2000 Profits: $- 400

Stock Ticker: MDKI
Employees: 320
Fiscal Year Ends: 12/31

SALARIES/BENEFITS:
Pension Plan: ESOP Stock Plan: Profit Sharing: Top Exec. Salary: $333,232   Bonus: $279,400
Savings Plan: Stock Purch. Plan: Second Exec. Salary: $168,923   Bonus: $117,078

OTHER THOUGHTS:
Apparent Top Female Officers:
Hot Spot for Advancement for Women/Minorities:

LOCATIONS: ("Y" = Yes)

West:	Southwest:	Midwest:	Southeast:	Northeast:	International:
		Y	Y	Y	

MEDQUIST INC

www.medquist.com

Industry Group Code: 514210 **Ranks within this company's industry group:** Sales: Profits:

Insurance/HMO/PPO:	Drugs:	Equipment/Supplies:	Hospitals/Clinics:	Services:	Health Care:
Insurance:	Manufacturer:	Manufacturer:	Acute Care:	Diagnostics:	Home Health:
Managed Care:	Distributor:	Distributor:	Sub-Acute Care:	Labs/Testing:	Long-Term Care:
Utilization Mgmt.:	Specialty Pharm.:	Leasing/Finance:	Outpatient Surgery:	Staffing:	Physical Therapy:
Payment Proc.:	Vitamins/Nutri.:	Information Sys.: Y	Phys. Rehab. Center:	Waste Disposal:	Phys. Practice Mgmt.:
	Clinical Trials:		Psychiatric Clinics:	Specialty Services: Y	

TYPES OF BUSINESS:
Data Processing-Transcription & Information Management

BRANDS/DIVISIONS/AFFILIATES:
Royal Philips Electronics
Dictation Tracking System
Quality Medical Transcription, Inc.
Medical Dictation Center, Inc.
Medical Transcription System
DocQment Enterprise Platform
Mediquest Dictation Tracking System

CONTACTS:
Note: Officers with more than one job title may be intentionally listed here more than once.
Stephen H. Rusckowski, CEO
Gregory M. Sebasky, Pres.
Brian J. Kearns, Exec. VP/CFO
John Kumpf, VP-Human Resources
Ethan Cohen, Exec. VP/Chief Tech. Officer
John M. Suender, Chief Legal Officer
Ronald F. Scarpone, Sr. VP-New Bus. Dev.

Phone:	Fax: 856-206-4020
Toll-Free: 800-206-4020	
Address: 1000 Bishops Gate Blvd., Ste.300, Mount Laurel, NJ 08054 US	

GROWTH PLANS/SPECIAL FEATURES:
MedQuist, Inc. is a leading national provider of electronic transcription and data management services to the health care industry. Through its proprietary software, open architecture environment and network of more than 10,000 trained transcriptionists, the company converts free-form medical dictation into electronically formatted patient records that health care providers use in connection with patient care and for other administrative purposes. The company's customized outsourcing devices enable clients to improve the accuracy of transcribed medical reports, reduce report turnaround times, shorten billing cycles and reduce overhead and other administrative costs. The company's client service centers, located throughout the U.S., are staffed with qualified support personnel and skilled medical transcriptionists, while its technical call center, in Atlanta, monitors, logs, tracks and charts systematic support and interaction 24 hours a day with its nationwide client base. MedQuist continues to implement advances in technology to improve the delivery of its services. Its Medical Transcription System is an integrated transcription and document management solution that addresses initial data capture, conversion of data into electronic format, editing and routing of electronically formatted reports to the client's host computer system. MedQuist's Dictation Tracking System enables the company and its clients to track the status of particular patient data and transcribed reports at any point in time. The firm also partners with WebMD, one of the most popular medical sites on the Internet. Its DocQment Enterprise Platform is a web-based document workflow management solution that integrates dictation, routing, speech recognition, transcription and document delivery. Royal Philips Electronics owns 71% of MedQuist.

The company provides an employee benefits package including medical and dental insurance, flexible spending accounts and long-term disability.

FINANCIALS:
Sales and profits are in thousands of dollars—add 000 to get the full amount. Year 2004 note: Complete fiscal 2004 results were not available for all companies at press time. For this company, year 2004 is for months.

2004 Sales: $ (months)   2004 Profits: $ (months)
2003 Sales: $ 2003 Profits: $
2002 Sales: $486,200   2002 Profits: $43,900
2001 Sales: $405,300   2001 Profits: $44,600
2000 Sales: $364,149   2000 Profits: $38,730

Stock Ticker: MEDQ.PK
Employees: 10,230
Fiscal Year Ends: 12/31

SALARIES/BENEFITS:
Pension Plan:	ESOP Stock Plan:	Profit Sharing:	Top Exec. Salary: $492,960	Bonus: $182,000
Savings Plan: Y	Stock Purch. Plan: Y		Second Exec. Salary: $369,200	Bonus: $110,760

OTHER THOUGHTS:
Apparent Top Female Officers:
Hot Spot for Advancement for Women/Minorities:

LOCATIONS: ("Y" = Yes)
West:	Southwest:	Midwest:	Southeast:	Northeast:	International:
Y	Y	Y	Y	Y	

Note: Financial information, benefits and other data can change quickly and may vary from those stated here.

MEDSTAR HEALTH

www.medstarhealth.org

Industry Group Code: 622110 Ranks within this company's industry group: Sales: 30 Profits:

Insurance/HMO/PPO:	Drugs:	Equipment/Supplies:	Hospitals/Clinics:		Services:		Health Care:	
Insurance:	Manufacturer:	Manufacturer:	Acute Care:	Y	Diagnostics:		Home Health:	Y
Managed Care:	Distributor:	Distributor:	Sub-Acute Care:	Y	Labs/Testing:		Long-Term Care:	Y
Utilization Mgmt.:	Specialty Pharm.:	Leasing/Finance:	Outpatient Surgery:		Staffing:		Physical Therapy:	
Payment Proc.:	Vitamins/Nutri.:	Information Sys.:	Phys. Rehab. Center:	Y	Waste Disposal:		Phys. Practice Mgmt.:	Y
	Clinical Trials:		Psychiatric Clinics:		Specialty Services:			

TYPES OF BUSINESS:
Hospitals
Assisted Living Services
Home Health Services
Ambulatory Centers
Rehabilitation Centers
Nursing Homes
Physician Network Management
Research

BRANDS/DIVISIONS/AFFILIATES:
MedStar Physician Partners
MedStar Health Visiting Nurse Association
MedStar Diabetes Institute
MedStar Research Institute
Franklin Square Hospital Center
Good Samaritan Hospital
Georgetown University Hospital
Union Memorial Hospital

CONTACTS:
Note: Officers with more than one job title may be intentionally listed here more than once.

John P. McDaniel, CEO
Kenneth A. Samet, Pres.
Kenneth A. Samet, COO
Michael J. Curran, Exec. VP/CFO
John D. Dayhoff, VP/Interim CIO
Robert J. Ryan, Sr. VP/General Counsel
Christine M. Swearingen, Sr. VP-Strategic Planning
John A. Marzano, Comm. & Public Affairs
Thomas J. Marchozzi, VP-Finance
Michael C. Rogers, Exec. VP-Corp. Services
William L. Thomas, Exec. VP-Medical Affairs
Steven S. Cohen, Sr. VP-Integrated Oper.
James R. Hyde, Chmn.

Phone: 410-772-6500 Fax: 410-715-3905
Toll-Free: 877-772-6644
Address: 5565 Sterrett Pl., Columbia, MD 21044 US

GROWTH PLANS/SPECIAL FEATURES:
MedStar Health is a not-for-profit, community-based health care organization primarily composed of seven major hospitals in the Baltimore/Washington, D.C. area: Franklin Square Hospital Center, Good Samaritan Hospital, Harbor Hospital and Union Memorial Hospital in Baltimore, and Washington Hospital Center, Georgetown University Hospital and National Rehabilitation Hospital in Washington, D.C., the last four of which were ranked in 2004 among America's Best Hospitals by U.S. News & World Report. MedStar serves roughly half a million patients annually and has 2,700 licensed beds. The hospital's services include primary, urgent and sub-acute care, medical education and research. MedStar also provides assisted living, home health, hospice and long-term care, and operates nursing homes, senior housing, adult day care, rehabilitation and ambulatory centers. The organization manages MedStar Physician Partners, a comprehensive physician network serving the region. Other subsidiaries include the MedStar Health Visiting Nurse Association, the MedStar Diabetes Institute and the MedStar Research Institute.

FINANCIALS:
Sales and profits are in thousands of dollars—add 000 to get the full amount. Year 2004 note: Complete fiscal 2004 results were not available for all companies at press time. For this company, year 2004 is for months.

2004 Sales: $ (months)
2003 Sales: $2,250,000
2002 Sales: $2,110,000
2001 Sales: $
2000 Sales: $

2004 Profits: $ (months)
2003 Profits: $
2002 Profits: $
2001 Profits: $
2000 Profits: $

Stock Ticker: Nonprofit
Employees: 22,000
Fiscal Year Ends: 6/30

SALARIES/BENEFITS:
Pension Plan: ESOP Stock Plan: Profit Sharing: Top Exec. Salary: $ Bonus: $
Savings Plan: Stock Purch. Plan: Second Exec. Salary: $ Bonus: $

OTHER THOUGHTS:
Apparent Top Female Officers: 1
Hot Spot for Advancement for Women/Minorities:

LOCATIONS: ("Y" = Yes)
West:	Southwest:	Midwest:	Southeast:	Northeast:	International:
				Y	

MEDTRONIC INC

www.medtronic.com

Industry Group Code: 339113   Ranks within this company's industry group: Sales: 68   Profits: 132

Insurance/HMO/PPO:	Drugs:	Equipment/Supplies:	Hospitals/Clinics:	Services:	Health Care:
Insurance: Managed Care: Utilization Mgmt.: Payment Proc.:	Manufacturer: Distributor: Specialty Pharm.: Vitamins/Nutri.: Clinical Trials:	Manufacturer: Y Distributor: Leasing/Finance: Information Sys.:	Acute Care: Sub-Acute Care: Outpatient Surgery: Phys. Rehab. Center: Psychiatric Clinics:	Diagnostics: Labs/Testing: Staffing: Waste Disposal: Specialty Services:	Home Health: Long-Term Care: Physical Therapy: Phys. Practice Mgmt.:

TYPES OF BUSINESS:
Equipment-Defibrillators and Pacing Products
Neurological Devices
Diabetes Devices
Ear, Nose and Throat Surgical Equipment
Pain Management Devices
Catheters and Stents
Cardiac Surgery Equipment

BRANDS/DIVISIONS/AFFILIATES:
Driver
Maximo
Marquis DR ICD
Synergy
Enterra
Gatekeeper Reflux Repair System
CD Horizon Sextant
METRx MicroDiscectomy System

CONTACTS:
Note: Officers with more than one job title may be intentionally listed here more than once.

Arthur D. Collins, Jr., CEO
William A. Hawkins, Pres.
William A. Hawkins, COO
Robert Ryan, CFO
Janet S. Fiola, VP-Human Resources
Jeffrey A. Balagna, Sr. VP-IT
Ronald E. Lund, General Counsel
Stephen H. Mahle, Sr. VP/Pres.-Cardiac Rhythm Mgmt.
Michael F. DeMane, Sr. VP/Pres.-Spinal, ENT and SNT

Phone: 763-514-4000   **Fax:** 763-514-4879
Toll-Free: 800-328-2518
Address: 710 Medtronic Pkwy. NE, Minneapolis, MN 55432 US

GROWTH PLANS/SPECIAL FEATURES:
Medtronic, a world leader in medical technology, has pioneered device-based therapies that restore and extend health and alleviate pain. The company operates in five business sectors: cardiac rhythm management; neurological and diabetes disorders; spinal, ear, nose and throat and surgical navigation technologies; vascular devices; and cardiac surgery. The company is the world's leading supplier of medical devices for cardiac rhythm management. These products consist mainly of pacemakers and implantable cardiac defibrillators. The neurological and diabetes segment develops, manufactures and markets devices for neurological disorders, diabetes, gastroenterological disorders and urological disorders. These devices include insulin monitors and pumps, electronic pain control devices and gastroenterological devices for the monitoring and treatment of incontinence, acid reflux and prostate conditions. The spinal, ear nose and throat and surgical navigation technologies segment produces devices for pain management, minimally invasive spinal surgery and ear, nose and throat surgical equipment. The vascular device segment produces coronary, endovascular and peripheral stents and related delivery systems, stent graft systems, distal embolic protection systems and a broad line of balloon angioplasty catheters, guide catheters, guide wires, diagnostic catheters and accessories. The cardiac surgery segment consists of positioning and stabilization systems for beating heart surgery; perfusion systems which warm, oxygenate and circulate a patient's blood during arrested heart surgery; and products for the repair and replacement of heart valves and surgical accessories. In recent news, Medtronic announced FDA approval for the world's first digital pacemaker, the company's Driver coronary splint and the Medtronic Maximo cardioverter defibrillator. In other news, the company is developing drug coated stents, cardiac implants and diagnostic devices using nanotechnology. The introduction of drug coated stents is expected double the stent market to $4.5 billion dollars by the end of 2005. Additionally, the company received FDA approval for its implantable deliberator using MEMS.

FINANCIALS:
Sales and profits are in thousands of dollars—add 000 to get the full amount. Year 2004 note: Complete fiscal 2004 results were not available for all companies at press time. For this company, year 2004 is for 12 months.

2004 Sales: $9,087,200 (12 months)   2004 Profits: $1,959,300 (12 months)
2003 Sales: $7,665,200   2003 Profits: $1,599,800
2002 Sales: $6,411,000   2002 Profits: $984,000
2001 Sales: $5,551,800   2001 Profits: $1,046,000
2000 Sales: $5,016,300   2000 Profits: $1,084,200

Stock Ticker: MDT
Employees: 30,900
Fiscal Year Ends: 4/30

SALARIES/BENEFITS:
Pension Plan: Y   ESOP Stock Plan: Y   Profit Sharing: Top Exec. Salary: $1,025,000   Bonus: $1,368,683
Savings Plan: Y   Stock Purch. Plan: Y   Second Exec. Salary: $485,000   Bonus: $500,000

OTHER THOUGHTS:
Apparent Top Female Officers: 1
Hot Spot for Advancement for Women/Minorities:

LOCATIONS: ("Y" = Yes)
West:	Southwest:	Midwest:	Southeast:	Northeast:	International:
Y	Y	Y	Y	Y	Y

MEDTRONIC MINIMED INC

www.minimed.com

Industry Group Code: 339113 Ranks within this company's industry group: Sales: 4 Profits: 2

Insurance/HMO/PPO:	Drugs:	Equipment/Supplies:	Hospitals/Clinics:	Services:	Health Care:
Insurance: Managed Care: Utilization Mgmt.: Payment Proc.:	Manufacturer: Distributor: Specialty Pharm.: Vitamins/Nutri.: Clinical Trials:	Manufacturer: Y Distributor: Leasing/Finance: Information Sys.:	Acute Care: Sub-Acute Care: Outpatient Surgery: Phys. Rehab. Center: Psychiatric Clinics:	Diagnostics: Labs/Testing: Staffing: Waste Disposal: Specialty Services:	Home Health: Long-Term Care: Physical Therapy: Phys. Practice Mgmt.:

TYPES OF BUSINESS:
Equipment-External Insulin Pumps & Related Products
Drug Delivery Microinfusion Systems
Diabetes Management Products

BRANDS/DIVISIONS/AFFILIATES:
Medtronic, Inc.
Medtronic CareLink Therapy Management System
Paradigm
CGMS System Gold
Guardian Continuous Glucose Monitor System

CONTACTS:
Note: Officers with more than one job title may be intentionally listed here more than once.
Arthur D. Collins, Jr., CEO
Brad Owings, VP-IT
Deanne McLaughlin, VP-Corp. Comm.
Arthur D. Collins, Jr., Chmn.

Phone: 818-362-5958 Fax:
Toll-Free: 800-933-3322
Address: 18000 Devonshire St., Northridge, CA 91325-1219 US

GROWTH PLANS/SPECIAL FEATURES:
Medtronic MiniMed, a subsidiary of Medtronic, Inc., designs, develops, manufactures and markets advanced microinfusion systems for the delivery of a variety of drugs, with a primary focus on the intensive management of diabetes. The company sells external insulin pumps and related disposables, which are designed to deliver small quantities of insulin in a controlled, programmable profile. Medtronic MiniMed has also developed an implantable insulin pump and is developing continuous subcutaneous glucose monitoring systems, which are approved for use only in Europe. The firm's Paradigm insulin pump recently underwent its third generation of upgrades. This new generation includes the web-based Medtronic CareLink Therapy Management System, which charts trends in A1C, BG and carbohydrates to optimize therapy. Medtronic MiniMed plans to use the Paradigm platform to launch the world's first sensor-augmented insulin pump system. The firm also offers a line of therapy management software that turns pump, meter and logbook data into treatment reports. In addition, the CGMS System Gold is often prescribed by health professionals because it provides a clearer picture of blood sugar levels than do fingersticks. The CGMS System Gold measures blood sugar levels every five minutes for a total of 288 readings a day. The company is currently planning to release the Guardian Continuous Glucose Monitor System, a blood glucose security system that warns the user of sudden drops in glucose levels.

Medtronic MiniMed offers its employees comprehensive insurance and health benefits as well as tuition reimbursement, flexible spending accounts, credit union membership and discounts on attractions and special events.

FINANCIALS:
Sales and profits are in thousands of dollars—add 000 to get the full amount. Year 2004 note: Complete fiscal 2004 results were not available for all companies at press time. For this company, year 2004 is for months.

2004 Sales: $ (months)
2003 Sales: $
2002 Sales: $
2001 Sales: $
2000 Sales: $

2004 Profits: $ (months)
2003 Profits: $
2002 Profits: $
2001 Profits: $
2000 Profits: $

Stock Ticker: Subsidiary
Employees: 1,539
Fiscal Year Ends: 4/30

SALARIES/BENEFITS:
Pension Plan: ESOP Stock Plan: Profit Sharing: Top Exec. Salary: $ Bonus: $
Savings Plan: Y   Stock Purch. Plan: Second Exec. Salary: $ Bonus: $

OTHER THOUGHTS:
Apparent Top Female Officers: 1
Hot Spot for Advancement for Women/Minorities:

LOCATIONS: ("Y" = Yes)
West:	Southwest:	Midwest:	Southeast:	Northeast:	International:
Y	Y	Y	Y	Y	Y

MEDTRONIC SOFAMOR DANEK

www.sofamordanek.com

Industry Group Code: 339113   Ranks within this company's industry group: Sales: Profits:

Insurance/HMO/PPO:	Drugs:	Equipment/Supplies:		Hospitals/Clinics:		Services:		Health Care:	
Insurance:	Manufacturer:	Manufacturer:	Y	Acute Care:		Diagnostics:		Home Health:	
Managed Care:	Distributor:	Distributor:		Sub-Acute Care:		Labs/Testing:		Long-Term Care:	
Utilization Mgmt.:	Specialty Pharm.:	Leasing/Finance:		Outpatient Surgery:		Staffing:		Physical Therapy:	
Payment Proc.:	Vitamins/Nutri.:	Information Sys.:		Phys. Rehab. Center:		Waste Disposal:		Phys. Practice Mgmt.:	
	Clinical Trials:			Psychiatric Clinics:		Specialty Services:			

TYPES OF BUSINESS:
Spinal Implants
Bone Grafts

BRANDS/DIVISIONS/AFFILIATES:
INFUSE Bone Graft
CD Horizon Eclipse Spinal System
METRx MicroDiscectomy System
CD Horizon Sextant System
Medtronic, Inc.

CONTACTS:
Note: Officers with more than one job title may be intentionally listed here more than once.
Michael F. DeMane, Pres.
Peter Wehly, Pres.-U.S. Sales
Richard W. Treharne, Sr. VP-Research & Dev.

Phone: 901-396-2695	Fax: 901-396-2699
Toll-Free: 800-876-3133	
Address: 1800 Pyramid Pl., Memphis, TN 38132 US	

GROWTH PLANS/SPECIAL FEATURES:

Medtronic Sofamor Danek, Inc., a subsidiary of Medtronic, Inc., is the world's largest producer of spinal implants. The firm offers the industry's broadest line of devices, instruments, computerized image guidance products and biomaterials used in the treatment of spine disorders such as herniated discs, congenital spine disorders, degenerative disc disease, tumors, fractures and stenosis. Sofamore Danek primarily produces a series of minimal-access spinal technologies (MAST) that allow safe, reproducible access to the spine with minimal disruption of vital muscles and surrounding structures. These techniques involve the use of advanced navigation and instrumentation to allow surgeons to operate with smaller incisions and less tissue damage than traditional surgeries, thus reducing pain and blood loss and improving recovery periods. Products used to treat spinal disorders and deformities include rods and pedical screws, plating systems, and interbody devices like spinal cages, bone dowels and bone wedges, which can be used in spinal fusion of both the thoracolumbar (mid to lower vertebrae) and cervical (upper spine and neck) regions of the spine. Products include the CD Horizon Sextant System for multi-level spinal fusion, the METRx MicroDiscectomy System to treat herniated discs, the CD Horizon Eclipse Spinal System to correct curvature of the spine in scoliosis patients and the INFUSE Bone Graft, which contains a recombinant human bone morphogenetic protein, or rhBMP-2, which induces the body to grow its own bone, eliminating the need for a painful second surgery to harvest bone from elsewhere in the body.

Sofamor Danek offers employees medical and dental insurance as well as on-site wellness screenings, massage therapy programs, on-site fitness centers, elder and child care assistance, adoption assistance and nursing rooms for new mothers.

FINANCIALS:
Sales and profits are in thousands of dollars—add 000 to get the full amount. Year 2004 note: Complete fiscal 2004 results were not available for all companies at press time. For this company, year 2004 is for months.

2004 Sales: $ (months)
2003 Sales: $
2002 Sales: $
2001 Sales: $
2000 Sales: $

2004 Profits: $ (months)
2003 Profits: $
2002 Profits: $
2001 Profits: $
2000 Profits: $

Stock Ticker: Subsidiary
Employees:
Fiscal Year Ends: 4/30

SALARIES/BENEFITS:
Pension Plan: Y	ESOP Stock Plan: Y	Profit Sharing:	Top Exec. Salary: $	Bonus: $
Savings Plan: Y	Stock Purch. Plan: Y		Second Exec. Salary: $	Bonus: $

OTHER THOUGHTS:
Apparent Top Female Officers:
Hot Spot for Advancement for Women/Minorities:

LOCATIONS: ("Y" = Yes)
West:	Southwest:	Midwest:	Southeast:	Northeast:	International:
			Y	Y	Y

Note: Financial information, benefits and other data can change quickly and may vary from those stated here.

MEDTRONIC VASCULAR

www.medtronicvascular.com

Industry Group Code: 339113   Ranks within this company's industry group: Sales: Profits:

Insurance/HMO/PPO:	Drugs:	Equipment/Supplies:	Hospitals/Clinics:	Services:	Health Care:
Insurance:	Manufacturer:	Manufacturer: Y	Acute Care:	Diagnostics:	Home Health:
Managed Care:	Distributor:	Distributor:	Sub-Acute Care:	Labs/Testing:	Long-Term Care:
Utilization Mgmt.:	Specialty Pharm.:	Leasing/Finance:	Outpatient Surgery:	Staffing:	Physical Therapy:
Payment Proc.:	Vitamins/Nutri.:	Information Sys.:	Phys. Rehab. Center:	Waste Disposal:	Phys. Practice Mgmt.:
	Clinical Trials:		Psychiatric Clinics:	Specialty Services:	

TYPES OF BUSINESS:
Medical Instruments
Coronary Products
Neurovascular Products
Peripheral Products

BRANDS/DIVISIONS/AFFILIATES:
Bridge
Solstice
Col-Sur P.A.D.
AneuRx
QS-10 Guidewire
GuardWire Plus
Medtronic
SE Biliary Stent Ststem

CONTACTS:
Note: Officers with more than one job title may be intentionally listed here more than once.

William A. Hawkins, Pres.
Katie M. Szyman, CFO
Kim McEachron, VP-Human Resources
Tony Semedo, VP-Research & Dev.
Katie M. Szyman, VP-IT
Mark Schlossberg, General Counsel
Mark Schlossberg, VP-Bus. Dev.
Katie M. Szyman, VP-Finance
Chris Hadland, VP-Quality Assurance
Sara Toyloy, VP-Regulatory Affairs
Alan Milinazzo, VP-Coronary & Peripheral Bus.
Pat Mackin, VP-Endovascular Bus.

Phone: 707-525-0111   Fax:
Toll-Free:
Address: 3576 Unocal Pl., Santa Rosa, CA 95403 US

GROWTH PLANS/SPECIAL FEATURES:

Medtronic Vascular, formerly Medtronic AVE, Inc., is a medical device company that manufactures technologies for use in coronary, peripheral and neurovascular conditions. The company develops coronary products that include stents, balloon catheters, guide catheters, diagnostic catheters and guidewires. Medtronic Vascular's peripheral technologies feature the Bridge Extra Support Renal Stent System, for use in patients with atherosclerotic disease of the renal arteries; the Bridge SE Biliary Stent System, a device indicated for palliation of malignant neoplasms in the biliary tree; and the Col-Sur P.A.D., a noninvasive approach to hemostasis. Neurovascular products include the company's Solstice system and the QS-10 Guidewire. The company also manufactures the GuardWire Plus Temporary Occlusion and Aspiration System, the first distal protection system available in the U.S. for use in diseased saphenous vein grafts. Medtronic Vascular's AneuRx stent graft was developed for the treatment of abdominal aortic aneurysm. Medtronic Vascular is a subsidiary of Medtronic, Inc.

The company offers its employees a comprehensive benefits package including elder care assistance, adoption assistance, rooms designated for nursing mothers and tuition reimbursement.

FINANCIALS:
Sales and profits are in thousands of dollars—add 000 to get the full amount. Year 2004 note: Complete fiscal 2004 results were not available for all companies at press time. For this company, year 2004 is for months.

2004 Sales: $ (months)   2004 Profits: $ (months)
2003 Sales: $ 2003 Profits: $
2002 Sales: $ 2002 Profits: $
2001 Sales: $ 2001 Profits: $
2000 Sales: $ 2000 Profits: $

Stock Ticker: Subsidiary
Employees: 1,265
Fiscal Year Ends: 4/30

SALARIES/BENEFITS:
Pension Plan: Y   ESOP Stock Plan: Profit Sharing: Top Exec. Salary: $ Bonus: $
Savings Plan: Y   Stock Purch. Plan: Y   Second Exec. Salary: $ Bonus: $

OTHER THOUGHTS:
Apparent Top Female Officers: 3
Hot Spot for Advancement for Women/Minorities: Y

LOCATIONS: ("Y" = Yes)

West:	Southwest:	Midwest:	Southeast:	Northeast:	International:
Y					

Note: Financial information, benefits and other data can change quickly and may vary from those stated here.

MEDTRONIC XOMED SURGICAL PRODUCTS INC www.xomed.com

Industry Group Code: 339113 Ranks within this company's industry group: Sales: Profits:

Insurance/HMO/PPO:	Drugs:	Equipment/Supplies:		Hospitals/Clinics:	Services:	Health Care:
Insurance:	Manufacturer:	Manufacturer:	Y	Acute Care:	Diagnostics:	Home Health:
Managed Care:	Distributor:	Distributor:	Y	Sub-Acute Care:	Labs/Testing:	Long-Term Care:
Utilization Mgmt.:	Specialty Pharm.:	Leasing/Finance:		Outpatient Surgery:	Staffing:	Physical Therapy:
Payment Proc.:	Vitamins/Nutri.:	Information Sys.:		Phys. Rehab. Center:	Waste Disposal:	Phys. Practice Mgmt.:
	Clinical Trials:			Psychiatric Clinics:	Specialty Services:	

TYPES OF BUSINESS:
Supplies-Ears, Nose and Throat Surgery
Wound Dressings

BRANDS/DIVISIONS/AFFILIATES:
Medtronic, Inc.
PowerSculpt Cosmetic System
TAB Tumescent Absorbent Bandage
FeatherTouch
HydroBrader
Meniett
MicroPlaner

CONTACTS:
Note: Officers with more than one job title may be intentionally listed here more than once.
Bob Blankemeyer, Pres.
Mike Nicoletta, COO
Timothy J. Kriewall, VP-Research & Dev.
Jamie A. Frias, VP/Legal Counsel
Gerald Bussell, VP-Global Oper.
Dean Rustad, VP-Finance
Mark J. Fletcher, Pres.-Ear, Nose & Throat
Brian Barry, Regulatory & Quality Affairs

Phone: 904-296-9600 Fax: 904-296-9666
Toll-Free: 800-874-5797
Address: 6743 Southpoint Dr. N., Jacksonville, FL 32216-0980 US

GROWTH PLANS/SPECIAL FEATURES:
Medtronic Xomed Surgical Products, Inc., a subsidiary of medical device manufacturer Medtronic, Inc., is a leading developer, manufacturer and marketer of surgical products for use by ear, nose and throat specialists. The company has six business lines: otology, head and neck; endoscopy, a minimally invasive internal procedure; plastic surgery; rhinology, having to do with the nose; and image guidance. The firm also manufactures the TAB Tumescent Absorbent Bandage line, a series of sponge wound dressings. In addition, the company developed the PowerSculpt Cosmetic System, which includes the MicroPlaner product for facial soft tissue shaving, the FeatherTouch for rhinoplasty and the HydroBrader for hydrobrasion procedures. The company also designed the Meniett, a portable pressure pulse generator, which treats Meniere's disease. The company's products are distributed in 69 countries worldwide.

FINANCIALS:
Sales and profits are in thousands of dollars—add 000 to get the full amount. Year 2004 note: Complete fiscal 2004 results were not available for all companies at press time. For this company, year 2004 is for months.

2004 Sales: $ (months)   2004 Profits: $ (months)
2003 Sales: $ 2003 Profits: $
2002 Sales: $ 2002 Profits: $
2001 Sales: $ 2001 Profits: $
2000 Sales: $ 2000 Profits: $

Stock Ticker: Subsidiary
Employees:
Fiscal Year Ends: 4/30

SALARIES/BENEFITS:
Pension Plan: Y   ESOP Stock Plan: Y   Profit Sharing: Top Exec. Salary: $ Bonus: $
Savings Plan: Y   Stock Purch. Plan: Y   Second Exec. Salary: $ Bonus: $

OTHER THOUGHTS:
Apparent Top Female Officers: 1
Hot Spot for Advancement for Women/Minorities:

LOCATIONS: ("Y" = Yes)
West:	Southwest:	Midwest:	Southeast:	Northeast:	International:
Y	Y	Y	Y	Y	Y

MEMORIAL HERMANN HEALTHCARE SYSTEM
www.memorialhermann.org

Industry Group Code: 622110 Ranks within this company's industry group: Sales: 26 Profits:

Insurance/HMO/PPO:	Drugs:	Equipment/Supplies:	Hospitals/Clinics:		Services:		Health Care:	
Insurance:	Manufacturer:	Manufacturer:	Acute Care:	Y	Diagnostics:		Home Health:	Y
Managed Care:	Distributor:	Distributor:	Sub-Acute Care:	Y	Labs/Testing:		Long-Term Care:	Y
Utilization Mgmt.:	Specialty Pharm.:	Leasing/Finance:	Outpatient Surgery:		Staffing:		Physical Therapy:	
Payment Proc.:	Vitamins/Nutri.:	Information Sys.:	Phys. Rehab. Center:	Y	Waste Disposal:		Phys. Practice Mgmt.:	
	Clinical Trials:		Psychiatric Clinics:		Specialty Services:	Y		

TYPES OF BUSINESS:
Hospitals
Long-Term Care
Retirement and Nursing Homes
Wellness Centers
Rehabilitation Services
Home Health Services
Air Ambulance Services
Sports Medicine

BRANDS/DIVISIONS/AFFILIATES:
Memorial Hermann Garden Spa
Houston Health Hour Radio Show
Lindig Men's Health Center and Resource Library
Mind/Body Institute for Clinical Wellness
Memorial Hermann Heart and Vascular Institute
Memorial Hermann Children's Hospital
Fort Bend Hospital
Katy Hospital

CONTACTS:
Note: Officers with more than one job title may be intentionally listed here more than once.
Daniel J. Wolterman, CEO
Daniel J. Wolterman, Pres.
Carrol Aulbaugh, Sr. VP-Finance
A. T. Blackshear, Jr., Chmn.

Phone: 713-448-5555 Fax: 713-448-5665
Toll-Free:
Address: 7737 Southwest Fwy., Ste. 200, Houston, TX 77074 US

GROWTH PLANS/SPECIAL FEATURES:
Memorial Hermann Healthcare System is a leading provider of health care in greater Houston and southeast Texas. The system consists of nine acute care hospitals, two long-term acute care hospitals, a physician network for primary and specialty care, retirement living and nursing homes, wellness centers, rehabilitation and home health programs, an air ambulance service and more than a dozen affiliates spread across southeast Texas. The acute care hospitals include Memorial Hermann Children's Hospital, Fort Bend Hospital, Memorial Hermann Hospital, Katy Hospital, Memorial City Hospital, Northwest Hospital, Southeast Hospital, Southwest Hospital and Woodlands Hospital. Together these hospitals contain 3,189 licensed beds and offer the full range of health care services, including a sports medicine center, residency programs, radiology, chemical dependency programs, nutrition programs, a vocational nursing program, infertility services, diabetes self-management programs and cancer treatment, to name just a few. The Memorial Hermann Garden Spa, Houston Health Hour Radio Show, Lindig Men's Health Center and Resource Library and the Mind/Body Institute for Clinical Wellness are also part of the system. The organization is currently undergoing a $420-million expansion program to build new patient towers, parking garages, labor and deliver beds and surgical suites, among other things. The physicians at Memorial Hermann Heart and Vascular Institute recently completed the city's first minimally invasive surgery to correct atrial fibrillation, one of only a few dozen such surgeries to have been performed worldwide.

Memorial Hermann provides residency programs, nursing internships, massage and spa therapy school and technical schools. It provides its employees with a comprehensive health care package, an employee assistance program, legal assistance, discounted auto and home insurance and tuition reimbursement, among other benefits.

FINANCIALS:
Sales and profits are in thousands of dollars—add 000 to get the full amount. Year 2004 note: Complete fiscal 2004 results were not available for all companies at press time. For this company, year 2004 is for months.

2004 Sales: $ (months)   2004 Profits: $ (months)
2003 Sales: $2,500,000   2003 Profits: $
2002 Sales: $2,250,000   2002 Profits: $
2001 Sales: $ 2001 Profits: $
2000 Sales: $ 2000 Profits: $

Stock Ticker: Nonprofit
Employees: 13,000
Fiscal Year Ends:

SALARIES/BENEFITS:
Pension Plan: Y   ESOP Stock Plan: Profit Sharing: Top Exec. Salary: $ Bonus: $
Savings Plan: Stock Purch. Plan: Second Exec. Salary: $ Bonus: $

OTHER THOUGHTS:
Apparent Top Female Officers: 1
Hot Spot for Advancement for Women/Minorities:

LOCATIONS: ("Y" = Yes)
West:	Southwest:	Midwest:	Southeast:	Northeast:	International:
	Y				

MEMORIAL SLOAN KETTERING CANCER CENTER   www.mskcc.org

Industry Group Code: 622110   Ranks within this company's industry group: Sales: 39   Profits: 4

Insurance/HMO/PPO:	Drugs:	Equipment/Supplies:	Hospitals/Clinics:		Services:		Health Care:	
Insurance: Managed Care: Utilization Mgmt.: Payment Proc.:	Manufacturer: Distributor: Specialty Pharm.: Vitamins/Nutri.: Clinical Trials:	Manufacturer: Distributor: Leasing/Finance: Information Sys.:	Acute Care: Sub-Acute Care: Outpatient Surgery: Phys. Rehab. Center: Psychiatric Clinics:	Y	Diagnostics: Labs/Testing: Staffing: Waste Disposal: Specialty Services:	Y	Home Health: Long-Term Care: Physical Therapy: Phys. Practice Mgmt.:	

TYPES OF BUSINESS:
Hospital
Research

BRANDS/DIVISIONS/AFFILIATES:
Memorial Hospital for Cancer and Allied Diseases
Sloan-Kettering Institute

CONTACTS:
Note: Officers with more than one job title may be intentionally listed here more than once.
Harold Varmus, CEO
Harold Varmus, Pres.
Christine Hickey, Dir.-Comm.
Douglas A. Warner, III, Chmn.

Phone: 212-639-2000   Fax: 212-639-3576
Toll-Free:
Address: 1275 York Ave., New York, NY 10021 US

GROWTH PLANS/SPECIAL FEATURES:

Memorial Sloan-Kettering Cancer Center, a not-for-profit organization, was formed in 1960 from the combination of Memorial Hospital for Cancer and Allied Diseases and Sloan-Kettering Institute, both located in Manhattan. Memorial Hospital has 427 beds and admitted 12,254 patients last year. The hospital also had 388,655 outpatient visits. Memorial has a separate international center and pediatrics center to address the specific needs of international patients and children. The Sloan-Kettering Institute functions as the hospital's research arm, with specific focus on genetics, biochemistry, structural biology, computational biology, immunology and therapeutics. The institute provides research training in conjunction with the Weill Medical College of Cornell University and the Rockefeller University for PhD and MD students. The institute's Office of Industrial Affairs is responsible for protecting and licensing inventions developed by the center's scientists, obtaining funding for laboratories, and negotiating and reviewing consulting agreements. The institute's Office of Community Affairs publishes a monthly newsletter informing local residents and patients of services and activities and is responsible for community outreach.

Memorial Sloan-Kettering Cancer Center provides its employees with a flexible benefits program, including several different medical plans, employee discounts, work/life balance programs and tuition reimbursement.

FINANCIALS:
Sales and profits are in thousands of dollars—add 000 to get the full amount. Year 2004 note: Complete fiscal 2004 results were not available for all companies at press time. For this company, year 2004 is for months.

2004 Sales: $ (months)
2003 Sales: $1,317,700
2002 Sales: $1,088,300
2001 Sales: $
2000 Sales: $

2004 Profits: $ (months)
2003 Profits: $422,700
2002 Profits: $-80,600
2001 Profits: $
2000 Profits: $

Stock Ticker: Nonprofit
Employees: 8,255
Fiscal Year Ends: 12/31

SALARIES/BENEFITS:
Pension Plan: Y   ESOP Stock Plan: Profit Sharing: Top Exec. Salary: $ Bonus: $
Savings Plan: Y   Stock Purch. Plan: Second Exec. Salary: $ Bonus: $

OTHER THOUGHTS:
Apparent Top Female Officers: 1
Hot Spot for Advancement for Women/Minorities:

LOCATIONS: ("Y" = Yes)
West:	Southwest:	Midwest:	Southeast:	Northeast:	International:
				Y	

MENTOR CORP

www.mentorcorp.com

Industry Group Code: 339113   Ranks within this company's industry group: Sales: 46   Profits: 31

Insurance/HMO/PPO:	Drugs:	Equipment/Supplies:		Hospitals/Clinics:	Services:	Health Care:
Insurance:	Manufacturer:	Manufacturer:	Y	Acute Care:	Diagnostics:	Home Health:
Managed Care:	Distributor:	Distributor:	Y	Sub-Acute Care:	Labs/Testing:	Long-Term Care:
Utilization Mgmt.:	Specialty Pharm.:	Leasing/Finance:		Outpatient Surgery:	Staffing:	Physical Therapy:
Payment Proc.:	Vitamins/Nutri.:	Information Sys.:		Phys. Rehab. Center:	Waste Disposal:	Phys. Practice Mgmt.:
	Clinical Trials:			Psychiatric Clinics:	Specialty Services:	

TYPES OF BUSINESS:
Supplies-Plastic Surgery Products
General Surgery Products
Urologic Products

BRANDS/DIVISIONS/AFFILIATES:
South Bay Medical
Mentor Medical, Ltd.
A-Life, Ltd.
Contour Profile Moderate Plus Gel

CONTACTS: Note: Officers with more than one job title may be intentionally listed here more than once.
Joshua H. Levine, CEO
Joshua H. Levine, Pres.
Loren L. McFarland, VP/CFO
Kathleen M. Beauchamp, VP-Mktg. & Sales
Cathryn S. Ullery, VP-Human Resources
Bobby K. Purkait, Sr. VP-Science & Tech.
A. Chris Fawzy, General Counsel
David J. Adornetto, VP-Oper.
Maher Michael, VP-Corp. Dev.
Christopher J. Conway, Chmn.

Phone: 805-879-6000   Fax: 805-681-6006
Toll-Free: 800-525-0245
Address: 201 Mentor Dr., Santa Barbara, CA 93111 US

GROWTH PLANS/SPECIAL FEATURES:
Mentor Corporation develops, manufactures and markets a broad range of products for plastic and reconstructive surgery, urology and general surgery in the U.S. and more than 60 other countries. Plastic surgery products or aesthetics include surgically implantable prostheses for cosmetic and reconstructive surgery, principally breast implants and tissue expanders. General surgery products include capital equipment and disposable products used in soft tissue aspiration. Urologic products include disposable products for the management of urinary incontinence; surgically implantable prostheses, principally penile implants for the treatment of chronic male sexual impotence; and brachytherapy seeds for the treatment of prostate cancer. The company also markets a variety of other disposable products used in the management of urinary incontinence, including leg bags and urine collection systems, organic odor eliminators, moisturizing skin creams and ointments. South Bay Medical, one of Mentor's subsidiaries, is a development-stage company focused on the development of a new technology for a computer-based workstation and automated cartridge-based needle loading system for use in brachytherapy procedures. Mentor Medical, Ltd. encompasses the company's manufacturing and sales operations for home health care products in the U.K. and provides the firm with a number of home care products such as urinary drainage bags and ostomy products. Subsidiary A-Life, Ltd., which has developed a hyaluronic acid-based dermal filler product, has manufacturing and R&D facilities in Edinburgh, Scotland and in California. The firm operates a state-of-the-art aesthetics manufacturing facility in Leiden, The Netherlands, the biggest of its kind in the world. In recent news, Mentor received European approval for its new Contour Profile Moderate Plus Gel breast implant.

The firm's employees enjoy medical, dental, life and disability insurance, as well as flexible spending accounts, employee assistance, credit union membership, tuition reimbursement and discounts on various attractions and services.

FINANCIALS: Sales and profits are in thousands of dollars—add 000 to get the full amount. Year 2004 note: Complete fiscal 2004 results were not available for all companies at press time. For this company, year 2004 is for 12 months.

2004 Sales: $422,168 (12 months)   2004 Profits: $54,779 (12 months)
2003 Sales: $382,400   2003 Profits: $55,900
2002 Sales: $321,100   2002 Profits: $41,800
2001 Sales: $268,900   2001 Profits: $32,100
2000 Sales: $249,300   2000 Profits: $36,500

Stock Ticker: MNT
Employees: 2,050
Fiscal Year Ends: 3/31

SALARIES/BENEFITS:
Pension Plan: ESOP Stock Plan: Profit Sharing: Top Exec. Salary: $425,724   Bonus: $304,289
Savings Plan: Y   Stock Purch. Plan: Second Exec. Salary: $344,768   Bonus: $226,125

OTHER THOUGHTS:
Apparent Top Female Officers: 2
Hot Spot for Advancement for Women/Minorities:

LOCATIONS: ("Y" = Yes)
West:	Southwest:	Midwest:	Southeast:	Northeast:	International:
Y	Y	Y			Y

Note: Financial information, benefits and other data can change quickly and may vary from those stated here.

MERCK & CO INC

www.merck.com

Industry Group Code: 325412   Ranks within this company's industry group: Sales: 5   Profits: 2

Insurance/HMO/PPO:	Drugs:	Equipment/Supplies:	Hospitals/Clinics:	Services:	Health Care:
Insurance:	Manufacturer: Y	Manufacturer:	Acute Care:	Diagnostics:	Home Health:
Managed Care: Y	Distributor:	Distributor:	Sub-Acute Care:	Labs/Testing:	Long-Term Care:
Utilization Mgmt.:	Specialty Pharm.:	Leasing/Finance:	Outpatient Surgery:	Staffing:	Physical Therapy:
Payment Proc.:	Vitamins/Nutri.:	Information Sys.:	Phys. Rehab. Center:	Waste Disposal:	Phys. Practice Mgmt.:
	Clinical Trials:		Psychiatric Clinics:	Specialty Services: Y	

TYPES OF BUSINESS:
Drugs-Manufacturer
Cholesterol Drugs
Hypertension Drugs
Heart Failure Drugs
Allergy Medicine
Asthma Medication
High Blood Pressure Medicine
Farm Animal Therapeutic and Preventative Agents

BRANDS/DIVISIONS/AFFILIATES:
Merck Institute for Science Education
Vasotec
Singulair
Zocor
Cozaar
Fosamax

CONTACTS:
Note: Officers with more than one job title may be intentionally listed here more than once.
Raymond V. Gilmartin, CEO
Raymond V. Gilmartin, Pres.
Judy C. Lewent, CFO/Sr. VP/Pres., Human Health-Asia
Marcia J. Avedon, Sr. VP-Human Resources
Peter S. Kim, Pres., Merck Research Laboratories
Richard T. Clark, Pres., Merck Mfg. Div.
Kenneth C. Frazier, General Counsel/Sr. VP
Bradley T. Sheares, Pres., U.S. Human Health
Margaret G. McGlynn, Pres., U.S. Human Health
Adel A.F. Mahmoud, Pres., Merck Vaccine Div.
David W. Anstice, Pres., Human Health
Raymond V. Gilmartin, Chmn.
Per Wold-Olsen, Pres., Human Health-Europe, Middle East, Africa

Phone: 908-423-1000   **Fax:** 908-735-1253
Toll-Free:
Address: One Merck Dr., Whitehouse Station, NJ 08889-0100 US

GROWTH PLANS/SPECIAL FEATURES:
Merck & Co., Inc. is a leading global research-driven pharmaceutical company that manufactures a broad range of products. Merck's products are sold in approximately 150 countries. The products include human therapeutic and preventative drugs generally sold by prescription. The company also makes medications used to control and alleviate disease in livestock, small animals and poultry. As one of the world's largest and most prestigious pharmaceuticals companies, Merck develops drugs that treat ailments including high cholesterol, hypertension and heart failure. These products generate approximately one-third of the company's sales. Merck's top-selling cholesterol drugs are Zocor and Mevacor, and its primary hypertension drugs are Vasotec and Prinivil. Singulair is offered as both seasonal allergy and asthma medicine, both of which are offered in tablets that are taken once a day. The seasonal allergy Singulair is a leukotriene blocker, and the asthma Singular is a non-steroid that controls asthma. The firm manufactures four key medicines: Zocor, a prescription drug which controls cholesterol levels; Cozaar and Hyzaar, high blood pressure medicines; and Fosamax, which prevents postmenopausal osteoporosis. The company also manufactures Propecia, a popular treatment for male pattern baldness. Merck & Co. is partnering with nanotech companies, including C Sixty, to research the applications of nanotechnology in the pharmaceutical industry. Merck and C Sixty are teaming up to produce anti-oxidants that may slow the progression of Lou Gehrig's disease. In August 2003, the firm spun off its Medco Health Solutions unit. Later, in 2003 and 2004, the firm cut its remaining workforce by about 4,400 people. In September 2004, Merck endured a major setback when it withdrew its best-selling Vioxx, a once-a-day medicine for both osteoarthritis and acute pain, from the market. The withdrawal of this drug has serious negative implications for the company.

Merck offers its employees on-site fitness facilities with personal trainers, day-care and summer camp programs and extensive training as well as scholarships, tuition reimbursement and financial planning assistance. The company also offers on-site auto maintenance and video rentals for employees at its headquarters location.

FINANCIALS:
Sales and profits are in thousands of dollars—add 000 to get the full amount. Year 2004 note: Complete fiscal 2004 results were not available for all companies at press time. For this company, year 2004 is for 9 months.

2004 Sales: $17,190,700 (9 months)	2004 Profits: $4,712,300 (9 months)	**Stock Ticker:** MRK
2003 Sales: $22,485,900	2003 Profits: $6,830,900	Employees: 30,828
2002 Sales: $21,445,800	2002 Profits: $7,149,500	Fiscal Year Ends: 12/31
2001 Sales: $	2001 Profits: $	
2000 Sales: $	2000 Profits: $	

SALARIES/BENEFITS:
Pension Plan: Y   ESOP Stock Plan: Y   Profit Sharing: Top Exec. Salary: $1,483,334   Bonus: $1,500,000
Savings Plan: Y   Stock Purch. Plan: Second Exec. Salary: $854,170   Bonus: $800,000

OTHER THOUGHTS:
Apparent Top Female Officers: 4
Hot Spot for Advancement for Women/Minorities: Y

LOCATIONS: ("Y" = Yes)
West:	Southwest:	Midwest:	Southeast:	Northeast:	International:
Y	Y	Y	Y	Y	Y

Note: Financial information, benefits and other data can change quickly and may vary from those stated here.

MERIDIAN BIOSCIENCE INC

www.meridianbioscience.com

Industry Group Code: 325413   Ranks within this company's industry group: Sales: 2   Profits: 1

Insurance/HMO/PPO:	Drugs:	Equipment/Supplies:		Hospitals/Clinics:	Services:	Health Care:
Insurance:	Manufacturer:	Manufacturer:	Y	Acute Care:	Diagnostics:	Home Health:
Managed Care:	Distributor:	Distributor:		Sub-Acute Care:	Labs/Testing:	Long-Term Care:
Utilization Mgmt.:	Specialty Pharm.:	Leasing/Finance:		Outpatient Surgery:	Staffing:	Physical Therapy:
Payment Proc.:	Vitamins/Nutri.:	Information Sys.:		Phys. Rehab. Center:	Waste Disposal:	Phys. Practice Mgmt.:
	Clinical Trials:			Psychiatric Clinics:	Specialty Services:	

TYPES OF BUSINESS:
Supplies-Diagnosis Kits
Contract Manufacturing
Bulk Antigens and Reagents
Biopharmaceuticals

BRANDS/DIVISIONS/AFFILIATES:
Viral Antigens, Inc.
BIODESIGN

CONTACTS:
Note: Officers with more than one job title may be intentionally listed here more than once.

William J. Motto, CEO
John A. Kraeutler, Pres.
John A. Kraeutler, COO
Melissa A. Lueke, VP/CFO
Gregory S. Ballish, VP-Sales & Mktg.
Marlene Cook, Dir.-Human Resources
Kenneth J. Kozak, VP-R&D
Lawrence J. Baldini, VP-Oper.
Brenda Hughes, Head-Investor Rel.
Richard L. Eberly, Exec. VP/Mgr.-Meridian Life Science
Susan D. Rolih, VP-Regulatory Affairs & Quality Assurance
Antonio A. Interno, Managing Dir.-Europe
William J. Motto, Chmn.

Phone: 513-271-3700 **Fax:** 513-271-3762
Toll-Free:
Address: 3471 River Hills Dr., Cincinnati, OH 45244 US

GROWTH PLANS/SPECIAL FEATURES:
Meridian Biosciences, Inc. is a fully integrated life sciences company that develops, manufactures and markets a broad range of diagnostic test kits; manufactures and distributes bulk antigens and reagents used by researchers and other manufacturers; and engages in the contract manufacture of proteins and other biologicals. The company's primary business is its diagnostics products, which are marketed to hospitals, reference laboratories, physician offices, nursing homes, veterinary laboratories and water treatment facilities in more than 60 countries worldwide by its U.S. and European operating segments. Meridian's diagnostics products are used principally in the detection of respiratory diseases, such as pneumonia, valley fever, flu and RSV; gastrointestinal diseases, such as stomach ulcers (H. pylori) and diarrhea; viral diseases, such as mononucleosis, herpes, chicken pox and shingles (Varicella Zoster); and parasitic diseases, such as Giardiasis, Cryptosporidiosis and Lyme disease. The company also has a new E. coli test, which can return results in 10 minutes, as opposed to 24 to 72 hours for some culture methods. These tests utilize a variety of technologies, including enzyme immunoassay, immunofluorescence, particle agglutinization/aggregation, immunodiffusion, complement fixation and chemical stains. Meridian's life science operating segment, which facilitates the research, development and manufacture of biopharmaceuticals and clinical diagnostics, consists of the Viral Antigens and BIODESIGN subsidiaries. In 2004, the company began manufacturing a recombinant protein that will be used by the National Institutes of Health to develop a vaccine for parvovirus.

FINANCIALS:
Sales and profits are in thousands of dollars—add 000 to get the full amount. Year 2004 note: Complete fiscal 2004 results were not available for all companies at press time. For this company, year 2004 is for 9 months.

2004 Sales: $57,362 (9 months)   2004 Profits: $6,241 (9 months)
2003 Sales: $65,864   2003 Profits: $7,018
2002 Sales: $59,100   2002 Profits: $5,000
2001 Sales: $56,500   2001 Profits: $-10,300
2000 Sales: $57,096   2000 Profits: $7,111

Stock Ticker: VIVO
Employees: 334
Fiscal Year Ends: 9/30

SALARIES/BENEFITS:
Pension Plan: ESOP Stock Plan: Profit Sharing: Top Exec. Salary: $395,000   Bonus: $251,813
Savings Plan: Y   Stock Purch. Plan: Second Exec. Salary: $294,000   Bonus: $187,425

OTHER THOUGHTS:
Apparent Top Female Officers: 4
Hot Spot for Advancement for Women/Minorities: Y

LOCATIONS: ("Y" = Yes)

West:	Southwest:	Midwest:	Southeast:	Northeast:	International:
		Y	Y	Y	Y

MERIDIAN MEDICAL TECHNOLOGIES INC
www.meridianmeds.com

Industry Group Code: 339113 **Ranks within this company's industry group:** Sales: Profits:

Insurance/HMO/PPO:	Drugs:	Equipment/Supplies:	Hospitals/Clinics:	Services:	Health Care:
Insurance:	Manufacturer:	Manufacturer: Y	Acute Care:	Diagnostics:	Home Health:
Managed Care:	Distributor:	Distributor:	Sub-Acute Care:	Labs/Testing:	Long-Term Care:
Utilization Mgmt.:	Specialty Pharm.:	Leasing/Finance:	Outpatient Surgery:	Staffing:	Physical Therapy:
Payment Proc.:	Vitamins/Nutri.:	Information Sys.:	Phys. Rehab. Center:	Waste Disposal:	Phys. Practice Mgmt.:
	Clinical Trials:		Psychiatric Clinics:	Specialty Services:	

TYPES OF BUSINESS:
Supplies-Allergic Reaction Auto-Injectors
Cardiopulmonary Diagnostics

BRANDS/DIVISIONS/AFFILIATES:
King Pharmaceuticals
EpiPen
CardioPocket
PRIME ECG
CardioBeeper
AtroPen
Morphine Auto-Injector
Mark I Nerve Agent Antidote Kit

CONTACTS:
Note: Officers with more than one job title may be intentionally listed here more than once.

James H. Miller, CEO
James H. Miller, Pres.
Thomas Handel, VP-Sales
Gerald Wannarka, Sr. VP/Chief Scientific Officer
J. Donald Ferry, Jr., Mgr.-Mfg.
Dennis O'Brien, Sr. VP-Oper.
Carl J. Rebert, Pres.-Cardiopulmonary Systems
Cristina D'Erasmo, VP-Military Contracts
Thomas Handel, VP-Homeland Security Pharmaceuticals
James H. Miller, Chmn.

Phone: 410-309-6830 **Fax:** 410-309-1475
Toll-Free: 800-638-8093
Address: 10240 Old Columbia Rd., Columbia, MD 21046 US

GROWTH PLANS/SPECIAL FEATURES:
Meridian Medical Technologies, Inc., a subsidiary of King Pharmaceuticals, is a worldwide leader in developing auto-injector drug delivery systems and manufactures non-invasive cardiopulmonary diagnostic equipment. Meridian delivers technology for medicine in early intervention home health care and emergency medical technologies and also provides product development and manufacturing support to the pharmaceutical and biotechnology industries. The company's drug delivery systems unit participates in the rapidly developing home and emergency markets for drugs using innovative technology. The firm is an innovator in auto-injector technology and currently produces EpiPen, the leading product for severe allergic reactions. Meridian markets a Morphine Auto-Injector as well as AtroPen, a pre-prepared injection of nerve agent antidote, and the Mark I Nerve Agent Antidote Kit. Meridian also markets CardioPocket (a pocket-size ECG transmitter), CardioBeeper (a personal heart monitor) and PRIME ECG (an electrocardiac mapping device). Meridian's principal customers are the U.S. armed forces and homeland defense first responders.

FINANCIALS:
Sales and profits are in thousands of dollars—add 000 to get the full amount. Year 2004 note: Complete fiscal 2004 results were not available for all companies at press time. For this company, year 2004 is for   months.

2004 Sales: $ (months)	2004 Profits: $ (months)	**Stock Ticker:** Subsidiary
2003 Sales: $	2003 Profits: $	Employees: 452
2002 Sales: $82,400	2002 Profits: $9,300	Fiscal Year Ends: 12/31
2001 Sales: $58,100	2001 Profits: $2,900	
2000 Sales: $54,600	2000 Profits: $2,300	

SALARIES/BENEFITS:
Pension Plan: Y	ESOP Stock Plan:	Profit Sharing:	Top Exec. Salary: $395,833	Bonus: $140,000
Savings Plan: Y	Stock Purch. Plan:		Second Exec. Salary: $169,333	Bonus: $40,000

OTHER THOUGHTS:
Apparent Top Female Officers: 1
Hot Spot for Advancement for Women/Minorities:

LOCATIONS: ("Y" = Yes)
West:	Southwest:	Midwest:	Southeast:	Northeast:	International:
		Y		Y	Y

MERIT MEDICAL SYSTEMS INC

www.merit.com

Industry Group Code: 339113 Ranks within this company's industry group: Sales: 77 Profits: 60

Insurance/HMO/PPO:	Drugs:	Equipment/Supplies:		Hospitals/Clinics:	Services:	Health Care:
Insurance: Managed Care: Utilization Mgmt.: Payment Proc.:	Manufacturer: Distributor: Specialty Pharm.: Vitamins/Nutri.: Clinical Trials:	Manufacturer: Distributor: Leasing/Finance: Information Sys.:	Y	Acute Care: Sub-Acute Care: Outpatient Surgery: Phys. Rehab. Center: Psychiatric Clinics:	Diagnostics: Labs/Testing: Staffing: Waste Disposal: Specialty Services:	Home Health: Long-Term Care: Physical Therapy: Phys. Practice Mgmt.:

TYPES OF BUSINESS:
Equipment-Cardiovascular
Diagnostics Products
Disposable Products

BRANDS/DIVISIONS/AFFILIATES:
Merit Sensor Systems

CONTACTS:
Note: Officers with more than one job title may be intentionally listed here more than once.

Fred P. Lampropoulos, CEO
Fred P. Lampropoulos, Pres.
B. Leigh Weintraub, COO
Kent W. Stanger, CFO
Larry R. Tolman, VP-Mktg.
Susan Kubiak, VP-Human Resources
B. Leigh Weintraub, VP-Oper.
Anne-Marie Wright, Dir.-Corp. Comm.
Anne-Marie Wright, Dir.-Investor Rel.
Kent W. Stanger, Treas.
Diana Upp, Pres., Merit Sensor Systems
Kent W. Stanger, Corp. Sec.
Darla Gill, Exec. VP-EMEA
Fred P. Lampropoulos, Chmn.

Phone: 801-253-1600 Fax: 801-253-1687
Toll-Free:
Address: 1600 W. Merit Pkwy., South Jordan, UT 84095 US

GROWTH PLANS/SPECIAL FEATURES:
Merit Medical Systems, Inc. is a world leader in the development, manufacture and distribution of disposable proprietary medical products used in interventional diagnostic and therapeutic procedures, particularly in cardiology and radiology. The company serves client hospitals in both domestic and international markets. Merit's strategy is to increase its market presence and opportunity through the development of its core strengths of customer-responsive product design and innovation. The company currently participates in a segment of the medical device industry that includes disposable products used in pressure monitoring, contrast and fluid management. The company serves hospital-based cardiologists, radiologists, technicians and nurses who practice in cardiac catheterization labs and special procedure labs. Merit has developed and introduced over 2,000 FDA-approved devices, including control syringes; inflation devices; specialty syringes; high-pressure tubing and connectors; waste handling and disposal products; a disposable blood pressure transducer; disposable hemostasis valves; manifolds and stopcocks; contrast management systems; angiography needles; blood containment devices; pericardiocentesis catheters and procedure trays; PTCA guide wires and extension wires; thrombolytic infusion catheters and accessories; diagnostic angiographic pigtail catheters; diagnostic cardiology and radiology catheters; sheath introducers; and diagnostic guide wires. These products are sold separately and in custom kits consisting primarily of selected combinations of products.

Employees at Merit enjoy medical and dental coverage, disability and group life insurance, a cafeteria plan and wellness fairs. Additionally, employees receive a Thanksgiving bonus and can join smoking cessation classes, a weight loss club, time management classes, a walking club or an English-as-a-second-language program.

FINANCIALS:
Sales and profits are in thousands of dollars—add 000 to get the full amount. Year 2004 note: Complete fiscal 2004 results were not available for all companies at press time. For this company, year 2004 is for 9 months.

2004 Sales: $112,059 (9 months)   2004 Profits: $13,635 (9 months)
2003 Sales: $135,954   2003 Profits: $17,295
2002 Sales: $116,200   2002 Profits: $11,300
2001 Sales: $104,000   2001 Profits: $6,700
2000 Sales: $91,400   2000 Profits: $800

Stock Ticker: MMSI
Employees: 1,210
Fiscal Year Ends: 12/31

SALARIES/BENEFITS:
Pension Plan: ESOP Stock Plan: Profit Sharing: Top Exec. Salary: $305,000   Bonus: $364,300
Savings Plan: Y   Stock Purch. Plan: Y   Second Exec. Salary: $250,000   Bonus: $168,750

OTHER THOUGHTS:
Apparent Top Female Officers: 4
Hot Spot for Advancement for Women/Minorities: Y

LOCATIONS: ("Y" = Yes)
West:	Southwest:	Midwest:	Southeast:	Northeast:	International:
Y	Y				Y

METROPOLITAN HEALTH NETWORKS

www.metcare.com

Industry Group Code: 524114 **Ranks within this company's industry group:** Sales: 54 Profits: 42

Insurance/HMO/PPO:	Drugs:	Equipment/Supplies:	Hospitals/Clinics:	Services:	Health Care:
Insurance:	Manufacturer:	Manufacturer:	Acute Care:	Diagnostics:	Home Health:
Managed Care: Y	Distributor:	Distributor:	Sub-Acute Care:	Labs/Testing:	Long-Term Care:
Utilization Mgmt.: Y	Specialty Pharm.:	Leasing/Finance:	Outpatient Surgery:	Staffing:	Physical Therapy:
Payment Proc.:	Vitamins/Nutri.:	Information Sys.:	Phys. Rehab. Center:	Waste Disposal:	Phys. Practice Mgmt.:
	Clinical Trials:		Psychiatric Clinics:	Specialty Services: Y	

TYPES OF BUSINESS:
Provider Service Network
HMO
Managed Care Risk Contracting
Disease Management
Pharmacy Benefits Management
Utilization Management

BRANDS/DIVISIONS/AFFILIATES:
MetHealth
Metcare
Metcare RX, Inc.

CONTACTS:
Note: Officers with more than one job title may be intentionally listed here more than once.

Michael M. Earley, CEO
Debra A. Finnel, Pres.
Debra A. Finnel, COO
David S. Gartner, CFO
Roberto L. Palenzuela, General Counsel
Michael M. Earley, Chmn.

Phone: 561-805-8500	Fax: 561-805-8501
Toll-Free: 888-663-8227	
Address: 500 Australian Ave., Ste. 400, West Palm Beach, FL 33401 US	

GROWTH PLANS/SPECIAL FEATURES:
Metropolitan Health Networks, Inc., also known as Metcare, a provider service network, specializes in managed care risk contracting. Previously, the firm owned and managed physician practices and provided ancillary services, but it reorganized in 2001 to become a health maintenance organization (HMO). Subsidiary MetHealth provides turnkey services to managed care companies on a full-risk basis and pharmacy management on behalf of physicians. Focused in the Southeast, it has a managed care network and infrastructure of experts in disease, quality and utilization management. Disease management involves managing costs and care of high-risk patients, thus producing better patient care. Quality management allows the company to measure its overall patient care against the best medical practice patterns. Utilization management encompasses the daily review of data created by encounters, referrals, hospital admissions and nursing home information. MetHealth has plans to administer self-insured health plans for large employers and point-of-service and preferred provider organization services to individual and small employers.

FINANCIALS:
Sales and profits are in thousands of dollars—add 000 to get the full amount. Year 2004 note: Complete fiscal 2004 results were not available for all companies at press time. For this company, year 2004 is for 9 months.

2004 Sales: $117,189 (9 months)	2004 Profits: $8,968 (9 months)	Stock Ticker: MDPA
2003 Sales: $143,874	2003 Profits: $4,402	Employees: 100
2002 Sales: $152,900	2002 Profits: $-17,100	Fiscal Year Ends: 12/31
2001 Sales: $131,500	2001 Profits: $1,000	
2000 Sales: $119,100	2000 Profits: $4,900	

SALARIES/BENEFITS:
Pension Plan:	ESOP Stock Plan:	Profit Sharing:	Top Exec. Salary: $249,026	Bonus: $118,000
Savings Plan:	Stock Purch. Plan:		Second Exec. Salary: $143,767	Bonus: $

OTHER THOUGHTS:
Apparent Top Female Officers: 1
Hot Spot for Advancement for Women/Minorities:

LOCATIONS: ("Y" = Yes)
West:	Southwest:	Midwest:	Southeast:	Northeast:	International:
			Y	Y	

METTLER-TOLEDO INTERNATIONAL

www.mt.com

Industry Group Code: 334500 **Ranks within this company's industry group:** Sales: 3 Profits: 3

Insurance/HMO/PPO:	Drugs:	Equipment/Supplies:	Hospitals/Clinics:	Services:	Health Care:
Insurance: Managed Care: Utilization Mgmt.: Payment Proc.:	Manufacturer: Distributor: Specialty Pharm.: Vitamins/Nutri.: Clinical Trials:	Manufacturer: Y Distributor: Leasing/Finance: Information Sys.:	Acute Care: Sub-Acute Care: Outpatient Surgery: Phys. Rehab. Center: Psychiatric Clinics:	Diagnostics: Labs/Testing: Staffing: Waste Disposal: Specialty Services: Y	Home Health: Long-Term Care: Physical Therapy: Phys. Practice Mgmt.:

TYPES OF BUSINESS:
Measurement Instruments
Supply Chain Solutions & Services
Repair & Maintenance Services

BRANDS/DIVISIONS/AFFILIATES:

CONTACTS:
Note: Officers with more than one job title may be intentionally listed here more than once.
Robert F. Spoerry, CEO
Robert F. Spoerry, Pres.
William P. Donnelly, CFO
Olivier A Filiol, Global Sales & Mktg.
Peter Burker, VP-Human Resources
Beat E. Luthi, VP-Laboratory Div.
Jean-Lucien Gloor, VP-Info. Systems
Mary T. Finnegan, Investor Rel./Treas.
Olivier A. Filliol, VP-Process Analytics Div.
Ken A. Peters, VP-North America
Urs Widmer, VP-Industrial Div.
Timothy P. Haynes, VP-Retail Div.
Robert F. Spoerry, Chmn.
Karl M. Lang, VP-Asia Pacific

Phone: 41-1-944-2211 **Fax:** 41-1-944-2255
Toll-Free:
Address: Im Langacher, Greifensee, Zurich, CH-8606 Switzerland

GROWTH PLANS/SPECIAL FEATURES:
Mettler-Toledo is one of the world's leading providers of precision measurement instruments. The greatest portion of the company's revenues comes from the sale of balances, pipettes and pH meters to laboratories in North America and Europe, but the firm has designed and manufactured instruments for dozens of applications and industries, including the food and beverage, textile, electronics, automotive, transportation and food retail industries, as well as providing instruments to universities and government agencies. Mettler-Toledo is a pioneer in the automated chemistry industry, shortening time-to-market for the chemical and pharmaceutical industries by accelerating synthesis, purification and process development of chemical compounds through automation. The company is also a leader in providing supply chain, inventory management and other solutions and services to supermarkets, specialty shops, convenience stores and butcher shops all over the world. Some of its products in this industry include retail and self-service scales, cash registers, wrapping machines for perishable goods, auto-labeling and security tags and retail software. For laboratories, Mettler-Toledo provides, among other things, mass comparators, weighing modules, halogen moisture analyzers, titrators, density meters and refractometers. In addition to selling measurement devices, the company offers a number of support services that include calibration, repair and maintenance, as well as compliance certification for such processes as meeting FDA regulations.

FINANCIALS:
Sales and profits are in thousands of dollars—add 000 to get the full amount. Year 2004 note: Complete fiscal 2004 results were not available for all companies at press time. For this company, year 2004 is for 9 months.

2004 Sales: $1,005,249 (9 months)   2004 Profits: $71,668 (9 months)
2003 Sales: $1,304,400   2003 Profits: $95,800
2002 Sales: $1,213,700   2002 Profits: $100,400
2001 Sales: $1,148,000   2001 Profits: $72,300
2000 Sales: $ 2000 Profits: $

Stock Ticker: MTD
Employees: 8,500
Fiscal Year Ends: 12/31

SALARIES/BENEFITS:
Pension Plan: Y   ESOP Stock Plan: Profit Sharing: Top Exec. Salary: $582,828   Bonus: $173,100
Savings Plan: Stock Purch. Plan: Second Exec. Salary: $235,263   Bonus: $64,062

OTHER THOUGHTS:
Apparent Top Female Officers: 1
Hot Spot for Advancement for Women/Minorities:

LOCATIONS: ("Y" = Yes)
West	Southwest	Midwest	Southeast	Northeast	International
Y		Y	Y	Y	Y

MICROTEK MEDICAL HOLDINGS INC
www.microtekmed.com

Industry Group Code: 339113   Ranks within this company's industry group: Sales: 92   Profits: 61

Insurance/HMO/PPO:	Drugs:	Equipment/Supplies:	Hospitals/Clinics:	Services:	Health Care:
Insurance:	Manufacturer:	Manufacturer: Y	Acute Care:	Diagnostics:	Home Health:
Managed Care:	Distributor:	Distributor:	Sub-Acute Care:	Labs/Testing:	Long-Term Care:
Utilization Mgmt.:	Specialty Pharm.:	Leasing/Finance:	Outpatient Surgery:	Staffing:	Physical Therapy:
Payment Proc.:	Vitamins/Nutri.:	Information Sys.:	Phys. Rehab. Center:	Waste Disposal:	Phys. Practice Mgmt.:
	Clinical Trials:		Psychiatric Clinics:	Specialty Services:	

TYPES OF BUSINESS:
Supplies-Assorted Health Care Products
Disposable Products
Hazardous Waste Products
Safety & Protection Products
Fluid Management Products

BRANDS/DIVISIONS/AFFILIATES:
Plasco, Inc.
OREX Technologies International
Microtek Medical, Inc.
Iosorb
LTS-Plus
CleanOp
Venodyne
OREX Processor

CONTACTS:
Note: Officers with more than one job title may be intentionally listed here more than once.

Dan R. Lee, CEO
Dan R. Lee, Pres.
J. Michael Mabry, Exec. VP/COO
Roger G. Wilson, CFO
Barbara J. Osborne, Exec. VP-Mktg. & Sales
John Mills, Investor Rel.
Roger G. Wilson, Treas.
J. Michael Mabry, Corp. Sec.
Dan R. Lee, Chmn.

Phone: 800-844-0988   Fax: 800-642-0255
Toll-Free: 800-824-3027
Address: 512 Lehmberg Rd., Columbus, MS 39702 US

GROWTH PLANS/SPECIAL FEATURES:
Microtek Medical Holdings, Inc. (MMHI) develops and markets materials for the control of medical and nuclear hazardous substances. Its Microtek Medical, Inc. (MMI) subsidiary develops, manufacturers and sells contamination control materials, fluid control products and safety products to health care professionals for use in environments such as operating rooms and outpatient surgical centers. These consist primarily of disposable equipment drapes, specialty patient drapes, Iosorb and LTS-Plus encapsulation products, CleanOp cleaning kits, Venodyne pneumatic pumps, decanters and wound evacuation products. Through Plasco, Inc., MMI offers a branded line of fluid management products and emergency medical products including a patented CPR shield system that prevents contamination from mouth-to-mouth resuscitation and a vacuum system used to immobilize or splint injured limbs. The company also engages in contract manufacturing and private labeling and is a supplier of OEM disposable medical devices. MMHI's OREX Technologies International (OTI) subsidiary develops and sells systems engineered for the subsequent disposal of contaminant control products. It focuses on seeking to commercialize its degradable OREX products and technology for use in the nuclear power generating industry. These products perform like traditional disposable and reusable products but can be dissolved in hot water in an OREX Processor and can then be disposed of through the municipal sewer system or other specialty engineered treatment and disposal systems.

FINANCIALS:
Sales and profits are in thousands of dollars—add 000 to get the full amount. Year 2004 note: Complete fiscal 2004 results were not available for all companies at press time. For this company, year 2004 is for 9 months.

2004 Sales: $93,438 (9 months)	2004 Profits: $5,600 (9 months)	**Stock Ticker:** MTMD
2003 Sales: $98,664	2003 Profits: $16,023	Employees: 1,813
2002 Sales: $86,700	2002 Profits: $8,400	Fiscal Year Ends: 12/31
2001 Sales: $81,000	2001 Profits: $4,800	
2000 Sales: $56,400	2000 Profits: $-12,100	

SALARIES/BENEFITS:
Pension Plan:	ESOP Stock Plan:	Profit Sharing:	Top Exec. Salary: $296,154	Bonus: $225,000
Savings Plan: Y	Stock Purch. Plan: Y		Second Exec. Salary: $170,096	Bonus: $85,000

OTHER THOUGHTS:
Apparent Top Female Officers: 1
Hot Spot for Advancement for Women/Minorities:

LOCATIONS: ("Y" = Yes)
West:	Southwest:	Midwest:	Southeast:	Northeast:	International:
	Y	Y	Y		Y

MID ATLANTIC MEDICAL SERVICES INC

www.mamsi.com

Industry Group Code: 524114 Ranks within this company's industry group: Sales: Profits:

Insurance/HMO/PPO:	Drugs:	Equipment/Supplies:	Hospitals/Clinics:	Services:	Health Care:
Insurance:	Manufacturer:	Manufacturer:	Acute Care:	Diagnostics:	Home Health: Y
Managed Care: Y	Distributor:	Distributor:	Sub-Acute Care:	Labs/Testing:	Long-Term Care:
Utilization Mgmt.:	Specialty Pharm.:	Leasing/Finance:	Outpatient Surgery: Y	Staffing:	Physical Therapy:
Payment Proc.:	Vitamins/Nutri.:	Information Sys.:	Phys. Rehab. Center:	Waste Disposal:	Phys. Practice Mgmt.:
	Clinical Trials:		Psychiatric Clinics:	Specialty Services:	

TYPES OF BUSINESS:
HMO/PPO
Life & Health Insurance
Home Health Care Services

BRANDS/DIVISIONS/AFFILIATES:
MAMSI Life and Health Insurance Company
Optimum Choice, Inc.
MD-Individual Practice Association, Inc.
Optimum Choice of the Carolinas, Inc.
HomeCall, Inc.
Alliance PPO, LLC
M.D. IPA Surgicenter, Inc.
UnitedHealth Group

CONTACTS:
Note: Officers with more than one job title may be intentionally listed here more than once.

Thomas P. Barbera, CEO
Thomas P. Barbera, Pres.
Robert E. Foss, CFO
Debbie J. Hulen, Sr. VP-Small Group Sales
Judy Graham, VP-Human Resources
Craig Magargel, VP-IT
Sharon C. Pavlos, General Counsel
Vera C. Dvorak, Exec. VP/Medical Dir.
Sharon C. Pavlos, Corp. Sec.
Mark D. Groban, Chmn.

Phone: 301-762-8205 **Fax:** 301-838-5682
Toll-Free: 800-544-2853
Address: 4 Taft Ct., Rockville, MD 20850-5310 US

GROWTH PLANS/SPECIAL FEATURES:

Mid Atlantic Medical Services, Inc. (MAMSI) and its subsidiaries comprise one of the largest managed care companies in the mid-Atlantic region of the United States. The firm was purchased in early 2004 for nearly $3 billion and is now a subsidiary of UnitedHealth Group, a health care company with more than 50 million clients. MAMSI's health care plans offer a wide variety of products and health care coverage options for individuals and corporations including PPOs, HMOs, dental, prescription drugs, vision and term life insurances. The company serves approximately 1.9 million clients in Maryland, Washington, D.C., Virginia, Delaware, West Virginia, northern North Carolina and southeast Pennsylvania. The company operates three health maintenance organizations: MD-Individual Practice Association, Inc., Optimum Choice, Inc. and Optimum Choice of the Carolinas, Inc. MAMSI also owns Alliance PPO, HomeCall, Inc., MAMSI Life and Health Insurance Co. and Mid Atlantic Psychiatric Services, Inc.

The company offers employees health, dental and group life coverage, as well as tuition reimbursement and credit union membership.

FINANCIALS:
Sales and profits are in thousands of dollars—add 000 to get the full amount. Year 2004 note: Complete fiscal 2004 results were not available for all companies at press time. For this company, year 2004 is for months.

2004 Sales: $ (months)   2004 Profits: $ (months)
2003 Sales: $ 2003 Profits: $
2002 Sales: $2,313,100   2002 Profits: $97,400
2001 Sales: $1,807,700   2001 Profits: $57,200
2000 Sales: $1,484,500   2000 Profits: $39,400

Stock Ticker: Subsidiary
Employees: 3,315
Fiscal Year Ends: 12/31

SALARIES/BENEFITS:
Pension Plan:	ESOP Stock Plan:	Profit Sharing:	Top Exec. Salary: $818,226	Bonus: $778,602
Savings Plan: Y	Stock Purch. Plan: Y		Second Exec. Salary: $635,202	Bonus: $559,977

OTHER THOUGHTS:
Apparent Top Female Officers: 4
Hot Spot for Advancement for Women/Minorities: Y

LOCATIONS: ("Y" = Yes)
West:	Southwest:	Midwest:	Southeast: Y	Northeast: Y	International:

Note: Financial information, benefits and other data can change quickly and may vary from those stated here.

MILLENNIUM PHARMACEUTICALS INC

www.mlnm.com

Industry Group Code: 325412 Ranks within this company's industry group: Sales: 37 Profits: 40

Insurance/HMO/PPO:	Drugs:	Equipment/Supplies:	Hospitals/Clinics:	Services:	Health Care:
Insurance:	Manufacturer: Y	Manufacturer:	Acute Care:	Diagnostics:	Home Health:
Managed Care:	Distributor:	Distributor:	Sub-Acute Care:	Labs/Testing: Y	Long-Term Care:
Utilization Mgmt.:	Specialty Pharm.:	Leasing/Finance:	Outpatient Surgery:	Staffing:	Physical Therapy:
Payment Proc.:	Vitamins/Nutri.:	Information Sys.:	Phys. Rehab. Center:	Waste Disposal:	Phys. Practice Mgmt.:
	Clinical Trials:		Psychiatric Clinics:	Specialty Services: Y	

TYPES OF BUSINESS:
Drugs-Gene-Based Discovery Platform
Small-Molecule Drugs
Diagnostic Products

BRANDS/DIVISIONS/AFFILIATES:
COR Therapeutics, Inc.
VELCADE
Integrilin

CONTACTS:
Note: Officers with more than one job title may be intentionally listed here more than once.
Mark J. Levin, CEO
Mark J. Levin, Pres.
Kevin Starr, COO
Marsha Fanucci, Sr. VP/CFO
Linda K. Pine, Sr. VP-Human Resources
Robert I. Tepper, VP-R&D
John B. Douglas, III, General Counsel
Clare Midgley, VP-Global Corp. Affairs
Kenneth Bate, Exec. VP-Commercial Oper.
Mark J. Levin, Chmn.

Phone: 617-679-7000   Fax: 617-374-7788
Toll-Free:
Address: 40 Landsowne St., Cambridge, MA 02139 US

GROWTH PLANS/SPECIAL FEATURES:

Millennium Pharmaceuticals researches and manufactures small-molecule, biotherapeutic and predictive medicine products. The company integrates large-scale genetics, genomics, high-throughput screening and informatics into a drug discovery platform that accelerates the development of therapeutic and diagnostic products. The company identifies important genes, determines their functions, validates drug and product development targets, formulates assays based on these targets and identifies product candidates. The company's research primarily emphasizes treatments for cancer, inflammation and metabolic diseases such as obesity. In addition, Millennium has significant programs in infectious diseases, cardiovascular diseases and diseases of the central nervous system. The firm focuses on developing small-molecule drugs, typically formulated into pills for oral consumption, as well as proteins and monoclonal antibodies, typically only available as injections. The company licenses its platform to various pharmaceutical and biotechnology firms in exchange for royalties from products developed with the technology. FDA-approved VELCADE, the first proteasome inhibitor to earn approval, is the first new treatment in over 10 years for multiple myeloma, a cancer of the blood. Through its merger with COR Therapeutics, Inc., Millennium acquired Integrilin, a drug that treats acute coronary problems. The firm also received substantial research and development capabilities in the areas of cardiovascular disease and oncology. In June 2004, Millennium announced a research agreement with Harvard University. Harvard has granted Millennium the rights to certain intellectual properties and inventions for developing proteasome inhibitors.

The firm's Millennium University offers employees a variety of in-house workshops and off-site seminars designed to enhance career development. Employees are eligible for bonus opportunities depending on Millennium's achievement of various goals as well as individual performance.

FINANCIALS:
Sales and profits are in thousands of dollars—add 000 to get the full amount. Year 2004 note: Complete fiscal 2004 results were not available for all companies at press time. For this company, year 2004 is for 9 months.

2004 Sales: $347,859 (9 months)   2004 Profits: $-157,590 (9 months)
2003 Sales: $433,687   2003 Profits: $-483,687
2002 Sales: $353,000   2002 Profits: $-590,200
2001 Sales: $246,200   2001 Profits: $-192,000
2000 Sales: $196,300   2000 Profits: $-309,600

Stock Ticker: MLNM
Employees: 1,530
Fiscal Year Ends: 12/31

SALARIES/BENEFITS:
Pension Plan: ESOP Stock Plan: Profit Sharing: Top Exec. Salary: $524,231   Bonus: $400,000
Savings Plan: Y   Stock Purch. Plan: Y   Second Exec. Salary: $500,000   Bonus: $250,000

OTHER THOUGHTS:
Apparent Top Female Officers: 3
Hot Spot for Advancement for Women/Minorities: Y

LOCATIONS: ("Y" = Yes)
West	Southwest	Midwest	Southeast	Northeast	International
Y				Y	Y

MIM CORP

www.mimcorp.net

Industry Group Code: 522320A **Ranks within this company's industry group:** Sales: 4 Profits: 4

Insurance/HMO/PPO:	Drugs:	Equipment/Supplies:	Hospitals/Clinics:	Services:	Health Care:
Insurance: Managed Care: Utilization Mgmt.: Y Payment Proc.: Y	Manufacturer: Distributor: Specialty Pharm.: Y Vitamins/Nutri.: Clinical Trials:	Manufacturer: Distributor: Leasing/Finance: Information Sys.:	Acute Care: Sub-Acute Care: Outpatient Surgery: Phys. Rehab. Center: Psychiatric Clinics:	Diagnostics: Labs/Testing: Staffing: Waste Disposal: Specialty Services: Y	Home Health: Long-Term Care: Physical Therapy: Phys. Practice Mgmt.:

TYPES OF BUSINESS:
Pharmacy Benefits Management
Online & Mail-Order Pharmacy Services
Disease Management
Home Infusion Services
Specialty Pharmacy Services

BRANDS/DIVISIONS/AFFILIATES:
BioScrip
Chronimed

CONTACTS:
Note: Officers with more than one job title may be intentionally listed here more than once.

Richard H. Friedman, CEO
Alfred Carfora, Pres.
Alfred Carfora, COO
James S. Lusk, CFO
Michael J. Sicilian, Exec. VP-Sales
Barry A. Posner, Exec. VP/General Counsel
Russel J. Corvese, VP-Oper.
Rachel Levine, VP-Investor Rel.
Richard H. Friedman, Chmn.

Phone: 914-460-1600 **Fax:** 914-460-1660
Toll-Free: 888-818-3939
Address: 100 Clearbrook Rd., Elmsford, NY 10523 US

GROWTH PLANS/SPECIAL FEATURES:
MIM Corp. is a pharmaceutical health care organization that provides pharmacy benefit management (PBM), specialty pharmaceutical management, distribution and other pharmacy-related health care solutions to individual patients or enrollees receiving health benefits through HMOs, indemnity plans, PPOs, managed care organizations and other plan sponsors. It operates throughout the U.S., with offices in New York, Rhode Island, Ohio, New Jersey and Tennessee. The company's specialty management and delivery services segment distributes biotech and other high-cost pharmaceuticals and provides clinically focused case and therapy management programs to members that are chronically ill or genetically impaired. Its BioScrip specialty pharmacy programs provide pharmacy case management, prior authorizations, infusion therapy, therapy assessment, patient enrollment, risk assessment, education, medication delivery, pharmacy data services and disease management for Crohn's disease, Gaucher's disease, growth hormone deficiency, HIV/AIDS, hemophilia, hepatitis C, immune deficiency, infertility, multiple sclerosis, oncology, psoriasis, rheumatoid arthritis and transplants. MIM's PBM services group offers plan sponsors, employers and third-party administrators services that ensure cost-effective drug delivery. Its services include formulary and benefit design, clinical services, drug use evaluation, pharmacy data services, disease management, behavioral health pharmacy services, capitated billing arrangements and a mail-order pharmacy. In August 2004, the company agreed to acquire Chronimed, a specialty pharmacy, for $80 million in cash and stock.

FINANCIALS:
Sales and profits are in thousands of dollars—add 000 to get the full amount. Year 2004 note: Complete fiscal 2004 results were not available for all companies at press time. For this company, year 2004 is for 9 months.

2004 Sales: $463,676 (9 months)   2004 Profits: $5,848 (9 months)
2003 Sales: $588,770   2003 Profits: $9,130
2002 Sales: $576,600   2002 Profits: $18,700
2001 Sales: $456,600   2001 Profits: $14,200
2000 Sales: $369,800   2000 Profits: $-1,800

Stock Ticker: MIMS
Employees: 480
Fiscal Year Ends: 12/31

SALARIES/BENEFITS:
Pension Plan: ESOP Stock Plan: Profit Sharing: Top Exec. Salary: $593,384   Bonus: $207,000
Savings Plan: Stock Purch. Plan: Second Exec. Salary: $328,508 Bonus: $40,000

OTHER THOUGHTS:
Apparent Top Female Officers: 1
Hot Spot for Advancement for Women/Minorities:

LOCATIONS: ("Y" = Yes)

West:	Southwest:	Midwest:	Southeast:	Northeast:	International:
		Y	Y	Y	

MINE SAFETY APPLIANCES CO

www.msanet.com

Industry Group Code: 339113   Ranks within this company's industry group: Sales: 33   Profits: 25

Insurance/HMO/PPO:	Drugs:	Equipment/Supplies:		Hospitals/Clinics:	Services:	Health Care:
Insurance: Managed Care: Utilization Mgmt.: Payment Proc.:	Manufacturer: Distributor: Specialty Pharm.: Vitamins/Nutri.: Clinical Trials:	Manufacturer: Distributor: Leasing/Finance: Information Sys.:	Y	Acute Care: Sub-Acute Care: Outpatient Surgery: Phys. Rehab. Center: Psychiatric Clinics:	Diagnostics: Labs/Testing: Staffing: Waste Disposal: Specialty Services:	Home Health: Long-Term Care: Physical Therapy: Phys. Practice Mgmt.:

TYPES OF BUSINESS:
Equipment/Supplies-Manufacturer
Safety and Health Equipment
Personal Protective Products
Respiratory Protective Equipment
Thermal Imaging Cameras
Combat Helmets

BRANDS/DIVISIONS/AFFILIATES:
MSA Safety Works
Sordin AB

GROWTH PLANS/SPECIAL FEATURES:
Mine Safety Appliances Company (MSA) is primarily engaged in the manufacture and sale of safety and health equipment. Operating 27 companies worldwide, it is the leading provider of safety products and services. Its principal products include respiratory protective equipment that is air-purifying, air-supplied and self-contained; instruments that monitor and analyze workplace environments and control industrial processes; thermal imaging cameras that enable firefighters and rescue workers to see through smoke and darkness; fall protection equipment; and personal protective products such as head, eye, face and hearing protectors, as well as combat helmets for the U.S. Army. MSA markets its products under the MSA Safety Works brand and builds its products to conform to governmental standards worldwide. The company maintains manufacturing and research operations internationally in 25 countries. In May 2004, MSA reached an agreement to acquire Sordin AB of Sweden, a manufacturer of passive and electronic hearing protection equipment.

CONTACTS:
Note: Officers with more than one job title may be intentionally listed here more than once.
John T. Ryan, III, CEO
Dennis L. Zeitler, CFO
Benedict DeMaria, VP-Human Resources
Douglas K. McClaine, General Counsel
Dennis L. Zeitler, Treas.
James H. Baillie, Pres.-Europe
William M. Lambert, Pres.-North America
John T. Ryan, III, Chmn.

Phone: 412-967-3000   **Fax:** 412-967-3326
Toll-Free: 800-672-2222
Address: 121 Gamma Dr., Pittsburgh, PA 15238 US

FINANCIALS:
Sales and profits are in thousands of dollars—add 000 to get the full amount. Year 2004 note: Complete fiscal 2004 results were not available for all companies at press time. For this company, year 2004 is for 9 months.

2004 Sales: $627,566 (9 months)	2004 Profits: $53,367 (9 months)	**Stock Ticker:** MSA
2003 Sales: $698,197	2003 Profits: $65,267	Employees: 4,300
2002 Sales: $564,400	2002 Profits: $35,100	Fiscal Year Ends: 12/31
2001 Sales: $545,700	2001 Profits: $31,600	
2000 Sales: $502,800	2000 Profits: $23,200	

SALARIES/BENEFITS:
Pension Plan: ESOP Stock Plan: Profit Sharing: Top Exec. Salary: $555,990   Bonus: $744,750
Savings Plan: Y   Stock Purch. Plan: Second Exec. Salary: $304,705   Bonus: $252,927

OTHER THOUGHTS:
Apparent Top Female Officers:
Hot Spot for Advancement for Women/Minorities:

LOCATIONS: ("Y" = Yes)
West:	Southwest:	Midwest:	Southeast:	Northeast:	International:
Y				Y	Y

MINNTECH CORP

www.minntech.com

Industry Group Code: 339113 **Ranks within this company's industry group:** Sales: Profits:

Insurance/HMO/PPO:	Drugs:	Equipment/Supplies:	Hospitals/Clinics:	Services:	Health Care:
Insurance:	Manufacturer:	Manufacturer: Y	Acute Care:	Diagnostics:	Home Health:
Managed Care:	Distributor:	Distributor:	Sub-Acute Care:	Labs/Testing:	Long-Term Care:
Utilization Mgmt.:	Specialty Pharm.:	Leasing/Finance:	Outpatient Surgery:	Staffing:	Physical Therapy:
Payment Proc.:	Vitamins/Nutri.:	Information Sys.:	Phys. Rehab. Center:	Waste Disposal:	Phys. Practice Mgmt.:
	Clinical Trials:		Psychiatric Clinics:	Specialty Services:	

TYPES OF BUSINESS:
Supplies-Kidney Dialysis Products
Sterilants
Filtration & Separation Products

BRANDS/DIVISIONS/AFFILIATES:
Minntech Renal Systems
Minntech International
Minntech Fibercor
Cantel Medical Corp.
Renalin 100 Cold Sterilant
Renatron II
RenaClear

CONTACTS:
Note: Officers with more than one job title may be intentionally listed here more than once.

Roy Malkin, CEO
Roy Malkin, Pres.
Denise Bauer, VP-Human Resources
Michael P. Peterson, VP-Research & Dev., Electro-Mechanical/Software
Jim McMillen, VP-Mfg.
Kevin Finkle, VP-Admin.
Kevin Finkle, VP-Finance
R. C. Kippenhan, VP-Research & Dev., Sterilants/Disinfectants
Craig Smith, VP-Quality Assurance & Regulatory Affairs
Paul E. Helms, Exec. VP
Nicholas Strout, VP-Int'l

Phone: 763-553-3300 **Fax:** 763-553-3387
Toll-Free: 800-328-3345
Address: 14605 28th Ave. N., Minneapolis, MN 55447-4822 US

GROWTH PLANS/SPECIAL FEATURES:
Minntech Corp., a subsidiary of Cantel Medical Corp. since 2001, develops, manufactures and markets medical supplies and devices, sterilants and filtration and separation products. The company's products are used primarily in kidney dialysis, open-heart surgery, endoscopy and in the preparation of pure water for medical or laboratory use. Products used in dialysis are marketed under the trade name Minntech Renal Systems. Its filtration and separation products are marketed to the pharmaceutical, medical, semiconductor and biotechnology industries under the name Minntech Fibercor. Minntech has also developed core technologies in electronics, fibers, plastics and chemical solutions. Minntech provides several leading product lines for the dialysis market, including the Renatron II, an automated dialyzer reprocessing system; Renalin 100 Cold Sterilant for increasing reprocessing efficiency; and the RenaClear dialyzer cleaning system. The company's reprocessing products help dialysis centers maximize the use of costly dialyzers while safeguarding their patients.

FINANCIALS:
Sales and profits are in thousands of dollars—add 000 to get the full amount. Year 2004 note: Complete fiscal 2004 results were not available for all companies at press time. For this company, year 2004 is for months.

2004 Sales: $ (months)	2004 Profits: $ (months)	**Stock Ticker:** Subsidiary
2003 Sales: $	2003 Profits: $	Employees: 376
2002 Sales: $	2002 Profits: $	Fiscal Year Ends: 7/31
2001 Sales: $76,600	2001 Profits: $2,200	
2000 Sales: $74,400	2000 Profits: $5,900	

SALARIES/BENEFITS:
| Pension Plan: | ESOP Stock Plan: | Profit Sharing: Y | Top Exec. Salary: $293,750 | Bonus: $198,750 |
| Savings Plan: Y | Stock Purch. Plan: | | Second Exec. Salary: $227,707 | Bonus: $105,495 |

OTHER THOUGHTS:
Apparent Top Female Officers: 1
Hot Spot for Advancement for Women/Minorities:

LOCATIONS: ("Y" = Yes)
West:	Southwest:	Midwest:	Southeast:	Northeast:	International:
		Y	Y	Y	Y

MISONIX INC

www.misonix.com

Industry Group Code: 339113   Ranks within this company's industry group: Sales: 120   Profits: 98

Insurance/HMO/PPO:	Drugs:	Equipment/Supplies:	Hospitals/Clinics:	Services:	Health Care:
Insurance:	Manufacturer:	Manufacturer: Y	Acute Care:	Diagnostics:	Home Health:
Managed Care:	Distributor:	Distributor:	Sub-Acute Care:	Labs/Testing:	Long-Term Care:
Utilization Mgmt.:	Specialty Pharm.:	Leasing/Finance:	Outpatient Surgery:	Staffing:	Physical Therapy:
Payment Proc.:	Vitamins/Nutri.:	Information Sys.:	Phys. Rehab. Center:	Waste Disposal:	Phys. Practice Mgmt.:
	Clinical Trials:		Psychiatric Clinics:	Specialty Services: Y	

TYPES OF BUSINESS:
Equipment-Ultrasonic
Air Pollution Products
Medical Devices
Filtration Equipment
Aftermarket Services

BRANDS/DIVISIONS/AFFILIATES:
Aura
Nebulizer
Sonomist
Sonora Medical Systems, Inc.
Mystaire
Sonicator

CONTACTS:
Note: Officers with more than one job title may be intentionally listed here more than once.
Michael A. McManus, Jr., CEO
Michael A. McManus, Jr., Pres.
Richard A. Zaremba, Sr. VP/CFO
Kenneth Coviello, Sr. VP-Medical Mktg. & Sales
Dan Voic, VP-Research & Dev.
Ronald Manna, VP-New Product Dev.
Dan Voic, VP-Eng.
Kenneth Coviello, Sr. VP-Oper.
Richard Zaremba, Treas.
Bernhard Berger, VP-Laboratory & Scientific Products
Ronald Manna, VP-Regulatory Affairs
Gary Gelman, Chmn.

Phone: 631-694-9555   **Fax:** 631-694-9412
Toll-Free: 800-645-9846
Address: 1938 New Hwy., Farmingdale, NY 11735 US

GROWTH PLANS/SPECIAL FEATURES:

Misonix, Inc., through its many subsidiaries, designs, manufactures and markets ultrasonic medical devices, ultrasonic equipment for use in the scientific and industrial markets and air pollution control products. The company's ultrasonic medical devices are used in neurology, urology, orthopedics, audiology and cosmetic surgery, for kidney stone pulverization, destruction of brain tumors, cutting and coagulation of small blood vessels and other applications. Misonix's Sonicator line of ultrasonic liquid processors and cell disrupters have a number of laboratory applications, including sample preparation, degassing, cleaning, soil testing, improving solubility, mixing, catalyzing reactions, creating emulsions and as a homogenizer. The company's other laboratory products include Aura ductless fume enclosures for filtration of gaseous contaminants; technology for controlling and eliminating hazardous fumes, noxious odors and powders used in fingerprinting, evidence drying and DNA testing; and biological safety cabinets for level 1-3 containment. Other ultrasonic applications include cleaners, soldering products and Nebulizer and Sonomist nozzles for atomizing liquids, applying fine coatings, customizing spray patterns and controlling droplet diameter. Finally, Misonix's Mystaire scrubbers remove airborne pollutants in the chemical processing, pharmaceutical, laboratory, waste treatment, metallurgical, industrial and nuclear industries. The company holds 39 distinct U.S. patents related to its various technologies. Majority-owned subsidiary Sonora Medical Systems is a refurbisher of high-performance ultrasound systems and replacement transducers for the medical diagnostic ultrasound industry, offering a range of aftermarket products, such as ultrasound probes and transducers, and services that can extend the life of ultrasound imaging systems beyond the usual five to seven years.

Misonix offers employees medical and dental insurance, as well as life insurance, short- and long-term disability insurance and a vision plan.

FINANCIALS:
Sales and profits are in thousands of dollars—add 000 to get the full amount. Year 2004 note: Complete fiscal 2004 results were not available for all companies at press time. For this company, year 2004 is for 12 months.

2004 Sales: $39,059 (12 months)   2004 Profits: $1,718 (12 months)
2003 Sales: $34,900   2003 Profits: $1,000
2002 Sales: $29,600   2002 Profits: $ 200
2001 Sales: $30,800   2001 Profits: $-4,500
2000 Sales: $29,000   2000 Profits: $2,500

Stock Ticker: MSON
Employees: 201
Fiscal Year Ends: 6/30

SALARIES/BENEFITS:
Pension Plan: ESOP Stock Plan: Profit Sharing: Top Exec. Salary: $275,000   Bonus: $250,000
Savings Plan: Y   Stock Purch. Plan: Second Exec. Salary: $157,878   Bonus: $30,000

OTHER THOUGHTS:
Apparent Top Female Officers:
Hot Spot for Advancement for Women/Minorities:

LOCATIONS: ("Y" = Yes)
West	Southwest	Midwest	Southeast	Northeast	International
Y				Y	Y

Note: Financial information, benefits and other data can change quickly and may vary from those stated here.

MIV THERAPEUTICS INC

www.mivtherapeutics.com

Industry Group Code: 339113 **Ranks within this company's industry group:** Sales: Profits: 116

Insurance/HMO/PPO:	Drugs:	Equipment/Supplies:		Hospitals/Clinics:	Services:	Health Care:
Insurance:	Manufacturer:	Manufacturer:	Y	Acute Care:	Diagnostics:	Home Health:
Managed Care:	Distributor:	Distributor:		Sub-Acute Care:	Labs/Testing:	Long-Term Care:
Utilization Mgmt.:	Specialty Pharm.:	Leasing/Finance:		Outpatient Surgery:	Staffing:	Physical Therapy:
Payment Proc.:	Vitamins/Nutri.:	Information Sys.:		Phys. Rehab. Center:	Waste Disposal:	Phys. Practice Mgmt.:
	Clinical Trials:			Psychiatric Clinics:	Specialty Services:	

TYPES OF BUSINESS:
Medical Equipment
Stents

BRANDS/DIVISIONS/AFFILIATES:
MIVI Technologies, Inc.
Stentgenix
M-I Vascular, Inc.
DBS Holdings, Inc.

CONTACTS: *Note: Officers with more than one job title may be intentionally listed here more than once.*
Alan P. Lindsay, CEO
Alan P. Lindsay, Pres.
Patrick A. McGowan, Exec. VP/CFO
Tom Troczynski, VP-Coating Tech.
Arc Rajtar, VP-Oper., MIVI Tech.

Phone: 604-301-9545 **Fax:** 604-301-9546
Toll-Free:
Address: 8765 Ash St., Unit 1, Vancouver, BC V6P 6T3 Canada

GROWTH PLANS/SPECIAL FEATURES:
MIV Therapeutics, Inc. aims to commercialize stents that feature biocompatible coatings. MIV Therapeutics is the new name for M-I Vascular, Inc. (following its acquisition of DBS Holdings), with major operations managed by its wholly-owned subsidiary, MIVI Technologies, Inc. The company seeks to expand production of laser-cut stainless steel coronary stents, specifically targeting distribution to international markets. MIVI Technologies' manufacturing facility has also been equipped to support the development of its next anticipated product: thin-film coated biocompatible stents (built on the company's current laser-cut platform) using dense, crystalline hydroxyapatite (HAp) to reduce the occurrence of restenosis (arterial reblockage following angioplasty). The development of a viable coated stent has been assisted by research at the University of British Columbia under a collaborative research and development agreement. A further aspect of this joint research is the application of HAp coating in a thicker, porous film to provide an adhesive layer suitable for drug delivery. Continued development, testing and approval protocols position the probable commercialization of coated stents for no earlier than mid-2005. MIVI Technologies anticipates that its current facilities and technologies will accommodate the semi-automated manufacturing, quality assurance testing and final packaging of the coated stent product. Additionally, MIV Therapeutics has entered into a joint venture with Endovasc to develop new stent technologies under the name Stentgenix. Now in its initial phase, this research seeks to apply Endovasc's ANGIOGENIX as a stent coating to stimulate angiogenesis, or new blood vessel growth. Stentgenix is also charged with developing new biodegradable and resorbable stents, which might significantly expand esophageal, renal, biliary, urinary and vascular stent applications.

FINANCIALS:
Sales and profits are in thousands of dollars—add 000 to get the full amount. Year 2004 note: Complete fiscal 2004 results were not available for all companies at press time. For this company, year 2004 is for 12 months.

2004 Sales: $ (12 months)	2004 Profits: $-3,500 (12 months)	**Stock Ticker:** Foreign
2003 Sales: $	2003 Profits: $-3,200	Employees: 6
2002 Sales: $	2002 Profits: $-3,900	Fiscal Year Ends: 5/31
2001 Sales: $	2001 Profits: $	
2000 Sales: $	2000 Profits: $	

SALARIES/BENEFITS:
Pension Plan:	ESOP Stock Plan:	Profit Sharing:	Top Exec. Salary: $138,710	Bonus: $
Savings Plan:	Stock Purch. Plan:		Second Exec. Salary: $64,166	Bonus: $

OTHER THOUGHTS:
Apparent Top Female Officers:
Hot Spot for Advancement for Women/Minorities:

LOCATIONS: ("Y" = Yes)
West:	Southwest:	Midwest:	Southeast:	Northeast:	International: Y

Note: Financial information, benefits and other data can change quickly and may vary from those stated here.

MOLECULAR DEVICES CORP
www.moleculardevices.com

Industry Group Code: 339113   Ranks within this company's industry group: Sales: 85   Profits: 77

Insurance/HMO/PPO:	Drugs:	Equipment/Supplies:	Hospitals/Clinics:	Services:	Health Care:
Insurance: Managed Care: Utilization Mgmt.: Payment Proc.:	Manufacturer: Distributor: Specialty Pharm.: Vitamins/Nutri.: Clinical Trials:	Manufacturer: Y Distributor: Leasing/Finance: Information Sys.:	Acute Care: Sub-Acute Care: Outpatient Surgery: Phys. Rehab. Center: Psychiatric Clinics:	Diagnostics: Labs/Testing: Staffing: Waste Disposal: Specialty Services:	Home Health: Long-Term Care: Physical Therapy: Phys. Practice Mgmt.:

TYPES OF BUSINESS:
Supplies-Drug Discovery Automation
Bioanalytical Measurement Systems

BRANDS/DIVISIONS/AFFILIATES:
SpectraMax
Gemini
Embla 96/384
Combi-12
FLIPR
SealChip
Threshold ImmunoLigand
Axon Instruments, Inc.

CONTACTS:
Note: Officers with more than one job title may be intentionally listed here more than once.

Joseph D. Keegan, CEO
Joseph D. Keegan, Pres.
Tim Harkness, CFO
Stephen J. Oldfield, VP-Worldwide Mktg.
Patricia C. Sharp, VP-Human Resources
Gillian M.K. Humphries, VP-Research
Andrew T. Zander, VP-Eng.
Robert J. Murray, VP-Oper.
Gillian M.K. Humphries, VP-Strategic Affairs
Tim Harkness, VP-Finance
Thomas J. O'Lenic, VP-North American Sales and Service
John S. Senaldi, VP/Mgr.-IonWorks
J. Richard Sportsman, VP-Assay and Reagent Research and Dev.
Joseph D. Keegan, Chmn.

Phone: 408-747-1700   **Fax:** 408-747-3601
Toll-Free: 800-635-5577
Address: 1311 Orleans Dr., Sunnyvale, CA 94089-1136 US

GROWTH PLANS/SPECIAL FEATURES:
Molecular Devices Corp. (MDC) is a leading supplier of high-performance bioanalytical measurement systems that accelerate and improve drug discovery and other life sciences research. Product offerings are divided into six categories: microplate readers and software, liquid handling systems, screening systems, electrophysiology systems, microscopy systems and reagents. Microplate readers include absorbance, multimode, luminescence or fluorescence readers for between one and 384 simultaneous samples. The firm's reader brands include SpectraMax and Gemini. The division also creates reader software, test validation packets and plate handling robots for sensitive or toxic testing. Liquid handling systems include plate washers and cell harvesters like the Embla 96/384 and the Combi-12. Screening systems include assay systems like the FLIPR brand and accompanying software in various sizes. Electrophysiology systems are ion channel screeners for drug discovery and development using patented SealChip electrodes. Microscopy includes screening and imaging systems that are hardware and software integrations for image capture and microscopic digital archives including time-lapse, multi-dimensional acquisition and 3D reconstruction. The firm's reagents are used in assay kits for calcium, membrane potential, IMAPs, ELISA cyclic GMP and the firm's specialty brands, Threshold ImmunoLigand and Total DNA. In recent news, MDC acquired Axon Instruments, Inc. and all of its intellectual property and patents.

FINANCIALS:
Sales and profits are in thousands of dollars—add 000 to get the full amount. Year 2004 note: Complete fiscal 2004 results were not available for all companies at press time. For this company, year 2004 is for 9 months.

2004 Sales: $101,044 (9 months)   2004 Profits: $2,666 (9 months)
2003 Sales: $115,581   2003 Profits: $7,742
2002 Sales: $102,200   2002 Profits: $6,800
2001 Sales: $92,200   2001 Profits: $-5,200
2000 Sales: $96,000   2000 Profits: $-4,900

Stock Ticker: MDCC
Employees: 106
Fiscal Year Ends: 12/31

SALARIES/BENEFITS:
Pension Plan:	ESOP Stock Plan:	Profit Sharing:	Top Exec. Salary: $377,445	Bonus: $468,084
Savings Plan: Y	Stock Purch. Plan: Y		Second Exec. Salary: $237,499	Bonus: $142,500

OTHER THOUGHTS:
Apparent Top Female Officers: 2
Hot Spot for Advancement for Women/Minorities:

LOCATIONS: ("Y" = Yes)
West:	Southwest:	Midwest:	Southeast:	Northeast:	International:
Y					Y

MONARCH DENTAL CORP

www.monarchdental.com

Industry Group Code: 621111   Ranks within this company's industry group: Sales: Profits:

Insurance/HMO/PPO:	Drugs:	Equipment/Supplies:	Hospitals/Clinics:	Services:	Health Care:
Insurance:	Manufacturer:	Manufacturer:	Acute Care:	Diagnostics:	Home Health:
Managed Care:	Distributor:	Distributor:	Sub-Acute Care:	Labs/Testing:	Long-Term Care:
Utilization Mgmt.:	Specialty Pharm.:	Leasing/Finance:	Outpatient Surgery:	Staffing:	Physical Therapy:
Payment Proc.:	Vitamins/Nutri.:	Information Sys.:	Phys. Rehab. Center:	Waste Disposal:	Phys. Practice Mgmt.: Y
	Clinical Trials:		Psychiatric Clinics:	Specialty Services:	

TYPES OF BUSINESS:
Dental Practice Management

BRANDS/DIVISIONS/AFFILIATES:
Bright Now! Dental, Inc.

CONTACTS:
Note: Officers with more than one job title may be intentionally listed here more than once.

Steven C. Bilt, CEO
Steven C. Bilt, Pres.
Bradley E. Schmidt, CFO
Timothy J. Kriske, VP-Oper.
Steven C. Bilt, Pres./CEO-Bright Now! Dental
Bradley E. Schmidt, CFO-Bright Now! Dental

Phone: 972-702-7446   Fax: 714-428-1300
Toll-Free:
Address: Tollway Plaza II, 15950 N. Dallas Pkwy., Ste. 825, Dallas, TX 75248 US

GROWTH PLANS/SPECIAL FEATURES:

Monarch Dental Corp., a wholly-owned subsidiary of Bright Now! Dental, Inc., provides management and administrative services to dental group practices in selected markets under long-term administrative services agreements. Practicing dentists at its 158 offices provide general dentistry services such as examinations, cleanings, fillings, bonding, placing crowns and fitting and placing fixed or removable prostheses. At many of the company's offices, dentists also provide specialty dental services such as orthodontics, cosmetic services, oral surgery, endodontics, periodontics and pediatric dentistry. Specialty dental services are typically offered through teams that rotate through several dental offices in a particular market. This enables the dental professional corporations managed by the company to capture revenue from services that would otherwise be referred to independent specialists. To drive patient volume, Monarch applies proven retailing principles including the extensive use of television, radio, print and outdoor advertising. These advertising and marketing programs emphasize that Monarch offers quality general and specialty dentistry services, convenient hours, payment plans and a choice of locations. Recently, Monarch opened new offices in Arlington and McKinney, Texas.

Monarch's employee benefits include heath, group life and disability insurance as well as vision care and flexible spending plans.

FINANCIALS:
Sales and profits are in thousands of dollars—add 000 to get the full amount. Year 2004 note: Complete fiscal 2004 results were not available for all companies at press time. For this company, year 2004 is for months.

2004 Sales: $ (months)   2004 Profits: $ (months)
2003 Sales: $ 2003 Profits: $
2002 Sales: $ 2002 Profits: $
2001 Sales: $211,900   2001 Profits: $-3,800
2000 Sales: $211,300   2000 Profits: $- 500

Stock Ticker: Subsidiary
Employees: 1,500
Fiscal Year Ends: 12/31

SALARIES/BENEFITS:
| Pension Plan: | ESOP Stock Plan: | Profit Sharing: | Top Exec. Salary: $450,000 | Bonus: $83,262 |
| Savings Plan: Y | Stock Purch. Plan: | | Second Exec. Salary: $208,154 | Bonus: $33,566 |

OTHER THOUGHTS:
Apparent Top Female Officers:
Hot Spot for Advancement for Women/Minorities:

LOCATIONS: ("Y" = Yes)
West:	Southwest:	Midwest:	Southeast:	Northeast:	International:
Y	Y	Y	Y		

MOORE MEDICAL CORP

www.mooremedical.com

Industry Group Code: 421450   **Ranks within this company's industry group:** Sales: 6   Profits: 6

Insurance/HMO/PPO:	Drugs:		Equipment/Supplies:		Hospitals/Clinics:	Services:	Health Care:
Insurance:	Manufacturer:		Manufacturer:		Acute Care:	Diagnostics:	Home Health:
Managed Care:	Distributor:	Y	Distributor:	Y	Sub-Acute Care:	Labs/Testing:	Long-Term Care:
Utilization Mgmt.:	Specialty Pharm.:		Leasing/Finance:		Outpatient Surgery:	Staffing:	Physical Therapy:
Payment Proc.:	Vitamins/Nutri.:		Information Sys.:	Y	Phys. Rehab. Center:	Waste Disposal:	Phys. Practice Mgmt.:
	Clinical Trials:				Psychiatric Clinics:	Specialty Services:	

TYPES OF BUSINESS:
Distribution-Assorted Health Care Products

BRANDS/DIVISIONS/AFFILIATES:
McKesson Corporation

CONTACTS:
Note: Officers with more than one job title may be intentionally listed here more than once.

Linda M. Autore, CEO
Linda M. Autore, Pres.
Ronald C. Flormann, Jr., VP-Mktg. & Sales
David Lafferty, CIO
Patrick Early, VP-Oper.

Phone: 860-826-3600   **Fax:** 860-225-4440
Toll-Free:
Address: 389 John Downey Dr., New Britain, CT 06050 US

GROWTH PLANS/SPECIAL FEATURES:

Moore Medical Corporation, a subsidiary of McKesson Corporation, is a multi-channel marketer and distributor of medical, surgical and pharmaceutical products to over 100,000 health care practices and facilities in non-hospital settings nationwide. Its primary customer groups include physicians, emergency medical technicians, schools, correctional institutions, municipalities, occupational/industrial health doctors and nurses and other specialty practice communities. The firm markets and serves its customers through direct mail, industry-specialized telephone support staff, field sales representatives and the Internet. Moore Medical purchases products primarily from manufacturers and other distributors and does not manufacture or assemble any products, with the exception of medical and first-aid kits. The largest product suppliers for the company are 3M, Becton Dickinson, GlaxoSmithKline, Johnson & Johnson, Kendall Healthcare Products Co., Laerdal Medical Corp., Microflex, Wyeth-Ayerst Labs, Graham Medical Products and Welch Allyn. McKesson acquired Moore Medical in April 2004.

FINANCIALS:
Sales and profits are in thousands of dollars—add 000 to get the full amount. Year 2004 note: Complete fiscal 2004 results were not available for all companies at press time. For this company, year 2004 is for months.

2004 Sales: $ (months)   2004 Profits: $ (months)
2003 Sales: $141,700   2003 Profits: $-1,500
2002 Sales: $137,800   2002 Profits: $1,000
2001 Sales: $132,800   2001 Profits: $-1,700
2000 Sales: $123,600   2000 Profits: $-4,500

Stock Ticker: Subsidiary
Employees: 315
Fiscal Year Ends: 12/31

SALARIES/BENEFITS:
Pension Plan: Y   ESOP Stock Plan: Profit Sharing: Top Exec. Salary: $295,550   Bonus: $27,957
Savings Plan: Stock Purch. Plan: Second Exec. Salary: $225,000   Bonus: $20,192

OTHER THOUGHTS:
Apparent Top Female Officers: 1
Hot Spot for Advancement for Women/Minorities:

LOCATIONS: ("Y" = Yes)
West: Y   Southwest: Midwest: Southeast: Y   Northeast: Y   International:

MORRISON MANAGEMENT SPECIALISTS INC

www.iammorrison.com

Industry Group Code: 722310 Ranks within this company's industry group: Sales: Profits:

Insurance/HMO/PPO:	Drugs:	Equipment/Supplies:	Hospitals/Clinics:	Services:	Health Care:
Insurance:	Manufacturer:	Manufacturer:	Acute Care:	Diagnostics:	Home Health:
Managed Care:	Distributor:	Distributor:	Sub-Acute Care:	Labs/Testing:	Long-Term Care:
Utilization Mgmt.:	Specialty Pharm.:	Leasing/Finance:	Outpatient Surgery:	Staffing:	Physical Therapy:
Payment Proc.:	Vitamins/Nutri.:	Information Sys.:	Phys. Rehab. Center:	Waste Disposal:	Phys. Practice Mgmt.:
	Clinical Trials:		Psychiatric Clinics:	Specialty Services: Y	

TYPES OF BUSINESS:
Nutrition/Health Care Facility-Based Cafeterias & Food Service
Human Resource Services

BRANDS/DIVISIONS/AFFILIATES:
Compass Group
Morrison Healthcare Food Services
Morrison Senior Dining
Morrison Human Resource Services
Crothall Services

CONTACTS:
Note: Officers with more than one job title may be intentionally listed here more than once.

Glenn A. Davenport, CEO
Glenn A. Davenport, Pres.
K. Wyatt Engwall, CFO
Scott MacLellan, Exec. VP-Sales
Chip Kent, Sr. VP-Human Resources & Learning
Tony Mitchell, Chief Tech. Officer
John E. Fountain, VP/General Counsel
George Levins, Sr. VP-Oper.
Ritch Brandon, VP-Mktg. & Strategy
Cheryl Webster, VP-Corp. Comm.
Richard C. Roberson, Sr. VP-Client Rel.
Amy Hartman, Dir.-Mktg. & Comm.
Jerry D. Underhill, Pres., Morrison Senior Dining

Phone: 404-845-3330 Fax: 404-845-3333
Toll-Free: 800-225-5368
Address: 5801 Peachtree Dunwoody Rd., Atlanta, GA 30342 US

GROWTH PLANS/SPECIAL FEATURES:

Morrison Management Specialists, Inc. is one of the largest U.S. health care and senior living food service companies and a subsidiary of U.K.-based Compass Group. The company is organized into two groups, Morrison Healthcare Food Services and Morrison Senior Dining, providing hospital culinary programs and senior living food services, respectively. Morrison Healthcare Food Services has contracts with approximately 350 acute care institutions, while Morrison Senior Dining currently works in 250 senior living communities. In addition to providing food services, Morrison helps clients manage costs, integrate their systems and create appealing food service environments. Morrison has branched out into other areas, forming Morrison Human Resource Services, which provides, among other things, employee training, worker's compensation administration and benefit and payroll administration. Morrison is also in a longstanding partnership with Crothall Services, another member of the Compass Group. Crothall handles complementary areas of health care facilities management.

Along with health coverage, Morrison, as part of the Compass Group, offers insurance for spouses and children, management incentive programs and service awards.

FINANCIALS:
Sales and profits are in thousands of dollars—add 000 to get the full amount. Year 2004 note: Complete fiscal 2004 results were not available for all companies at press time. For this company, year 2004 is for months.

2004 Sales: $ (months)   2004 Profits: $ (months)
2003 Sales: $ 2003 Profits: $
2002 Sales: $ 2002 Profits: $
2001 Sales: $ 2001 Profits: $
2000 Sales: $ 2000 Profits: $

Stock Ticker: Subsidiary
Employees: 14,000
Fiscal Year Ends: 9/30

SALARIES/BENEFITS:
Pension Plan: ESOP Stock Plan: Profit Sharing: Top Exec. Salary: $393,000   Bonus: $225,000
Savings Plan: Y   Stock Purch. Plan: Second Exec. Salary: $199,238 Bonus: $80,000

OTHER THOUGHTS:
Apparent Top Female Officers: 2
Hot Spot for Advancement for Women/Minorities:

LOCATIONS: ("Y" = Yes)

West:	Southwest:	Midwest:	Southeast:	Northeast:	International:
Y	Y	Y	Y	Y	Y

MYLAN LABORATORIES INC

www.mylan.com

Industry Group Code: 325416   Ranks within this company's industry group: Sales: 3   Profits: 2

Insurance/HMO/PPO:	Drugs:	Equipment/Supplies:	Hospitals/Clinics:	Services:	Health Care:
Insurance:	Manufacturer: Y	Manufacturer:	Acute Care:	Diagnostics:	Home Health:
Managed Care:	Distributor: Y	Distributor:	Sub-Acute Care:	Labs/Testing:	Long-Term Care:
Utilization Mgmt.:	Specialty Pharm.: Y	Leasing/Finance:	Outpatient Surgery:	Staffing:	Physical Therapy:
Payment Proc.:	Vitamins/Nutri.:	Information Sys.:	Phys. Rehab. Center:	Waste Disposal:	Phys. Practice Mgmt.:
	Clinical Trials:		Psychiatric Clinics:	Specialty Services:	

TYPES OF BUSINESS:
Drugs-Generic
Branded Pharmaceutical Development

BRANDS/DIVISIONS/AFFILIATES:
Mylan Bertek Pharmaceuticals
Mylan Pharmaceuticals
Mylan Technologies
UDL Laboratories
Maxzide
Nifedipine ER
Digitek
King Pharmaceuticals

CONTACTS:
Note: Officers with more than one job title may be intentionally listed here more than once.

Robert J. Coury, CEO
Louis J. DeBone, Pres.
Louis J. DeBone, COO
Edward J. Borkowski, CFO
Collette Taylor, VP-Human Resources
John P. O'Donnell, Chief Scientific Officer
David B. Springgate, VP-IT
Mark Fitch, VP-Mfg. Oper.
Roger L. Foster, Sr. VP/General Counsel
Margaret A. McKenna, Chief Bus. Dev. Officer
Thomas S. Clark, VP-Corp. Affairs
J. Mark Morgan, VP-Finance
James J. Mauzey, Sr. VP/Pres., Mylan Bertek Pharmaceuticals
John P. O'Donnell, Exec. VP-Mylan Pharmaceuticals
Harry A. Korman, VP/Pres., UDL Laboratories
Sharad K. Govil, VP/Pres., Mylan Technologies
Milan Puskar, Chmn.

Phone: 724-514-1800   Fax: 724-514-1870
Toll-Free:
Address: 1500 Corporate Dr., Ste. 400, Canonsburg, PA 15317 US

GROWTH PLANS/SPECIAL FEATURES:

Mylan Laboratories, Inc. develops, markets and distributes generic and branded prescription drugs, operating through four primary subsidiaries: generics units Mylan Pharmacuticals, Mylan Technologies and UDL Laboratories, and branded pharmaceuticals company Mylan Bertek Pharmaceuticals. Over 80% of Mylan's revenues relate to its generic products, with the company's portfolio covering a range of dosage forms including immediate- and extended-release oral tablets and capsules, as well as transdermal patches. The generics companies additionally repackage and market products in unit dose form for institutional customers. Among Mylan's generics are Nifedipine ER (equivalent to Procardia), used for the treatment of hypertension and angina, and Tizanidine Hydrochloride tablets (equivalent to Zanaflex), used as a short-acting drug for spasticity. The company recently announced FDA approval to market Levothyroxine Sodium tablets as a bioequivalent and therapeutically equivalent product to Levoxyl. In addition to generics, Mylan is engaged in developing and marketing branded pharmaceuticals through its Mylan Bertek Pharmaceuticals subsidiary. Mylan Bertek operates as a stand-alone proprietary pharmaceutical company with independent clinical development, sales and marketing efforts, and is intended to serve as a transitional company that will enable Mylan to grow from a dedicated generics manufacturer to a proprietary brand-based company. The company's branded portfolio includes Maxzide, Digitek and Nitrek for the treatment of various heart conditions and Avita, Mentax and Anticin for skin conditions. Components for drug delivery systems and dressings, including medical and wound care films, transdermal backing materials, release liners and skin-contact adhesive laminates, are developed by Mylan Technologies and used across company product lines. In July 2004, Mylan Laboratories and King Pharmaceuticals entered into a $4-billion stock-for-stock agreement, through which Mylan will acquire King and its portfolio of branded drugs and products in development. Pending regulatory approval, the transaction is anticipated to close by the end of 2004.

Mylan offers its employees stock options, life insurance and supplemental medical coverage.

FINANCIALS:
Sales and profits are in thousands of dollars—add 000 to get the full amount. Year 2004 note: Complete fiscal 2004 results were not available for all companies at press time. For this company, year 2004 is for 12 months.

2004 Sales: $1,374,617 (12 months)
2003 Sales: $1,269,200
2002 Sales: $1,104,100
2001 Sales: $846,700
2000 Sales: $790,100

2004 Profits: $334,609 (12 months)
2003 Profits: $272,400
2002 Profits: $260,300
2001 Profits: $37,100
2000 Profits: $154,200

Stock Ticker: MYL
Employees: 2,800
Fiscal Year Ends: 3/31

SALARIES/BENEFITS:
Pension Plan: ESOP Stock Plan: Profit Sharing: Y   Top Exec. Salary: $1,100,008   Bonus: $2,000,000
Savings Plan: Y   Stock Purch. Plan: Second Exec. Salary: $600,028   Bonus: $625,000

OTHER THOUGHTS:
Apparent Top Female Officers: 2
Hot Spot for Advancement for Women/Minorities:

LOCATIONS: ("Y" = Yes)
West:	Southwest:	Midwest:	Southeast:	Northeast:	International:
		Y	Y	Y	

Note: Financial information, benefits and other data can change quickly and may vary from those stated here.

NANOBIO CORPORATION

www.nanobio.com

Industry Group Code: 325414   Ranks within this company's industry group: Sales: Profits:

Insurance/HMO/PPO:	Drugs:	Equipment/Supplies:	Hospitals/Clinics:	Services:	Health Care:
Insurance:	Manufacturer: Y	Manufacturer:	Acute Care:	Diagnostics:	Home Health:
Managed Care:	Distributor:	Distributor:	Sub-Acute Care:	Labs/Testing:	Long-Term Care:
Utilization Mgmt.:	Specialty Pharm.:	Leasing/Finance:	Outpatient Surgery:	Staffing:	Physical Therapy:
Payment Proc.:	Vitamins/Nutri.:	Information Sys.:	Phys. Rehab. Center:	Waste Disposal:	Phys. Practice Mgmt.:
	Clinical Trials:		Psychiatric Clinics:	Specialty Services: Y	

TYPES OF BUSINESS:
Biological Pharmaceuticals
Antimicrobial Products
Nanoemulsion Technology

BRANDS/DIVISIONS/AFFILIATES:
NanoStat

CONTACTS:
Note: Officers with more than one job title may be intentionally listed here more than once.

James R. Nold, CFO
James R. Baker, Jr., Chief Science Officer
James R. Baker, Jr., Chmn.

Phone: 734-302-4000   Fax: 734-302-9150
Toll-Free:
Address: P.O. Box 8110, Ann Arbor, MI 48107 US

GROWTH PLANS/SPECIAL FEATURES:
NanoBio Corp. is a biopharmaceutical company whose mission is to develop and commercialize high-value, over-the-counter pharmaceutical products enabled by its patented NanoStat antimicrobial nanoemulsion technology. The technology's researcher/inventor is Dr. James R. Baker, Jr., the firm's Chief Science Officer. NanoBio's initial commercial product pipeline consists of eight promising pharmaceuticals. The two near-term NanoStat products, currently in advanced clinical development, are treatments for cold sores and nail fungus. Treatments for genital herpes, shingles and vaginal infection are in the final stages of preclinical development. At the exploratory stage are products that address the prevention of SARS, genital herpes virus transmission and AIDS transmission. The technology also has the potential for facilitating a wide range of additional products. The company owns a comprehensive portfolio of intellectual property rights that include patents, proprietary formulations and processes, confidential data and trademarks, which gives it a strong competitive advantage in introducing novel and efficacious antimicrobial products. The research resulting in these patents was performed over a period of five years at the University of Michigan Medical Center with funding from the Defense Advanced Research Programs Agency within the U.S. Department of Defense. These patents, related international patents and other University of Michigan nanoemulsion inventions and patent applications are licensed to NanoBio by the college on an exclusive, worldwide basis. NanoBio holds exclusive intellectual property rights for virucidal, fungicidal, sporicidal and bactericidal applications in a wide spectrum of products, including personal care products, medical products and anti-bioterrorism applications. In addition to the licensed portfolio of emulsion technology, NanoBio's research team continues to discover new applications, methods, processes and compositions of matters relating to the field of antimicrobial emulsions.

FINANCIALS:
Sales and profits are in thousands of dollars—add 000 to get the full amount. Year 2004 note: Complete fiscal 2004 results were not available for all companies at press time. For this company, year 2004 is for   months.

2004 Sales: $ (months)   2004 Profits: $ (months)
2003 Sales: $ 2003 Profits: $
2002 Sales: $ 2002 Profits: $
2001 Sales: $ 2001 Profits: $
2000 Sales: $ 2000 Profits: $

Stock Ticker: Private
Employees:
Fiscal Year Ends:

SALARIES/BENEFITS:
Pension Plan: ESOP Stock Plan: Profit Sharing: Top Exec. Salary: $ Bonus: $
Savings Plan: Stock Purch. Plan: Second Exec. Salary: $ Bonus: $

OTHER THOUGHTS:
Apparent Top Female Officers:
Hot Spot for Advancement for Women/Minorities:

LOCATIONS: ("Y" = Yes)
| West: | Southwest: | Midwest: Y | Southeast: | Northeast: | International: |

NATIONAL DENTEX CORP

www.nadx.com

Industry Group Code: 339113   Ranks within this company's industry group: Sales: 91   Profits: 84

Insurance/HMO/PPO:	Drugs:	Equipment/Supplies:		Hospitals/Clinics:	Services:		Health Care:	
Insurance:	Manufacturer:	Manufacturer:	Y	Acute Care:	Diagnostics:		Home Health:	
Managed Care:	Distributor:	Distributor:		Sub-Acute Care:	Labs/Testing:	Y	Long-Term Care:	
Utilization Mgmt.:	Specialty Pharm.:	Leasing/Finance:		Outpatient Surgery:	Staffing:		Physical Therapy:	
Payment Proc.:	Vitamins/Nutri.:	Information Sys.:		Phys. Rehab. Center:	Waste Disposal:		Phys. Practice Mgmt.:	
	Clinical Trials:			Psychiatric Clinics:	Specialty Services:			

TYPES OF BUSINESS:
Supplies-Dental
Dental Prosthetic Appliances
Dental Laboratories

BRANDS/DIVISIONS/AFFILIATES:
Salem Dental
Top Quality Partials
Midtown Dental
Thoele Dental
D.H. Baker Dental Laboratory

CONTACTS:
Note: Officers with more than one job title may be intentionally listed here more than once.
David L. Brown, CEO
David L. Brown, Pres.
Richard F. Becker, Jr., CFO
Lynn D. Dine, VP-Research & Dev.
Richard G. Mariacher, VP-Tech. Svcs.
James F. Dodd, III, VP-Corp. Dev.
Richard F. Becker, Jr., VP-Investor Rel.
Richard F. Becker, Jr., Treas.
Donald E. Merz, Sr. VP
Arthur B. Chambagne, Group VP
Eloy V. Sepulveda, Group VP
Wayne M. Coll, Corp. Controller
David V. Harkins, Chmn.

Phone: 508-358-4422   **Fax:** 508-358-6199
Toll-Free:
Address: 526 Boston Post Rd., Wayland, MA 01778 US

GROWTH PLANS/SPECIAL FEATURES:
National Dentex Corporation designs, manufactures, markets and sells custom dental prosthetic appliances such as crowns, bridges and dentures. The company owns and operates 40 dental laboratories consisting of 38 full-service labs and two branch labs located in 29 states. National Dentex's products are produced by trained technicians working primarily with work orders and cases (consisting of impressions, models and occlusal registrations of a patient's teeth) provided by the over 20,000 dentists in the company's customer base. Each of the company's local dental laboratories markets and sells its products through its own direct sales force. The branch labs are smaller than the main laboratories and thus offer fewer products. When one of the branches is unable to fill an order, it sends it on to one of the full-service laboratories. National Dentex's products are grouped into three main categories: restorative products (crowns and bridges), reconstructive products (dentures) and cosmetic products (veneers and crowns). The company has used funds raised from its IPO in 1993 to pay for a steady stream of acquisitions since then, its most recent purchases including Salem Dental, Top Quality Partials, Midtown Dental and Thoele Dental in 2003, and D.H. Baker Dental Laboratory, in Traverse City, Michigan, in August 2004.

The company offers employees medical, dental and life insurance, as well as educational assistance.

FINANCIALS:
Sales and profits are in thousands of dollars—add 000 to get the full amount. Year 2004 note: Complete fiscal 2004 results were not available for all companies at press time. For this company, year 2004 is for 9 months.

2004 Sales: $73,504 (9 months)	2004 Profits: $4,258 (9 months)	
2003 Sales: $99,274	2003 Profits: $5,757	**Stock Ticker:** NADX
2002 Sales: $95,200	2002 Profits: $5,900	Employees: 1,621
2001 Sales: $85,700	2001 Profits: $6,000	Fiscal Year Ends: 12/31
2000 Sales: $75,700	2000 Profits: $6,000	

SALARIES/BENEFITS:
Pension Plan:	ESOP Stock Plan:	Profit Sharing:	Top Exec. Salary: $273,385	Bonus: $65,000
Savings Plan: Y	Stock Purch. Plan: Y		Second Exec. Salary: $169,192	Bonus: $70,812

OTHER THOUGHTS:
Apparent Top Female Officers:
Hot Spot for Advancement for Women/Minorities:

LOCATIONS: ("Y" = Yes)
West:	Southwest:	Midwest:	Southeast:	Northeast:	International:
Y	Y	Y	Y	Y	

NATIONAL HEALTHCARE CORP

www.nhccare.com

Industry Group Code: 623110   **Ranks within this company's industry group:** Sales: 8   Profits: 5

Insurance/HMO/PPO:	Drugs:	Equipment/Supplies:	Hospitals/Clinics:		Services:		Health Care:	
Insurance:	Manufacturer:	Manufacturer:	Acute Care:		Diagnostics:		Home Health:	Y
Managed Care:	Distributor:	Distributor:	Sub-Acute Care:	Y	Labs/Testing:		Long-Term Care:	Y
Utilization Mgmt.:	Specialty Pharm.: Y	Leasing/Finance:	Outpatient Surgery:		Staffing:		Physical Therapy:	Y
Payment Proc.:	Vitamins/Nutri.:	Information Sys.:	Phys. Rehab. Center:	Y	Waste Disposal:		Phys. Practice Mgmt.:	
	Clinical Trials:		Psychiatric Clinics:		Specialty Services:	Y		

TYPES OF BUSINESS:
Long-Term & Home Health Care
Rehabilitative Services
Pharmacy Operations
Managed Care Contracts
Medical Specialty Units
Assisted Living Projects
Nutritional Support Services

BRANDS/DIVISIONS/AFFILIATES:
National Health Investors, Inc.
National Health Realty, Inc.

CONTACTS:
Note: Officers with more than one job title may be intentionally listed here more than once.
Robert G. Adams, CEO
Robert G. Adams, Pres.
David L. Lassiter, Human Resources
Richard F. LaRoche, Jr., General Counsel
Steven A. Strawn, VP-Oper.
Kenneth D. DenBesten, VP-Finance
Joanne G. Batey, VP-Home Care
D. Gerald Coggin, VP-Gov't & Rehabilitative Services
Julia W. Powell, VP-Patient Services
Richard F. LaRoche, Jr., Corp. Sec.
W. Andrew Adams, Chmn.

Phone: 615-890-2020   **Fax:** 615-890-0123
Toll-Free:
Address: 100 Vine St., Murfreesboro, TN 37130 US

GROWTH PLANS/SPECIAL FEATURES:
National HealthCare Corporation (NHC) operates long-term health care centers and home health care programs primarily in the southeastern and midwestern regions of the United States. Approximately 90% of the company's revenue comes from its health care services, with the remainder coming from its National Health Realty and National Health Investors subsidiaries. NHC's health services can be divided into seven segments: long-term health care centers, home care programs, rehabilitative services, medical specialty units, pharmacy operations, assisted living projects and managed care contracts. The firm services 76 long-term health care centers, 32 home care programs, six independent living centers and assisted living centers at 19 locations. NHC also maintains specialized care units such as Alzheimer's disease care units, sub-acute nursing units and a number of in-house pharmacies. Similar specialty units and freestanding projects are under development or consideration at a number of NHC's centers. The company's health care centers provide sub-acute, skilled and intermediate nursing and rehabilitative care, including physical, occupational and speech therapies. Most of the company's retirement centers are constructed adjacent to NHC's health care properties. Apart from its health care services, NHC is engaged in nutritional support services and advisory services businesses.

FINANCIALS:
Sales and profits are in thousands of dollars—add 000 to get the full amount. Year 2004 note: Complete fiscal 2004 results were not available for all companies at press time. For this company, year 2004 is for 9 months.

2004 Sales: $370,797 (9 months)	2004 Profits: $15,195 (9 months)	**Stock Ticker:** NHC
2003 Sales: $472,864	2003 Profits: $19,952	**Employees:** 12,000
2002 Sales: $407,400	2002 Profits: $16,400	**Fiscal Year Ends:** 12/31
2001 Sales: $378,400	2001 Profits: $13,200	
2000 Sales: $462,400	2000 Profits: $10,200	

SALARIES/BENEFITS:
Pension Plan:	ESOP Stock Plan: Y	Profit Sharing:	Top Exec. Salary: $140,194	Bonus: $461,600
Savings Plan: Y	Stock Purch. Plan:		Second Exec. Salary: $115,105	Bonus: $70,560

OTHER THOUGHTS:
Apparent Top Female Officers: 2
Hot Spot for Advancement for Women/Minorities:

LOCATIONS: ("Y" = Yes)
West:	Southwest:	Midwest:	Southeast:	Northeast:	International:
		Y	Y	Y	

NATIONAL HOME HEALTH CARE CORP

www.nhhc.net

Industry Group Code: 621610 Ranks within this company's industry group: Sales: 12 Profits: 9

Insurance/HMO/PPO:	Drugs:	Equipment/Supplies:	Hospitals/Clinics:	Services:		Health Care:	
Insurance:	Manufacturer:	Manufacturer:	Acute Care:	Diagnostics:		Home Health:	Y
Managed Care:	Distributor:	Distributor:	Sub-Acute Care:	Labs/Testing:		Long-Term Care:	
Utilization Mgmt.:	Specialty Pharm.:	Leasing/Finance:	Outpatient Surgery:	Staffing:	Y	Physical Therapy:	Y
Payment Proc.:	Vitamins/Nutri.:	Information Sys.:	Phys. Rehab. Center:	Waste Disposal:		Phys. Practice Mgmt.:	
	Clinical Trials:		Psychiatric Clinics:	Specialty Services:	Y		

TYPES OF BUSINESS:
Home Health Care
Disease Management Services
Physical, Occupational & Speech Therapies
Staffing Services
Medical Social Services
Mental Health Services

BRANDS/DIVISIONS/AFFILIATES:
Health Acquisition Corp.
New England Home Care, Inc.
Impressive Staffing Corp.
New Jersey Staffing Works Corp.
Allen Health Care
Accredited Health Services, Inc.
Connecticut Staffing Works Corp.
Medical Resources Home Health Corp.

CONTACTS:
Note: Officers with more than one job title may be intentionally listed here more than once.
Steven Fialkow, CEO
Steven Fialkow, Pres.
Robert P. Heller, CFO
Robert P. Heller, Treas.
Frederick H. Fialkow, Chmn.

Phone: 914-722-9000   Fax: 914-722-9239
Toll-Free:
Address: 700 White Plains Rd., Ste. 275, Scarsdale, NY 10583 US

GROWTH PLANS/SPECIAL FEATURES:
National Home Health Care Corporation (NHHC) is a provider of home health care services through seven operating subsidiaries: Health Acquisition Corp. (which operates in New York), New England Home Care, Inc. (operating in Connecticut), Accredited Health Services, Inc. (New Jersey), Connecticut Staffing Works Corp., Impressive Staffing Corp. (New York), New Jersey Staffing Works Corp. and Medical Resources Home Health Corp. (Massachusetts). Health Acquisition Corp., operating as Allen Health Care, provides its services through registered nurses, personal care aides, home health aides and homemakers. All personnel are licensed or agency-certified and can be engaged on a full-time, part-time or live-in basis. New England Home Care is Medicare-certified and provides services including skilled nursing; physical, occupational and speech therapies; medical social services; and home health aide services. The company also offers specialty services such as mental health and wellness, perinatal/high-risk pregnancy and disease management. Accredited Health Services provides home health aide services. Connecticut Staffing Works conducts health care staffing operations, providing temporary staffing to hospitals, skilled nursing facilities, home health organizations and schools and other institutions. Additional subsidiaries conduct health care staffing operations in various states. The company's main customers are federal and state-funded public assistance programs such as Medicare and Medicaid, insurance companies and private parties. NHHC also derives revenues from subcontracts with certified home health care agencies and long-term health care provider programs.

FINANCIALS:
Sales and profits are in thousands of dollars—add 000 to get the full amount. Year 2004 note: Complete fiscal 2004 results were not available for all companies at press time. For this company, year 2004 is for 12 months.

2004 Sales: $94,592 (12 months)   2004 Profits: $4,720 (12 months)
2003 Sales: $97,200   2003 Profits: $5,800
2002 Sales: $82,200   2002 Profits: $5,300
2001 Sales: $74,500   2001 Profits: $4,200
2000 Sales: $55,600   2000 Profits: $4,100

Stock Ticker: NHHC
Employees: 3,350
Fiscal Year Ends: 7/31

SALARIES/BENEFITS:
Pension Plan: ESOP Stock Plan: Profit Sharing: Top Exec. Salary: $398,612   Bonus: $208,158
Savings Plan: Y Stock Purch. Plan: Second Exec. Salary: $335,075 Bonus: $190,438

OTHER THOUGHTS:
Apparent Top Female Officers:
Hot Spot for Advancement for Women/Minorities:

LOCATIONS: ("Y" = Yes)
West:	Southwest:	Midwest:	Southeast:	Northeast:	International:
				Y	

NATIONAL MEDICAL HEALTH CARD SYSTEMS INC

www.nmhc.com

Industry Group Code: 522320A   Ranks within this company's industry group: Sales: 5   Profits: 5

Insurance/HMO/PPO:	Drugs:	Equipment/Supplies:	Hospitals/Clinics:	Services:	Health Care:
Insurance:	Manufacturer:	Manufacturer:	Acute Care:	Diagnostics:	Home Health:
Managed Care:	Distributor:	Distributor:	Sub-Acute Care:	Labs/Testing:	Long-Term Care:
Utilization Mgmt.: Y	Specialty Pharm.: Y	Leasing/Finance:	Outpatient Surgery:	Staffing:	Physical Therapy:
Payment Proc.:	Vitamins/Nutri.:	Information Sys.: Y	Phys. Rehab. Center:	Waste Disposal:	Phys. Practice Mgmt.:
	Clinical Trials:		Psychiatric Clinics:	Specialty Services: Y	

TYPES OF BUSINESS:
Pharmacy Benefits Management
Mail-Order & Specialty Pharmacies
Health Information Systems

BRANDS/DIVISIONS/AFFILIATES:
Integrail, Inc.
NMHCRX Mail Order, Inc.
Ascend Specialty Pharmacy Services, Inc.
New Mountain Partners

CONTACTS:
Note: Officers with more than one job title may be intentionally listed here more than once.

James F. Smith, CEO
James F. Smith, Pres.
Stuart F. Fleischer, CFO
Tery Baskin, Chief Mktg. Officer
Bill Masters, CIO
Jonathan I. Friedman, VP-Legal Affairs & Compliance
Tery Baskin, Exec. VP-Bus. Dev.
David Gershen, Treas.
Agnes Hall, Pres., NMHCRX
Mark A. Adkison, Pres., Ascend Specialty Pharmacy Services
James Bigl, Chmn.

Phone: 516-626-0007   Fax: 516-484-0679
Toll-Free: 800-251-3883
Address: 26 Harbor Park Dr., Port Washington, NY 11050 US

GROWTH PLANS/SPECIAL FEATURES:
National Medical Health Card Systems, Inc. (NMHC) provides pharmacy benefit management (PBM) services for corporations, labor organizations, third-party administrators, managed care companies and local governments. Its programs are designed to assist pharmacy benefit plan sponsors by monitoring the cost and quality of prescription drugs and related services. The company's program components are integrated and managed through proprietary system protocols. In addition, the company operates a health information company through subsidiary Integrail, Inc.; a mail-service pharmacy through subsidiary NMHCRX Mail Order, Inc.; and a specialty pharmacy through subsidiary Ascend Specialty Pharmacy Services, Inc. In recent news, NMHC completed an $80-million strategic investment from New Mountain Partners, a New York-based private equity investment fund, which now owns 66% of NMHC's outstanding equity. The cash raised from the deal will be directed towards acquisition opportunities in the PBM and specialty pharmacy sectors. In other news, the company was ranked number six on Fortune Magazine's 2004 list of America's 100 Fastest Growing Companies.

FINANCIALS:
Sales and profits are in thousands of dollars—add 000 to get the full amount. Year 2004 note: Complete fiscal 2004 results were not available for all companies at press time. For this company, year 2004 is for 12 months.

2004 Sales: $651,098 (12 months)	2004 Profits: $7,953 (12 months)	Stock Ticker: NMHC
2003 Sales: $573,300	2003 Profits: $6,400	Employees: 394
2002 Sales: $459,800	2002 Profits: $4,500	Fiscal Year Ends: 6/30
2001 Sales: $272,100	2001 Profits: $1,200	
2000 Sales: $172,300	2000 Profits: $1,600	

SALARIES/BENEFITS:
Pension Plan: ESOP Stock Plan: Profit Sharing: Top Exec. Salary: $343,612   Bonus: $357,500
Savings Plan: Stock Purch. Plan: Second Exec. Salary: $326,669 Bonus: $753,500

OTHER THOUGHTS:
Apparent Top Female Officers: 1
Hot Spot for Advancement for Women/Minorities:

LOCATIONS: ("Y" = Yes)
West:	Southwest:	Midwest:	Southeast:	Northeast:	International:
	Y		Y	Y	

NEIGHBORCARE INC

www.neighborcare.com

Industry Group Code: 446110A   Ranks within this company's industry group: Sales: 3   Profits: 4

Insurance/HMO/PPO:	Drugs:	Equipment/Supplies:	Hospitals/Clinics:	Services:	Health Care:
Insurance:	Manufacturer:	Manufacturer:	Acute Care:	Diagnostics:	Home Health:
Managed Care:	Distributor:	Distributor:	Sub-Acute Care:	Labs/Testing:	Long-Term Care:
Utilization Mgmt.:	Specialty Pharm.: Y	Leasing/Finance:	Outpatient Surgery:	Staffing:	Physical Therapy:
Payment Proc.:	Vitamins/Nutri.:	Information Sys.:	Phys. Rehab. Center:	Waste Disposal:	Phys. Practice Mgmt.:
	Clinical Trials:		Psychiatric Clinics:	Specialty Services: Y	

TYPES OF BUSINESS:
Pharmacy & Medical Supply Services
Consulting Services
Group Purchasing Programs

BRANDS/DIVISIONS/AFFILIATES:
Genesis Health Ventures, Inc.
Tidewater Healthcare Shared Services Group, Inc.
Quest Total Care Pharmacy
Medicine Centre, LLC
NeighborCare At Home

CONTACTS: Note: Officers with more than one job title may be intentionally listed here more than once.
John J. Arlotta, CEO
John J. Arlotta, Pres.
Robert A. Smith, COO
Richard W. Hunt, Sr. VP/CFO
Steve Duvall, Sr. VP-Sales & Acct. Mgmt.
Kathleen F. Ayres, Sr. VP-Human Resources
Walt Meffert, Sr. VP-IT
John F. Gaither, Jr., Sr. VP/General Counsel
Tim Stefan, Pres.-Tidewater Group Purchasing
Michael Azzaro, Sr. VP-NeighborCare At Home
Charles P. Feeney, Sr. VP-Purchasing
Nancy Losben, Sr. VP-Clinical Services
John J. Arlotta, Chmn.
J. Robert Dunlap, Sr. VP-Materials Mgmt. & Logistics

Phone: 410-528-7300   Fax: 410-528-7473
Toll-Free:
Address: 601 E. Pratt St., 3rd Fl., Baltimore, MD 21202 US

GROWTH PLANS/SPECIAL FEATURES:

NeighborCare, Inc., a spin-off of Genesis Health Ventures, Inc., is a provider of institutional pharmacy services, supplying approximately 246,000 beds in long-term care facilities in 32 states and the District of Columbia. Its operations consist of 62 institutional pharmacies, 32 community-based professional retail pharmacies and 20 on-site pharmacies, which are located in customers' facilities and serve only customers of that facility. In addition, it operates 16 home infusion, respiratory and medical equipment distribution centers. The company's pharmacies maintain 24-hour, seven-days-a-week, on-call service for emergency dispensing and delivery or for consultation with the facility's staff or the resident's attending physician. NeighborCare also owns and operates Tidewater Healthcare Shared Services Group, Inc., one of the largest long-term care group purchasing companies in the country. Tidewater provides purchasing and shared service programs specially designed to meet the needs of elder care centers and other long-term care facilities. In 2004, NeighborCare acquired Quest Total Care Pharmacy and Medicine Centre, LLC, long-term care pharmacies serving skilled nursing and assisted living facilities in Texas and Connecticut, respectively.

NeighborCare offers its workforce tuition reimbursement, employee assistance and comprehensive medical and dental plans.

FINANCIALS: Sales and profits are in thousands of dollars—add 000 to get the full amount. Year 2004 note: Complete fiscal 2004 results were not available for all companies at press time. For this company, year 2004 is for 9 months.

2004 Sales: $1,066,134 (9 months)   2004 Profits: $-4,272   (9 months)
2003 Sales: $2,649,000   2003 Profits: $32,700   Stock Ticker: NCRX
2002 Sales: $2,623,700   2002 Profits: $72,800   Employees: 6,000
2001 Sales: $2,569,900   2001 Profits: $292,600   Fiscal Year Ends: 9/30
2000 Sales: $2,433,900   2000 Profits: $-840,900

SALARIES/BENEFITS:
Pension Plan: ESOP Stock Plan: Profit Sharing: Y   Top Exec. Salary: $850,000   Bonus: $1,221,410
Savings Plan: Y   Stock Purch. Plan: Second Exec. Salary: $400,001   Bonus: $715,875

OTHER THOUGHTS:
Apparent Top Female Officers: 2
Hot Spot for Advancement for Women/Minorities:

LOCATIONS: ("Y" = Yes)
West:	Southwest:	Midwest:	Southeast:	Northeast:	International:
Y	Y	Y	Y	Y	

NEKTAR THERAPEUTICS

www.nektar.com

Industry Group Code: 339113 Ranks within this company's industry group: Sales: 88 Profits: 134

Insurance/HMO/PPO:	Drugs:	Equipment/Supplies:	Hospitals/Clinics:	Services:	Health Care:
Insurance:	Manufacturer:	Manufacturer: Y	Acute Care:	Diagnostics:	Home Health:
Managed Care:	Distributor:	Distributor:	Sub-Acute Care:	Labs/Testing:	Long-Term Care:
Utilization Mgmt.:	Specialty Pharm.:	Leasing/Finance:	Outpatient Surgery:	Staffing:	Physical Therapy:
Payment Proc.:	Vitamins/Nutri.:	Information Sys.:	Phys. Rehab. Center:	Waste Disposal:	Phys. Practice Mgmt.:
	Clinical Trials:		Psychiatric Clinics:	Specialty Services:	

TYPES OF BUSINESS:
Equipment-Deep Lung Drug Delivery System
PEG-Based Delivery Systems
Molecular and Particle Engineering Technology

BRANDS/DIVISIONS/AFFILIATES:
Inhale Therapeutic Systems, Inc.
Bradford Particle Design
Shearwater Corp.

CONTACTS:
Note: Officers with more than one job title may be intentionally listed here more than once.
Ajit S. Gill, CEO
Ajit S. Gill, Pres.
Ajay Bansal, CFO
Elizabeth Frisby, VP-Human Resources
John S. Patton, Chief Scientific Officer
Brigid Makes, VP-Oper. Mgmt.
Christopher J. Searcy, VP-Corp. Dev.
Robert J. Gerety, VP-Proprietary Products Group
Michael D. Bentley, VP-Research, Molecule Eng.
Andy Clark, Chief Scientist/Sr. Fellow
Peter York, Chief Scientist
Robert B. Chess, Chmn.

Phone: 650-631-3100   Fax: 650-631-3150
Toll-Free:
Address: 150 Industrial Rd., San Carlos, CA 94070 US

GROWTH PLANS/SPECIAL FEATURES:
Nektar Therapeutics is the product of three pharmaceutical companies: Shearwater Corp., Inhale Therapeutic Systems, Inc. and Bradford Particle Design. The company's goal is to help its pharmaceutical and biotechnology partners solve complex development challenges to create novel therapeutics. Nektar uses three distinct methods to achieve this goal: molecule engineering, particle engineering and delivery solutions. The molecular engineering division encompasses a suite of technologies, including advanced PEGylation and PEG-based delivery systems like hydrogels and solubilizing agents. These technologies can improve drug performance by optimizing pharmacokinetics, increasing bioavailability and protecting the drugs from immune response. The particle engineering division uses its expertise in pulmonary particle technology and supercritical fluid technology to design and manufacture optimal drug particles. In addition, the unit uses proprietary particle engineering methods designed to obtain precision and consistency in particle formulation; improve dissolution for poorly soluble compounds; and increase bioavailability through high-surface-area particles. The delivery solutions division is focused on the formulation of molecules for multiple delivery platforms, with a special focus on pulmonary delivery of both large- and small-molecule drugs. Nektar has five approved products on the market, with another 15 in various stages of clinical trials. Most of these are collaborations with other pharmaceutical companies, including Amgen, Celltech, Pfizer, Roche and Schering-Plough.

Nektar Therapeutics offers its employees medical, dental, vision and life insurance, flexible spending accounts and tuition reimbursement.

FINANCIALS:
Sales and profits are in thousands of dollars—add 000 to get the full amount. Year 2004 note: Complete fiscal 2004 results were not available for all companies at press time. For this company, year 2004 is for 9 months.

2004 Sales: $82,904 (9 months)	2004 Profits: $-82,616 (9 months)	Stock Ticker: NKTR
2003 Sales: $106,257	2003 Profits: $-65,890	Employees: 668
2002 Sales: $94,800	2002 Profits: $-107,500	Fiscal Year Ends: 12/31
2001 Sales: $77,500	2001 Profits: $-250,000	
2000 Sales: $51,600	2000 Profits: $-97,400	

SALARIES/BENEFITS:
Pension Plan: Y   ESOP Stock Plan: Profit Sharing: Top Exec. Salary: $474,461   Bonus: $250,903
Savings Plan: Y   Stock Purch. Plan: Y   Second Exec. Salary: $321,000   Bonus: $170,067

OTHER THOUGHTS:
Apparent Top Female Officers: 2
Hot Spot for Advancement for Women/Minorities:

LOCATIONS: ("Y" = Yes)
West:	Southwest:	Midwest:	Southeast:	Northeast:	International:
Y			Y		Y

NEW YORK CITY HEALTH AND HOSPITALS CORPORATION

www.ci.nyc.ny.us

Industry Group Code: 622110   Ranks within this company's industry group: Sales: 13   Profits:

Insurance/HMO/PPO:	Drugs:	Equipment/Supplies:	Hospitals/Clinics:		Services:		Health Care:	
Insurance: Managed Care: Y Utilization Mgmt.: Payment Proc.:	Manufacturer: Distributor: Specialty Pharm.: Vitamins/Nutri.: Clinical Trials:	Manufacturer: Distributor: Leasing/Finance: Information Sys.:	Acute Care: Sub-Acute Care: Outpatient Surgery: Phys. Rehab. Center: Psychiatric Clinics:	Y Y	Diagnostics: Labs/Testing: Staffing: Waste Disposal: Specialty Services:		Home Health: Long-Term Care: Physical Therapy: Phys. Practice Mgmt.:	Y Y

TYPES OF BUSINESS:
Hospitals-General
Community Health Clinics
HMO
Long-Term Care Facilities
Home Health Care

BRANDS/DIVISIONS/AFFILIATES:
MetroPlus
HHC Health and Home Care
Harlem Hospital Center

CONTACTS:
Note: Officers with more than one job title may be intentionally listed here more than once.
Benjamin Chu, CEO
Benjamin Chu, Pres.
Alan D. Aviles, General Counsel
Frank J. Cirillo, VP-Oper.
LaRay Brown, VP-Planning & Community Health
Marlene Zurack, VP-Finance
Edwin Mendez-Santiago, Vice-Chmn.
Van Dunn, Sr. VP-Medical & Professional Affairs
Charlynn Goins, Chmn.

Phone: 212-788-3321   Fax: 212-788-0040
Toll-Free:
Address: 125 Worth St., Ste. 514, New York, NY 10013 US

GROWTH PLANS/SPECIAL FEATURES:
New York City Health and Hospitals Corporations (HHC) operates 11 acute care hospitals, more than 100 community health clinics, long-term care facilities, a home health care agency and MetroPlus, a health maintenance organization. HHC provides health care to all five boroughs of New York, serving 1.3 million New Yorkers annually and caring for nearly 500,000 people with no health insurance. The firm also runs medical stations in New York correctional facilities. HHC Health and Home Care, a division of HHC, is a home health agency for Manhattan, Queens and the Bronx. Services include nursing, physical therapy, speech-language pathology, housekeepers, home health aides, personal care workers and medical supply. HHC is beginning a major modernization and expansion of Harlem Hospital Center that will last five years and cost $225.5 million. The changes will expand the hospital as well as renovate 183,000 square feet of existing space. In the course of the renovation, three antiquated and obsolete buildings will be demolished.

FINANCIALS:
Sales and profits are in thousands of dollars—add 000 to get the full amount. Year 2004 note: Complete fiscal 2004 results were not available for all companies at press time. For this company, year 2004 is for months.

2004 Sales: $ (months)	2004 Profits: $ (months)	
2003 Sales: $4,200,000	2003 Profits: $	Stock Ticker: Government-Owned
2002 Sales: $4,300,000	2002 Profits: $	Employees:
2001 Sales: $	2001 Profits: $	Fiscal Year Ends: 6/30
2000 Sales: $	2000 Profits: $	

SALARIES/BENEFITS:
Pension Plan:	ESOP Stock Plan:	Profit Sharing:	Top Exec. Salary: $	Bonus: $
Savings Plan:	Stock Purch. Plan:		Second Exec. Salary: $	Bonus: $

OTHER THOUGHTS:
Apparent Top Female Officers: 2
Hot Spot for Advancement for Women/Minorities:

LOCATIONS: ("Y" = Yes)
West:	Southwest:	Midwest:	Southeast:	Northeast:	International:
				Y	

NEW YORK HEALTH CARE INC

www.nyhc.com

Industry Group Code: 621610 **Ranks within this company's industry group:** Sales: 13 Profits: 13

Insurance/HMO/PPO:	Drugs:	Equipment/Supplies:	Hospitals/Clinics:	Services:	Health Care:
Insurance:	Manufacturer: Y	Manufacturer:	Acute Care:	Diagnostics:	Home Health: Y
Managed Care:	Distributor:	Distributor:	Sub-Acute Care:	Labs/Testing:	Long-Term Care:
Utilization Mgmt.:	Specialty Pharm.:	Leasing/Finance:	Outpatient Surgery:	Staffing:	Physical Therapy:
Payment Proc.:	Vitamins/Nutri.:	Information Sys.:	Phys. Rehab. Center:	Waste Disposal:	Phys. Practice Mgmt.:
	Clinical Trials:		Psychiatric Clinics:	Specialty Services:	

TYPES OF BUSINESS:
Home Health Care
Nursing & Assisted Living Services
Biotherapeutic Agents

BRANDS/DIVISIONS/AFFILIATES:
BioBalance Corp.
PROBACTRIX

CONTACTS:
Note: Officers with more than one job title may be intentionally listed here more than once.
Jerry Braun, CEO
Jerry Braun, Pres.
Jacob Rosenberg, COO
Jacob Rosenberg, CFO
Ben Wilhelm, Dir.-Info. Svcs.
Anthony Acquaviva, Comptroller
Jacob Rosenberg, Corp. Sec.
Dennis O'Donnell, Pres., BioBalance Corp.

Phone: 718-375-6700 **Fax:** 718-375-1555
Toll-Free:
Address: 1850 McDonald Ave., Brooklyn, NY 11223 US

GROWTH PLANS/SPECIAL FEATURES:
New York Health Care, Inc. operates through two business segments: a licensed home health care agency that provides nursing and assisted living services to homebound clients; and a manufacturer and marketer of proprietary biotherapeutic agents for the treatment of gastrointestinal disorders. Home care services include meal preparation, light housekeeping, standard nursing services, physical therapy and medicine administration. The firm's staff is fluent in Spanish, Mandarin and Cantonese Chinese, Yiddish and Russian. New York Health Care is approved by the New York State Department of Health to train home health aides, by the New York Department of Social Services to train personal care aides and by the Board of Nursing in New Jersey to train certified home health aides. The biotherapeutic segment works through the firm's BioBalance Corporation subsidiary, which was acquired in 2003. BioBalance is a development-stage specialty pharmaceutical company focused on the development of patented biotherapeutic agents for gastrointestinal disorders. Its sole product, PROBACTRIX, is under review by the FDA to be recognized as a medicinal food, which has much less stringent regulations than a drug. In recent news, the firm announced plans to sell off all of its home health business for $2.7 million to a company controlled by the current CEO and COO, who have both tendered their resignation from the company. The sale is subject to a number of conditions including obtaining shareholder and regulatory approvals.

FINANCIALS:
Sales and profits are in thousands of dollars—add 000 to get the full amount. Year 2004 note: Complete fiscal 2004 results were not available for all companies at press time. For this company, year 2004 is for 6 months.

2004 Sales: $23,677 (6 months)	2004 Profits: $-2,389 (6 months)	**Stock Ticker:** BBAL
2003 Sales: $45,060	2003 Profits: $-22,052	Employees: 1,848
2002 Sales: $38,900	2002 Profits: $ 400	Fiscal Year Ends: 12/31
2001 Sales: $34,300	2001 Profits: $ 400	
2000 Sales: $29,400	2000 Profits: $-1,200	

SALARIES/BENEFITS:
Pension Plan:	ESOP Stock Plan:	Profit Sharing:	Top Exec. Salary: $333,872	Bonus: $35,000
Savings Plan: Y	Stock Purch. Plan:		Second Exec. Salary: $257,557	Bonus: $30,000

OTHER THOUGHTS:
Apparent Top Female Officers:
Hot Spot for Advancement for Women/Minorities:

LOCATIONS: ("Y" = Yes)
West:	Southwest:	Midwest:	Southeast:	Northeast: Y	International:

NEW YORK-PRESBYTERIAN HEALTHCARE SYSTEM

www.nypsystem.org

Industry Group Code: 622110   Ranks within this company's industry group: Sales: 6   Profits:

Insurance/HMO/PPO:	Drugs:	Equipment/Supplies:	Hospitals/Clinics:		Services:		Health Care:	
Insurance:	Manufacturer:	Manufacturer:	Acute Care:	Y	Diagnostics:		Home Health:	
Managed Care:	Distributor:	Distributor:	Sub-Acute Care:	Y	Labs/Testing:		Long-Term Care:	Y
Utilization Mgmt.:	Specialty Pharm.:	Leasing/Finance:	Outpatient Surgery:	Y	Staffing:		Physical Therapy:	Y
Payment Proc.:	Vitamins/Nutri.:	Information Sys.:	Phys. Rehab. Center:	Y	Waste Disposal:		Phys. Practice Mgmt.:	
	Clinical Trials:		Psychiatric Clinics:		Specialty Services:	Y		

TYPES OF BUSINESS:
Hospitals
Nursing Homes

BRANDS/DIVISIONS/AFFILIATES:
New York-Presbyterian Hospital

CONTACTS: Note: Officers with more than one job title may be intentionally listed here more than once.
Herbert Pardes, CEO
Herbert Pardes, Pres.
Richard D'Aquila, Sr. VP/COO
Phyllis R.F. Lantos, Sr. VP/CFO/Treas.
David A. Feinberg, VP-Mktg.
G. Thomas Ferguson, Sr. VP-Human Resources
Thomas Corredine, VP-Info. Systems
Maxine Fass, Sr. VP/General Counsel
Emme Deland, Sr. VP-Strategic Dev.
Myrna A. Manners, VP-Public Affairs
Mark E. Laramore, VP-Finance
Michael A. Berman, Exec. VP/Hospital Dir.
Steven J. Corwin, Sr. VP/Chief Medical Officer
Steven Kurz, VP-Patient Accounts
John J. Mack, Chmn.
Jose Nunez, VP-Int'l

Phone: 212-305-2500   **Fax:** 212-746-8235
Toll-Free: 877-697-9355
Address: 525 E. 68th St., New York, NY 10021-4870 US

GROWTH PLANS/SPECIAL FEATURES:
The New York-Presbyterian Healthcare System is a not-for-profit partnership of top-quality hospitals, specialty institutes and continuing care centers serving New York, New Jersey and Connecticut. In total the system includes 33 hospitals, 15 nursing homes and three specialty institutes, all of which are affiliated with two Ivy League medical schools: Columbia University College of Physicians & Surgeons and Weill Medical College of Cornell University. The system had a combined 493,027 inpatient discharges last year, 5,154,529 outpatient visits and a total of 14,184 licensed beds. The system's flagship hospital and founder is New York-Presbyterian Hospital, which was formed in 1997 from the merger of The Presbyterian Hospital and The New York Hospital, the second oldest hospital in the United States, dating from 1771. New York-Presbyterian Hospital's five campuses are the primary teaching sites for both Columbia's and Cornell's medical colleges. The hospital has leading specialists in every field of medicine and several well-regarded centers of excellence, including AIDS care, aesthetic laser surgery, gene therapy, reproductive medicine, trauma, vascular medicine and women's health.

The New York-Presbyterian Healthcare System employs more than 2,500 volunteers through the New York Weil Cornell Center, the Columbia University Center and the Allen Pavilion. Volunteers are needed in every area, from ambulatory care clinics and radiology, to adult recreation, child literacy and food services. Volunteers enjoy various benefits including tax deductions, discounted theater tickets and a letter of commendation to future employers.

FINANCIALS: Sales and profits are in thousands of dollars—add 000 to get the full amount. Year 2004 note: Complete fiscal 2004 results were not available for all companies at press time. For this company, year 2004 is for ___ months.

2004 Sales: $ (months)   2004 Profits: $ (months)
2003 Sales: $7,060,000   2003 Profits: $
2002 Sales: $6,580,000   2002 Profits: $
2001 Sales: $ 2001 Profits: $
2000 Sales: $ 2000 Profits: $

Stock Ticker: Nonprofit
Employees: 53,562
Fiscal Year Ends:

SALARIES/BENEFITS:
| Pension Plan: | ESOP Stock Plan: | Profit Sharing: | Top Exec. Salary: $ | Bonus: $ |
| Savings Plan: | Stock Purch. Plan: | | Second Exec. Salary: $ | Bonus: $ |

OTHER THOUGHTS:
Apparent Top Female Officers: 4
Hot Spot for Advancement for Women/Minorities: Y

LOCATIONS: ("Y" = Yes)
West:	Southwest:	Midwest:	Southeast:	Northeast:	International:
				Y	

NMT MEDICAL INC

www.nmtmedical.com

Industry Group Code: 339113 **Ranks within this company's industry group:** Sales: 131 Profits: 112

Insurance/HMO/PPO:	Drugs:	Equipment/Supplies:	Hospitals/Clinics:	Services:	Health Care:
Insurance: Managed Care: Utilization Mgmt.: Payment Proc.:	Manufacturer: Distributor: Specialty Pharm.: Vitamins/Nutri.: Clinical Trials:	Manufacturer: Y Distributor: Leasing/Finance: Information Sys.:	Acute Care: Sub-Acute Care: Outpatient Surgery: Phys. Rehab. Center: Psychiatric Clinics:	Diagnostics: Labs/Testing: Staffing: Waste Disposal: Specialty Services:	Home Health: Long-Term Care: Physical Therapy: Phys. Practice Mgmt.:

TYPES OF BUSINESS:
Equipment-Surgery
Cardiovascular Devices
Neurosurgical Products

BRANDS/DIVISIONS/AFFILIATES:
STARFlex

CONTACTS:
Note: Officers with more than one job title may be intentionally listed here more than once.
John A. Ahern, CEO
John A. Ahern, Pres.
Richard E. Davis, VP/CFO
Geoff Fournie, Dir.-European Sales & Mktg.
Richard E. Davis, Corp. Sec.
John A. Ahern, Chmn.

Phone: 617-737-0930 **Fax:** 617-737-0924
Toll-Free: 800-666-6484
Address: 27 Wormwood St., Boston, MA 02210 US

GROWTH PLANS/SPECIAL FEATURES:
NMT Medical, Inc. designs, develops and markets innovative medical devices that allow non-surgical closure of defects in the walls of a heart. The company's products provide alternative approaches to existing complex treatments; shorten procedures, hospitalization and recovery times; and lower overall treatment costs. NMT's cardiovascular business unit provides the interventional cardiologist with proprietary, catheter-based implant technologies designed to minimize or prevent the risk of embolic events. The cardiovascular division also serves the pediatric interventional cardiologist with a broad range of cardiac septal repair implants delivered with non-surgical catheter techniques. The company's neurosciences division serves the needs of neurosurgeons with a wide range of implantable and disposable products, including cerebral spinal fluid shunts and external drainage products. STARFlex, the firm's newest implant, has a self-adjusting, flexible spring system that can automatically adjust to different shapes and locations of a defect, allowing the implant to lie flat against the septum. Its smaller-sized closing device allows physicians to leave a smaller amount of metal behind in the body.

FINANCIALS:
Sales and profits are in thousands of dollars—add 000 to get the full amount. Year 2004 note: Complete fiscal 2004 results were not available for all companies at press time. For this company, year 2004 is for 9 months.

2004 Sales: $16,441 (9 months)	2004 Profits: $-766 (9 months)	**Stock Ticker:** NMTI
2003 Sales: $22,961	2003 Profits: $-1,150	Employees: 101
2002 Sales: $25,000	2002 Profits: $11,100	Fiscal Year Ends: 12/31
2001 Sales: $39,200	2001 Profits: $19,200	
2000 Sales: $36,500	2000 Profits: $-9,600	

SALARIES/BENEFITS:
Pension Plan: ESOP Stock Plan: Profit Sharing: Top Exec. Salary: $350,000 Bonus: $90,000
Savings Plan: Y Stock Purch. Plan: Y   Second Exec. Salary: $246,875 Bonus: $91,000

OTHER THOUGHTS:
Apparent Top Female Officers:
Hot Spot for Advancement for Women/Minorities:

LOCATIONS: ("Y" = Yes)
West:	Southwest:	Midwest:	Southeast:	Northeast:	International:
				Y	

NOVAMED INC

www.novamed.com

Industry Group Code: 621490   Ranks within this company's industry group: Sales: 17   Profits: 14

Insurance/HMO/PPO:	Drugs:	Equipment/Supplies:		Hospitals/Clinics:		Services:		Health Care:	
Insurance:	Manufacturer:	Manufacturer:	Y	Acute Care:		Diagnostics:		Home Health:	
Managed Care:	Distributor:	Distributor:	Y	Sub-Acute Care:		Labs/Testing:		Long-Term Care:	
Utilization Mgmt.:	Specialty Pharm.:	Leasing/Finance:		Outpatient Surgery:	Y	Staffing:		Physical Therapy:	
Payment Proc.:	Vitamins/Nutri.:	Information Sys.:		Phys. Rehab. Center:		Waste Disposal:		Phys. Practice Mgmt.:	
	Clinical Trials:			Psychiatric Clinics:		Specialty Services:	Y		

TYPES OF BUSINESS:
Outpatient Surgery
Eye-Care Services
Laser Vision Correction
Corrective Lenses Labs
Eye-Care Products Distribution

BRANDS/DIVISIONS/AFFILIATES:
NovaMed Eyecare, Inc.

CONTACTS: Note: Officers with more than one job title may be intentionally listed here more than once.
Stephen J. Winjum, CEO
Stephen J. Winjum, Pres.
Scott T. Macomber, Exec. VP/CFO
John W. Lawrence, Jr., VP/General Counsel
E. Michele Vickery, Exec. VP-Oper.
Robert C. Goettling, Sr. VP-Corp. Dev.
John P. Hart, VP/Corp. Controller
Daniel S. Durrie, Dir.-Refractive Surgery
Frank L. Soppa, VP-Optical Services Group
Stephen J. Winjum, Chmn.

Phone: 312-664-4100 **Fax:** 312-664-4250
Toll-Free: 800-388-4133
Address: 980 N. Michigan Ave., Ste. 1620, Chicago, IL 60611 US

GROWTH PLANS/SPECIAL FEATURES:
NovaMed, Inc., formerly NovaMed Eyecare, Inc., is an owner and operator of ambulatory surgery centers (ASCs), with a focus on developing and operating ASCs in joint ownership with physicians. The company owns and operates 22 primarily practice-based ASCs. Most of these are single-specialty ophthalmic surgical facilities where eye-care professionals perform surgical procedures, primarily cataract and laser vision correction (LVC). NovaMed also provides excimer lasers and other services to eye-care professionals through fixed-site laser agreements. In addition, the company owns and operates an optical laboratory business that specializes in surfacing, finishing and distributing corrective eyeglass lenses, selling them to over 350 ophthalmologists, optometrists, opticians and optical retail chains. The company's recent name change reflects NovaMed's desire to expand its surgical facilities business into additional medical specialties, exploring opportunities to acquire ASCs offering differing types of medical specialties and to add new specialties to existing ASCs.

FINANCIALS: Sales and profits are in thousands of dollars—add 000 to get the full amount. Year 2004 note: Complete fiscal 2004 results were not available for all companies at press time. For this company, year 2004 is for 9 months.

2004 Sales: $47,098 (9 months)
2003 Sales: $55,506
2002 Sales: $53,800
2001 Sales: $70,100
2000 Sales: $67,800

2004 Profits: $3,240 (9 months)
2003 Profits: $3,491
2002 Profits: $ 300
2001 Profits: $-32,600
2000 Profits: $5,300

Stock Ticker: NOVA
Employees: 341
Fiscal Year Ends: 12/31

SALARIES/BENEFITS:
| Pension Plan: | ESOP Stock Plan: | Profit Sharing: | Top Exec. Salary: $343,269 | Bonus: $154,000 |
| Savings Plan: | Stock Purch. Plan: | | Second Exec. Salary: $237,308 | Bonus: $74,480 |

OTHER THOUGHTS:
Apparent Top Female Officers: 1
Hot Spot for Advancement for Women/Minorities:

LOCATIONS: ("Y" = Yes)
West:	Southwest:	Midwest:	Southeast:	Northeast:	International:
Y	Y	Y	Y	Y	

NOVAMETRIX MEDICAL SYSTEMS INC

www.novametrix.com

Industry Group Code: 339113   **Ranks within this company's industry group:** Sales: Profits:

Insurance/HMO/PPO:	Drugs:	Equipment/Supplies:		Hospitals/Clinics:	Services:		Health Care:
Insurance: Managed Care: Utilization Mgmt.: Payment Proc.:	Manufacturer: Distributor: Specialty Pharm.: Vitamins/Nutri.: Clinical Trials:	Manufacturer: Distributor: Leasing/Finance: Information Sys.:	Y	Acute Care: Sub-Acute Care: Outpatient Surgery: Phys. Rehab. Center: Psychiatric Clinics:	Diagnostics: Labs/Testing: Staffing: Waste Disposal: Specialty Services:	Y	Home Health: Long-Term Care: Physical Therapy: Phys. Practice Mgmt.:

TYPES OF BUSINESS:
Equipment-Patient Monitoring Systems
Non-Invasive Heart & Lung Monitors & Sensors
Developmental Care Products & Services

BRANDS/DIVISIONS/AFFILIATES:
Respironics, Inc.
Children's Medical Ventures

GROWTH PLANS/SPECIAL FEATURES:
Novametrix Medical Systems, Inc., a subsidiary of Respironics, Inc., is a leading developer, manufacturer and marketer of non-invasive heart and lung monitors and sensors, as well as developmental care products and services to the critical care marketplace. The company produces a number of non-invasive monitoring devices that measure cardiopulmonary patient parameters such as cardiac output, pulmonary dead space and carbon dioxide production. Novametrix also manufactures pulse oximeters, devices that measure a patient's pulse rate and blood oxygen levels. Its oximeters incorporate reusable sensors that come with an unconditional guarantee. Subsidiary Children's Medical Ventures is a leading provider of developmental care products and services to neonatal and pediatric departments in hospitals. It offers a wide and growing assortment of developmental care and baby care products that assist clinicians in providing improved quality of care for premature and sick babies.

CONTACTS:
Note: Officers with more than one job title may be intentionally listed here more than once.

William J. Lacourciere, CEO
Thomas M. Patton, Pres.
Thomas M. Patton, COO
Joseph A. Vincent, Exec. VP/CFO
William J. Lacourciere, Chmn.

Phone: 203-265-7701   **Fax:** 203-284-0753
Toll-Free:
Address: 5 Technology Dr., Wallingford, CT 06492-1926 US

FINANCIALS:
Sales and profits are in thousands of dollars—add 000 to get the full amount. Year 2004 note: Complete fiscal 2004 results were not available for all companies at press time. For this company, year 2004 is for months.

2004 Sales: $ (months)	2004 Profits: $ (months)	**Stock Ticker:** Subsidiary
2003 Sales: $	2003 Profits: $	**Employees:** 246
2002 Sales: $	2002 Profits: $	**Fiscal Year Ends:** 4/30
2001 Sales: $54,700	2001 Profits: $ 600	
2000 Sales: $43,700	2000 Profits: $2,500	

SALARIES/BENEFITS:
| Pension Plan: | ESOP Stock Plan: | Profit Sharing: | Top Exec. Salary: $294,049 | Bonus: $ |
| Savings Plan: | Stock Purch. Plan: | | Second Exec. Salary: $188,987 | Bonus: $ |

OTHER THOUGHTS:
Apparent Top Female Officers:
Hot Spot for Advancement for Women/Minorities:

LOCATIONS: ("Y" = Yes)
West:	Southwest:	Midwest:	Southeast:	Northeast:	International:
Y				Y	

Plunkett's Health Care Industry Almanac 2005   535

NOVARTIS AG
www.novartis.com
Industry Group Code: 325412   Ranks within this company's industry group: Sales: 4   Profits: 3

Insurance/HMO/PPO:	Drugs:	Equipment/Supplies:	Hospitals/Clinics:	Services:	Health Care:
Insurance:	Manufacturer: Y	Manufacturer: Y	Acute Care:	Diagnostics:	Home Health:
Managed Care:	Distributor:	Distributor:	Sub-Acute Care:	Labs/Testing:	Long-Term Care:
Utilization Mgmt.:	Specialty Pharm.:	Leasing/Finance:	Outpatient Surgery:	Staffing:	Physical Therapy:
Payment Proc.:	Vitamins/Nutri.: Y	Information Sys.:	Phys. Rehab. Center:	Waste Disposal:	Phys. Practice Mgmt.:
	Clinical Trials:		Psychiatric Clinics:	Specialty Services:	

TYPES OF BUSINESS:
Drugs-Diversified
Therapeutic Drug Discovery
Therapeutic Drug Manufacturing
Generic Drugs
Over-the-Counter Drugs
Ophthalmic Products
Nutritional Products
Animal Health Products

BRANDS/DIVISIONS/AFFILIATES:
CIBA Vision
Grand Laboratories, Inc.
ImmTech Biologics, Inc.
Novartis Institute for Biomedical Research, Inc.

CONTACTS: Note: Officers with more than one job title may be intentionally listed here more than once.
Daniel Vasella, CEO
Daniel Vasella, Pres.
Alex Gorsky, COO
Raymund Breu, CFO
Jurgen Brokatzky-Geiger, Head-Human Resources
Urs Barlocher, Dir.-Legal & General Affairs
Steven Kelmar, Head-Public Affairs and Corp. Comm.
Thomas Ebeling, CEO-Pharmaceuticals
Paul Choffat, CEO-Consumer Health
Marc Fishman, Pres., Novartis Institutes for Biomedical Research
Ingrid Duplain, Corp. Sec.
Daniel Vasella, Chmn.

Phone: 41-61-324-1111   Fax: 41-61-324-8001
Toll-Free:
Address: Lichtstrasse 35, Basel, CH-4002 Switzerland

GROWTH PLANS/SPECIAL FEATURES:
Novartis is engaged in research and development focused on pharmaceuticals, consumer health, generics, eye care and animal health. It operates in two principle business segments: pharmaceuticals, encompassing the oncology, transplantation, ophthalmics and mature products divisions; and consumer health, which includes generics, over-the-counter drugs, animal health, medical nutrition, infant and baby products and CIBA Vision. Through its pharmaceuticals division, Novartis develops, manufactures and markets prescription medicines. Its generics division competes in two segments: finished dosage forms and active pharmaceutical ingredients and their intermediates. Finished dosage forms are sold to pharmacies, hospitals and other health care outlets, while active ingredients and their intermediates for pharmaceutical and biotechnological substances are sold to industrial customers. The consumer health segment operates in over-the-counter self-medication, health and functional nutrition in addition to medical nutrition units. CIBA Vision is a world leader in the research, development and manufacturing of eye care products, namely soft contact lenses, lens care products and ophthalmic surgical products. Through its animal health division, Novartis enhances and extends the life of companion animals and improves the health and productivity of farm animals. This business unit owns Grand Laboratories, Inc. and ImmTech Biologics, Inc., both engaged in the development of vaccines for cattle and pigs. Novartis has established the Novartis Institute for Biomedical Research, Inc. in Cambridge, Massachusetts, where U.S. and Japanese research operations are held. All other worldwide research activities are performed in Europe. In August 2004, the company agreed to acquire Canadian generics pharmaceutical manufacturer, Sabex Holdings, for $565 million in cash.

The company offers its employees medical, dental and vision insurance, in addition to child care and elderly care support and tuition reimbursement. Novartis also offers health and fitness programs.

FINANCIALS: Sales and profits are in thousands of dollars—add 000 to get the full amount. Year 2004 note: Complete fiscal 2004 results were not available for all companies at press time. For this company, year 2004 is for 6 months.

2004 Sales: $13,612,000 (6 months)   2004 Profits: $1,289,000 (6 months)
2003 Sales: $24,864,000   2003 Profits: $5,016,000
2002 Sales: $23,151,000   2002 Profits: $3,546,000
2001 Sales: $19,070,000   2001 Profits: $5,225,000
2000 Sales: $21,312,500   2000 Profits: $4,291,666

Stock Ticker: Foreign
Employees: 78,541
Fiscal Year Ends: 12/31

SALARIES/BENEFITS:
Pension Plan: Y   ESOP Stock Plan: Y   Profit Sharing: Top Exec. Salary: $ Bonus: $
Savings Plan: Stock Purch. Plan: Second Exec. Salary: $ Bonus: $

OTHER THOUGHTS:
Apparent Top Female Officers: 1
Hot Spot for Advancement for Women/Minorities:

LOCATIONS: ("Y" = Yes)
West:	Southwest:	Midwest:	Southeast:	Northeast:	International:
		Y	Y	Y	Y

Note: Financial information, benefits and other data can change quickly and may vary from those stated here.

NOVATION LLC

www.novationco.com

Industry Group Code: 561400 **Ranks within this company's industry group:** Sales: Profits:

Insurance/HMO/PPO:	Drugs:		Equipment/Supplies:		Hospitals/Clinics:	Services:		Health Care:	
Insurance:	Manufacturer:		Manufacturer:		Acute Care:	Diagnostics:		Home Health:	
Managed Care:	Distributor:	Y	Distributor:	Y	Sub-Acute Care:	Labs/Testing:		Long-Term Care:	
Utilization Mgmt.:	Specialty Pharm.:		Leasing/Finance:		Outpatient Surgery:	Staffing:		Physical Therapy:	
Payment Proc.:	Vitamins/Nutri.:		Information Sys.:		Phys. Rehab. Center:	Waste Disposal:		Phys. Practice Mgmt.:	
	Clinical Trials:				Psychiatric Clinics:	Specialty Services:	Y		

TYPES OF BUSINESS:
Medical Supplies Distributor
Pharmaceuticals Distributor
Supply Chain Management
Health Care Consulting
Health Care Publications

BRANDS/DIVISIONS/AFFILIATES:
Marketplace@Novation
NOVAPLUS

CONTACTS:
Note: Officers with more than one job title may be intentionally listed here more than once.
Mark McKenna, CEO
Mark McKenna, Pres.
Jody Hatcher, Sr. VP-Mktg.
Mike Hobbs, VP-Customization & Dev.
Veronica S. Lewis, General Counsel/Compliance Officer
Mike Woodhouse, Dir.-Financial Services
Eldon Petersen, Group Sr. VP
Jo Klein, VP
Maryann S. Restino, VP-Contract & Program Services
Larry McComber, VP-Contract & Program Services
Larry Dooley, VP-Supplier Rel.

Phone: 888-766-8283 **Fax:**
Toll-Free:
Address: 125 E. John Carpenter Fwy., Ste. 1400, Irving, TX 75062 US

GROWTH PLANS/SPECIAL FEATURES:
Novation, LLC is a leading medical supply chain management company. The firm specializes in providing services to the Veteran's Administration, operator of the VA hospitals, and United Healthcare, one of the nation's leading health benefits services, supplying a total of 2,300 health care organizations. The company, through its over 500 suppliers, is able to provide 75% of the products that these organizations use in their medical practices, including medical and surgical supplies, pharmaceuticals, diagnostic imaging machines, business products, laboratory products, dietary and food products and capital equipment and related services. The company's NOVAPLUS is the private label of the VA and United Healthcare, offering over 1,300 items. In addition, Novation offers e-commerce services for its customers and suppliers, a health care management consultancy, a service delivery team and a variety of publications. Marketplace@Novation is a members-only, Internet-based solution that allows health care suppliers to provide products at a lower price. The company's health care consultancy service teaches organizations how to reduce cost and increase safety. The service delivery division manages the relationships between various facilities and their suppliers and helps to implement cost-reduction strategies. Novation also publishes newsletters, product shortages and recalls, industry news and the latest in clinical information.

FINANCIALS:
Sales and profits are in thousands of dollars—add 000 to get the full amount. Year 2004 note: Complete fiscal 2004 results were not available for all companies at press time. For this company, year 2004 is for   months.

2004 Sales: $ (months)   2004 Profits: $ (months)
2003 Sales: $ 2003 Profits: $
2002 Sales: $ 2002 Profits: $
2001 Sales: $ 2001 Profits: $
2000 Sales: $ 2000 Profits: $

Stock Ticker: Private
Employees:
Fiscal Year Ends: 12/31

SALARIES/BENEFITS:
Pension Plan: ESOP Stock Plan: Profit Sharing: Top Exec. Salary: $ Bonus: $
Savings Plan: Stock Purch. Plan: Second Exec. Salary: $ Bonus: $

OTHER THOUGHTS:
Apparent Top Female Officers: 4
Hot Spot for Advancement for Women/Minorities: Y

LOCATIONS: ("Y" = Yes)
West:	Southwest:	Midwest:	Southeast:	Northeast:	International:
Y	Y	Y	Y	Y	

NOVO-NORDISK AS

www.novonordisk.com

Industry Group Code: 325412 **Ranks within this company's industry group:** Sales: 17 Profits: 14

Insurance/HMO/PPO:	Drugs:	Equipment/Supplies:	Hospitals/Clinics:	Services:	Health Care:
Insurance:	Manufacturer: Y	Manufacturer: Y	Acute Care:	Diagnostics:	Home Health:
Managed Care:	Distributor:	Distributor:	Sub-Acute Care:	Labs/Testing:	Long-Term Care:
Utilization Mgmt.:	Specialty Pharm.:	Leasing/Finance:	Outpatient Surgery:	Staffing:	Physical Therapy:
Payment Proc.:	Vitamins/Nutri.:	Information Sys.:	Phys. Rehab. Center:	Waste Disposal:	Phys. Practice Mgmt.:
	Clinical Trials:		Psychiatric Clinics:	Specialty Services: Y	

TYPES OF BUSINESS:
Drugs-Diabetes
Hormone Replacement Therapy
Growth Disorder Drugs
Hemophilia Drugs
Insulin Delivery Systems
Educational Services

BRANDS/DIVISIONS/AFFILIATES:
NovoPen
NovoSeven
Norditropin SimpleXx
Activelle
Kliogest
Trisequens
Estrofem
Vagifem

CONTACTS:
Note: Officers with more than one job title may be intentionally listed here more than once.

Lars R. Sorensen, CEO
Lars R. Sorensen, Pres.
Kare Schultz, Exec. VP/COO
Jesper Brandgaard, Exec. VP/CFO
Lise Kingo, Exec. VP-Human Resources
Mads K. Thomsen, Exec. VP/Chief Science Officer
Lars A. Jorgensen, Exec. VP-Bus. Dev.
Michael Shalmi, VP-Biopharmaceuticals United States

Phone: 45-4444-8888	Fax: 45-4449-0555
Toll-Free:	
Address: 2880 Novo Alle, Basgvaerd, DK-2880 Denmark	

GROWTH PLANS/SPECIAL FEATURES:

Novo-Nordisk AS focuses on developing treatments for diabetes, hemostasis management, growth hormone therapy and hormone replacement therapy. With its affiliates, the company markets its products in 68 countries. The firm is a world leader in insulin manufacturing and has the broadest diabetes product line in the world. NovoPen, a pen-like, multiple-dose injector, allows patients to easily inject themselves with insulin or hormones. Novo-Nordisk's growth hormone replacement product, Norditropin SimpleXx, is a premixed liquid growth hormone designed to provide the most flexible and accurate dosing. The company's NovoSeven product, a treatment for hemophilia, is a recombinant coagulation factor that enables coagulation to proceed in the absence of natural factors. The firm also manufactures post-menopausal hormone replacement therapy products, including Activelle, Kliogest, Trisequens, Estrofem and Vagifem. In addition, the company offers educational services and training materials for both patients and health care professionals. The company is investing in companies that use nanotechnology for biotech applications. Such applications include labs-on-a-chip, genomics and drug delivery. The company has a licensing agreement with ZymoGenetics for microarrays. In recent news, Novo-Nordisk received approval from the European Union for the use of its NovoSeven product for two additional conditions.

Novo-Nordisk offers its U.S. employees health, life, dental, auto and supplemental insurance, as well as tuition reimbursement.

FINANCIALS:
Sales and profits are in thousands of dollars—add 000 to get the full amount. Year 2004 note: Complete fiscal 2004 results were not available for all companies at press time. For this company, year 2004 is for 6 months.

2004 Sales: $2,212,000 (6 months)	2004 Profits: $195,000 (6 months)	**Stock Ticker:** Foreign
2003 Sales: $4,501,000	2003 Profits: $824,000	Employees: 18,800
2002 Sales: $3,554,000	2002 Profits: $578,000	Fiscal Year Ends: 12/31
2001 Sales: $2,839,000	2001 Profits: $461,000	
2000 Sales: $2,437,000	2000 Profits: $417,000	

SALARIES/BENEFITS:
Pension Plan:	ESOP Stock Plan:	Profit Sharing:	Top Exec. Salary: $	Bonus: $
Savings Plan: Y	Stock Purch. Plan:		Second Exec. Salary: $	Bonus: $

OTHER THOUGHTS:
Apparent Top Female Officers: 1
Hot Spot for Advancement for Women/Minorities

LOCATIONS: ("Y" = Yes)
West:	Southwest:	Midwest:	Southeast:	Northeast:	International:
Y	Y	Y	Y	Y	Y

NOVOSTE CORPORATION

www.novoste.com

Industry Group Code: 339113   Ranks within this company's industry group: Sales: 106   Profits: 110

Insurance/HMO/PPO:	Drugs:	Equipment/Supplies:		Hospitals/Clinics:	Services:	Health Care:
Insurance: Managed Care: Utilization Mgmt.: Payment Proc.:	Manufacturer: Distributor: Specialty Pharm.: Vitamins/Nutri.: Clinical Trials:	Manufacturer: Distributor: Leasing/Finance: Information Sys.:	Y Y	Acute Care: Sub-Acute Care: Outpatient Surgery: Phys. Rehab. Center: Psychiatric Clinics:	Diagnostics: Labs/Testing: Staffing: Waste Disposal: Specialty Services:	Home Health: Long-Term Care: Physical Therapy: Phys. Practice Mgmt.:

TYPES OF BUSINESS:
Vascular Brachytherapy
Radiation Therapy Devices

BRANDS/DIVISIONS/AFFILIATES:
Beta-Cath
CORONA
BRAVO

CONTACTS:
Note: Officers with more than one job title may be intentionally listed here more than once.

Alfred J. Novak, CEO
Alfred J. Novak, Pres.
Robert N. Wood, Jr., VP-Global Sales
Susan D. Smith, VP-Human Resources
Daniel G. Hall, VP/General Counsel
Subhash C. Sarda, VP-Finance
Adam G. Lowe, VP-Quality Assurance
Daniel G. Hall, Corp. Sec.
Andrew Green, VP-Regulatory & Clinical Affairs
Thomas D. Weldon, Chmn.

Phone: 770-717-0904   Fax: 770-717-1283
Toll-Free: 800-668-6783
Address: 3890 Steve Reynolds Blvd., Norcross, GA 30093 US

GROWTH PLANS/SPECIAL FEATURES:
Novoste Corporation is a world leader in the new field of vascular brachytherapy (VBT). VBT is a form of radiation therapy delivered inside an artery to prevent it from re-closing, which occurs when scar tissue grows inside an artery and limits blood flow after procedures such as angioplasty, often resulting in the need for additional procedures to re-open the vessel. The company's Beta-Cath system is a hand-held device designed to hydraulically deliver beta radiation through a closed-end catheter to the site of a treated blockage. The FDA has approved 30-, 40- and 60-mm radiation source train versions, which are designed to treat lesions of various lengths, as well as the next-generation 3.5F catheter, which has a smaller profile than the original 5.0F version, allowing it to treat blockages in smaller passageways. Novoste has been focusing its research efforts on modifying the Beta-Cath system for use in peripheral applications, such as arterial-venous shunts and the femoral arteries. The company is investigating its CORONA system to treat non-thrombotic arterial-venous dialysis graft stenosis, a condition that occurs when the grafts used for long-term dialysis become clogged. The BRAVO (beta radiation for treatment of arterial-venous graft outflow) trial is currently underway to determine whether the CORONA system will prove effective at keeping these dialysis grafts clear and functional. The system is also being developed to treat reduced blood flow to the legs, though that trial has been suspended due to the likelihood that commercial approval would not be attained for at least three years. Novoste's products are commercially available in the U.S. as well as in the European Union and several other countries.

FINANCIALS:
Sales and profits are in thousands of dollars—add 000 to get the full amount. Year 2004 note: Complete fiscal 2004 results were not available for all companies at press time. For this company, year 2004 is for 9 months.

2004 Sales: $18,730 (9 months)	2004 Profits: $-13,658 (9 months)	**Stock Ticker:** NOVT
2003 Sales: $62,901	2003 Profits: $- 868	Employees: 198
2002 Sales: $69,000	2002 Profits: $-13,100	Fiscal Year Ends: 12/31
2001 Sales: $69,908	2001 Profits: $-5,109	
2000 Sales: $6,530	2000 Profits: $-33,073	

SALARIES/BENEFITS:
Pension Plan:	ESOP Stock Plan:	Profit Sharing:	Top Exec. Salary: $350,000	Bonus: $123,452
Savings Plan: Y	Stock Purch. Plan:		Second Exec. Salary: $233,649	Bonus: $56,612

OTHER THOUGHTS:
Apparent Top Female Officers: 1
Hot Spot for Advancement for Women/Minorities:

LOCATIONS: ("Y" = Yes)
West:	Southwest:	Midwest:	Southeast:	Northeast:	International:
			Y		

NYER MEDICAL GROUP INC

www.nyermedicalgroup.com

Industry Group Code: 421450 Ranks within this company's industry group: Sales: 7 Profits: 5

Insurance/HMO/PPO:	Drugs:	Equipment/Supplies:	Hospitals/Clinics:	Services:	Health Care:
Insurance:	Manufacturer:	Manufacturer:	Acute Care:	Diagnostics:	Home Health:
Managed Care:	Distributor:	Distributor: Y	Sub-Acute Care:	Labs/Testing:	Long-Term Care:
Utilization Mgmt.:	Specialty Pharm.: Y	Leasing/Finance:	Outpatient Surgery:	Staffing:	Physical Therapy:
Payment Proc.:	Vitamins/Nutri.:	Information Sys.:	Phys. Rehab. Center:	Waste Disposal:	Phys. Practice Mgmt.:
	Clinical Trials:		Psychiatric Clinics:	Specialty Services: Y	

TYPES OF BUSINESS:
Distribution-Medical Equipment
Home Health Supplies
Surgical/Laboratory Supplies
Fire, Police & Rescue Equipment
Drug Stores
Online Medical Supply Sales
Emergency Medical Services Supplies

BRANDS/DIVISIONS/AFFILIATES:
ADCO Surgical Supply, Inc.
Eaton Apothecary
Nyer Internet, Inc.
Conway Associates, Inc.
SCBA, Inc.
D.A.W., Inc.
www.medicalmailorder.com
www.physicianequipment.com

CONTACTS:
Note: Officers with more than one job title may be intentionally listed here more than once.

Karen L. Wright, CEO
Karen L. Wright, Pres.
William J. Clifford, Jr., VP-Sales
Karen L. Wright, VP-Oper.
Samuel Nyer, VP-Mergers & Acquisitions
Michael Curry, VP
David Dumouchel, VP/Pres., Eaton Apothecary
Wayne Gunter, VP
Samuel Nyer, Chmn.

Phone: 207-942-5273 Fax: 207-941-9392
Toll-Free:
Address: 1292 Hammond St., Bangor, ME 04401 US

GROWTH PLANS/SPECIAL FEATURES:

Nyer Medical Group, Inc. (NMG) operates medical supply subsidiaries and a chain of pharmacies. Its ADCO Surgical Supply, Inc. and ADCO South Medical Supplies, Inc. subsidiaries sell surgical and medical equipment and supplies, wholesale and retail, to health care facilities throughout New England and Florida. ADCO also delivers blood glucose meters, test strips, lancets and penlets, control solutions and alcohol prep pads to diabetics in their homes. Nyer Internet, Inc. sells medical equipment and supplies over the Internet. Nyer Internet's web site, www.medicalmailorder.com, directs consumers through an online medical mall and store directories to locate the site that best suits their needs. The firm also runs www.physicianequipment.com and continues to develop new sites in order to expand its virtual mall. Conway Associates, Inc., 80%-owned by the company, sells equipment, supplies and novelty items to emergency medical services and fire and police departments throughout most of New England. SBCA, Inc. repairs and services self-contained breathing apparatuses for fire departments. Doing business under the name Eaton Apothecary, subsidiary D.A.W., Inc. operates a chain of 11 pharmacy drug stores located in the greater Boston area. In February 2004, NMG closed its subsidiary Anton Investments, Inc.

FINANCIALS:
Sales and profits are in thousands of dollars—add 000 to get the full amount. Year 2004 note: Complete fiscal 2004 results were not available for all companies at press time. For this company, year 2004 is for 12 months.

2004 Sales: $61,687 (12 months) 2004 Profits: $-425 (12 months)
2003 Sales: $59,900 2003 Profits: $500
2002 Sales: $54,100 2002 Profits: $200
2001 Sales: $23,900 2001 Profits: $-200
2000 Sales: $42,000 2000 Profits: $-600

Stock Ticker: NYER
Employees: 241
Fiscal Year Ends: 6/30

SALARIES/BENEFITS:
Pension Plan: ESOP Stock Plan: Profit Sharing: Top Exec. Salary: $140,000 Bonus: $42,000
Savings Plan: Stock Purch. Plan: Y   Second Exec. Salary: $128,700 Bonus: $26,000

OTHER THOUGHTS:
Apparent Top Female Officers: 1
Hot Spot for Advancement for Women/Minorities:

LOCATIONS: ("Y" = Yes)
West:	Southwest:	Midwest:	Southeast:	Northeast:	International:
Y			Y	Y	

OCA INC

www.ocai.com

Industry Group Code: 621111 **Ranks within this company's industry group:** Sales: 6 Profits: 3

Insurance/HMO/PPO:	Drugs:	Equipment/Supplies:	Hospitals/Clinics:	Services:	Health Care:
Insurance:	Manufacturer:	Manufacturer:	Acute Care:	Diagnostics:	Home Health:
Managed Care:	Distributor:	Distributor:	Sub-Acute Care:	Labs/Testing:	Long-Term Care:
Utilization Mgmt.:	Specialty Pharm.:	Leasing/Finance:	Outpatient Surgery:	Staffing:	Physical Therapy:
Payment Proc.:	Vitamins/Nutri.:	Information Sys.:	Phys. Rehab. Center:	Waste Disposal:	Phys. Practice Mgmt.: Y
	Clinical Trials:		Psychiatric Clinics:	Specialty Services:	

TYPES OF BUSINESS:
Dental Practice Management
Orthodontics Practice Management

BRANDS/DIVISIONS/AFFILIATES:
Orthodontic Centers of America

CONTACTS:
Note: Officers with more than one job title may be intentionally listed here more than once.

Bartholomew F. Palmisano, Sr., CEO
Bartholomew F. Palmisano, Sr., Pres.
Bartholomew F. Palmisano, Jr., COO
Thomas J. Sandeman, CFO
David E. Verret, Sr. VP-Finance
Dennis J.L. Buchman, Sr.VP-Doctor Relations
Bartholomew F. Palmisano, Jr., Corp. Sec.
Bartholomew F. Palmisano, Sr., Chmn.

Phone: 504-834-4392 **Fax:** 504-834-3663
Toll-Free: 866-765-8583
Address: 3850 N. Causeway Blvd., Ste. 970, Metairie, LA 70002 US

GROWTH PLANS/SPECIAL FEATURES:

OCA, Inc., formerly Orthodontic Centers of America, is the leading provider of integrated business services to orthodontic and pediatric dental practices throughout the U.S. and Puerto Rico, as well as parts of Japan, Mexico and Spain. Its services include marketing and advertising, management information systems, staffing, supplies and inventory, scheduling, billing, financial reporting, accounting and other administrative and business services. The company works with affiliated orthodontists and dentists under long-term contracts, with terms ranging from 20 to 40 years. OCA's marketing and advertising plans use television, radio and print advertising and internal marketing promotions, helping orthodontists and dentists to generate significantly greater patient volume. In addition, the company's operating systems and office designs enable doctors to treat more patients per day. The firm's operating strategy emphasizes high-quality patient care, competitive patient fees and convenient payment plans, operating efficiency through innovative office designs and superior service through information technology.

The company offers an employee benefits package that includes medical, dental and vision insurance. Other incentives include bonuses, stock options and paid vacation.

FINANCIALS:
Sales and profits are in thousands of dollars—add 000 to get the full amount. Year 2004 note: Complete fiscal 2004 results were not available for all companies at press time. For this company, year 2004 is for 6 months.

2004 Sales: $215,214 (6 months) 2004 Profits: $-65,133 (6 months)
2003 Sales: $375,380   2003 Profits: $49,065
2002 Sales: $439,600   2002 Profits: $58,200
2001 Sales: $351,000   2001 Profits: $61,100
2000 Sales: $268,800   2000 Profits: $-2,900

Stock Ticker: OCA
Employees: 3,296
Fiscal Year Ends: 12/31

SALARIES/BENEFITS:
Pension Plan: ESOP Stock Plan: Profit Sharing: Top Exec. Salary: $230,000   Bonus: $15,000
Savings Plan: Y   Stock Purch. Plan: Second Exec. Salary: $200,000   Bonus: $

OTHER THOUGHTS:
Apparent Top Female Officers: 1
Hot Spot for Advancement for Women/Minorities:

LOCATIONS: ("Y" = Yes)
West:	Southwest:	Midwest:	Southeast:	Northeast:	International:
Y	Y	Y	Y	Y	Y

OCCUPATIONAL HEALTH + REHABILITATION INC
www.ohplus.com

Industry Group Code: 621340   Ranks within this company's industry group: Sales: 3   Profits: 2

Insurance/HMO/PPO:	Drugs:	Equipment/Supplies:	Hospitals/Clinics:	Services:		Health Care:	
Insurance:	Manufacturer:	Manufacturer:	Acute Care:	Diagnostics:		Home Health:	
Managed Care:	Distributor:	Distributor:	Sub-Acute Care:	Labs/Testing:	Y	Long-Term Care:	
Utilization Mgmt.:	Specialty Pharm.:	Leasing/Finance:	Outpatient Surgery:	Staffing:		Physical Therapy:	Y
Payment Proc.:	Vitamins/Nutri.:	Information Sys.:	Phys. Rehab. Center:	Waste Disposal:		Phys. Practice Mgmt.:	
	Clinical Trials:		Psychiatric Clinics:	Specialty Services:	Y		

TYPES OF BUSINESS:
Occupational Health Care Provider
Regulatory Compliance Services
Workplace Health Services
Pre-Placement Examinations
Medical Surveillance Services
Work-Site Safety Programs
Drug and Alcohol Testing

BRANDS/DIVISIONS/AFFILIATES:
Baptist Care Centers

GROWTH PLANS/SPECIAL FEATURES:
Occupational Health + Rehabilitation, Inc. (OHR) is a leading national occupational health care provider specializing in the prevention, treatment and management of work-related injuries and illnesses, as well as regulatory compliance services. The firm operates 36 occupational health centers serving over 15,000 employer clients in 10 states. OHR also delivers workplace health services at employer locations throughout the United States. These services improve the health status of employees, reduce workers' compensation costs and assist employers in their compliance with state and federal regulations concerning governing workplace health and safety. Prevention and compliance services include pre-placement examinations, medical surveillance services, fitness-for-duty and return-to-work evaluations, drug and alcohol testing, physical exams and work-site safety programs. OHR intends to expand its network of delivery sites through joint ventures, acquisitions and start-up centers. The company recently acquired ownership of Baptist Hospital's five Baptist Care Centers in Nashville and Murfreesboro, Tennessee, and is opening a new center in Augusta, Maine.

CONTACTS: Note: Officers with more than one job title may be intentionally listed here more than once.
John C. Garbarino, CEO
John C. Garbarino, Pres.
Lynne M. Rosen, COO
Keith G. Frey, CFO
Peter D. Senger, Corp. Dir.-Sales
Mark S. Flieger, Sr. VP-Info. Systems
Lynne M. Rosen, Sr. VP-Oper.
H. Nicholas Kirby, Sr. VP-Corp. Dev.
Thomas J. Ward, VP-Missouri & Tennessee Oper.
Patti E. Walkover, VP-Reimbursement & Payor Contracting
Mary E. Kenney, VP-Northeast Oper.
William B. Patterson, Chief Medical Officer

Phone: 781-741-5175   Fax: 781-741-5499
Toll-Free:
Address: 175 Derby St., Ste. 36, Hingham, MA 02043 US

FINANCIALS:
Sales and profits are in thousands of dollars—add 000 to get the full amount. Year 2004 note: Complete fiscal 2004 results were not available for all companies at press time. For this company, year 2004 is for 6 months.

2004 Sales: $28,500 (6 months)   2004 Profits: $ 422 (6 months)
2003 Sales: $53,538   2003 Profits: $- 231
2002 Sales: $56,900   2002 Profits: $ 100
2001 Sales: $57,000   2001 Profits: $4,100
2000 Sales: $43,700   2000 Profits: $1,200

Stock Ticker: OHRI
Employees: 524
Fiscal Year Ends: 12/31

SALARIES/BENEFITS:
Pension Plan: ESOP Stock Plan: Profit Sharing: Top Exec. Salary: $226,646   Bonus: $10,000
Savings Plan: Y   Stock Purch. Plan: Second Exec. Salary: $182,685   Bonus: $10,000

OTHER THOUGHTS:
Apparent Top Female Officers: 3
Hot Spot for Advancement for Women/Minorities: Y

LOCATIONS: ("Y" = Yes)
West:	Southwest:	Midwest:	Southeast:	Northeast:	International:
		Y	Y	Y	

OCULAR SCIENCES INC

www.ocularsciences.com

Industry Group Code: 339113   Ranks within this company's industry group: Sales: 55   Profits: 49

Insurance/HMO/PPO:	Drugs:	Equipment/Supplies:		Hospitals/Clinics:	Services:	Health Care:
Insurance:	Manufacturer:	Manufacturer:	Y	Acute Care:	Diagnostics:	Home Health:
Managed Care:	Distributor:	Distributor:	Y	Sub-Acute Care:	Labs/Testing:	Long-Term Care:
Utilization Mgmt.:	Specialty Pharm.:	Leasing/Finance:		Outpatient Surgery:	Staffing:	Physical Therapy:
Payment Proc.:	Vitamins/Nutri.:	Information Sys.:		Phys. Rehab. Center:	Waste Disposal:	Phys. Practice Mgmt.:
	Clinical Trials:			Psychiatric Clinics:	Specialty Services:	

TYPES OF BUSINESS:
Supplies-Soft Contact Lenses
Reusable & Disposable Contact Lenses

BRANDS/DIVISIONS/AFFILIATES:
Biomedics
Hydron
Edge
Ultraflex
SmartChoice
Hydrogenics
ProActive
Sunsoft

CONTACTS: Note: Officers with more than one job title may be intentionally listed here more than once.
Stephen J. Fanning, CEO
Stephen J. Fanning, Pres.
Steven M. Neil, Exec. VP/CFO
Gary E. Paladin, VP-Global Mktg.
Greg A. Zimmerman, VP-Human Resources
J. Christopher Marmo, VP-Research & Dev.
Ken Hurley, VP-IT
Linda A. Hoffman, VP-Oper.
John A. Weber, Exec. VP-Worldwide Oper.
Richard P. Franz, VP-Professional Rel.
Bradley S. Jones, VP-U.S. Sales
John D. Fruth, Chmn.
James M. Welch, Pres.-Int'l Div.

Phone: 925-969-7000   **Fax:** 888-301-0264
Toll-Free:
Address: 1855 Gateway Blvd., Ste. 700, Concord, CA 94520 US

GROWTH PLANS/SPECIAL FEATURES:
Ocular Sciences, Inc. is a global manufacturer and marketer of soft contact lenses. The company manufactures a broad line of soft contact lenses for annual and quarterly planned replacement, as well as semimonthly and monthly disposable replacement regimens. Disposables constitute most of the firm's sales. Ocular Sciences believes that eye care practitioners significantly influence a patient's selection of contact lenses and therefore markets its lenses exclusively to eye care practitioners, both in private practices and in retail optical chains. Accordingly, the firm does not sell to mail-order companies, pharmacies or other distribution channels that do not provide the regular eye examinations necessary to maintain overall ocular health. Ocular Sciences' marketing strategies are designed to assist eye care practitioners in retaining their patients and monitoring their patients' ocular health, creating a significant incentive for practitioners to prescribe its lenses. The company's lenses are made from flexible polymers, and most contain an ultraviolet absorber. Ocular Sciences also offers specialty lenses including toric lenses to correct astigmatisms, multifocal lenses and rigid gas permeable cosmetic, aspheric, sports and extended-wear lenses. The firm's products are marketed under the Hydron, Edge, Ultraflex, SmartChoice, Biomedics, Hydrogenics, ProActive, Sunsoft, Lunelle and Rythmic brand names. Its Biomedics 55 Premier is the first disposable lens to correct for spherical aberration in the eye. In July 2004, Ocular Sciences announced that it would be acquired by the Cooper Companies, Inc., a leading global supplier of specialty contact lenses.

FINANCIALS: Sales and profits are in thousands of dollars—add 000 to get the full amount. Year 2004 note: Complete fiscal 2004 results were not available for all companies at press time. For this company, year 2004 is for 9 months.

2004 Sales: $251,622 (9 months)   2004 Profits: $25,179 (9 months)
2003 Sales: $310,563   2003 Profits: $26,554
2002 Sales: $267,100   2002 Profits: $7,200
2001 Sales: $253,900   2001 Profits: $6,500
2000 Sales: $177,000   2000 Profits: $38,900

Stock Ticker: OCLR
Employees: 2,591
Fiscal Year Ends: 12/31

SALARIES/BENEFITS:
Pension Plan: ESOP Stock Plan: Profit Sharing: Top Exec. Salary: $400,000   Bonus: $316,875
Savings Plan: Y   Stock Purch. Plan: Second Exec. Salary: $244,265   Bonus: $275,074

OTHER THOUGHTS:
Apparent Top Female Officers: 1
Hot Spot for Advancement for Women/Minorities:

LOCATIONS: ("Y" = Yes)

West:	Southwest:	Midwest:	Southeast:	Northeast:	International:
Y	Y		Y		Y

ODYSSEY HEALTHCARE INC

www.odyssey-healthcare.net

Industry Group Code: 621610 Ranks within this company's industry group: Sales: 7 Profits: 4

Insurance/HMO/PPO:	Drugs:	Equipment/Supplies:	Hospitals/Clinics:	Services:	Health Care:
Insurance:	Manufacturer:	Manufacturer:	Acute Care:	Diagnostics:	Home Health:
Managed Care:	Distributor:	Distributor:	Sub-Acute Care:	Labs/Testing:	Long-Term Care: Y
Utilization Mgmt.:	Specialty Pharm.:	Leasing/Finance:	Outpatient Surgery:	Staffing:	Physical Therapy: Y
Payment Proc.:	Vitamins/Nutri.:	Information Sys.:	Phys. Rehab. Center:	Waste Disposal:	Phys. Practice Mgmt.:
	Clinical Trials:		Psychiatric Clinics:	Specialty Services: Y	

TYPES OF BUSINESS:
Hospice Care Services
Physical Therapy

BRANDS/DIVISIONS/AFFILIATES:
Crown of Texas Hospice

CONTACTS:
Note: Officers with more than one job title may be intentionally listed here more than once.

David C. Gasmire, CEO
David C. Gasmire, Pres.
Deborah A. Hoffpauir, Sr. VP/COO
Doug Cannon, Sr. VP/CFO
Brenda A. Belger, Sr. VP-Human Resources
Doug Cannon, Treas./Corp. Sec.
Kathleen A. Ventre, Sr. VP-Clinical & Regulatory Affairs
Richard R. Burnham, Chmn.

Phone: 214-922-9711 **Fax:** 214-922-9752
Toll-Free: 888-922-9711
Address: 717 N. Harwood St., Ste. 1500, Dallas, TX 75201 US

GROWTH PLANS/SPECIAL FEATURES:
Odyssey HealthCare, Inc. is one of the largest providers of hospice care in the U.S. in terms of average daily census and number of locations. The company has hospice office locations in 30 states and six inpatient facilities in Nevada, Arizona, Texas and Georgia. The firm's goal is to improve the quality of life of terminally ill patients and their families. Odyssey assigns each of its patients to an interdisciplinary team, which assesses the clinical, psychosocial and spiritual needs of the patient and his or her family; develops a plan of care; and delivers, monitors and coordinates that plan. This team typically includes a physician, a patient care manager, one or more nurses, one or more home health aides, a medical social worker, a chaplain, a homemaker and one or more specially trained volunteers. Odyssey provides symptom-relieving medication and medical supplies and equipment associated with the terminal illness, such as bandages, catheters, oxygen, hospital bed, wheelchair and walkers, at no cost to the patient. Services, which are available 24 hours a day, include nursing care, home care aides, spiritual support, counseling and physical, occupational and speech therapy services to help the patient remain independent. The firm also contracts with hospitals and long-term care facilities to provide inpatient hospice care on an as-needed basis. Odyssey's strategic advantages in the hospice industry include active cost management and centralized corporate services, as well as comprehensive compliance and quality improvement programs, made possible by its large size. The company continues to grow rapidly through acquisitions, having recently acquired two Crown of Texas Hospice companies that together serve approximately 400 patients.

Employee benefits at Odyssey include PPO or HMO medical, dental, vision and life insurance, employee referral bonuses, employee recognition programs and tuition reimbursement.

FINANCIALS:
Sales and profits are in thousands of dollars—add 000 to get the full amount. Year 2004 note: Complete fiscal 2004 results were not available for all companies at press time. For this company, year 2004 is for 9 months.

2004 Sales: $196,005 (9 months)   2004 Profits: $22,622 (9 months)
2003 Sales: $274,309   2003 Profits: $31,207
2002 Sales: $194,500   2002 Profits: $21,100
2001 Sales: $130,200   2001 Profits: $12,900
2000 Sales: $85,300   2000 Profits: $3,100

Stock Ticker: ODSY
Employees: 3,904
Fiscal Year Ends: 12/31

SALARIES/BENEFITS:
| Pension Plan: | ESOP Stock Plan: | Profit Sharing: | Top Exec. Salary: $460,764 | Bonus: $266,900 |
| Savings Plan: Y | Stock Purch. Plan: Y | | Second Exec. Salary: $348,131 | Bonus: $201,627 |

OTHER THOUGHTS:
Apparent Top Female Officers: 3
Hot Spot for Advancement for Women/Minorities: Y

LOCATIONS: ("Y" = Yes)
West:	Southwest:	Midwest:	Southeast:	Northeast:	International:
Y	Y	Y	Y	Y	

OHIOHEALTH CORPORATION

www.ohiohealth.com

Industry Group Code: 622110 Ranks within this company's industry group: Sales: 40 Profits:

Insurance/HMO/PPO:	Drugs:	Equipment/Supplies:	Hospitals/Clinics:		Services:		Health Care:	
Insurance: Y	Manufacturer:	Manufacturer:	Acute Care:	Y	Diagnostics:		Home Health:	Y
Managed Care:	Distributor:	Distributor:	Sub-Acute Care:		Labs/Testing:		Long-Term Care:	Y
Utilization Mgmt.:	Specialty Pharm.:	Leasing/Finance:	Outpatient Surgery:	Y	Staffing:		Physical Therapy:	
Payment Proc.:	Vitamins/Nutri.:	Information Sys.:	Phys. Rehab. Center:	Y	Waste Disposal:		Phys. Practice Mgmt.:	
	Clinical Trials:		Psychiatric Clinics:		Specialty Services:			

TYPES OF BUSINESS:
Hospitals-General
Health Insurance
Home Health Care
Hospice Services
Long-Term Care
Surgery Centers
Rehabilitation Services

BRANDS/DIVISIONS/AFFILIATES:
HomeReach
WorkHealth
OhioHealth Group
HealthReach PPO
Doctors Hospital Nelsonville
Grant Medical Center
Hardin Memorial Hospital
Southern Ohio Medical Center

GROWTH PLANS/SPECIAL FEATURES:
OhioHealth Corporation, founded in 1891, is a collection of 14 acute care hospitals in Ohio, eight of which are owned by the company and six directly affiliated with it. The firm has a relationship with nearly 4,000 physicians and has more than 2,000 acute care beds along with outpatient health care, surgery centers, home health services, long-term care facilities and hospice services. OhioHealth also owns HomeReach, a provider of home health care; WorkHealth, for workers' compensation and rehabilitation services; and OhioHealth Group, a joint venture with the Medical Group of Ohio that manages HealthReach PPO. Hospitals owned by OhioHealth include Doctors Hospital Nelsonville, Doctors Hospital, Grant Medical Center, Hardin Memorial Hospital, Marion General Hospital, Riverside Methodist Hospital and Southern Ohio Medical Center.

CONTACTS:
Note: Officers with more than one job title may be intentionally listed here more than once.

David Blom, CEO
David Blom, Pres.
Robert P. Millen, COO
Mike Louge, CFO
Debra P. Moore, VP-Human Resources
Bill Winnenberg, CIO
Steve Garlock, Sr. VP-Oper.
Cheryl Herbert, VP-Bus. Dev.
Susan Besanceney, Pres., OhioHealth Foundation
David Morehead, Sr. VP/Chief Medical Officer
Keith R. Vesper, VP-Mission & Ministry

Phone: 614-544-5424 Fax: 614-566-6938
Toll-Free:
Address: 1087 Dennison Ave., Columbus, OH 43201 US

FINANCIALS:
Sales and profits are in thousands of dollars—add 000 to get the full amount. Year 2004 note: Complete fiscal 2004 results were not available for all companies at press time. For this company, year 2004 is for months.

2004 Sales: $ (months) 2004 Profits: $ (months)
2003 Sales: $1,036,000 2003 Profits: $
2002 Sales: $1,955,000 2002 Profits: $
2001 Sales: $ 2001 Profits: $
2000 Sales: $ 2000 Profits: $

Stock Ticker: Nonprofit
Employees: 15,000
Fiscal Year Ends: 6/31

SALARIES/BENEFITS:
Pension Plan: ESOP Stock Plan: Profit Sharing: Top Exec. Salary: $ Bonus: $
Savings Plan: Stock Purch. Plan: Second Exec. Salary: $ Bonus: $

OTHER THOUGHTS:
Apparent Top Female Officers: 3
Hot Spot for Advancement for Women/Minorities: Y

LOCATIONS: ("Y" = Yes)
West:	Southwest:	Midwest:	Southeast:	Northeast:	International:
		Y			

OMNICARE INC

www.omnicare.com

Industry Group Code: 446110A Ranks within this company's industry group: Sales: 2 Profits: 2

Insurance/HMO/PPO:	Drugs:	Equipment/Supplies:	Hospitals/Clinics:	Services:	Health Care:
Insurance:	Manufacturer:	Manufacturer:	Acute Care:	Diagnostics:	Home Health:
Managed Care:	Distributor: Y	Distributor: Y	Sub-Acute Care:	Labs/Testing: Y	Long-Term Care:
Utilization Mgmt.:	Specialty Pharm.: Y	Leasing/Finance:	Outpatient Surgery:	Staffing:	Physical Therapy:
Payment Proc.: Y	Vitamins/Nutri.:	Information Sys.: Y	Phys. Rehab. Center:	Waste Disposal:	Phys. Practice Mgmt.:
	Clinical Trials:		Psychiatric Clinics:	Specialty Services: Y	

TYPES OF BUSINESS:
Specialty Pharmacies
Infusion Therapy
Consulting Services
Pharmaceutical Research
Medical Records Services
Billing Services
Pharmaceutical Distribution
Software Information Systems

BRANDS/DIVISIONS/AFFILIATES:
Omnicare Clinical Research
CompScript, Inc.

CONTACTS:
Note: Officers with more than one job title may be intentionally listed here more than once.

Joel F. Gemunder, CEO
Joel F. Gemunder, Pres.
David W. Froesel, Jr., Sr. VP/CFO
Jack M. Clark, Sr. VP-Sales & Mktg.
D. Michael Laney, VP-MIS
Peter Laterza, VP/General Counsel
Patrick E. Keefe, Exec. VP-Oper.
Tracy Finn, VP-Strategic Planning & Dev.
Thomas R. Marsh, Treas.
W. Gary Erwin, Pres.-Senior Health Outcomes
Timothy E. Bien, Sr. VP-Professional Services
David Morra, VP/CEO-Omnicare Clinical Research
Thomas W. Ludeke, Pres., Accu-Med Services, Inc.
Edward Hutton, Chmn.
Timothy E. Bien, Sr. VP-Purchasing

Phone: 859-392-3300 Fax: 859-392-3333
Toll-Free:
Address: 1600 RiverCenter II, 100 E. RiverCenter Blvd., Covington, KY 41011 US

GROWTH PLANS/SPECIAL FEATURES:
Omnicare, Inc. is a leading provider of pharmaceuticals and related pharmacy services to long-term care institutions such as skilled nursing facilities, assisted living facilities and retirement centers, as well as hospitals and other institutional health care facilities. The firm's main business segment, pharmacy services, provides pharmaceutical distribution, related pharmacy consulting, data management services and medical supplies to long-term care facilities. Services include purchasing, repackaging and dispensing pharmaceuticals, computerized medical record keeping and third-party billing for residents in the institutions. Omnicare also provides infusion therapy services, distribution of medical supplies and clinical and financial software information systems to nursing facilities. Omnicare's second operating segment involves comprehensive product development and research services to client companies in the pharmaceutical, biotechnology, medical device and diagnostics industries. This segment operates in 29 countries around the world. Another business segment, contract research organization services, or CRO services, is a leading international provider of comprehensive product development and research services to client companies in the pharmaceutical, biotechnology, medical device and diagnostics industries. Subsidiary Omnicare Clinical Research has expertise in various fields including cardiovascular, anti-infectives, oncology, central nervous system and geriatrics areas. Another subdivision, CompScript, provides services to institutions across the United States. Omnicare is currently attempting an acquisition of NeighborCare, Inc. but is facing multiple difficulties.
Employees at Omnicare enjoy benefits including tuition assistance, training and health plan options.

FINANCIALS:
Sales and profits are in thousands of dollars—add 000 to get the full amount. Year 2004 note: Complete fiscal 2004 results were not available for all companies at press time. For this company, year 2004 is for 9 months.

2004 Sales: $3,046,809 (9 months)	2004 Profits: $179,831 (9 months)	**Stock Ticker: OCR**
2003 Sales: $3,499,174	2003 Profits: $194,368	Employees: 12,100
2002 Sales: $2,606,500	2002 Profits: $125,900	Fiscal Year Ends: 12/31
2001 Sales: $2,159,100	2001 Profits: $74,300	
2000 Sales: $1,971,300	2000 Profits: $48,800	

SALARIES/BENEFITS:
Pension Plan: Y   ESOP Stock Plan: Profit Sharing: Top Exec. Salary: $1,254,167   Bonus: $2,089,749
Savings Plan: Y   Stock Purch. Plan: Y   Second Exec. Salary: $381,583   Bonus: $229,178

OTHER THOUGHTS:
Apparent Top Female Officers: 1
Hot Spot for Advancement for Women/Minorities:

LOCATIONS: ("Y" = Yes)
West:	Southwest:	Midwest:	Southeast:	Northeast:	International:
Y	Y	Y	Y	Y	Y

OPTICARE HEALTH SYSTEMS

www.opticare.com

Industry Group Code: 621490   **Ranks within this company's industry group:** Sales: 12   Profits: 19

Insurance/HMO/PPO:	Drugs:	Equipment/Supplies:	Hospitals/Clinics:	Services:	Health Care:
Insurance:	Manufacturer: Y	Manufacturer:	Acute Care:	Diagnostics:	Home Health:
Managed Care:	Distributor:	Distributor:	Sub-Acute Care:	Labs/Testing:	Long-Term Care:
Utilization Mgmt.:	Specialty Pharm.:	Leasing/Finance:	Outpatient Surgery: Y	Staffing:	Physical Therapy:
Payment Proc.: Y	Vitamins/Nutri.:	Information Sys.: Y	Phys. Rehab. Center:	Waste Disposal:	Phys. Practice Mgmt.:
	Clinical Trials:		Psychiatric Clinics:	Specialty Services: Y	

TYPES OF BUSINESS:
Integrated Eye Care Services
Laser Vision Correction
Managed Care Services
Practice Management Software
Claims Payment Administration
Ambulatory Surgery Facilities
Wholesale Buying Services

BRANDS/DIVISIONS/AFFILIATES:
Eye Care for a Lifetime
Connecticut Vision Correction
Doctor's Express
TLC
OcuCare Systems, Inc.

CONTACTS:
Note: Officers with more than one job title may be intentionally listed here more than once.

Dean J. Yimoyines, CEO
Christopher J. Walls, Pres.
William A. Blaskiewicz, VP/CFO
James Carmona, Jr., CIO
Christopher J. Walls, Chief Admin. Officer
Christopher J. Walls, General Counsel
Gordon A. Bishop, Pres.-Consumer Vision Div.
Jason Harrold, Pres.-Managed Care Div.
Dean J. Yimoyines, Chmn.

Phone: 203-596-2236   **Fax:** 203-596-2230
Toll-Free:
Address: 87 Grandview Ave., Waterbury, CT 06708 US

GROWTH PLANS/SPECIAL FEATURES:
OptiCare Health Systems, Inc. is an integrated eye care services company focused on providing managed care and professional eye care services. The firm operates in three segments covering virtually every major sector of the eye care market: managed care, professional services and other integrated services. The managed care division contracts with insurers, managed care plans and other third-party payers to manage claims payment administration of eye health benefits. The professional services division provides laser and ambulatory surgery facilities; develops and sells integrated practice management systems (including web-based software solutions); and provides support services to eye care professionals throughout the country. The company's third division owns, operates and contracts with integrated eye health centers and professional optometric practices in Connecticut and North Carolina, in addition to providing wholesale buying services to eye care professionals nationwide. OptiCare's trademarks include Eye Care for a Lifetime, Connecticut Vision Correction, Doctor's Express and TLC. In October 2004, OptiCare announce it would acquire OcuCare Systems, Inc., which provides comprehensive vision network management and administrative services to an array of managed care organizations and single-specialty networks.

FINANCIALS:
Sales and profits are in thousands of dollars—add 000 to get the full amount. Year 2004 note: Complete fiscal 2004 results were not available for all companies at press time. For this company, year 2004 is for 6 months.

2004 Sales: $60,332 (6 months)	2004 Profits: $-1,920 (6 months)	**Stock Ticker:** OPT
2003 Sales: $125,702	2003 Profits: $-12,353	**Employees:** 482
2002 Sales: $91,500	2002 Profits: $ 800	**Fiscal Year Ends:** 12/31
2001 Sales: $112,500	2001 Profits: $3,000	
2000 Sales: $127,900	2000 Profits: $-14,200	

SALARIES/BENEFITS:
Pension Plan:	ESOP Stock Plan:	Profit Sharing:	Top Exec. Salary: $345,000	Bonus: $93,500
Savings Plan: Y	Stock Purch. Plan:		Second Exec. Salary: $150,000	Bonus: $50,000

OTHER THOUGHTS:
Apparent Top Female Officers:
Hot Spot for Advancement for Women/Minorities:

LOCATIONS: ("Y" = Yes)
West:	Southwest:	Midwest:	Southeast:	Northeast: Y	International:

OPTION CARE INC

www.optioncare.com

Industry Group Code: 621610 Ranks within this company's industry group: Sales: 4 Profits: 6

Insurance/HMO/PPO:	Drugs:	Equipment/Supplies:	Hospitals/Clinics:	Services:	Health Care:
Insurance: Managed Care: Utilization Mgmt.: Payment Proc.:	Manufacturer: Distributor: Specialty Pharm.: Y Vitamins/Nutri.: Clinical Trials:	Manufacturer: Distributor: Y Leasing/Finance: Y Information Sys.: Y	Acute Care: Sub-Acute Care: Outpatient Surgery: Phys. Rehab. Center: Psychiatric Clinics:	Diagnostics: Labs/Testing: Staffing: Waste Disposal: Specialty Services: Y	Home Health: Y Long-Term Care: Physical Therapy: Phys. Practice Mgmt.:

TYPES OF BUSINESS:
Home Health Care
Home Health Care Data Management
Infusion Therapy
Home Health Equipment
Specialty Pharmacy Services
Software Products

BRANDS/DIVISIONS/AFFILIATES:
Management by Information, Inc.

CONTACTS:
Note: Officers with more than one job title may be intentionally listed here more than once.
Rajat Rai, CEO
Richard M. Smith, Pres.
Richard M. Smith, COO
Paul Mastrapa, Sr. VP/CFO
Irwin Halperin, Sr. VP-Sales
Kent Kerkhof, Sr. VP-Network Mgmt.
Bruce Kutinsky, Sr. VP-Specialty Pharmacy Services
John N. Kapoor, Chmn.

Phone: 847-615-1690 **Fax:** 847-615-1794
Toll-Free: 800-879-6137
Address: 485 Half Day Rd., Ste. 300, Buffalo Grove, IL 60089 US

GROWTH PLANS/SPECIAL FEATURES:

Option Care, Inc. provides pharmacy services to patients with acute and chronic conditions at the patient's home or alternative settings, such as a physician's office. The company works under contractual agreements with managed care organizations and other payors, providing home infusion therapy, specialty pharmacy services and other related health care services. It provides services locally through a nationwide network of 128 owned and franchised pharmacy locations. Through subsidiary Management by Information, Inc., the corporation receives franchise royalties and license or rental fees for software products. Option Care plans to strengthen its position as the leading national provider of infusion therapy by investing in sales execution to new and existing referral sources and through selective acquisitions that expand its geographic coverage into new markets. The firm's specialty pharmacy strategy involves expanding its relationships with biotech and other pharmaceutical manufacturers in order to acquire distribution rights to existing and new products, as well as developing its existing relationships and entering into new agreements with managed care organizations to lower the cost of injectable drugs at the physician's office. Operating under the OptionMed name, its specialty pharmacy in Miramar, Florida serves as a central management and distribution point for the delivery of specialty pharmaceuticals to physician offices. The company also has a national specialty care pharmacy in Ann Arbor, Michigan to provide a central distribution channel for certain specialty pharmaceuticals. Option Care provides specialty pharmacy services to treat growth hormone deficiency, respiratory diseases, hepatitis C, multiple sclerosis, hemophilia, immune deficiency and cancer.

The firm offers its employees health, dental and vision plans in addition to stock options.

FINANCIALS:
Sales and profits are in thousands of dollars—add 000 to get the full amount. Year 2004 note: Complete fiscal 2004 results were not available for all companies at press time. For this company, year 2004 is for 9 months.

2004 Sales: $301,751 (9 months)	2004 Profits: $13,616 (9 months)	**Stock Ticker:** OPTN
2003 Sales: $335,440	2003 Profits: $8,718	Employees: 1,792
2002 Sales: $320,500	2002 Profits: $14,100	Fiscal Year Ends: 12/31
2001 Sales: $217,100	2001 Profits: $10,000	
2000 Sales: $141,300	2000 Profits: $7,500	

SALARIES/BENEFITS:
Pension Plan:	ESOP Stock Plan:	Profit Sharing:	Top Exec. Salary: $324,327	Bonus: $100,625
Savings Plan: Y	Stock Purch. Plan:		Second Exec. Salary: $245,346	Bonus: $48,808

OTHER THOUGHTS:
Apparent Top Female Officers:
Hot Spot for Advancement for Women/Minorities:

LOCATIONS: ("Y" = Yes)
West:	Southwest:	Midwest:	Southeast:	Northeast:	International:
Y	Y	Y	Y	Y	

Note: Financial information, benefits and other data can change quickly and may vary from those stated here.

ORGANOGENESIS INC

www.organogenesis.com

Industry Group Code: 325414 Ranks within this company's industry group: Sales: Profits:

Insurance/HMO/PPO:	Drugs:	Equipment/Supplies:	Hospitals/Clinics:	Services:	Health Care:
Insurance: Managed Care: Utilization Mgmt.: Payment Proc.:	Manufacturer: Distributor: Specialty Pharm.: Vitamins/Nutri.: Clinical Trials:	Manufacturer: Y Distributor: Leasing/Finance: Information Sys.:	Acute Care: Sub-Acute Care: Outpatient Surgery: Phys. Rehab. Center: Psychiatric Clinics:	Diagnostics: Labs/Testing: Staffing: Waste Disposal: Specialty Services:	Home Health: Long-Term Care: Physical Therapy: Phys. Practice Mgmt.:

TYPES OF BUSINESS:
Tissue Replacement Products
Wound Dressing Products

BRANDS/DIVISIONS/AFFILIATES:
Apligraph
FortaFlex
FortaPerm
FortaGen
CuffPatch
PuraPly
TESTSKIN II

GROWTH PLANS/SPECIAL FEATURES:
Organogenesis, Inc. is a tissue-engineering firm that designs, develops and manufactures medical products containing living cells or natural connective tissue. The firm develops and manufactures the only mass-produced medical product containing living human cells marketed in the U.S. The Apligraf living cell substitute, the company's lead product, is designed for the treatment of venous leg ulcers due to poor blood circulation and for diabetic foot ulcers without tendon, muscle, capsule or bone exposure. Apligraf contains living human skin cells, fibroblasts and keratinocytes, which are organized in an epidermal and dermal layer. Organogenesis also markets the Fortaflex line of products, including FortaPerm for tissue support, FortaGen for tissue repair, CuffPatch for tissue reinforcement and PuraPly for wound management. The company's other product, TESTSKIN II, is a realistic model of human skin, used for in vitro research and testing. The firm recently completed its court-approved reorganization plan, allowing it to emerge from Chapter 11 protection.

CONTACTS:
Note: Officers with more than one job title may be intentionally listed here more than once.
Geoff MacKay, CEO
Geoff MacKay, Pres.
Santino Costanzo, VP-Sales
Alan Ades, Chmn.

Phone: 781-575-0775 **Fax:** 781-575-0440
Toll-Free:
Address: 150 Dan Rd., Canton, MA 02021 US

FINANCIALS:
Sales and profits are in thousands of dollars—add 000 to get the full amount. Year 2004 note: Complete fiscal 2004 results were not available for all companies at press time. For this company, year 2004 is for months.

2004 Sales: $ (months)   2004 Profits: $ (months)
2003 Sales: $ 2003 Profits: $
2002 Sales: $ 2002 Profits: $
2001 Sales: $10,300   2001 Profits: $-30,100
2000 Sales: $10,200   2000 Profits: $-28,600

Stock Ticker: Private
Employees: 182
Fiscal Year Ends: 12/31

SALARIES/BENEFITS:
Pension Plan: ESOP Stock Plan: Profit Sharing: Top Exec. Salary: $277,420   Bonus: $56,000
Savings Plan: Y   Stock Purch. Plan: Second Exec. Salary: $229,836 Bonus: $30,000

OTHER THOUGHTS:
Apparent Top Female Officers:
Hot Spot for Advancement for Women/Minorities:

LOCATIONS: ("Y" = Yes)
West:	Southwest:	Midwest:	Southeast:	Northeast:	International:
				Y	

Note: Financial information, benefits and other data can change quickly and may vary from those stated here.

ORTHOFIX INTERNATIONAL NV

www.orthofix.com

Industry Group Code: 339113 Ranks within this company's industry group: Sales: 63 Profits: 51

Insurance/HMO/PPO:	Drugs:	Equipment/Supplies:	Hospitals/Clinics:	Services:	Health Care:
Insurance: Managed Care: Utilization Mgmt.: Payment Proc.:	Manufacturer: Distributor: Specialty Pharm.: Vitamins/Nutri.: Clinical Trials:	Manufacturer: Y Distributor: Y Leasing/Finance: Information Sys.:	Acute Care: Sub-Acute Care: Outpatient Surgery: Phys. Rehab. Center: Psychiatric Clinics:	Diagnostics: Labs/Testing: Staffing: Waste Disposal: Specialty Services:	Home Health: Long-Term Care: Physical Therapy: Phys. Practice Mgmt.:

TYPES OF BUSINESS:
Medical Equipment-Orthopedic

BRANDS/DIVISIONS/AFFILIATES:
Orthofix
ProCallus
Orthotrac
XCaliber
OASIS
EZBrace
Spinal-Stim
Breg

CONTACTS:
Note: Officers with more than one job title may be intentionally listed here more than once.

Charles Federico, CEO
Charles Federico, Pres.
Thomas Hein, CFO
Peter W. Clarke, Corp. Sec.
Gary Henley, Sr. VP/Pres.-Americas Div.
Bradley R. Mason, VP/Pres., Breg, Inc.
Edgar Wallner, Vice-Chmn.
Robert Gaines-Cooper, Chmn.
Galvin Mould, VP-Int'l

Phone: 599-9-465-8525 Fax: 599-9-461-6978
Toll-Free:
Address: 7 Abraham de Veerstraat, Curacao, Netherlands Antilles

GROWTH PLANS/SPECIAL FEATURES:
Orthofix International NV designs, develops, manufactures, markets and distributes medical equipment used principally by musculoskeletal medical specialists for orthopedic applications including minimally invasive surgical equipment, as well as non-surgical products. The company has multiple trademarked products including Orthofix, ProCallus, Orthotrac, XCaliber, OASIS, EZBrace, Spinal-Stim, Physio-Stim, Breg, Polar Care and Pain Care. Sales are divided into two segments, orthopedic and non-orthopedic. Orthopedic products account for approximately 90% of revenues and are divided into three market sectors: spine, bone reconstruction and trauma. Sales of non-orthopedic products include airway management, women's care and other products and account for 10% of the firm's revenues. Orthofix's most successful products are external and internal fixation devices used in fracture treatment, limb lengthening and bone reconstruction; non-invasive stimulation products used to increase healing for spinal fusions and non-union fractures; and bracing products used for ligament injury prevention, pain management and protection of surgical repair for faster healing. Other products include a device for enhancing venous circulation, cold therapy, pain management products, bone cement and devices for bone cement removal, and a bone substitute compound. Orthofix has facilities in the United States, the United Kingdom, Italy, Mexico and the Seychelles and distributes products in the United States, the United Kingdom, Ireland, Italy, Germany, Switzerland, Austria, France, Belgium, Mexico and Brazil.

FINANCIALS:
Sales and profits are in thousands of dollars—add 000 to get the full amount. Year 2004 note: Complete fiscal 2004 results were not available for all companies at press time. For this company, year 2004 is for 6 months.

2004 Sales: $141,533 (6 months)   2004 Profits: $25,990 (6 months)
2003 Sales: $203,707   2003 Profits: $24,730
2002 Sales: $177,595   2002 Profits: $25,913
2001 Sales: $ 2001 Profits: $
2000 Sales: $ 2000 Profits: $

Stock Ticker: Foreign
Employees: 988
Fiscal Year Ends: 12/31

SALARIES/BENEFITS:
| Pension Plan: | ESOP Stock Plan: | Profit Sharing: | Top Exec. Salary: $450,944 | Bonus: $171,755 |
| Savings Plan: | Stock Purch. Plan: | | Second Exec. Salary: $239,099 | Bonus: $100,000 |

OTHER THOUGHTS:
Apparent Top Female Officers:
Hot Spot for Advancement for Women/Minorities:

LOCATIONS: ("Y" = Yes)
West:	Southwest:	Midwest:	Southeast:	Northeast:	International:
Y			Y	Y	Y

OSTEOTECH INC

www.osteotech.com

Industry Group Code: 339113   Ranks within this company's industry group: Sales: 95   Profits: 71

Insurance/HMO/PPO:	Drugs:	Equipment/Supplies:		Hospitals/Clinics:	Services:		Health Care:	
Insurance:	Manufacturer:	Manufacturer:	Y	Acute Care:	Diagnostics:		Home Health:	
Managed Care:	Distributor:	Distributor:		Sub-Acute Care:	Labs/Testing:		Long-Term Care:	
Utilization Mgmt.:	Specialty Pharm.:	Leasing/Finance:		Outpatient Surgery:	Staffing:		Physical Therapy:	
Payment Proc.:	Vitamins/Nutri.:	Information Sys.:		Phys. Rehab. Center:	Waste Disposal:		Phys. Practice Mgmt.:	
	Clinical Trials:			Psychiatric Clinics:	Specialty Services:	Y		

TYPES OF BUSINESS:
Supplies-Processed Bone
Musculoskeletal System Repair Products & Services
Allograft Bone Tissue

BRANDS/DIVISIONS/AFFILIATES:
Grafton Demineralized Bone Matrix
Bio-d
OsteoPure
Ovation
VBR
Affirm
Sentinel

CONTACTS: Note: Officers with more than one job title may be intentionally listed here more than once.
Richard W. Bauer, CEO
Sam Owusu-Akyaw, Pres.
Sam Owusu-Akyaw, COO
Michael J. Jeffries, Exec. VP/CFO
Robert M. Wynalek, Sr. VP-Sales & Mktg.
Jeffrey M. Rosen, VP-Human Resources
James L. Russell, Exec. VP/Chief Scientific Officer
Thomas L. Cobb, VP-Oper.
Mark H. Burroughs, VP-Finance/Treas.
Michael J. Jeffries, Corp. Sec.
Marilyn C. Murray, VP-Quality Assurance & Regulatory
Donald D. Johnston, Chmn.
Richard Russo, Exec. VP/General Mgr.-Int'l
Robert W. Honneffer, VP-Supply Chain

Phone: 732-542-2800   Fax: 732-542-9312
Toll-Free:
Address: 51 James Way, Eatontown, NJ 07724 US

GROWTH PLANS/SPECIAL FEATURES:
Osteotech, Inc. provides services and products primarily focused on the repair and healing of the musculoskeletal system and marketed to the orthopedic, spinal, neurological, oral/maxillofacial, dental and general surgery markets in the United States and Europe. The firm is a leading processor and developer of human bone and bone connective tissue, or allograft bone tissue, forms. This allograft bone tissue is procured by independent tissue banks or other tissue recovery organizations, primarily through the donation of tissue from deceased donors, and is used for transplantation. Osteotech's two main operating segments are the Grafton Demineralized Bone Matrix (DBM) segment and the base allograft bone tissue segment. The Grafton DBM segment processes and markets this product using its advanced, proprietary demineralization process. The base tissue segment processes mineralized weight-bearing tissue, as well as bio-implants, the Bio-d threaded cortical bone dowel and OsteoPure femoral head bone tissue, among other products. The company also provides ceramic and titanium plasma spray coating services and ceramic products used as bone graft substitutes, in addition to metal spinal implant products, including the Ovation and VBR lines. In addition, Osteotech maintains a distribution agreement with Alphatec Manufacturing to market the Sentinal pedicle screw system and the Affirm cervical plating system.

FINANCIALS:
Sales and profits are in thousands of dollars—add 000 to get the full amount. Year 2004 note: Complete fiscal 2004 results were not available for all companies at press time. For this company, year 2004 is for 9 months.

2004 Sales: $68,134 (9 months)	2004 Profits: $- 660 (9 months)	**Stock Ticker:** OSTE
2003 Sales: $94,433	2003 Profits: $10,867	Employees: 367
2002 Sales: $83,400	2002 Profits: $-1,300	Fiscal Year Ends: 12/31
2001 Sales: $77,800	2001 Profits: $-4,400	
2000 Sales: $75,700	2000 Profits: $4,800	

SALARIES/BENEFITS:
Pension Plan:	ESOP Stock Plan:	Profit Sharing:	Top Exec. Salary: $386,250	Bonus: $152,284
Savings Plan: Y	Stock Purch. Plan:		Second Exec. Salary: $236,750	Bonus: $301,092

OTHER THOUGHTS:
Apparent Top Female Officers: 1
Hot Spot for Advancement for Women/Minorities:

LOCATIONS: ("Y" = Yes)

West:	Southwest:	Midwest:	Southeast:	Northeast:	International:
				Y	Y

OUTLOOK POINTE CORP

www.outlookpointe.com

Industry Group Code: 623110 **Ranks within this company's industry group:** Sales: Profits:

Insurance/HMO/PPO:	Drugs:	Equipment/Supplies:	Hospitals/Clinics:	Services:	Health Care:
Insurance:	Manufacturer:	Manufacturer:	Acute Care:	Diagnostics:	Home Health:
Managed Care:	Distributor:	Distributor:	Sub-Acute Care:	Labs/Testing:	Long-Term Care: Y
Utilization Mgmt.:	Specialty Pharm.:	Leasing/Finance:	Outpatient Surgery:	Staffing:	Physical Therapy: Y
Payment Proc.:	Vitamins/Nutri.:	Information Sys.:	Phys. Rehab. Center:	Waste Disposal:	Phys. Practice Mgmt.:
	Clinical Trials:		Psychiatric Clinics:	Specialty Services:	

TYPES OF BUSINESS:
Assisted Living Facilities
Wellness Programs
Therapy Services

BRANDS/DIVISIONS/AFFILIATES:
Balanced Gold

CONTACTS:
Note: Officers with more than one job title may be intentionally listed here more than once.
Jim Fields, CEO
Jim Fields, Pres.
Diane M. Borger, Treas.

Phone: 717-796-6100 **Fax:** 717-796-6150
Toll-Free:
Address: 1215 Manor Dr., Mechanicsburg, PA 17055 US

GROWTH PLANS/SPECIAL FEATURES:
Outlook Pointe Corp. develops, manages and operates assisted living facilities to meet the needs of upper-middle-, middle- and moderate-income populations in non-urban, secondary markets. The company operates 37 such facilities in Arkansas, North Carolina, Ohio, Pennsylvania, Virginia, Tennessee and West Virginia. These facilities provide a care continuum consisting of preventative care and wellness, medical rehabilitation, dementia and Alzheimer's care and, in certain markets, extended care. Outlook Pointe's philosophy includes the belief that providing health care services coupled with wellness and preventative therapy will strengthen residents, improve their health and forestall the deterioration that generally accompanies aging, thus extending their lives and lengths of stay in assisted living facilities. Balanced Gold, the firm's wellness-oriented program, has been developed to proactively address resident care needs, stabilizing and improving residents' cognitive, emotional and physical well-being through participation in exercise classes, gardening, intellectually stimulating games, religious studies and social events. The company also offers physical, occupational and speech therapy services, which are available for both residents and outpatients, and Alzheimer's and dementia care according to patients' needs. In addition, Outlook Pointe provides adult day care and respite care.

FINANCIALS:
Sales and profits are in thousands of dollars—add 000 to get the full amount. Year 2004 note: Complete fiscal 2004 results were not available for all companies at press time. For this company, year 2004 is for months.

2004 Sales: $ (months)   2004 Profits: $ (months)
2003 Sales: $ 2003 Profits: $
2002 Sales: $ 2002 Profits: $
2001 Sales: $56,800   2001 Profits: $-46,100
2000 Sales: $60,700   2000 Profits: $-21,600

Stock Ticker: Private
Employees: 2,100
Fiscal Year Ends: 6/30

SALARIES/BENEFITS:
| Pension Plan: | ESOP Stock Plan: | Profit Sharing: | Top Exec. Salary: $235,504 | Bonus: $105,000 |
| Savings Plan: | Stock Purch. Plan: | | Second Exec. Salary: $180,000 | Bonus: $65,000 |

OTHER THOUGHTS:
Apparent Top Female Officers: 1
Hot Spot for Advancement for Women/Minorities:

LOCATIONS: ("Y" = Yes)
West:	Southwest:	Midwest:	Southeast:	Northeast:	International:
		Y	Y	Y	

OWENS & MINOR INC

www.owens-minor.com

Industry Group Code: 421450 **Ranks within this company's industry group:** Sales: 1 Profits: 4

Insurance/HMO/PPO:	Drugs:	Equipment/Supplies:	Hospitals/Clinics:	Services:	Health Care:
Insurance:	Manufacturer:	Manufacturer:	Acute Care:	Diagnostics:	Home Health:
Managed Care:	Distributor:	Distributor: Y	Sub-Acute Care:	Labs/Testing:	Long-Term Care:
Utilization Mgmt.:	Specialty Pharm.:	Leasing/Finance:	Outpatient Surgery:	Staffing:	Physical Therapy:
Payment Proc.:	Vitamins/Nutri.:	Information Sys.:	Phys. Rehab. Center:	Waste Disposal:	Phys. Practice Mgmt.:
	Clinical Trials:		Psychiatric Clinics:	Specialty Services: Y	

TYPES OF BUSINESS:
Distribution-Medical & Surgical Equipment
Supply Chain Management
Logistics Services

BRANDS/DIVISIONS/AFFILIATES:
CostTrack
WISDOM
OM DIRECT
SurgiTrack
Pandac
FOCUS

CONTACTS:
Note: Officers with more than one job title may be intentionally listed here more than once.

G. Gilmer Minor, III, CEO
Craig R. Smith, Pres.
Craig R. Smith, COO
Jeffrey Kaczka, Sr. VP/CFO
Timothy Callahan, Sr. VP-Sales & Mktg.
Erika T. Davis, Sr. VP-Human Resources
David R. Guzman, Sr. VP/CIO
Grace R. den Harling, General Counsel
Charles C. Colpo, Sr. VP-Oper.
Hue Thomas, III, VP-Corp. Rel.
Richard F. Bozard, Treas.
Henry A. Berling, Exec. VP
Hugh F. Gouldthorpe, Jr., VP-Quality & Comm.
Drew St. J. Carneal, Corp. Sec.
G. Gilmer Minor, III, Chmn.

Phone: 804-747-9794 **Fax:** 804-270-7281
Toll-Free:
Address: 4800 Cox Rd., Glen Allen, VA 23060-6292 US

GROWTH PLANS/SPECIAL FEATURES:
Owens & Minor, Inc. (O&M) is one of the largest distributors of medical and surgical supplies in the U.S. The company serves hospitals, integrated health care systems and group purchasing organizations, stocking and distributing approximately 120,000 finished medical and surgical products from almost 1,500 suppliers. It sells to 4,000 customers from 41 distribution centers nationwide. The company's customers are primarily acute care hospitals and hospital-based systems but also include alternate care facilities such as clinics, surgery centers, rehabilitation facilities, nursing homes, physician's offices and home health care providers. The majority of O&M's sales consist of dressings, endoscopic products, intravenous products, disposable gloves, needles and syringes, sterile procedure trays, surgical products and gowns, urological products and wound closure products. In addition, the company helps customers control health care costs and improve inventory management through services in supply chain management, logistics and technology. FOCUS is the company's product standardization and consolidation program that moves market share to its most efficient suppliers. CostTrack separates product and process costs to clearly reflect the cost of individual distribution activities. Pandac and SurgiTrack are both programs that help with operating room equipment management. Online services and order forms are available through OM DIRECT and WISDOM.

FINANCIALS:
Sales and profits are in thousands of dollars—add 000 to get the full amount. Year 2004 note: Complete fiscal 2004 results were not available for all companies at press time. For this company, year 2004 is for 9 months.

2004 Sales: $3,359,836 (9 months)   2004 Profits: $45,147 (9 months)
2003 Sales: $4,244,067   2003 Profits: $53,641
2002 Sales: $3,959,800   2002 Profits: $47,300
2001 Sales: $3,815,000   2001 Profits: $23,000
2000 Sales: $3,503,600   2000 Profits: $33,100

Stock Ticker: OMI
Employees: 3,245
Fiscal Year Ends: 12/31

SALARIES/BENEFITS:
Pension Plan: Y   ESOP Stock Plan: Y   Profit Sharing: Top Exec. Salary: $751,583   Bonus: $500,000
Savings Plan: Y   Stock Purch. Plan: Second Exec. Salary: $552,635   Bonus: $311,145

OTHER THOUGHTS:
Apparent Top Female Officers: 2
Hot Spot for Advancement for Women/Minorities:

LOCATIONS: ("Y" = Yes)
West:	Southwest:	Midwest:	Southeast:	Northeast:	International:
Y	Y	Y	Y	Y	

OXFORD HEALTH PLANS INC

www.oxhp.com

Industry Group Code: 524114 Ranks within this company's industry group: Sales: 20 Profits: 8

Insurance/HMO/PPO:	Drugs:	Equipment/Supplies:	Hospitals/Clinics:	Services:	Health Care:
Insurance:	Manufacturer:	Manufacturer:	Acute Care:	Diagnostics:	Home Health:
Managed Care: Y	Distributor:	Distributor:	Sub-Acute Care:	Labs/Testing:	Long-Term Care:
Utilization Mgmt.: Y	Specialty Pharm.:	Leasing/Finance:	Outpatient Surgery:	Staffing:	Physical Therapy:
Payment Proc.:	Vitamins/Nutri.:	Information Sys.:	Phys. Rehab. Center:	Waste Disposal:	Phys. Practice Mgmt.:
	Clinical Trials:		Psychiatric Clinics:	Specialty Services:	

TYPES OF BUSINESS:
HMO/PPO
Health Benefit Plans
Employee Benefit Plans
Health & Life Insurance

BRANDS/DIVISIONS/AFFILIATES:
UnitedHealth Group
MedSpan Health Options, Inc.
Oxford Health Insurance, Inc.
Oxford Health Plans, Inc.
Investors Guaranty Life Insurance Company
oxfordhealth.com
Freedom
Liberty

CONTACTS:
Note: Officers with more than one job title may be intentionally listed here more than once.

Charles G. Berg, CEO
Charles G. Berg, Pres.
Kurt B. Thompson, Exec. VP/CFO
Kevin R. Hill, Exec. VP-Sales
Steve Black, CIO
Daniel N. Gregoire, Exec. VP/General Counsel
Steve Black, Exec. VP-Oper.
Kevin R. Hill, Exec. VP-Bus. Strategy
Lee deStefano, VP-Investor Rel.
Kent J. Thiry, Chmn.

Phone: 203-459-6000 **Fax:** 203-459-6464
Toll-Free: 800-889-7658
Address: 48 Monroe Tpke., Trumbull, CT 06611 US

GROWTH PLANS/SPECIAL FEATURES:
Oxford Health Plans, Inc., a subsidiary of UnitedHealth Group, provides health benefit plans to about 1.6 million members primarily in New York, New Jersey and Connecticut. The firm provides the Freedom and Liberty point-of-service plans, HMO plans, PPO plans, Medicare plans and third-party administration of employer-funded benefit plans or self-funded health plans. The company operates through its HMO subsidiaries (Oxford Health Plans, Inc. of New York, New Jersey and Connecticut and MedSpan Health Options, Inc.) and through its insurance subsidiaries (Oxford Health Insurance, Inc. and Investors Guaranty Life Insurance Company). Through its web site, www.oxfordhealth.com, prospective enrollees, members, benefit administrators, employer groups, providers and brokers can view benefit packages, obtain rate quotes and enroll members in certain services. The company focuses on developing new products and benefit packages, expanding geographically, managing health care costs in order to reduce health care prices and achieving administrative efficiencies by increasing the level of electronic transactions and automation. Recently, Oxford Health increased its Medicare coverage area to include eight counties in northern and central New Jersey, as well as the lower Hudson Valley in New York. Oxford merged with UnitedHealth in July 2004.

The firm provides its employees with reward and recognition programs, college tuition reimbursement, flexible work options and fitness center benefits.

FINANCIALS:
Sales and profits are in thousands of dollars—add 000 to get the full amount. Year 2004 note: Complete fiscal 2004 results were not available for all companies at press time. For this company, year 2004 is for 3 months.

2004 Sales: $1,411,200 (3 months)	2004 Profits: $86,600 (3 months)	
2003 Sales: $5,452,444	2003 Profits: $351,853	**Stock Ticker:** Subsidiary
2002 Sales: $4,963,400	2002 Profits: $222,000	Employees: 3,200
2001 Sales: $4,421,200	2001 Profits: $322,400	Fiscal Year Ends: 12/31
2000 Sales: $4,111,800	2000 Profits: $265,100	

SALARIES/BENEFITS:
Pension Plan: ESOP Stock Plan: Profit Sharing: Top Exec. Salary: $800,962 Bonus: $800,000
Savings Plan: Y Stock Purch. Plan: Second Exec. Salary: $500,000 Bonus: $350,000

OTHER THOUGHTS:
Apparent Top Female Officers:
Hot Spot for Advancement for Women/Minorities:

LOCATIONS: ("Y" = Yes)
West	Southwest	Midwest	Southeast	Northeast	International
			Y	Y	

PACIFICARE HEALTH SYSTEMS INC
www.pacificare.com

Industry Group Code: 524114   Ranks within this company's industry group: Sales: 10   Profits: 13

Insurance/HMO/PPO:		Drugs:		Equipment/Supplies:		Hospitals/Clinics:		Services:		Health Care:	
Insurance:		Manufacturer:	Y	Manufacturer:		Acute Care:		Diagnostics:		Home Health:	
Managed Care:	Y	Distributor:		Distributor:		Sub-Acute Care:		Labs/Testing:		Long-Term Care:	
Utilization Mgmt.:		Specialty Pharm.:		Leasing/Finance:		Outpatient Surgery:		Staffing:		Physical Therapy:	
Payment Proc.:		Vitamins/Nutri.:		Information Sys.:		Phys. Rehab. Center:		Waste Disposal:		Phys. Practice Mgmt.:	
		Clinical Trials:				Psychiatric Clinics:		Specialty Services:	Y		

TYPES OF BUSINESS:
HMO/PPO
Managed Care Products & Services
Dental Plans
Behavioral Health
Wellness Program
Insurance
Management Services

BRANDS/DIVISIONS/AFFILIATES:
PacifiCare Behavioral Health of California, Inc.
PacifiCare Life Assurance Company
PacifiCare Life and Health Insurance Company
Prescription Solutions
California Dental Health Plan
Secure Horizons Medicare Supplement Plan
SHUSA
American Medical Security Group

CONTACTS: Note: Officers with more than one job title may be intentionally listed here more than once.
Howard G. Phantstiel, CEO
Howard G. Phantstiel, Pres.
Gregory W. Scott, Exec. VP/CFO
Judy Ehrenreich, Sr. VP-Human Resources
Joseph Konowiecki, Exec. VP/General Counsel
Nick Franklin, Sr. VP-Public Affairs
Sharon Garrett, Exec. Enterprise Services
Brad Bowlus, Pres./CEO-Health Plans Div.
Jacqueline Kosecoff, Exec. VP-Pharmaceutical Services
Katherine F. Feeny, Exec. VP-Senior Solutions
Howard Phanstiel, Chmn.

Phone: 714-952-1121	Fax: 714-226-3581
Toll-Free:	
Address: 5995 Plaza Dr., Cypress, CA 90630 US	

GROWTH PLANS/SPECIAL FEATURES:
PacifiCare Health Systems, Inc. is a managed health care services company that serves approximately 3 million HMO members in eight states and Guam and offers a variety of specialty managed health care products. The company's commercial plans offer a comprehensive range of products to employer groups and individuals, including HMO, preferred provider organization (PPO) and point-of-service (POS) plans. PacifiCare offers Medicare risk management through SHUSA, a division that provides management services and best practices to HMOs and health care delivery systems. Subsidiary Prescription Solutions offers pharmacy benefit management services and a variety of cost and quality management capabilities. Other subsidiaries, including PacifiCare Life and Health Insurance Company and PacifiCare Life Assurance Company, offer managed health care products that have been integrated with the company's existing HMO products to form multi-option health benefits programs. PacifiCare Behavioral Health of California, Inc. provides behavioral health care services directly to customers in California. California Dental Health Plan offers prepaid dental and optometry benefits. The company recently broadened its reach by offering Secure Horizons Medicare Supplement plans in Georgia, Illinois, Kansas, Michigan, Missouri and Ohio. In September 2004, the company agreed to acquire American Medical Security Group for $502 million in cash.

Among various employee benefits, the company provides educational assistance, child care subsidies and health improvement programs. PacifiCare Health Systems also offers $250 per year to employees for personal choice expenses that can go toward health club memberships, classes, financial planning or charity.

FINANCIALS:
Sales and profits are in thousands of dollars—add 000 to get the full amount. Year 2004 note: Complete fiscal 2004 results were not available for all companies at press time. For this company, year 2004 is for 9 months.

2004 Sales: $9,117,197 (9 months)
2003 Sales: $11,008,511
2002 Sales: $10,894,000
2001 Sales: $11,560,000
2000 Sales: $11,467,900

2004 Profits: $231,193 (9 months)
2003 Profits: $242,748
2002 Profits: $-758,000
2001 Profits: $19,000
2000 Profits: $161,000

Stock Ticker: PHS
Employees: 7,700
Fiscal Year Ends: 9/30

SALARIES/BENEFITS:
Pension Plan:	ESOP Stock Plan:	Profit Sharing:	Top Exec. Salary: $976,155	Bonus: $2,000,000
Savings Plan: Y	Stock Purch. Plan:		Second Exec. Salary: $642,308	Bonus: $690,000

OTHER THOUGHTS:
Apparent Top Female Officers: 4
Hot Spot for Advancement for Women/Minorities: Y

LOCATIONS: ("Y" = Yes)
West:	Southwest:	Midwest:	Southeast:	Northeast:	International:
Y	Y	Y	Y		Y

PALOMAR MEDICAL TECHNOLOGIES INC   www.palmed.com

Industry Group Code: 339113 Ranks within this company's industry group: Sales: 121 Profits: 92

Insurance/HMO/PPO:	Drugs:	Equipment/Supplies:	Hospitals/Clinics:	Services:	Health Care:
Insurance:	Manufacturer:	Manufacturer: Y	Acute Care:	Diagnostics:	Home Health:
Managed Care:	Distributor:	Distributor:	Sub-Acute Care:	Labs/Testing:	Long-Term Care:
Utilization Mgmt.:	Specialty Pharm.:	Leasing/Finance:	Outpatient Surgery:	Staffing:	Physical Therapy:
Payment Proc.:	Vitamins/Nutri.:	Information Sys.:	Phys. Rehab. Center:	Waste Disposal:	Phys. Practice Mgmt.:
	Clinical Trials:		Psychiatric Clinics:	Specialty Services:	

TYPES OF BUSINESS:
Equipment-Laser Hair Removal Systems
Tattoo & Lesion Removal Systems

BRANDS/DIVISIONS/AFFILIATES:
Polamar Medical Products, Inc.
Esthetica Partners, Inc.
EsteLux
SLP 1000
LightSheer
EpiLaser
Q-Yag 5
MediLux

CONTACTS: Note: Officers with more than one job title may be intentionally listed here more than once.
Joseph P. Caruso, CEO
Joseph P. Caruso, Pres.
Michael DiToro, VP-Mktg.
Kathy Freitas, VP-Human Resources
Gregory Altshuler, VP-Research
Michael H. Smotrich, Chief Tech. Officer
Patricia A. Davis, VP/General Counsel
Steven Armstrong, VP-Oper.
Robert Brody, VP-Bus. Dev.
Paul S. Weiner, VP-Investor Rel.
Douglas Baraw, VP/Chief Acct. Officer
Patricia A. Davis, Corp. Sec.
Paul F. Wiener, VP-Sales
Michail Pankratov, VP-Clinical & Consumer Affairs
Louis P. Valente, Chmn.

Phone: 781-993-2300   Fax: 781-993-2330
Toll-Free: 800-725-6627
Address: 82 Cambridge St., Ste. 1, Burlington, MA 01803 US

GROWTH PLANS/SPECIAL FEATURES:
Palomar Medical Technologies, Inc. is focused on lasers and light-based products for use in dermatology and cosmetic procedures, with an emphasis on hair removal and research and development relating to that and other cosmetic products. The firm currently has two operating subsidiaries, Palomar Medical Products, Inc. and Esthetica Partners, Inc. Palomar's principal products include the EsteLux light-based system, featuring a fast coverage rate and a long pulse width, especially effective for large areas like legs and backs; and the SLP 1000 diode laser system, which uses super-long pulse technology to provide hair removal and vascular treatments for virtually all skin types. This system is compact and easy-to-use and provides safe and effective treatment. Palomar was also the first company to receive FDA approval for a diode laser for hair removal and leg vein treatment, the LightSheer system. Other products include the EpiLaser for permanent hair reduction and the Q-Yag 5 system for tattoo and pigmented lesion removal. The Q-Yag 5 is smaller and lighter than other systems, making it desirable for mobile and small physician offices. MediLux and StarLux are the higher-powered versions of EsteLux. Palomar has been trying to bring its technologies to a broader consumer market. To this effect it has reached agreements with the Gillette Company to develop a home-use hair removal device for women and with Johnson & Johnson Consumer Companies to develop home-use devices for reducing or reshaping body fat, reducing wrinkles and reducing or preventing acne.

FINANCIALS: Sales and profits are in thousands of dollars—add 000 to get the full amount. Year 2004 note: Complete fiscal 2004 results were not available for all companies at press time. For this company, year 2004 is for 9 months.

2004 Sales: $38,011 (9 months)	2004 Profits: $5,272 (9 months)	Stock Ticker: PMTI
2003 Sales: $34,773	2003 Profits: $3,369	Employees: 119
2002 Sales: $25,400	2002 Profits: $ 39	Fiscal Year Ends: 12/31
2001 Sales: $16,700	2001 Profits: $-5,500	
2000 Sales: $13,200	2000 Profits: $-9,600	

SALARIES/BENEFITS:
Pension Plan:	ESOP Stock Plan:	Profit Sharing:	Top Exec. Salary: $250,000	Bonus: $112,500
Savings Plan: Y	Stock Purch. Plan:		Second Exec. Salary: $165,000	Bonus: $74,250

OTHER THOUGHTS:
Apparent Top Female Officers: 2
Hot Spot for Advancement for Women/Minorities:

LOCATIONS: ("Y" = Yes)
West:	Southwest:	Midwest:	Southeast:	Northeast: Y	International:

PAR PHARMACEUTICAL COMPANIES INC
www.parpharm.com

Industry Group Code: 325412 **Ranks within this company's industry group:** Sales: 34 Profits: 25

Insurance/HMO/PPO:	Drugs:		Equipment/Supplies:	Hospitals/Clinics:	Services:	Health Care:
Insurance:	Manufacturer:	Y	Manufacturer:	Acute Care:	Diagnostics:	Home Health:
Managed Care:	Distributor:		Distributor:	Sub-Acute Care:	Labs/Testing:	Long-Term Care:
Utilization Mgmt.:	Specialty Pharm.:		Leasing/Finance:	Outpatient Surgery:	Staffing:	Physical Therapy:
Payment Proc.:	Vitamins/Nutri.:		Information Sys.:	Phys. Rehab. Center:	Waste Disposal:	Phys. Practice Mgmt.:
	Clinical Trials:			Psychiatric Clinics:	Specialty Services:	

TYPES OF BUSINESS:
Drugs-Generic
Intermediate Ingredients

BRANDS/DIVISIONS/AFFILIATES:
Pharmaceutical Resources, Inc.
Par Pharmaceutical, Inc.
FineTech
Kali Laboratories, Inc.

CONTACTS:
Note: Officers with more than one job title may be intentionally listed here more than once.

Scott L. Tarriff, CEO
Scott L. Tarriff, Pres.
Dennis J. O'Connor, VP/CFO
Shankar Hariharan, Exec. VP/Chief Scientific Officer
Thomas Haughey, VP/General Counsel
Arie Gutman, Pres., FineTech
Mark Auerbach, Chmn.

Phone: 845-425-7100 **Fax:** 845-425-7907
Toll-Free:
Address: One Ram Ridge Rd., Spring Valley, NY 10977-6714 US

GROWTH PLANS/SPECIAL FEATURES:
Par Pharmaceutical Companies, Inc. (formerly Pharmaceutical Resources, Inc.) develops, manufactures and markets generic pharmaceuticals through its principal subsidiary, Par Pharmaceutical, Inc. The company's current portfolio consists of 73 prescription and over-the-counter drugs, available in varying dosage strengths for a total of more than 170 products. Products include treatments for central nervous system disorders, cardiovascular drugs, analgesics and anti-inflammatory products, anti-bacterials, anti-diabetics, antihistamines, anti-virals, cholesterol-lowering drugs and ovulation stimulants. Among these are generic versions of Advil, Daypro, Glucophage, Zantac, Clomid, Prozac, Halcion and Prilosec. Through its FineTech subsidiary, Par Pharmaceutical also develops and utilizes synthetic chemical processes to design and develop intermediate ingredients for the pharmaceutical manufacturing industry. The company is also developing a line of proprietary specialty pharmaceuticals and expects to market the first of these in 2005. Par Pharmaceutical recently completed the acquisition of Kali Laboratories, Inc. for $135 million in cash and warrants, more than doubling the size of Par's existing research and development capabilities in the process. Par now has 35 Abbreviated New Drug Applications (ANDAs) currently awaiting approval by the U.S. FDA, with a total of more than 60 drug products in development.

FINANCIALS:
Sales and profits are in thousands of dollars—add 000 to get the full amount. Year 2004 note: Complete fiscal 2004 results were not available for all companies at press time. For this company, year 2004 is for 6 months.

2004 Sales: $424,298 (6 months)	2004 Profits: $60,066 (6 months)	**Stock Ticker:** PRX
2003 Sales: $646,023	2003 Profits: $122,533	Employees: 531
2002 Sales: $381,600	2002 Profits: $79,500	Fiscal Year Ends: 12/31
2001 Sales: $271,000	2001 Profits: $53,900	
2000 Sales: $85,022	2000 Profits: $-929	

SALARIES/BENEFITS:
Pension Plan: Y	ESOP Stock Plan:	Profit Sharing:	Top Exec. Salary: $401,538	Bonus: $450,000
Savings Plan: Y	Stock Purch. Plan: Y		Second Exec. Salary: $300,000	Bonus: $225,000

OTHER THOUGHTS:
Apparent Top Female Officers:
Hot Spot for Advancement for Women/Minorities:

LOCATIONS: ("Y" = Yes)
West:	Southwest:	Midwest:	Southeast:	Northeast:	International:
				Y	Y

PARTNERS HEALTHCARE SYSTEM

www.partners.org

Industry Group Code: 622110 Ranks within this company's industry group: Sales: 12 Profits: 14

Insurance/HMO/PPO:	Drugs:	Equipment/Supplies:	Hospitals/Clinics:		Services:		Health Care:	
Insurance: Managed Care: Utilization Mgmt.: Payment Proc.:	Manufacturer: Distributor: Specialty Pharm.: Vitamins/Nutri.: Clinical Trials:	Manufacturer: Distributor: Leasing/Finance: Information Sys.:	Acute Care: Sub-Acute Care: Outpatient Surgery: Phys. Rehab. Center: Psychiatric Clinics:	Y	Diagnostics: Labs/Testing: Staffing: Waste Disposal: Specialty Services:		Home Health: Long-Term Care: Physical Therapy: Phys. Practice Mgmt.:	Y Y Y

TYPES OF BUSINESS:
Hospitals-General
Home & Long-Term Care
Medical Schools
Private Practices
Teaching Hospitals
Mental Health Hospitals

BRANDS/DIVISIONS/AFFILIATES:
Massachusetts General Hospital
Brigham and Women's Hospital
Partners Community HealthCare
Dana-Farber/Partners CancerCare
MGH Institute of Health Professions
Harvard Medical School
Faulkner Hospital
North Shore Medical Center

GROWTH PLANS/SPECIAL FEATURES:
Partners HealthCare is the largest health care system in Massachusetts. The firm was founded as the umbrella corporation of Massachusetts General Hospital and Brigham and Women's Hospital and has since grown to include primary physicians, specialist caregivers, acute care hospitals, medical schools and long-term elderly care. Other company members include Partners Community HealthCare, a network of more than 1,000 physicians; the Dana-Farber/Partners CancerCare, a joint venture with Dana Farber Cancer Institute; MGH Institute of Health Professions; and Harvard Medical School. Partners member hospitals are the Faulkner Hospital, a nonprofit, community teaching hospital with 150 beds; the North Shore Medical Center; the McLean Hospital for the treatment of mental illness and chemical dependency; and Newton-Wellesley, the premier community teaching hospital in Massachusetts. The firm also runs Partners Continuing Care, an elderly care facility for home and community care. Partners is a nonprofit organization supported in part by charitable contributions.

CONTACTS:
Note: Officers with more than one job title may be intentionally listed here more than once.
James J. Mongan, CEO
James J. Mongan, Pres.
Thomas P. Glynn, COO
John Glaser, CIO
John M. Connors, Jr., Chmn.

Phone: 617-278-1000 **Fax:** 617-278-1049
Toll-Free:
Address: Prudential Tower, 800 Boylston St., Ste. 1150, Boston, MA 02199-8001 US

FINANCIALS:
Sales and profits are in thousands of dollars—add 000 to get the full amount. Year 2004 note: Complete fiscal 2004 results were not available for all companies at press time. For this company, year 2004 is for months.

2004 Sales: $ (months)   2004 Profits: $ (months)
2003 Sales: $4,561,200   2003 Profits: $85,600
2002 Sales: $4,217,600   2002 Profits: $55,700
2001 Sales: $ 2001 Profits: $
2000 Sales: $ 2000 Profits: $

Stock Ticker: Nonprofit
Employees:
Fiscal Year Ends: 9/30

SALARIES/BENEFITS:
Pension Plan: ESOP Stock Plan: Profit Sharing: Top Exec. Salary: $ Bonus: $
Savings Plan: Stock Purch. Plan: Second Exec. Salary: $ Bonus: $

OTHER THOUGHTS:
Apparent Top Female Officers:
Hot Spot for Advancement for Women/Minorities:

LOCATIONS: ("Y" = Yes)
West:	Southwest:	Midwest:	Southeast:	Northeast:	International:
				Y	

Note: Financial information, benefits and other data can change quickly and may vary from those stated here.

PATIENT CARE INC

www.patientcare.com

Industry Group Code: 621610 **Ranks within this company's industry group:** Sales: Profits:

Insurance/HMO/PPO:	Drugs:	Equipment/Supplies:	Hospitals/Clinics:	Services:	Health Care:
Insurance: Managed Care: Utilization Mgmt.: Payment Proc.:	Manufacturer: Distributor: Specialty Pharm.: Vitamins/Nutri.: Clinical Trials:	Manufacturer: Distributor: Leasing/Finance: Information Sys.:	Acute Care: Sub-Acute Care: Outpatient Surgery: Phys. Rehab. Center: Psychiatric Clinics:	Diagnostics: Labs/Testing: Staffing: Waste Disposal: Specialty Services:	Home Health: Y Long-Term Care: Physical Therapy: Phys. Practice Mgmt.:

TYPES OF BUSINESS:
Home Health Care

BRANDS/DIVISIONS/AFFILIATES:
Rush Home Care Network
Tri-Hospital Home Health and Hospice

CONTACTS:
Note: Officers with more than one job title may be intentionally listed here more than once.
Arthur Stratton, CEO
Arthur Stratton, Chmn.

Phone: 973-669-5222   **Fax:** 973-325-2590
Toll-Free: 800-541-8676
Address: 100 Executive Dr., Ste. 130, West Orange, NJ 07052 US

GROWTH PLANS/SPECIAL FEATURES:
Patient Care, Inc. is a provider of home health care services predominantly in the Northeast, with additional agency locations in the Southeast. The company has 27 branches in New York, New Jersey, Massachusetts, Connecticut, Florida, Georgia, Illinois, Ohio and Pennsylvania. The firm offers qualified professionals who are available to provide customized home health care services ranging from one- to two-hour visits every week to 24-hour live-in aid. When service is requested, the company first sends a field nurse supervisor to assess the physical and social needs of the potential client and then assigns the most qualified and appropriate member of the staff possible. Available services include personal care, such as basic hygienic assistance; housekeeping, such as cooking, cleaning and errands; and socialization, providing supportive companionship. JCAHO (the Joint Commission on Accreditation of Healthcare Organizations) certifies all Patient Care locations. As well, most of its offices are certified Medicare agencies and accredited by various regional health care supervisory boards. In recent news, Patient Care acquired Rush Home Care Network in Chicago, Illinois and Tri-Hospital Home Health and Hospice in West Orange, New Jersey.

FINANCIALS:
Sales and profits are in thousands of dollars—add 000 to get the full amount. Year 2004 note: Complete fiscal 2004 results were not available for all companies at press time. For this company, year 2004 is for   months.

2004 Sales: $ (months)
2003 Sales: $
2002 Sales: $314,200
2001 Sales: $477,100
2000 Sales: $500,685

2004 Profits: $ (months)
2003 Profits: $
2002 Profits: $-1,800
2001 Profits: $-10,400
2000 Profits: $20,584

Stock Ticker: Private
Employees: 6,000
Fiscal Year Ends: 12/31

SALARIES/BENEFITS:
Pension Plan: ESOP Stock Plan: Profit Sharing: Top Exec. Salary: $629,820   Bonus: $582,165
Savings Plan: Stock Purch. Plan: Second Exec. Salary: $347,154   Bonus: $237,390

OTHER THOUGHTS:
Apparent Top Female Officers:
Hot Spot for Advancement for Women/Minorities: Y

LOCATIONS: ("Y" = Yes)

West:	Southwest:	Midwest:	Southeast:	Northeast:	International:
		Y	Y	Y	

Note: Financial information, benefits and other data can change quickly and may vary from those stated here.

PATTERSON COMPANIES INC

www.pattersondental.com

Industry Group Code: 421450 Ranks within this company's industry group: Sales: 4 Profits: 2

Insurance/HMO/PPO:	Drugs:	Equipment/Supplies:	Hospitals/Clinics:	Services:	Health Care:
Insurance:	Manufacturer:	Manufacturer: Y	Acute Care:	Diagnostics:	Home Health:
Managed Care:	Distributor:	Distributor: Y	Sub-Acute Care:	Labs/Testing:	Long-Term Care:
Utilization Mgmt.:	Specialty Pharm.:	Leasing/Finance: Y	Outpatient Surgery:	Staffing:	Physical Therapy:
Payment Proc.: Y	Vitamins/Nutri.:	Information Sys.:	Phys. Rehab. Center:	Waste Disposal:	Phys. Practice Mgmt.:
	Clinical Trials:		Psychiatric Clinics:	Specialty Services: Y	

TYPES OF BUSINESS:
Distribution-Dental Products
Private-Label Dental Products
Inventory Management
Dental Office Design
Equipment Installation & Services
Equipment Financing
Rehabilitation Supplies
Veterinary Supplies

BRANDS/DIVISIONS/AFFILIATES:
Patterson Dental Company
Direct Dental Supply Co.
Patterson Dental Supply, Inc.
AOC Vertriebs GmbH
AbilityOne Products Corp.
Webster Veterinary Supply, Inc.
PDC Funding Company, LLC
Milburn Distributions, Inc.

CONTACTS:
Note: Officers with more than one job title may be intentionally listed here more than once.

Peter L. Frechette, CEO
James W. Wiltz, Pres.
James W. Wiltz, COO
R. Stephen Armstrong, Exec. VP/CFO
Cree Z. Hanna, VP-Human Resources
Lynn E. Askew, VP-MIS
Matthew L. Levitt, General Counsel
Gary D. Johnson, VP-Oper.
R. Stephen Armstrong, Treas.
Jeffrey H. Webster, Pres., Webster Veterinary Supply, Inc.
Scott R. Kabbes, Pres., Patterson Dental Supply
Howard A. Schwartz, Pres., AbilityOne Products Corp.
Peter L. Frechette, Chmn.

Phone: 651-686-1600 **Fax:** 651-686-9331
Toll-Free: 800-328-5536
Address: 1031 Mendota Heights Rd., St. Paul, MN 55120-1401 US

GROWTH PLANS/SPECIAL FEATURES:

Patterson Companies, Inc., formerly Patterson Dental Company, is a leading full-service distributor of dental products, companion pet aids and rehabilitative products. The company has several subsidiaries including Direct Dental Supply Co., Patterson Dental Canada, Inc., Patterson Dental Supply, Inc., Webster Veterinary Supply, Inc., PDC Funding Company, LLC, Webster Management, LP, AbilityOne Products Corp., AbilityOne Corporation, Sammons Preston Canada, Inc., J.A. Preston Corporation, AbilityOne Homecraft, Ltd., AbilityOne, Ltd., AbilityOne Kinetec S.A. and AOC Vertriebs GmbH. Patterson Dental Supply is one of the two largest distributors of dental products in North America and supplies dentists, dental laboratories, institutions and other health care professionals with necessary instruments. Dental products include consumables such as x-ray film, restorative materials, hand instruments, sterilization products as well as advanced-technology dental equipment, practice management, clinical software, patient education systems and office forms and stationery. Webster Veterinary Supply is the leading distributor of veterinary supplies to companion-pet veterinary clinics in the eastern United States and the second-largest nationally. It provides products such as consumable supplies, equipment, diagnostic supplies, vaccines and pharmaceuticals for the treatment and prevention of diseases in dogs, cats, horses and other small animals. Patterson is the world's leading distributor of rehabilitative medical supplies and non-wheelchair assistive products through AbilityOne Products Corp. The subsidiary offers over 15,000 rehabilitation products from more than 1,500 suppliers and manufacturers for physical and occupational therapists. Patterson recently acquired the largest distributor of equine veterinary supplies in the United States, Milburn Distributions, Inc. Milburn will be operated as part of Patterson's Webster Veterinary Supply unit.

Patterson offers its employees an educational assistance program, health benefits, disability and accidental death insurance, an employee assistance program and discount purchase programs.

FINANCIALS:
Sales and profits are in thousands of dollars—add 000 to get the full amount. Year 2004 note: Complete fiscal 2004 results were not available for all companies at press time. For this company, year 2004 is for 12 months.

2004 Sales: $1,969,349 (12 months)   2004 Profits: $149,465 (12 months)
2003 Sales: $1,657,000   2003 Profits: $119,700
2002 Sales: $1,415,500   2002 Profits: $95,300
2001 Sales: $1,156,500   2001 Profits: $76,500
2000 Sales: $1,045,900   2000 Profits: $64,500

Stock Ticker: PDCO
Employees: 5,750
Fiscal Year Ends: 4/30

SALARIES/BENEFITS:
Pension Plan: ESOP Stock Plan: Y   Profit Sharing: Top Exec. Salary: $399,265   Bonus: $381,612
Savings Plan: Y   Stock Purch. Plan: Y   Second Exec. Salary: $317,001   Bonus: $273,000

OTHER THOUGHTS:
Apparent Top Female Officers: 2
Hot Spot for Advancement for Women/Minorities:

LOCATIONS: ("Y" = Yes)
West:	Southwest:	Midwest:	Southeast:	Northeast:	International:
Y	Y	Y	Y	Y	Y

Note: Financial information, benefits and other data can change quickly and may vary from those stated here.

PDI INC

www.pdi-inc.com

Industry Group Code: 541613 Ranks within this company's industry group: Sales: 1 Profits: 1

Insurance/HMO/PPO:	Drugs:	Equipment/Supplies:	Hospitals/Clinics:	Services:	Health Care:
Insurance: Managed Care: Utilization Mgmt.: Payment Proc.:	Manufacturer: Distributor: Specialty Pharm.: Vitamins/Nutri.: Clinical Trials:	Manufacturer: Distributor: Leasing/Finance: Information Sys.:	Acute Care: Sub-Acute Care: Outpatient Surgery: Phys. Rehab. Center: Psychiatric Clinics:	Diagnostics: Labs/Testing: Staffing: Waste Disposal: Specialty Services: Y	Home Health: Long-Term Care: Physical Therapy: Phys. Practice Mgmt.:

TYPES OF BUSINESS:
Marketing & Advertising-Sales Campaigns for Drugmakers
Contract Sales Organization
Pharmaceutical Sales Support
Marketing Research

BRANDS/DIVISIONS/AFFILIATES:
Pharmakon LLC

CONTACTS:
Note: Officers with more than one job title may be intentionally listed here more than once.
Charles T. Saldarini, CEO
Bernard C. Boyle, CFO
Robert R. Higgins, Exec. VP-Sales & Mktg.
Nancy McCarthy, Exec. VP-Human Resources
Beth R. Jacobson, General Counsel
Deborah Schnell, VP-Bus. Dev.
Steve P. Cotugno, Exec. VP-Investor Rel.
Bernard C. Boyle, Treas.
Stephen P. Cotugno, Exec. VP-Corp. Dev.
Christopher Tama, Exec. VP-Pharmaceutical Products
Lloyd X. Fishman, Exec. VP-Medical Devices & Diagnostics
Bernard C. Boyle, Corp. Sec.
John P. Dugan, Chmn.

Phone: 201-258-8450 **Fax:** 201-258-8400
Toll-Free: 800-242-7494
Address: Saddle River Executive Ctr., 1 Rte. 17 S., Saddle River, NJ 07458-1937 US

GROWTH PLANS/SPECIAL FEATURES:
PDI, Inc. is a sales and marketing company serving the pharmaceutical, biotechnology and medical services and diagnostics (MDD) industries. The firm provides product-specific programs designed to maximize profitability throughout a product's lifecycle, from pre-launch through maturity. The company is recognized as an industry leader based on its expertise in sales, brand management, product marketing, marketing research, medical education, medical affairs and managed market and trade relations. PDI creates and executes sales and marketing programs designed for clients' products, which it promotes for fees or percentages of sales, as well as products the company itself distributes, licenses or owns outright. Clients engage PDI on a contractual basis to design and implement product detailing programs for both prescription and over-the-counter products. PDI has designed and executed customized sales and marketing programs for many of the industry's largest companies, including Bayer, GlaxoSmithKline, Johnson & Johnson, Pfizer and Allergan. The firm's medical education and communications group creates custom programs to inform its clients' potential customers about the benefits of its clients' products. Such programs may include teleconferences, audio seminars, publication planning and continuing medical education programs. In addition, PDI offers qualitative and quantitative marketing research to health care providers, patients and managed care customers in the U.S. and globally. In August 2004, PDI acquired Pharmakon, L.L.C. a healthcare communications company that markets ethical pharmaceutical and biotechnology products.

FINANCIALS:
Sales and profits are in thousands of dollars—add 000 to get the full amount. Year 2004 note: Complete fiscal 2004 results were not available for all companies at press time. For this company, year 2004 is for 9 months.

2004 Sales: $276,632 (9 months) 2004 Profits: $16,485 (9 months)
2003 Sales: $317,448   2003 Profits: $12,258
2002 Sales: $284,000   2002 Profits: $-30,800
2001 Sales: $696,600   2001 Profits: $6,400
2000 Sales: $416,900   2000 Profits: $27,000

Stock Ticker: PDII
Employees: 3,884
Fiscal Year Ends: 12/31

SALARIES/BENEFITS:
Pension Plan: ESOP Stock Plan: Profit Sharing: Top Exec. Salary: $376,486   Bonus: $752,972
Savings Plan: Y   Stock Purch. Plan: Second Exec. Salary: $289,620 Bonus: $477,875

OTHER THOUGHTS:
Apparent Top Female Officers: 3
Hot Spot for Advancement for Women/Minorities: Y

LOCATIONS: ("Y" = Yes)
West:	Southwest:	Midwest:	Southeast:	Northeast:	International:
Y				Y	

PEDIATRIC SERVICES OF AMERICA INC

www.psakids.com

Industry Group Code: 621610   Ranks within this company's industry group: Sales: 8   Profits: 10

Insurance/HMO/PPO:	Drugs:	Equipment/Supplies:	Hospitals/Clinics:	Services:	Health Care:
Insurance:	Manufacturer:	Manufacturer:	Acute Care:	Diagnostics:	Home Health: Y
Managed Care:	Distributor:	Distributor:	Sub-Acute Care:	Labs/Testing:	Long-Term Care:
Utilization Mgmt.:	Specialty Pharm.:	Leasing/Finance: Y	Outpatient Surgery:	Staffing:	Physical Therapy: Y
Payment Proc.:	Vitamins/Nutri.:	Information Sys.:	Phys. Rehab. Center:	Waste Disposal:	Phys. Practice Mgmt.:
	Clinical Trials:		Psychiatric Clinics:	Specialty Services: Y	

TYPES OF BUSINESS:
Home Health Care-Pediatric
Case Management Services
Medical Equipment Rental & Sales
Pharmaceutical Services
Infusion Therapy Services
Pediatric Rehabilitation Services
Pediatric Outpatient Treatment

BRANDS/DIVISIONS/AFFILIATES:

CONTACTS:
Note: Officers with more than one job title may be intentionally listed here more than once.
Edward K. Wissing, Interim CEO
Joseph D. Sansone, Pres.
James M. McNeill, Sr. VP/CFO
Ken Wilson, VP-Mktg. & Sales
James M. McNeill, Treas.
Joseph P. Harrelson, VP-PPEC Oper.
James M. McNeill, Corp. Sec.
Edward K. Wissing, Chmn.

Phone: 770-441-1580   Fax: 770-263-9340
Toll-Free: 800-950-1580
Address: 310 Technology Pkwy., Norcross, GA 30092-2929 US

GROWTH PLANS/SPECIAL FEATURES:
Pediatric Services of America, Inc. (PSA) is a leading provider of children's health care and related services. The company provides children's health care services through over 120 branch offices located in 22 states, including satellite offices and branch office start-ups. Services and equipment include nursing, respiratory therapy, rental and sale of durable home medical equipment, pharmaceutical services and infusion therapy services. The firm also provides pediatric rehabilitation services, day treatment centers for medically fragile children, well care services and special needs educational services for pediatric patients. Additionally, PSA offers case management services to assist the family and patient by coordinating between the insurer or other payor, the physician, the hospital and other health care providers. These services are designed to provide a high-quality, lower-cost alternative to prolonged hospitalization. PSA also offers respiratory, infusion therapy and related services for adults. Pediatric nursing services consist of private duty home care for patients with conditions such as digestive and absorptive diseases, congenital heart defects, cancer, cerebral palsy, hemophilia and post-surgical needs. Personnel monitor the child's condition, administer medications and treatment regimens, provide feeding and pain management and provide daily care, including baths and skin care. Physical and other forms of therapy are also conducted. The company also rents and sells medical equipment such as ventilators, liquid oxygen systems and apnea monitors.

PSA offers its employees benefits including flexible schedules, flexible benefit plans, group health and dental insurance, training and support, relocation opportunities and credit union membership.

FINANCIALS:
Sales and profits are in thousands of dollars—add 000 to get the full amount. Year 2004 note: Complete fiscal 2004 results were not available for all companies at press time. For this company, year 2004 is for 9 months.

2004 Sales: $179,276 (9 months)	2004 Profits: $4,192 (9 months)	
2003 Sales: $215,592	2003 Profits: $5,126	Stock Ticker: PSAI
2002 Sales: $197,500	2002 Profits: $14,100	Employees: 4,800
2001 Sales: $184,100	2001 Profits: $5,500	Fiscal Year Ends: 9/30
2000 Sales: $186,366	2000 Profits: $28,645	

SALARIES/BENEFITS:
Pension Plan:	ESOP Stock Plan:	Profit Sharing:	Top Exec. Salary: $378,000	Bonus: $140,000
Savings Plan: Y	Stock Purch. Plan: Y		Second Exec. Salary: $215,250	Bonus: $125,000

OTHER THOUGHTS:
Apparent Top Female Officers:
Hot Spot for Advancement for Women/Minorities:

LOCATIONS: ("Y" = Yes)
West:	Southwest:	Midwest:	Southeast:	Northeast:	International:
Y	Y	Y	Y	Y	

PEDIATRIX MEDICAL GROUP INC

www.pediatrix.com

Industry Group Code: 621111   **Ranks within this company's industry group:** Sales: 3   Profits: 1

Insurance/HMO/PPO:	Drugs:	Equipment/Supplies:	Hospitals/Clinics:	Services:		Health Care:	
Insurance:	Manufacturer:	Manufacturer:	Acute Care:	Diagnostics:		Home Health:	
Managed Care:	Distributor:	Distributor:	Sub-Acute Care:	Labs/Testing:	Y	Long-Term Care:	
Utilization Mgmt.:	Specialty Pharm.:	Leasing/Finance:	Outpatient Surgery:	Staffing:	Y	Physical Therapy:	
Payment Proc.:	Vitamins/Nutri.:	Information Sys.:	Phys. Rehab. Center:	Waste Disposal:		Phys. Practice Mgmt.:	Y
	Clinical Trials:		Psychiatric Clinics:	Specialty Services:	Y		

TYPES OF BUSINESS:
Hospital-Based Pediatrician Practice Management
Pediatric Intensive Care Units
Neonatal Intensive Care Units
Perinatal Physician Services
Staffing Services
Laboratory Services

BRANDS/DIVISIONS/AFFILIATES:
Pediatrix Screening, Inc.
Atlanta Neonatal Physician Group
www.natalu.com

CONTACTS:
Note: Officers with more than one job title may be intentionally listed here more than once.
Roger J. Medel, CEO
Joseph M. Calabro, Pres.
Joseph M. Calabro, COO
Karl B. Wagner, VP/CFO
Robert C. Bryant, Sr. VP/CIO
Thomas W. Hawkins, Sr. VP/General Counsel
David Clark, Sr. VP-Oper.
John F. Rizzo, Sr. VP-Bus. Dev.
Robert J. Balcom, Regional Pres.-Central Region
Eric Kurzweil, Regional Pres.-Mountain Region
Frederick V. Miller, Regional Pres.-Atlantic Region
Michael Pokroy, Regional Pres.-Pacific Region

Phone: 954-384-0175   **Fax:** 954-233-3202
Toll-Free: 800-243-3839
Address: 1301 Concord Terrace, Sunrise, FL 33323 US

GROWTH PLANS/SPECIAL FEATURES:

Pediatrix Medical Group, Inc. (PMG) is the nation's leading provider of physician services at hospital-based neonatal intensive care units (NICUs) staffed by neonatologists, pediatricians with additional training to care for newborn infants with low birth weight and other medical complications. The firm is also the nation's leading provider of perinatal physician services. Perinatologists are obstetricians with additional training to care for women with high-risk or complicated pregnancies and their fetuses. PMG also provides physician services at hospital-based pediatric intensive care units (PICUs) and pediatrics departments in hospitals including 24-hour coverage with on-site or on-call physicians. These doctors are also available to provide pediatric support to other areas of hospitals on an as-needed basis. The firm provides services in 30 states and Puerto Rico. The company also staffs and manages perinatal practices, which involves the operation of outpatient offices as well as the management of inpatient maternal-fetal care. PMG's database compiles patient information into best-practice models for its members. The firm's web site, www.natalu.com, is an online community for neonatal and perinatal clinical discussion, education and professional development. Pediatrix Screening, a subsidiary, operates the nation's largest independent laboratory specializing in newborn metabolic screening. In recent news, Pediatrix acquired the Atlanta Neonatal Physician Group, which staffs Atlanta Medical Center's NICU. In addition, the company has expanded its practice in Texas through the acquisition of a Houston-based neonatal physicians group.
Pediatrix offers its employees preventative health care checkups, credit union membership and prescription, dental, vision and life insurance. The firm's employee assistance program provides confidential counseling for employees.

FINANCIALS:
Sales and profits are in thousands of dollars—add 000 to get the full amount. Year 2004 note: Complete fiscal 2004 results were not available for all companies at press time. For this company, year 2004 is for 9 months.

2004 Sales: $458,636 (9 months)	2004 Profits: $72,494 (9 months)	**Stock Ticker:** PDX
2003 Sales: $551,197	2003 Profits: $84,328	**Employees:** 2,678
2002 Sales: $465,500	2002 Profits: $68,800	**Fiscal Year Ends:** 12/31
2001 Sales: $354,600	2001 Profits: $30,400	
2000 Sales: $243,100	2000 Profits: $11,000	

SALARIES/BENEFITS:
Pension Plan:	ESOP Stock Plan:	Profit Sharing:	Top Exec. Salary: $600,000	Bonus: $600,000
Savings Plan: Y	Stock Purch. Plan: Y		Second Exec. Salary: $350,000	Bonus: $500,000

OTHER THOUGHTS:
Apparent Top Female Officers:
Hot Spot for Advancement for Women/Minorities:

LOCATIONS: ("Y" = Yes)
West:	Southwest:	Midwest:	Southeast:	Northeast:	International:
Y	Y	Y	Y	Y	Y

PER SE TECHNOLOGIES INC

www.per-se.com

Industry Group Code: 511200   Ranks within this company's industry group: Sales: 4   Profits: 5

Insurance/HMO/PPO:	Drugs:	Equipment/Supplies:	Hospitals/Clinics:	Services:	Health Care:
Insurance:	Manufacturer:	Manufacturer:	Acute Care:	Diagnostics:	Home Health:
Managed Care:	Distributor:	Distributor:	Sub-Acute Care:	Labs/Testing:	Long-Term Care:
Utilization Mgmt.:	Specialty Pharm.:	Leasing/Finance:	Outpatient Surgery:	Staffing:	Physical Therapy:
Payment Proc.:	Vitamins/Nutri.:	Information Sys.: Y	Phys. Rehab. Center:	Waste Disposal:	Phys. Practice Mgmt.: Y
	Clinical Trials:		Psychiatric Clinics:	Specialty Services: Y	

TYPES OF BUSINESS:
Physician Practice Management
Business Management Outsourcing
Health Care Application Software
Online Data Exchange

BRANDS/DIVISIONS/AFFILIATES:
Per-Se Exchange

CONTACTS:
Note: Officers with more than one job title may be intentionally listed here more than once.
Philip M. Pead, CEO
Philip M. Pead, Pres.
Chris E. Perkins, Exec. VP/CFO
Frank B. Murphy, Pres.-Physician Services Div.
Karen B. Andrews, Pres.-Application Software Div.
William N. Dagher, Pres.-e-Health Solutions Div.
Philip M. Pead, Chmn.

Phone: 770-237-4300   Fax: 770-237-6525
Toll-Free: 877-737-3773
Address: 1145 Santuary Pkwy., Ste. 200, Alpharetta, GA 30004 US

GROWTH PLANS/SPECIAL FEATURES:
Per-Se Technologies, Inc. provides integrated business management outsourcing services, application software and Internet-enabled connectivity for the health care industry. Its physicians services division provides business management outsourcing services to the hospital-affiliated physician practice market, physicians in academic settings and other large physician practices. Services focus on management of revenue cycles and include clinical data collection, data input, medical coding, billing, contract management and cash collection. Per-Se also provides enterprise-wide financial, clinical and administrative software to acute health care organizations, including patient financial management software and patient and staff scheduling systems. The e-health solutions segment provides connectivity and business intelligence solutions to health care providers and payers, helping to reduce administrative costs and enhance revenue cycle management. The Per-Se Exchange is the third-largest electronic clearinghouse in the health care industry.

FINANCIALS:
Sales and profits are in thousands of dollars—add 000 to get the full amount. Year 2004 note: Complete fiscal 2004 results were not available for all companies at press time. For this company, year 2004 is for 9 months.

2004 Sales: $263,383 (9 months)	2004 Profits: $12,131 (9 months)	**Stock Ticker:** PSTI
2003 Sales: $335,200	2003 Profits: $12,000	Employees: 4,800
2002 Sales: $354,100	2002 Profits: $8,000	Fiscal Year Ends: 12/31
2001 Sales: $328,900	2001 Profits: $-6,300	
2000 Sales: $310,000	2000 Profits: $-48,200	

SALARIES/BENEFITS:
Pension Plan:	ESOP Stock Plan:	Profit Sharing:	Top Exec. Salary: $365,385	Bonus: $108,000
Savings Plan: Y	Stock Purch. Plan:		Second Exec. Salary: $250,000	Bonus: $222,000

OTHER THOUGHTS:
Apparent Top Female Officers: 1
Hot Spot for Advancement for Women/Minorities:

LOCATIONS: ("Y" = Yes)
West:	Southwest:	Midwest:	Southeast: Y	Northeast:	International: Y

PERKINELMER INC

www.perkinelmer.com

Industry Group Code: 334500 **Ranks within this company's industry group:** Sales: 2 Profits: 4

Insurance/HMO/PPO:	Drugs:	Equipment/Supplies:		Hospitals/Clinics:	Services:		Health Care:
Insurance: Managed Care: Utilization Mgmt.: Payment Proc.:	Manufacturer: Distributor: Specialty Pharm.: Vitamins/Nutri.: Clinical Trials:	Manufacturer: Distributor: Leasing/Finance: Information Sys.:	Y	Acute Care: Sub-Acute Care: Outpatient Surgery: Phys. Rehab. Center: Psychiatric Clinics:	Diagnostics: Labs/Testing: Staffing: Waste Disposal: Specialty Services:	Y	Home Health: Long-Term Care: Physical Therapy: Phys. Practice Mgmt.:

TYPES OF BUSINESS:
Medical Equipment-Assorted Instruments
Mechanical Components
Optoelectronics
Technical Services
Life Science Systems
Fluid Science Components
Engineering Services
Testing Services

BRANDS/DIVISIONS/AFFILIATES:
Aanalyst
UltraVIEW
EnVision
Belfab
ColdBlue
Cermax Xenon
Callisto
DELFIA Xpress

CONTACTS:
Note: Officers with more than one job title may be intentionally listed here more than once.

Gregory L. Summe, CEO
Gregory L. Summe, Pres.
John P. Murphy, Exec. VP/COO
Robert F. Friel, CFO
Richard F. Walsh, Sr. VP-Human Resources
Neil Cook, Chief Scientific Officer
Terrence L. Carlson, General Counsel
Robert F. Friel, Exec. VP-Bus. Dev.
Jeffrey D. Capello, Chief Acct. Officer/VP-Finance
Peter B. Coggins, Sr. VP/Pres.-Life & Analytical Sciences
John A. Roush, Pres.-Optoelectronics
Robert A. Barrett, Sr. VP/Pres.-Fluid Sciences
Gregory L. Summe, Chmn.

Phone: 781-237-5100	Fax:
Toll-Free:	
Address: 45 William St., Wellesley, MA 02481 US	

GROWTH PLANS/SPECIAL FEATURES:
PerkinElmer, Inc. is a leading provider of scientific instruments, consumables and services to the pharmaceutical, biomedical, environmental testing, chemical and general industrial markets. The firm designs, manufactures, markets and services products and systems within three business units: life and analytical sciences, optoelectronics and fluid sciences. The life and analytical sciences unit is a provider of drug discovery, genetic screening, environmental and chemical analysis tools and instrumentation. Principal products of this segment include EnVision, the first modular multi-label plate reader designed for use in high-throughput screening laboratories; the AAnalyst series of atomic absorption spectrometers; DELFIA Xpress, a fast and flexible random access analyzer for maternal health clinics and laboratories; and UltraVIEW, a fully automated, high-resolution, live cell imaging system. The optoelectronics segment provides a broad range of digital imaging, sensor and specialty lighting components used in the biomedical, consumer products and other specialty end markets. It is a leading supplier of amorphous silicon digital x-ray detectors used in medical imaging and radiation therapy, and its optical sensor products are used in sample detection in life sciences instruments, luggage screening, laser printers, security and fire detection systems, HVAC controls, document sorting and smart weaponry. New product releases by the segment include Cermax Xenon lamps for home theater and HDTV applications, an amorphous silicon flat-panel detector for oncology and ColdBlue, a cooled imaging system offering improved sensitivity and detection of very faint signals, used in protein quantification and fluorescent microscopy. The fluid sciences segment offers critical fluid control and containment systems for highly demanding environments such as turbine engines and semiconductor fabrication facilities. This segment offers its products under brand names including Belfab, Callisto, Centurion and PressureScience.

FINANCIALS:
Sales and profits are in thousands of dollars—add 000 to get the full amount. Year 2004 note: Complete fiscal 2004 results were not available for all companies at press time. For this company, year 2004 is for 9 months.

2004 Sales: $1,208,625 (9 months)	2004 Profits: $58,120 (9 months)	**Stock Ticker:** PKI
2003 Sales: $1,535,200	2003 Profits: $52,900	Employees: 10,700
2002 Sales: $1,505,000	2002 Profits: $-151,900	Fiscal Year Ends: 12/31
2001 Sales: $1,330,100	2001 Profits: $34,500	
2000 Sales: $1,695,267	2000 Profits: $90,520	

SALARIES/BENEFITS:
Pension Plan:	ESOP Stock Plan:	Profit Sharing:	Top Exec. Salary: $950,000	Bonus: $1,755,600
Savings Plan: Y	Stock Purch. Plan:		Second Exec. Salary: $450,000	Bonus: $606,375

OTHER THOUGHTS:
Apparent Top Female Officers:
Hot Spot for Advancement for Women/Minorities:

LOCATIONS: ("Y" = Yes)

West:	Southwest:	Midwest:	Southeast:	Northeast:	International:
Y	Y	Y	Y	Y	Y

Plunkett's Health Care Industry Almanac 2005 565

PETMED EXPRESS INC
www.1800petmeds.com

Industry Group Code: 422210   **Ranks within this company's industry group:** Sales: 6   Profits: 5

Insurance/HMO/PPO:	Drugs:		Equipment/Supplies:	Hospitals/Clinics:	Services:	Health Care:
Insurance:	Manufacturer:		Manufacturer:	Acute Care:	Diagnostics:	Home Health:
Managed Care:	Distributor:		Distributor:	Sub-Acute Care:	Labs/Testing:	Long-Term Care:
Utilization Mgmt.:	Specialty Pharm.:	Y	Leasing/Finance:	Outpatient Surgery:	Staffing:	Physical Therapy:
Payment Proc.:	Vitamins/Nutri.:		Information Sys.:	Phys. Rehab. Center:	Waste Disposal:	Phys. Practice Mgmt.:
	Clinical Trials:			Psychiatric Clinics:	Specialty Services:	

TYPES OF BUSINESS:
Pet Pharmacy

BRANDS/DIVISIONS/AFFILIATES:
1-800-PetMeds

CONTACTS: *Note: Officers with more than one job title may be intentionally listed here more than once.*
Menderes Akdag, CEO
Marc Puleo, Pres.
Bruce Rosenbloom, CFO
Marc Puleo, Chmn.

Phone: 954-979-4788   **Fax:**
Toll-Free:
Address: 1441 SW 29th Ave., Pompano Beach, FL 33069 US

GROWTH PLANS/SPECIAL FEATURES:

PetMed Express, Inc. is a nationwide pet pharmacy that markets its products under the brand name 1-800-PetMeds through national television, online and direct-mail advertising campaigns. The company markets prescription and non-prescription pet medications and health and nutritional supplements for dogs and cats directly to consumers, offering an alternative option to conventional pet stores. Marketing directly to customers allows increased convenience, price reduction and quicker delivery. The firm offers a broad selection of name-brand products for dogs and cats, including Frontline, Advantage, Heartguard, Sentinel, Interceptor, Program, Revolution and Rimadyl, at a discount of up to 25% off the prices charged by veterinarians. Non-prescription medications include flea and tick control, bone and joint care products, vitamins and nutritional supplements and hygiene products. Prescription medications include heartworm treatments, thyroid and arthritis medications, antibiotics and other proprietary medications and generic substitutes. Approximately 1,250,000 customers have purchased from PetMed within the last two years, with approximately 51% of customers residing in California, Florida, Texas, New York, New Jersey, Pennsylvania and Virginia.

FINANCIALS: Sales and profits are in thousands of dollars—add 000 to get the full amount. Year 2004 note: Complete fiscal 2004 results were not available for all companies at press time. For this company, year 2004 is for 12 months.

2004 Sales: $93,994 (12 months)	2004 Profits: $5,813 (12 months)	**Stock Ticker:** PETS
2003 Sales: $54,975	2003 Profits: $3,258	**Employees:** 148
2002 Sales: $32,026	2002 Profits: $ 825	**Fiscal Year Ends:** 3/31
2001 Sales: $32,000	2001 Profits: $-2,800	
2000 Sales: $	2000 Profits: $	

SALARIES/BENEFITS:
| Pension Plan: | ESOP Stock Plan: | Profit Sharing: | Top Exec. Salary: $201,731 | Bonus: $ |
| Savings Plan: | Stock Purch. Plan: | | Second Exec. Salary: $146,154 | Bonus: $50,000 |

OTHER THOUGHTS:
Apparent Top Female Officers:
Hot Spot for Advancement for Women/Minorities:

LOCATIONS: ("Y" = Yes)
West:	Southwest:	Midwest:	Southeast:	Northeast:	International:
Y	Y	Y	Y	Y	

Note: Financial information, benefits and other data can change quickly and may vary from those stated here.

PFIZER INC

Industry Group Code: 325412 **Ranks within this company's industry group:** Sales: 1 Profits: 4

www.pfizer.com

Insurance/HMO/PPO:	Drugs:		Equipment/Supplies:		Hospitals/Clinics:	Services:	Health Care:
Insurance:	Manufacturer:	Y	Manufacturer:	Y	Acute Care:	Diagnostics:	Home Health:
Managed Care:	Distributor:		Distributor:		Sub-Acute Care:	Labs/Testing:	Long-Term Care:
Utilization Mgmt.:	Specialty Pharm.:		Leasing/Finance:		Outpatient Surgery:	Staffing:	Physical Therapy:
Payment Proc.:	Vitamins/Nutri.:		Information Sys.:		Phys. Rehab. Center:	Waste Disposal:	Phys. Practice Mgmt.:
	Clinical Trials:				Psychiatric Clinics:	Specialty Services:	

TYPES OF BUSINESS:
Drugs-Diversified
Prescription Pharmaceuticals
Over-the-Counter Drugs
Animal Vaccines

BRANDS/DIVISIONS/AFFILIATES:
Pharmacia Corporation
Diflucan
Zoloft
Neurontin
Benadryl
Zithromax
Visine
Rolaids

CONTACTS:
Note: Officers with more than one job title may be intentionally listed here more than once.
Henry A. McKinnell, Jr., CEO
David L. Shedlarz, CFO
Yvonne R. Jackson, Sr. VP-Human Resources
Peter B. Corr, Sr. VP-Science & Tech.
John W. Mitchell, VP-Global Mfg.
Jeffrey B. Kindler, General Counsel
Frederick W. Telling, VP-Corp. Strategic Planning
Chuck Hardwick, Sr. VP-Corp. Affairs
Karen Katen, Pres. Pfizer Global Pharmaceuticals
John L. LaMattina, Sr. VP/Pres.-Pfizer Global Research & Dev.
Henry A. McKinnell, Jr., Chmn.

Phone: 212-573-2323 **Fax:** 212-573-7851
Toll-Free:
Address: 235 E. 42nd St., New York, NY 10017-5755 US

GROWTH PLANS/SPECIAL FEATURES:
Pfizer, Inc. is a research-based, global pharmaceutical company. The firm operates in two business segments, pharmaceuticals and over-the-counter drugs. Pfizer's pharmaceutical division includes prescription pharmaceuticals for treating cardiovascular diseases, infectious diseases, central nervous system disorders, diabetes, erectile dysfunction, allergies, arthritis and other disorders. Major drugs offered by the company include Zoloft and Neurontin for the treatment of central nervous system disorders; Diflucan for the treatment of various fungal infections; Viracept for treatment of HIV infections; and Zithromax, an oral or injectable antibiotic. The pharmaceutical segment also develops products for livestock as well as companion animals. The firm's Revolution topical liquid is the first medicine that can protect against external parasites, gastrointestinal worms and heartworms. In addition, the company's Capsugel subsidiary is one of the world's largest producers of two-piece capsules used in manufacturing prescription and over-the-counter pharmaceuticals and nutritional supplements. Pfizer's consumer products segment markets many of the world's best-known consumer health brands, including Benadryl, Rolaids, Zantac 75, Visine, Cortizone and BenGay. In a major development, Pfizer acquired Pharmacia Corporation for $60 billion, making it the largest pharmaceutical company in the U.S., Europe, Japan and Latin America. The combined entity is the largest privately funded biomedical research firm in the world, with a research and development pipeline of some 120 chemical entities, as well as over 80 additional projects for product development. Continuing operations under the Pfizer name, the company plans to file 20 new drug applications in the next five years. In recent news, Pfizer has formed partnerships with and invested in a number of nanotechnology companies working in biotech. These companies include BioTrove, ChondroGene and Perlegen Sciences Inc.

Pfizer offers its workforce medical, vision and dental plans, tuition reimbursement, adoption assistance, a matching gift program, child care assistance, a referral program, educational loans and four-year college scholarships for children of employees.

FINANCIALS:
Sales and profits are in thousands of dollars—add 000 to get the full amount. Year 2004 note: Complete fiscal 2004 results were not available for all companies at press time. For this company, year 2004 is for 9 months.

2004 Sales: $37,593,000 (9 months) 2004 Profits: $8,536,000 (9 months)
2003 Sales: $45,188,000 2003 Profits: $3,910,000
2002 Sales: $32,373,000 2002 Profits: $9,126,000
2001 Sales: $32,259,000 2001 Profits: $7,788,000
2000 Sales: $29,574,000 2000 Profits: $3,726,000

Stock Ticker: PFE
Employees: 112,000
Fiscal Year Ends: 12/31

SALARIES/BENEFITS:
Pension Plan: Y ESOP Stock Plan: Profit Sharing: Top Exec. Salary: $2,042,700 Bonus: $4,607,400
Savings Plan: Y Stock Purch. Plan: Second Exec. Salary: $1,086,700 Bonus: $1,434,400

OTHER THOUGHTS:
Apparent Top Female Officers: 1
Hot Spot for Advancement for Women/Minorities:

LOCATIONS: ("Y" = Yes)
West:	Southwest:	Midwest:	Southeast:	Northeast:	International:
Y	Y	Y	Y	Y	Y

Note: Financial information, benefits and other data can change quickly and may vary from those stated here.

PHARMACEUTICAL PRODUCT DEVELOPMENT INC   www.ppdi.com

Industry Group Code: 541710   Ranks within this company's industry group: Sales: 4   Profits: 4

Insurance/HMO/PPO:	Drugs:	Equipment/Supplies:	Hospitals/Clinics:	Services:	Health Care:
Insurance:	Manufacturer:	Manufacturer:	Acute Care:	Diagnostics:	Home Health:
Managed Care:	Distributor:	Distributor:	Sub-Acute Care:	Labs/Testing: Y	Long-Term Care:
Utilization Mgmt.:	Specialty Pharm.:	Leasing/Finance:	Outpatient Surgery:	Staffing:	Physical Therapy:
Payment Proc.:	Vitamins/Nutri.:	Information Sys.: Y	Phys. Rehab. Center:	Waste Disposal:	Phys. Practice Mgmt.:
	Clinical Trials: Y		Psychiatric Clinics:	Specialty Services: Y	

TYPES OF BUSINESS:
Contract Research Services
Drug Discovery & Development Services
Clinical Data Consulting Services
Marketing Support Services
Drug Development Software

BRANDS/DIVISIONS/AFFILIATES:
PPD Development
PPD Discovery
CSS Informatics
PPD Medical Communications
PPD Virtual
eLoader 3.5
PPD Medical Device

CONTACTS:
Note: Officers with more than one job title may be intentionally listed here more than once.
Fredric N. Eshelman, CEO
Fred B. Davenport, Jr., Pres.
Linda Baddour, CFO
Steadman Harrison, Sr. Dir.-Research
Colin Shannon, VP-Clinical Oper.
Paul S. Covington, Exec. VP-Dev.
Paul S. Covington, Treas.
Fred B. Davenport, Jr., Corp. Sec.
Ernest Mario, Chmn.
Francis J. Casieri, Sr. VP-Global Bus. Dev.

Phone: 910-251-0081   Fax: 910-762-5820
Toll-Free:
Address: 3151 S. 17th St., Wilmington, NC 28412 US

GROWTH PLANS/SPECIAL FEATURES:
Pharmaceutical Product Development, Inc. (PPD) is a global provider of drug discovery and development services to pharmaceutical and biotechnology companies. The company's PPD Discovery subsidiary is engaged in discovery sciences in pharmaceutical research and development. PPD Development, another subsidiary, is engaged in life science contract research organization services, providing integrated product development resources. PPD Development also operates PPD Medical Communications, which provides medical information and marketing support services to health care providers and consumers on behalf of pharmaceutical and biotechnology companies. CSS Informatics provides clinical data consulting services and software solutions for pharmaceutical and biotechnology companies, government and drug development service providers. It recently released eLoader 3.5, an enhanced version of its specialized software product for trial protocol. PPD also manages PPD Virtual, which provides virtual drug development consulting and management via an innovative risk-sharing model to pharmaceutical companies, biotechnology firms and academic research institutions. The firm recently launched PPD Medical Device, another division of PPD Development, providing services to the medical device industry with experience in developing stents, devices and therapies in the areas of interventional cardiology, endovascular, neurology and orthopedic disorders as well as wound care.

PPD offers its employees a range of health plans and life, dental and vision insurance, as well as a legal advisory plan and a medical spending account. The firm also offers special-needs services varied by location, including counseling services, on-site child care, dry cleaning pickup and delivery and access to a credit union.

FINANCIALS:
Sales and profits are in thousands of dollars—add 000 to get the full amount. Year 2004 note: Complete fiscal 2004 results were not available for all companies at press time. For this company, year 2004 is for 9 months.

2004 Sales: $534,362 (9 months)   2004 Profits: $62,832 (9 months)
2003 Sales: $726,983   2003 Profits: $46,310
2002 Sales: $562,600   2002 Profits: $39,900
2001 Sales: $431,500   2001 Profits: $49,200
2000 Sales: $345,300   2000 Profits: $32,300

Stock Ticker: PPDI
Employees: 5,700
Fiscal Year Ends: 12/31

SALARIES/BENEFITS:
Pension Plan: Y   ESOP Stock Plan: Profit Sharing: Top Exec. Salary: $623,479   Bonus: $525,000
Savings Plan: Y   Stock Purch. Plan: Second Exec. Salary: $327,825   Bonus: $180,000

OTHER THOUGHTS:
Apparent Top Female Officers: 1
Hot Spot for Advancement for Women/Minorities:

LOCATIONS: ("Y" = Yes)
West	Southwest	Midwest	Southeast	Northeast	International
Y			Y	Y	Y

PHARMACOPEIA INC

www.pharmacopeia.com

Industry Group Code: 541710 Ranks within this company's industry group: Sales: 7 Profits: 7

Insurance/HMO/PPO:	Drugs:	Equipment/Supplies:	Hospitals/Clinics:	Services:	Health Care:
Insurance: Managed Care: Utilization Mgmt.: Payment Proc.:	Manufacturer: Distributor: Specialty Pharm.: Vitamins/Nutri.: Clinical Trials:	Manufacturer: Distributor: Leasing/Finance: Information Sys.: Y	Acute Care: Sub-Acute Care: Outpatient Surgery: Phys. Rehab. Center: Psychiatric Clinics:	Diagnostics: Labs/Testing: Y Staffing: Waste Disposal: Specialty Services: Y	Home Health: Long-Term Care: Physical Therapy: Phys. Practice Mgmt.:

TYPES OF BUSINESS:
Research & Development-Drug Discovery Support
Molecular Combinational Chemistry
Molecular Modeling and Simulation Software
Chemical Databases

BRANDS/DIVISIONS/AFFILIATES:
Pharmacopeia Drug Discovery
ECLiPS
Accelrys
GCG Wisconsin Package
Failed Reactions Database
BIOSTER

CONTACTS:
Note: Officers with more than one job title may be intentionally listed here more than once.

Joseph A. Mollica, CEO
Joseph A. Mollica, Pres.
Stephen A. Spearman, Exec. VP/COO
John J. Hanlon, CFO
William J. DeLorbe, Exec. VP-Human Resources
Michael G. Lenahan, General Counsel
Arthur E. Roke, Chief Acc. Officer/VP-Finance
Mark J. Emkjer, Pres., Accelrys
Scott D. Kahn, Chief Science Officer, Accelrys
Joseph A. Mollica, Chmn.

Phone: 609-452-3600 Fax: 609-452-3672
Toll-Free:
Address: P.O. Box 5350, Princeton, NJ 08543 US

GROWTH PLANS/SPECIAL FEATURES:

Pharmacopeia, Inc. is engaged in the design, development and marketing of products and services that are intended to improve and accelerate drug discovery and chemical development. The company's drug discovery segment integrates proprietary small-molecule combinatorial and medicinal chemistry, high-throughput screening, in-vitro pharmacology, computational methods and informatics to discover and optimize potential drugs. The subsidiary's ECLiPS encoding technology enables it to generate thousands of small-molecule compounds at a fraction of the cost of traditional chemical synthesis methods. Pharmacopeia Drug Discovery's customers include AstraZeneca, Novartis, Schering AG and Antigenics. The company's Accelrys subsidiary develops and commercializes molecular modeling and simulation software, cheminformatics and decision support systems and bioinformatics tools. Accelrys's modeling technology simulates subatomic, interatomic and intermolecular interactions and a wide range of corresponding properties, including molecular structure and activity. The subsidiary's GCG Wisconsin Package software features gene sequence comparison, DNA/RNA secondary structure prediction, evolutionary analysis and protein analysis. Accelrys also offers a number of chemical databases, including the Failed Reactions Database, which offers data on reactions that afford unexpected results; and BIOSTER, which features a compilation of thousands of bio-analogous molecule pairs. The subsidiary's customers include Bristol Myers Squibb, Amgen, Monsanto and Unilever. In recent news, Pharmacopeia announced plans to spin off its Pharmacopeia Drug Discovery unit into a separate company. Additionally, as part of the spin off, Pharmacopeia will change its name to Accelrys, Inc.

FINANCIALS:
Sales and profits are in thousands of dollars—add 000 to get the full amount. Year 2004 note: Complete fiscal 2004 results were not available for all companies at press time. For this company, year 2004 is for months.

2004 Sales: $ (months) 2004 Profits: $ (months)
2003 Sales: $115,064 2003 Profits: $-3,497
2002 Sales: $124,400 2002 Profits: $-11,600
2001 Sales: $122,300 2001 Profits: $-14,300
2000 Sales: $119,400 2000 Profits: $1,200

Stock Ticker: ACCL
Employees: 713
Fiscal Year Ends: 12/31

SALARIES/BENEFITS:
Pension Plan: ESOP Stock Plan: Profit Sharing: Top Exec. Salary: $530,000 Bonus: $242,500
Savings Plan: Y Stock Purch. Plan: Y   Second Exec. Salary: $325,000 Bonus: $151,200

OTHER THOUGHTS:
Apparent Top Female Officers:
Hot Spot for Advancement for Women/Minorities:

LOCATIONS: ("Y" = Yes)
West	Southwest	Midwest	Southeast	Northeast	International
Y				Y	Y

PHC INC

www.phc-inc.com

Industry Group Code: 621490 **Ranks within this company's industry group:** Sales: 18 Profits: 16

Insurance/HMO/PPO:	Drugs:	Equipment/Supplies:	Hospitals/Clinics:		Services:		Health Care:
Insurance:	Manufacturer:	Manufacturer:	Acute Care:		Diagnostics:		Home Health:
Managed Care:	Distributor:	Distributor:	Sub-Acute Care:	Y	Labs/Testing:		Long-Term Care:
Utilization Mgmt.:	Specialty Pharm.:	Leasing/Finance:	Outpatient Surgery:		Staffing:		Physical Therapy:
Payment Proc.:	Vitamins/Nutri.:	Information Sys.:	Phys. Rehab. Center:		Waste Disposal:		Phys. Practice Mgmt.:
	Clinical Trials: Y		Psychiatric Clinics:		Specialty Services:	Y	

TYPES OF BUSINESS:
Clinics-Psychiatric
Substance Abuse Treatment Services
Behavioral Health Services
Specialty Care and Sub-Acute Facilities
Clinical Research

BRANDS/DIVISIONS/AFFILIATES:
Pioneer Behavioral Health
Pioneer Pharmaceutical Research
behavioralhealthonline.com

CONTACTS:
Note: Officers with more than one job title may be intentionally listed here more than once.
Bruce A. Shear, CEO
Bruce A. Shear, Pres.
Michael R. Cornelison, Exec. VP/COO
Paula C. Wurts, CFO
Paula C. Wurts, Treas.
Robert H. Boswell, Sr. VP

Phone: 978-536-2777 **Fax:** 978-536-2677
Toll-Free: 800-543-2447
Address: 200 Lake St., Ste. 102, Peabody, MA 01960 US

GROWTH PLANS/SPECIAL FEATURES:
PHC, Inc., doing business as Pioneer Behavioral Health, is a national health care company that provides psychiatric services primarily to individuals who have alcohol and drug dependency and related disorders and to individuals in the gaming and trucking industry. The firm operates substance abuse treatment centers in Utah and Virginia; three outpatient psychiatric facilities in Michigan, Utah and Nevada; and two inpatient psychiatric facilities in Utah and Michigan. PHC also operates a web site, behavioralhealthonline.com, which provides education, training and material to professionals, in addition to Internet support for its subsidiaries. Its 24-hour help line and 24-hour crisis stabilization rapid-response team help clients and their families during extreme crisis through counseling and medical attention. PHC's substance abuse facilities provide specialty treatment to patients who typically have poor recovery prognoses and are prone to relapse. The company targets its programs and services at safety-sensitive industries such as transportation, heavy equipment, law enforcement, gaming and health services. Psychiatric facilities provide inpatient care and intensive outpatient treatment to children, adolescents and adults. The company's mental health clinics provide services to employees of major employers as well as to managed care, Medicare and Medicaid clients. The firm's clinical trials division, Pioneer Pharmaceutical Research (PPR), has research sites in Michigan and Arizona.

FINANCIALS:
Sales and profits are in thousands of dollars—add 000 to get the full amount. Year 2004 note: Complete fiscal 2004 results were not available for all companies at press time. For this company, year 2004 is for 12 months.

2004 Sales: $26,648 (12 months)   2004 Profits: $-257 (12 months)
2003 Sales: $23,833   2003 Profits: $977
2002 Sales: $22,700   2002 Profits: $1,100
2001 Sales: $22,700   2001 Profits: $-5,200
2000 Sales: $20,400   2000 Profits: $-600

Stock Ticker: PIHC
Employees: 404
Fiscal Year Ends: 6/30

SALARIES/BENEFITS:
| Pension Plan: | ESOP Stock Plan: | Profit Sharing: | Top Exec. Salary: $306,771 | Bonus: $2,500 |
| Savings Plan: | Stock Purch. Plan: Y | | Second Exec. Salary: $152,937 | Bonus: $40,147 |

OTHER THOUGHTS:
Apparent Top Female Officers: 1
Hot Spot for Advancement for Women/Minorities:

LOCATIONS: ("Y" = Yes)
West:	Southwest:	Midwest:	Southeast:	Northeast:	International:
Y		Y		Y	

PHILIPS MEDICAL SYSTEMS

www.medical.philips.com

Industry Group Code: 339113   Ranks within this company's industry group: Sales: Profits:

Insurance/HMO/PPO:	Drugs:	Equipment/Supplies:		Hospitals/Clinics:	Services:		Health Care:
Insurance:	Manufacturer:	Manufacturer:	Y	Acute Care:	Diagnostics:		Home Health:
Managed Care:	Distributor:	Distributor:		Sub-Acute Care:	Labs/Testing:		Long-Term Care:
Utilization Mgmt.:	Specialty Pharm.:	Leasing/Finance:	Y	Outpatient Surgery:	Staffing:		Physical Therapy:
Payment Proc.:	Vitamins/Nutri.:	Information Sys.:		Phys. Rehab. Center:	Waste Disposal:		Phys. Practice Mgmt.:
	Clinical Trials:			Psychiatric Clinics:	Specialty Services:	Y	

TYPES OF BUSINESS:
Manufacturing-Medical Equipment
Diagnostic & Treatment Equipment
Imaging Equipment
Equipment Financing & Leasing
Equipment Repair & Maintenance
Clinical Investment Consulting

BRANDS/DIVISIONS/AFFILIATES:
Royal Philips Electronics
Philips Medcare
ADAC Laboratories
Marconi Medical Systems
ATL Ultrasound
DigitalDiagnost
Integris Allura
iE33 Intelligent Echocardiography System

CONTACTS:
Note: Officers with more than one job title may be intentionally listed here more than once.
Jouko Karvinen, CEO
Jouko Karvinen, Pres.

Phone: 978-687-1501   Fax: 978-689-8295
Toll-Free: 800-722-7900
Address: 3000 Minuteman Rd., Andover, MA 01810-1099 US

GROWTH PLANS/SPECIAL FEATURES:
Philips Medical Systems (PMS), a subsidiary of electronics giant Royal Philips Electronics, manufactures medical diagnostic and treatment equipment. PMS has a broad range of products and business lines, including x-ray, ultrasound, computed tomography (CT), positron emission tomography (PET), cardiac and monitoring systems (CMS), cardiovascular x-ray, magnetic resonance imaging (MRI) and nuclear medicine. Companies PMS has acquired in its effort to expand into the medical market, include industry leaders such as ATL Ultrasound, the health care solutions group of Agilent Technologies, Marconi Medical Systems and ADAC Laboratories, carry out much of its business. PMS entered the clinical support and financing business through its acquisition of Medcare Corporation, which now operates under the name Philips Medcare. It provides on-site equipment training, asset management, biomedical maintenance, clinical investment consulting and equipment financing and leasing. Additionally, PMS offers clinical information technology solutions for cardiology and radiology image and information management. The company is a leader in the fields of x-ray, cardiovascular and ultrasound imaging and diagnostic systems, with products under the brand names DigitalDiagnost, Integris Allura and SonoCT, respectively. In October 2004, PMS introduced the iE33 Intelligent Echocardiography System, the first premium echocardiography system to feature fully integrated 2D and 3D cardiac quantification software.

FINANCIALS:
Sales and profits are in thousands of dollars—add 000 to get the full amount. Year 2004 note: Complete fiscal 2004 results were not available for all companies at press time. For this company, year 2004 is for months.

2004 Sales: $ (months)   2004 Profits: $ (months)
2003 Sales: $ 2003 Profits: $
2002 Sales: $229,400   2002 Profits: $
2001 Sales: $ 2001 Profits: $
2000 Sales: $ 2000 Profits: $

Stock Ticker: Subsidiary
Employees: 1,538
Fiscal Year Ends: 12/31

SALARIES/BENEFITS:
Pension Plan: ESOP Stock Plan: Profit Sharing: Top Exec. Salary: $ Bonus: $
Savings Plan: Stock Purch. Plan: Second Exec. Salary: $ Bonus: $

OTHER THOUGHTS:
Apparent Top Female Officers:
Hot Spot for Advancement for Women/Minorities:

LOCATIONS: ("Y" = Yes)
West:	Southwest:	Midwest:	Southeast:	Northeast:	International:
				Y	Y

PLANVISTA CORP

www.planvista.com

Industry Group Code: 522320   Ranks within this company's industry group: Sales: 2   Profits:

Insurance/HMO/PPO:	Drugs:	Equipment/Supplies:	Hospitals/Clinics:	Services:	Health Care:
Insurance:	Manufacturer:	Manufacturer:	Acute Care:	Diagnostics:	Home Health:
Managed Care:	Distributor:	Distributor:	Sub-Acute Care:	Labs/Testing:	Long-Term Care:
Utilization Mgmt.: Y	Specialty Pharm.:	Leasing/Finance:	Outpatient Surgery:	Staffing:	Physical Therapy:
Payment Proc.: Y	Vitamins/Nutri.:	Information Sys.: Y	Phys. Rehab. Center:	Waste Disposal:	Phys. Practice Mgmt.:
	Clinical Trials:		Psychiatric Clinics:	Specialty Services: Y	

TYPES OF BUSINESS:
Payment Processing-Medical
Risk Management Services
Administrative Services
Utilization Management Services

BRANDS/DIVISIONS/AFFILIATES:
HealthPlan Services
PlanServ
PayerServ
PlanVista Solutions, Inc.
ClaimPassXL
National Preferred Provider Network
ProxyMed

CONTACTS:
Note: Officers with more than one job title may be intentionally listed here more than once.

Phillip S. Dingle, CEO
Jeffrey L. Markle, Pres.
Jeffrey L. Markle, COO
Donald W. Schmeling, CFO
James T. Kearns, Sr. VP-Oper.
David C. Reilly, Sr. VP-Strategic Planning
Robert A. Martin, Sr. VP-PlanServ & PayerServ
Phillip S. Dingle, Chmn.

Phone: 813-353-2300   Fax: 813-353-2310
Toll-Free: 866-813-7877
Address: 4010 Boy Scout Blvd., Tampa, FL 33607 US

GROWTH PLANS/SPECIAL FEATURES:
PlanVista Corp., a subsidiary of ProxyMed, provides medical cost management services to health care providers. PlanVista's customers include health care payers such as self-insured employers, medical insurance carriers, health maintenance organizations (HMOs), third-party administrators, other entities that pay claims on behalf of health plans and participating health care services providers, which include individual providers and provider networks (preferred provider organizations, or PPOs). The company provides health care payers with access to its preferred provider network, the National Preferred Provider Network (NPPN), which offers payers discounts on participating provider medical services. PlanVista's NPPN is made up of more than 30 local PPO networks and independent physician associations, as well as directly contracted independent physicians. The company's other programs include PayerServ, which helps payers manage their network relationships; and PlanServ, which provides claim re-pricing and network and data management outsourcing services. PlanVista also offers a claims re-pricing and processing system, ClaimPassXL

FINANCIALS:
Sales and profits are in thousands of dollars—add 000 to get the full amount. Year 2004 note: Complete fiscal 2004 results were not available for all companies at press time. For this company, year 2004 is for months.

2004 Sales: $ (months)   2004 Profits: $ (months)
2003 Sales: $33,100   2003 Profits: $
2002 Sales: $33,100   2002 Profits: $4,200
2001 Sales: $32,900   2001 Profits: $-45,300
2000 Sales: $27,000   2000 Profits: $-104,500

Stock Ticker: Subsidiary
Employees: 150
Fiscal Year Ends: 12/31

SALARIES/BENEFITS:
Pension Plan: ESOP Stock Plan: Profit Sharing: Top Exec. Salary: $222,115   Bonus: $50,000
Savings Plan: Y   Stock Purch. Plan: Second Exec. Salary: $186,846   Bonus: $90,000

OTHER THOUGHTS:
Apparent Top Female Officers:
Hot Spot for Advancement for Women/Minorities:

LOCATIONS: ("Y" = Yes)
West:	Southwest:	Midwest:	Southeast:	Northeast:	International:
			Y	Y	

POLYMEDICA CORPORATION

www.polymedica.com

Industry Group Code: 339113 Ranks within this company's industry group: Sales: 50 Profits: 50

Insurance/HMO/PPO:	Drugs:	Equipment/Supplies:	Hospitals/Clinics:	Services:	Health Care:
Insurance:	Manufacturer: Y	Manufacturer: Y	Acute Care:	Diagnostics:	Home Health:
Managed Care:	Distributor: Y	Distributor: Y	Sub-Acute Care:	Labs/Testing:	Long-Term Care:
Utilization Mgmt.:	Specialty Pharm.:	Leasing/Finance:	Outpatient Surgery:	Staffing:	Physical Therapy:
Payment Proc.:	Vitamins/Nutri.:	Information Sys.:	Phys. Rehab. Center:	Waste Disposal:	Phys. Practice Mgmt.:
	Clinical Trials:		Psychiatric Clinics:	Specialty Services:	

TYPES OF BUSINESS:
Equipment-Insulin & Related Products
Diabetes Testing Supplies
Prescription Respiratory Products
Prescription Oral Medications
Urology & Suppository Products
Home Diagnostic Kits

BRANDS/DIVISIONS/AFFILIATES:
Liberty Diabetes
Liberty Respiratory
AZO

CONTACTS:
Note: Officers with more than one job title may be intentionally listed here more than once.
Patrick T. Ryan, CEO
Patrick T. Ryan, Pres.
Stephen C. Farrell, Sr. VP/COO
Fred H. Croninger, III, CFO
John K.P. Stone, III, Sr. VP/General Counsel
Bruce L. Haskin, Treas.
William B. Eck, Sr. VP/Chief of Health Care Affairs
Samuel L. Shanaman, Chmn.

Phone: 781-933-2020 Fax: 781-938-6950
Toll-Free:
Address: 11 State St., Woburn, MA 01801 US

GROWTH PLANS/SPECIAL FEATURES:
PolyMedica is a leading provider of direct-to-consumer medical products, conducting business through its pharmaceuticals segment, Liberty Diabetes and Liberty Respiratory. Liberty Diabetes sells insulin, syringes and other products primarily to Medicare-eligible customers suffering from diabetes and related chronic diseases. Its direct-mail program serves approximately 625,000 customers throughout the country. Liberty Respiratory delivers prescription respiratory medications and supplies to approximately 65,000 primarily Medicare-eligible customers suffering from chronic obstructive pulmonary disease. The pharmaceuticals segment provides prescription oral medications not covered by Medicare and sells prescription urology and suppository products, over-the-counter female urinary discomfort products and AZO home medical diagnostic kits. These products are sold to Liberty Diabetes and Liberty Respiratory customers, as well as to large U.S. drug distributors, drug store chains, supermarkets and mass merchandisers.

FINANCIALS:
Sales and profits are in thousands of dollars—add 000 to get the full amount. Year 2004 note: Complete fiscal 2004 results were not available for all companies at press time. For this company, year 2004 is for 12 months.

2004 Sales: $419,694 (12 months)   2004 Profits: $37,932 (12 months)
2003 Sales: $356,200   2003 Profits: $25,600
2002 Sales: $279,700   2002 Profits: $30,400
2001 Sales: $220,000   2001 Profits: $22,800
2000 Sales: $156,900   2000 Profits: $15,100

Stock Ticker: PLMD
Employees: 1,716
Fiscal Year Ends: 3/31

SALARIES/BENEFITS:
Pension Plan: ESOP Stock Plan: Profit Sharing: Top Exec. Salary: $433,038   Bonus: $748,219
Savings Plan: Y   Stock Purch. Plan: Second Exec. Salary: $373,846   Bonus: $600,000

OTHER THOUGHTS:
Apparent Top Female Officers:
Hot Spot for Advancement for Women/Minorities:

LOCATIONS: ("Y" = Yes)
| West: | Southwest: | Midwest: | Southeast: Y | Northeast: Y | International: |

Note: Financial information, benefits and other data can change quickly and may vary from those stated here.

ság
PREMERA BLUE CROSS

www.premera.com

Industry Group Code: 524114   Ranks within this company's industry group: Sales: 28   Profits: 43

Insurance/HMO/PPO:	Drugs:	Equipment/Supplies:	Hospitals/Clinics:	Services:	Health Care:
Insurance: Y Managed Care: Utilization Mgmt.: Payment Proc.:	Manufacturer: Distributor: Specialty Pharm.: Vitamins/Nutri.: Clinical Trials:	Manufacturer: Distributor: Leasing/Finance: Information Sys.:	Acute Care: Sub-Acute Care: Outpatient Surgery: Phys. Rehab. Center: Psychiatric Clinics:	Diagnostics: Labs/Testing: Staffing: Waste Disposal: Specialty Services:	Home Health: Long-Term Care: Physical Therapy: Phys. Practice Mgmt.:

TYPES OF BUSINESS:
Insurance-Health

BRANDS/DIVISIONS/AFFILIATES:
Dimension

CONTACTS:
Note: Officers with more than one job title may be intentionally listed here more than once.

H.R. Brereton Barlow, CEO
H.R. Brereton Barlow, Pres.
Kent Marquardt, CFO
Heyward Donigan, Exec. VP-Mktg.
Alan Smit, CIO
Yori Milo, General Counsel
Karen Bartlett, VP-Oper.
Brian Ancell, VP-Strategy
John L. Castiglia, Chief Medical Officer

Phone: 425-918-4000   Fax: 425-918-5575
Toll-Free: 800-722-1471
Address: 7001 220th SW, Mountlake Terrace, WA 98043 US

GROWTH PLANS/SPECIAL FEATURES:

Premera Blue Cross, the second-largest private company in Washington, is a not-for-profit health insurance provider for Washington and Alaska. The firm has 1.2 million members in Washington and 108,000 members in Alaska, with revenues of $2.4 billion and a network of 21,038 health care providers and 120 hospitals. Premera health plans include preferred provider organization (PPO) plans, exclusive provider organization (EPO) plans, Medicare supplemental, indemnity coverage, dental and long-term care. Premera recently launched a collection of products under the Dimension brand that allow business customers to tailor health plans with features from HMOs, PPOs or managed indemnity plans. Employers are then able to decide which doctor and hospital network to support along with what out-of-network coverage, deductibles, copays and pharmacy benefits will be offered. In other news, Premera's request to change to a for-profit, publicly traded company was denied by the Washington state insurance commission.

Employees of Premera receive medical, dental and life insurance, along with dependant care reimbursement accounts, an educational assistance program, on-site training, an employee assistance program and legal assistance.

FINANCIALS:
Sales and profits are in thousands of dollars—add 000 to get the full amount. Year 2004 note: Complete fiscal 2004 results were not available for all companies at press time. For this company, year 2004 is for months.

2004 Sales: $ (months)   2004 Profits: $ (months)
2003 Sales: $2,800,000   2003 Profits: $3,300
2002 Sales: $ 2002 Profits: $
2001 Sales: $ 2001 Profits: $
2000 Sales: $ 2000 Profits: $

Stock Ticker: Nonprofit
Employees:
Fiscal Year Ends: 12/31

SALARIES/BENEFITS:
Pension Plan: ESOP Stock Plan: Profit Sharing: Top Exec. Salary: $ Bonus: $
Savings Plan: Y   Stock Purch. Plan: Second Exec. Salary: $ Bonus: $

OTHER THOUGHTS:
Apparent Top Female Officers: 1
Hot Spot for Advancement for Women/Minorities:

LOCATIONS: ("Y" = Yes)
| West: Y | Southwest: | Midwest: | Southeast: | Northeast: | International: |

Note: Financial information, benefits and other data can change quickly and may vary from those stated here.

PREMIER INC

www.premierinc.com

Industry Group Code: 561400   **Ranks within this company's industry group:** Sales: Profits:

Insurance/HMO/PPO:		Drugs:		Equipment/Supplies:		Hospitals/Clinics:		Services:		Health Care:	
Insurance:	Y	Manufacturer:		Manufacturer:		Acute Care:		Diagnostics:		Home Health:	
Managed Care:		Distributor:		Distributor:	Y	Sub-Acute Care:		Labs/Testing:		Long-Term Care:	
Utilization Mgmt.:		Specialty Pharm.:		Leasing/Finance:		Outpatient Surgery:		Staffing:		Physical Therapy:	
Payment Proc.:		Vitamins/Nutri.:		Information Sys.:	Y	Phys. Rehab. Center:		Waste Disposal:		Phys. Practice Mgmt.:	
		Clinical Trials:				Psychiatric Clinics:		Specialty Services:	Y		

TYPES OF BUSINESS:
Medical Supply Distribution
Supply Chain Management
Health Care Consulting
Insurance Services
IT Services

BRANDS/DIVISIONS/AFFILIATES:
Premier Sourcing Partners
Premier Insurance Management

GROWTH PLANS/SPECIAL FEATURES:
Premier, Inc. is primarily a medical supply chain management and health care consulting company. The firm is a joint venture owned by more than 200 independent hospitals, with nearly 1,500 affiliated hospitals and clinics nationwide. Premier purchases more than $14 billion in medical supplies and equipment per year. These products include facilities, food and dietary, imaging, information technology, medical and surgical and pharmacy supplies. The company also supplies low-cost insurance and medical IT services through its Premier Insurance Management and Premier Sourcing Partners subsidiaries. In addition, Premier offers a wide range of consulting services including IT, risk management, financial, safety support, pharmaceutical analysis, patient satisfaction and employee retention services. The company also acts as an industry advocate in the areas of state and national government.

Premier offers its employees a comprehensive medical and insurance benefits package and tuition reimbursement.

CONTACTS:
Note: Officers with more than one job title may be intentionally listed here more than once.

Richard A. Norling, CEO
Ann Rhoads, CFO
Jena E. Abernathy, Sr. VP-Human Resources
Larry D. Grandia, Exec. VP-IT
Jeffrey W. Maysent, General Counsel
Hunter Kome, VP-Corp. Comm.
Robert L. Hamon, Sr. VP-Group Purchasing Services
Stephen La Neve, Sr. VP-Bus. Partner Rel.
Jack L. Cox, Sr. VP-Medical
Larry Abramson, Sr. VP-Supply Chain

Phone: 858-481-2727   **Fax:** 858-481-8919
Toll-Free:
Address: 12225 Camino Real, San Diego, CA 92130 US

FINANCIALS:
Sales and profits are in thousands of dollars—add 000 to get the full amount. Year 2004 note: Complete fiscal 2004 results were not available for all companies at press time. For this company, year 2004 is for months.

2004 Sales: $ (months)   2004 Profits: $ (months)
2003 Sales: $ 2003 Profits: $
2002 Sales: $ 2002 Profits: $
2001 Sales: $ 2001 Profits: $
2000 Sales: $ 2000 Profits: $

Stock Ticker: Joint Venture
Employees:
Fiscal Year Ends: 12/31

SALARIES/BENEFITS:
Pension Plan: ESOP Stock Plan: Profit Sharing: Top Exec. Salary: $ Bonus: $
Savings Plan: Y   Stock Purch. Plan: Second Exec. Salary: $ Bonus: $

OTHER THOUGHTS:
Apparent Top Female Officers: 2
Hot Spot for Advancement for Women/Minorities:

LOCATIONS: ("Y" = Yes)
West:	Southwest:	Midwest:	Southeast:	Northeast:	International:
Y		Y	Y		

PRIMEDEX HEALTH SYSTEMS INC
www.radnetonline.com

Industry Group Code: 621511   Ranks within this company's industry group: Sales: 7   Profits: 6

Insurance/HMO/PPO:	Drugs:	Equipment/Supplies:	Hospitals/Clinics:	Services:		Health Care:
Insurance:	Manufacturer:	Manufacturer:	Acute Care:	Diagnostics:	Y	Home Health:
Managed Care:	Distributor:	Distributor:	Sub-Acute Care:	Labs/Testing:		Long-Term Care:
Utilization Mgmt.:	Specialty Pharm.:	Leasing/Finance:	Outpatient Surgery:	Staffing:		Physical Therapy:
Payment Proc.:	Vitamins/Nutri.:	Information Sys.:	Phys. Rehab. Center:	Waste Disposal:		Phys. Practice Mgmt.:
	Clinical Trials:		Psychiatric Clinics:	Specialty Services:		

TYPES OF BUSINESS:
Diagnostics Services
Medical Imaging

BRANDS/DIVISIONS/AFFILIATES:
RadNet Management, Inc.

GROWTH PLANS/SPECIAL FEATURES:
Primedex Health Systems, Inc. operates a network of 55 diagnostic imaging centers in California, which offer medical imaging services to the public, including MRI, CT, PET, ultrasound, mammography, nuclear medicine and general diagnostic radiology. RadNet Management, Inc. manages the centers. Patients are generally referred to the centers by their treating physicians and may be affiliated with an IPA, HMO, PPO or similar organization. The most common imaging procedures are x-ray, fluoroscopy, endoscopy and modalities such as CT scans and digital image processing. The centers also offer open MRI, allowing studies with patients not typically compatible with conventional MRI, such as infants and pediatric, claustrophobic or obese patients.

CONTACTS:
Note: Officers with more than one job title may be intentionally listed here more than once.
Howard G. Berger, CEO
Howard G. Berger, Pres.
Norman R. Hames, VP/COO
Howard G. Berger, CFO
Jeffrey L. Linden, General Counsel
Howard G. Berger, Treas.
John V. Crues, III, VP
Michael J. Krane, VP-Medical
Norman R. Hames, Corp. Sec.

Phone: 310-478-7808   **Fax:** 310-445-2980
Toll-Free:
Address: 1516 Cotner Ave., Los Angeles, CA 90025 US

FINANCIALS:
Sales and profits are in thousands of dollars—add 000 to get the full amount. Year 2004 note: Complete fiscal 2004 results were not available for all companies at press time. For this company, year 2004 is for 9 months.

2004 Sales: $103,800 (9 months)	2004 Profits: $-7,719 (9 months)	**Stock Ticker:** PMDX
2003 Sales: $140,259	2003 Profits: $-2,267	Employees: 1,224
2002 Sales: $139,300	2002 Profits: $-5,600	Fiscal Year Ends: 10/31
2001 Sales: $111,800	2001 Profits: $14,500	
2000 Sales: $88,000	2000 Profits: $2,600	

SALARIES/BENEFITS:
Pension Plan:	ESOP Stock Plan:	Profit Sharing:	Top Exec. Salary: $363,000	Bonus: $
Savings Plan: Y	Stock Purch. Plan:		Second Exec. Salary: $328,846	Bonus: $

OTHER THOUGHTS:
Apparent Top Female Officers:
Hot Spot for Advancement for Women/Minorities:

LOCATIONS: ("Y" = Yes)
West:	Southwest:	Midwest:	Southeast:	Northeast:	International:
Y					

PRIORITY HEALTHCARE CORP
www.priorityhealthcare.com

Industry Group Code: 446110A Ranks within this company's industry group: Sales: 4 Profits: 3

Insurance/HMO/PPO:	Drugs:	Equipment/Supplies:	Hospitals/Clinics:	Services:	Health Care:
Insurance:	Manufacturer:	Manufacturer:	Acute Care:	Diagnostics:	Home Health:
Managed Care:	Distributor: Y	Distributor:	Sub-Acute Care:	Labs/Testing:	Long-Term Care:
Utilization Mgmt.:	Specialty Pharm.: Y	Leasing/Finance:	Outpatient Surgery:	Staffing:	Physical Therapy:
Payment Proc.:	Vitamins/Nutri.:	Information Sys.:	Phys. Rehab. Center:	Waste Disposal:	Phys. Practice Mgmt.:
	Clinical Trials:		Psychiatric Clinics:	Specialty Services:	

TYPES OF BUSINESS:
Drugs-Specialty Pharmacy
Alternative-Site Drug Distribution
Disease Treatment Programs
Specialty Biopharmaceuticals

BRANDS/DIVISIONS/AFFILIATES:
Priority Healthcare Pharmacy
Integrity Healthcare Services

CONTACTS: Note: Officers with more than one job title may be intentionally listed here more than once.
Steven D. Cosler, CEO
Steven D. Cosler, Pres.
Tracy Nolan, Exec. VP/COO
Donald J. Perfetto, Exec. VP/CFO
Kim K. Rondeau, VP-Mktg. & Sales
Rebecca M. Shanahan, Exec. VP-Admin.
Rebecca M. Shanahan, General Counsel
William M. Woodard, VP-Strategic Alliances
Stephen M. Saft, Treas.
Melissa E. McIntyre, VP-Strategic Program Dev.
Donald J. Perfetto, Exec. VP-Special Projects
Barbara J. Luttrell, VP-Admin.
William E. Bindley, Chmn.

Phone: 407-804-6700 **Fax:** 407-804-5675
Toll-Free: 800-892-9622
Address: 250 Technology Park, Ste. 124, Lake Mary, FL 32746 US

GROWTH PLANS/SPECIAL FEATURES:
Priority Healthcare Corp. is a national distributor of specialty pharmaceuticals and related medical supplies to the alternative-site health care market. The firm is also a provider of patient-specific, self-administered biopharmaceuticals and disease treatment programs to individuals with chronic diseases. Priority sells specialty pharmaceuticals and medical supplies to outpatient renal care centers and office-based physicians in oncology and other specialty markets. The firm also offers value-added services to meet the specific needs of these markets, including shipping refrigerated pharmaceuticals overnight in special packaging and offering automated order entry services and customized distribution for group accounts. The company services over 4,000 customers in all 50 states from distribution centers in Nevada and Ohio. Priority fills individual patient prescriptions, primarily for self-administered biopharmaceuticals, at licensed pharmacies in Florida, Massachusetts, Pennsylvania, Delaware, New York and Tennessee. The company also provides disease treatment programs for hepatitis, cancer, hemophilia, human growth deficiency, rheumatoid arthritis, Crohn's disease, infertility, pulmonary hypertension, pain management, multiple sclerosis and others. In July 2004, Priority Healthcare acquired Integrity Healthcare Services, a specialty infusion pharmacy with 23 branches in 16 states.

Priority Healthcare offers its employees tuition reimbursement, group medical and life insurance, stock options and discount programs, such as a Costco corporate membership.

FINANCIALS: Sales and profits are in thousands of dollars—add 000 to get the full amount. Year 2004 note: Complete fiscal 2004 results were not available for all companies at press time. For this company, year 2004 is for 9 months.

2004 Sales: $1,279,854 (9 months)   2004 Profits: $37,044 (9 months)
2003 Sales: $1,461,811   2003 Profits: $50,600
2002 Sales: $1,200,400   2002 Profits: $43,600
2001 Sales: $805,100   2001 Profits: $27,700
2000 Sales: $584,700   2000 Profits: $28,100

Stock Ticker: PHCC
Employees: 810
Fiscal Year Ends: 12/31

SALARIES/BENEFITS:
Pension Plan: ESOP Stock Plan: Profit Sharing: Y   Top Exec. Salary: $498,641   Bonus: $331,293
Savings Plan: Y Stock Purch. Plan: Y   Second Exec. Salary: $320,633 Bonus: $110,334

OTHER THOUGHTS:
Apparent Top Female Officers: 4
Hot Spot for Advancement for Women/Minorities: Y

LOCATIONS: ("Y" = Yes)
West:	Southwest:	Midwest:	Southeast:	Northeast:	International:
Y	Y	Y	Y	Y	

PROVIDENCE HEALTH SYSTEM

www.providence.org

Industry Group Code: 622110   Ranks within this company's industry group: Sales: 15   Profits: 9

Insurance/HMO/PPO:	Drugs:	Equipment/Supplies:	Hospitals/Clinics:		Services:		Health Care:	
Insurance: Managed Care: Utilization Mgmt.: Payment Proc.:	Manufacturer: Distributor: Specialty Pharm.: Vitamins/Nutri.: Clinical Trials:	Manufacturer: Distributor: Leasing/Finance: Information Sys.:	Acute Care: Sub-Acute Care: Outpatient Surgery: Phys. Rehab. Center: Psychiatric Clinics:	Y	Diagnostics: Labs/Testing: Staffing: Waste Disposal: Specialty Services:		Home Health: Long-Term Care: Physical Therapy: Phys. Practice Mgmt.:	Y

TYPES OF BUSINESS:
Hospitals-General
Assisted Living Facilities

BRANDS/DIVISIONS/AFFILIATES:
Providence St. Peter Hospital
Little Company of Mary
Sisters of Providence
Providence Milwaukie Hospital
Little Company of Mary Hospital
San Pedro Peninsula Hospital
Providence Valdez Medical Center
Providence Holy Cross

CONTACTS:
Note: Officers with more than one job title may be intentionally listed here more than once.
Hank Walker, CEO
Hank Walker, Pres.
John Koster, COO
Mike Butler, CFO
Sue Byington, VP-Human Resources
Rick Skinner, CIO
Jan Jones, VP-Admin.
Jeff Rogers, General Counsel
Adrienne McDunn, VP-Strategy
Cheryl Sjoblom, VP-Corp. Comm.
Ron Oldfield, VP-Finance
Rocky Fredrickson, Chief Medical Officer
Chuck Hawley, VP-Gov't Affairs, Ethics & Theology

Phone: 206-464-3355   Fax: 206-464-3355
Toll-Free:
Address: 506 2nd Ave., Ste. 1200, Seattle, WA 98104 US

GROWTH PLANS/SPECIAL FEATURES:
Providence Health System is a not-for-profit collection of health facilities in the Pacific Northwest run by two catholic charities: the Sisters of Providence and the Little Company of Mary. The firm operates 17 acute care hospitals, 12 freestanding long-term care facilities and 19 low-income and assisted living facilities in Alaska, Washington, Oregon and Southern California. In total the company operates 3,719 acute and 1,741 long-term licensed beds. Hospitals under the system include Providence Alaska Medical Center, Providence Kodiak Island Medical Center and Providence Seward Medical Center in Alaska; Providence St. Peter Hospital and Providence Centralia Hospital in Washington; Providence Hood River Memorial Hospital, Providence Seaside Hospital, Providence Milwaukie Hospital and Providence Newberg Hospital in Oregon; and Little Company of Mary Hospital and San Pedro Peninsula Hospital in California. The firm has plans to open the new Providence Valdez Medical Center in early 2005, as well as to expand the emergency center of Providence Holy Cross.

Providence provides employees with medical, dental and vision insurance, along with flexible reimbursement accounts and tuition reimbursement.

FINANCIALS:
Sales and profits are in thousands of dollars—add 000 to get the full amount. Year 2004 note: Complete fiscal 2004 results were not available for all companies at press time. For this company, year 2004 is for   months.

2004 Sales: $ (months)   2004 Profits: $ (months)
2003 Sales: $3,780,200   2003 Profits: $176,600
2002 Sales: $3,528,600   2002 Profits: $
2001 Sales: $ 2001 Profits: $
2000 Sales: $ 2000 Profits: $

Stock Ticker: Nonprofit
Employees: 32,526
Fiscal Year Ends: 12/31

SALARIES/BENEFITS:
Pension Plan: ESOP Stock Plan: Profit Sharing: Top Exec. Salary: $ Bonus: $
Savings Plan: Y Stock Purch. Plan: Second Exec. Salary: $ Bonus: $

OTHER THOUGHTS:
Apparent Top Female Officers: 4
Hot Spot for Advancement for Women/Minorities: Y

LOCATIONS: ("Y" = Yes)
West: Y   Southwest: Midwest: Southeast: Northeast: International:

PROVINCE HEALTHCARE CO
www.provincehealthcare.com

Industry Group Code: 622110   Ranks within this company's industry group: Sales: 41   Profits: 16

Insurance/HMO/PPO:	Drugs:	Equipment/Supplies:	Hospitals/Clinics:		Services:		Health Care:	
Insurance:	Manufacturer:	Manufacturer:	Acute Care:	Y	Diagnostics:	Y	Home Health:	Y
Managed Care:	Distributor:	Distributor:	Sub-Acute Care:	Y	Labs/Testing:	Y	Long-Term Care:	
Utilization Mgmt.:	Specialty Pharm.:	Leasing/Finance:	Outpatient Surgery:	Y	Staffing:		Physical Therapy:	Y
Payment Proc.:	Vitamins/Nutri.:	Information Sys.:	Phys. Rehab. Center:	Y	Waste Disposal:		Phys. Practice Mgmt.:	
	Clinical Trials:		Psychiatric Clinics:		Specialty Services:	Y		

TYPES OF BUSINESS:
Hospitals-General
Management Services
Skilled Nursing
Outpatient & Ancillary Services

BRANDS/DIVISIONS/AFFILIATES:
Lifepoint Hospitals, Inc.

CONTACTS:
Note: Officers with more than one job title may be intentionally listed here more than once.

Martin S. Rash, CEO
Daniel S. Slipkovich, Pres.
Daniel S. Slipkovich, COO
Christopher T. Hannon, Sr. VP/CFO
Howard T. Wall, III, Sr. VP/General Counsel
Sam Moody, Sr. VP-Oper.
J. Thomas Anderson, Sr. VP-Acquisitions & Dev.
Thomas A. Salerno, Regional VP-Western Div.
Thomas A. Pemberton, Regional VP-Eastern Div.
Carl W. Gower, Regional VP-Central Div.
Howard T. Wall, III, Corp. Sec.
Martin S. Rash, Chmn.

Phone: 615-370-1377   **Fax:** 615-376-4856
Toll-Free:
Address: 105 Westwood Pl., Ste. 400, Brentwood, TN 37027 US

GROWTH PLANS/SPECIAL FEATURES:
Province Healthcare Company owns and operates acute care hospitals located in rural markets throughout the U.S. The firm operates 19 general acute care hospitals in 13 states with about 2,260 licensed beds. One of its affiliates provides management services to 38 primarily rural hospitals in 14 states with a total of 3,130 licensed beds. The company targets hospitals for acquisition that are the sole or primary provider of health care in their communities. After an acquisition, Province implements a number of strategies to improve financial performance, including improving hospital operations, expanding the breadth of services offered and recruiting physicians to increase market share. The company's acute care hospitals typically provide a full range of services commonly available in hospitals, such as internal medicine, general surgery, cardiology, oncology, orthopedics, obstetrics, rehabilitation, sub-acute care and diagnostic and emergency services. The hospitals also provide outpatient and ancillary health care services, such as laboratory, radiology, respiratory therapy, home health care and physical therapy. Some of the firm's hospitals also have a limited number of psychiatric beds. Province provides capital resources and makes available a variety of management services to its owned and leased hospitals in Alabama, Arizona, California, Colorado, Florida, Indiana, Louisiana, Mississippi, Nevada, Pennsylvania, New Mexico, Virginia and Texas. In August 2004, Lifepoint Hospitals, Inc. agreed to acquire Province for $1.03 billion in cash, stocks and debt assumption.

FINANCIALS:
Sales and profits are in thousands of dollars—add 000 to get the full amount. Year 2004 note: Complete fiscal 2004 results were not available for all companies at press time. For this company, year 2004 is for 9 months.

2004 Sales: $644,426 (9 months)	2004 Profits: $41,289 (9 months)	
2003 Sales: $761,978	2003 Profits: $31,619	**Stock Ticker:** PRV
2002 Sales: $704,300	2002 Profits: $36,100	Employees: 5,848
2001 Sales: $530,700	2001 Profits: $32,900	Fiscal Year Ends: 12/31
2000 Sales: $469,900	2000 Profits: $19,900	

SALARIES/BENEFITS:
Pension Plan: Y   ESOP Stock Plan: Profit Sharing: Top Exec. Salary: $624,000   Bonus: $624,000
Savings Plan: Y   Stock Purch. Plan: Second Exec. Salary: $520,000   Bonus: $520,000

OTHER THOUGHTS:
Apparent Top Female Officers:
Hot Spot for Advancement for Women/Minorities:

LOCATIONS: ("Y" = Yes)
West:	Southwest:	Midwest:	Southeast:	Northeast:	International:
Y	Y	Y	Y	Y	

PSS WORLD MEDICAL INC

www.pssd.com

Industry Group Code: 421450 Ranks within this company's industry group: Sales: 5 Profits: 7

Insurance/HMO/PPO:	Drugs:	Equipment/Supplies:	Hospitals/Clinics:	Services:	Health Care:
Insurance:	Manufacturer:	Manufacturer:	Acute Care:	Diagnostics:	Home Health:
Managed Care:	Distributor: Y	Distributor: Y	Sub-Acute Care:	Labs/Testing:	Long-Term Care:
Utilization Mgmt.:	Specialty Pharm.:	Leasing/Finance:	Outpatient Surgery:	Staffing:	Physical Therapy:
Payment Proc.:	Vitamins/Nutri.:	Information Sys.:	Phys. Rehab. Center:	Waste Disposal:	Phys. Practice Mgmt.:
	Clinical Trials:		Psychiatric Clinics:	Specialty Services:	

TYPES OF BUSINESS:
Distribution-Medical Supplies & Equipment
Distribution-Pharmaceuticals

BRANDS/DIVISIONS/AFFILIATES:
WorldMed International, Inc.
Gulf South Medical Supply, Inc.
Taylor Medical, Inc.
Highpoint Healthcare Distribution
Advantage Medical Products, LLC

CONTACTS:
Note: Officers with more than one job title may be intentionally listed here more than once.
David A. Smith, CEO
David A. Smith, Pres.
David M. Bronson, Exec. VP/CFO
John F. Sasen, Sr., Exec. VP/Chief Mktg. Officer
Jeffrey H. Anthony, Sr. VP-Human Resources
David H. Ramsey, VP/CIO
Jeffrey H. Anthony, Sr. VP-Corp. Dev.
Robert C. Weiner, VP-Investor Rel.
David Klamer, VP/Treas.
Kevin P. English, VP-Finance
Gary A. Corless, Exec. VP/Pres.-Physician Sales & Service
Tony E. Oglesby, Pres./CEO-Gulf South Medical Supply, Inc.
Mary Jennings, VP-Compliance & Tax
Clark A. Johnson, Chmn.

Phone: 904-332-3000   **Fax:** 904-332-3213
Toll-Free:
Address: 4345 Southpoint Blvd., Jacksonville, FL 32216 US

GROWTH PLANS/SPECIAL FEATURES:
PSS World Medical, Inc. is a specialty marketer and distributor of medical products to physicians, alternate-site imaging centers, long-term care providers, home care providers and hospitals through 33 service centers to customers in all 50 states. Through strategic acquisitions and internal growth, the company has become a leader in the market segments it serves. PSS's physician sales and services division is a leading distributor of medical supplies, equipment and pharmaceuticals to over 50% of office-based physician practices in the U.S. The firm's other main division, Gulf South Medical Supply, Inc. (GSMS), is a leading national distributor of medical supplies and related products to the nursing and long-term care industry, currently operating 14 centers and serving accounts in all 50 states. GSMS's market includes a large number of independent operators, small to mid-sized local and regional chains and several national chains. It also owns Highpoint Healthcare Distribution, a Texas-based marketing and distribution organization that serves the long-term, assisted living and home health markets in Texas, Oklahoma and Kansas. GSMS subsidiary Advantage Medical Products, LLC, based in Louisiana, distributes medical supplies and equipment to the long-term care industry.

The firm offers its employees health, dental, vision and life insurance, an employee assistance program, a legal access plan, short- and long-term disability and flexible spending accounts.

FINANCIALS:
Sales and profits are in thousands of dollars—add 000 to get the full amount. Year 2004 note: Complete fiscal 2004 results were not available for all companies at press time. For this company, year 2004 is for 12 months.

2004 Sales: $1,349,917 (12 months)   2004 Profits: $27,539 (12 months)
2003 Sales: $1,177,900   2003 Profits: $-54,800
2002 Sales: $1,815,800   2002 Profits: $-81,200
2001 Sales: $1,814,800   2001 Profits: $-36,100
2000 Sales: $1,804,000   2000 Profits: $20,700

Stock Ticker: PSSI
Employees: 2,954
Fiscal Year Ends: 3/31

SALARIES/BENEFITS:
Pension Plan:	ESOP Stock Plan: Y	Profit Sharing:	Top Exec. Salary: $522,500	Bonus: $630,768
Savings Plan: Y	Stock Purch. Plan: Y		Second Exec. Salary: $309,000	Bonus: $376,997

OTHER THOUGHTS:
Apparent Top Female Officers: 1
Hot Spot for Advancement for Women/Minorities:

LOCATIONS: ("Y" = Yes)
West:	Southwest:	Midwest:	Southeast:	Northeast:	International:
Y	Y	Y	Y	Y	Y

PSYCHIATRIC SOLUTIONS INC

www.psysolutions.com

Industry Group Code: 622210 **Ranks within this company's industry group:** Sales: 3 Profits: 3

Insurance/HMO/PPO:	Drugs:	Equipment/Supplies:	Hospitals/Clinics:	Services:	Health Care:
Insurance: Managed Care: Utilization Mgmt.: Payment Proc.:	Manufacturer: Distributor: Specialty Pharm.: Vitamins/Nutri.: Clinical Trials:	Manufacturer: Distributor: Leasing/Finance: Information Sys.:	Acute Care: Sub-Acute Care: Outpatient Surgery: Phys. Rehab. Center: Psychiatric Clinics:	Diagnostics: Labs/Testing: Staffing: Waste Disposal: Specialty Services:	Home Health: Long-Term Care: Physical Therapy: Phys. Practice Mgmt.:

TYPES OF BUSINESS:
Clinics-Psychiatric
Substance Abuse Treatment

BRANDS/DIVISIONS/AFFILIATES:
SunStone

CONTACTS:
Note: Officers with more than one job title may be intentionally listed here more than once.

Joey A. Jacobs, CEO
Joey A. Jacobs, Pres.
Jack Salberg, COO
Steven T. Davidson, Chief Dev. Officer
Brent Turner, VP-Investor Rel.
Brent Turner, VP/Treas.
Steven T. Davidson, Corp. Sec.
Jack E. Polson, Chief Acc. Officer
Joey A. Jacobs, Chmn.

Phone: 615-312-5700 **Fax:** 615-312-5711
Toll-Free:
Address: 840 Crescent Centre Dr., Ste. 460, Franklin, TN 37067 US

GROWTH PLANS/SPECIAL FEATURES:
Psychiatric Solutions, Inc. is a leading provider of behavioral health care services in the U.S. The company owns and operates 34 inpatient behavioral health care facilities with over 4,000 beds, and its SunStone division manages 43 units for third-party acute care hospitals and 11 for government agencies. It also has a contract to provide mental health case management services to approximately 4,300 children and adults with serious mental illness in the Nashville, Tennessee area. All of these facilities provide 24-hour nursing observation and care, daily interventions and oversight by a psychiatrist and intensive treatment by a physician-led team of mental health professionals. Through its managed and freestanding psychiatric facilities, Psychiatric Solutions offers a comprehensive array of behavioral health programs to children, adolescents and adults, working closely with counselors, therapists, social workers, psychiatrists, physicians, emergency rooms and law enforcement. Many of the company's facilities have mobile assessment teams who travel to prospective clients in order to determine if they meet criteria for inpatient care, and some provide outpatient care or a less intensive level of care to those who do not qualify. Services offered include acute psychiatric care, partial hospitalization, rehabilitation care, detoxification, vocational training and treatment for chemical dependency, acute eating disorders, developmentally delayed disorders and neurological disorders.

FINANCIALS:
Sales and profits are in thousands of dollars—add 000 to get the full amount. Year 2004 note: Complete fiscal 2004 results were not available for all companies at press time. For this company, year 2004 is for 6 months.

2004 Sales: $228,094 (6 months)   2004 Profits: $5,071 (6 months)
2003 Sales: $293,665   2003 Profits: $5,216
2002 Sales: $113,912   2002 Profits: $5,684
2001 Sales: $43,999   2001 Profits: $2,578
2000 Sales: $ 2000 Profits: $

Stock Ticker: PSYS
Employees: 4,810
Fiscal Year Ends: 12/31

SALARIES/BENEFITS:
Pension Plan: ESOP Stock Plan: Profit Sharing: Top Exec. Salary: $325,000   Bonus: $125,000
Savings Plan: Y   Stock Purch. Plan: Second Exec. Salary: $275,258   Bonus: $100,000

OTHER THOUGHTS:
Apparent Top Female Officers:
Hot Spot for Advancement for Women/Minorities:

LOCATIONS: ("Y" = Yes)
West:	Southwest:	Midwest:	Southeast:	Northeast:	International:
Y	Y	Y	Y	Y	

Note: Financial information, benefits and other data can change quickly and may vary from those stated here.

QUALITY SYSTEMS INC

www.qsii.com

Industry Group Code: 511200 **Ranks within this company's industry group:** Sales: 9 Profits: 7

Insurance/HMO/PPO:	Drugs:	Equipment/Supplies:	Hospitals/Clinics:	Services:	Health Care:
Insurance: Managed Care: Utilization Mgmt.: Payment Proc.:	Manufacturer: Distributor: Specialty Pharm.: Vitamins/Nutri.: Clinical Trials:	Manufacturer: Distributor: Leasing/Finance: Information Sys.: Y	Acute Care: Sub-Acute Care: Outpatient Surgery: Phys. Rehab. Center: Psychiatric Clinics:	Diagnostics: Labs/Testing: Staffing: Waste Disposal: Specialty Services:	Home Health: Long-Term Care: Physical Therapy: Phys. Practice Mgmt.:

TYPES OF BUSINESS:
Software-Practice Management

BRANDS/DIVISIONS/AFFILIATES:
Clinical Product Suite
NextGen Healthcare Information Systems, Inc.
Electronic Medical Records
Enterprise Practice Management
Enterprise Appointment Scheduling
Enterprise Master Patient Index
Image Control System
Managed Care Server

CONTACTS:
Note: Officers with more than one job title may be intentionally listed here more than once.
Louis E. Silverman, CEO
Louis E. Silverman, Pres.
Paul Holt, CFO
Patrick Cline, Pres., NextGen Healthcare Information Systems
Greg Flynn, Exec. VP-Quality Systems Div.
Sheldon Razin, Chmn.

Phone: 714-731-7171 **Fax:** 949-255-2605
Toll-Free: 800-888-7955
Address: 18191 Von Karman Ave., Ste. 450, Irvine, CA 92612 US

GROWTH PLANS/SPECIAL FEATURES:
Quality Systems, Inc. develops and markets health care information systems that automate medical and dental practices, practice networks, management service organizations, ambulatory care centers, community health centers and medical and dental schools. These include systems designed to streamline patient records and administrative functions such as billing and scheduling. The company's QSI division focuses on developing, marketing and supporting software suites for dental and niche medical practices. Its Clinical Product Suite uses a Windows NT operating system and incorporates clinical tools including periodontal charting and digital imaging of x-ray and inter-oral camera images. Subsidiary NextGen Healthcare Information Systems, Inc. develops and sells proprietary electronic medical records software and practice management systems. Its NextGen product line includes Electronic Medical Records, Enterprise Practice Management, Enterprise Appointment Scheduling, Enterprise Master Patient Index, Image Control System, Managed Care Server, Electronic Data Interchange, System Interfaces, Internet Operability, patient-centric and provider-centric web portal solutions and a handheld product.

FINANCIALS:
Sales and profits are in thousands of dollars—add 000 to get the full amount. Year 2004 note: Complete fiscal 2004 results were not available for all companies at press time. For this company, year 2004 is for 12 months.

2004 Sales: $70,934 (12 months)   2004 Profits: $10,400 (12 months)
2003 Sales: $54,769   2003 Profits: $7,035
2002 Sales: $44,422   2002 Profits: $5,268
2001 Sales: $39,900   2001 Profits: $3,500
2000 Sales: $ 2000 Profits: $

Stock Ticker: QSII
Employees: 327
Fiscal Year Ends: 3/31

SALARIES/BENEFITS:
Pension Plan: ESOP Stock Plan: Profit Sharing: Top Exec. Salary: $278,500   Bonus: $196,500
Savings Plan: Y   Stock Purch. Plan: Second Exec. Salary: $257,500   Bonus: $139,250

OTHER THOUGHTS:
Apparent Top Female Officers:
Hot Spot for Advancement for Women/Minorities:

LOCATIONS: ("Y" = Yes)
West	Southwest	Midwest	Southeast	Northeast	International
Y			Y	Y	

QUEST DIAGNOSTICS INC
www.questdiagnostics.com

Industry Group Code: 621511 Ranks within this company's industry group: Sales: 1 Profits: 1

Insurance/HMO/PPO:	Drugs:	Equipment/Supplies:	Hospitals/Clinics:	Services:		Health Care:	
Insurance:	Manufacturer:	Manufacturer:	Acute Care:	Diagnostics:	Y	Home Health:	
Managed Care:	Distributor:	Distributor:	Sub-Acute Care:	Labs/Testing:	Y	Long-Term Care:	
Utilization Mgmt.:	Specialty Pharm.:	Leasing/Finance:	Outpatient Surgery:	Staffing:		Physical Therapy:	
Payment Proc.:	Vitamins/Nutri.:	Information Sys.:	Phys. Rehab. Center:	Waste Disposal:		Phys. Practice Mgmt.:	
	Clinical Trials:		Psychiatric Clinics:	Specialty Services:			

TYPES OF BUSINESS:
Services-Testing & Diagnostics
Clinical Laboratory Testing
Clinical Trials Testing

BRANDS/DIVISIONS/AFFILIATES:
ImmunoCAP
ThinPrep Pap
HEPTIMAX
Nichols Institute
Bio-Intact PTH
eMaxx
MedPlus
Cardio CRP

CONTACTS:
Note: Officers with more than one job title may be intentionally listed here more than once.

Surya N. Mohapatra, CEO
Surya N. Mohapatra, Pres.
Robert A. Hagemann, Sr. VP/CFO
Gerald C. Marrone, CIO
Michael E. Prevoznik, General Counsel/VP-Legal & Compliance
Gary Samuels, VP-Corp. Comm.
Laura Park, Dir.-Investor Rel.
Sirisha Gummaregula, Corp. Sec.
David M. Zewe, Sr. VP-Diagnostic Testing Oper.
Surya N. Mohapatra, Chmn.

Phone: 201-393-5000 Fax: 201-462-4715
Toll-Free: 800-222-0446
Address: One Malcolm Ave., Teterboro, NJ 07608 US

GROWTH PLANS/SPECIAL FEATURES:
Quest Diagnostics, Inc. is one of the largest clinical laboratory testing companies in the U.S., offering a broad array of diagnostic testing and related services to the health care industry. The firm's testing operations consist of routine, esoteric and clinical trials testing. Quest offers patients and physicians comprehensive access to diagnostic testing services through its national network of 2,000 patient service centers, approximately 155 rapid-response laboratories, more than 30 regional laboratories and esoteric testing laboratories on both coasts. Routine tests measure various important bodily health parameters such as the functions of the kidney, heart, liver, thyroid and other organs. Tests in this category include blood cholesterol level tests, complete blood cell counts, pap smears, HIV-related tests, urinalyses, pregnancy and prenatal tests and substance-abuse tests, including the company's ImmunoCAP and ThinPrep Pap tests. Esoteric tests require more sophisticated equipment and technology, professional attention and highly skilled personnel. The firm's tests in this field include Cardio CRP and HEPTIMAX. Quest's Nichols Institute, located in San Juan Capistrano, California, is one of the leading esoteric clinical testing laboratories in the world. Esoteric tests involve a number of medical fields including endocrinology, genetics, immunology, microbiology, oncology, serology and special chemistry. Clinical trial testing primarily involves assessing the safety and efficacy of new drugs to meet FDA requirements, with services including Bio-Intact PTH. Quest recently announced an agreement with Express Scripts, one of the largest pharmacy benefit management companies in North America, to construct an eletronic percription system run by the firm's subsidiaries eMaxx and MedPlus.

Quest offers its employees medical and dental plans, short- and long-term disability, life insurance, educational assistance, adoption assistance, free lab testing, annual development training and access to a credit union.

FINANCIALS:
Sales and profits are in thousands of dollars—add 000 to get the full amount. Year 2004 note: Complete fiscal 2004 results were not available for all companies at press time. For this company, year 2004 is for 9 months.

2004 Sales: $3,843,313 (9 months)   2004 Profits: $373,122 (9 months)
2003 Sales: $4,737,958   2003 Profits: $436,717
2002 Sales: $4,108,100   2002 Profits: $322,200
2001 Sales: $3,627,800   2001 Profits: $162,300
2000 Sales: $3,421,200   2000 Profits: $102,100

Stock Ticker: DGX
Employees: 37,200
Fiscal Year Ends: 12/31

SALARIES/BENEFITS:
Pension Plan: ESOP Stock Plan: Profit Sharing: Top Exec. Salary: $1,091,525   Bonus: $1,243,901
Savings Plan: Y   Stock Purch. Plan: Y   Second Exec. Salary: $597,846   Bonus: $586,647

OTHER THOUGHTS:
Apparent Top Female Officers: 1
Hot Spot for Advancement for Women/Minorities:

LOCATIONS: ("Y" = Yes)
West:	Southwest:	Midwest:	Southeast:	Northeast:	International:
Y	Y	Y	Y	Y	Y

Note: Financial information, benefits and other data can change quickly and may vary from those stated here.

QUIDEL CORP

www.quidel.com

Industry Group Code: 339113 Ranks within this company's industry group: Sales: 94 Profits: 58

Insurance/HMO/PPO:	Drugs:	Equipment/Supplies:		Hospitals/Clinics:	Services:	Health Care:
Insurance:	Manufacturer:	Manufacturer:	Y	Acute Care:	Diagnostics:	Home Health:
Managed Care:	Distributor:	Distributor:		Sub-Acute Care:	Labs/Testing:	Long-Term Care:
Utilization Mgmt.:	Specialty Pharm.:	Leasing/Finance:		Outpatient Surgery:	Staffing:	Physical Therapy:
Payment Proc.:	Vitamins/Nutri.:	Information Sys.:	Y	Phys. Rehab. Center:	Waste Disposal:	Phys. Practice Mgmt.:
	Clinical Trials:			Psychiatric Clinics:	Specialty Services:	

TYPES OF BUSINESS:
Equipment/Supplies-Manufacturer
Point-of-Care Diagnostic Tests

GROWTH PLANS/SPECIAL FEATURES:

Quidel Corporation is a leader in discovering, manufacturing and marketing point-of-care rapid diagnostic tests for the detection and management of a variety of medical conditions and illnesses, including pregnancy, infectious diseases, autoimmune disorders, osteoporosis and urinalysis. Products are sold to hospitals, clinical labs, physicians' offices and wellness screening centers. They utilize immunoassay technology, enzymology, biochemistry and LTF technology in dipstick, lateral flow cassette, microwall plate and LTF format. Currently, the firm manufactures testing products for influenza, strep, mononucleosis, H. pylori, chlamydia, pregnancy, vaginosis and bone health, under the QuickVue, Advance, RapidVue, BlueTest, Metra, QUS-2 and Semi-Q brand names. In addition, the company's UrinQuick urinalysis instrument uses software and optic systems to increase ease of interpretation, detecting the presence of 10 important health markers that assist in the diagnosis of diabetes, liver and kidney disease, urinary tract infections and other ailments. Quidel is also working to develop new tests for strep A, influenza and vaginal pH, as well as a new LTF immunoassay platform.

Quidel's employees benefit from comprehensive medical, dental and vision coverage, life insurance and an employee assistance program.

BRANDS/DIVISIONS/AFFILIATES:
QuickVue
UrinQuick
Advance
RapidVue
BlueTest
Metra
QUS-2
Semi-Q

CONTACTS: Note: Officers with more than one job title may be intentionally listed here more than once.
Caren L. Mason, CEO
Caren L. Mason, Pres.
Mark E. Paiz, Sr. VP/COO
Paul E. Landers, CFO
Paul E. Landers, Sr. VP-Admin.
Paul E. Landers, Sr. VP-Finance
Paul E. Landers, Corp. Sec.
Mark A. Pulido, Chmn.

Phone: 858-552-1100 **Fax:**
Toll-Free: 800-874-1517
Address: 10165 McKellar Ct., San Diego, CA 92121 US

FINANCIALS:
Sales and profits are in thousands of dollars—add 000 to get the full amount. Year 2004 note: Complete fiscal 2004 results were not available for all companies at press time. For this company, year 2004 is for 9 months.

2004 Sales: $48,169 (9 months)   2004 Profits: $-5,643 (9 months)
2003 Sales: $95,105   2003 Profits: $19,651
2002 Sales: $74,600   2002 Profits: $1,300
2001 Sales: $74,100   2001 Profits: $900
2000 Sales: $68,400   2000 Profits: $-5,800

Stock Ticker: QDEL
Employees: 280
Fiscal Year Ends: 12/31

SALARIES/BENEFITS:
| Pension Plan: | ESOP Stock Plan: | Profit Sharing: | Top Exec. Salary: $400,010 | Bonus: $200,005 |
| Savings Plan: Y | Stock Purch. Plan: Y | | Second Exec. Salary: $213,509 | Bonus: $107,308 |

OTHER THOUGHTS:
Apparent Top Female Officers: 1
Hot Spot for Advancement for Women/Minorities:

LOCATIONS: ("Y" = Yes)
West:	Southwest:	Midwest:	Southeast:	Northeast:	International:
Y					Y

QUINTILES TRANSNATIONAL CORP

www.quintiles.com

Industry Group Code: 541710   Ranks within this company's industry group: Sales: 1   Profits: 1

Insurance/HMO/PPO:	Drugs:	Equipment/Supplies:	Hospitals/Clinics:	Services:	Health Care:
Insurance:	Manufacturer:	Manufacturer:	Acute Care:	Diagnostics:	Home Health:
Managed Care:	Distributor:	Distributor:	Sub-Acute Care:	Labs/Testing: Y	Long-Term Care:
Utilization Mgmt.:	Specialty Pharm.:	Leasing/Finance:	Outpatient Surgery:	Staffing:	Physical Therapy:
Payment Proc.:	Vitamins/Nutri.:	Information Sys.:	Phys. Rehab. Center:	Waste Disposal:	Phys. Practice Mgmt.:
	Clinical Trials: Y		Psychiatric Clinics:	Specialty Services: Y	

TYPES OF BUSINESS:
Research & Development
Sales & Marketing Services

BRANDS/DIVISIONS/AFFILIATES:
PharmaBio Development
Innovex
Pharma Services Holding

CONTACTS:
Note: Officers with more than one job title may be intentionally listed here more than once.

Dennis B. Gillings, CEO
John Ratliff, CFO/Exec. VP
Mike Mortimer, Exec. VP-Global Human Resources
Oppel Greef, Exec. VP-Global Prod. Dev. Services
John S. Russell, Chief Admin. Officer/Exec. VP
John S. Russell, General Counsel
Ron Wooten, Exec. VP-Corp. Dev.
Hywel Evans, Pres., Quintiles Europe
Dennis B. Gillings, Chmn.

Phone: 919-998-2000   **Fax:** 919-998-9113
Toll-Free:
Address: 4709 Creekstone Dr., Ste. 200, Durham, NC 27703 US

GROWTH PLANS/SPECIAL FEATURES:

Quintiles Transnational Corporation is a leading provider of full-service contract research, sales and marketing services to the global pharmaceutical, biotechnology and medical device industries. The company provides a broad range of contract services to speed the process from development to peak sales of a new drug or medical device. Quintiles operates in three primary business segments: the product development group, the commercialization group and the PharmaBio development group. The product development group provides a full range of drug development services from strategic planning and preclinical services to regulatory submission and approval. The commercial services group, which operates under the Innovex brand, engages in sales force deployment and strategic marketing services as well as consulting services and training for its customers. The PharmaBio development group works with the other service groups to enter into strategic transactions that it believes will position the company to explore new opportunities and areas for potential growth. PharmaBio also acquires the rights to market pharmaceutical products. In September 2003 Pharma Services Holding, Inc. was created for the purpose of taking Quintiles private. Pharma Services currently owns all of Quintiles' common stock.

Quintiles Transnational offers its employees a comprehensive benefits package including on-the-job training, recreational activities and community support activities.

FINANCIALS:
Sales and profits are in thousands of dollars—add 000 to get the full amount. Year 2004 note: Complete fiscal 2004 results were not available for all companies at press time. For this company, year 2004 is for __ months.

2004 Sales: $ (months)	2004 Profits: $ (months)
2003 Sales: $2,046,000	2003 Profits: $297,000
2002 Sales: $1,992,400	2002 Profits: $127,400
2001 Sales: $1,619,900	2001 Profits: $-33,900
2000 Sales: $1,659,900	2000 Profits: $418,900

Stock Ticker: Private
Employees: 15,991
Fiscal Year Ends: 12/31

SALARIES/BENEFITS:
Pension Plan: ESOP Stock Plan: Profit Sharing: Top Exec. Salary: $706,061   Bonus: $825,000
Savings Plan: Y   Stock Purch. Plan: Second Exec. Salary: $471,224   Bonus: $709,000

OTHER THOUGHTS:
Apparent Top Female Officers:
Hot Spot for Advancement for Women/Minorities:

LOCATIONS: ("Y" = Yes)
West:	Southwest:	Midwest:	Southeast:	Northeast:	International:
Y	Y	Y	Y	Y	Y

QUOVADX INC

Industry Group Code: 511200 **Ranks within this company's industry group:** Sales: 7 Profits: 11

www.quovadx.com

Insurance/HMO/PPO:	Drugs:	Equipment/Supplies:	Hospitals/Clinics:	Services:	Health Care:
Insurance: Managed Care: Utilization Mgmt.: Payment Proc.:	Manufacturer: Distributor: Specialty Pharm.: Vitamins/Nutri.: Clinical Trials:	Manufacturer: Distributor: Leasing/Finance: Information Sys.: Y	Acute Care: Sub-Acute Care: Outpatient Surgery: Phys. Rehab. Center: Psychiatric Clinics:	Diagnostics: Labs/Testing: Staffing: Waste Disposal: Specialty Services:	Home Health: Long-Term Care: Physical Therapy: Phys. Practice Mgmt.:

TYPES OF BUSINESS:
Health Care Information Management Software
Customer Relationship Management Software
Consulting Services

BRANDS/DIVISIONS/AFFILIATES:
QDX Platform V
Rogue Wave C++
Adaptive Applications
QDX Cash Accelerator
QDX Quick Trials
QDX Enterprise Data Exchange
QDX Care Management System
QDX Phoenix Solution Sourcing

CONTACTS:
Note: Officers with more than one job title may be intentionally listed here more than once.

Harvey A. Wagner, CEO
Harvey A. Wagner, Pres.
Melvin L. Keating, Acting CFO
Mark S. Rangell, Sr. VP-Mktg.
Linda Wackwitz, Exec. VP/General Counsel
Thomas H. Zajac, Exec. VP/Pres.-CareScience Div.
Ronald A. Paulus, Chief Health Care Officer
Afshin Cangarlu, Exec. VP/Pres.-Integration Solutions Div.
Cory Isaacson, Exec. VP/Pres.-Rogue Wave Software Div.
Jeffrey M. Krauss, Chmn.

Phone: 303-488-2019 **Fax:** 303-488-9738
Toll-Free:
Address: 6400 S. Fiddler's Green Cir., Ste. 1000, Englewood, CO 80111 US

GROWTH PLANS/SPECIAL FEATURES:
Quovadx, Inc. provides software and services, including an integrated suite of application development tools and vertical enterprise applications for companies in health care, financial services, software, telecommunications, public sector, manufacturing and life sciences. The company has compiled a set of strategic software tools based on eXtensible Markup Language (XML) technology. QDX Platform V, its integrated software tool suite, allows customers to leverage processes and data in existing legacy applications and databases while they develop new composite applications. It contains application development tools, business process management tools and integration tools. Quovadx also offers the Rogue Wave C++ toolkit, which offers multiplatform support, support for distributed applications, enterprise scalability and easy customization. The company's Adaptive Applications, built on QDX Platform V, serve the health care industry with the QDX Cash Accelerator, QDX Enterprise Data Exchange, QDX Care Management System, QDX Phoenix Solution Sourcing, QDX Medical Management, QUOVADX Life Sciences Adaptive Framework and QDX Quick Trials. These applications facilitate payment, information exchange and clinical trials and reduce medical errors. In addition, Quovadx adds extensive professional service capabilities, including consulting, implementation, hosting, transaction services and operations management. The company's products and services are used by over 20,000 organizations worldwide.

FINANCIALS:
Sales and profits are in thousands of dollars—add 000 to get the full amount. Year 2004 note: Complete fiscal 2004 results were not available for all companies at press time. For this company, year 2004 is for 9 months.

2004 Sales: $66,231 (9 months)   2004 Profits: $-22,286 (9 months)
2003 Sales: $71,595   2003 Profits: $-14,694
2002 Sales: $63,700   2002 Profits: $-104,100
2001 Sales: $51,400   2001 Profits: $-4,300
2000 Sales: $10,681   2000 Profits: $-17,317

Stock Ticker: QVDX
Employees: 628
Fiscal Year Ends: 12/31

SALARIES/BENEFITS:
Pension Plan: ESOP Stock Plan: Profit Sharing: Top Exec. Salary: $374,808   Bonus: $125,000
Savings Plan: Y   Stock Purch. Plan: Y   Second Exec. Salary: $262,404   Bonus: $100,000

OTHER THOUGHTS:
Apparent Top Female Officers: 1
Hot Spot for Advancement for Women/Minorities:

LOCATIONS: ("Y" = Yes)

West:	Southwest:	Midwest:	Southeast:	Northeast:	International:
Y	Y		Y	Y	Y

RADIOLOGIX INC

www.radiologix.com

Industry Group Code: 621511 Ranks within this company's industry group: Sales: 6 Profits: 8

Insurance/HMO/PPO:	Drugs:	Equipment/Supplies:	Hospitals/Clinics:	Services:		Health Care:	
Insurance: Managed Care: Utilization Mgmt.: Payment Proc.:	Manufacturer: Distributor: Specialty Pharm.: Vitamins/Nutri.: Clinical Trials:	Manufacturer: Distributor: Leasing/Finance: Information Sys.:	Acute Care: Sub-Acute Care: Outpatient Surgery: Phys. Rehab. Center: Psychiatric Clinics:	Diagnostics: Labs/Testing: Staffing: Waste Disposal: Specialty Services:	Y	Home Health: Long-Term Care: Physical Therapy: Phys. Practice Mgmt.:	

TYPES OF BUSINESS:
Diagnostic Imaging Center Management

BRANDS/DIVISIONS/AFFILIATES:

CONTACTS:
Note: Officers with more than one job title may be intentionally listed here more than once.

Marvin S. Cadwell, Interim CEO
Marvin S. Cadwell, Interim Pres.
Sami S. Abbasi, Exec. VP/COO
Richard J. Sabolik, Sr. VP/CFO
Michael L. Silhol, Sr. VP/General Counsel
Marvin S. Cadwell, Chmn.

Phone: 214-303-2776 Fax: 214-303-2777
Toll-Free:
Address: 3600 JP Morgan Chase Tower, 2200 Ross Ave., Dallas, TX 75201 US

GROWTH PLANS/SPECIAL FEATURES:
Radiologix, Inc. is a leading national provider of diagnostic imaging services through its ownership and operation of freestanding, outpatient diagnostic imaging centers. The firm utilizes sophisticated technology and technical expertise to perform a broad range of imaging procedures, including MRI, computed tomography, positron emission tomography (PET), nuclear medicine, ultrasound, mammography, bone density (DEXA), x-ray and fluoroscopy. Radiologix operates 107 diagnostic imaging centers located in 15 states, with a concentration in markets located in Maryland, California, New York and Texas. The centers' 514 diagnostic units perform approximately 1.6 million imaging procedures per year. The firm also provides administrative, management and information services to certain radiology practices that provide professional services in connection with its diagnostic imaging centers and to hospitals and radiology practices with which it operates joint ventures. Referrals for diagnostic imaging services at Radiologix's centers primarily come from primary care physicians and specialists, with payment coming from commercial third parties, government agencies such as Medicare and Medicaid, private individuals and organizations.

Radiologix offers its employees benefits including health, dental and vision coverage, a prescription drug program, an employee assistance program and tuition reimbursement.

FINANCIALS:
Sales and profits are in thousands of dollars—add 000 to get the full amount. Year 2004 note: Complete fiscal 2004 results were not available for all companies at press time. For this company, year 2004 is for 9 months.

2004 Sales: $199,224 (9 months)   2004 Profits: $-10,203 (9 months)
2003 Sales: $257,014   2003 Profits: $-7,963
2002 Sales: $283,900   2002 Profits: $10,800
2001 Sales: $276,700   2001 Profits: $13,900
2000 Sales: $246,700   2000 Profits: $4,300

Stock Ticker: RGX
Employees: 2,500
Fiscal Year Ends: 12/31

SALARIES/BENEFITS:
Pension Plan: ESOP Stock Plan: Profit Sharing: Top Exec. Salary: $375,692   Bonus: $100,000
Savings Plan: Y   Stock Purch. Plan: Second Exec. Salary: $314,500   Bonus: $75,000

OTHER THOUGHTS:
Apparent Top Female Officers:
Hot Spot for Advancement for Women/Minorities:

LOCATIONS: ("Y" = Yes)
West:	Southwest:	Midwest:	Southeast:	Northeast:	International:
Y	Y	Y	Y	Y	

REGENCE GROUP (THE)

www.regence.com

Industry Group Code: 524114 Ranks within this company's industry group: Sales: 16 Profits:

Insurance/HMO/PPO:	Drugs:	Equipment/Supplies:	Hospitals/Clinics:	Services:	Health Care:
Insurance: Y	Manufacturer:	Manufacturer:	Acute Care:	Diagnostics:	Home Health:
Managed Care:	Distributor:	Distributor:	Sub-Acute Care:	Labs/Testing:	Long-Term Care:
Utilization Mgmt.:	Specialty Pharm.:	Leasing/Finance:	Outpatient Surgery:	Staffing:	Physical Therapy:
Payment Proc.:	Vitamins/Nutri.:	Information Sys.:	Phys. Rehab. Center:	Waste Disposal:	Phys. Practice Mgmt.:
	Clinical Trials:		Psychiatric Clinics:	Specialty Services:	

TYPES OF BUSINESS:
Health Insurance
Life Insurance

BRANDS/DIVISIONS/AFFILIATES:
Regence BlueShield of Idaho
Regence BlueCross BlueShield of Oregon
Regence BlueCross BlueShield of Utah
Regence BlueShield of Washington
Regence Life & Health Insurance

CONTACTS: Note: Officers with more than one job title may be intentionally listed here more than once.
Mark Ganz, Pres.
Steve Hooker, CFO
Mohan Niar, Chief Mktg. Officer
Tom Kennedy, VP-Human Resources
Cheron Vail, CIO
Kerry Barnett, Chief Legal Officer
Kerry Barnett, VP-Corp. Comm.
Dan Mallea, Controller
Jeff Robertson, Exec. VP-Health Care Services
Steven Gaspar, Chief Actuarial Officer

Phone: 503-225-5221 Fax: 503-225-5274
Toll-Free:
Address: 200 SW Market St., Portland, OR 97201 US

GROWTH PLANS/SPECIAL FEATURES:
The Regence Group Plans, the largest group of Blue Cross Blue Shield companies in the northwestern United States, provides health insurance and related services in Idaho, Oregon, Utah and Washington. The firm offers multiple health insurance policies, which cover a variety of medical and dental emergencies and routine visits. The company's main insurance subsidiaries are Regence BlueShield of Idaho, Regence BlueCross BlueShield of Oregon, Regence BlueCross BlueShield of Utah and Regence BlueShield of Washington. The four companies work interchangeably, offering coverage for customers across state lines. All together, the firm provides health insurance coverage to nearly 3 million people, with more than $6.5 billion in revenue. The company also provides life, disability and short-term medical insurance through its Regence Life & Health Insurance subsidiary.

Regence employees are given their choice of medical, dental and life insurance plans, legal and financial assistance, pre-tax commute reimbursement accounts, on-site fitness centers, child care and credit union access.

FINANCIALS: Sales and profits are in thousands of dollars—add 000 to get the full amount. Year 2004 note: Complete fiscal 2004 results were not available for all companies at press time. For this company, year 2004 is for months.

2004 Sales: $ (months) 2004 Profits: $ (months)
2003 Sales: $6,700,000 2003 Profits: $
2002 Sales: $6,250,100 2002 Profits: $
2001 Sales: $ 2001 Profits: $
2000 Sales: $ 2000 Profits: $

Stock Ticker: Private
Employees: 6,000
Fiscal Year Ends: 12/31

SALARIES/BENEFITS:
Pension Plan: ESOP Stock Plan: Profit Sharing: Top Exec. Salary: $ Bonus: $
Savings Plan: Y Stock Purch. Plan: Second Exec. Salary: $ Bonus: $

OTHER THOUGHTS:
Apparent Top Female Officers: 2
Hot Spot for Advancement for Women/Minorities:

LOCATIONS: ("Y" = Yes)
West	Southwest	Midwest	Southeast	Northeast	International
Y					

REGENT ASSISTED LIVING INC

www.regentassistedliving.com

Industry Group Code: 623110 Ranks within this company's industry group: Sales: 14 Profits:

Insurance/HMO/PPO:	Drugs:	Equipment/Supplies:	Hospitals/Clinics:	Services:	Health Care:
Insurance:	Manufacturer:	Manufacturer:	Acute Care:	Diagnostics:	Home Health:
Managed Care:	Distributor:	Distributor:	Sub-Acute Care:	Labs/Testing:	Long-Term Care: Y
Utilization Mgmt.:	Specialty Pharm.:	Leasing/Finance:	Outpatient Surgery:	Staffing:	Physical Therapy:
Payment Proc.:	Vitamins/Nutri.:	Information Sys.:	Phys. Rehab. Center:	Waste Disposal:	Phys. Practice Mgmt.:
	Clinical Trials:		Psychiatric Clinics:	Specialty Services:	

TYPES OF BUSINESS:
Long-Term Health Care/Assisted Living Communities

BRANDS/DIVISIONS/AFFILIATES:

CONTACTS:
Note: Officers with more than one job title may be intentionally listed here more than once.

Walter C. Bowen, CEO
Walter C. Bowen, Pres.
Steven L. Gish, CFO
Steven L. Gish, Treas.
Walter C. Bowen, Chmn.

Phone: 503-227-4000 Fax: 503-274-4685
Toll-Free: 888-853-7468
Address: 121 SW Morrison St., Ste. 1000, Portland, OR 97204 US

GROWTH PLANS/SPECIAL FEATURES:

Regent Assisted Living, Inc. owns and operates nine assisted living communities across the West and Southwest: one each in Arizona, Utah, Idaho and Washington, two in California and three in Oregon. Assisted living services are part of a spectrum of long-term care services that include a combination of housing, personal services such as meals, laundry, housekeeping and transportation and health care, including Alzheimer's care, for elderly individuals requiring assistance with the activities of daily living. Assistance with banking, shopping and pet care is also available. The company's growth strategy has been based upon the premise that high-quality assisted living services can be more appropriately and efficiently provided in its prototypical-designed communities rather than in an existing facility that could be converted for use. However, in recent years Regent Assistant Living has undergone considerable reductions. After a massive expansion from its IPO in 1995, when it operated four communities with a total of 565 beds, to 2000, when it had grown to a peak of 30 communities with 2,996 beds, the company has incurred unforeseen operating costs, problems in obtaining licenses and difficulty in maintaining occupancy. These have all contributed to the company's downsizing of its workforce, sale of some its property and leasing out of many of its management functions to other assisted living companies, particularly Emeritus Corporation.

FINANCIALS:
Sales and profits are in thousands of dollars—add 000 to get the full amount. Year 2004 note: Complete fiscal 2004 results were not available for all companies at press time. For this company, year 2004 is for months.

2004 Sales: $ (months)   2004 Profits: $ (months)
2003 Sales: $19,100   2003 Profits: $
2002 Sales: $ 2002 Profits: $
2001 Sales: $64,000   2001 Profits: $-1,300
2000 Sales: $64,909   2000 Profits: $-6,466

Stock Ticker: RGNT.PK
Employees: 900
Fiscal Year Ends: 12/31

SALARIES/BENEFITS:

| Pension Plan: | ESOP Stock Plan: | Profit Sharing: | Top Exec. Salary: $150,000 | Bonus: $ |
| Savings Plan: Y | Stock Purch. Plan: | | Second Exec. Salary: $133,750 | Bonus: $ |

OTHER THOUGHTS:
Apparent Top Female Officers:
Hot Spot for Advancement for Women/Minorities:

LOCATIONS: ("Y" = Yes)

West:	Southwest:	Midwest:	Southeast:	Northeast:	International:
Y	Y				

REHABCARE GROUP INC

www.rehabcare.com

Industry Group Code: 621340 Ranks within this company's industry group: Sales: 2 Profits: 3

Insurance/HMO/PPO:	Drugs:	Equipment/Supplies:	Hospitals/Clinics:		Services:		Health Care:	
Insurance:	Manufacturer:	Manufacturer:	Acute Care:		Diagnostics:		Home Health:	
Managed Care:	Distributor:	Distributor:	Sub-Acute Care:	Y	Labs/Testing:		Long-Term Care:	
Utilization Mgmt.:	Specialty Pharm.:	Leasing/Finance:	Outpatient Surgery:		Staffing:	Y	Physical Therapy:	
Payment Proc.:	Vitamins/Nutri.:	Information Sys.:	Phys. Rehab. Center:	Y	Waste Disposal:		Phys. Practice Mgmt.:	
	Clinical Trials:		Psychiatric Clinics:		Specialty Services:			

TYPES OF BUSINESS:
Contract Rehabilitation Services
Acute Care Facilities
Skilled Nursing Services
Outpatient Therapy Programs
Staffing Services

BRANDS/DIVISIONS/AFFILIATES:
Healthcare Staffing Solutions, Inc.
DiversiCare Rehab Services
StarMed Staffing, Inc.
Rehabilitative Care Systems of America
Therapeutic Systems, Ltd.
AllStaff, Inc.

CONTACTS:
Note: Officers with more than one job title may be intentionally listed here more than once.

John H. Short, CEO
John H. Short, Pres.
Vincent L. Germanese, CFO
Patricia K. Fish, Sr. VP-Human Resources
Betty Cammarata, VP-Investor Rel.
Vincent L. Germanese, Corp. Sec.
H. Edwin Trusheim, Chmn.

Phone: 314-863-7422 Fax: 314-863-0769
Toll-Free: 800-677-1238
Address: 7733 Forsyth Blvd., 17th Fl., St. Louis, MO 63105 US

GROWTH PLANS/SPECIAL FEATURES:

RehabCare Group, Inc. provides comprehensive medical rehabilitation, sub-acute and outpatient therapy programs on a multi-year contract basis. The company also provides therapists to hospitals and long-term care and rehabilitation facilities on both an interim and permanent basis. These health care staffing services enable clients to manage fixed labor costs, turnover and other temporary staffing needs. The firm uses its expertise and experience to provide its clients with efficient, cost-effective rehabilitation services in whatever setting is most economically feasible. At the same time, RehabCare focuses on establishing long-term relationships with its clients. Historically, the company has sought to broaden its service offerings through both internal growth and strategic acquisitions. Key acquisitions include DiversiCare Rehab Services, Healthcare Staffing Solutions, Inc., AllStaff, Inc., StarMed Staffing, Inc., Therapeutic Systems, Ltd. and Rehabilitative Care Systems of America. The firm has experienced major success in increasing the renewal rate for its unit contracts, which increases stability and earnings. RehabCare believes that the introduction of a prospective payment system for skilled nursing facilities has increased demand for its management systems and expertise, particularly with regard to controlling costs.

RehabCare Group offers its employees dental, vision and life insurance, as well as continuing education assistance. The company offers several programs for tuition and school loan assistance.

FINANCIALS:
Sales and profits are in thousands of dollars—add 000 to get the full amount. Year 2004 note: Complete fiscal 2004 results were not available for all companies at press time. For this company, year 2004 is for 9 months.

2004 Sales: $288,718 (9 months)   2004 Profits: $16,884 (9 months)
2003 Sales: $539,322   2003 Profits: $-13,699
2002 Sales: $562,600   2002 Profits: $24,400
2001 Sales: $542,300   2001 Profits: $21,000
2000 Sales: $452,400   2000 Profits: $23,500

Stock Ticker: RHB
Employees: 13,100
Fiscal Year Ends: 12/31

SALARIES/BENEFITS:

Pension Plan: ESOP Stock Plan: Profit Sharing: Top Exec. Salary: $281,667   Bonus: $24,959
Savings Plan: Y   Stock Purch. Plan: Second Exec. Salary: $263,457   Bonus: $75,000

OTHER THOUGHTS:
Apparent Top Female Officers: 2
Hot Spot for Advancement for Women/Minorities:

LOCATIONS: ("Y" = Yes)

West:	Southwest:	Midwest:	Southeast:	Northeast:	International:
Y	Y	Y	Y	Y	

RENAL CARE GROUP INC

www.renalcaregroup.com

Industry Group Code: 621490 Ranks within this company's industry group: Sales: 4 Profits: 4

Insurance/HMO/PPO:	Drugs:	Equipment/Supplies:	Hospitals/Clinics:	Services:	Health Care:
Insurance:	Manufacturer:	Manufacturer:	Acute Care:	Diagnostics:	Home Health:
Managed Care:	Distributor:	Distributor:	Sub-Acute Care: Y	Labs/Testing:	Long-Term Care:
Utilization Mgmt.:	Specialty Pharm.:	Leasing/Finance:	Outpatient Surgery:	Staffing:	Physical Therapy:
Payment Proc.:	Vitamins/Nutri.:	Information Sys.:	Phys. Rehab. Center:	Waste Disposal:	Phys. Practice Mgmt.:
	Clinical Trials:		Psychiatric Clinics:	Specialty Services: Y	

TYPES OF BUSINESS:
Kidney Dialysis Centers
Nephrology Services
Dialysis Care Staffing/Leasing

BRANDS/DIVISIONS/AFFILIATES:

CONTACTS: Note: Officers with more than one job title may be intentionally listed here more than once.
Gary A. Brukardt, CEO
Gary A. Brukardt, Pres.
Timothy J. Balch, COO
R. Dirk Allison, Exec. VP/CFO
John Anderson, VP-Human Resources
David M. Maloney, Sr. VP/CIO
Harlan Cleaver, Chief Tech. Officer
John Anderson, VP-Admin.
Douglas B. Chappell, General Counsel
Carolyn E. Latham, VP-Clinical Oper.
Robert Stillwell, Sr. VP-Strategic Dev.
LeAnne Zumwalt, VP-Investor Rel.
R. Dirk Allison, Treas.
Joe McLellan, VP-Mergers & Acquisitions
Christi Griffin, VP/Asst. General Counsel
Dawn Sharp, Compliance Officer
Rebecca Wingard, VP-Quality
William P. Johnston, Chmn.

Phone: 615-345-5500 **Fax:** 615-345-5505
Toll-Free:
Address: 2100 W. End Ave., Ste. 800, Nashville, TN 37203 US

GROWTH PLANS/SPECIAL FEATURES:
Renal Care Group, Inc. (RCG) provides dialysis services to patients with chronic kidney failure, also known as end-stage renal disease (ESRD). The company has provided dialysis and ancillary services to over 21,000 patients through 390 outpatient dialysis centers in 30 states, in addition to providing acute dialysis services to more than 190 hospitals. In RCG's technologically advanced outpatient dialysis facilities ESRD patients receive treatments, generally three times per week. The firm's centers typically consist of 10 to 30 dialysis stations, a nurses' station, a patient waiting area, examination rooms, a supply room, a water treatment space, a dialyzer reprocessing room and staff work areas, offices and a lounge. Many centers also have areas for training patients in home dialysis, and some provide inpatient dialysis services to hospitals in their service areas. RCG provides equipment, supplies and personnel to perform hemodialysis and peritoneal dialysis, usually required for patients with acute renal failure resulting from accidents and medical and surgical complications. Additionally, RCG manages the dialysis programs at Vanderbilt University Medical Center and is the owner or managing partner at various other programs, including St. Louis University Hospital, Northwestern Memorial Hospital of Chicago and the Cleveland Clinic Foundation. The firm's presence in Pennsylvania includes the dialysis program of Delaware Valley Nephrology in Philadelphia, Pennsylvania.

FINANCIALS:
Sales and profits are in thousands of dollars—add 000 to get the full amount. Year 2004 note: Complete fiscal 2004 results were not available for all companies at press time. For this company, year 2004 is for 9 months.

2004 Sales: $743,039 (9 months)	2004 Profits: $74,110 (9 months)	**Stock Ticker: RCI**
2003 Sales: $1,105,319	2003 Profits: $102,056	Employees: 6,749
2002 Sales: $903,400	2002 Profits: $92,500	Fiscal Year Ends: 12/31
2001 Sales: $755,100	2001 Profits: $76,600	
2000 Sales: $622,600	2000 Profits: $51,500	

SALARIES/BENEFITS:
Pension Plan:	ESOP Stock Plan:	Profit Sharing:	Top Exec. Salary: $501,000	Bonus: $461,250
Savings Plan: Y	Stock Purch. Plan: Y		Second Exec. Salary: $389,231	Bonus: $433,000

OTHER THOUGHTS:
Apparent Top Female Officers: 5
Hot Spot for Advancement for Women/Minorities: Y

LOCATIONS: ("Y" = Yes)
West:	Southwest:	Midwest:	Southeast:	Northeast:	International:
Y	Y	Y	Y	Y	

Note: Financial information, benefits and other data can change quickly and may vary from those stated here.

RES CARE INC

www.rescare.com

Industry Group Code: 622210   Ranks within this company's industry group: Sales: 2 Profits: 2

Insurance/HMO/PPO:	Drugs:	Equipment/Supplies:	Hospitals/Clinics:	Services:	Health Care:
Insurance:	Manufacturer:	Manufacturer:	Acute Care:	Diagnostics:	Home Health: Y
Managed Care:	Distributor:	Distributor:	Sub-Acute Care:	Labs/Testing:	Long-Term Care: Y
Utilization Mgmt.:	Specialty Pharm.:	Leasing/Finance:	Outpatient Surgery:	Staffing:	Physical Therapy: Y
Payment Proc.:	Vitamins/Nutri.:	Information Sys.:	Phys. Rehab. Center:	Waste Disposal:	Phys. Practice Mgmt.:
	Clinical Trials:		Psychiatric Clinics:	Specialty Services: Y	

TYPES OF BUSINESS:
Clinics-Psychiatric
Developmental Disabilities Support Services
Youth Services
Residential Treatment Programs
Technical Consultation & Training

BRANDS/DIVISIONS/AFFILIATES:
ResCare Premier
Citadel Group (The)
Alternative Youth Services
Youthtrack
ResCare Training Technologies

CONTACTS:
Note: Officers with more than one job title may be intentionally listed here more than once.

Ronald G. Geary, CEO
Ronald G. Geary, Pres.
L. Bryan Shaul, CFO
Nina P. Seigle, Chief People Officer
L. Bryan Shaul, Exec. VP-Admin.
David S. Waskey, General Counsel
Paul G. Dunn, Chief Dev. Officer
Nel Taylor, Chief Comm. Officer
Kelley Abell, Chief Gov't Rel. Officer
William J Ballard, Pres.-Youth Services
Ralph G. Gronefeld, Jr., Pres.-Persons with Disabilities Div.
Vincent F. Doran, Pres.-Training Services Div.
Katherine W. Gilchrist, VP-Persons with Disabilities Div.
Ronald G. Geary, Chmn.

Phone: 502-394-2100   **Fax:** 502-394-2206
Toll-Free:
Address: 10140 Linn Station Rd., Louisville, KY 40223 US

GROWTH PLANS/SPECIAL FEATURES:
ResCare, Inc. provides residential, training, educational and support services to people with disabilities and youth with special needs. The company offers in-home services, supported living, group homes, large facilities and vocational day programs for people with developmental disabilities such as mental retardation, mental illness and acquired brain injuries. ResCare serves more than 28,900 disabled adults and children in 32 states, Washington, D.C., Canada and Puerto Rico. The division for youth services offers educational and treatment programs for adolescents who can no longer live in their homes through its Alternative Youth Services units and its contract with the federal Job Corps program. The company's Youthtrack program offers secure and non-secure residential treatment programs for pre-adjudicated and adjudicated delinquent youth up to age 18. ResCare Premier, a segment of ResCare, facilitates the transition from medically based treatment settings to a rehabilitative lifestyle for people with acquired brain injury. The Citadel Group, a ResCare subsidiary, provides for people with chronic and severe mental illness through community-oriented programs. ResCare Training Technologies provides training, consultation and technical assistance to organizations that offer support and services to people with disabilities.

FINANCIALS:
Sales and profits are in thousands of dollars—add 000 to get the full amount. Year 2004 note: Complete fiscal 2004 results were not available for all companies at press time. For this company, year 2004 is for 9 months.

2004 Sales: $751,511 (9 months)	2004 Profits: $14,602 (9 months)	**Stock Ticker:** RSCR
2003 Sales: $961,333	2003 Profits: $13,387	Employees: 29,000
2002 Sales: $919,700	2002 Profits: $2,700	Fiscal Year Ends: 12/31
2001 Sales: $895,200	2001 Profits: $-4,400	
2000 Sales: $865,800	2000 Profits: $14,200	

SALARIES/BENEFITS:
Pension Plan: ESOP Stock Plan: Profit Sharing: Top Exec. Salary: $364,948   Bonus: $133,174
Savings Plan: Y   Stock Purch. Plan: Second Exec. Salary: $283,064   Bonus: $

OTHER THOUGHTS:
Apparent Top Female Officers: 4
Hot Spot for Advancement for Women/Minorities: Y

LOCATIONS: ("Y" = Yes)
West:	Southwest:	Midwest:	Southeast:	Northeast:	International:
Y	Y	Y	Y	Y	Y

RESMED INC

www.resmed.com

Industry Group Code: 339113   **Ranks within this company's industry group:** Sales: 57   Profits: 37

Insurance/HMO/PPO:	Drugs:	Equipment/Supplies:		Hospitals/Clinics:	Services:	Health Care:
Insurance:	Manufacturer:	Manufacturer:	Y	Acute Care:	Diagnostics:	Home Health:
Managed Care:	Distributor:	Distributor:	Y	Sub-Acute Care:	Labs/Testing:	Long-Term Care:
Utilization Mgmt.:	Specialty Pharm.:	Leasing/Finance:		Outpatient Surgery:	Staffing:	Physical Therapy:
Payment Proc.:	Vitamins/Nutri.:	Information Sys.:		Phys. Rehab. Center:	Waste Disposal:	Phys. Practice Mgmt.:
	Clinical Trials:			Psychiatric Clinics:	Specialty Services:	

TYPES OF BUSINESS:
Supplies-Flow Generators (Sleep Disordered Breathing)
Diagnostic Products

BRANDS/DIVISIONS/AFFILIATES:
Comfort
Mirage
ResControl

CONTACTS:
Note: Officers with more than one job title may be intentionally listed here more than once.

Peter C. Farrell, CEO
Adrian M. Smith, CFO
Keith Serzen, VP-Mktg. & Sales
Connie Garett, VP-Global Human Resources
Curt Kenyon, Sr. VP-Telemedicine & Informatics
David Pendarvis, General Counsel
Elliott Glick, VP-Oper., U.S.
Deirdre Stewart, VP-Strategic Clinical Initiatives
Adrian M. Smith, Sr. VP-Finance
Kieran T. Gallahue, Pres./COO-Americas
Walter Flicker, Corp. Sec.
Dana Voien, VP-Telemedicine & Channel Mgmt.
Ann Tisthammer, VP-Clinical Education & Training
Peter C. Farrell, Chmn.

Phone: 858-746-2400   **Fax:** 858-880-1618
Toll-Free: 800-424-0737
Address: 14040 Danielson St., Poway, CA 92064-6857 US

GROWTH PLANS/SPECIAL FEATURES:
ResMed, Inc. is a leading developer, manufacturer and distributor of medical equipment for treating, diagnosing and managing sleep disordered breathing, or SDB. SDB includes obstructive sleep apnea (OSA) and other related respiratory disorders that occur during sleep. The company was originally founded to commercialize a Continuous Positive Airway Pressure (CPAP) treatment for OSA, which was the first successful noninvasive treatment for the disorder. CPAP systems deliver pressurized air, typically through a nasal mask, to prevent collapse of the upper airway during sleep. Since the introduction of nasal CPAP, the company has developed a number of innovative products for SDB, including Comfort flow generators, ResControl diagnostic products, Mirage mask systems, headgear and other accessories. ResMed's growth has been fueled by a productive research and development effort, geographic expansion and increased awareness of SDB as a significant health concern. The company's business strategy includes expanding into new clinical applications by seeking to identify new uses for its technologies. Studies have established a link between OSA and stroke and congestive heart failure (CHF), and ResMed is in the process of developing a device for the treatment of Cheyne-Stokes breathing in CHF patients.

FINANCIALS:
Sales and profits are in thousands of dollars—add 000 to get the full amount. Year 2004 note: Complete fiscal 2004 results were not available for all companies at press time. For this company, year 2004 is for 12 months.

2004 Sales: $339,338 (12 months)	2004 Profits: $57,284 (12 months)	**Stock Ticker:** RMD
2003 Sales: $273,600	2003 Profits: $45,700	**Employees:** 1,520
2002 Sales: $204,100	2002 Profits: $37,500	**Fiscal Year Ends:** 6/30
2001 Sales: $155,200	2001 Profits: $11,600	
2000 Sales: $115,600	2000 Profits: $22,200	

SALARIES/BENEFITS:
Pension Plan: Y   ESOP Stock Plan: Profit Sharing: Top Exec. Salary: $413,125   Bonus: $273,534
Savings Plan: Stock Purch. Plan: Second Exec. Salary: $300,000   Bonus: $155,726

OTHER THOUGHTS:
Apparent Top Female Officers: 4
Hot Spot for Advancement for Women/Minorities: Y

LOCATIONS: ("Y" = Yes)
West:	Southwest:	Midwest:	Southeast:	Northeast:	International:
Y					Y

RESPIRONICS INC

www.respironics.com

Industry Group Code: 339113 **Ranks within this company's industry group:** Sales: 34 Profits: 35

Insurance/HMO/PPO:	Drugs:	Equipment/Supplies:		Hospitals/Clinics:	Services:	Health Care:
Insurance: Managed Care: Utilization Mgmt.: Payment Proc.:	Manufacturer: Distributor: Specialty Pharm.: Vitamins/Nutri.: Clinical Trials:	Manufacturer: Distributor: Leasing/Finance: Information Sys.:	Y	Acute Care: Sub-Acute Care: Outpatient Surgery: Phys. Rehab. Center: Psychiatric Clinics:	Diagnostics: Labs/Testing: Staffing: Waste Disposal: Specialty Services:	Home Health: Long-Term Care: Physical Therapy: Phys. Practice Mgmt.:

TYPES OF BUSINESS:
Equipment/Supplies-Respiratory Devices

BRANDS/DIVISIONS/AFFILIATES:
Power Programs for Managing Diseases
Western Biomedical Technologies
Profile Therapeutics plc

CONTACTS:
Note: Officers with more than one job title may be intentionally listed here more than once.

John Miclot, CEO
John Miclot, Pres.
Craig B. Reynolds, Exec. VP/COO
Daniel J. Bevevino, VP/CFO
Susan A. Lloyd, VP-Respiratory Drug Delivery Div.
Paul L. Woodring, Pres.-Hospital Div.
William Post, Pres.-Home Care Div.
Gerald E. McGinnis, Chmn.
Geoffrey C. Waters, Pres.-Int'l Div.

Phone: 724-387-5200   **Fax:**
Toll-Free: 800-345-6443
Address: 1010 Murry Ridge Ln., Murrysville, PA 15668 US

GROWTH PLANS/SPECIAL FEATURES:

Respironics, Inc. is a leading developer, manufacturer and marketer of medical devices that are used for the treatment of patients suffering from sleep and respiratory disorders. The company's home care products include sleep apnea products, including continuous positive airway pressure devices and bi-level positive airway pressure devices; bi-level non-invasive ventilation products that provide positive airway pressure to supplement the patient's own breathing; invasive portable volume ventilation products; oxygen products including oxygen concentrators and oximeters; and infant management and developmental care products. Its hospital products include non-invasive and invasive therapeutic devices that assist or control a patient's ventilation, cardio-respiratory monitoring products that provide information about a patient's condition and respiratory drug delivery products, including nebulizers, peak flow meters and spacers. Respironics sells and occasionally rents its products primarily to home medical equipment service providers and hospital distributors, who in turn resell and rent them to end-users. The company's marketing strategy includes the Power Programs for Managing Diseases, designed to provide home care providers, physicians, hospitals and sub-acute facilities with technical support, training, educational tools and products. The Power Programs are focused on sleep management, chronic respiratory management, total ventilation solutions, respiratory drug delivery and neonatal and infant care. In 2004, the firm acquired Western Biomedical Technologies and Profile Therapeutics plc, expanding its presence in the global sleep and respiratory markets.

The company compensates its employees with medical and dental benefits, wellness programs, fitness centers, educational reimbursement, awards and access to a credit union. Some employees have the option to telecommute from home.

FINANCIALS:
Sales and profits are in thousands of dollars—add 000 to get the full amount. Year 2004 note: Complete fiscal 2004 results were not available for all companies at press time. For this company, year 2004 is for 12 months.

2004 Sales: $759,550 (12 months)   2004 Profits: $65,020 (12 months)
2003 Sales: $629,800   2003 Profits: $46,600
2002 Sales: $494,900   2002 Profits: $38,400
2001 Sales: $422,400   2001 Profits: $33,600
2000 Sales: $368,200   2000 Profits: $5,800

Stock Ticker: RESP
Employees: 3,000
Fiscal Year Ends: 6/30

SALARIES/BENEFITS:
Pension Plan: ESOP Stock Plan: Profit Sharing: Y   Top Exec. Salary: $600,000   Bonus: $456,800
Savings Plan: Y   Stock Purch. Plan: Y   Second Exec. Salary: $430,769   Bonus: $315,478

OTHER THOUGHTS:
Apparent Top Female Officers: 1
Hot Spot for Advancement for Women/Minorities:

LOCATIONS: ("Y" = Yes)

West:	Southwest:	Midwest:	Southeast:	Northeast:	International:
Y	Y		Y	Y	Y

RITA MEDICAL SYSTEMS INC

www.ritamedical.com

Industry Group Code: 339113 Ranks within this company's industry group: Sales: 133 Profits: 125

Insurance/HMO/PPO:	Drugs:	Equipment/Supplies:		Hospitals/Clinics:	Services:	Health Care:
Insurance:	Manufacturer:	Manufacturer:	Y	Acute Care:	Diagnostics:	Home Health:
Managed Care:	Distributor:	Distributor:	Y	Sub-Acute Care:	Labs/Testing:	Long-Term Care:
Utilization Mgmt.:	Specialty Pharm.:	Leasing/Finance:		Outpatient Surgery:	Staffing:	Physical Therapy:
Payment Proc.:	Vitamins/Nutri.:	Information Sys.:		Phys. Rehab. Center:	Waste Disposal:	Phys. Practice Mgmt.:
	Clinical Trials:			Psychiatric Clinics:	Specialty Services:	

TYPES OF BUSINESS:
Equipment-Implantable Ports & Specialty Catheters
Vascular & Spinal Access Systems
Specialty Device Distribution

BRANDS/DIVISIONS/AFFILIATES:
Horizon Medical Products, Inc.
RITA System

CONTACTS:
Note: Officers with more than one job title may be intentionally listed here more than once.
Joseph M. DeVivo, CEO
Joseph M. DeVivo, Pres.
Donald Stewart, CFO/VP-Finance
Trent Reutiman, VP-U.S. Sales
Darrin Uecker, CTO
Donald Stewart, VP-Admin.
Stephen Pedroff, VP-Mktg. Comm.
Lynn Saccoliti, VP-Reimbursement
Juan J. Soto, VP-Int'l Sales
Marshall B. Hunt, Chmn.

Phone: 650-314-3400   Fax: 650-390-8505
Toll-Free:
Address: 967 N. Shoreline Blvd., Mountain View, CA 94043 US

GROWTH PLANS/SPECIAL FEATURES:
RITA Medical Systems, Inc. develops, manufactures and markets medical products for cancer patients. These products include radio frequency ablation systems for treating malignant tumors and percutaneous vascular and spinal access systems. Other oncology product lines include implantable ports, tunneled central venous catheters and stem-cell transplant catheters for use primarily in cancer treatment protocols. RITA's proprietary tumor treatment system is an electrosurgical delivery method that uses radio frequency waves to heat human tissue to temperatures high enough to kill malignant cells. The RITA System includes radio frequency generators and a family of electrosurgical devices that deliver controlled thermal energy to targeted tissue. The company was the first to receive FDA clearance for the treatment of unresectable liver lesions, as well as the first to receive FDA approval for the palliation of pain associated with metastatic lesions involving bone. In recent news, RITA completed a merger with Horizon Medical Products, Inc., also a provider of medical oncology devices.

RITA offers its full-time employees medical, dental, vision, life and long-term disability insurance, flexible spending accounts and an employee referral bonus. Free snacks, beverages and a health club membership are also offered.

FINANCIALS:
Sales and profits are in thousands of dollars—add 000 to get the full amount. Year 2004 note: Complete fiscal 2004 results were not available for all companies at press time. For this company, year 2004 is for 9 months.

2004 Sales: $17,254 (9 months)   2004 Profits: $-7,431 (9 months)
2003 Sales: $16,607   2003 Profits: $-11,079
2002 Sales: $17,393   2002 Profits: $-13,499
2001 Sales: $ 2001 Profits: $
2000 Sales: $ 2000 Profits: $

Stock Ticker: RITA
Employees: 77
Fiscal Year Ends: 12/31

SALARIES/BENEFITS:
Pension Plan: ESOP Stock Plan: Profit Sharing: Top Exec. Salary: $196,381   Bonus: $27,500
Savings Plan: Y Stock Purch. Plan: Y   Second Exec. Salary: $174,247 Bonus: $539,738

OTHER THOUGHTS:
Apparent Top Female Officers: 1
Hot Spot for Advancement for Women/Minorities:

LOCATIONS: ("Y" = Yes)
West	Southwest	Midwest	Southeast	Northeast	International
Y			Y		

RITE AID CORPORATION

www.riteaid.com

Industry Group Code: 446110   Ranks within this company's industry group: Sales: 3   Profits: 5

Insurance/HMO/PPO:	Drugs:	Equipment/Supplies:	Hospitals/Clinics:	Services:	Health Care:
Insurance:	Manufacturer:	Manufacturer:	Acute Care:	Diagnostics:	Home Health:
Managed Care:	Distributor:	Distributor:	Sub-Acute Care:	Labs/Testing:	Long-Term Care:
Utilization Mgmt.:	Specialty Pharm.: Y	Leasing/Finance:	Outpatient Surgery:	Staffing:	Physical Therapy:
Payment Proc.:	Vitamins/Nutri.:	Information Sys.:	Phys. Rehab. Center:	Waste Disposal:	Phys. Practice Mgmt.:
	Clinical Trials:		Psychiatric Clinics:	Specialty Services:	

TYPES OF BUSINESS:
Drug Stores, Retail

BRANDS/DIVISIONS/AFFILIATES:
FLAVORx

CONTACTS:
Note: Officers with more than one job title may be intentionally listed here more than once.

Mary F. Sammons, CEO
Mary F. Sammons, Pres.
John Standley, CFO
James P. Mastrian, Sr. Exec. VP-Mktg.
Keith W. Lovett, Sr. VP-Human Resources & Labor Rel.
Don P. Davis, Sr. VP/CIO
John Standley, Sr. Exec. VP/Chief Admin. Officer
Robert Sari, Sr. VP/General Counsel
Mark Panzer, Sr. Exec. VP-Store Oper.
Christopher Hall, Sr. VP-Real Estate & Planning
Karen Rugen, Sr. VP-Corp. Comm. & Public Affairs
Kevin Twomey, Sr. VP/Chief Acct. Officer
Tony Bellezza, Sr. VP/Chief Compliance Officer
Doug Donley, VP/Corp. Controller
Philip J. Keough, IV, Sr. VP-Pharmacy Oper.
John Learish, Sr. VP-Mktg.
Robert G. Miller, Chmn.
James P. Mastrian, Sr. Exec. VP-Logistics & Pharmacy Services

Phone: 717-761-2633   Fax:
Toll-Free: 800-748-3243
Address: 30 Hunter Ln., Camp Hill, PA 17011 US

GROWTH PLANS/SPECIAL FEATURES:
Rite Aid Corp. is one of the leading retail drug store chains in the U.S. The company currently operates approximately 3,400 drug stores in 28 states and the District of Columbia. The stores sell prescription drugs and other merchandise such as non-prescription medications, health and beauty aids, personal care items, cosmetics, household items, beverages, convenience foods, greeting cards, seasonal merchandise and numerous other everyday products. Rite Aid offers over 24,000 products, approximately 2,100 of which are private-label. Most stores also offer one-hour photo processing, and 38% have a drive-thru pharmacy. The company maintains a strategic alliance with General Nutrition Companies, Inc. (GNC), which operates stores within almost a third of Rite Aid stores. However, the pharmacy remains the core of the firm's business, with prescription drugs representing over 63% of sales. Rite Aid's pharmacies offer a service in which FLAVORx flavoring can be added to all prescription and over-the-counter syrups and liquid medications. Customers can choose from 20 different flavorings.

Rite Aid offers employee benefits including health, dental and vision plans, basic and dependent life insurance, an employee assistance program, product discounts and credit union membership.

FINANCIALS:
Sales and profits are in thousands of dollars—add 000 to get the full amount. Year 2004 note: Complete fiscal 2004 results were not available for all companies at press time. For this company, year 2004 is for 12 months.

2004 Sales: $16,600,449 (12 months)   2004 Profits: $83,311   (12 months)
2003 Sales: $15,800,900   2003 Profits: $-112,100
2002 Sales: $15,171,000   2002 Profits: $-828,000
2001 Sales: $14,516,900   2001 Profits: $-1,589,200
2000 Sales: $13,338,947   2000 Profits: $-1,133,043

Stock Ticker: RAD
Employees: 72,500
Fiscal Year Ends: 2/28

SALARIES/BENEFITS:
Pension Plan: ESOP Stock Plan: Profit Sharing: Top Exec. Salary: $1,240,000   Bonus: $1,498,161
Savings Plan: Y   Stock Purch. Plan: Y   Second Exec. Salary: $1,240,000 Bonus: $1,498,161

OTHER THOUGHTS:
Apparent Top Female Officers: 2
Hot Spot for Advancement for Women/Minorities:

LOCATIONS: ("Y" = Yes)
West:	Southwest:	Midwest:	Southeast:	Northeast:	International:
Y	Y	Y	Y	Y	

ROCHE GROUP

www.roche.com

Industry Group Code: 325412 **Ranks within this company's industry group:** Sales: 3 Profits: 9

Insurance/HMO/PPO:	Drugs:	Equipment/Supplies:	Hospitals/Clinics:	Services:	Health Care:
Insurance:	Manufacturer: Y	Manufacturer:	Acute Care:	Diagnostics: Y	Home Health:
Managed Care:	Distributor:	Distributor:	Sub-Acute Care:	Labs/Testing:	Long-Term Care:
Utilization Mgmt.:	Specialty Pharm.:	Leasing/Finance:	Outpatient Surgery:	Staffing:	Physical Therapy:
Payment Proc.:	Vitamins/Nutri.:	Information Sys.:	Phys. Rehab. Center:	Waste Disposal:	Phys. Practice Mgmt.:
	Clinical Trials:		Psychiatric Clinics:	Specialty Services:	

TYPES OF BUSINESS:
Drugs, Manufacturing
Consumer Health Products
Diagnostics
Cancer Drugs
Virology Products

BRANDS/DIVISIONS/AFFILIATES:
Roche Holding, Ltd.
F. Hoffmann-La Roche, Ltd.
Aleve
Rennie
Avastin
Herceptin
Chugai Pharmaceuticals
Genentech

CONTACTS:
Note: Officers with more than one job title may be intentionally listed here more than once.
Franz B. Humer, CEO
Erich Hunziker, CFO
Jonathan Knowles, Head-Global Research
William M. Burns, Head-Pharmaceuticals Div.
Heino von Prondzynski, Head-Diagnostics Div.
Richard T. Laube, Head-Roche Consumer Health
Gottlieb Keller, Head-Corp. Services
Franz B. Humer, Chmn.

Phone: 41-61-688-1111	Fax: 41-61-691-9391
Toll-Free:	
Address: Grenzacherstrasse 124, Basel, 4070 Switzerland	

GROWTH PLANS/SPECIAL FEATURES:
Roche Group is one of the world's largest health care concerns, occupying an industry-leading position in the global diagnostics market and ranking as one of the top suppliers of pharmaceuticals, with particular market penetration in the areas of cancer drugs as well as virology and transplantation medicine. Roche's consumer health products are sold around the world, ranging from vitamins to pain relievers (such as Aleve) to antacids (like leading U.K. brand Rennie). Group operations presently extend to some 150 countries, with additional alliances and research and development agreements with corporate and institutional partners furthering Roche's collective reach. Among the company's related corporate interests are majority ownership holdings in Bay Area biotechnology research company Genentech and Japanese pharmaceutical firm Chugai. Pharmaceuticals are the Roche Group's primary source of revenues, with over 90% of pharmaceutical sales transacted through prescription drug units. Among the company's products are cancer drugs Avastin, Xeloda, Herceptin and Mab-Thera/Rituxan, antibiotic Rocephin, HIV/AIDS treatments Viracept, Invirase and Fuzeon (developed with Trimeris) and Tamiflu, which is used to prevent and treat influenza. Roche has invested heavily in diagnostics, both through internal resource development and through selective acquisitions. Roche companies presently control proprietary diagnostic technologies across a range of areas, including advanced DNA tests, leading consumer diabetes monitoring devices and applied sciences methodologies for laboratory research. In recent news, Roche announced plans to construct two new biotechnology centers, one at the company's Basel, Switzerland headquarters and one in Penzberg, Germany. Scheduled for completion by 2007, the new facilities are anticipated to support the production of monoclonal antibodies, including anti-cancer medicines Avastin and Herceptin. In July 2004, Roche agreed to sell its over-the-counter drugs unit to Bayer.

FINANCIALS:
Sales and profits are in thousands of dollars—add 000 to get the full amount. Year 2004 note: Complete fiscal 2004 results were not available for all companies at press time. For this company, year 2004 is for months.

2004 Sales: $ (months)	2004 Profits: $ (months)	
2003 Sales: $25,132,100	2003 Profits: $2,470,500	Stock Ticker: Foreign
2002 Sales: $21,422,800	2002 Profits: $-2,901,500	Employees: 65,357
2001 Sales: $15,637,600	2001 Profits: $2,209,700	Fiscal Year Ends: 12/31
2000 Sales: $	2000 Profits: $	

SALARIES/BENEFITS:
Pension Plan:	ESOP Stock Plan:	Profit Sharing:	Top Exec. Salary: $	Bonus: $
Savings Plan:	Stock Purch. Plan:		Second Exec. Salary: $	Bonus: $

OTHER THOUGHTS:
Apparent Top Female Officers:
Hot Spot for Advancement for Women/Minorities:

LOCATIONS: ("Y" = Yes)
West:	Southwest:	Midwest:	Southeast:	Northeast:	International:
Y		Y	Y	Y	Y

ROTECH HEALTHCARE INC

www.rotech.com

Industry Group Code: 339113 Ranks within this company's industry group: Sales: 36 Profits: 74

Insurance/HMO/PPO:	Drugs:	Equipment/Supplies:	Hospitals/Clinics:	Services:	Health Care:
Insurance:	Manufacturer:	Manufacturer:	Acute Care:	Diagnostics:	Home Health:
Managed Care:	Distributor:	Distributor: Y	Sub-Acute Care:	Labs/Testing:	Long-Term Care:
Utilization Mgmt.:	Specialty Pharm.:	Leasing/Finance:	Outpatient Surgery:	Staffing:	Physical Therapy:
Payment Proc.:	Vitamins/Nutri.:	Information Sys.:	Phys. Rehab. Center:	Waste Disposal:	Phys. Practice Mgmt.:
	Clinical Trials:		Psychiatric Clinics:	Specialty Services:	

TYPES OF BUSINESS:
Home Medical Equipment
Respiratory Equipment

BRANDS/DIVISIONS/AFFILIATES:
Rotech Medical Corporation

CONTACTS:
Note: Officers with more than one job title may be intentionally listed here more than once.

Philip L. Carter, CEO
Philip L. Carter, Pres.
Michael R. Dobbs, COO
Barry Stewart, CFO
J. Chad Brown, Chief Sales Officer
Albert A. Prast, CIO
Albert A. Prast, Chief Tech. Officer
Rebecca L. Myers, Chief Legal Officer
Arthur J. Reimers, Chmn.

Phone: 407-822-4600 Fax:
Toll-Free:
Address: 2600 Technology Dr., Ste. 300, Orlando, FL 32804 US

GROWTH PLANS/SPECIAL FEATURES:

Rotech Healthcare, Inc., created as the holding company for the assets of Rotech Medical Corporation after it emerged from bankruptcy in 2002, is one of the largest providers of home medical equipment and related products and services in the U.S. The firm offers respiratory therapy and durable home medical equipment and related services in 48 states through approximately 500 operating centers. Rotech provides equipment and services, mainly to older patients with breathing disorders such as chronic obstructive pulmonary diseases, or COPD, which includes chronic bronchitis and emphysema, obstructive sleep apnea and other cardiopulmonary disorders. Company revenues are principally derived from respiratory equipment rental and related services, making up 83.9% of Rotech's revenues. Respiratory equipment includes oxygen concentrator rentals, liquid oxygen systems, portable oxygen systems, ventilator therapy systems, nebulizer equipment, sleep disorder breathing therapy systems and the sale of nebulizer medications. Rotech also rents and sells durable medical equipment, including hospital beds, wheelchairs, walkers, patient aids and ancillary supplies, which generate about 14% of revenues annually.

FINANCIALS:
Sales and profits are in thousands of dollars—add 000 to get the full amount. Year 2004 note: Complete fiscal 2004 results were not available for all companies at press time. For this company, year 2004 is for 6 months.

2004 Sales: $267,411 (6 months)
2003 Sales: $581,221
2002 Sales: $617,800
2001 Sales: $
2000 Sales: $

2004 Profits: $19,433 (6 months)
2003 Profits: $8,413
2002 Profits: $-119,400
2001 Profits: $
2000 Profits: $

Stock Ticker: ROHI
Employees: 4,400
Fiscal Year Ends: 12/31

SALARIES/BENEFITS:
Pension Plan: Y ESOP Stock Plan: Profit Sharing: Top Exec. Salary: $716,346 Bonus: $
Savings Plan: Y Stock Purch. Plan: Second Exec. Salary: $369,231 Bonus: $180,000

OTHER THOUGHTS:
Apparent Top Female Officers: 1
Hot Spot for Advancement for Women/Minorities:

LOCATIONS: ("Y" = Yes)

West:	Southwest:	Midwest:	Southeast:	Northeast:	International:
Y	Y	Y	Y	Y	

SAFEGUARD HEALTH ENTERPRISES INC

www.safeguard.net

Industry Group Code: 524114A **Ranks within this company's industry group:** Sales: 3 Profits: 2

Insurance/HMO/PPO:	Drugs:	Equipment/Supplies:	Hospitals/Clinics:	Services:	Health Care:
Insurance: Y	Manufacturer:	Manufacturer:	Acute Care:	Diagnostics:	Home Health:
Managed Care: Y	Distributor:	Distributor:	Sub-Acute Care:	Labs/Testing:	Long-Term Care:
Utilization Mgmt.:	Specialty Pharm.:	Leasing/Finance:	Outpatient Surgery:	Staffing:	Physical Therapy:
Payment Proc.:	Vitamins/Nutri.:	Information Sys.:	Phys. Rehab. Center:	Waste Disposal:	Phys. Practice Mgmt.:
	Clinical Trials:		Psychiatric Clinics:	Specialty Services:	

TYPES OF BUSINESS:
HMO/PPO
Vision & Life Insurance Products
Administrative Services
Dental Benefit Plans

BRANDS/DIVISIONS/AFFILIATES:
Health Net Vision, Inc.
SafeGuard Health Plans, Inc.
Health Net Dental, Inc.

CONTACTS:
Note: Officers with more than one job title may be intentionally listed here more than once.
James E. Buncher, CEO
James E. Buncher, Pres.
Stephen J. Baker, Exec. VP/COO
Dennis L. Gates, Sr. VP/CFO
Kenneth E. Keating, VP-Mktg. & Sales
Ronald I. Brendzel, Sr. VP/General Counsel
Ronald I. Brendzel, Corp. Sec.
Steven J. Baileys, Chmn.

Phone: 949-425-4300 **Fax:** 949-425-4308
Toll-Free: 800-880-1800
Address: 95 Enterprise, Aliso Viejo, CA 92656 US

GROWTH PLANS/SPECIAL FEATURES:
SafeGuard Health Enterprises, Inc. provides a wide range of dental benefit plans, including health maintenance organization (HMO) plan designs and preferred provider organization (PPO) and indemnity plan designs, to government and private sector employers, associations and individuals. In addition, the firm offers vision benefit plans, administrative services and PPO services. Currently, SafeGuard has group contracts with about 4,500 employer or association groups and delivers dental or vision services to approximately 750,000 covered individuals. The firm conducts its business through several subsidiaries, one of which is an insurance company and several of which are dental HMO plans. The company's primary operations are in California, Texas and Florida. SafeGuard's dental HMO plan designs typically cover basic dental procedures, such as examinations, x-rays, cleanings and fillings, as well as more extensive procedures provided by a general dentist, such as root canals and crowns. These plans also cover procedures performed by specialists contracted with the company, including oral surgery, periodontics and orthodontics. PPO/indemnity plan designs generally cover the same procedures as HMO plans, but individuals are required to make a co-insurance payment at the time of each service. Under the firm's defined benefit dental plans, subscribers and dependents are reimbursed a fixed amount for each procedure performed. In April 2004, SafeGuard merged subsidiaries Health Net Dental, Inc. and Health Net Vision, Inc., purchased from Health Net, Inc., into SafeGuard Health Plans, Inc. As a result of the transaction, SafeGuard is now one of the largest dental and vision benefits providers in California.

Full-time employees receive a benefits package including medical, dental, vision and life insurance, as well as an employee assistance program. Promotions within the organization are commonplace.

FINANCIALS:
Sales and profits are in thousands of dollars—add 000 to get the full amount. Year 2004 note: Complete fiscal 2004 results were not available for all companies at press time. For this company, year 2004 is for months.

2004 Sales: $ (months)   2004 Profits: $ (months)
2003 Sales: $104,891   2003 Profits: $7,813
2002 Sales: $83,000   2002 Profits: $1,400
2001 Sales: $84,800   2001 Profits: $12,500
2000 Sales: $97,300   2000 Profits: $-9,000

Stock Ticker: Private
Employees: 360
Fiscal Year Ends: 12/31

SALARIES/BENEFITS:
| Pension Plan: | ESOP Stock Plan: | Profit Sharing: | Top Exec. Salary: $250,000 | Bonus: $25,000 |
| Savings Plan: Y | Stock Purch. Plan: | | Second Exec. Salary: $220,000 | Bonus: $20,000 |

OTHER THOUGHTS:
Apparent Top Female Officers:
Hot Spot for Advancement for Women/Minorities:

LOCATIONS: ("Y" = Yes)
West:	Southwest:	Midwest:	Southeast:	Northeast:	International:
Y	Y		Y		

SANOFI-SYNTHELABO

www.sanofi-synthelabo.fr

Industry Group Code: 325412 Ranks within this company's industry group: Sales: 13 Profits: 7

Insurance/HMO/PPO:	Drugs:	Equipment/Supplies:	Hospitals/Clinics:	Services:	Health Care:
Insurance:	Manufacturer: Y	Manufacturer:	Acute Care:	Diagnostics:	Home Health:
Managed Care:	Distributor:	Distributor:	Sub-Acute Care:	Labs/Testing:	Long-Term Care:
Utilization Mgmt.:	Specialty Pharm.:	Leasing/Finance:	Outpatient Surgery:	Staffing:	Physical Therapy:
Payment Proc.:	Vitamins/Nutri.:	Information Sys.:	Phys. Rehab. Center:	Waste Disposal:	Phys. Practice Mgmt.:
	Clinical Trials:		Psychiatric Clinics:	Specialty Services:	

TYPES OF BUSINESS:
Pharmaceuticals, Manufacturing

BRANDS/DIVISIONS/AFFILIATES:
Aprovel
Plavix
Arixtra
Depakine
Stilnox
Xatral
Eloxatin
Aventis

CONTACTS:
Note: Officers with more than one job title may be intentionally listed here more than once.

Jean-Francois Dehecq, CEO
Marie-Helene Laimay, CFO
Jean-Claude Armbruster, Sr. VP-Human Resources
Gerard Le Fur, Exec. VP-Science
Jean-Pierre Kerjouan, General Counsel
Hanspeter Spek, VP-Oper.
Jean-Claude Leroy, Sr. VP-Strategy
Pierre-Jean Lepienne, Exec. VP-Corp. Affairs
Christian Lajoux, Sr. VP-Europe
Gilles Lhernould, Sr. VP-Industrial Affairs
Gordon Proctor, Sr. VP-Intercontinental
Timothy Rothwell, Sr. VP-North America
Jean-Francois Dehecq, Chmn.

Phone: 33-1-53-77-4000 **Fax:** 33-1-53-77-4296
Toll-Free:
Address: 174 Ave. de France, Paris, 75013 France

GROWTH PLANS/SPECIAL FEATURES:
Sanofi-Synthelabo is an international pharmaceutical group engaged in the research, development, manufacture and marketing of pharmaceutical products for sale principally in the prescription market. The company has four major business areas: cardiovascular, central nervous system (CNS), internal medicine and oncology. The company's cardiovascular products include two of the fastest-growing products on the cardiovascular market today: the blood pressure medication Aprovel and the anti-clotting agent Plavix, as well as one of its newest products, the anti-thrombosis Arixtra. The company's CNS medicines include Stilnox, the world's leading prescription insomnia medication, and Depakine, one of the leading treatments for epilepsy. The company's internal medicine products include Xatral, a leading treatment for benign prostatic hypertrophy. Sanofi's lead product in this strategic market is the cancer drug Eloxatin, which is marketed in Europe as a first-line treatment against colorectal cancer and in the United States as a second-line treatment in combination with 5-FU/LV. The company currently has 56 compounds in development, 25 of which are in Phases II and III. Sanofi sells its products in 100 countries on five continents. In recent news, the firm has a proposed acquisition of Aventis, which would make Sanofi one of the world's third-largest pharmaceutical companies.

FINANCIALS:
Sales and profits are in thousands of dollars—add 000 to get the full amount. Year 2004 note: Complete fiscal 2004 results were not available for all companies at press time. For this company, year 2004 is for 6 months.

2004 Sales: $5,461,000 (6 months)	2004 Profits: $694,000 (6 months)	**Stock Ticker:** Foreign
2003 Sales: $10,118,000	2003 Profits: $2,610,000	Employees: 33,086
2002 Sales: $7,823,000	2002 Profits: $1,847,000	Fiscal Year Ends: 12/31
2001 Sales: $5,747,100	2001 Profits: $1,404,000	
2000 Sales: $	2000 Profits: $	

SALARIES/BENEFITS:
Pension Plan:	ESOP Stock Plan:	Profit Sharing: Y	Top Exec. Salary: $	Bonus: $
Savings Plan:	Stock Purch. Plan: Y		Second Exec. Salary: $	Bonus: $

OTHER THOUGHTS:
Apparent Top Female Officers: 1
Hot Spot for Advancement for Women/Minorities:

LOCATIONS: ("Y" = Yes)
West:	Southwest:	Midwest:	Southeast:	Northeast:	International:
				Y	Y

SCHERING AG

www.schering.de

Industry Group Code: 325412   Ranks within this company's industry group: Sales: 16   Profits: 18

Insurance/HMO/PPO:	Drugs:	Equipment/Supplies:	Hospitals/Clinics:	Services:	Health Care:
Insurance:	Manufacturer: Y	Manufacturer:	Acute Care:	Diagnostics:	Home Health:
Managed Care:	Distributor:	Distributor:	Sub-Acute Care:	Labs/Testing:	Long-Term Care:
Utilization Mgmt.:	Specialty Pharm.:	Leasing/Finance:	Outpatient Surgery:	Staffing:	Physical Therapy:
Payment Proc.:	Vitamins/Nutri.:	Information Sys.:	Phys. Rehab. Center:	Waste Disposal:	Phys. Practice Mgmt.:
	Clinical Trials:		Psychiatric Clinics:	Specialty Services:	

TYPES OF BUSINESS:
Drug Development & Manufacturing
Gynecology & Andrology Treatments
Cancer Treatments
Multiple Sclerosis Treatments
Circulatory Disorder Treatments
Diagnostic & Radiopharmaceutical Agents
Skin Treatments
Proteomics

BRANDS/DIVISIONS/AFFILIATES:
Yasmin
Angeliq
Testoviron
Androcur
Betaseron
Fludara
Illomedin
Betapace

CONTACTS: Note: Officers with more than one job title may be intentionally listed here more than once.
Jorge Spiekerkotter, Head-Finance
Ulrich Kostlin, Head-Mktg. & Sales
Jorge Spiekerkotter, Head-Human Resources
Gunter Stock, Head-Research
Jorge Spiekerkotter, Head-IT
Jorge Spiekerkotter, Head-Admin.
Hubertus Erlen, Head-Strategy & Bus. Dev.
Christof Ehrhart, Head-Corp. Comm.
Peter Vogt, Head-Investor Rel.
Jorge Spiekerkotter, Head-Latin America
Lutz Lingnau, Head-North America
Lutz Lingnau, Head-Specialized Therapeutics & Dermatology
Gunter Stock, Head-Gynecology & Andrology/Diagnostics
Hubertus Erlen, Chmn.-Exec. Board
Ulrich Kostlin, Head-Europe & Africa
Ulrich Kostlin, Head-Supply Chain & Environment

Phone: 49-30-468-1111   Fax: 49-30-468-15305
Toll-Free:
Address: Mullerstrasse 178, Berlin, 13353 Germany

GROWTH PLANS/SPECIAL FEATURES:
Schering AG is a leading global research-based pharmaceutical company operating through more than 140 subsidiaries. The firm concentrates its activities on four business areas: gynecology and andrology, specialized therapeutics, diagnostics and radiopharmaceuticals, and dermatology. The company's gynecology and andrology products include birth control pills (Yasmin), hormone therapy (Angeliq and Menostar) and other contraceptives for women (Mirena), as well as products for the treatment of testosterone deficiency in men (Testoviron, Testogel and Nebido) and prostate cancer (Androcur). The firm is also developing a hormonal method to control male fertility. Schering's specialized therapeutic products are for people with life-threatening diseases, such as multiple sclerosis (Betaseron/Betaferon, which is the firm's top-selling product), leukemia (Fludara), solid tumors (Androcur and Bonefos), peripheral circulatory disorders (Illomedin), arrhythmia (Betapace) and primary pulmonary hypertension (Ventavis). The company is working on molecular approaches, such as antibodies for leukemia therapy (MabCampath/Campath and Leukine), anti-angiogenesis for treating tumors and gene therapy for biological bypasses. Schering's diagnostics and radiopharmaceuticals products include a range of imaging contrast media, such as Magnevist, a general MRI contrast agent; Resovist, a liver-specific MRI contrast agent; Gadovist, a central nervous system MRI contrast agent; and Ultravist and Iopamiron, x-ray contrast media. This segment also includes a range of radiopharmaceuticals, which can be used for early diagnosis or targeted therapy, such as Flucis, a diagnostic agent for positron emission tomography, which can be used in diagnosing and examining the progression of various tumors in the head, throat and lung areas, as well as for melanomas. The company's dermatology products treat acne (Skinoren Creme and Gel), eczema (Advantan), rosacea, psoriasis (Psorcutan Beta) and mycosis.

FINANCIALS: Sales and profits are in thousands of dollars—add 000 to get the full amount. Year 2004 note: Complete fiscal 2004 results were not available for all companies at press time. For this company, year 2004 is for 6 months.

2004 Sales: $2,947,000 (6 months)   2004 Profits: $319,000 (6 months)
2003 Sales: $6,070,000   2003 Profits: $557,000
2002 Sales: $5,267,000   2002 Profits: $910,000
2001 Sales: $4,310,000   2001 Profits: $372,000
2000 Sales: $ 2000 Profits: $

Stock Ticker: Foreign
Employees: 26,245
Fiscal Year Ends: 12/31

SALARIES/BENEFITS:
Pension Plan: ESOP Stock Plan: Profit Sharing: Top Exec. Salary: $ Bonus: $
Savings Plan: Stock Purch. Plan: Second Exec. Salary: $ Bonus: $

OTHER THOUGHTS:
Apparent Top Female Officers:
Hot Spot for Advancement for Women/Minorities:

LOCATIONS: ("Y" = Yes)
West:	Southwest:	Midwest:	Southeast:	Northeast:	International:
				Y	Y

SCHERING-PLOUGH CORP

www.sch-plough.com

Industry Group Code: 325412   Ranks within this company's industry group: Sales: 15   Profits: 37

Insurance/HMO/PPO:	Drugs:	Equipment/Supplies:	Hospitals/Clinics:	Services:	Health Care:
Insurance:	Manufacturer: Y	Manufacturer:	Acute Care:	Diagnostics:	Home Health:
Managed Care:	Distributor:	Distributor:	Sub-Acute Care:	Labs/Testing:	Long-Term Care:
Utilization Mgmt.:	Specialty Pharm.:	Leasing/Finance:	Outpatient Surgery:	Staffing:	Physical Therapy:
Payment Proc.:	Vitamins/Nutri.:	Information Sys.:	Phys. Rehab. Center:	Waste Disposal:	Phys. Practice Mgmt.:
	Clinical Trials:		Psychiatric Clinics:	Specialty Services:	

TYPES OF BUSINESS:
Drugs-Allergies & Respiratory
Anti-Infective/Anti-Cancer Drugs
Dermatologicals
Cardiovascular Drugs
Animal Health Products
Over-the-Counter Drugs

BRANDS/DIVISIONS/AFFILIATES:
Schering-Plough Pharmaceuticals
Schering-Plough Healthcare Products
Schering-Plough Animal Health
Schering-Plough Research Institute
Afrin
Tinactin
Dr. Scholl's
Coppertone

CONTACTS:
Note: Officers with more than one job title may be intentionally listed here more than once.

Fred Hassan, CEO
Fred Hassan, Pres.
Robert J. Bertolini, CFO/Exec. VP
C. Ron Cheeley, Sr. VP-Global Human Resources
Cecil B. Pickett, VP/Pres., Schering-Plough Research Institute
Lisa W. DeBerardine, VP-Strategic Planning & Financial Forecasting
Thomas H. Kelly, VP & Controller
Raul E. Kohan, Pres. Animal Health/Group Head-Global Specialty Op
Brett Saunders, Sr. VP-Global Compliance & Business Practices
Daniel A. Nichols, Staff VP-Taxes
Douglas J. Gingerella, VP-Corp. Audits
Fred Hassan, Chmn.
Carrie S. Cox, Exec. VP/Pres.-Global Pharmaceuticals

Phone: 908-298-4000   Fax: 908-298-7653
Toll-Free:
Address: 2000 Galloping Hill Rd., Kenilworth, NJ 07033-0530 US

GROWTH PLANS/SPECIAL FEATURES:
Schering-Plough Corporation engages in the discovery, development, manufacture and marketing of pharmaceutical products through its pharmaceuticals, health care products and animal health subsidiaries. Schering-Plough Pharmaceuticals manufactures and markets allergy, respiratory, anti-infective, anti-cancer, dermatological, central nervous system and cardiovascular prescription pharmaceuticals. Schering-Plough HealthCare Products markets a number of over-the-counter drugs, as well as foot care and sun care products, including Clear Away wart remover; Dr. Scholl's foot care products; Lotrimin and Tinactin antifungals; A & D ointment; Afrin nasal decongestant; Chlor-Trimeton antihistamine; Coricidin and Drixoral cold and decongestant products; Correctol laxative; and Bain De Soleil, Coppertone and Solarcaine sun care products. Schering-Plough Animal Health develops and markets a broad range of pharmaceuticals and biologicals for companion animals and animals involved in food production. Animal health products include Cepravin and Nuflor antimicrobials; Banamine, a non-steroidal anti-inflammatory; Ralgro, a growth promotant implant; Otomax, an otic product; and a broad range of vaccines, parasiticides, sutures, bandages and nutritional products. The company's research arm, Schering-Plough Research Institute, has pioneered many new technologies in genomics and gene therapy, both in support of drug discovery and as tools in stratifying target groups for treatment. While Schering-Plough continues to pursue an aggressive internal reorganization (since his arrival in April 2003 CEO Fred Hassan has effectively replaced every member of the company's executive management staff), the company has re-affirmed its commitment to research and development for an advance pipeline of breakthrough pharmaceuticals and biomedical technologies. Schering-Plough has also expressed its intention to pursue additional collaborative enterprises and to engage in targeted in-license of its technologies in an effort to speed product flow from the research lab to the marketplace.

FINANCIALS:
Sales and profits are in thousands of dollars—add 000 to get the full amount. Year 2004 note: Complete fiscal 2004 results were not available for all companies at press time. For this company, year 2004 is for 9 months.

2004 Sales: $6,088,000 (9 months)   2004 Profits: $-112,000 (9 months)
2003 Sales: $8,334,000   2003 Profits: $-92,000
2002 Sales: $10,180,000   2002 Profits: $1,974,000
2001 Sales: $9,802,000   2001 Profits: $1,943,000
2000 Sales: $9,815,000   2000 Profits: $2,423,000

Stock Ticker: SGP
Employees: 30,500
Fiscal Year Ends: 12/31

SALARIES/BENEFITS:
Pension Plan: Y   ESOP Stock Plan: Profit Sharing: Top Exec. Salary: $1,046,154   Bonus: $1,872,000
Savings Plan: Y   Stock Purch. Plan: Second Exec. Salary: $699,500   Bonus: $55,000

OTHER THOUGHTS:
Apparent Top Female Officers: 1
Hot Spot for Advancement for Women/Minorities:

LOCATIONS: ("Y" = Yes)
West:	Southwest:	Midwest:	Southeast:	Northeast:	International:
Y	Y	Y	Y	Y	Y

SCHICK TECHNOLOGIES INC

www.schicktech.com

Industry Group Code: 339113   Ranks within this company's industry group: Sales: 126   Profits: 69

Insurance/HMO/PPO:	Drugs:	Equipment/Supplies:	Hospitals/Clinics:	Services:	Health Care:
Insurance:	Manufacturer:	Manufacturer: Y	Acute Care:	Diagnostics:	Home Health:
Managed Care:	Distributor:	Distributor:	Sub-Acute Care:	Labs/Testing:	Long-Term Care:
Utilization Mgmt.:	Specialty Pharm.:	Leasing/Finance:	Outpatient Surgery:	Staffing:	Physical Therapy:
Payment Proc.:	Vitamins/Nutri.:	Information Sys.:	Phys. Rehab. Center:	Waste Disposal:	Phys. Practice Mgmt.:
	Clinical Trials:		Psychiatric Clinics:	Specialty Services:	

TYPES OF BUSINESS:
Equipment-Medical & Dental Digital-Imaging Products
Dental X-Ray Devices

BRANDS/DIVISIONS/AFFILIATES:
CDR
CDR Wireless
CDRPan
accuDEXA

CONTACTS:
Note: Officers with more than one job title may be intentionally listed here more than once.
Jeffrey T. Slovin, CEO
Jeffrey T. Slovin, Pres.
Michael Stone, Exec. VP-Sales & Mktg.
Ari Neugroschl, VP-MIS
Stan Manelkern, VP-Eng.
Will Autz, VP-Mfg.
Ronald Rosner, VP-Admin.
Zvi N. Raskin, General Counsel
William Rogers, VP-Oper.
Eli Schick, Dir.-Investor Rel.
Ronald Rosner, Dir.-Finance
Zvi N. Raskin, Corp. Sec.
William K. Hood, Chmn.

Phone: 718-937-5765   Fax: 718-937-5962
Toll-Free:
Address: 30-00 47th Ave., Long Island City, NY 11101 US

GROWTH PLANS/SPECIAL FEATURES:
Schick Technologies, Inc. designs, develops and manufactures digital radiographic imaging systems and devices for the dental and medical markets. The firm's products, which are based on proprietary digital imaging technologies, create instant high-resolution radiographs with reduced levels of radiation. The CDR system, which has become a leading product in the field over the past decade, uses an intra-oral sensor to produce instant, full-size, high-resolution dental x-ray images on a color computer monitor without the use of film or the need for chemical development, while reducing the radiation dose by up to 90% compared to conventional x-rays. The firm also manufactures and sells CDR Wireless, a wireless radiography sensor for use with an existing CDR system, and CDRPan, a digital panoramic imaging device. In the field of medical radiography, the company manufactures and sells the accuDEXA bone densitometer, which assesses bone mineral density and fracture risk. Core products are based primarily on proprietary active-pixel sensor imaging technology, in addition to enhanced charged coupled device technology.

FINANCIALS:
Sales and profits are in thousands of dollars—add 000 to get the full amount. Year 2004 note: Complete fiscal 2004 results were not available for all companies at press time. For this company, year 2004 is for 12 months.

2004 Sales: $39,393 (12 months)	2004 Profits: $18,109 (12 months)	Stock Ticker: SCHK
2003 Sales: $29,817	2003 Profits: $11,825	Employees: 133
2002 Sales: $24,400	2002 Profits: $3,100	Fiscal Year Ends: 3/31
2001 Sales: $21,300	2001 Profits: $-1,600	
2000 Sales: $22,000	2000 Profits: $-12,300	

SALARIES/BENEFITS:
Pension Plan:	ESOP Stock Plan:	Profit Sharing:	Top Exec. Salary: $266,185	Bonus: $100,000
Savings Plan: Y	Stock Purch. Plan:		Second Exec. Salary: $266,378	Bonus: $100,000

OTHER THOUGHTS:
Apparent Top Female Officers:
Hot Spot for Advancement for Women/Minorities:

LOCATIONS: ("Y" = Yes)
West:	Southwest:	Midwest:	Southeast:	Northeast: Y	International:

SENTARA HEALTHCARE

www.sentara.com

Industry Group Code: 622110 **Ranks within this company's industry group:** Sales: 38 Profits:

Insurance/HMO/PPO:	Drugs:	Equipment/Supplies:	Hospitals/Clinics:	Services:	Health Care:
Insurance:	Manufacturer:	Manufacturer:	Acute Care: Y	Diagnostics:	Home Health: Y
Managed Care: Y	Distributor:	Distributor:	Sub-Acute Care: Y	Labs/Testing:	Long-Term Care: Y
Utilization Mgmt.:	Specialty Pharm.:	Leasing/Finance:	Outpatient Surgery: Y	Staffing:	Physical Therapy: Y
Payment Proc.:	Vitamins/Nutri.:	Information Sys.:	Phys. Rehab. Center: Y	Waste Disposal:	Phys. Practice Mgmt.:
	Clinical Trials:		Psychiatric Clinics:	Specialty Services: Y	

TYPES OF BUSINESS:
Hospitals-General
Health Insurance
Primary Care Practices
Hospice Services
Air Medical Transport
Rehabilitation Services
Physical Therapy Services
Organ Transplant Center

BRANDS/DIVISIONS/AFFILIATES:
Nightingale
Life Care
Mobile Meals
Sentara CarePlex
Sentara Norfolk General
Sentara Leigh
Sentara Virginia Beach
Sentara Bayside

CONTACTS:
Note: Officers with more than one job title may be intentionally listed here more than once.

David L. Bernd, CEO
Howard Kern, Pres.
Howard Kern, COO
Robert A. Broermann, CFO
Michael V. Taylor, VP-Human Resources
Bertram Reese, CIO
Megan Perry, VP-Admin.
Rodney F. Hochman, Chief Medical Officer
Donald V. Jellig, Pres.-Sentara Enterprises
Douglas M. Thompson, VP-Reinvesting Decision Support
Michael M. Dudley, Sr. VP/Pres.-Sentara Health Plans
David L. Bernd, Chmn.

Phone: 757-455-7000 **Fax:** 757-455-7164
Toll-Free: 800-736-8272
Address: 6015 Poplar Hall Dr., Norfolk, VA 23502 US

GROWTH PLANS/SPECIAL FEATURES:

Sentara Healthcare, founded in 1888, is a not-for-profit health care provider in Virginia and North Carolina, with more than 70 care sites including six hospitals and over 1,500 licensed beds. Hospitals include Sentara Norfolk General, Sentara Leigh, Sentara Virginia Beach, Sentara Bayside, Sentara CarePlex and Sentara Williamsburg Community Hospitals. The firm also offers home health and hospice services, physical therapy and rehabilitation services, ground and air medical transport, mobile diagnostic vans and two on-site fitness facilities. The company's air transport system, Nightingale, is the region's only air ambulance service. Care sites include 25 primary care practices, two outpatient care campuses, seven nursing centers and three assisted living centers. Sentara offers a full range of health coverage plans including commercial plans, a Medicaid HMO and workers' compensation. The firm also operates the region's comprehensive solid organ transplant center, which has conducted more than 1,400 total heart, lung and kidney transplants, including 200 heart transplants since 1989. Long-term life assistance, provided through the Life Care division, includes seven nursing centers, three assisted living centers, an adult day care center, the Mobile Meals program and the only program for all-inclusive care for the elderly (PACE) in the state. Sentara is the only health care system on the East Coast to be ranked in the nation's top 10 facilities in Modern Healthcare magazine for six consecutive years.

Sentara offers employees life, medical, dental and vision insurance, health care spending accounts, a tuition assistance program, an employee assistance program and access to the Sentara Hampton Health and Fitness Center.

FINANCIALS:
Sales and profits are in thousands of dollars—add 000 to get the full amount. Year 2004 note: Complete fiscal 2004 results were not available for all companies at press time. For this company, year 2004 is for 12 months.

2004 Sales: $1,500,000 (12 months)   2004 Profits: $ (12 months)
2003 Sales: $1,530,000   2003 Profits: $
2002 Sales: $1,600,000   2002 Profits: $
2001 Sales: $ 2001 Profits: $
2000 Sales: $ 2000 Profits: $

Stock Ticker: Nonprofit
Employees: 15,000
Fiscal Year Ends: 3/31

SALARIES/BENEFITS:
Pension Plan: ESOP Stock Plan: Profit Sharing: Top Exec. Salary: $ Bonus: $
Savings Plan: Y   Stock Purch. Plan: Second Exec. Salary: $ Bonus: $

OTHER THOUGHTS:
Apparent Top Female Officers: 1
Hot Spot for Advancement for Women/Minorities:

LOCATIONS: ("Y" = Yes)
| West: | Southwest: | Midwest: | Southeast: | Northeast: Y | International: |

SEPRACOR INC

www.sepracor.com

Industry Group Code: 325412 **Ranks within this company's industry group:** Sales: 41 Profits: 39

Insurance/HMO/PPO:	Drugs:	Equipment/Supplies:	Hospitals/Clinics:	Services:	Health Care:
Insurance:	Manufacturer: Y	Manufacturer:	Acute Care:	Diagnostics:	Home Health:
Managed Care:	Distributor:	Distributor:	Sub-Acute Care:	Labs/Testing:	Long-Term Care:
Utilization Mgmt.:	Specialty Pharm.:	Leasing/Finance:	Outpatient Surgery:	Staffing:	Physical Therapy:
Payment Proc.:	Vitamins/Nutri.:	Information Sys.:	Phys. Rehab. Center:	Waste Disposal:	Phys. Practice Mgmt.:
	Clinical Trials:		Psychiatric Clinics:	Specialty Services:	

TYPES OF BUSINESS:
Drugs-New & Improved
Respiratory Treatments
Central Nervous System Disorder Treatments

BRANDS/DIVISIONS/AFFILIATES:
XOPENEX
ESTORRA
ALLEGRA
CLARINEX
XUSA/XYZAL
ZYRTEC

CONTACTS:
Note: Officers with more than one job title may be intentionally listed here more than once.
Timothy J. Barberich, CEO
William J. O'Shea, Pres.
William J. O'Shea, COO
David P. Southwell, Exec. VP/CFO
Mark H.N. Corrigan, Exec. VP-Research & Dev.
Robert F. Scumaci, Exec. VP-Admin.
Douglas E. Reedich, Sr. VP-Legal Affairs/Chief Patent Counsel
Robert F. Scumaci, Exec. VP-Finance/Treas.
David P. Sothwell, Corp. Sec.
Timothy J. Barberich, Chmn.

Phone: 508-481-6700 **Fax:** 508-357-7499
Toll-Free:
Address: 84 Waterford Dr., Marlborough, MA 01752 US

GROWTH PLANS/SPECIAL FEATURES:
Sepracor, Inc. is a research-based pharmaceutical company whose goal is to discover, develop and market products that are directed toward serving unmet medical needs, particularly in the treatment of respiratory and central nervous system disorders. The company also develops and markets improved versions of widely prescribed drugs. These versions, known as improved chemical entities, feature enhancements such as reduced side effects, increased therapeutic efficacy, improved dosage forms and in some cases additional indications. Serpacor's lead product is XOPENEX, an inhalation solution used in nebulizers for patients with asthma or chronic obstructive pulmonary disease (COPD). The company has submitted a New Drug Application for a metered-dose inhaler of the same drug. It also recently received an approvable letter for ESTORRA-brand eszopiclone, a drug for the treatment of insomnia. In addition, the company has two products in clinical trials and three more in concept studies, for COPD, hypertension, spasticity and sleep apnea. Sepracor markets its own and other companies' products through its sales force, co-promotion agreements and out-licensing partnerships. Due to the company's patents relating to the chemicals desloratadine, fexofenadine and levocetirizine, Sepracor has out-licensing agreements with Schering-Plough for CLARINEX, Aventis for ALLEGRA and UCB Farchim SA for its XUSAL/XYZAL and ZYRTEC products, all of which are allergy medications.

Sepracor offers its employees tuition reimbursement, adoption reimbursement and a comprehensive health plan.

FINANCIALS:
Sales and profits are in thousands of dollars—add 000 to get the full amount. Year 2004 note: Complete fiscal 2004 results were not available for all companies at press time. For this company, year 2004 is for 9 months.

2004 Sales: $249,526 (9 months)	2004 Profits: $-261,933 (9 months)	**Stock Ticker:** SEPR
2003 Sales: $344,040	2003 Profits: $-135,936	Employees: 983
2002 Sales: $239,000	2002 Profits: $-276,500	Fiscal Year Ends: 12/31
2001 Sales: $152,100	2001 Profits: $-224,000	
2000 Sales: $85,200	2000 Profits: $-204,000	

SALARIES/BENEFITS:
Pension Plan:	ESOP Stock Plan: Y	Profit Sharing:	Top Exec. Salary: $455,965	Bonus: $228,247
Savings Plan: Y	Stock Purch. Plan: Y		Second Exec. Salary: $403,433	Bonus: $212,048

OTHER THOUGHTS:
Apparent Top Female Officers:
Hot Spot for Advancement for Women/Minorities:

LOCATIONS: ("Y" = Yes)
West:	Southwest:	Midwest:	Southeast:	Northeast: Y	International: Y

SEROLOGICALS CORP

www.serologicals.com

Industry Group Code: 621991 Ranks within this company's industry group: Sales: 1 Profits: 1

Insurance/HMO/PPO:	Drugs:	Equipment/Supplies:	Hospitals/Clinics:	Services:	Health Care:
Insurance:	Manufacturer: Y	Manufacturer:	Acute Care:	Diagnostics:	Home Health:
Managed Care:	Distributor:	Distributor:	Sub-Acute Care:	Labs/Testing: Y	Long-Term Care:
Utilization Mgmt.:	Specialty Pharm.:	Leasing/Finance:	Outpatient Surgery:	Staffing:	Physical Therapy:
Payment Proc.:	Vitamins/Nutri.:	Information Sys.:	Phys. Rehab. Center:	Waste Disposal:	Phys. Practice Mgmt.:
	Clinical Trials: Y		Psychiatric Clinics:	Specialty Services: Y	

TYPES OF BUSINESS:
Drugs-Specialty Human Antibody-Based Products
Biological Products
Blood Proteins
Media Supplements
Reagents
Diagnostic Kits

BRANDS/DIVISIONS/AFFILIATES:
Chemicon International, Inc.
Serologicals, Ltd.
Serologicals Proteins, Inc.
Intergen Company
EX-CYTE
Trypsin
AltaGen Biosciences
Sierra BioSource

CONTACTS:
Note: Officers with more than one job title may be intentionally listed here more than once.

David A. Dodd, CEO
David A. Dodd, Pres.
Harold W. Ingalls, CFO
Robert P. Collins, VP-Human Resources
Dennis W. Harris, Chief Scientific Officer
M. Dwain Wilcox, VP-Global Info. Services
James J. Kramer, VP-Global Mfg. Oper.
Phillip A. Theodore, VP/General Counsel
David L. Bellitt, VP-Global Commercial Oper.
Dennis W. Harris, VP-Bus. Dev.
Harold W. Ingalls, VP-Finance
Jeffrey D. Linton, Pres., Chemicon International
Dennis W. Harris, VP-R&D
Phillip A. Theodore, Corp. Sec.
Sue Sutton-Jones, VP-Global Quality Tech. & Regulatory Systems
Desmond H. O'Connell, Jr., Chmn.

Phone: 678-728-2000 **Fax:** 678-728-2299
Toll-Free: 800-842-9099
Address: 5655 Spalding Dr., Norcross, GA 30092 US

GROWTH PLANS/SPECIAL FEATURES:

Serologicals Corp. is a leading provider of biological products and enabling technologies to life sciences companies for use in the areas of neurobiology, cell signaling, oncology, angiogenesis, apoptosis, developmental biology, cellular physiology, hematology, immunology, cardiology, molecular biology and infectious diseases. Through subsidiaries Serologicals, Ltd. in the U.K. and Serologicals Proteins and Intergen Company in the U.S., the company offers a wide selection of media supplements, such as EX-CYTE growth enhancement media supplement for maximum productivity in cell cultures, and cell dissociation reagents like Trypsin and DNase. It also produces monoclonal antibodies for diagnostic laboratories, plasma and serum biodiagnostic products, buffer additives and detection proteins. Chemicon International, Inc., a division of Serologicals, supplies specialty reagents, diagnostic kits and a line of molecular biology products to the biomedical research community. Chemicon develops, manufactures, markets and distributes over 6,000 products. Though Serologicals began as a collection center for human plasma, in the last few years it has sold all its collection centers and exited the therapeutic plasma business. In recent news, the company acquired AltaGen Biosciences, parent company of Sierra BioSource. This will enable Serologicals to more broadly address the cell culture market by providing custom research and development services and custom media formulation. The company has also been issued a patent on a purification process that inactivates the prions causing mad cow disease.

Employees of Serologicals receive medical coverage, tuition reimbursement, employee assistance and a 401(k) in the U.S. or pension plan in the U.K.

FINANCIALS:
Sales and profits are in thousands of dollars—add 000 to get the full amount. Year 2004 note: Complete fiscal 2004 results were not available for all companies at press time. For this company, year 2004 is for 9 months.

2004 Sales: $126,761 (9 months)   2004 Profits: $14,120 (9 months)
2003 Sales: $146,915   2003 Profits: $1,506
2002 Sales: $145,500   2002 Profits: $13,900
2001 Sales: $109,800   2001 Profits: $17,100
2000 Sales: $147,800   2000 Profits: $12,900

Stock Ticker: SERO
Employees: 677
Fiscal Year Ends: 12/31

SALARIES/BENEFITS:
Pension Plan: Y   ESOP Stock Plan: Profit Sharing: Top Exec. Salary: $384,461   Bonus: $87,300
Savings Plan: Y   Stock Purch. Plan: Y   Second Exec. Salary: $269,769   Bonus: $81,938

OTHER THOUGHTS:
Apparent Top Female Officers: 1
Hot Spot for Advancement for Women/Minorities:

LOCATIONS: ("Y" = Yes)

West:	Southwest:	Midwest:	Southeast:	Northeast:	International:
Y		Y	Y	Y	Y

SERONO SA

www.serono.com

Industry Group Code: 325412 Ranks within this company's industry group: Sales: 22 Profits: 19

Insurance/HMO/PPO:	Drugs:	Equipment/Supplies:	Hospitals/Clinics:	Services:	Health Care:
Insurance:	Manufacturer: Y	Manufacturer:	Acute Care:	Diagnostics:	Home Health:
Managed Care:	Distributor:	Distributor:	Sub-Acute Care:	Labs/Testing:	Long-Term Care:
Utilization Mgmt.:	Specialty Pharm.:	Leasing/Finance:	Outpatient Surgery:	Staffing:	Physical Therapy:
Payment Proc.:	Vitamins/Nutri.:	Information Sys.:	Phys. Rehab. Center:	Waste Disposal:	Phys. Practice Mgmt.:
	Clinical Trials:		Psychiatric Clinics:	Specialty Services:	

TYPES OF BUSINESS:
Drugs-Manufacturing
Drugs-Fertility
Drugs-Neurology
Drugs-Growth & Metabolism
Drugs-Dermatology

BRANDS/DIVISIONS/AFFILIATES:
GONAL-f
Ovidrel/Ovitrelle
Luveris
Crinone
Cetrotide
Rebif
Saizen
Serostim

CONTACTS: Note: Officers with more than one job title may be intentionally listed here more than once.
Ernesto Bertarelli, CEO
Stuart Grant, CFO
Jacques Theurillat, Pres.-European & Int'l Sales & Mktg.
Francois Naef, Sr. Exec. VP-Human Resources
Andrew Galazka, Sr. VP-Scientific Affairs
Frank Latrille, Sr. Exec. VP-Global Prod. Dev.
Roland Baumann, Head-Corp. Admin.
Leon Bushara, Sr. Exec. VP-Bus. Dev.
Djan Yagtug, VP-Corp. Comm.
Jacques Theurillat, Deputy CEO
Roland Baumann, Sr. Exec. VP/Compliance Officer
Giampiero de Luca, Chief Intellectual Property Counsel
Georges Muller, Chmn.

Phone: 41-22-739-3000 **Fax:** 41-22-731-2179
Toll-Free:
Address: 15bis, chemin des Mines, Case postale 54, Geneva, CH-1211 20 Switzerland

GROWTH PLANS/SPECIAL FEATURES:
Serono SA is the world's third largest biotechnology company, working to develop products in the therapeutic areas of reproductive health, neurology, growth and metabolism and dermatology. The company currently markets GONAL-f, Ovidrel/Ovitrelle, Luveris, Crinone and Cetrotide for female infertility; Rebif and Rebiject for Multiple Sclerosis; Saizen for Growth Hormone deficiency; Serostim and SeroJet for AIDS wasting; and Raptiva for psoriasis. Many more candidates are in preclinical or clinical trials for treatment of diabetes, obesity, lupus, rheumatoid arthritis, hepatitis C and B-cell lymphomas. In addition to offering a number of fertility products, Serono recently launched www.fertility.com, a patient website for people who have concerns about their fertility or are seeking or undergoing treatment. The website provides comprehensive facts and describes therapy throughout each stage of the patient journey, from initial concerns to a potential pregnancy. Serono does business in Europe, Asia and Latin and North America, and is involved in numerous partnerships with companies all over the world. In May 2004 the company's U.S. subsidiary, Serono, Inc., released Zorbitive for use in patients with short bowel syndrome, a potentially life-threatening condition.

FINANCIALS: Sales and profits are in thousands of dollars—add 000 to get the full amount. Year 2004 note: Complete fiscal 2004 results were not available for all companies at press time. For this company, year 2004 is for 6 months.

2004 Sales: $1,095,700 (6 months)   2004 Profits: $240,100 (6 months)
2003 Sales: $1,858,000   2003 Profits: $390,000
2002 Sales: $1,546,500   2002 Profits: $320,800
2001 Sales: $1,376,500   2001 Profits: $316,700
2000 Sales: $ 2000 Profits: $

Stock Ticker: Foreign
Employees: 4,597
Fiscal Year Ends: 12/31

SALARIES/BENEFITS:
| Pension Plan: Y | ESOP Stock Plan: Y | Profit Sharing: | Top Exec. Salary: $ | Bonus: $ |
| Savings Plan: | Stock Purch. Plan: Y | | Second Exec. Salary: $ | Bonus: $ |

OTHER THOUGHTS:
Apparent Top Female Officers:
Hot Spot for Advancement for Women/Minorities:

LOCATIONS: ("Y" = Yes)
West:	Southwest:	Midwest:	Southeast:	Northeast:	International:
				Y	Y

SHIRE PHARMACEUTICALS PLC

www.shire.com

Industry Group Code: 325412   Ranks within this company's industry group: Sales: 26   Profits: 20

Insurance/HMO/PPO:	Drugs:	Equipment/Supplies:	Hospitals/Clinics:	Services:	Health Care:
Insurance:	Manufacturer: Y	Manufacturer:	Acute Care:	Diagnostics:	Home Health:
Managed Care:	Distributor:	Distributor:	Sub-Acute Care:	Labs/Testing:	Long-Term Care:
Utilization Mgmt.:	Specialty Pharm.:	Leasing/Finance:	Outpatient Surgery:	Staffing:	Physical Therapy:
Payment Proc.:	Vitamins/Nutri.:	Information Sys.:	Phys. Rehab. Center:	Waste Disposal:	Phys. Practice Mgmt.:
	Clinical Trials:		Psychiatric Clinics:	Specialty Services:	

TYPES OF BUSINESS:
Drugs-Diversified
Drug Delivery Technology
Small-Molecule Drugs

BRANDS/DIVISIONS/AFFILIATES:
Adderall XR
Carbatrol
Shire Laboratories
Agrylin
Pentasa
Reminyl
Proamatine
3TC

CONTACTS:
Note: Officers with more than one job title may be intentionally listed here more than once.

Matthew Emmens, CEO
Angus Russell, CFO/Group Finance Dir.
Anita Graham, Exec. VP-Human Resources
Eliseo Salinas, Chief Scientific Officer
Tatjana May, General Counsel
Jeff Devlin, Dir.-Corp. Affairs
Eliseo Salinas, Exec. VP-Research & Dev.
James Cavanaugh, Chmn.
Joseph Rus, Dir.-Int'l
John Lee, Exec. VP-Supply Chain

Phone: 44-1256-894000   Fax: 44-1256-894708
Toll-Free:
Address: Hampshire International Business Park/Chineham, Basingstoke, Hampshire RG24 8EP UK

GROWTH PLANS/SPECIAL FEATURES:
Shire Pharmaceuticals is an international specialty pharmaceutical company with a strategic focus on four therapeutic areas: central nervous system disorders, metabolic diseases, cancer and gastrointestinal disorders. The company's focus is supported by three technology platforms: lead optimization for small molecules, drug delivery and biologics. Shire's revenues come primarily from sales of products by its own sales and marketing operations, licensing fees, development fees and royalties. Sales and marketing operations are principally in the U.S., Canada, the U.K., Ireland, France, Germany, Italy and Spain. Shire's principal products in the U.S. include Adderall XR and Adderall for the treatment of attention deficit hyperactivity disorder; Agrylin for the treatment of elevated blood platelets; Pentasa for the treatment of ulcerative colitis; Carbatrol for the treatment of epilepsy; and Proamatine for the treatment of postural hypotension. In addition, the company receives royalties on sales of Reminyl for the treatment of Alzheimer's disease, marketed by Johnson & Johnson. In the U.K. and Ireland, the Calcichew range (used primarily as adjuncts in the treatment of osteoporosis) and Reminyl are co-promoted by Janssen-Cilag. Products in Canada include 3TC for the treatment of HIV/AIDS, Combivir and Heptovir (all marketed in partnership with GlaxoSmithKline); Amatine; Second Look, a breast cancer diagnostics product; and Fluviral S/F, a vaccine for the prevention of influenza. In recent news, the company acquired the worldwide sales and marketing rights to Methypatch, a methylphenidate transdermal delivery system for the once-daily treatment of attention deficit hyperactivity disorder, from Noven Pharmaceuticals, as well as five products from DRAXIS Health, Inc. and certain international rights to Vaniqa from Women First Healthcare, Inc.

FINANCIALS:
Sales and profits are in thousands of dollars—add 000 to get the full amount. Year 2004 note: Complete fiscal 2004 results were not available for all companies at press time. For this company, year 2004 is for 6 months.

2004 Sales: $647,300 (6 months)	2004 Profits: $164,200 (6 months)	**Stock Ticker:** Foreign
2003 Sales: $1,237,101	2003 Profits: $276,051	Employees: 1,814
2002 Sales: $1,037,300	2002 Profits: $250,600	Fiscal Year Ends: 12/31
2001 Sales: $877,600	2001 Profits: $38,800	
2000 Sales: $517,600	2000 Profits: $76,200	

SALARIES/BENEFITS:
Pension Plan: Y   ESOP Stock Plan: Profit Sharing: Top Exec. Salary: $730,000   Bonus: $385,000
Savings Plan: Stock Purch. Plan: Y   Second Exec. Salary: $557,000   Bonus: $267,000

OTHER THOUGHTS:
Apparent Top Female Officers: 2
Hot Spot for Advancement for Women/Minorities:

LOCATIONS: ("Y" = Yes)
West:	Southwest:	Midwest:	Southeast:	Northeast:	International:
Y	Y	Y	Y	Y	Y

SHL TELEMEDICINE

www.shl-telemedicine.com

Industry Group Code: 513390D   Ranks within this company's industry group: Sales: Profits:

Insurance/HMO/PPO:	Drugs:	Equipment/Supplies:	Hospitals/Clinics:	Services:	Health Care:
Insurance: Managed Care: Utilization Mgmt.: Payment Proc.:	Manufacturer: Distributor: Specialty Pharm.: Vitamins/Nutri.: Clinical Trials:	Manufacturer: Y Distributor: Leasing/Finance: Information Sys.:	Acute Care: Sub-Acute Care: Outpatient Surgery: Phys. Rehab. Center: Psychiatric Clinics:	Diagnostics: Y Labs/Testing: Staffing: Waste Disposal: Specialty Services: Y	Home Health: Long-Term Care: Physical Therapy: Phys. Practice Mgmt.:

TYPES OF BUSINESS:
Services-Cardiovascular Disease Diagnostics and Therapy
Personal Telemedicine Systems
Medical Call Center Services
Cardiac Testing Services
Remote Cardiac Monitoring
Nuclear Cardiology Diagnostics
Outpatient Diagnostic Imaging

BRANDS/DIVISIONS/AFFILIATES:
Raytel Medical Corp.
Philips Telemedicine Services
CardioBeeper
CardioPocket
TeleBreather
TelePress
Watchman
TeleWeight

CONTACTS:
Note: Officers with more than one job title may be intentionally listed here more than once.

Yoram Alroy, CEO
Erez Alroy, Co-Pres.
Erez Termachey, CFO
Irit Alroy, Exec. VP-Tech. Dev.
Eli Oren, Mgr.-Product Dev.
Ronen Elad, General Mgr.-Oper., Israel
Erez Nachtomy, Exec. VP-Bus. Dev.
Yariv Alroy, Co-Pres.
Katz Yoshida, Exec. VP-Bus. Dev.
Michal Golovner, Mgr.-Medical Affairs
Yoram Alroy, Chmn.

Phone: 972-3-5612212   Fax: 972-3-6242414
Toll-Free:
Address: Ashdar Bldg., 90 Igal Alon St., Tel Aviv, 67891 Israel

GROWTH PLANS/SPECIAL FEATURES:
SHL Telemedicine, Ltd. specializes in developing and marketing advanced personal telemedicine systems, which provide transmission of medical data by an individual from a remote location to a medical call center, as well as providing medical call center services. The company operates in the U.S. through its Raytel Medical Corp. subsidiary, a cardiovascular health care services provider. Throughout Europe, the firm mainly operates through Philips Telemedicine Services (PTS). PTS focuses on providing personal telemedicine services related to ailments of the heart. Bikurofe, another subsidiary, is Israel's leading nationwide operator of 24/7 medical call center and house-call services. SHL's client base consists of approximately 250,000 clients, providing a reliable recurring revenue stream. Subscribers who do not call the center within pre-arranged time periods are automatically contacted, ensuring consistent monitoring patterns and on-going interaction with clients. Some of the firm's services and products include MC Interactives, a sophisticated medical record database management application used as the company's monitor center's core software package; CardioVision, which serves as the backbone of the remote emergency cardiac diagnostic service in conjunction with MC Interactives; Telepress, a blood pressure reader/transmitter; LidoPen, a lidocaine auto-injector; CardioPocket, an electrocardiogram (ECG) heart monitoring transmitter wallet; Watchman, an emergency communication system built into a wristwatch; CardioBeeper, a heart monitoring handheld ECG transmitter; TeleWeight high-precision medical scales; and TeleBreather, a pulmonary data transmitter. In November 2003, the firm reached an agreement whereby it will acquire full ownership and control of Philips Heartcare Telemedicine Systems, the European telemedicine service that was previously owned 80% by Philips and 20% by SHL.

FINANCIALS:
Sales and profits are in thousands of dollars—add 000 to get the full amount. Year 2004 note: Complete fiscal 2004 results were not available for all companies at press time. For this company, year 2004 is for months.

2004 Sales: $ (months)   2004 Profits: $ (months)
2003 Sales: $ 2003 Profits: $
2002 Sales: $89,804   2002 Profits: $1,411
2001 Sales: $30,615   2001 Profits: $12,056
2000 Sales: $ 2000 Profits: $

Stock Ticker: Foreign
Employees: 1,389
Fiscal Year Ends: 9/30

SALARIES/BENEFITS:
Pension Plan: ESOP Stock Plan: Profit Sharing: Top Exec. Salary: $ Bonus: $
Savings Plan: Stock Purch. Plan: Second Exec. Salary: $ Bonus: $

OTHER THOUGHTS:
Apparent Top Female Officers:
Hot Spot for Advancement for Women/Minorities:

LOCATIONS: ("Y" = Yes)
| West: | Southwest: | Midwest: | Southeast: | Northeast: | International: Y |

Note: Financial information, benefits and other data can change quickly and may vary from those stated here.

SIEMENS MEDICAL SOLUTIONS
www.siemensmedical.com

Industry Group Code: 339113 **Ranks within this company's industry group:** Sales: Profits:

Insurance/HMO/PPO:	Drugs:	Equipment/Supplies:	Hospitals/Clinics:	Services:	Health Care:
Insurance:	Manufacturer:	Manufacturer: Y	Acute Care:	Diagnostics:	Home Health:
Managed Care:	Distributor:	Distributor:	Sub-Acute Care:	Labs/Testing:	Long-Term Care:
Utilization Mgmt.:	Specialty Pharm.:	Leasing/Finance:	Outpatient Surgery:	Staffing:	Physical Therapy:
Payment Proc.:	Vitamins/Nutri.:	Information Sys.: Y	Phys. Rehab. Center:	Waste Disposal:	Phys. Practice Mgmt.:
	Clinical Trials:		Psychiatric Clinics:	Specialty Services: Y	

TYPES OF BUSINESS:
Medical Equipment Manufacturing
Information Systems
Health Care Management Consulting
Ultrasound Systems
Hearing Aids

BRANDS/DIVISIONS/AFFILIATES:
Siemens AG
Soarian
TRIANO
Sonoline
Acuson
Somatom Sensation 16

CONTACTS:
Note: Officers with more than one job title may be intentionally listed here more than once.
Erich R. Reinhardt, CEO
Erich R. Reinhardt, Pres.
Johannes Naerger, VP/CFO
John Kijewski, Sr. VP-Tech. Services
Louise F. Morgan, Head-Global Solutions Div.
Melanie Schmude, Dir.-Int'l Public Rel.
Gail Latimer, Chief Nursing Officer

Phone: 49-91-31-840 **Fax:** 49-91-31-8437-54
Toll-Free:
Address: Henkestrasse 127, Erlangen, 91052 Germany

GROWTH PLANS/SPECIAL FEATURES:
Siemens Medical Solutions (SMS), a business segment of Siemens AG, is one of the largest suppliers to the health care industry, with operations around the world in over 138 countries. The firm is known for innovative medical technologies, health care information systems, management consulting and support services. It manufactures and markets a wide range of medical equipment including MRI systems, radiation therapy equipment and patient monitoring systems. With 75% of all of the company's products less than five years old, the firm devotes 10% of its budget to research and development and launches numerous new products every year. SMS's ultrasound division is the world's largest supplier of ultrasound systems and the worldwide leader in the production and sale of general imaging systems. It produces imaging equipment for cardiology, gynecology, radiology and urology under the Sonoline and Acuson brand-name product lines. Through its health services division, the health care industry's leading applications service provider, the firm offers information technology to doctors, hospitals and clinics. Through the hearing instruments division, SMS is a leading maker of hearing aids. Some of SMS's cutting-edge products include the Somatom Sensation 16 spiral CT scanner, an imaging system that enables previously unavailable applications such as virtual flight through the heart or intestine, and TRIANO, the firm's newest generation of hearing aid, made up of a combination of three microphones that permit directional hearing.

SMS offer employees work/life initiatives including child care discounts, emergency child care, mothers' rooms, financial planning resources, tuition reimbursement and flexible spending accounts, along with health, vision, hearing, life and prescription insurance.

FINANCIALS:
Sales and profits are in thousands of dollars—add 000 to get the full amount. Year 2004 note: Complete fiscal 2004 results were not available for all companies at press time. For this company, year 2004 is for months.

2004 Sales: $ (months)   2004 Profits: $ (months)
2003 Sales: $ 2003 Profits: $
2002 Sales: $ 2002 Profits: $
2001 Sales: $ 2001 Profits: $
2000 Sales: $ 2000 Profits: $

Stock Ticker: Foreign
Employees:
Fiscal Year Ends: 9/30

SALARIES/BENEFITS:
Pension Plan: Y   ESOP Stock Plan: Profit Sharing: Top Exec. Salary: $ Bonus: $
Savings Plan: Y   Stock Purch. Plan: Second Exec. Salary: $ Bonus: $

OTHER THOUGHTS:
Apparent Top Female Officers: 3
Hot Spot for Advancement for Women/Minorities: Y

LOCATIONS: ("Y" = Yes)
West:	Southwest:	Midwest:	Southeast:	Northeast:	International:
				Y	Y

SIERRA HEALTH SERVICES INC

www.sierrahealth.com

Industry Group Code: 524114   Ranks within this company's industry group: Sales: 40   Profits: 29

Insurance/HMO/PPO:	Drugs:	Equipment/Supplies:	Hospitals/Clinics:	Services:	Health Care:
Insurance:	Manufacturer:	Manufacturer:	Acute Care:	Diagnostics:	Home Health:
Managed Care: Y	Distributor:	Distributor:	Sub-Acute Care:	Labs/Testing:	Long-Term Care:
Utilization Mgmt.: Y	Specialty Pharm.: Y	Leasing/Finance:	Outpatient Surgery:	Staffing:	Physical Therapy:
Payment Proc.:	Vitamins/Nutri.:	Information Sys.:	Phys. Rehab. Center:	Waste Disposal:	Phys. Practice Mgmt.:
	Clinical Trials:		Psychiatric Clinics:	Specialty Services:	

TYPES OF BUSINESS:
HMO
PPO
Health Insurance
Administrative Services
Workers' Compensation Management
Health Care Services
Hospice Health Programs
Testing & Diagnostic Services

BRANDS/DIVISIONS/AFFILIATES:
Southwest Medical Associates
Health Plan of Nevada, Inc.
Sierra Health-Care Options

CONTACTS:
Note: Officers with more than one job title may be intentionally listed here more than once.

Anthony M. Marlon, CEO
Erin E. MacDonald, Chief of Staff
Paul H. Palmer, CFO
Daniel A. Kruger, VP-Human Resources
Robert L. Schaich, VP/CIO
Frank E. Collins, Sr. VP-Legal & Admin.
Peter O'Neill, Public & Investor Rel.
Paul H. Palmer, Treas.
Christine A. Peterson, Chief Medical Officer
William R. Godfrey, Exec. VP-Admin. Services
Jonathan W. Bunker, Pres.-Managed Health Care Div.
Michael A. Montalvo, VP-Customer Service
Anthony M. Marlon, Chmn.

Phone: 702-242-7000   Fax: 702-242-9711
Toll-Free:
Address: 2724 N. Tenaya Way, Las Vegas, NV 89128 US

GROWTH PLANS/SPECIAL FEATURES:
Through its numerous subsidiaries, Sierra Health Services, Inc. provides and delivers managed care benefit plans for individuals, government programs and employers. The company's subsidiaries include health maintenance organizations, managed indemnity plans, workers' compensation medical management programs, a third-party administrative services program for employer-funded health benefit plans and an administrator of managed care federal contracts for the U.S. Department of Defense's TRICARE subsidiary. Sierra Health Services also offers behavioral health care services and hospice health programs. The company has a significant presence in Nevada, where its Southwest Medical Associates subsidiary is the largest multi-specialty medical group in the state. In addition, Health Plan of Nevada, Inc. is the state's largest HMO. The firm also has a large presence in Texas, where it provides HMO products to more than 81,000 members. Combined, Sierra's subsidiaries provide health care-related products to more than 1.2 million members. Through subsidiary Sierra Health-Care Options, the firm offers administrative service products, including utilization review and PPO services, to large employer groups that are usually self-insured. Moreover, Sierra provides ancillary products and services that complement its managed health care and workers' compensation product lines. These ancillary products and services include outpatient surgical care, diagnostic testing, x-rays, vision services and mental health and substance abuse services.

Sierra offers its employees a variety of internal training and development programs designed to enhance computer skills, management techniques and general professional development.

FINANCIALS:
Sales and profits are in thousands of dollars—add 000 to get the full amount. Year 2004 note: Complete fiscal 2004 results were not available for all companies at press time. For this company, year 2004 is for 9 months.

2004 Sales: $1,242,709 (9 months)   2004 Profits: $94,777 (9 months)
2003 Sales: $1,485,079   2003 Profits: $62,326
2002 Sales: $1,278,600   2002 Profits: $36,400
2001 Sales: $1,291,500   2001 Profits: $3,500
2000 Sales: $1,393,000   2000 Profits: $-199,900

Stock Ticker: SIE
Employees: 3,600
Fiscal Year Ends: 12/31

SALARIES/BENEFITS:
Pension Plan: ESOP Stock Plan: Profit Sharing: Top Exec. Salary: $995,246   Bonus: $2,035,000
Savings Plan: Y   Stock Purch. Plan: Y   Second Exec. Salary: $317,172   Bonus: $590,100

OTHER THOUGHTS:
Apparent Top Female Officers: 2
Hot Spot for Advancement for Women/Minorities:

LOCATIONS: ("Y" = Yes)
West	Southwest	Midwest	Southeast	Northeast	International
Y	Y				

Note: Financial information, benefits and other data can change quickly and may vary from those stated here.

SIGMA ALDRICH CORP

www.sigmaaldrich.com

Industry Group Code: 325000   Ranks within this company's industry group: Sales: 2   Profits: 1

Insurance/HMO/PPO:	Drugs:	Equipment/Supplies:	Hospitals/Clinics:	Services:	Health Care:
Insurance: Managed Care: Utilization Mgmt.: Payment Proc.:	Manufacturer: Distributor: Specialty Pharm.: Vitamins/Nutri.: Clinical Trials:	Manufacturer: Y Distributor: Leasing/Finance: Information Sys.:	Acute Care: Sub-Acute Care: Outpatient Surgery: Phys. Rehab. Center: Psychiatric Clinics:	Diagnostics: Labs/Testing: Staffing: Waste Disposal: Specialty Services:	Home Health: Long-Term Care: Physical Therapy: Phys. Practice Mgmt.:

TYPES OF BUSINESS:
Chemicals Manufacturer
Organic & Inorganic Chemicals
Radio-Labeled Chemicals
Photovoltaic Materials
Chromatography Products
Fuel Cell & Battery Materials
DNA Synthesis Technology
Immunoassays

BRANDS/DIVISIONS/AFFILIATES:
Nafion

CONTACTS:
Note: Officers with more than one job title may be intentionally listed here more than once.

David R. Harvey, CEO
Jai Nagarkatti, Pres.
Jai Nagarkatti, COO
Michael R. Hogan, CFO
Patty Fish, VP-Human Resources
David A. Smoller, VP-R&D
Larry S. Blazevich, VP-Info. Systems
Michael R. Hogan, Chief Admin. Officer
Kirk A. Richter, Treas.
Jai P. Nagarkatti, Pres.-Scientific Research
James W. Meteer, VP-Process Improvement
David W. Julien, Pres.-Biotech.
Franklin D. Wicks, Pres.-Fine Chemicals
David R. Harvey, Chmn.

Phone: 314-771-5765   Fax: 314-286-7874
Toll-Free: 800-521-8956
Address: 3050 Spruce St., St. Louis, MO 63103 US

GROWTH PLANS/SPECIAL FEATURES:
Sigma-Aldrich develops and manufactures more than 85,000 chemical products and materials used for scientific and genomic research, biotechnology, pharmaceutical development, the diagnosis of disease and chemical manufacturing. Additional applications for its products include molecular biology, cell biology, cell culture, protein analysis and chromatography, DNA sequencing and gene studies. The company currently operates in 34 countries and distributes its products in more than 150 countries. Customers of the company primarily consist of life science companies, university and government institutions, hospitals, nonprofit organizations and pharmaceutical, diagnostic and biotechnology companies. The company's scientific research unit researches biochemicals, organic chemicals and reagents. The company's biotechnology unit markets immunochemistry, cell culture, molecular biology, cell signaling and neuroscience products. Its fine chemicals unit is a top supplier of large-scale organic chemicals and biochemicals. Sigma-Aldrich also offers a broad range of products for advanced battery and fuel cell research including precious metal catalysts for electrolytes, conducting polymers, plasticizers and binders, acids, carbonates, and other liquid electrolytes. Its products include a number of solid polymeric electrolyte (SPE) materials such as Nafion, as well as ceramic electrolytes for solid oxide fuel cells (SOFCs) like yttria-stabilized zirconia (YSZ). It also supplies the highest purity electrochemical grade lithium salts and related compounds for advanced lithium ion batteries, as well as photovoltaic materials.

FINANCIALS:
Sales and profits are in thousands of dollars—add 000 to get the full amount. Year 2004 note: Complete fiscal 2004 results were not available for all companies at press time. For this company, year 2004 is for 9 months.

2004 Sales: $1,057,300 (9 months)   2004 Profits: $178,200 (9 months)
2003 Sales: $1,298,146   2003 Profits: $193,102
2002 Sales: $1,207,000   2002 Profits: $130,700
2001 Sales: $1,179,400   2001 Profits: $140,700
2000 Sales: $1,096,300   2000 Profits: $320,200

Stock Ticker: SIAL
Employees: 5,920
Fiscal Year Ends: 12/31

SALARIES/BENEFITS:
Pension Plan: Y   ESOP Stock Plan: Profit Sharing: Top Exec. Salary: $725,000   Bonus: $298,401
Savings Plan: Y   Stock Purch. Plan: Second Exec. Salary: $430,000   Bonus: $132,870

OTHER THOUGHTS:
Apparent Top Female Officers: 1
Hot Spot for Advancement for Women/Minorities:

LOCATIONS: ("Y" = Yes)

West:	Southwest:	Midwest:	Southeast:	Northeast:	International:
Y	Y	Y	Y	Y	Y

SIGNATURE EYEWEAR INC

www.signatureeyewear.com

Industry Group Code: 333314 **Ranks within this company's industry group:** Sales: 2 Profits: 2

Insurance/HMO/PPO:	Drugs:	Equipment/Supplies:		Hospitals/Clinics:	Services:	Health Care:
Insurance:	Manufacturer:	Manufacturer:	Y	Acute Care:	Diagnostics:	Home Health:
Managed Care:	Distributor:	Distributor:	Y	Sub-Acute Care:	Labs/Testing:	Long-Term Care:
Utilization Mgmt.:	Specialty Pharm.:	Leasing/Finance:		Outpatient Surgery:	Staffing:	Physical Therapy:
Payment Proc.:	Vitamins/Nutri.:	Information Sys.:		Phys. Rehab. Center:	Waste Disposal:	Phys. Practice Mgmt.:
	Clinical Trials:			Psychiatric Clinics:	Specialty Services:	

TYPES OF BUSINESS:
Optical Instruments & Lens Manufacturing
Prescription Eyeglass & Sunglass Frames

BRANDS/DIVISIONS/AFFILIATES:
Signature Eyewear Collection
Dakota Smith
Laura Ashley Eyewear
Eddie Bauer Eyewear
Intuition
bebe eyes
Hart Schaffner & Marx Eyewear
Lifescape

CONTACTS:
Note: Officers with more than one job title may be intentionally listed here more than once.

Michael Prince, CEO
Michael Prince, CFO
Raul Khantzis, VP-Int'l Sales
Sheptanya Page, Dir.-Human Resources
Kevin D. Seifert, VP-Oper.
Jill Gardner, VP-Design
Marie Welsch, VP-Corp. Accounts
Richard M. Torre, Chmn.

Phone: 310-330-2700 **Fax:**
Toll-Free:
Address: 498 N. Oak St., Inglewood, CA 90302 US

GROWTH PLANS/SPECIAL FEATURES:
Signature Eyewear, Inc. (SEI) and its subsidiaries design, market and distribute prescription eyeglass frames and sunglasses. The company operates primarily under exclusive licenses for Laura Ashley Eyewear, Eddie Bauer Eyewear, bebe eyes, Hart Schaffner & Marx Eyewear, Dakota Smith and Nicole Miller Eyewear, as well as through its proprietary Signature Eyewear Collections, which include Intuition and Lifescape. Its best-selling product lines are Laura Ashley and Eddie Bauer. SEI distributes its products to independent optical retailers in the U.S.; internationally through exclusive distributors and a direct sales force in Western Europe; and through its account managers to major optical retail chains, including Pearle Vision, LensCrafters and U.S. Vision. SEI's development process includes identifying a market niche, obtaining the rights to a carefully selected brand name, producing a comprehensive marketing plan, developing unique in-store displays and creating innovative sales and merchandising programs for independent optical retailers and retail chains. To stem the tide of recent operating losses, the company has undergone a recapitalization that included obtaining a new credit facility, issuing preferred stock and initiating management, board and accountant changes.

FINANCIALS:
Sales and profits are in thousands of dollars—add 000 to get the full amount. Year 2004 note: Complete fiscal 2004 results were not available for all companies at press time. For this company, year 2004 is for 9 months.

2004 Sales: $17,634 (9 months)
2003 Sales: $24,420
2002 Sales: $33,121
2001 Sales: $61,138
2000 Sales: $51,932

2004 Profits: $ 120 (9 months)
2003 Profits: $3,463
2002 Profits: $-4,115
2001 Profits: $ 500
2000 Profits: $-9,439

Stock Ticker: SEYE
Employees: 123
Fiscal Year Ends: 10/31

SALARIES/BENEFITS:
Pension Plan: ESOP Stock Plan: Profit Sharing: Top Exec. Salary: $228,462   Bonus: $
Savings Plan: Y   Stock Purch. Plan: Second Exec. Salary: $215,000   Bonus: $25,000

OTHER THOUGHTS:
Apparent Top Female Officers: 3
Hot Spot for Advancement for Women/Minorities: Y

LOCATIONS: ("Y" = Yes)
West:	Southwest:	Midwest:	Southeast:	Northeast:	International:
Y					Y

SISTERS OF MERCY HEALTH SYSTEMS

www.smhs.com

Industry Group Code: 622110 Ranks within this company's industry group: Sales: 21 Profits:

Insurance/HMO/PPO:	Drugs:	Equipment/Supplies:	Hospitals/Clinics:		Services:		Health Care:	
Insurance:	Manufacturer:	Manufacturer:	Acute Care:	Y	Diagnostics:		Home Health:	
Managed Care:	Distributor:	Distributor:	Sub-Acute Care:	Y	Labs/Testing:		Long-Term Care:	Y
Utilization Mgmt.:	Specialty Pharm.:	Leasing/Finance:	Outpatient Surgery:	Y	Staffing:		Physical Therapy:	
Payment Proc.:	Vitamins/Nutri.:	Information Sys.:	Phys. Rehab. Center:		Waste Disposal:		Phys. Practice Mgmt.:	
	Clinical Trials:		Psychiatric Clinics:		Specialty Services:	Y		

TYPES OF BUSINESS:
Hospitals-General
Outpatient Care
Health Classes
Long-Term Care

BRANDS/DIVISIONS/AFFILIATES:

GROWTH PLANS/SPECIAL FEATURES:
The Sisters of Mercy Health System (Mercy), established in 1986, is one of the largest Catholic health care systems in the U.S. and serves as the parent corporation of a variety of health care facilities and services sponsored by the Sisters of Mercy of the St. Louis Regional Community. The firm has more than 4,000 licensed beds, including 18 acute care hospitals, a heart hospital, outpatient care facilities, skilled nursing, long-term residential care facilities and stand-alone clinics. Mercy operates in seven states: Arkansas, Kansas, Louisiana, Mississippi, Missouri, Oklahoma and Texas. The company also offers a variety of free and inexpensive classes at its hospitals, including a healing-through-the-arts program, babysitter skills, massage classes, infant care, CPR/first aid classes and substance abuse and terminal illness support groups.

CONTACTS:
Note: Officers with more than one job title may be intentionally listed here more than once.
Ron Ashworth, CEO
Ron Ashworth, Pres.
John Sullivan, COO
Dick Escue, CIO
Barb Meyer, VP-Corp. Comm.
Julie Hurtubise, Controller
Lynn Britton, Sr. VP
Mike McCurry, VP-Resource Optimization
Shannon Sock, VP-Health Care Solutions
Diana Silvey, Exec. Dir.-Community Outreach Services

Phone: 314-579-6100 Fax: 314-628-3723
Toll-Free:
Address: 14528 S. Outer Forty, Ste. 100, Chesterfield, MO 63017 US

FINANCIALS:
Sales and profits are in thousands of dollars—add 000 to get the full amount. Year 2004 note: Complete fiscal 2004 results were not available for all companies at press time. For this company, year 2004 is for months.

2004 Sales: $ (months)	2004 Profits: $ (months)	
2003 Sales: $2,721,900	2003 Profits: $	Stock Ticker: Nonprofit
2002 Sales: $2,392,100	2002 Profits: $	Employees: 26,000
2001 Sales: $	2001 Profits: $	Fiscal Year Ends: 12/31
2000 Sales: $	2000 Profits: $	

SALARIES/BENEFITS:
Pension Plan: ESOP Stock Plan: Profit Sharing: Top Exec. Salary: $ Bonus: $
Savings Plan: Stock Purch. Plan: Second Exec. Salary: $ Bonus: $

OTHER THOUGHTS:
Apparent Top Female Officers: 5
Hot Spot for Advancement for Women/Minorities: Y

LOCATIONS: ("Y" = Yes)
West:	Southwest:	Midwest:	Southeast:	Northeast:	International:
	Y	Y	Y		

SMITH & NEPHEW PLC

www.smith-nephew.com

Industry Group Code: 339113 Ranks within this company's industry group: Sales: 11 Profits: 11

Insurance/HMO/PPO:	Drugs:	Equipment/Supplies:	Hospitals/Clinics:	Services:	Health Care:
Insurance:	Manufacturer:	Manufacturer: Y	Acute Care:	Diagnostics:	Home Health:
Managed Care:	Distributor:	Distributor:	Sub-Acute Care:	Labs/Testing:	Long-Term Care:
Utilization Mgmt.:	Specialty Pharm.:	Leasing/Finance:	Outpatient Surgery:	Staffing:	Physical Therapy:
Payment Proc.:	Vitamins/Nutri.:	Information Sys.:	Phys. Rehab. Center:	Waste Disposal:	Phys. Practice Mgmt.:
	Clinical Trials:		Psychiatric Clinics:	Specialty Services:	

TYPES OF BUSINESS:
Medical Device Manufacturing
Orthopedic Products
Endoscopy Products
Wound Management Products

BRANDS/DIVISIONS/AFFILIATES:
Smith & Nephew Group
GENESIS II
PROFIX
SPECTRON
REFLECTION
Midland Medical Technologies

CONTACTS:
Note: Officers with more than one job title may be intentionally listed here more than once.
Christopher O'Donnell, CEO
Paul Williams, VP-Human Resources
Peter Arnold, Chief Tech. Officer
Jim Ralston, General Counsel
Peter Hooley, VP-Finance
Jim Dick, Pres.-Wound Mgmt.
Peter Huntley, Group Dir.-Indirect Markets
David Ilingworth, Pres.-Orthopedics
Jim Taylor, Pres.-Endoscopy
Dudley Eustace, Chmn.

Phone: 4420-7401-7646 Fax: 4420-7930-3353
Toll-Free:
Address: 15 Adam St, London, WC2N 6LA UK

GROWTH PLANS/SPECIAL FEATURES:
Smith & Nephew plc is the parent company of the Smith & Nephew Group, an international medical devices business organized into three global business units: orthopedics, endoscopy and advanced wound management. Orthopedic products include reconstructive joint implants, trauma products and associated clinical therapies. Reconstructive joint implants are hip, knee and shoulder joints as well as ancillary products like bone cement and mixing systems used in cemented reconstructive joint surgery. Trauma products consist of internal and external fixation devices, used in the stabilization of severe fractures. Clinical therapies include products applied in an orthopedic office or clinic setting such as growth stimulators and a joint fluid therapy product. Product lines include the GENESIS II and PROFIX knee replacements, SPECTRON cemented hip system and the REFLECTION acetabular cup system. Smith & Nephew's endoscopy business, headquartered in Andover, Massachusetts, develops and markets a range of minimally invasive surgery techniques and educational programs to treat and repair soft tissues, articulating joints, spinal discs and vascular structures. The business focuses principally on the arthroscopy sector of the endoscopy market. Arthroscopy is the minimally invasive surgery of joints, in particular the knee, hip and shoulder. Products include fluid management instruments, digital image capture, central control, multimedia broadcasting, scopes, light sources and monitors, radiofrequency wands, electromechanical and mechanical blades, and hand instruments. The company's advanced wound management business supplies products for chronic and acute skin wounds from initial wound bed preparation to full wound closure. These products are targeted particularly at chronic wounds connected with the elderly population, such as pressure sores, venous leg ulcers, diabetic foot ulcers, burns and complex surgical wounds. Smith & Nephew recently completed the acquisition of Midland Medical Technologies, the global market leader in metal-on-metal hip resurfacing.

FINANCIALS:
Sales and profits are in thousands of dollars—add 000 to get the full amount. Year 2004 note: Complete fiscal 2004 results were not available for all companies at press time. For this company, year 2004 is for 3 months.

2004 Sales: $556,600 (3 months)   2004 Profits: $73,700 (3 months)
2003 Sales: $2,102,500   2003 Profits: $264,100
2002 Sales: $1,788,600   2002 Profits: $180,600
2001 Sales: $ 2001 Profits: $
2000 Sales: $ 2000 Profits: $

Stock Ticker: Foreign
Employees: 7,451
Fiscal Year Ends: 12/31

SALARIES/BENEFITS:
Pension Plan: ESOP Stock Plan: Profit Sharing: Top Exec. Salary: $ Bonus: $
Savings Plan: Stock Purch. Plan: Second Exec. Salary: $ Bonus: $

OTHER THOUGHTS:
Apparent Top Female Officers:
Hot Spot for Advancement for Women/Minorities:

LOCATIONS: ("Y" = Yes)
West:	Southwest:	Midwest:	Southeast:	Northeast:	International:
			Y	Y	Y

Note: Financial information, benefits and other data can change quickly and may vary from those stated here.

SOLA INTERNATIONAL INC

www.sola.com

Industry Group Code: 339113 Ranks within this company's industry group: Sales: 37 Profits: 91

Insurance/HMO/PPO:	Drugs:	Equipment/Supplies:	Hospitals/Clinics:	Services:	Health Care:
Insurance:	Manufacturer:	Manufacturer: Y	Acute Care:	Diagnostics:	Home Health:
Managed Care:	Distributor:	Distributor:	Sub-Acute Care:	Labs/Testing:	Long-Term Care:
Utilization Mgmt.:	Specialty Pharm.:	Leasing/Finance:	Outpatient Surgery:	Staffing:	Physical Therapy:
Payment Proc.:	Vitamins/Nutri.:	Information Sys.:	Phys. Rehab. Center:	Waste Disposal:	Phys. Practice Mgmt.:
	Clinical Trials:		Psychiatric Clinics:	Specialty Services:	

TYPES OF BUSINESS:
Supplies-Eyeglass Lenses
Lens Coatings & Treatments

BRANDS/DIVISIONS/AFFILIATES:
Transitions
Teflon EasyCare
AO Compact
Percepta
AO ProEasy
SOLAOne
SOLAMax

CONTACTS: Note: Officers with more than one job title may be intentionally listed here more than once.
Jeremy C. Bishop, CEO
Jeremy C. Bishop, Pres.
Ronald F. Dutt, CFO
Simon Edwards, VP-Research & Dev.
Ronald F. Dutt, Exec. VP-Finance/Treas.
Barry J. Packham, Exec. VP-North America
Mark Ashcroft, Exec. VP-Europe
David Cross, VP-Asia Pacific
Gaetano Sciuto, VP-Sunlens Div.
Maurice J. Cunniffe, Chmn.

Phone: 858-509-9899 Fax: 858-509-9898
Toll-Free:
Address: 10590 W. Ocean Air Dr., Ste. 300, San Diego, CA 92130 US

GROWTH PLANS/SPECIAL FEATURES:
SOLA International, Inc. is a worldwide leader in the development of eyeglass lens designs and materials. The company has sales operations in 28 countries and distributes its products in more than 50 markets worldwide, primarily in North America, Europe and Asia. It sells over 1 million pairs of lenses per week, with one in four U.S. eyeglass wearers using SOLA lenses. SOLA focuses on value-added products with advanced design characteristics, lens coatings and treatments and thin and lightweight materials. It manufactures both plastic and glass lenses, with plastic making up approximately 96% of sales. The company's Percepta, AO Compact, SOLAMax, AO ProEasy and SOLAOne progressive lenses correct for varying distances without utilizing the segment lines of bifocals and trifocals, thus avoiding image jumps when moving from one distance zone to another. Its Transitions photochromic lenses change tint depending on the amount of light available. The company also markets and produces a variety of lens coatings and treatments, including anti-scratch and anti-reflective coatings. Its Teflon EasyCare lenses, developed through an agreement with DuPont, are anti-scratch, anti-reflective, anti-static and hydrophobic-coated.

FINANCIALS: Sales and profits are in thousands of dollars—add 000 to get the full amount. Year 2004 note: Complete fiscal 2004 results were not available for all companies at press time. For this company, year 2004 is for 12 months.

2004 Sales: $650,109 (12 months)   2004 Profits: $-13,480 (12 months)
2003 Sales: $562,700   2003 Profits: $3,966   Stock Ticker: SOL
2002 Sales: $529,500   2002 Profits: $19,100   Employees: 6,634
2001 Sales: $545,400   2001 Profits: $-66,500   Fiscal Year Ends: 3/31
2000 Sales: $543,400   2000 Profits: $700

SALARIES/BENEFITS:
Pension Plan: Y   ESOP Stock Plan: Profit Sharing: Top Exec. Salary: $525,000   Bonus: $229,500
Savings Plan: Y   Stock Purch. Plan: Second Exec. Salary: $313,500 Bonus: $104,490

OTHER THOUGHTS:
Apparent Top Female Officers:
Hot Spot for Advancement for Women/Minorities:

LOCATIONS: ("Y" = Yes)
West:	Southwest:	Midwest:	Southeast:	Northeast:	International:
Y		Y	Y		Y

Note: Financial information, benefits and other data can change quickly and may vary from those stated here.

SOLUCIENT LLC

www.solucient.com

Industry Group Code: 511200   Ranks within this company's industry group: Sales: 11   Profits:

Insurance/HMO/PPO:	Drugs:	Equipment/Supplies:	Hospitals/Clinics:	Services:	Health Care:
Insurance: Managed Care: Utilization Mgmt.: Y Payment Proc.:	Manufacturer: Distributor: Specialty Pharm.: Vitamins/Nutri.: Clinical Trials:	Manufacturer: Distributor: Leasing/Finance: Information Sys.: Y	Acute Care: Sub-Acute Care: Outpatient Surgery: Phys. Rehab. Center: Psychiatric Clinics:	Diagnostics: Labs/Testing: Staffing: Waste Disposal: Specialty Services:	Home Health: Long-Term Care: Physical Therapy: Phys. Practice Mgmt.:

TYPES OF BUSINESS:
Computer Software-Health Care
Research Databases
Decision Support Systems

BRANDS/DIVISIONS/AFFILIATES:
Peer-A-Med
Veronis Suhler Stevenson Partners
VNU N.V.
VHA, Inc.
Market Planner Plus (The)
HealthViewPlus
InpatientView
AstroSachs

CONTACTS:
Note: Officers with more than one job title may be intentionally listed here more than once.

Charles E. Leonard, CEO
Gregg Bennett, Pres.
Ted Stone, Sr. VP/CFO
Al Vega, Sr. VP-Sales
Mary Oleksiuk, Sr. VP-Human Resources
Gary Pickens, Chief Research Officer
Ken Whitaker, Sr. VP-Product Dev.
Len Dintzer, Sr. VP-Oper. & Client Fulfillment
Mary Oleksiuk, Sr. VP-Comm. & Learning
Jagruti Oza, Exec. VP/General Mgr.
Amy Mosser, Sr. VP/General Mgr.-Shared Resources
Maureen McLaughlin, VP/General Mgr.-Pharmaceutical
Pauline Reisner, Sr. VP/Mgr.-Data Assets & Custom Solutions
Charles E. Leonard, Chmn.
Graham Harries, Chief Exec.-Int'l

Phone: 847-475-7526   **Fax:** 847-475-7830
Toll-Free: 800-366-7526
Address: 1800 Sherman Ave., Evanston, IL 60201 US

GROWTH PLANS/SPECIAL FEATURES:

Solucient, LLC is a leading health care information content company that develops and markets integrated clinical information systems and products. The firm, a joint venture of Veronis Suhler Stevenson Partners, VNU N.V. and VHA, Inc., has products ranging from standardized databases to highly focused decision support systems, which assist customers in evaluating the efficacy and economics of health care delivery. Solucient maintains the health care industry's leading database, representing 77.5% of all discharges. The company's client base of more than 5,500 customers includes over 3,000 hospitals and 18 of the 20 largest pharmaceutical manufacturers. Solucient offers a range of information products used in all areas of health care, including providers, pharmaceuticals, managed care and employers. Providers, such as hospitals, rely on Solucient to measure and analyze the cost and quality of medical interventions, thereby improving strategic decision-making. Solucient offers the pharmaceutical segment of the health care industry data management, planning and direct-to-consumer information. Companies also employ Solucient's databases and products to analyze potential markets for their products. Managed care organizations use the firm's targeted claim analysis systems to avoid overpayments to providers, and organizations use Solucient's information and analysis of medical resource usage and outcomes to lower medical costs and understand health care resource use. In addition, Solucient offers benefit plan and health care claim information, which allows employers to improve performance, decision-making and management. Solucient's product titles include InpatientView, HealthViewPlus, Astro Sachs, ProviderView and the Market Planner Plus. In recent news, the company launched Peer-A-Med, an enhanced cost information and risk-adjusted episode treatment group analysis tool.

The company offers its employees flexible spending accounts and medical, vision, dental and prescription drug plans.

FINANCIALS:
Sales and profits are in thousands of dollars—add 000 to get the full amount. Year 2004 note: Complete fiscal 2004 results were not available for all companies at press time. For this company, year 2004 is for months.

2004 Sales: $ (months)
2003 Sales: $50,000
2002 Sales: $100,000
2001 Sales: $63,000
2000 Sales: $82,900

2004 Profits: $ (months)
2003 Profits: $
2002 Profits: $
2001 Profits: $-48,600
2000 Profits: $-37,000

Stock Ticker: Joint Venture
Employees: 600
Fiscal Year Ends: 12/31

SALARIES/BENEFITS:
Pension Plan: ESOP Stock Plan: Profit Sharing: Top Exec. Salary: $ Bonus: $
Savings Plan: Y   Stock Purch. Plan: Second Exec. Salary: $ Bonus: $

OTHER THOUGHTS:
Apparent Top Female Officers: 4
Hot Spot for Advancement for Women/Minorities: Y

LOCATIONS: ("Y" = Yes)
West:	Southwest:	Midwest:	Southeast:	Northeast:	International:
Y		Y		Y	Y

SONIC INNOVATIONS INC

www.sonici.com

Industry Group Code: 339113 **Ranks within this company's industry group:** Sales: 97 Profits: 101

Insurance/HMO/PPO:	Drugs:	Equipment/Supplies:	Hospitals/Clinics:	Services:	Health Care:
Insurance:	Manufacturer:	Manufacturer: Y	Acute Care:	Diagnostics:	Home Health:
Managed Care:	Distributor:	Distributor: Y	Sub-Acute Care:	Labs/Testing:	Long-Term Care:
Utilization Mgmt.:	Specialty Pharm.:	Leasing/Finance:	Outpatient Surgery:	Staffing:	Physical Therapy:
Payment Proc.:	Vitamins/Nutri.:	Information Sys.:	Phys. Rehab. Center:	Waste Disposal:	Phys. Practice Mgmt.:
	Clinical Trials:		Psychiatric Clinics:	Specialty Services:	

TYPES OF BUSINESS:
Hearing Aids

BRANDS/DIVISIONS/AFFILIATES:
Altair
Adesso
Natura
Tribute
Conforma
Quartet
OMNI-ReSound ApS

CONTACTS:
Note: Officers with more than one job title may be intentionally listed here more than once.

Andrew G. Raguskus, CEO
Andrew G. Raguskus, Pres.
Stephen L. Wilson, Sr. VP/CFO
Robert P. Wolf, VP-Mktg. & Sales
Gregory N. Koskowich, VP-Research & Dev.
Weston O. Ison, VP-Oper. & Quality
Jerry L. Dabell, VP-Bus. Dev.
Daniel Roussel, Pres.-European Oper.
Jorgen Heide, VP-Licensing Div.
Michael A. James, Sr. VP-Worldwide Commercial Oper.
Kevin J. Ryan, Chmn.
Jorgen Heide, VP-Int'l

Phone: 801-365-2800 **Fax:** 801-365-3000
Toll-Free: 888-678-4327
Address: 2795 E. Cottonwood Pkwy., Salt Lake City, UT 84121 US

GROWTH PLANS/SPECIAL FEATURES:

Sonic Innovations, Inc. designs, develops, manufactures and markets advanced digital hearing aids. The firm's patented digital signal processing (DSP) platform is the smallest single-chip platform ever installed in a hearing aid. Sonic's Natura, Altair, Tribute and Quartet product lines are among the smallest products available today and conform to the five common models for hearing aids: behind-the-ear, in-the-ear, in-the-canal, mini-canal and completely-in-the-canal (CIC). Its Conforma and Adesso programmable, instant-fit CIC models, are the smallest digital hearing aids available today. Outside the U.S., Sonic sells finished hearing aids and hearing aid kits primarily to distributors. Subsidiary OMNI-ReSound ApS, acquired in 2002, is a Denmark-based distributor of hearing aid and tinnitus products. The company holds 15 U.S. patents, with 27 applications pending. Sonic's proprietary DSP platform contains a set of algorithms that pre-process incoming sound and present it to the impaired cochlea in a way that helps to restore natural loudness perception and preserves cues necessary for speech understanding. This platform also processes sound at a faster rate than other digital hearing aids. The DSP chip contains up to nine independent compression channels programmable with one-decibel accuracy, allowing the products to be personalized for each hearing loss with unprecedented accuracy.

Sonic offers employees competitive salaries, a health and dental plan and flexible work schedules.

FINANCIALS:
Sales and profits are in thousands of dollars—add 000 to get the full amount. Year 2004 note: Complete fiscal 2004 results were not available for all companies at press time. For this company, year 2004 is for 9 months.

2004 Sales: $73,100 (9 months)   2004 Profits: $1,552 (9 months)
2003 Sales: $87,690   2003 Profits: $ 376
2002 Sales: $68,000   2002 Profits: $ 32
2001 Sales: $57,300   2001 Profits: $-5,600
2000 Sales: $51,700   2000 Profits: $-3,200

Stock Ticker: SNCI
Employees: 586
Fiscal Year Ends: 12/31

SALARIES/BENEFITS:
Pension Plan: ESOP Stock Plan: Profit Sharing: Top Exec. Salary: $284,769   Bonus: $143,000
Savings Plan: Y   Stock Purch. Plan: Y   Second Exec. Salary: $246,154   Bonus: $64,067

OTHER THOUGHTS:
Apparent Top Female Officers:
Hot Spot for Advancement for Women/Minorities:

LOCATIONS: ("Y" = Yes)
West:	Southwest:	Midwest:	Southeast:	Northeast:	International:
Y		Y			Y

SPAN AMERICA MEDICAL SYSTEMS INC

www.spanamerica.com

Industry Group Code: 339113 Ranks within this company's industry group: Sales: 118 Profits: 97

Insurance/HMO/PPO:	Drugs:	Equipment/Supplies:	Hospitals/Clinics:	Services:	Health Care:
Insurance:	Manufacturer:	Manufacturer: Y	Acute Care:	Diagnostics:	Home Health:
Managed Care:	Distributor: Y	Distributor: Y	Sub-Acute Care:	Labs/Testing:	Long-Term Care:
Utilization Mgmt.:	Specialty Pharm.:	Leasing/Finance:	Outpatient Surgery:	Staffing:	Physical Therapy:
Payment Proc.:	Vitamins/Nutri.:	Information Sys.:	Phys. Rehab. Center:	Waste Disposal:	Phys. Practice Mgmt.:
	Clinical Trials:		Psychiatric Clinics:	Specialty Services:	

TYPES OF BUSINESS:
Supplies-Therapeutic Mattresses
Polyurethane Foam Products
Wound Management Products
Intravenous Catheters
Skin Care Products

BRANDS/DIVISIONS/AFFILIATES:
PressureGuard
Secure IV
Geo-Matt
Span+Aids
Louisville Bedding Products, Inc.
TerryFoam
SELAN+ Zinc Oxide
PressureGuard Easy Air

CONTACTS:
Note: Officers with more than one job title may be intentionally listed here more than once.

James D. Ferguson, CEO
James D. Ferguson, Pres.
Richard C. Coggins, CFO
Clyde A. Shew, VP-Medical Sales & Mktg.
James R. O'Reagan, VP-Research & Dev.
Erick C. Herlong, VP-Oper.
Richard C. Coggins, VP-Finance
Robert E. Ackley, VP-Custom Products
Richard C. Coggins, Corp. Sec.
Wanda J. Totton, VP-Quality

Phone: 864-288-8877 Fax: 864-288-8692
Toll-Free: 800-888-6752
Address: 70 Commerce Center, Greenville, SC 29606 US

GROWTH PLANS/SPECIAL FEATURES:
Span-America Medical Systems, Inc. manufactures and distributes a variety of polyurethane foam products for the medical, industrial and custom products markets under the brand names PressureGuard, Geo-Mattress, Geo-Matt, Span-Aids, Isch-Dish and Selan. The company's principal medical products consist of support surfaces, including polyurethane foam mattress overlays, powered and non-powered therapeutic replacement mattresses and patient positioning and seating products. These products are designed to provide patients with greater comfort and to assist in treating patients who have or are susceptible to pressure ulcers. The company's products are marketed to all health care settings, including acute care hospitals, long-term care facilities and home health care providers, primarily in North America. The company's patient positioning product line includes more than 300 items that aid in relieving the basic patient positioning problems of elevation, immobilization, muscle contracture and foot or leg rotation. Consumer products include pillows, terryfoam products, consumer bedding and mattress overlays. These products are distributed exclusively thorough Louisville Bedding Products, Inc. The industrial product line consists primarily of foam packaging and cushioning materials, as well as foam products used for flotation, sound insulation and gaskets. The company also produces peripheral intravenous catheters under the brand name Secure IV. In addition, the firm produces SELAN+ Zinc Oxide creams and lotions for use in treating rashes and other skin conditions caused by skin overlap and incontinence.

FINANCIALS:
Sales and profits are in thousands of dollars—add 000 to get the full amount. Year 2004 note: Complete fiscal 2004 results were not available for all companies at press time. For this company, year 2004 is for 9 months.

2004 Sales: $36,277 (9 months)	2004 Profits: $1,389 (9 months)	Stock Ticker: SPAN
2003 Sales: $41,575	2003 Profits: $1,399	Employees: 264
2002 Sales: $33,500	2002 Profits: $1,700	Fiscal Year Ends: 9/30
2001 Sales: $29,100	2001 Profits: $1,300	
2000 Sales: $26,600	2000 Profits: $1,000	

SALARIES/BENEFITS:
Pension Plan:	ESOP Stock Plan:	Profit Sharing:	Top Exec. Salary: $201,667	Bonus: $58,880
Savings Plan: Y	Stock Purch. Plan:		Second Exec. Salary: $145,513	Bonus: $35,829

OTHER THOUGHTS:
Apparent Top Female Officers: 1
Hot Spot for Advancement for Women/Minorities:

LOCATIONS: ("Y" = Yes)
West:	Southwest:	Midwest:	Southeast:	Northeast:	International:
Y			Y	Y	

SPECIALTY LABORATORIES INC

www.specialtylabs.com

Industry Group Code: 621511 Ranks within this company's industry group: Sales: 8 Profits: 7

Insurance/HMO/PPO:	Drugs:	Equipment/Supplies:	Hospitals/Clinics:	Services:		Health Care:	
Insurance: Managed Care: Utilization Mgmt.: Payment Proc.:	Manufacturer: Distributor: Specialty Pharm.: Vitamins/Nutri.: Clinical Trials:	Manufacturer: Distributor: Leasing/Finance: Information Sys.:	Acute Care: Sub-Acute Care: Outpatient Surgery: Phys. Rehab. Center: Psychiatric Clinics:	Diagnostics: Labs/Testing: Staffing: Waste Disposal: Specialty Services:	Y	Home Health: Long-Term Care: Physical Therapy: Phys. Practice Mgmt.:	

TYPES OF BUSINESS:
Clinical Reference Laboratory
Assays

BRANDS/DIVISIONS/AFFILIATES:

CONTACTS:
Note: Officers with more than one job title may be intentionally listed here more than once.
Douglas S. Harrington, CEO
Kevin R. Sayer, Exec. VP/CFO
Dan R. Angress, Sr. VP-Mktg. & Client Support
Cynthia K. French, VP/Chief Science Officer
Robert M. Harman, VP/CIO
Nicholas R. Simmons, VP/General Counsel
Cheryl G. Gallarda, VP-Bus. Oper.
Thomas J. Kosco, VP-Corp. Dev.
Michael C. Dugan, VP/Co-Laboratory Dir.
Mark R. Willig, VP-Sales
Douglas S. Harrington, Co-Laboratory Dir.
Maryam Sadri, Laboratory Oper.
Richard E. Belluzzo, Chmn.

Phone: 310-828-6543 **Fax:** 310-828-6634
Toll-Free: 800-421-7110
Address: 2211 Michigan Ave., Santa Monica, CA 90404-3900 US

GROWTH PLANS/SPECIAL FEATURES:

Specialty Laboratories, Inc. (SL) is a leading research-based clinical laboratory, predominantly focused on developing and performing esoteric clinical laboratory tests, referred to as assays. The firm offers a comprehensive menu of 2,500 assays, many of which were developed through its internal research and development efforts. These esoteric assays are complex, comprehensive and unique tests used to diagnose, evaluate and monitor patients in the areas of allergy and immunology, cardiology and coagulation, endocrinology, gastroenterology, genetics, infectious disease, nephrology, neurology, OB/GYN, oncology/hematology, pathology, pediatrics, rheumatology and toxicology. They are often performed on sophisticated instruments by highly skilled personnel and therefore offered by a limited number of clinical laboratories. Assays include procedures in the areas of molecular diagnostics, protein chemistry, cellular immunology and advanced microbiology. Commonly ordered assays include viral and bacterial detection and drug therapy monitoring assays, autoimmune panels and complex cancer evaluations.

FINANCIALS:
Sales and profits are in thousands of dollars—add 000 to get the full amount. Year 2004 note: Complete fiscal 2004 results were not available for all companies at press time. For this company, year 2004 is for 9 months.

2004 Sales: $89,194 (9 months)	2004 Profits: $-5,603 (9 months)	
2003 Sales: $119,653	2003 Profits: $-6,361	**Stock Ticker:** SP
2002 Sales: $140,200	2002 Profits: $-13,400	Employees: 683
2001 Sales: $175,200	2001 Profits: $13,100	Fiscal Year Ends: 12/31
2000 Sales: $153,200	2000 Profits: $8,700	

SALARIES/BENEFITS:
Pension Plan:	ESOP Stock Plan:	Profit Sharing:	Top Exec. Salary: $422,908	Bonus: $252,000
Savings Plan: Y	Stock Purch. Plan:		Second Exec. Salary: $262,000	Bonus: $120,120

OTHER THOUGHTS:
Apparent Top Female Officers: 3
Hot Spot for Advancement for Women/Minorities: Y

LOCATIONS: ("Y" = Yes)
West:	Southwest:	Midwest:	Southeast:	Northeast:	International:
Y				Y	

SPECTRANETICS CORP

www.spectranetics.com

Industry Group Code: 339113   Ranks within this company's industry group: Sales: 128   Profits: 99

Insurance/HMO/PPO:	Drugs:	Equipment/Supplies:		Hospitals/Clinics:	Services:	Health Care:
Insurance:	Manufacturer:	Manufacturer:	Y	Acute Care:	Diagnostics:	Home Health:
Managed Care:	Distributor:	Distributor:		Sub-Acute Care:	Labs/Testing:	Long-Term Care:
Utilization Mgmt.:	Specialty Pharm.:	Leasing/Finance:		Outpatient Surgery:	Staffing:	Physical Therapy:
Payment Proc.:	Vitamins/Nutri.:	Information Sys.:		Phys. Rehab. Center:	Waste Disposal:	Phys. Practice Mgmt.:
	Clinical Trials:			Psychiatric Clinics:	Specialty Services:	

TYPES OF BUSINESS:
Equipment-Atherosclerosis Treatments
Excimer Lasers Systems

BRANDS/DIVISIONS/AFFILIATES:
CVX-300
LACI
Extended FAMILI

CONTACTS: Note: Officers with more than one job title may be intentionally listed here more than once.
John G. Schulte, CEO
John G. Schulte, Pres.
Guy A. Childs, VP/CFO
Christopher Reiser, VP-Clinical Research
Christopher Reiser, VP-Tech.
Lawrence E. Martel, VP-Oper.
Paul C. Samek, VP-Finance
Adrian E. Elfe, VP-Quality Assurance & Regulatory Affairs
Emile J. Geisenheimer, Chmn.

Phone: 719-633-8333   **Fax:** 719-633-8791
Toll-Free: 800-633-0960
Address: 96 Talamine Ct., Colorado Springs, CO 80907-5186 US

GROWTH PLANS/SPECIAL FEATURES:
Spectranetics Corp. develops, manufactures and markets a proprietary excimer laser system and related accessory products for the treatment of certain coronary and vascular conditions. Excimer laser technology delivers comparatively cool ultraviolet light in short, controlled energy pulses to ablate or remove tissue. The firm's laser system includes the CVX-300 laser unit and various fiber-optic delivery devices, including disposable catheters and sheaths. This is the only excimer laser system approved in the U.S. and Europe for use in multiple, minimally invasive cardiovascular applications. The system is used in atherectomy procedures to open clogged or obstructed arteries, as well as to remove lead wires from patients with pacemakers or implantable cardioverter-defibrillators. The company also has approval to market its products in several key international markets, including Japan. Since it received FDA approval in 1993, over 50,000 patients have been treated with Spectranetics' excimer laser technology. The firm believes this system offers benefits including reduced procedure time, ease of use, small size and easy set-up. Spectranetics recently received FDA approval for the use of its LACI system (Laser Angioplasty for Critical Limb Ischemia), designed to treat patients suffering from total blockages in their leg arteries. The company also recently commenced an FDA-approved clinical trial of Extended FAMILI (Flow in Acute Myocardial Infarction after Laser Intervention), for treating heart-attack patients.

FINANCIALS: Sales and profits are in thousands of dollars—add 000 to get the full amount. Year 2004 note: Complete fiscal 2004 results were not available for all companies at press time. For this company, year 2004 is for 6 months.

2004 Sales: $16,444 (6 months)
2003 Sales: $27,869
2002 Sales: $28,100
2001 Sales: $27,800
2000 Sales: $26,900

2004 Profits: $ 536 (6 months)
2003 Profits: $ 929
2002 Profits: $-1,600
2001 Profits: $ 600
2000 Profits: $-8,700

Stock Ticker: SPNC
Employees: 144
Fiscal Year Ends: 12/31

SALARIES/BENEFITS:
Pension Plan: ESOP Stock Plan: Profit Sharing: Top Exec. Salary: $282,692   Bonus: $121,875
Savings Plan: Y   Stock Purch. Plan: Second Exec. Salary: $214,292   Bonus: $81,250

OTHER THOUGHTS:
Apparent Top Female Officers:
Hot Spot for Advancement for Women/Minorities:

LOCATIONS: ("Y" = Yes)
West:	Southwest:	Midwest:	Southeast:	Northeast:	International:
Y					Y

SPECTRUM HEALTH

www.spectrum-health.org

Industry Group Code: 622110 **Ranks within this company's industry group:** Sales: 37 Profits:

Insurance/HMO/PPO:	Drugs:	Equipment/Supplies:	Hospitals/Clinics:		Services:		Health Care:	
Insurance:	Manufacturer:	Manufacturer:	Acute Care:	Y	Diagnostics:		Home Health:	
Managed Care: Y	Distributor:	Distributor:	Sub-Acute Care:	Y	Labs/Testing:		Long-Term Care:	Y
Utilization Mgmt.:	Specialty Pharm.:	Leasing/Finance:	Outpatient Surgery:	Y	Staffing:		Physical Therapy:	
Payment Proc.:	Vitamins/Nutri.:	Information Sys.:	Phys. Rehab. Center:	Y	Waste Disposal:		Phys. Practice Mgmt.:	
	Clinical Trials:		Psychiatric Clinics:		Specialty Services:			

TYPES OF BUSINESS:
Hospitals-General
Burn Center
Poison Center
Trauma Center
Neonatal Center
HMO
Long-Term Care
Outpatient Centers

BRANDS/DIVISIONS/AFFILIATES:
Renucci Hospitality House
DeVos Children's Hospital
Priority Health
Kent Community Campus

GROWTH PLANS/SPECIAL FEATURES:
Spectrum Health is a health system in western Michigan with more than 140 service areas and a total of 2,000 beds, including a Level 1 trauma center, a neonatal center, a burn center, a poison center and the Renucci Hospitality House. The firm also operates nine acute care hospitals that provide diagnostic, outpatient, inpatient and emergency care, including the DeVos Children's Hospital, the only children's hospital in west Michigan, and Kent Community Campus, which provides long-term care for patients recovering from major illnesses and complex medical conditions. In addition to Spectrum's primary care locations, the firm operates over 100 outpatient sites for diagnostics, treatment, imaging services, surgery, rehabilitation and laboratory services. The company's operations also include Priority Health, an HMO. In recent news, Spectrum was named one of the Top 100 Cardiovascular Hospitals in the U.S. by Solucient.

CONTACTS:
Note: Officers with more than one job title may be intentionally listed here more than once.
Richard C. Breon, CEO
Richard C. Breon, Pres.
Michael P. Freed, CFO
Patrick O'Hare, CIO
Bruce Rossman, VP-Corp. Comm.
Shawn M. Ulreich, Chief Nursing Officer
Matt Van Vranken, Pres.-Spectrum Health Hospitals

Phone: 616-391-1774 **Fax:** 616-391-2780
Toll-Free: 888-989-7999
Address: 100 Michigan St. NE, Grand Rapids, MI 49503 US

FINANCIALS:
Sales and profits are in thousands of dollars—add 000 to get the full amount. Year 2004 note: Complete fiscal 2004 results were not available for all companies at press time. For this company, year 2004 is for 12 months.

2004 Sales: $1,867,800 (12 months)   2004 Profits: $ (12 months)
2003 Sales: $1,537,600   2003 Profits: $
2002 Sales: $1,372,900   2002 Profits: $
2001 Sales: $ 2001 Profits: $
2000 Sales: $ 2000 Profits: $

Stock Ticker: Nonprofit
Employees: 14,000
Fiscal Year Ends: 6/30

SALARIES/BENEFITS:
Pension Plan: ESOP Stock Plan: Profit Sharing: Top Exec. Salary: $ Bonus: $
Savings Plan: Stock Purch. Plan: Second Exec. Salary: $ Bonus: $

OTHER THOUGHTS:
Apparent Top Female Officers:
Hot Spot for Advancement for Women/Minorities:

LOCATIONS: ("Y" = Yes)
West:	Southwest:	Midwest:	Southeast:	Northeast:	International:
		Y			

Note: Financial information, benefits and other data can change quickly and may vary from those stated here.

SRI/SURGICAL EXPRESS INC

www.surgicalexpress.com

Industry Group Code: 339113 **Ranks within this company's industry group:** Sales: 98 Profits: 107

Insurance/HMO/PPO:	Drugs:	Equipment/Supplies:	Hospitals/Clinics:	Services:	Health Care:
Insurance:	Manufacturer:	Manufacturer:	Acute Care:	Diagnostics:	Home Health:
Managed Care:	Distributor: Y	Distributor:	Sub-Acute Care:	Labs/Testing:	Long-Term Care:
Utilization Mgmt.:	Specialty Pharm.:	Leasing/Finance:	Outpatient Surgery:	Staffing:	Physical Therapy:
Payment Proc.:	Vitamins/Nutri.:	Information Sys.:	Phys. Rehab. Center:	Waste Disposal:	Phys. Practice Mgmt.:
	Clinical Trials:		Psychiatric Clinics:	Specialty Services: Y	

TYPES OF BUSINESS:
Supplies-Surgery
Surgical Delivery Services
Disposable Accessory Kits

BRANDS/DIVISIONS/AFFILIATES:

CONTACTS:
Note: Officers with more than one job title may be intentionally listed here more than once.
Alex H. Edwards, Pres.
Charles L. Pope, CFO
Gene Kirtser, VP-Mktg.
Gene Kirtser, VP-Bus. Dev.

Phone: 813-891-9550 **Fax:** 813-925-8388
Toll-Free:
Address: 12425 Race Track Rd., Tampa, FL 33626 US

GROWTH PLANS/SPECIAL FEATURES:
SRI/Surgical Express, Inc. supplies hospitals and surgery centers with a comprehensive daily delivery surgical supply service, reducing hospital and surgery centers' processing costs and their investment in surgical products. SRI offers daily delivery and retrieval of its reusable surgical products, including gowns, towels, drapes, basins and instruments. The company collects, sorts, cleans, inspects, packages, sterilizes and delivers its products on a just-in-time basis. It complements its products with cost-effective disposable accessory packs and individual sterile disposable items. SRI also offers an integrated closed-loop reprocessing service that uses two of the most technologically advanced reusable textiles for gowns and drapes: a Gore surgical barrier fabric, which is breathable yet liquid-proof and provides a viral and bacterial barrier; and an advanced microfiber polyester surgical fabric, which is liquid- and bacteria-resistant. SRI continues to develop additional instrument procedure programs, including one for laparoscopic procedures. The firm serves a base of approximately 400 hospitals and centers in 25 states.

The firm's employee benefits include health, dental, vision and life insurance, a prescription program, savings bonds, educational assistance and paid jury duty.

FINANCIALS:
Sales and profits are in thousands of dollars—add 000 to get the full amount. Year 2004 note: Complete fiscal 2004 results were not available for all companies at press time. For this company, year 2004 is for 9 months.

2004 Sales: $69,064 (9 months)	2004 Profits: $ 198 (9 months)	**Stock Ticker:** STRC
2003 Sales: $86,474	2003 Profits: $- 499	Employees: 922
2002 Sales: $86,600	2002 Profits: $2,500	Fiscal Year Ends: 12/31
2001 Sales: $86,400	2001 Profits: $5,100	
2000 Sales: $77,800	2000 Profits: $4,600	

SALARIES/BENEFITS:
Pension Plan:	ESOP Stock Plan:	Profit Sharing:	Top Exec. Salary: $300,000	Bonus: $50,000
Savings Plan: Y	Stock Purch. Plan:		Second Exec. Salary: $192,308	Bonus: $32,000

OTHER THOUGHTS:
Apparent Top Female Officers:
Hot Spot for Advancement for Women/Minorities:

LOCATIONS: ("Y" = Yes)
West:	Southwest:	Midwest:	Southeast:	Northeast:	International:
Y	Y	Y	Y	Y	

SSL INTERNATIONAL

www.ssl-international.com

Industry Group Code: 339113 **Ranks within this company's industry group:** Sales: 28 Profits: 39

Insurance/HMO/PPO:	Drugs:	Equipment/Supplies:	Hospitals/Clinics:	Services:	Health Care:
Insurance:	Manufacturer: Y	Manufacturer: Y	Acute Care:	Diagnostics:	Home Health:
Managed Care:	Distributor:	Distributor:	Sub-Acute Care:	Labs/Testing:	Long-Term Care:
Utilization Mgmt.:	Specialty Pharm.:	Leasing/Finance:	Outpatient Surgery:	Staffing:	Physical Therapy:
Payment Proc.:	Vitamins/Nutri.:	Information Sys.:	Phys. Rehab. Center:	Waste Disposal:	Phys. Practice Mgmt.:
	Clinical Trials:		Psychiatric Clinics:	Specialty Services:	

TYPES OF BUSINESS:
Health Care Products
Condoms
Footcare Products
Oral Analgesics
Cough Medicine
Mother & Baby Products

BRANDS/DIVISIONS/AFFILIATES:
Durex
Scholl
Syndol
Meltus
Sauber
Mister Baby

GROWTH PLANS/SPECIAL FEATURES:
SSL International plc, based in London, manufactures and distributes health care products under the Durex, Scholl, Syndol, Meltus, Sauber and Mister Baby name brands. The firm sells its products in more than 35 countries and has manufacturing capabilities in Thailand, Spain and the U.K., as well as joint-venture manufacturing in India and China. Durex is the market leader in branded condoms with a 24% market share. The Scholl brand offers both footcare and footwear and includes products for blisters and corns, foot odor and aching feet, as well as exfoliating and moisturizing foot skincare products. Syndol is the U.K.'s fastest-growing adult oral analgesic. Meltus offers both child- and adult-strength cough medicine and has recently been reintroduced to the U.K. market. Sauber makes and markets compression hosiery and women's deodorant products. Mister Baby offers a range of mother and baby products, such as bottles and toys, sold in southern Europe. The firm has recently sold several of it companies, including its medical and industrial gloves division; Silipos, which consisted of gel-based products for prosthetic, orthopedic and skin care applications; and the Regent Infection Control business.

CONTACTS:
Note: Officers with more than one job title may be intentionally listed here more than once.
Gary Watts, CEO
Jan Young, VP-Corp. Comm.

Phone: 020-7367-5760   **Fax:** 020-7367-5790
Toll-Free:
Address: 35 New Bridge St., London, EC4V 6BW UK

FINANCIALS:
Sales and profits are in thousands of dollars—add 000 to get the full amount. Year 2004 note: Complete fiscal 2004 results were not available for all companies at press time. For this company, year 2004 is for months.

2004 Sales: $ (months)	2004 Profits: $ (months)	
2003 Sales: $982,000	2003 Profits: $39,000	**Stock Ticker:** Foreign
2002 Sales: $844,500	2002 Profits: $-19,000	Employees: 6,928
2001 Sales: $	2001 Profits: $	Fiscal Year Ends:
2000 Sales: $	2000 Profits: $	

SALARIES/BENEFITS:
| Pension Plan: | ESOP Stock Plan: | Profit Sharing: | Top Exec. Salary: $ | Bonus: $ |
| Savings Plan: | Stock Purch. Plan: | | Second Exec. Salary: $ | Bonus: $ |

OTHER THOUGHTS:
Apparent Top Female Officers: 1
Hot Spot for Advancement for Women/Minorities:

LOCATIONS: ("Y" = Yes)
| West: | Southwest: | Midwest: | Southeast: | Northeast: | International: Y |

SSM HEALTH CARE SYSTEM INC

www.ssmhc.com

Industry Group Code: 622110   Ranks within this company's industry group: Sales: 33   Profits:

Insurance/HMO/PPO:	Drugs:	Equipment/Supplies:	Hospitals/Clinics:		Services:		Health Care:	
Insurance:	Manufacturer:	Manufacturer:	Acute Care:	Y	Diagnostics:		Home Health:	
Managed Care: Y	Distributor:	Distributor:	Sub-Acute Care:		Labs/Testing:		Long-Term Care:	Y
Utilization Mgmt.:	Specialty Pharm.:	Leasing/Finance:	Outpatient Surgery:		Staffing:		Physical Therapy:	
Payment Proc.:	Vitamins/Nutri.:	Information Sys.:	Phys. Rehab. Center:		Waste Disposal:		Phys. Practice Mgmt.:	
	Clinical Trials:		Psychiatric Clinics:		Specialty Services:			

TYPES OF BUSINESS:
Hospitals-General
Nursing Homes
HMO

BRANDS/DIVISIONS/AFFILIATES:
Franciscan Sisters of Mary
Premier Medical Insurance Group, Inc.

GROWTH PLANS/SPECIAL FEATURES:
SSM Health Care (SSMHC), sponsored by the Franciscan Sisters of Mary, is one of the largest Catholic health systems in the country. The firm owns and manages 20 acute care hospitals and three nursing homes in Missouri, Illinois, Wisconsin and Oklahoma, with a total of 5,321 licensed beds. SSMHC also owns an interest in Premier Medical Insurance Group, Inc., one of Wisconsin's largest health maintenance organizations. SSMHC has been active for more than 125 years, beginning in 1877 when five catholic nuns fleeing religious persecution in Germany settled in St. Louis, Missouri in the midst of a smallpox epidemic and established a community hospital.

CONTACTS:
Note: Officers with more than one job title may be intentionally listed here more than once.

Mary Jean Ryan, CEO
Mary Jean Ryan, Pres.
William C. Schoenhard, COO
Steven M. Barney, Sr. VP-Human Resources
Thomas K. Langston, VP-IT
William P. Thomson, VP-Strategy
Kris A. Zimmer, Sr. VP-Finance
Dixie L. Platt, Sr. VP-Mission & External Affairs
James Sanger, Regional Pres.
Mary Stamonn-Harrison, Regional Pres.
Ronald L. Levy, Regional Pres.

Phone: 314-994-7800   Fax: 314-994-7900
Toll-Free:
Address: 477 N. Lindbergh Blvd., St. Louis, MO 63141 US

FINANCIALS:
Sales and profits are in thousands of dollars—add 000 to get the full amount. Year 2004 note: Complete fiscal 2004 results were not available for all companies at press time. For this company, year 2004 is for months.

2004 Sales: $ (months)	2004 Profits: $ (months)	Stock Ticker: Nonprofit
2003 Sales: $1,900,000	2003 Profits: $	Employees: 23,300
2002 Sales: $1,832,300	2002 Profits: $	Fiscal Year Ends: 12/31
2001 Sales: $	2001 Profits: $	
2000 Sales: $	2000 Profits: $	

SALARIES/BENEFITS:
Pension Plan: ESOP Stock Plan: Profit Sharing: Top Exec. Salary: $ Bonus: $
Savings Plan: Stock Purch. Plan: Second Exec. Salary: $ Bonus: $

OTHER THOUGHTS:
Apparent Top Female Officers: 4
Hot Spot for Advancement for Women/Minorities: Y

LOCATIONS: ("Y" = Yes)
| West: | Southwest: | Midwest: Y | Southeast: Y | Northeast: | International: |

ST JUDE CHILDRENS RESEARCH HOSPITAL
www.stjude.org

Industry Group Code: 622110 Ranks within this company's industry group: Sales: 43 Profits: 18

Insurance/HMO/PPO:	Drugs:	Equipment/Supplies:	Hospitals/Clinics:	Services:	Health Care:
Insurance:	Manufacturer:	Manufacturer:	Acute Care: Y	Diagnostics:	Home Health:
Managed Care:	Distributor:	Distributor:	Sub-Acute Care:	Labs/Testing:	Long-Term Care:
Utilization Mgmt.:	Specialty Pharm.:	Leasing/Finance:	Outpatient Surgery:	Staffing:	Physical Therapy:
Payment Proc.:	Vitamins/Nutri.:	Information Sys.:	Phys. Rehab. Center:	Waste Disposal:	Phys. Practice Mgmt.:
	Clinical Trials:		Psychiatric Clinics:	Specialty Services: Y	

TYPES OF BUSINESS:
Pediatric Cancer Research & Treatment

BRANDS/DIVISIONS/AFFILIATES:
ALSAC
Children's Infection Defense Center
International Outreach Program

CONTACTS:
Note: Officers with more than one job title may be intentionally listed here more than once.
Arthur W. Nienhuis, CEO
John P. Moses, Pres.
John Nash, COO
Michael Canarios, VP/CFO
John P. Moses, Chmn.

Phone: 901-495-3300 **Fax:** 901-495-3103
Toll-Free:
Address: 332 N. Lauderdale, Memphis, TN 38105 US

GROWTH PLANS/SPECIAL FEATURES:
St. Jude Children's Research Hospital, located in Memphis, Tennessee, is one of the world's premier centers for research and treatment of catastrophic diseases in children, primarily pediatric cancers. St. Jude's fundraising arm, ALSAC (American Lebanese Syrian Associated Charities), the fourth-largest health care charity in the country, covers costs of treatment not covered by insurance and all costs of treatment for those who have no insurance, including lodging, travel and food. The hospital sees about 4,600 patients yearly from every state and more than 60 countries. St. Jude has been on the cutting edge of research since its founding by entertainer Danny Thomas in 1962. The hospital developed a groundbreaking combination therapy for children with acute lymphoblastic leukemia, the most common form of childhood cancer, which changed leukemia therapy worldwide and increased the survival rate from 4% at the hospital's opening to 80% today. St. Jude has also developed groundbreaking treatments that have dramatically increased survival rates for brain tumors, solid tumors, Hodgkin disease, non-Hodgkin lymphoma and many other catastrophic diseases, including a unique procedure allowing children to receive bone-marrow transplants from a parent without an exact match. Current research at the hospital is focused on work in bone-marrow transplantation, gene therapy, biochemistry of cancerous cells, DNA research and a new HIV vaccine currently being tested to trigger an immune response capable of preventing HIV infection. In 1996, St. Jude's Dr. Peter Doherty won the Nobel Prize for Medicine for his work on the development and function of the immune system. St. Jude is currently undergoing a five-year, $1-billion expansion which includes the establishment of the Children's Infection Defense Center and the expansion of the International Outreach Program.

FINANCIALS:
Sales and profits are in thousands of dollars—add 000 to get the full amount. Year 2004 note: Complete fiscal 2004 results were not available for all companies at press time. For this company, year 2004 is for months.

2004 Sales: $ (months) 2004 Profits: $ (months)
2003 Sales: $450,800 2003 Profits: $17,900
2002 Sales: $324,600 2002 Profits: $
2001 Sales: $ 2001 Profits: $
2000 Sales: $ 2000 Profits: $

Stock Ticker: Nonprofit
Employees: 2,500
Fiscal Year Ends:

SALARIES/BENEFITS:
Pension Plan: ESOP Stock Plan: Profit Sharing: Top Exec. Salary: $ Bonus: $
Savings Plan: Stock Purch. Plan: Second Exec. Salary: $ Bonus: $

OTHER THOUGHTS:
Apparent Top Female Officers:
Hot Spot for Advancement for Women/Minorities:

LOCATIONS: ("Y" = Yes)
West	Southwest	Midwest	Southeast	Northeast	International
			Y		

ST JUDE MEDICAL INC

www.sjm.com

Industry Group Code: 339113 **Ranks within this company's industry group:** Sales: 14 Profits: 8

Insurance/HMO/PPO:	Drugs:	Equipment/Supplies:	Hospitals/Clinics:	Services:	Health Care:
Insurance:	Manufacturer:	Manufacturer: Y	Acute Care:	Diagnostics:	Home Health:
Managed Care:	Distributor:	Distributor:	Sub-Acute Care:	Labs/Testing:	Long-Term Care:
Utilization Mgmt.:	Specialty Pharm.:	Leasing/Finance:	Outpatient Surgery:	Staffing:	Physical Therapy:
Payment Proc.:	Vitamins/Nutri.:	Information Sys.:	Phys. Rehab. Center:	Waste Disposal:	Phys. Practice Mgmt.:
	Clinical Trials:		Psychiatric Clinics:	Specialty Services: Y	

TYPES OF BUSINESS:
Equipment-Mechanical Heart Valves
Cardiac Rhythm Management
Specialty Catheters
Heart Valve Disease Management

BRANDS/DIVISIONS/AFFILIATES:
Daig
Epicor Medical, Inc.
Endocardial Solutions
Irvine Biomedical, Inc.

CONTACTS:
Note: Officers with more than one job title may be intentionally listed here more than once.

Daniel J. Starks, CEO
Daniel J. Starks, Pres.
John C. Heinmiller, Exec. VP/CFO
Michael T. Rousseau, Pres.-U.S. Sales
Eric N. Falkenberg, Sr. VP-Research & Dev.
Jeri L. Lose, VP-IT/CIO
Thomas R. Northenscold, VP-Admin.
Kevin T. O'Malley, VP/General Counsel
Peter L. Grove, VP-Corp. Rel.
Laura C. Merriam, Dir.-Investor Rel.
Paul R. Buckman, Pres.-Cardiology
George J. Fazio, Pres.-Cardiac Surgery
Daniel J. Starks, Chmn.
Joseph H. McCullough, Pres.-Int'l

Phone: 651-483-2000 **Fax:** 651-482-8318
Toll-Free: 800-328-9634
Address: One Lillehei Plaza, St. Paul, MN 55117-9983 US

GROWTH PLANS/SPECIAL FEATURES:

St. Jude Medical, Inc. designs, manufactures and markets medical devices and provides services for the cardiovascular segment of the medical industry. St. Jude Medical engages in clinical research, physical training and education, patient follow-up and patient education. Products include catheters, pacemakers, implantable cardioverter defibrillators and mechanical and tissue heart valves. St. Jude Medical operates in three main segments. The cardiac rhythm management segment develops, manufactures and distributes products related to heart rhythm maintenance. The cardiac surgery unit specializes in the manufacture and distribution of products related to heart surgery, such as anastomotic connectors. The Daig division works with the cardiac rhythm management segment, specializing in catheter technologies. The U.S. sales division focuses on marketing St. Jude Medical products domestically, while the international division markets the products in more than 120 countries through a combination of direct sales personnel, independent manufacturers' representatives and distribution organizations. In recent news, the company reached an agreement to acquire Endocardial Solutions for approximately $273 million, expanding its electrophysiology product line. This follows St. Jude Medical's recent acquisition of Epicor Medical, Inc., a developer of devices to treat atrial fibrillation, and an agreement to acquire Irvine Biomedical, Inc., a developer of electrophysiology catheter products.

St. Jude Medical offers its employees vision insurance, tuition reimbursement and training classes.

FINANCIALS:
Sales and profits are in thousands of dollars—add 000 to get the full amount. Year 2004 note: Complete fiscal 2004 results were not available for all companies at press time. For this company, year 2004 is for 9 months.

2004 Sales: $1,683,497 (9 months)   2004 Profits: $285,175 (9 months)
2003 Sales: $1,932,500   2003 Profits: $339,400
2002 Sales: $1,589,900   2002 Profits: $276,300
2001 Sales: $1,347,400   2001 Profits: $172,600
2000 Sales: $1,178,800   2000 Profits: $129,100

Stock Ticker: STJ
Employees: 7,391
Fiscal Year Ends: 12/31

SALARIES/BENEFITS:
Pension Plan: Y   ESOP Stock Plan: Profit Sharing: Y   Top Exec. Salary: $722,885   Bonus: $715,656
Savings Plan: Y   Stock Purch. Plan: Y   Second Exec. Salary: $675,769   Bonus: $669,012

OTHER THOUGHTS:
Apparent Top Female Officers: 2
Hot Spot for Advancement for Women/Minorities:

LOCATIONS: ("Y" = Yes)
West:	Southwest:	Midwest:	Southeast:	Northeast:	International:
Y	Y	Y	Y	Y	Y

STAAR SURGICAL CO

www.staar.com

Industry Group Code: 339113   Ranks within this company's industry group: Sales: 111   Profits: 122

Insurance/HMO/PPO:	Drugs:	Equipment/Supplies:		Hospitals/Clinics:	Services:	Health Care:
Insurance: Managed Care: Utilization Mgmt.: Payment Proc.:	Manufacturer: Distributor: Specialty Pharm.: Vitamins/Nutri.: Clinical Trials:	Manufacturer: Distributor: Leasing/Finance: Information Sys.:	Y	Acute Care: Sub-Acute Care: Outpatient Surgery: Phys. Rehab. Center: Psychiatric Clinics:	Diagnostics: Labs/Testing: Staffing: Waste Disposal: Specialty Services:	Home Health: Long-Term Care: Physical Therapy: Phys. Practice Mgmt.:

TYPES OF BUSINESS:
Equipment-Ophthalmic Surgery
Intraocular Lenses

BRANDS/DIVISIONS/AFFILIATES:
Collamer
Cruise Control
SonicWAVE
AquaFlow
STAARVISC II

CONTACTS:
Note: Officers with more than one job title may be intentionally listed here more than once.

David Bailey, CEO
David Bailey, Pres.
John Bily, CFO
Nick Curtis, Sr. VP-Mktg. & Sales
Tom Paul, VP-Research & Dev.
James Farnworth, VP-Quality, Regulatory & Clinical Affairs
David Bailey, Chmn.

Phone: 626-303-7902   Fax: 626-303-2962
Toll-Free:
Address: 1911 Walker Ave., Monrovia, CA 91016 US

GROWTH PLANS/SPECIAL FEATURES:
STAAR Surgical Co. was created to develop, produce and market medical devices used by ophthalmologists and other eye care professionals to improve or correct vision in patients with refractive conditions, cataracts and glaucoma. The company's main product is a line of foldable silicone and Collamer intraocular lenses (IOLs), used after minimally invasive small-incision cataract extraction and to treat astigmatic abnormalities, myopia and hypermyopia. The lens is folded and implanted into the eye behind the iris and in front of the natural lens using minimally invasive techniques. This procedure is performed with topical anesthesia on an outpatient basis, with visual recovery within one to 24 hours. In addition to these, STAAR's products include the SonicWAVE phacoemulsification system, STAARVISC II viscoelastic material, Cruise Control filter and the AquaFlow collagen glaucoma drainage device. These products are designed to improve patient outcomes, minimize patient risk and discomfort and simplify ophthalmic procedures and post-operative care. Products are sold worldwide, primarily to ophthalmologists, surgical centers, hospitals, managed care providers, health maintenance organizations and group purchasing organizations.

FINANCIALS:
Sales and profits are in thousands of dollars—add 000 to get the full amount. Year 2004 note: Complete fiscal 2004 results were not available for all companies at press time. For this company, year 2004 is for 9 months.

2004 Sales: $37,733 (9 months)   2004 Profits: $-6,948 (9 months)
2003 Sales: $50,458   2003 Profits: $-8,357
2002 Sales: $47,900   2002 Profits: $-17,200
2001 Sales: $50,200   2001 Profits: $-14,800
2000 Sales: $54,400   2000 Profits: $-18,900

Stock Ticker: STAA
Employees: 258
Fiscal Year Ends: 12/31

SALARIES/BENEFITS:
Pension Plan: ESOP Stock Plan: Profit Sharing: Top Exec. Salary: $361,212   Bonus: $200,000
Savings Plan: Y Stock Purch. Plan: Second Exec. Salary: $318,537 Bonus: $141,352

OTHER THOUGHTS:
Apparent Top Female Officers:
Hot Spot for Advancement for Women/Minorities:

LOCATIONS: ("Y" = Yes)

West:	Southwest:	Midwest:	Southeast:	Northeast:	International:
Y					Y

Note: Financial information, benefits and other data can change quickly and may vary from those stated here.

STERIS CORP

www.steris.com

Industry Group Code: 339113 Ranks within this company's industry group: Sales: 29 Profits: 20

Insurance/HMO/PPO:	Drugs:	Equipment/Supplies:	Hospitals/Clinics:	Services:	Health Care:
Insurance:	Manufacturer:	Manufacturer: Y	Acute Care:	Diagnostics:	Home Health:
Managed Care:	Distributor:	Distributor:	Sub-Acute Care:	Labs/Testing:	Long-Term Care:
Utilization Mgmt.:	Specialty Pharm.:	Leasing/Finance:	Outpatient Surgery:	Staffing:	Physical Therapy:
Payment Proc.:	Vitamins/Nutri.:	Information Sys.:	Phys. Rehab. Center:	Waste Disposal:	Phys. Practice Mgmt.:
	Clinical Trials:		Psychiatric Clinics:	Specialty Services: Y	

TYPES OF BUSINESS:
Equipment-Sterilization Systems
Contamination Control Products
Surgical Support Systems
Sterilization Services

BRANDS/DIVISIONS/AFFILIATES:
STERIS SYSTEM 1
STERIS Isomedix Services
Finn-Aqua
Amsco
Reliance
Basil
Detach
Lyovac

CONTACTS:
Note: Officers with more than one job title may be intentionally listed here more than once.

Les C. Vinney, CEO
Les C. Vinney, Pres.
Laurie Brlas, CFO
Charles L. Immel, Sr. VP-Mktg. & Sales
Gerard J. Reis, Human Resources
Peter A. Burke, Chief Tech. Officer
David L. Crandall, VP-Mfg. & Distribution
Gerard J. Reis, Sr. VP-Corp. Admin.
William L. Aamoth, Corp. Treas.
Charles L. Immel, Pres.-Health Care Group
Gerard J. Reis, Pres.-Defense & Industrial
Jerry E. Robertson, Chmn.

Phone: 440-354-2600 **Fax:** 440-354-7043
Toll-Free: 800-548-4873
Address: 5960 Heisley Rd., Mentor, OH 44060-1834 US

GROWTH PLANS/SPECIAL FEATURES:

Steris Corp. develops, manufactures and markets infection prevention, contamination prevention, microbial reduction and therapy support systems, products, services and technologies for health care, scientific, research, food and industrial customers throughout the world. The firm is a leader in low-temperature sterilization, high-temperature sterilization, washing and decontamination systems, surgical tables, surgical lights, and associated consumables and service. The company is divided into three segments: health care, life sciences and STERIS Isomedix Services. The health care segment provides an integrated offering of equipment, consumables and services to hospitals and alternative sites, enabling them to improve the safety, efficiency and effectiveness of ambulatory and acute care environments. The health care segment includes products such as the company's STERIS SYSTEM 1, a complete system for just-in-time sterile processing at or near the site of patient care. This segment also provides various equipment maintenance programs to support effective operation of health care equipment. The life sciences segment offers a broad range of systems and products that includes several trusted brand names such as Finn-Aqua and Amsco sterilizers, Reliance and Basil washers, Detach automated cage and bedding processing systems, Vaporized Hydrogen Peroxide (VHP) bio-decontamination systems and Lyovac freeze dryers, as well as consumable products for contamination prevention, surface cleaning and sterility assurance. STERIS Isomedix Services provides contract sterilization, microbial reduction and materials modification services to medical supply, consumer and industrial customers. This business provides services to manufacturers of pre-packaged products, such as single-use medical devices. In recent news, STERIS acquired Albert Browne, Ltd., a privately held manufacturer of chemical indicators based in the U.K.

FINANCIALS:
Sales and profits are in thousands of dollars—add 000 to get the full amount. Year 2004 note: Complete fiscal 2004 results were not available for all companies at press time. For this company, year 2004 is for 12 months.

2004 Sales: $1,087,012 (12 months)	2004 Profits: $94,243 (12 months)	**Stock Ticker:** STE
2003 Sales: $972,100	2003 Profits: $79,400	**Employees:** 5,100
2002 Sales: $866,700	2002 Profits: $46,200	**Fiscal Year Ends:** 3/31
2001 Sales: $800,100	2001 Profits: $1,300	
2000 Sales: $760,600	2000 Profits: $10,500	

SALARIES/BENEFITS:
Pension Plan: Y ESOP Stock Plan: Profit Sharing: Top Exec. Salary: $660,418 Bonus: $506,730
Savings Plan: Stock Purch. Plan: Second Exec. Salary: $286,567 Bonus: $130,000

OTHER THOUGHTS:
Apparent Top Female Officers: 1
Hot Spot for Advancement for Women/Minorities:

LOCATIONS: ("Y" = Yes)

West:	Southwest:	Midwest:	Southeast:	Northeast:	International:
Y	Y	Y	Y	Y	Y

STRYKER CORP

www.strykercorp.com

Industry Group Code: 339113 Ranks within this company's industry group: Sales: 7 Profits: 6

Insurance/HMO/PPO:	Drugs:	Equipment/Supplies:		Hospitals/Clinics:		Services:		Health Care:	
Insurance:	Manufacturer:	Manufacturer:	Y	Acute Care:		Diagnostics:		Home Health:	
Managed Care:	Distributor:	Distributor:		Sub-Acute Care:		Labs/Testing:		Long-Term Care:	
Utilization Mgmt.:	Specialty Pharm.:	Leasing/Finance:		Outpatient Surgery:	Y	Staffing:		Physical Therapy:	Y
Payment Proc.:	Vitamins/Nutri.:	Information Sys.:		Phys. Rehab. Center:		Waste Disposal:		Phys. Practice Mgmt.:	
	Clinical Trials:			Psychiatric Clinics:		Specialty Services:			

TYPES OF BUSINESS:
Equipment-Surgical Instruments
Powered Surgical Instruments
Endoscopic Systems
Patient Care & Handling Equipment
Outpatient Physical Therapy Services
Orthopedic Implants
Biotechnical Engineering

BRANDS/DIVISIONS/AFFILIATES:
Stryker Howmedica Osteonics
Stryker MedSurg
Stryker Biotech
Physiotherapy Associates
Duracon Total Knee System
Ambulatory Surgery Center Program
Gamma Locking Nail System
Stryker Leibinger

CONTACTS:
Note: Officers with more than one job title may be intentionally listed here more than once.

John W. Brown, CEO
John W. Brown, Pres.
Dean H. Bergy, VP/CFO
Michael W. Rude, VP-Human Resources
Thomas R. Winkel, VP-Admin.
Curtis E. Hall, General Counsel
J. Patrick Anderson, VP-Bus. Dev.
Christopher F. Homrich, VP/Treas.
Edward P. Lipes, VP/Group Pres., Howmedica Osteonics
Stephen S. Johnson, VP/Group Pres., MedSurg
Eric Lum, VP-Tax
Mark A. Phillip, Pres., Stryker Biotech
John W. Brown, Chmn.
James E. Kemler, VP/Group Pres.-Int'l

Phone: 269-385-2600 Fax: 269-385-1062
Toll-Free:
Address: 2725 Fairfield Rd., Kalamazoo, MI 49002 US

GROWTH PLANS/SPECIAL FEATURES:
Stryker Corporation develops, manufactures and markets specialty surgical and medical products, including orthopedic implants, powered surgical instruments, endoscopic systems and patient care and handling equipment for the global market. Stryker also provides outpatient physical therapy services in the U.S. The company's five operating groups are Stryker Howmedica Osteonics; Stryker MedSurg (medical/surgery); Stryker Biotech, Stryker Spine and Stryker Trauma; Physiotherapy Associates; and international. Stryker Howmedica Osteonics develops and manufactures orthopedic reconstructive products. Stryker MedSurg consists of four divisions that design, manufacture and sell surgical products and medical equipment: Stryker Instruments, Stryker Endoscopy, Stryker Medical and Stryker Leibinger. Stryker Biotech, Spine and Trauma are interrelated divisions that develop products to treat muscolo-skeletal injuries. The Physiotherapy Associates division conducts physical, occupational and speech therapy services. The international division is composed of several sales and distribution divisions in Europe, Japan, Asia Pacific, Canada and Latin America. Stryker's products include the Duracon Total Knee System, Gamma Locking Nail System, Leibinger Resorbable Plating System, Hermes Voice Control System, Neptune Waste Management System and Zoom Motorized Stretcher. Stryker's other services include the Ambulatory Surgery Center Program, financial services, nurse education and practice and hospital marketing services. In recent news, Stryker moved to acquire SpineCore, Inc., a privately owned developer of artificial lumbar and cervical discs.

Most of the company's divisions offer employees fitness centers, subsidized cafeterias and a casual dress code. Other benefits include medical, dental and vision insurance, adoption assistance, tuition reimbursement and service and performance awards.

FINANCIALS:
Sales and profits are in thousands of dollars—add 000 to get the full amount. Year 2004 note: Complete fiscal 2004 results were not available for all companies at press time. For this company, year 2004 is for 9 months.

2004 Sales: $3,106,800 (9 months) 2004 Profits: $303,800 (9 months)
2003 Sales: $3,625,300   2003 Profits: $453,500
2002 Sales: $3,011,600   2002 Profits: $345,600
2001 Sales: $2,602,300   2001 Profits: $267,000
2000 Sales: $2,289,400   2000 Profits: $221,000

Stock Ticker: SYK
Employees: 14,762
Fiscal Year Ends: 12/31

SALARIES/BENEFITS:
Pension Plan: Y ESOP Stock Plan: Profit Sharing: Top Exec. Salary: $925,000 Bonus: $1,000,000
Savings Plan: Y Stock Purch. Plan: Y   Second Exec. Salary: $510,000 Bonus: $490,000

OTHER THOUGHTS:
Apparent Top Female Officers:
Hot Spot for Advancement for Women/Minorities:

LOCATIONS: ("Y" = Yes)
West:	Southwest:	Midwest:	Southeast:	Northeast:	International:
Y		Y	Y	Y	Y

SUN HEALTHCARE GROUP

www.sunh.com

Industry Group Code: 623110   **Ranks within this company's industry group:** Sales: 7   Profits: 7

Insurance/HMO/PPO:	Drugs:	Equipment/Supplies:	Hospitals/Clinics:		Services:		Health Care:	
Insurance:	Manufacturer:	Manufacturer:	Acute Care:		Diagnostics:		Home Health:	Y
Managed Care:	Distributor:	Distributor:	Sub-Acute Care:	Y	Labs/Testing:	Y	Long-Term Care:	Y
Utilization Mgmt.:	Specialty Pharm.:	Leasing/Finance:	Outpatient Surgery:		Staffing:	Y	Physical Therapy:	Y
Payment Proc.:	Vitamins/Nutri.:	Information Sys.:	Phys. Rehab. Center:	Y	Waste Disposal:		Phys. Practice Mgmt.:	
	Clinical Trials:		Psychiatric Clinics:		Specialty Services:			

TYPES OF BUSINESS:
Long-Term Care
Sub-Acute Care
Assisted Living Services
Temporary Medical Staffing
Mobile Radiology
Medical Laboratory Services
Home Health Care Services

BRANDS/DIVISIONS/AFFILIATES:
SunBridge Healthcare Corp.
SunDance Rehabilitation Corp.

CONTACTS:
Note: Officers with more than one job title may be intentionally listed here more than once.
Richard K. Matros, CEO
Kevin W. Pendergest, CFO
Heidi J. Fisher, Sr. VP-Human Resources
Steven E. Roseman, General Counsel
Craig Hayes, Interim Treas.
Chauncey J. Hunker, Compliance Officer
Tracy Gregg, Pres., SunDance Rehabilitation
Jennifer L. Clarke, Pres.-Home Health & Health Care Services
Gay Kelley, Pres., CareerStaff Unlimited
Richard K. Matros, Chmn.

Phone: 949-255-7100   **Fax:** 949-255-7054
Toll-Free: 800-729-6600
Address: 18831 Von Karman, Ste. 400, Irvine, CA 92612 US

GROWTH PLANS/SPECIAL FEATURES:
Sun Healthcare Group, Inc., through its subsidiaries, is one of the largest providers of long-term, sub-acute and related specialty health care services in the U.S. The firm operates in two principal business segments: inpatient services and rehabilitation therapy services. Through SunBridge Healthcare Corp. and others, Sun operates 108 long-term, sub-acute and assisted living facilities in 14 states. These facilities provide inpatient skilled nursing and custodial services as well as rehabilitative, restorative and transitional medical services. Specialized care is available for patients with Alzheimer's disease. Rehabilitation services are provided through SunDance Rehabilitation Corp. at over 500 facilities in 40 states. These services include speech pathology, physical therapy and occupational therapy. Sun is also a nationwide provider of temporary medical staffing, as well as a provider of mobile radiology, medical laboratory and home health care services in certain locations. In 2003, Sun Healthcare sold its pharmaceutical operation, SunScript, to Omnicare, Inc.

FINANCIALS:
Sales and profits are in thousands of dollars—add 000 to get the full amount. Year 2004 note: Complete fiscal 2004 results were not available for all companies at press time. For this company, year 2004 is for 9 months.

2004 Sales: $619,609 (9 months)	2004 Profits: $-14,216 (9 months)	
2003 Sales: $834,043	2003 Profits: $ 354	**Stock Ticker:** SUNH
2002 Sales: $1,900,000	2002 Profits: $1,047,400	Employees: 16,800
2001 Sales: $2,075,200	2001 Profits: $-69,400	Fiscal Year Ends: 12/31
2000 Sales: $2,458,900	2000 Profits: $-545,700	

SALARIES/BENEFITS:
Pension Plan: ESOP Stock Plan: Profit Sharing: Top Exec. Salary: $653,695   Bonus: $812,500
Savings Plan: Y   Stock Purch. Plan: Second Exec. Salary: $428,134   Bonus: $531,250

OTHER THOUGHTS:
Apparent Top Female Officers: 4
Hot Spot for Advancement for Women/Minorities: Y

LOCATIONS: ("Y" = Yes)
West:	Southwest:	Midwest:	Southeast:	Northeast:	International:
Y	Y	Y	Y	Y	

SUNRISE MEDICAL INC

www.sunrisemedical.com

Industry Group Code: 339113   Ranks within this company's industry group: Sales: Profits:

Insurance/HMO/PPO:	Drugs:	Equipment/Supplies:		Hospitals/Clinics:	Services:		Health Care:	
Insurance:	Manufacturer:	Manufacturer:	Y	Acute Care:	Diagnostics:		Home Health:	
Managed Care:	Distributor:	Distributor:		Sub-Acute Care:	Labs/Testing:		Long-Term Care:	
Utilization Mgmt.:	Specialty Pharm.:	Leasing/Finance:		Outpatient Surgery:	Staffing:		Physical Therapy:	
Payment Proc.:	Vitamins/Nutri.:	Information Sys.:		Phys. Rehab. Center:	Waste Disposal:		Phys. Practice Mgmt.:	
	Clinical Trials:			Psychiatric Clinics:	Specialty Services:	Y		

TYPES OF BUSINESS:

Supplies-Wheelchairs
Home Respiratory Devices
Ambulatory & Bath Safety Aids
Therapeutic Mattresses & Support Surfaces
Patient-Room Beds & Furnishings
Speech Communication Devices

BRANDS/DIVISIONS/AFFILIATES:

Quickie
Zippie
Quickie Chameleon
DeVilbiss
DynaVox
Sunrise Medical Education

CONTACTS:
Note: Officers with more than one job title may be intentionally listed here more than once.

Michael N. Hammes, CEO
Michael N. Hammes, Pres.
Raymond Huggenberger, COO
James L. Fetter, CFO
Heather Hand, Human Resources
Raymond Huggenberger, Pres.-Global Oper.
Michael N. Hammes, Chmn.

Phone: 760-930-1500   **Fax:** 760-930-1575
Toll-Free: 800-333-4000
Address: 2382 Faraday Ave., Ste. 200, Carlsbad, CA 92008-7220 US

GROWTH PLANS/SPECIAL FEATURES:

Sunrise Medical, Inc. designs, manufactures and markets medical products that address the recovery, rehabilitation and respiratory needs of patients in institutional and home care settings. The firm's products include custom manual and power wheelchairs and related seating systems; ambulatory, bathing and lifting products; health care beds and furniture; and therapeutic mattresses. Sunrise's broad range of wheelchairs includes the Quickie line, which is designed for sports such as tennis and basketball, and the Zippie line, designed for children. Recently, the company introduced Quickie Chameleon, the newest addition to its line of manual folding wheelchairs. The Quickie Chameleon line, which features depth- and angle-adjustable seating, interchangeable parts and footrests that swing in and out, enables dealers to customize each consumer's chair. Additionally, the company's DeVilbiss subsidiary manufactures and markets a broad array of home respiratory products, including aerosol products, oxygen concentrators and sleep therapy products. DynaVox, another subsidiary, markets speech communication devices. These devices feature dynamic touch-screen technology, predictive natural language software and a life-like voice synthesizer to speak for people with speech disorders. The Sunrise Medical Education department conducts seminars around the country that provide technical and clinical information for respiratory therapists, nurses, physicians and physical therapists.

FINANCIALS:
Sales and profits are in thousands of dollars—add 000 to get the full amount. Year 2004 note: Complete fiscal 2004 results were not available for all companies at press time. For this company, year 2004 is for months.

2004 Sales: $ (months)   2004 Profits: $ (months)
2003 Sales: $ 2003 Profits: $
2002 Sales: $ 2002 Profits: $
2001 Sales: $ 2001 Profits: $
2000 Sales: $ 2000 Profits: $

Stock Ticker: Private
Employees: 4,470
Fiscal Year Ends: 6/30

SALARIES/BENEFITS:

Pension Plan:	ESOP Stock Plan:	Profit Sharing:	Top Exec. Salary: $	Bonus: $
Savings Plan: Y	Stock Purch. Plan:		Second Exec. Salary: $	Bonus: $

OTHER THOUGHTS:

Apparent Top Female Officers: 1
Hot Spot for Advancement for Women/Minorities:

LOCATIONS: ("Y" = Yes)

West:	Southwest:	Midwest:	Southeast:	Northeast:	International:
Y		Y	Y	Y	Y

SUNRISE SENIOR LIVING

www.sunrise-al.com

Industry Group Code: 623110 Ranks within this company's industry group: Sales: 6 Profits: 3

Insurance/HMO/PPO:	Drugs:	Equipment/Supplies:	Hospitals/Clinics:	Services:	Health Care:
Insurance: Managed Care: Utilization Mgmt.: Payment Proc.:	Manufacturer: Distributor: Specialty Pharm.: Vitamins/Nutri.: Clinical Trials:	Manufacturer: Distributor: Leasing/Finance: Information Sys.:	Acute Care: Sub-Acute Care: Outpatient Surgery: Phys. Rehab. Center: Psychiatric Clinics:	Diagnostics: Labs/Testing: Staffing: Waste Disposal: Specialty Services: Y	Home Health: Long-Term Care: Y Physical Therapy: Phys. Practice Mgmt.:

TYPES OF BUSINESS:
Long-Term Health Care
Assisted Living Centers
Independent Living Centers
Nursing Homes

BRANDS/DIVISIONS/AFFILIATES:
Marriott Senior Living Services
Sunrise Assisted Living

CONTACTS:
Note: Officers with more than one job title may be intentionally listed here more than once.
Paul J. Klaassen, CEO
Thomas B. Newell, Pres.
Tiffany L. Tomasso, COO
Larry E. Hulse, Sr. VP/CFO
Jeffery M. Jasnoff, Sr. VP-Human Resources
John F. Gaul, General Counsel
Kenneth J. Abod, Sr. VP/Treas.
Teresa M. Klaassen, Exec. VP/Chief Cultural Officer
Christian B.A. Slavin, Exec. VP/Pres., Sunrise Properties
Brian C. Swinton, Exec. VP/Pres., Sunrise Senior Ventures, Inc.
Paul J. Klaassen, Chmn.

Phone: 703-273-7500   Fax: 703-744-1601
Toll-Free: 888-434-4648
Address: 7902 Westpark Dr., McLean, VA 22102 US

GROWTH PLANS/SPECIAL FEATURES:

Sunrise Senior Living, formerly Sunrise Assisted Living, Inc., offers a full range of services based upon individual resident needs, typically in apartment-like assisted living environments. The firm has more than 350 homes in operation or under construction in 33 U.S. states, the U.K. and Canada, with a resident capacity of approximately 40,000. Upon move-in, Sunrise assists the resident in determining the level of care required and developing an individualized service plan, including selection of resident accommodations and the appropriate level of care. The plan is periodically reviewed and updated by Sunrise. The range of services offered includes basic care, consisting of assistance with activities of daily living; plus care, consisting of more frequent and intensive care; and reminiscence care, consisting of programs and services to help cognitively impaired residents, including residents with Alzheimer's disease. The firm targets sites for development located in major metropolitan areas and their surrounding suburban communities, considering factors such as population, age demographics and estimated level of market demand. In a major strategy shift, the firm has been selling its properties to outside investors while retaining management contracts. This will convert Sunrise into an operating entity rather than a direct owner. In recent news, the company acquired Marriott Senior Living Services, boosting its total capacity from 17,000 residents to more than 42,000. As a result, Sunrise now operates nursing homes and several independent (rather than assisted) living complexes. Sunrise also announced that construction has begun on four assisted living communities in the U.K. and Germany in partnership with Pramerica Real Estate Investors, Ltd.

Sunrise offers its employees benefits including medical and dental coverage, flexible spending accounts, life insurance, short- and long-term disability insurance, a scholarship program, tuition reimbursement, a service recognition program and a meal discount program.

FINANCIALS:
Sales and profits are in thousands of dollars—add 000 to get the full amount. Year 2004 note: Complete fiscal 2004 results were not available for all companies at press time. For this company, year 2004 is for 9 months.

2004 Sales: $1,082,341 (9 months)   2004 Profits: $37,975 (9 months)
2003 Sales: $1,188,300   2003 Profits: $62,200
2002 Sales: $505,900   2002 Profits: $54,600
2001 Sales: $428,200   2001 Profits: $49,100
2000 Sales: $344,800   2000 Profits: $24,300

Stock Ticker: SRZ
Employees: 31,038
Fiscal Year Ends: 12/31

SALARIES/BENEFITS:
Pension Plan: ESOP Stock Plan: Profit Sharing: Top Exec. Salary: $420,910   Bonus: $146,865
Savings Plan: Y   Stock Purch. Plan: Y   Second Exec. Salary: $339,769   Bonus: $87,500

OTHER THOUGHTS:
Apparent Top Female Officers: 2
Hot Spot for Advancement for Women/Minorities:

LOCATIONS: ("Y" = Yes)
West:	Southwest:	Midwest:	Southeast:	Northeast:	International:
Y	Y	Y	Y	Y	Y

SUPERIOR CONSULTANT HOLDINGS CORP
www.superiorconsultant.com

Industry Group Code: 541512   Ranks within this company's industry group: Sales: 2   Profits: 1

Insurance/HMO/PPO:	Drugs:	Equipment/Supplies:	Hospitals/Clinics:	Services:	Health Care:
Insurance:	Manufacturer:	Manufacturer:	Acute Care:	Diagnostics:	Home Health:
Managed Care:	Distributor:	Distributor:	Sub-Acute Care:	Labs/Testing:	Long-Term Care:
Utilization Mgmt.:	Specialty Pharm.:	Leasing/Finance:	Outpatient Surgery:	Staffing:	Physical Therapy:
Payment Proc.:	Vitamins/Nutri.:	Information Sys.: Y	Phys. Rehab. Center:	Waste Disposal:	Phys. Practice Mgmt.:
	Clinical Trials:		Psychiatric Clinics:	Specialty Services: Y	

TYPES OF BUSINESS:
Computer Consulting
IT Outsourcing
Health Care Consulting

BRANDS/DIVISIONS/AFFILIATES:
Superior Consulting Company, Inc.

CONTACTS:
Note: Officers with more than one job title may be intentionally listed here more than once.
Richard D. Helppie, CEO
George S. Huntzinger, Pres.
George S. Huntzinger, COO
Richard R. Sorenson, CFO
Charles O. Bracken, Exec. VP
John L. Silverman, Chmn.

Phone: 248-386-8300   **Fax:** 248-386-8301
Toll-Free: 877-878-9895
Address: 17570 W. Twelve Mile Rd., Southfield, MI 48076 US

GROWTH PLANS/SPECIAL FEATURES:
Superior Consultant Holdings Corp. is a technology services company that provides IT services to the health care industry, connecting online technologies to business processes that have traditionally been conducted offline. The firm's primary operating subsidiary, Superior Consulting Company, Inc., offers IT outsourcing, management and consulting services to health care organizations, including health plans and technology providers, with special emphasis on hospital systems and integrated delivery networks. The firm has 20 years of expertise in clinical, financial and administrative systems consulting, including planning, selection and implementation. Clients can choose any combination of support, including full outsourcing with data center consolidation, 24-hour network monitoring and help desk, as well as facility management, unification and interim management of business process and IT operations. Superior's major offerings are designed to address cost pressures, resource restraints and regulatory requirements. The company's services are delivered through primary market offerings including strategic business consulting, revenue cycle, IT excellence, compliance, digital trust, patient safety and supply chain. Superior's comprehensive solution center in Alpharetta, Georgia provides clients with education, demonstrations and hands-on experience with advanced technologies.

Employee benefits at Superior include vision coverage, flexible spending accounts, a medical reimbursement account and an employee assistance program.

FINANCIALS:
Sales and profits are in thousands of dollars—add 000 to get the full amount. Year 2004 note: Complete fiscal 2004 results were not available for all companies at press time. For this company, year 2004 is for 6 months.

2004 Sales: $55,058 (6 months)   2004 Profits: $ 532   (6 months)
2003 Sales: $99,540   2003 Profits: $-1,755
2002 Sales: $92,600   2002 Profits: $-17,500
2001 Sales: $86,721   2001 Profits: $-17,565
2000 Sales: $99,237   2000 Profits: $-57,553

Stock Ticker: SUPC
Employees: 609
Fiscal Year Ends: 12/31

SALARIES/BENEFITS:
| Pension Plan: | ESOP Stock Plan: | Profit Sharing: | Top Exec. Salary: $309,245 | Bonus: $ |
| Savings Plan: | Stock Purch. Plan: | | Second Exec. Salary: $306,093 | Bonus: $20,000 |

OTHER THOUGHTS:
Apparent Top Female Officers:
Hot Spot for Advancement for Women/Minorities:

LOCATIONS: ("Y" = Yes)
West:	Southwest:	Midwest:	Southeast:	Northeast:	International:
Y		Y	Y	Y	

SUTTER HEALTH

www.sutterhealth.org

Industry Group Code: 622110　　Ranks within this company's industry group: Sales: 8　Profits:

Insurance/HMO/PPO:	Drugs:	Equipment/Supplies:	Hospitals/Clinics:		Services:		Health Care:	
Insurance:	Manufacturer:	Manufacturer:	Acute Care:	Y	Diagnostics:		Home Health:	Y
Managed Care:	Distributor:	Distributor:	Sub-Acute Care:	Y	Labs/Testing:		Long-Term Care:	Y
Utilization Mgmt.:	Specialty Pharm.:	Leasing/Finance:	Outpatient Surgery:		Staffing:		Physical Therapy:	
Payment Proc.:	Vitamins/Nutri.:	Information Sys.:	Phys. Rehab. Center:		Waste Disposal:		Phys. Practice Mgmt.:	
	Clinical Trials:		Psychiatric Clinics:		Specialty Services:	Y		

TYPES OF BUSINESS:
Hospitals-General
Home Health Services
Training Programs
Medical Research Facilities
Hospice Networks
Occupational Health Networks
Long-Term Care
Radiosurgery

BRANDS/DIVISIONS/AFFILIATES:
Sutter GammaKnife
Samuel Merritt College

GROWTH PLANS/SPECIAL FEATURES:
Sutter Health, Inc. is one of the nation's largest not-for-profit health care systems. Through its affiliates, the firm serves 20 northern California counties and Hawaii with more than 3,600 affiliated doctors. The firm operates 37 health care facilities, including 24 acute care hospitals. Sutter Health also has physician and nurse training programs, medical research facilities, home health companies, hospice and occupational health networks and long-term care centers. The Sutter Health network also operates several research institutes and specialty clinical services. Specialty services include pregnancy information and classes, cancer survival services, heart health services, visiting nurse and hospice care, direct medical billing services and Sutter GammaKnife, a radiosurgery department focused on brain abnormalities. The company also sponsors the Samuel Merritt College for nursing and health professional training.

CONTACTS:
Note: Officers with more than one job title may be intentionally listed here more than once.

Van R. Johnson, CEO
Van R. Johnson, Pres.
Patrick E. Fry, COO
Ralph E. Andersen, Chmn.

Phone: 916-733-8800　　**Fax:** 916-286-6841
Toll-Free:
Address: 2200 River Plaza Dr., Sacramento, CA 93833 US

FINANCIALS:
Sales and profits are in thousands of dollars—add 000 to get the full amount. Year 2004 note: Complete fiscal 2004 results were not available for all companies at press time. For this company, year 2004 is for months.

2004 Sales: $ (months)　　2004 Profits: $ (months)
2003 Sales: $5,672,000　　2003 Profits: $
2002 Sales: $4,931,000　　2002 Profits: $284,000
2001 Sales: $　　2001 Profits: $
2000 Sales: $　　2000 Profits: $

Stock Ticker: Nonprofit
Employees: 41,000
Fiscal Year Ends: 12/31

SALARIES/BENEFITS:
Pension Plan:　　ESOP Stock Plan:　　Profit Sharing:　　Top Exec. Salary: $　　Bonus: $
Savings Plan:　　Stock Purch. Plan:　　　　Second Exec. Salary: $　　Bonus: $

OTHER THOUGHTS:
Apparent Top Female Officers:
Hot Spot for Advancement for Women/Minorities:

LOCATIONS: ("Y" = Yes)
West	Southwest	Midwest	Southeast	Northeast	International
Y					

SYBRON DENTAL SPECIALTIES INC

www.sybrondental.com

Industry Group Code: 339113 Ranks within this company's industry group: Sales: 38 Profits: 29

Insurance/HMO/PPO:	Drugs:	Equipment/Supplies:	Hospitals/Clinics:	Services:	Health Care:
Insurance: Managed Care: Utilization Mgmt.: Payment Proc.:	Manufacturer: Distributor: Specialty Pharm.: Vitamins/Nutri.: Clinical Trials:	Manufacturer: Y Distributor: Leasing/Finance: Information Sys.:	Acute Care: Sub-Acute Care: Outpatient Surgery: Phys. Rehab. Center: Psychiatric Clinics:	Diagnostics: Labs/Testing: Staffing: Waste Disposal: Specialty Services:	Home Health: Long-Term Care: Physical Therapy: Phys. Practice Mgmt.:

TYPES OF BUSINESS:
Dental Products
Orthodontic Products
Infection Control Products

BRANDS/DIVISIONS/AFFILIATES:
Innova LifeSciences Corporation
Kerr
Belle
Metrex
Ormco
Pinnacle
Demetron
Hawe

GROWTH PLANS/SPECIAL FEATURES:
Sybron Dental Specialties, Inc. and its subsidiaries form a leading manufacturer of consumable products for the dental and orthodontic professions. The firm operates in three business segments: professional dental, which develops, manufactures, markets and distributes a comprehensive line of products to the dental industry worldwide; orthodontics, which engineers and distributes orthodontic and endodontic products used in root canal therapy; and infection control products, marketed to dental and medical professionals. Infection control products include surface disinfectants, cleaners, detergents and hand-hygiene products. Products are marketed under brand names including Kerr, Belle, Metrex, Ormco, Pinnacle, Demetron and Hawe. The company's business strategy includes product innovation, ongoing cost reduction and selective acquisitions. Sybron recently acquired Innova LifeSciences Corporation, a Canadian manufacturer of medical devices.

CONTACTS:
Note: Officers with more than one job title may be intentionally listed here more than once.

Floyd W. Pickrell, CEO
Floyd W. Pickrell, Pres.
Gregory D. Waller, CFO
John A. Trapani, VP-Human Resources
Michael R. DePrez, CIO
Stephen J. Tomassi, General Counsel
Michael R. DePrez, Exec. VP-Oper.
Frances Zee, VP-Regulatory Affairs & Quality Assurance
Steven J. Semmelmayer, Pres., Kerr Corp.
A. J. LaSota, VP/General Mgr.-Metrex
Daniel E. Even, Pres., Ormco
Kenneth F. Yontz, Chmn.

Phone: 714-516-7400 Fax:
Toll-Free: 800-537-7824
Address: 1717 W. Collins Ave., Orange, CA 92867 US

FINANCIALS:
Sales and profits are in thousands of dollars—add 000 to get the full amount. Year 2004 note: Complete fiscal 2004 results were not available for all companies at press time. For this company, year 2004 is for 9 months.

2004 Sales: $428,926 (9 months) 2004 Profits: $45,987 (9 months)
2003 Sales: $526,391 2003 Profits: $57,452
2002 Sales: $456,700 2002 Profits: $31,600
2001 Sales: $439,500 2001 Profits: $39,100
2000 Sales: $423,100 2000 Profits: $41,600

Stock Ticker: SYD
Employees: 4,200
Fiscal Year Ends: 9/30

SALARIES/BENEFITS:
Pension Plan: ESOP Stock Plan: Profit Sharing: Top Exec. Salary: $550,000 Bonus: $991,100
Savings Plan: Y Stock Purch. Plan: Second Exec. Salary: $250,000 Bonus: $331,500

OTHER THOUGHTS:
Apparent Top Female Officers: 1
Hot Spot for Advancement for Women/Minorities:

LOCATIONS: ("Y" = Yes)
West:	Southwest:	Midwest:	Southeast:	Northeast:	International:
Y		Y		Y	Y

SYMMETRY MEDICAL INC

www.symmetrymedical.com

Industry Group Code: 339113 Ranks within this company's industry group: Sales: 83 Profits: 83

Insurance/HMO/PPO:	Drugs:	Equipment/Supplies:	Hospitals/Clinics:	Services:	Health Care:
Insurance:	Manufacturer:	Manufacturer: Y	Acute Care:	Diagnostics:	Home Health:
Managed Care:	Distributor:	Distributor:	Sub-Acute Care:	Labs/Testing:	Long-Term Care:
Utilization Mgmt.:	Specialty Pharm.:	Leasing/Finance:	Outpatient Surgery:	Staffing:	Physical Therapy:
Payment Proc.:	Vitamins/Nutri.:	Information Sys.:	Phys. Rehab. Center:	Waste Disposal:	Phys. Practice Mgmt.:
	Clinical Trials:		Psychiatric Clinics:	Specialty Services: Y	

TYPES OF BUSINESS:
Medical Devices-Joint Replacement Parts
Orthopedic Implants
Medical Cases
Design and Development Services

BRANDS/DIVISIONS/AFFILIATES:
Symmetry Jet
Symmetry Othy
Symmetry PolyVac
Symmetry Thornton
Symmetry UltreXX
Othy
UltreXX
Total Solutions

CONTACTS:
Note: Officers with more than one job title may be intentionally listed here more than once.
Brian Moore, CEO
Brian Moore, Pres.
Fred Hite, CFO
Andrew Miclot, VP-Mktg. & Sales
Andrew Miclot, VP-Bus. Dev.

Phone: 574-268-2252 **Fax:** 574-267-4551
Toll-Free:
Address: 220 W. Market St., Warsaw, IN 46580 US

GROWTH PLANS/SPECIAL FEATURES:
Symmetry Medical, Inc. is a medical instrument provider that makes orthopedic implants including hip and knee replacement parts and the surgical instruments used to implant them. The firm has nine manufacturing subsidiaries in the U.S. and Europe. The Symmetry Jet subsidiary forges, creates and fully finishes orthopedic implants. Symmetry Othy is a supplier of custom and standard surgical instruments internationally. Symmetry PolyVac manufactures metal, plastic and hybrid medical cases in Manchester, New Hampshire and Lille, France. Symmetry Thornton, based in Sheffield, England, has supplied orthopedic components for over 100 years, specializing in precision forging, casting, rapid prototyping, machining and full finishing for implants. Symmetry UltreXX manufacturers and supplies precision spinal and trauma instruments and implants to original equipment manufacturers internationally. Symmetry Medical's design and development center offers independent or co-development design services, prototypes and project management. It has produced over 300 instruments and medical cases for specific client needs. The firm offers all of its products under the Othy, UltreXX and Total Solutions brands.

FINANCIALS:
Sales and profits are in thousands of dollars—add 000 to get the full amount. Year 2004 note: Complete fiscal 2004 results were not available for all companies at press time. For this company, year 2004 is for months.

2004 Sales: $ (months)   2004 Profits: $ (months)
2003 Sales: $122,000   2003 Profits: $5,900
2002 Sales: $65,400   2002 Profits: $ 200
2001 Sales: $ 2001 Profits: $
2000 Sales: $ 2000 Profits: $

Stock Ticker: SMA
Employees: 1,464
Fiscal Year Ends: 12/31

SALARIES/BENEFITS:
Pension Plan: ESOP Stock Plan: Profit Sharing: Top Exec. Salary: $ Bonus: $
Savings Plan: Stock Purch. Plan: Second Exec. Salary: $ Bonus: $

OTHER THOUGHTS:
Apparent Top Female Officers:
Hot Spot for Advancement for Women/Minorities:

LOCATIONS: ("Y" = Yes)

West:	Southwest:	Midwest:	Southeast:	Northeast:	International:
		Y			Y

SYNOVIS LIFE TECHNOLOGIES INC

www.synovislife.com

Industry Group Code: 339113   Ranks within this company's industry group: Sales: 108   Profits: 88

Insurance/HMO/PPO:	Drugs:	Equipment/Supplies:		Hospitals/Clinics:		Services:		Health Care:	
Insurance:	Manufacturer:	Manufacturer:	Y	Acute Care:		Diagnostics:		Home Health:	
Managed Care:	Distributor:	Distributor:		Sub-Acute Care:		Labs/Testing:		Long-Term Care:	
Utilization Mgmt.:	Specialty Pharm.:	Leasing/Finance:		Outpatient Surgery:		Staffing:		Physical Therapy:	
Payment Proc.:	Vitamins/Nutri.:	Information Sys.:		Phys. Rehab. Center:		Waste Disposal:		Phys. Practice Mgmt.:	
	Clinical Trials:			Psychiatric Clinics:		Specialty Services:	Y		

TYPES OF BUSINESS:
Supplies-Surgery
Implantable Biomaterials
Contract Manufacturing

BRANDS/DIVISIONS/AFFILIATES:
Synovis Surgical Innovations
Synovis Micro Companies Alliance
Synovis Interventional Solutions
Synovis Precision Engineering
Microvascular Anastomotis Coupler
Vascu-Guard
Peri-Strips
Ocu-Guard

CONTACTS: Note: Officers with more than one job title may be intentionally listed here more than once.
Karen G. Larson, CEO
Karen G. Larson, Pres.
Connie L. Magnuson, CFO
David Buche, VP-Mktg. & Sales
B. Nicholas Oray, VP-R&D
Evan Johnston, VP-Oper.
Connie L. Magnuson, VP-Finance/Corp. Sec.
Mary L. Frick, VP-Regulatory Affairs & Quality Assurance
Michael K. Campbell, Pres., Synovis Micro Companies Alliance
Fariborz Boor Boor, Pres., Synovis Interventional Solutions
Timothy M. Scanlan, Chmn.

Phone: 651-603-3700   **Fax:** 651-642-9018
Toll-Free: 800-255-4018
Address: 2575 University Ave. W., St. Paul, MN 55114 US

GROWTH PLANS/SPECIAL FEATURES:
Synovis Life Technologies, Inc. develops, manufactures and markets branded proprietary and patented specialty medical products for use in thoracic, cardiac, neuro-, vascular and ophthalmic surgery. The company operates in two business segments: the surgical device business and the interventional business. Through subsidiaries Synovis Surgical Innovations and Synovis Micro Companies Alliance, the surgical device business develops, manufactures and markets implantable biomaterial products, devices for microsurgery and surgical tools that reduce risks of critical surgeries, lead to better patient outcomes and lower costs. The interventional business provides the services of concept development, engineering, rapid prototyping and manufacturing of complex micro-wire forms and polymer components used in many interventional devices in the cardiac rhythm management, neurostimulation and vascular markets. Subsidiaries Synovis Interventional Solutions and Synovis Precision Engineering operate this segment. The company's surgical device product lines and associated products include Ocu-Guard, Peri-Strips, Vascu-Guard, Dura-Guard, Veritas Collagen Matrix, Flo-Thru Intraluminal Shunt Flo-Rester and Microvascular Anastomotis Coupler. Peri-Strips provide reinforcement at the surgical staple line to prevent potentially fatal fluid leaks, most significantly in gastric bypass surgery, a treatment for morbid obesity. The Microvascular Anastomotis Coupler system enables microsurgeons to perform highly effective anastomotic surgical procedures faster, easier and as or more dependably than traditional suture or sleeve anastomosis. In recent news, the company procured market approval for the Navi-Guide steerable stylet, a single-use disposable device designed to assist physicians with implanting pacemaker leads in the heart, as well as expanded clearance for applications of Peri-Strips.

FINANCIALS:
Sales and profits are in thousands of dollars—add 000 to get the full amount. Year 2004 note: Complete fiscal 2004 results were not available for all companies at press time. For this company, year 2004 is for 9 months.

2004 Sales: $40,407 (9 months)	2004 Profits: $1,089 (9 months)	**Stock Ticker:** SYNO
2003 Sales: $58,000	2003 Profits: $5,000	Employees: 425
2002 Sales: $39,962	2002 Profits: $3,041	Fiscal Year Ends: 10/31
2001 Sales: $28,500	2001 Profits: $1,800	
2000 Sales: $21,926	2000 Profits: $589	

SALARIES/BENEFITS:
Pension Plan:	ESOP Stock Plan:	Profit Sharing:	Top Exec. Salary: $300,000	Bonus: $73,400
Savings Plan: Y	Stock Purch. Plan:		Second Exec. Salary: $185,000	Bonus: $25,720

OTHER THOUGHTS:
Apparent Top Female Officers: 3
Hot Spot for Advancement for Women/Minorities: Y

LOCATIONS: ("Y" = Yes)
West:	Southwest:	Midwest:	Southeast:	Northeast:	International:
		Y			

TEAM HEALTH

www.teamhealth.com

Industry Group Code: 621111 **Ranks within this company's industry group:** Sales: 2 Profits: 8

Insurance/HMO/PPO:	Drugs:	Equipment/Supplies:	Hospitals/Clinics:	Services:	Health Care:
Insurance: Managed Care: Utilization Mgmt.: Payment Proc.:	Manufacturer: Distributor: Specialty Pharm.: Vitamins/Nutri.: Clinical Trials:	Manufacturer: Distributor: Leasing/Finance: Information Sys.:	Acute Care: Sub-Acute Care: Outpatient Surgery: Phys. Rehab. Center: Psychiatric Clinics:	Diagnostics: Labs/Testing: Staffing: Y Waste Disposal: Specialty Services:	Home Health: Long-Term Care: Physical Therapy: Phys. Practice Mgmt.:

TYPES OF BUSINESS:
Hospital Staffing

BRANDS/DIVISIONS/AFFILIATES:
Spectrum Healthcare Resources
Cornerstone Equity Investors
Madison Dearborn Capital Partners

GROWTH PLANS/SPECIAL FEATURES:
Team Health is the leading provider of clinical outsourcing services in the U.S. The firm has more than 7,000 health care professionals, including 3,000 physicians, who serve at 450 care facilities in 45 states, both permanently and as temporary assistance. The health care professionals provide a variety of staffing and management services, including emergency medicine, radiology, anesthesia, urgent care and pediatrics. Clients of the firm include civilian and military hospitals, surgical centers, imaging centers and private clinics. Team Health operates through a chain of regional affiliates that are all physician-managed. The company is controlled by Cornerstone Equity Investors and Madison Dearborn Capital Partners, which each own about 40%. In recent news, Team Health acquired Spectrum Healthcare Resources, a major provider of permanent staffing services to military health care facilities.

CONTACTS:
Note: Officers with more than one job title may be intentionally listed here more than once.

Lynn Massingale, CEO
Gregory Roth, Pres.
Gregory Roth, COO
David Jones, CFO
Harry Herman, CIO
Robert Joyner, General Counsel
Michael J. Shea, VP-Bus. Dev.
Robert Abramowski, Exec. VP-Finance
Stephen Sherlin, Chief Compliance Officer
Gar LaSalle, Chief Medical Officer
Kent Bristow, Sr. VP
Jonathan D. Grimes, Pres.-Team Health East

Phone: 865-693-1000 **Fax:** 865-539-8003
Toll-Free: 800-818-1498
Address: 1900 Winston Rd., Knoxville, TN 37919 US

FINANCIALS:
Sales and profits are in thousands of dollars—add 000 to get the full amount. Year 2004 note: Complete fiscal 2004 results were not available for all companies at press time. For this company, year 2004 is for months.

2004 Sales: $ (months)   2004 Profits: $ (months)
2003 Sales: $1,479,000   2003 Profits: $-2,800
2002 Sales: $1,230,700   2002 Profits: $16,100
2001 Sales: $ 2001 Profits: $
2000 Sales: $ 2000 Profits: $

Stock Ticker: Private
Employees: 6,700
Fiscal Year Ends: 12/31

SALARIES/BENEFITS:
Pension Plan: ESOP Stock Plan: Profit Sharing: Top Exec. Salary: $ Bonus: $
Savings Plan: Stock Purch. Plan: Second Exec. Salary: $ Bonus: $

OTHER THOUGHTS:
Apparent Top Female Officers: 1
Hot Spot for Advancement for Women/Minorities:

LOCATIONS: ("Y" = Yes)
West:	Southwest:	Midwest:	Southeast:	Northeast:	International:
Y	Y	Y	Y	Y	

TECHNE CORP

www.techne-corp.com

Industry Group Code: 339113 **Ranks within this company's industry group:** Sales: 73 Profits: 38

Insurance/HMO/PPO:	Drugs:		Equipment/Supplies:		Hospitals/Clinics:	Services:	Health Care:
Insurance:	Manufacturer:	Y	Manufacturer:	Y	Acute Care:	Diagnostics:	Home Health:
Managed Care:	Distributor:		Distributor:	Y	Sub-Acute Care:	Labs/Testing:	Long-Term Care:
Utilization Mgmt.:	Specialty Pharm.:		Leasing/Finance:		Outpatient Surgery:	Staffing:	Physical Therapy:
Payment Proc.:	Vitamins/Nutri.:		Information Sys.:		Phys. Rehab. Center:	Waste Disposal:	Phys. Practice Mgmt.:
	Clinical Trials:				Psychiatric Clinics:	Specialty Services:	

TYPES OF BUSINESS:
Supplies-Cytokines, Antibodies & Assay Kits
Biotechnology Products
Hematology Products

BRANDS/DIVISIONS/AFFILIATES:
Research and Diagnostic Systems, Inc.
R&D Systems Europe, Ltd.
R&D Systems GmbH
Whole Blood Flow Cytometry Control
Whole Blood Glucose/Hemoglobin Control

CONTACTS:
Note: Officers with more than one job title may be intentionally listed here more than once.

Thomas E. Oland, CEO
Thomas E. Oland, Pres.
Lea Simoane, Dir.-Human Resources
Monica Tsang, VP-Research
Timothy M. Heaney, General Counsel
Thomas E. Oland, Treas.
James A. Weatherbee, VP/Chief Scientific Officer
Thomas C. Detwiler, VP-Scientific & Regulatory Affairs
Marcel Veronneau, VP-Hematology Oper.
Timothy M. Heaney, Corp. Sec.
Thomas E. Oland, Chmn.

Phone: 612-379-8854 **Fax:** 612-379-6580
Toll-Free: 800-343-7475
Address: 614 McKinley Pl. NE, Minneapolis, MN 55413-2610 US

GROWTH PLANS/SPECIAL FEATURES:
Techne Corp. is a holding company that operates via two subsidiaries: Research and Diagnostic Systems, Inc. (R&D Systems) and R&D Systems Europe, Ltd. (R&D Europe). R&D Systems is a specialty manufacturer of biological products. Its two major operating segments are hematology controls, which are utilized in clinical and hospital laboratories to monitor the accuracy of blood analysis instruments, and biotechnology products, including purified proteins and antibodies that are sold exclusively to the research market. The firm's biotechnology division, part of R&D Systems, produces highly purified, biologically active proteins. Techne's products include laboratory kits and reagents, ELISA/assay kits, proteases, substrates and inhibitors. R&D Europe also distributes biotechnology products and has a German sales subsidiary, R&D Systems GmbH. Techne also produces controls and calibrators for a variety of medical brands including Abbott Cell-Dyn, ABX, Beckman Coulter, Danam, Hycel, Roche and TOA Sysmex instruments. The company's Whole Blood Flow Cytometry Control is a control for flow cytometry instruments, which are used to identify and quantify white blood cells by their surface antigens. The Whole Blood Glucose/Hemoglobin Control product is designed to monitor instruments that measure glucose and hemoglobin in the blood. R&D Systems is currently engaged in ongoing research and development in all of its major product lines: hematology controls and calibrators, biotechnology cytokines, antibodies, assays and other related products. New products this year include Human VEGF sets, containing the basic components required to measure natural and recombinant human Vascular Endothelial Growth Factor; mouse immunoassays; and several other laboratory assistance tools.

FINANCIALS:
Sales and profits are in thousands of dollars—add 000 to get the full amount. Year 2004 note: Complete fiscal 2004 results were not available for all companies at press time. For this company, year 2004 is for 12 months.

2004 Sales: $161,257 (12 months)   2004 Profits: $52,928 (12 months)
2003 Sales: $145,000   2003 Profits: $45,400
2002 Sales: $130,900   2002 Profits: $27,100
2001 Sales: $115,400   2001 Profits: $34,000
2000 Sales: $103,800   2000 Profits: $26,600

Stock Ticker: TECH
Employees: 524
Fiscal Year Ends: 6/30

SALARIES/BENEFITS:
Pension Plan: ESOP Stock Plan: Profit Sharing: Y   Top Exec. Salary: $225,000   Bonus: $39,820
Savings Plan: Y   Stock Purch. Plan: Y   Second Exec. Salary: $221,000   Bonus: $39,480

OTHER THOUGHTS:
Apparent Top Female Officers: 3
Hot Spot for Advancement for Women/Minorities: Y

LOCATIONS: ("Y" = Yes)

West:	Southwest:	Midwest:	Southeast:	Northeast:	International:
		Y			Y

Note: Financial information, benefits and other data can change quickly and may vary from those stated here.

TELEX COMMUNICATIONS INC

www.telex.com

Industry Group Code: 334200 Ranks within this company's industry group: Sales: Profits:

Insurance/HMO/PPO:	Drugs:	Equipment/Supplies:		Hospitals/Clinics:	Services:	Health Care:
Insurance:	Manufacturer:	Manufacturer:	Y	Acute Care:	Diagnostics:	Home Health:
Managed Care:	Distributor:	Distributor:		Sub-Acute Care:	Labs/Testing:	Long-Term Care:
Utilization Mgmt.:	Specialty Pharm.:	Leasing/Finance:		Outpatient Surgery:	Staffing:	Physical Therapy:
Payment Proc.:	Vitamins/Nutri.:	Information Sys.:		Phys. Rehab. Center:	Waste Disposal:	Phys. Practice Mgmt.:
	Clinical Trials:			Psychiatric Clinics:	Specialty Services:	

TYPES OF BUSINESS:
Communications Equipment-Sound & Entertainment
Multimedia Communications Equipment
Specialty Hearing Assistance Technology

BRANDS/DIVISIONS/AFFILIATES:
Dynacord
Electro-Voice
Klark-Teknik
Midas Consoles
RTS
EVI
Telex

GROWTH PLANS/SPECIAL FEATURES:
Telex Communications, Inc., formed from the merger of Telex and EVI, designs, manufactures and markets sophisticated audio, wireless and multimedia communications equipment to commercial, professional and industrial customers. Telex manufactures a comprehensive range of products worldwide for professional audio systems and wireless product markets, including wired and wireless microphones, wired and wireless intercom systems, mixing consoles, signal processors, amplifiers, loudspeaker systems, headphones and headsets, digital duplication products, talking book players, antennas, land mobile communication systems, personal computer speech recognition systems, speech dictation microphone systems and wireless assistive listening systems.

CONTACTS:
Note: Officers with more than one job title may be intentionally listed here more than once.

Raymond V. Malpocher, CEO
Raymond V. Malpocher, Pres.
Greg Richter, CFO
Mathias von Heydekampf, Pres.-Worldwide Pro Audio
Joseph Vaughan, Pres.-Audio & Wireless Tech.
Edgar S. Woolard, Jr., Chmn.
Greg Richter, VP-Int'l

Phone: 952-884-4051	Fax: 952-884-0043
Toll-Free:	
Address: 12000 Portland Ave. S., Burnsville, MN 55337 US	

FINANCIALS:
Sales and profits are in thousands of dollars—add 000 to get the full amount. Year 2004 note: Complete fiscal 2004 results were not available for all companies at press time. For this company, year 2004 is for 9 months.

2004 Sales: $222,369 (9 months)   2004 Profits: $9,973 (9 months)
2003 Sales: $ 2003 Profits: $
2002 Sales: $266,500   2002 Profits: $-30,100
2001 Sales: $284,500   2001 Profits: $61,000
2000 Sales: $328,900   2000 Profits: $-18,000

Stock Ticker: Private
Employees: 1,983
Fiscal Year Ends: 12/31

SALARIES/BENEFITS:
Pension Plan: ESOP Stock Plan: Profit Sharing: Top Exec. Salary: $382,693   Bonus: $380,000
Savings Plan: Y   Stock Purch. Plan: Second Exec. Salary: $244,332   Bonus: $306,000

OTHER THOUGHTS:
Apparent Top Female Officers:
Hot Spot for Advancement for Women/Minorities:

LOCATIONS: ("Y" = Yes)
West:	Southwest:	Midwest:	Southeast:	Northeast:	International:
		Y	Y		Y

ural
TENET HEALTHCARE CORPORATION
www.tenethealth.com

Industry Group Code: 622110 Ranks within this company's industry group: Sales: 3 Profits: 21

Insurance/HMO/PPO:	Drugs:	Equipment/Supplies:	Hospitals/Clinics:		Services:		Health Care:	
Insurance:	Manufacturer:	Manufacturer:	Acute Care:	Y	Diagnostics:		Home Health:	
Managed Care:	Distributor:	Distributor:	Sub-Acute Care:	Y	Labs/Testing:		Long-Term Care:	
Utilization Mgmt.:	Specialty Pharm.:	Leasing/Finance:	Outpatient Surgery:	Y	Staffing:		Physical Therapy:	Y
Payment Proc.:	Vitamins/Nutri.:	Information Sys.:	Phys. Rehab. Center:	Y	Waste Disposal:		Phys. Practice Mgmt.:	
	Clinical Trials:		Psychiatric Clinics:		Specialty Services:			

TYPES OF BUSINESS:
Hospitals-General
Specialty Care Facilities
Outpatient Centers
Home Health Agencies

BRANDS/DIVISIONS/AFFILIATES:

CONTACTS: *Note: Officers with more than one job title may be intentionally listed here more than once.*
Trevor Fetter, CEO
Trevor Fetter, Pres.
Reynold J. Jennings, COO
Stephen D. Farber, CFO
Joseph A. Bosch, Sr. VP-Human Resources
Stephen F. Brown, Exec. VP/CIO
E. Peter Urbanowicz, General Counsel
Tim Pullen, Exec. VP/Chief Acc. Officer
W. Randolph Smith, Pres.-Western Div.
Edward A. Kangas, Chmn.

Phone: 805-563-7000   **Fax:** 805-563-7070
Toll-Free:
Address: 3820 State St., Santa Barbara, CA 93105 US

GROWTH PLANS/SPECIAL FEATURES:

Tenet Healthcare Corporation, through its subsidiaries, is a nationwide provider of health care services. The company's 101 general acute care hospitals contain 25,116 licensed beds, serving urban and rural communities in 15 states. The majority of the firm's beds are concentrated in California, Florida and Texas, which reduces management and marketing expenses and improves relations with managed care providers. Each of the company's general hospitals offers acute care services, operating and recovery rooms, radiology services, respiratory therapy services, clinical laboratories and pharmacies; most also offer intensive care, critical care or coronary care units, physical therapy and orthopedic, oncology and outpatient services. In addition, some of the hospitals offer specialty procedures such as heart, lung, liver and kidney transplants; gamma-knife brain surgery; and bone marrow transplants. Tenet recently agreed to sell three Massachusetts hospitals, 12 California hospitals, one Texas hospital and one Louisiana hospital, opening up two new facilities in Texas and Tennessee.

Tenet's employees receive comprehensive medical and dental benefits, an employee assistance program and credit union services. Additionally, registered nurses are elegible for the company's student loan repayment program.

FINANCIALS: Sales and profits are in thousands of dollars—add 000 to get the full amount. Year 2004 note: Complete fiscal 2004 results were not available for all companies at press time. For this company, year 2004 is for 9 months.

2004 Sales: $7,544,000 (9 months)	2004 Profits: $-72,000 (9 months)	**Stock Ticker:** THC
2003 Sales: $13,212,000	2003 Profits: $-1,477,000	**Employees:** 109,759
2002 Sales: $13,913,000	2002 Profits: $785,000	**Fiscal Year Ends:** 12/31
2001 Sales: $12,053,000	2001 Profits: $643,000	
2000 Sales: $11,414,000	2000 Profits: $302,000	

SALARIES/BENEFITS:

Pension Plan: Y	ESOP Stock Plan:	Profit Sharing:	Top Exec. Salary: $848,539	Bonus: $262,500
Savings Plan: Y	Stock Purch. Plan: Y		Second Exec. Salary: $602,308	Bonus: $89,937

OTHER THOUGHTS:
Apparent Top Female Officers:
Hot Spot for Advancement for Women/Minorities:

LOCATIONS: ("Y" = Yes)

West:	Southwest:	Midwest:	Southeast:	Northeast:	International:
Y	Y	Y	Y	Y	

Note: Financial information, benefits and other data can change quickly and may vary from those stated here.

TEVA PHARMACEUTICAL INDUSTRIES

www.tevapharm.com

Industry Group Code: 325416   Ranks within this company's industry group: Sales: 1   Profits: 1

Insurance/HMO/PPO:	Drugs:		Equipment/Supplies:	Hospitals/Clinics:	Services:	Health Care:
Insurance:	Manufacturer:	Y	Manufacturer:	Acute Care:	Diagnostics:	Home Health:
Managed Care:	Distributor:		Distributor:	Sub-Acute Care:	Labs/Testing:	Long-Term Care:
Utilization Mgmt.:	Specialty Pharm.:		Leasing/Finance:	Outpatient Surgery:	Staffing:	Physical Therapy:
Payment Proc.:	Vitamins/Nutri.:		Information Sys.:	Phys. Rehab. Center:	Waste Disposal:	Phys. Practice Mgmt.:
	Clinical Trials:			Psychiatric Clinics:	Specialty Services:	

TYPES OF BUSINESS:
Drugs-Generic
Active Pharmaceutical Ingredients

BRANDS/DIVISIONS/AFFILIATES:
Teva North America
Teva Pharmaceuticals USA
Sicor, Inc.
Pharmachemie BV
Bupropion

CONTACTS: *Note: Officers with more than one job title may be intentionally listed here more than once.*
Israel Makov, CEO
Israel Makov, Pres.
Dan S. Suesskind, CFO
Aharon Agmon, VP-Int'l Sales
Haim Benjamini, VP-Human Resources
Christopher Pelloni, VP-Generic Research & Dev.
Rodney Kasan, VP/Chief Tech. Officer
Ben-Zion Weiner, Group VP-Global Products
Uzi Karniel, General Counsel/Corp. Sec.
Jacob Winter, VP-Global Oper.
Eli Shohet, VP-Bus. Dev.
William A. Fletcher, Pres., Teva North America
David Reisman, VP-Israel Pharmaceutical Oper.
Meron Mann, Group VP-Europe
Aharon Schwartz, VP-Strategic Bus. Planning & New Ventures
Chaim Hurvitz, Group VP-Int'l

Phone: 972-3-926-7267   **Fax:** 972-3-923-4050
Toll-Free:
Address: 5 Basel St., Petach Tikva, 49131 Israel

GROWTH PLANS/SPECIAL FEATURES:

Teva Pharmaceutical Industries, Ltd., based in Israel, is a global pharmaceutical company, with a leading position in Israel in the production, distribution and sale of pharmaceutical products, as well as operating manufacturing and marketing facilities in North America and Europe. The firm primarily focuses on human pharmaceuticals (HP) and active pharmaceutical ingredients (API). The HP segment produces generic drugs in all major therapeutics and steriles in a variety of dosage forms. Teva also manufactures innovative drugs in niche markets through its research and development efforts. Subsidiary Teva Pharmaceuticals USA is one of the most successful manufacturers and distributors of generic drugs in the U.S. In addition, Pharmachemie BV has the largest market share in generics in The Netherlands. The API segment distributes ingredients to manufacturers worldwide, in addition to supporting its own pharmaceutical products. Teva is currently focusing its research and development on neurological disorders and auto-immune diseases. The company is developing novel treatments for multiple sclerosis (MS), Parkinson's disease, Alzheimer's disease, epilepsy and lupus. The firm's Copaxone is a branded treatment for MS, currently marketed and sold in 42 countries including the U.S. In January 2004, Teva completed its acquisition of Sicor, Inc., expanding its customer base and product portfolio. In other news, the company announced the commercial launch of Bupropion, a generic equivalent of Wellbutrin.

FINANCIALS: Sales and profits are in thousands of dollars—add 000 to get the full amount. Year 2004 note: Complete fiscal 2004 results were not available for all companies at press time. For this company, year 2004 is for 6 months.

2004 Sales: $2,228,800 (6 months)   2004 Profits: $-197,800 (6 months)
2003 Sales: $3,276,400   2003 Profits: $691,000
2002 Sales: $2,518,600   2002 Profits: $410,300
2001 Sales: $2,077,400   2001 Profits: $278,200
2000 Sales: $1,749,000   2000 Profits: $46,858

Stock Ticker: Foreign
Employees: 10,960
Fiscal Year Ends: 12/31

SALARIES/BENEFITS:
Pension Plan: Y   ESOP Stock Plan: Profit Sharing: Top Exec. Salary: $ Bonus: $
Savings Plan: Stock Purch. Plan: Second Exec. Salary: $ Bonus: $

OTHER THOUGHTS:
Apparent Top Female Officers:
Hot Spot for Advancement for Women/Minorities:

LOCATIONS: ("Y" = Yes)
West:	Southwest:	Midwest:	Southeast:	Northeast:	International:
Y		Y		Y	Y

Note: Financial information, benefits and other data can change quickly and may vary from those stated here.

TEXAS HEALTH RESOURCES

www.texashealth.org

Industry Group Code: 622110 **Ranks within this company's industry group:** Sales: 34 Profits:

Insurance/HMO/PPO:	Drugs:	Equipment/Supplies:	Hospitals/Clinics:		Services:		Health Care:	
Insurance:	Manufacturer:	Manufacturer:	Acute Care:	Y	Diagnostics:		Home Health:	
Managed Care:	Distributor:	Distributor:	Sub-Acute Care:	Y	Labs/Testing:		Long-Term Care:	
Utilization Mgmt.:	Specialty Pharm.:	Leasing/Finance:	Outpatient Surgery:		Staffing:		Physical Therapy:	
Payment Proc.:	Vitamins/Nutri.:	Information Sys.:	Phys. Rehab. Center:		Waste Disposal:		Phys. Practice Mgmt.:	
	Clinical Trials:		Psychiatric Clinics:		Specialty Services:	Y		

TYPES OF BUSINESS:
Hospitals-General
Medical Research

BRANDS/DIVISIONS/AFFILIATES:
Harris Methodist Health System
Presbyterian Healthcare Resources
Arlington Memorial Hospital
Texas Health Research Institute

CONTACTS:
Note: Officers with more than one job title may be intentionally listed here more than once.

Doug Hawthorne, CEO
Doug Hawthorne, Pres.
Ron Bourland, CFO
Oscar Amparan, VP-Oper.
Dave Ashworth, VP-Strategy
Ferdinand Velasco, Chief Medical Info. Officer

Phone: 817-462-7900 **Fax:** 817-462-6996
Toll-Free:
Address: 611 Ryan Plaza Dr., Ste. 900, Arlington, TX 76011 US

GROWTH PLANS/SPECIAL FEATURES:

Texas Health Resources (THR) is one of the largest faith-based, nonprofit health care delivery systems in the U.S. The firm serves more than 5.4 million people living in north-central Texas through three hospital systems. THR was formed in 1997 when Harris Methodist Health System and Presbyterian Healthcare Resources united; Arlington Memorial Hospital joined later the same year. Together, the company has 14 acute-care hospitals, which account for half of the firm's health care sites and have a total of 2,405 hospital beds that are watched by more than 3,200 physicians. Arlington Memorial Hospital is an acute-care, full-service, 369-bed hospital in northern Texas with more than 550 staffed physicians. Harris Methodist Hospitals is a collection of seven hospitals and three care facilities in three northeastern Texas counties. The Presbyterian Healthcare system serves five Texas counties with six hospitals and 10 care facilities. The firm's Texas Health Research Institute subsidiary conducts medical research, offers educational programs and develops projects for the prevention, diagnosis and treatment of diseases. The firm offers e-mail and Internet access to all of its long-term patients.

THR provides employees with medical, dental, vision and life insurance, as well as flexible scheduling, community time off, a credit union and child care at some facilities.

FINANCIALS:
Sales and profits are in thousands of dollars—add 000 to get the full amount. Year 2004 note: Complete fiscal 2004 results were not available for all companies at press time. For this company, year 2004 is for months.

2004 Sales: $ (months)   2004 Profits: $ (months)
2003 Sales: $1,900,000   2003 Profits: $ **Stock Ticker:** Nonprofit
2002 Sales: $1,700,000   2002 Profits: $ **Employees:** 16,800
2001 Sales: $ 2001 Profits: $ **Fiscal Year Ends:** 12/31
2000 Sales: $ 2000 Profits: $

SALARIES/BENEFITS:
Pension Plan:	ESOP Stock Plan:	Profit Sharing:	Top Exec. Salary: $	Bonus: $
Savings Plan:	Stock Purch. Plan:		Second Exec. Salary: $	Bonus: $

OTHER THOUGHTS:
Apparent Top Female Officers:
Hot Spot for Advancement for Women/Minorities:

LOCATIONS: ("Y" = Yes)
West:	Southwest:	Midwest:	Southeast:	Northeast:	International:
Y	Y	Y	Y	Y	

THERAGENICS CORP

www.theragenics.com

Industry Group Code: 339113 Ranks within this company's industry group: Sales: 119 Profits: 104

Insurance/HMO/PPO:	Drugs:	Equipment/Supplies:		Hospitals/Clinics:	Services:	Health Care:
Insurance: Managed Care: Utilization Mgmt.: Payment Proc.:	Manufacturer: Distributor: Specialty Pharm.: Vitamins/Nutri.: Clinical Trials:	Manufacturer: Distributor: Leasing/Finance: Information Sys.:	Y	Acute Care: Sub-Acute Care: Outpatient Surgery: Phys. Rehab. Center: Psychiatric Clinics:	Diagnostics: Labs/Testing: Staffing: Waste Disposal: Specialty Services:	Home Health: Long-Term Care: Physical Therapy: Phys. Practice Mgmt.:

TYPES OF BUSINESS:
Implantable Radiation Devices

BRANDS/DIVISIONS/AFFILIATES:
TheraSeed
TheraSource
IsoSeed

CONTACTS:
Note: Officers with more than one job title may be intentionally listed here more than once.

M. Christine Jacobs, CEO
M. Christine Jacobs, Pres.
James A. MacLennan, CFO
Bruce W. Smith, Exec. VP-Acquisitions, Strategy & Dev.
James A. MacLennan, Treas.
R. Michael O'Bannon, Exec. VP-Organizational Dev.
M. Christine Jacobs, Chmn.

Phone: 770-271-0233 **Fax:** 770-831-5294
Toll-Free:
Address: 5203 Bristol Industrial Way, Buford, GA 30518 US

GROWTH PLANS/SPECIAL FEATURES:

Theragenics Corp. produces and sells implanted radioactive devices for the treatment of cancer and other complications. TheraSeed, an implant the size of a grain of rice, is used primarily in treating localized prostate cancer with a one-time, minimally invasive procedure. The implant emits radiation within the immediate prostate area, killing the tumor while sparing surrounding organs form significant radiation exposure. Theragenics is the world's leading producer of Palladium-103, the radioactive isotope that supplies the therapeutic radiation for its TheraSeed implants. The product was sold previously through an exclusive distributor, but it is now sold directly to physicians and non-exclusive third-party distributors. The firm also researches and develops uses for the isotope in the treatment of macular degeneration and other diseases. The company recently initiated a clinical study of its TheraSource intravascular brachytherapy system, which is designed to prevent restenosis following treatment of peripheral vascular disease by balloon angioplasty. Theragenics has acquired the IsoSeed business of BEBIG Isotopen-und Medizintechnik GmbH. IsoSeed is an iodine-based medical device used to treat prostate cancer.

Theragenics offers employees medical, dental and life insurance, as well as an on-site wellness center.

FINANCIALS:
Sales and profits are in thousands of dollars—add 000 to get the full amount. Year 2004 note: Complete fiscal 2004 results were not available for all companies at press time. For this company, year 2004 is for 9 months.

2004 Sales: $24,735 (9 months)	2004 Profits: $-3,022 (9 months)	
2003 Sales: $35,600	2003 Profits: $- 300	**Stock Ticker:** TGX
2002 Sales: $41,900	2002 Profits: $5,600	**Employees:** 177
2001 Sales: $50,000	2001 Profits: $15,100	**Fiscal Year Ends:** 12/31
2000 Sales: $44,000	2000 Profits: $18,700	

SALARIES/BENEFITS:
Pension Plan:	ESOP Stock Plan:	Profit Sharing:	Top Exec. Salary: $390,000	Bonus: $257,400
Savings Plan: Y	Stock Purch. Plan: Y		Second Exec. Salary: $250,000	Bonus: $7,000

OTHER THOUGHTS:
Apparent Top Female Officers: 1
Hot Spot for Advancement for Women/Minorities:

LOCATIONS: ("Y" = Yes)
West:	Southwest:	Midwest:	Southeast:	Northeast:	International:
			Y		

THERASENSE INC

www.therasense.com

Industry Group Code: 339113 **Ranks within this company's industry group:** Sales: 61 Profits: 119

Insurance/HMO/PPO:	Drugs:	Equipment/Supplies:		Hospitals/Clinics:	Services:	Health Care:
Insurance: Managed Care: Utilization Mgmt.: Payment Proc.:	Manufacturer: Distributor: Specialty Pharm.: Vitamins/Nutri.: Clinical Trials:	Manufacturer: Distributor: Leasing/Finance: Information Sys.:	Y Y Y	Acute Care: Sub-Acute Care: Outpatient Surgery: Phys. Rehab. Center: Psychiatric Clinics:	Diagnostics: Labs/Testing: Staffing: Waste Disposal: Specialty Services:	Home Health: Long-Term Care: Physical Therapy: Phys. Practice Mgmt.:

TYPES OF BUSINESS:
Glucose Measurement Devices
Data Management Software

BRANDS/DIVISIONS/AFFILIATES:
Abbott Laboratories
Disetronic Injection Systems
Nipro Corp.
FreeStyle Flash
FreeStyle Tracker
FreeStyle

CONTACTS:
Note: Officers with more than one job title may be intentionally listed here more than once.
Mark Lortz, CEO
Mark Lortz, Pres.
Mark Lortz, Chmn.

Phone: 510-749-5400 **Fax:** 510-749-5401
Toll-Free: 888-522-5226
Address: 1360 S. Loop Rd., Alameda, CA 94502 US

GROWTH PLANS/SPECIAL FEATURES:
TheraSense, Inc., a subsidiary of Abbot Laboratories since April 2004, develops, manufactures and sells simple glucose self-monitoring systems that dramatically reduce the pain of testing. The firm's main product, FreeStyle, employs patented technology to accurately measure glucose concentrations from a tiny 0.3-microliter sample of blood, as opposed to competitive products that require up to 10 microliters of blood. Such a small blood sample can come from the forearm, thigh, calf, upper arm or hand and avoids the pain of drawing a larger sample exclusively from the fingertip. TheraSense also provides the FreeStyle Tracker, a system that incorporates a blood glucose meter and management software into a PDA. Its newest device, the FreeStyle Flash, features a faster testing time and is only three inches long. The company's direct sales force promotes FreeStyle in the U.S. to health care professionals that advise patients on the management of their diabetes, while its contract sales force focuses on high-volume pharmacies. The firm also sells throughout Canada. Its Disetronic Injection Systems subsidiary distributes FreeStyle to various European countries, while Nipro Corp. distributes to Japan. The company also intends to investigate alternative applications for its FreeStyle technology, such as biochemicals testing, immunoassays and DNA sensors.

TheraSense offers its employees medical, dental, vision, life, disability and accidental death and dismemberment insurance.

FINANCIALS:
Sales and profits are in thousands of dollars—add 000 to get the full amount. Year 2004 note: Complete fiscal 2004 results were not available for all companies at press time. For this company, year 2004 is for ___ months.

2004 Sales: $ (months)	2004 Profits: $ (months)	**Stock Ticker:** Subsidiary
2003 Sales: $210,900	2003 Profits: $-4,800	Employees: 513
2002 Sales: $177,700	2002 Profits: $-29,200	Fiscal Year Ends: 12/31
2001 Sales: $71,900	2001 Profits: $-52,900	
2000 Sales: $5,500	2000 Profits: $-43,600	

SALARIES/BENEFITS:
Pension Plan:	ESOP Stock Plan:	Profit Sharing:	Top Exec. Salary: $353,173	Bonus: $43,700
Savings Plan: Y	Stock Purch. Plan: Y		Second Exec. Salary: $254,615	Bonus: $20,000

OTHER THOUGHTS:
Apparent Top Female Officers:
Hot Spot for Advancement for Women/Minorities: Y

LOCATIONS: ("Y" = Yes)
West:	Southwest:	Midwest:	Southeast:	Northeast:	International:
Y					Y

THERMO ELECTRON CORP

www.thermo.com

Industry Group Code: 334500   Ranks within this company's industry group: Sales: 1   Profits: 1

Insurance/HMO/PPO:	Drugs:	Equipment/Supplies:		Hospitals/Clinics:	Services:	Health Care:
Insurance:	Manufacturer:	Manufacturer:	Y	Acute Care:	Diagnostics:	Home Health:
Managed Care:	Distributor:	Distributor:		Sub-Acute Care:	Labs/Testing:	Long-Term Care:
Utilization Mgmt.:	Specialty Pharm.:	Leasing/Finance:		Outpatient Surgery:	Staffing:	Physical Therapy:
Payment Proc.:	Vitamins/Nutri.:	Information Sys.:		Phys. Rehab. Center:	Waste Disposal:	Phys. Practice Mgmt.:
	Clinical Trials:			Psychiatric Clinics:	Specialty Services:	

TYPES OF BUSINESS:
Measurement & Detection Equipment-Manufacturer
Analytical Instruments
Mammography Units
Infection Control Products
General Purpose X-Ray Systems
Alternative Energy Sources
Optical & Semiconductor Systems
Spectroscopy Systems

BRANDS/DIVISIONS/AFFILIATES:
NOW Flu A&B
NOW RSV

CONTACTS:
Note: Officers with more than one job title may be intentionally listed here more than once.

Marijn E. Dekkers, CEO
Marijn E. Dekkers, Pres.
Peter M. Wilver, VP/CFO
Daniel F. Kelly, VP-Mktg.
Stephen G. Sheehan, VP-Human Resources
Marc N. Casper, Pres.-Life & Laboratory Sciences
Seth H. Hoogasian, General Counsel
Peter M. Wilver, VP-Financial Oper.
J. Timothy Corcoran, VP-Corp. Comm.
J. Timothy Corcoran, VP-Investor Rel.
Kenneth J. Apicerno, Treas.
Barry S. Howe, Pres.-Measurement & Control
Guy Broadbent, Pres.-Optical Tech.
Thomas J. Burke, VP-Global Bus. Services
Seth H. Hoogasian, Corp. Sec.
Jim P. Manzi, Chmn.

Phone: 781-622-1000   Fax: 781-622-1207
Toll-Free:
Address: 81 Wyman St., Waltham, MA 02454-9046 US

GROWTH PLANS/SPECIAL FEATURES:
Thermo Electron Corporation is a global leader in the development, manufacture and sale of instrument systems, components and solutions used in virtually every industry to monitor, collect and analyze data. Thermo operates in three principal sectors: life sciences, optical technologies and measurement and control. The life sciences division addresses the biotechnology and pharmaceutical markets, as well as the clinical laboratory and health care industries, through four divisions: bioscience technologies, analytical instruments, informatics and clinical diagnostics. The optical technologies segment produces optical and semiconductor equipment systems that control and apply light for a variety of uses, including biomedical and telecommunications applications. The measurement and control segment provides a broad range of real-time, online sensors, monitors and control systems, including spectroscopy, process instruments and environmental instruments. In September 2004, Thermo announced that it would begin distributing its NOW Flu A&B and NOW RSV test kits for the rapid diagnosis of influenza and respiratory syncytial virus (RSV) in hospital and physician office laboratories in the U.S. and select overseas markets.

FINANCIALS:
Sales and profits are in thousands of dollars—add 000 to get the full amount. Year 2004 note: Complete fiscal 2004 results were not available for all companies at press time. For this company, year 2004 is for 9 months.

2004 Sales: $1,592,656 (9 months)   2004 Profits: $240,738 (9 months)
2003 Sales: $2,097,135   2003 Profits: $200,009
2002 Sales: $2,086,400   2002 Profits: $309,700
2001 Sales: $2,188,200   2001 Profits: $- 700
2000 Sales: $2,280,500   2000 Profits: $-36,100

Stock Ticker: TMO
Employees: 10,800
Fiscal Year Ends: 12/31

SALARIES/BENEFITS:
Pension Plan: Y   ESOP Stock Plan: Profit Sharing: Top Exec. Salary: $804,103   Bonus: $820,800
Savings Plan: Y   Stock Purch. Plan: Y   Second Exec. Salary: $794,872   Bonus: $820,800

OTHER THOUGHTS:
Apparent Top Female Officers:
Hot Spot for Advancement for Women/Minorities:

LOCATIONS: ("Y" = Yes)
West:	Southwest:	Midwest:	Southeast:	Northeast:	International:
Y	Y	Y	Y	Y	Y

THORATEC CORPORATION

www.thoratec.com

Industry Group Code: 339113 Ranks within this company's industry group: Sales: 72 Profits: 114

Insurance/HMO/PPO:	Drugs:	Equipment/Supplies:	Hospitals/Clinics:	Services:	Health Care:
Insurance:	Manufacturer:	Manufacturer: Y	Acute Care:	Diagnostics:	Home Health:
Managed Care:	Distributor:	Distributor:	Sub-Acute Care:	Labs/Testing:	Long-Term Care:
Utilization Mgmt.:	Specialty Pharm.:	Leasing/Finance:	Outpatient Surgery:	Staffing:	Physical Therapy:
Payment Proc.:	Vitamins/Nutri.:	Information Sys.:	Phys. Rehab. Center:	Waste Disposal:	Phys. Practice Mgmt.:
	Clinical Trials:		Psychiatric Clinics:	Specialty Services:	

TYPES OF BUSINESS:
Equipment-Heart Transplant Substitutes
Circulatory Support Products
Vascular Graft Products
Point-of-Care Diagnostic Products

BRANDS/DIVISIONS/AFFILIATES:
Thoratec VAD
International Technidyne Corp.
Thermo Cardiosystems
Thoratec IVAD

CONTACTS: Note: Officers with more than one job title may be intentionally listed here more than once.
D. Keith Grossman, CEO
D. Keith Grossman, Pres.
M. Wayne Boylston, Sr. VP/CFO
Beth A. Taylor, Human Resources Admin.
David J. Farrar, VP-Research & Dev.
David A. Lehman, General Counsel
Joseph G. Sharpe, VP-Oper.
Jon R. Shear, VP-Bus. Dev.
Donald A. Middlebrook, VP-Regulatory Affairs & Quality Assurance
Jeffrey W. Nelson, Pres.-Cardiovascular Div.
Lawrence Cohen, Pres., International Technidyne Corp.

Phone: 925-847-8600 Fax: 925-847-8574
Toll-Free: 800-528-2577
Address: 6035 Stoneridge Dr., Pleasanton, CA 94588 US

GROWTH PLANS/SPECIAL FEATURES:
Thoratec Corp. is the leading manufacturer of circulatory support products for patients with congestive heart failure (CHF). Products are divided into three categories: circulatory support products, which are products for the short- and long-term treatment of CHF; vascular graft products, which are small-diameter grafts for vascular access and coronary bypass surgery; and point-of-care diagnostics, which are blood test systems to improve patient management, reduce health care costs and improve patient outcomes. The firm was the first company to receive approval from the FDA to commercially market a ventricular assist device (VAD) to treat patients with late-stage heart failure. These VADs are used to perform some or all of the pumping function of the heart. Thoratec offers the widest range of products to serve this market. The firm's VADs have treated approximately 8,500 patients, can be implanted or worn outside the body and are suitable for the treatment of patients of varying sizes and ages for different durations. The company is pursuing approval to use its VADs in other applications, including as an alternative to maximum drug therapy. Through British subsidiary International Technidyne Corp., the firm provides a family of single-use skin incision devices used to provide blood samples. Following its merger with Thermo Cardiosystems, a manufacturer of cardiac assist, blood coagulation testing and skin incision devices, Thoratec substantially increased its size and become the leading provider of circulatory support products worldwide. Thoratec recently received premarket approval from the FDA for the Thoratec Implantable Ventricular Assist Device (IVAD).

Thoratec offers its employees benefits including a comprehensive health plan, education assistance, a referral program and stock options.

FINANCIALS:
Sales and profits are in thousands of dollars—add 000 to get the full amount. Year 2004 note: Complete fiscal 2004 results were not available for all companies at press time. For this company, year 2004 is for 6 months.

2004 Sales: $83,395 (6 months)   2004 Profits: $1,500 (6 months)
2003 Sales: $149,916   2003 Profits: $-2,182
2002 Sales: $130,800   2002 Profits: $ 500
2001 Sales: $113,400   2001 Profits: $-87,900
2000 Sales: $30,400   2000 Profits: $-1,700

Stock Ticker: THOR
Employees: 802
Fiscal Year Ends: 12/31

SALARIES/BENEFITS:
Pension Plan: ESOP Stock Plan: Profit Sharing: Top Exec. Salary: $410,577   Bonus: $315,900
Savings Plan: Y Stock Purch. Plan: Second Exec. Salary: $259,904   Bonus: $157,223

OTHER THOUGHTS:
Apparent Top Female Officers: 1
Hot Spot for Advancement for Women/Minorities:

LOCATIONS: ("Y" = Yes)
West:	Southwest:	Midwest:	Southeast:	Northeast:	International:
Y				Y	Y

Note: Financial information, benefits and other data can change quickly and may vary from those stated here.

TLC VISION CORPORATION

www.tlcv.com

Industry Group Code: 621490 Ranks within this company's industry group: Sales: 8 Profits: 18

Insurance/HMO/PPO:	Drugs:	Equipment/Supplies:	Hospitals/Clinics:	Services:	Health Care:
Insurance:	Manufacturer:	Manufacturer: Y	Acute Care:	Diagnostics:	Home Health:
Managed Care:	Distributor:	Distributor:	Sub-Acute Care:	Labs/Testing:	Long-Term Care:
Utilization Mgmt.:	Specialty Pharm.:	Leasing/Finance:	Outpatient Surgery: Y	Staffing:	Physical Therapy:
Payment Proc.:	Vitamins/Nutri.:	Information Sys.: Y	Phys. Rehab. Center:	Waste Disposal:	Phys. Practice Mgmt.:
	Clinical Trials:		Psychiatric Clinics:	Specialty Services:	

TYPES OF BUSINESS:
Eye Clinics
Laser Vision Correction Services
Blood Filtration Equipment
Management Software & Systems

BRANDS/DIVISIONS/AFFILIATES:
Laser Vision Centers, Inc.
TLC Laser Eye Centers, Inc.
CustomLASIK
OccuLogix, LP
Rheopheresis

CONTACTS:
Note: Officers with more than one job title may be intentionally listed here more than once.

James C. Wachtman, CEO
James C. Wachtman, Pres.
Steven P. Rasche, CFO
Jay Peters, Chief Mktg. Officer
Paul Frederick, Exec. VP-Human Resources
Henry Lynn, VP-Info. Systems
Robert W. May, General Counsel
Rikki Bradley, VP-Oper. & Clinical Services
William P. Leonard, Exec. VP-Eastern Zone
Rob Thornhill, Exec. VP-Western Zone
Robert W. May, Corp. Sec.
Elias Vamvakas, Chmn.

Phone: 905-602-2020 Fax: 905-602-2025
Toll-Free: 800-852-1033
Address: 5280 Solar Dr., Ste. 300, Mississauga, Ontario L4W 5M8 Canada

GROWTH PLANS/SPECIAL FEATURES:

TLC Vision Corporation is a leading provider of laser vision correction services in North America. TLC owns and manages about 130 eye care centers, which, together with TLC's network of over 12,500 eye care doctors, provide laser vision correction of common refractive vision disorders, including myopia, hyperopia and astigmatism. TLC physicians use excimer lasers to perform eye surgery, using either photorefractive keratectomy (PRK) or laser in-situ keratomileusis (LASIK). More than 90% of the excimer laser procedures performed at the company's eye care centers are LASIK, which TLC doctors believe is more precise than PRK. TLC uses its proprietary management and administrative software in all of the company eye clinics. The software helps to provide a potential surgical candidate with current information on affiliated doctors throughout North America, direct a candidate to the closest eye care center, track calls and procedures, coordinate patients and doctor scheduling and produce financial and surgical outcome reporting and analysis. Additionally, TLC has introduced a new online consumer consultation feature on its web site, which allows consumers to book their consultation appointment. The firm has a joint venture with Vascular Sciences Corporation, OccuLogix, LP, which intends to commercialize Vascular Sciences' Rheopheresis blood filtration process for age-related macular degeneration (AMD).

The company offers its employees comprehensive medical, dental, life and disability insurance.

FINANCIALS:
Sales and profits are in thousands of dollars—add 000 to get the full amount. Year 2004 note: Complete fiscal 2004 results were not available for all companies at press time. For this company, year 2004 is for 9 months.

2004 Sales: $186,480 (9 months) 2004 Profits: $17,613 (9 months)
2003 Sales: $195,680 2003 Profits: $-9,399
2002 Sales: $100,200 2002 Profits: $-43,300
2001 Sales: $174,000 2001 Profits: $-34,800
2000 Sales: $201,200 2000 Profits: $-5,900

Stock Ticker: TLCV
Employees: 854
Fiscal Year Ends: 12/31

SALARIES/BENEFITS:
Pension Plan: ESOP Stock Plan: Profit Sharing: Top Exec. Salary: $218,750   Bonus: $37,500
Savings Plan: Y Stock Purch. Plan: Y   Second Exec. Salary: $140,000   Bonus: $37,500

OTHER THOUGHTS:
Apparent Top Female Officers: 1
Hot Spot for Advancement for Women/Minorities:

LOCATIONS: ("Y" = Yes)
West:	Southwest:	Midwest:	Southeast:	Northeast:	International:
Y	Y	Y	Y	Y	Y

TOSHIBA CORPORATION

www.toshiba.com

Industry Group Code: 334111 Ranks within this company's industry group: Sales: 1 Profits: 1

Insurance/HMO/PPO:	Drugs:	Equipment/Supplies:		Hospitals/Clinics:	Services:	Health Care:	
Insurance:	Manufacturer:	Manufacturer:	Y	Acute Care:	Diagnostics:	Home Health:	
Managed Care:	Distributor:	Distributor:		Sub-Acute Care:	Labs/Testing:	Long-Term Care:	
Utilization Mgmt.:	Specialty Pharm.:	Leasing/Finance:		Outpatient Surgery:	Staffing:	Physical Therapy:	
Payment Proc.:	Vitamins/Nutri.:	Information Sys.:	Y	Phys. Rehab. Center:	Waste Disposal:	Phys. Practice Mgmt.:	
	Clinical Trials:			Psychiatric Clinics:	Specialty Services:		

TYPES OF BUSINESS:
Computers and Storage Devices Manufacturing
Medical Equipment
Telecommunications Equipment
Energy Power Plant Systems
Consumer Electronics
Semiconductors
Transportation Systems
Air Traffic Control Systems

BRANDS/DIVISIONS/AFFILIATES:

CONTACTS:
Note: Officers with more than one job title may be intentionally listed here more than once.
Tadashi Okamura, CEO
Tadashi Okamura, Pres.
Yasuo Morimoto, Corp. Sr. Exec. VP
Takeshi Iida, Corp. Sr. Exec. VP
Makoto Nakagawa, Corp. Sr. Exec. VP
Taizo Nishimuro, Chmn.

Phone: 81-3-3457-4511 Fax: 81-3-3455-1631
Toll-Free:
Address: 1-1, Shibaura 1-chome, Minato-ku, Tokyo, 105-8001 Japan

GROWTH PLANS/SPECIAL FEATURES:
Toshiba is a global leader in the manufacture of consumer, industrial, medical and communications electronics. The company has recently recategorized its component in-house and group companies into four autonomous business divisions: digital products, including mobile communications, digital media networks (consumer DVD recorders, LCD TVs, etc.) and personal computers; electronic devices, including semiconductors and display devices; social infrastructure, overseeing industrial and power systems, social network and infrastructure systems (such as automated letter processing systems and ATMs), elevator systems and medical technologies; and home appliances, managing white goods, as well as battery manufacturing, lighting systems and network services. With highly diversified products and clients, it is not surprising that recent advances at Toshiba range from web acceleration protocols and wireless home media stations to non-fluorochloro-hydrocarbon refrigerators and nuclear reactor inspection technologies. The company's power systems division also offers thermal, geothermal and hydroelectric power generation systems. Among Toshiba's many breakthroughs is the development, in partnership with Sony, of a 45-nanometer large-scale integration (LSI) CMOS process technology, a chip-based DNA detection and analysis system, experimental applications utilizing nanosensitive materials in high-density storage devices and the development of solid-state quantum computer technologies, which use semiconductor nanocrystals without the requirement of extensive micromachining or nanofabrication. The company has announced that its short-term core business development efforts will focus on digital products and electronic devices.

FINANCIALS:
Sales and profits are in thousands of dollars—add 000 to get the full amount. Year 2004 note: Complete fiscal 2004 results were not available for all companies at press time. For this company, year 2004 is for 12 months.

2004 Sales: $52,815,600 (12 months)   2004 Profits: $272,900 (12 months)
2003 Sales: $47,191,800   2003 Profits: $154,400
2002 Sales: $40,665,600   2002 Profits: $-1,915,000
2001 Sales: $47,110,900   2001 Profits: $761,300
2000 Sales: $54,492,500   2000 Profits: $-265,400

Stock Ticker: Foreign
Employees: 166,651
Fiscal Year Ends: 3/31

SALARIES/BENEFITS:
Pension Plan: ESOP Stock Plan: Profit Sharing: Top Exec. Salary: $ Bonus: $
Savings Plan: Stock Purch. Plan: Second Exec. Salary: $ Bonus: $

OTHER THOUGHTS:
Apparent Top Female Officers:
Hot Spot for Advancement for Women/Minorities:

LOCATIONS: ("Y" = Yes)

West:	Southwest:	Midwest:	Southeast:	Northeast:	International:
Y	Y			Y	Y

TRANSCEND SERVICES INC
www.transcendservices.com

Industry Group Code: 514210 Ranks within this company's industry group: Sales: 1 Profits: 1

Insurance/HMO/PPO:	Drugs:	Equipment/Supplies:	Hospitals/Clinics:	Services:	Health Care:
Insurance:	Manufacturer:	Manufacturer:	Acute Care:	Diagnostics:	Home Health:
Managed Care:	Distributor:	Distributor:	Sub-Acute Care:	Labs/Testing:	Long-Term Care:
Utilization Mgmt.:	Specialty Pharm.:	Leasing/Finance:	Outpatient Surgery:	Staffing:	Physical Therapy:
Payment Proc.:	Vitamins/Nutri.:	Information Sys.:	Phys. Rehab. Center:	Waste Disposal:	Phys. Practice Mgmt.:
	Clinical Trials:		Psychiatric Clinics:	Specialty Services: Y	

TYPES OF BUSINESS:
Data Processing Services
Internet-Based Medical Transcription Services

BRANDS/DIVISIONS/AFFILIATES:

CONTACTS:
Note: Officers with more than one job title may be intentionally listed here more than once.

Larry G. Gerdes, CEO
Thomas C. Binion, Pres.
Thomas C. Binion, COO
Joe Bleser, CFO
Dominick DeRosa, VP-Mktg. & Sales
Carl Hawkins, CIO
Larry G. Gerdes, Treas.
Bob Alexander, VP-Customer Service
Joe Bleser, Corp. Sec.

Phone: 404-836-8000 Fax: 404-836-8009
Toll-Free: 800-555-8727
Address: 945 E. Paces Ferry Rd., Ste. 1475, Atlanta, GA 30326 US

GROWTH PLANS/SPECIAL FEATURES:

Transcend Services, Inc. is one of the four largest transcription service providers in the United States and one of only several national companies that operates on a single, Internet-based technology. The firm provides medical transcription services to the health care industry through its web-based voice and data distribution technology and home-based medical transcription professionals who document patient care by converting physicians' voice recordings into electronic medical record documents. Physicians may access the company's technology from any phone, where they can dictate patient medical records information. This information is captured digitally in the firm's central voice hub in Atlanta, Georgia, where the digital files are compressed, encrypted and stored. After transcription, documents are returned to the Atlanta hub over the Internet. The documents may then be accessed by remote quality assurance personnel and delivered electronically to the health care provider. These operations are available around the clock, every day of the year. Generally documents are produced and delivered within 24 hours, with faster service available at a premium cost. The company is now strategically focused solely on providing medical transcription services, having sold its coding and abstracting software subsidiary in May 2002. Customers include hospitals, hospital systems, multi-specialty clinics and physician group practices.

Transcend Services offers its employees flexible hours, competitive rates, production-based incentive pay and a benefits package that includes medical, dental and life insurance.

FINANCIALS:
Sales and profits are in thousands of dollars—add 000 to get the full amount. Year 2004 note: Complete fiscal 2004 results were not available for all companies at press time. For this company, year 2004 is for 9 months.

2004 Sales: $11,296 (9 months)   2004 Profits: $ 195 (9 months)
2003 Sales: $14,663   2003 Profits: $1,020
2002 Sales: $12,200   2002 Profits: $ 900
2001 Sales: $13,800   2001 Profits: $- 600
2000 Sales: $26,300   2000 Profits: $- 700

Stock Ticker: TRCR
Employees: 373
Fiscal Year Ends: 12/31

SALARIES/BENEFITS:
Pension Plan: ESOP Stock Plan: Profit Sharing: Top Exec. Salary: $220,000   Bonus: $
Savings Plan: Y   Stock Purch. Plan: Second Exec. Salary: $165,000   Bonus: $

OTHER THOUGHTS:
Apparent Top Female Officers:
Hot Spot for Advancement for Women/Minorities:

LOCATIONS: ("Y" = Yes)
West:	Southwest:	Midwest:	Southeast:	Northeast:	International:
Y	Y	Y	Y	Y	

… continued

TRIAD HOSPITALS INC

www.triadhospitals.com

Industry Group Code: 622110   Ranks within this company's industry group: Sales: 14   Profits: 12

Insurance/HMO/PPO:	Drugs:	Equipment/Supplies:	Hospitals/Clinics:		Services:		Health Care:	
Insurance:	Manufacturer:	Manufacturer:	Acute Care:	Y	Diagnostics:		Home Health:	
Managed Care:	Distributor:	Distributor:	Sub-Acute Care:		Labs/Testing:		Long-Term Care:	
Utilization Mgmt.:	Specialty Pharm.:	Leasing/Finance:	Outpatient Surgery:	Y	Staffing:		Physical Therapy:	
Payment Proc.:	Vitamins/Nutri.:	Information Sys.:	Phys. Rehab. Center:		Waste Disposal:		Phys. Practice Mgmt.:	
	Clinical Trials:		Psychiatric Clinics:		Specialty Services:	Y		

TYPES OF BUSINESS:
Hospitals-General
Ambulatory Surgery Centers
Management & Consulting Services

BRANDS/DIVISIONS/AFFILIATES:
Quorum Health Group

CONTACTS:
Note: Officers with more than one job title may be intentionally listed here more than once.

James D. Shelton, CEO
James D. Shelton, Pres.
Michael J. Parsons, COO
Burke W. Whitman, CFO
Rick Thomason, VP-Human Resources
Thomas H. Frazier, VP-Admin.
Rebecca Hurley, General Counsel
Daniel J. Moen, Exec. VP- Dev. & Mgmt. Services
James R. Bedenbaugh, Treas.
William L. Anderson, Div. Pres.
Kevin R. Andrews, Div. Pres.
R. Brian Deaver, Pres.- Ambulatory Surgery Div.
Marsha D. Powers, Div. Pres.
James D. Shelton, Chmn.

Phone: 214-473-7000   Fax: 214-473-9411
Toll-Free: 800-238-6006
Address: 5800 Tennyson Pkwy., Plano, TX 75024 US

GROWTH PLANS/SPECIAL FEATURES:
Triad Hospitals, Inc. is one of the largest publicly owned hospital companies in the U.S. and provides health care services through hospitals and surgery centers located in small cities and selected high-growth urban markets in the southwestern, western and south-central U.S. Triad's facilities, located in Alabama, Alaska, Arizona, Arkansas, California, Indiana, Kansas, Louisiana, Mississippi, Missouri, Nevada, New Mexico, Ohio, Oklahoma, Oregon, South Carolina, Texas and West Virginia, include 56 general acute care hospitals and 16 ambulatory surgery centers. The firm is also a minority investor in three joint ventures that own seven general acute care hospitals in Georgia and Nevada. Triad also offers a variety of management services available to health care facilities, including ethics and compliance programs, national supply and equipment purchasing and leasing contracts, accounting, financial and clinical systems, governmental reimbursement assistance, information systems, legal support, personnel management and internal audit, access to regional managed care networks and resource management. Through subsidiary Quorum Health Group, the company provides management and consulting services to acute care hospitals, serving approximately 200 hospitals throughout the U.S. Triad recently announced plans to sell its hospital in San Leandro, California to Eden Township Healthcare District. The hospital is a 122-bed acute care facility and the only California hospital the firm owns. Under the terms of the agreement, there will be no change in emergency or acute care services at San Leandro Hospital for at least three years.

FINANCIALS:
Sales and profits are in thousands of dollars—add 000 to get the full amount. Year 2004 note: Complete fiscal 2004 results were not available for all companies at press time. For this company, year 2004 is for 9 months.

2004 Sales: $3,310,700 (9 months)   2004 Profits: $141,800 (9 months)
2003 Sales: $3,865,900   2003 Profits: $95,200
2002 Sales: $3,541,100   2002 Profits: $141,500
2001 Sales: $2,669,500   2001 Profits: $2,800
2000 Sales: $1,235,500   2000 Profits: $4,400

Stock Ticker: TRI
Employees: 36,000
Fiscal Year Ends: 12/31

SALARIES/BENEFITS:
Pension Plan: ESOP Stock Plan: Profit Sharing: Top Exec. Salary: $976,240   Bonus: $731,250
Savings Plan: Stock Purch. Plan: Y   Second Exec. Salary: $487,744   Bonus: $243,934

OTHER THOUGHTS:
Apparent Top Female Officers: 2
Hot Spot for Advancement for Women/Minorities

LOCATIONS: ("Y" = Yes)
West:	Southwest:	Midwest:	Southeast:	Northeast:	International:
Y	Y	Y	Y	Y	

TRINITY HEALTH COMPANY

www.trinity-health.org

Industry Group Code: 622110 **Ranks within this company's industry group:** Sales: 10 Profits: 20

Insurance/HMO/PPO:	Drugs:	Equipment/Supplies:	Hospitals/Clinics:		Services:		Health Care:	
Insurance:	Manufacturer:	Manufacturer:	Acute Care:	Y	Diagnostics:		Home Health:	Y
Managed Care: Y	Distributor:	Distributor:	Sub-Acute Care:	Y	Labs/Testing:		Long-Term Care:	Y
Utilization Mgmt.:	Specialty Pharm.:	Leasing/Finance:	Outpatient Surgery:		Staffing:		Physical Therapy:	
Payment Proc.:	Vitamins/Nutri.:	Information Sys.:	Phys. Rehab. Center:		Waste Disposal:		Phys. Practice Mgmt.:	
	Clinical Trials:		Psychiatric Clinics:		Specialty Services:	Y		

TYPES OF BUSINESS:
Hospitals
Assisted Living Facilities
Hospice Programs
Senior Housing Communities
Management & Consulting Services
HMO
Building & Design Services

BRANDS/DIVISIONS/AFFILIATES:
Catholic Health Ministries
Trinity Health International
Trinity Health Plans
Care Choice
Trinity Design

CONTACTS:
Note: Officers with more than one job title may be intentionally listed here more than once.
Judy Pelham, CEO
Judy Pelham, Pres.
Edgar T. Carlson, COO
James Hendricks, Chmn.

Phone: 248-489-5004   **Fax:** 248-489-6039
Toll-Free:
Address: 27870 Cabot Dr., Novi, MI 48377-2920 US

GROWTH PLANS/SPECIAL FEATURES:

Trinity Health Company, sponsored by Catholic Health Ministries, is the country's third-largest Catholic health system, with more than 6,500 acute-care and non-acute-care beds in 45 hospitals. The firm also has 372 outpatient facilities, numerous assisted living facilities, home health services, hospice programs and senior housing communities in seven states. Trinity operates in California, Idaho, Indiana, Iowa, Maryland, Michigan, Ohio and internationally. The company's Trinity Health International subsidiary provides management, training, consulting and technical assistance to health care organizations and governments in more than 40 countries around the world through more than 160 projects. Other subsidiaries include Trinity Health Plans, which operates Care Choice HMOs in six southeast Michigan counties, and Trinity Design, which offers health care facility building and design services. In recent news, Trinity Health received the National Committee of Quality Health Care's National Quality Health Care Award for 2004.

Trinity Health offers employees health and dental coverage, employee and dependant life insurance, flexible spending accounts, tuition reimbursement and adoption assistance.

FINANCIALS:
Sales and profits are in thousands of dollars—add 000 to get the full amount. Year 2004 note: Complete fiscal 2004 results were not available for all companies at press time. For this company, year 2004 is for months.

2004 Sales: $ (months)	2004 Profits: $ (months)	**Stock Ticker:** Nonprofit
2003 Sales: $4,956,700	2003 Profits: $-235,900	Employees: 43,900
2002 Sales: $4,696,600	2002 Profits: $5,400	Fiscal Year Ends: 6/30
2001 Sales: $	2001 Profits: $	
2000 Sales: $	2000 Profits: $	

SALARIES/BENEFITS:
Pension Plan: Y	ESOP Stock Plan:	Profit Sharing:	Top Exec. Salary: $	Bonus: $
Savings Plan: Y	Stock Purch. Plan:		Second Exec. Salary: $	Bonus: $

OTHER THOUGHTS:
Apparent Top Female Officers: 1
Hot Spot for Advancement for Women/Minorities:

LOCATIONS: ("Y" = Yes)
West:	Southwest:	Midwest:	Southeast:	Northeast:	International:
Y		Y		Y	Y

TRIPATH IMAGING INC

www.tripathimaging.com

Industry Group Code: 339113 Ranks within this company's industry group: Sales: 110 Profits: 123

Insurance/HMO/PPO:	Drugs:	Equipment/Supplies:	Hospitals/Clinics:	Services:	Health Care:
Insurance:	Manufacturer:	Manufacturer: Y	Acute Care:	Diagnostics:	Home Health:
Managed Care:	Distributor:	Distributor:	Sub-Acute Care:	Labs/Testing:	Long-Term Care:
Utilization Mgmt.:	Specialty Pharm.:	Leasing/Finance:	Outpatient Surgery:	Staffing:	Physical Therapy:
Payment Proc.:	Vitamins/Nutri.:	Information Sys.:	Phys. Rehab. Center:	Waste Disposal:	Phys. Practice Mgmt.:
	Clinical Trials:		Psychiatric Clinics:	Specialty Services:	

TYPES OF BUSINESS:
Automated Diagnostic Devices
Cervical Cancer Screening Products

BRANDS/DIVISIONS/AFFILIATES:
AutoCyte
PrepStain
FocalPoint SlideProfiler
SurePath
TriPath Oncology

CONTACTS:
Note: Officers with more than one job title may be intentionally listed here more than once.
Paul R. Sohmer, CEO
Paul R. Sohmer, Pres.
Stephen P. Hall, CFO
Pat W. Kennedy, General Counsel
Ray Swanson, Sr. VP-Commercial Oper.
Johnny D. Powers, VP/Mgr.-TriPath Oncology

Phone: 336-222-9707 Fax: 336-222-8819
Toll-Free: 800-426-2176
Address: 780 Plantation Dr., Burlington, NC 27215 US

GROWTH PLANS/SPECIAL FEATURES:
TriPath Imaging, Inc. manufactures proprietary products for all phases of cervical cancer treatment, including detection, diagnosis, staging and management. TriPath is organized into two operating units: commercial operations and TriPath Oncology. The commercial operations unit manages the market introduction, sales, service, manufacturing and ongoing development of the firm's products. TriPath Oncology, a wholly-owned subsidiary, manages the development of molecular diagnostic and pharmacogenomic tests for cancer. TriPath products include the SurePath system, a liquid-based cytology sample collection, preservation and transport system; PrepStain, an automated slide preparation system that produces slides for cervical cancer testing; and the FocalPoint SlideProfiler system, a slide screening system that analyzes cervical cell samples for abnormalities. The company also produces the AutoCyte pathology workstation, which allows for digital imaging of pathology specimens.

TriPath offers its employees a competitive health and insurance package plus stock options.

FINANCIALS:
Sales and profits are in thousands of dollars—add 000 to get the full amount. Year 2004 note: Complete fiscal 2004 results were not available for all companies at press time. For this company, year 2004 is for 9 months.

2004 Sales: $50,259 (9 months)   2004 Profits: $ 297 (9 months)
2003 Sales: $53,764   2003 Profits: $-8,538
2002 Sales: $37,500   2002 Profits: $-18,100
2001 Sales: $27,000   2001 Profits: $-21,700
2000 Sales: $32,700   2000 Profits: $-17,000

Stock Ticker: TPTH
Employees: 280
Fiscal Year Ends: 12/31

SALARIES/BENEFITS:
| Pension Plan: | ESOP Stock Plan: Y | Profit Sharing: | Top Exec. Salary: $391,731 | Bonus: $199,000 |
| Savings Plan: Y | Stock Purch. Plan: | | Second Exec. Salary: $240,206 | Bonus: $100,800 |

OTHER THOUGHTS:
Apparent Top Female Officers: 1
Hot Spot for Advancement for Women/Minorities:

LOCATIONS: ("Y" = Yes)
West:	Southwest:	Midwest:	Southeast:	Northeast:	International:
Y				Y	

TRIPOS INC

www.tripos.com

Industry Group Code: 511200   Ranks within this company's industry group: Sales: 10   Profits: 8

Insurance/HMO/PPO:	Drugs:	Equipment/Supplies:	Hospitals/Clinics:	Services:	Health Care:
Insurance:	Manufacturer:	Manufacturer:	Acute Care:	Diagnostics:	Home Health:
Managed Care:	Distributor:	Distributor:	Sub-Acute Care:	Labs/Testing:	Long-Term Care:
Utilization Mgmt.:	Specialty Pharm.:	Leasing/Finance:	Outpatient Surgery:	Staffing:	Physical Therapy:
Payment Proc.:	Vitamins/Nutri.:	Information Sys.: Y	Phys. Rehab. Center:	Waste Disposal:	Phys. Practice Mgmt.:
	Clinical Trials:		Psychiatric Clinics:	Specialty Services: Y	

TYPES OF BUSINESS:
Research-Pharmaceuticals
Clinical Software
Consulting Services
Chemical Compound Libraries
Integrated Data Systems

BRANDS/DIVISIONS/AFFILIATES:
SYBYL
LITHIUM
SARNavigator
LeadQuest

GROWTH PLANS/SPECIAL FEATURES:
Tripos, Inc., through its many subsidiaries worldwide, is a leader in discovery services, informatics and products for life science organizations. Its products and services are used primarily in the preclinical phases of new pharmaceutical development, the equivalent pre-approval phase of agrochemical product development and the product discovery phases of chemical research. The company's discovery informatics products include SYBYL, a virtual discovery laboratory; LITHIUM software for creating 3-D molecular models; and SARNavigator, a data analysis tool. In addition, Tripos produces custom IT solutions for customers, designed to reduce the amount of time involved in drug discovery. It also owns LeadQuest, a group of compound libraries designed to be drug-like. Tripos is involved in many collaborations, most recently inclluding partnerships with the European Molecular Biology Laboratory and German Cancer Research Centre, Bayer Healthcare AG and Schering AG.

CONTACTS:
Note: Officers with more than one job title may be intentionally listed here more than once.
John P. McAlister, III, CEO
John P. McAlister, III, Pres.
B. James Rubin, Sr. VP/CFO/Corp. Sec.
Dieter Schmidt-Base, Sr. VP-Worldwide Sales
Richard D. Cramer, III, Chief Scientific Officer/Sr. VP-Science
Mark Allen, VP-Oper., Tripos Receptor Research
Mary P. Woodward, Sr. VP-Strategic Dev.
John D. Yingling, VP/Chief Acc. Officer
Trevor W. Heritage, Sr. VP/Mgr.-Discovery Informatics
Peter Hecht, Sr. VP-Discovery Research Oper.
Edward Hodgkin, VP-Mktg. & Bus. Dev.
Ralph S. Lobdell, Chmn.

Phone: 314-647-1099   Fax: 314-647-9241
Toll-Free: 800-323-2960
Address: 1699 S. Hanley Rd., St. Louis, MO 63144-2913 US

FINANCIALS:
Sales and profits are in thousands of dollars—add 000 to get the full amount. Year 2004 note: Complete fiscal 2004 results were not available for all companies at press time. For this company, year 2004 is for 9 months.

2004 Sales: $47,463 (9 months)	2004 Profits: $- 14 (9 months)	Stock Ticker: TRPS
2003 Sales: $54,148	2003 Profits: $2,100	Employees: 358
2002 Sales: $51,100	2002 Profits: $ 900	Fiscal Year Ends: 12/31
2001 Sales: $49,100	2001 Profits: $5,900	
2000 Sales: $29,000	2000 Profits: $-2,100	

SALARIES/BENEFITS:
| Pension Plan: | ESOP Stock Plan: | Profit Sharing: | Top Exec. Salary: $325,000 | Bonus: $76,050 |
| Savings Plan: Y | Stock Purch. Plan: Y | | Second Exec. Salary: $205,833 | Bonus: $44,480 |

OTHER THOUGHTS:
Apparent Top Female Officers: 1
Hot Spot for Advancement for Women/Minorities:

LOCATIONS: ("Y" = Yes)
| West: | Southwest: | Midwest: Y | Southeast: | Northeast: | International: Y |

TUFTS ASSOCIATED HEALTH PLANS   www.tufts-healthplan.com

Industry Group Code: 524114   Ranks within this company's industry group: Sales: 30   Profits: 30

Insurance/HMO/PPO:		Drugs:	Equipment/Supplies:	Hospitals/Clinics:	Services:	Health Care:
Insurance:		Manufacturer:	Manufacturer:	Acute Care:	Diagnostics:	Home Health:
Managed Care:	Y	Distributor:	Distributor:	Sub-Acute Care:	Labs/Testing:	Long-Term Care:
Utilization Mgmt.:		Specialty Pharm.:	Leasing/Finance:	Outpatient Surgery:	Staffing:	Physical Therapy:
Payment Proc.:		Vitamins/Nutri.:	Information Sys.:	Phys. Rehab. Center:	Waste Disposal:	Phys. Practice Mgmt.:
		Clinical Trials:		Psychiatric Clinics:	Specialty Services:	

Insurance/HMO/PPO: Insurance: Y (Managed Care: Y)

TYPES OF BUSINESS:
Insurance-Health
Insurance-Life

BRANDS/DIVISIONS/AFFILIATES:
Tufts Associated Health Maintenance Organization
Tufts Insurance Company
Tufts Benefit Administrators, Inc.
Tufts Total Health Plan
Tufts Preferred Provider Option
Secure Horizons

CONTACTS:
Note: Officers with more than one job title may be intentionally listed here more than once.
Nancy L. Leaming, CEO
Nancy L. Leaming, Pres.
Richard Hallworth, COO
J. Andy Hilbert, CFO
Keven J. Counihan, VP-Mktg. & Sales
Tricia Trebino, CIO
James Roosevelt Jr., General Counsel
Jon M. Kingsdale, VP-Planning
Philip R. Boulter, Chief Medical Officer

Phone: Fax: 781-466-8504
Toll-Free: 800-208-8013
Address: 333 Wyman St., P.O. Box 9112, Waltham, MA 02454-9112 US

GROWTH PLANS/SPECIAL FEATURES:
Tufts Associated Health Plans serves a collection of subsidiaries, including Tufts Associated Health Maintenance Organization (TAHMO) and the Tufts Insurance Company with administrative, management, advertising and marketing services. TAHMO is a not-for-profit HMO with 747,000 customers. It was founded in 1979, and offers health care coverage, including HMOs, PPOs, POSs and other plans, to corporations, groups and individuals through employer groups. The subsidiary has 85 hospitals and 20,326 physicians in network and $2.3 billion in total revenue. Other health insurance subsidiaries include Secure Horizons, a health plan specifically designed for seniors as a Medicare supplemental plan offering comprehensive health benefits, including preventive care; The Tufts Total Health Plan for POS plans that offer a choice between two levels of coverage and others. The Tufts Insurance Company supplies life insurance to more than 800,000 customers. Tufts Benefit Administrators, Inc. offers third party administrative services for the Tufts Preferred Provider Option and indemnity plans. Tufts Health Plan has recently been named one of the top ten health plans in the country for clinical effectiveness by the National Committee for Quality Assurance.

FINANCIALS:
Sales and profits are in thousands of dollars—add 000 to get the full amount. Year 2004 note: Complete fiscal 2004 results were not available for all companies at press time. For this company, year 2004 is for months.

2004 Sales: $ (months)	2004 Profits: $ (months)	**Stock Ticker:** Private
2003 Sales: $2,300,000	2003 Profits: $56,900	Employees: 2,500
2002 Sales: $2,329,400	2002 Profits: $	Fiscal Year Ends: 12/31
2001 Sales: $	2001 Profits: $	
2000 Sales: $	2000 Profits: $	

SALARIES/BENEFITS:
Pension Plan: ESOP Stock Plan: Profit Sharing: Top Exec. Salary: $ Bonus: $
Savings Plan: Stock Purch. Plan: Second Exec. Salary: $ Bonus: $

OTHER THOUGHTS:
Apparent Top Female Officers: 2
Hot Spot for Advancement for Women/Minorities:

LOCATIONS: ("Y" = Yes)
West:	Southwest:	Midwest:	Southeast:	Northeast:	International:
				Y	

Note: Financial information, benefits and other data can change quickly and may vary from those stated here.

TYCO HEALTHCARE GROUP

www.tycohealthcare.com

Industry Group Code: 339113 Ranks within this company's industry group: Sales: Profits:

Insurance/HMO/PPO:	Drugs:	Equipment/Supplies:	Hospitals/Clinics:	Services:	Health Care:
Insurance:	Manufacturer: Y	Manufacturer: Y	Acute Care:	Diagnostics:	Home Health:
Managed Care:	Distributor:	Distributor:	Sub-Acute Care:	Labs/Testing:	Long-Term Care:
Utilization Mgmt.:	Specialty Pharm.:	Leasing/Finance:	Outpatient Surgery:	Staffing:	Physical Therapy:
Payment Proc.:	Vitamins/Nutri.:	Information Sys.:	Phys. Rehab. Center:	Waste Disposal:	Phys. Practice Mgmt.:
	Clinical Trials:		Psychiatric Clinics:	Specialty Services:	

TYPES OF BUSINESS:
Medical Supplies, Manufacturing
Pharmaceuticals
Chemicals
Surgical Products
Imaging Products
Respiratory Products
Diagnostic Products

BRANDS/DIVISIONS/AFFILIATES:
Tyco International, Ltd.
U.S. Surgical
Valleylab
Kendall
Mallinckodt
Nellcor
Ludlow Tape
UniPatch

CONTACTS: Note: Officers with more than one job title may be intentionally listed here more than once.
Richard Meelia, CEO
Richard Meelia, Pres.
Chuck Dockendorff, CFO

Phone:	Fax:
Toll-Free: 800-962-9888	
Address: 15 Hampshire St., Mansfield, MA 02048 US	

GROWTH PLANS/SPECIAL FEATURES:
Tyco Healthcare Group, a subsidiary of Tyco International, Ltd., is one of the largest manufacturers, distributors and service suppliers of medical devices in the world, producing thousands of safety, security, health and communication products. The firm divides into surgical, medical, imaging, respiratory, pharmaceutical and other assistance units. The surgical unit is divided into U.S. Surgical (USS) and Valleylab. USS is primarily a manufacturer of wound closure products and advanced surgical devices. Its sub-units include Auto Suture, Syneture, U.S. Sports Medicine and U.S. Women's Healthcare. Valleylab designs, develops, and manufactures energy-based surgical treatment systems for electrosurgery and ultrasonic surgery systems. The firm's medical unit includes Kendall and UniPatch. Kendall manufactures medical equipment including sharps disposal and nursing care products. Unipatch markets stimulating eletrode patches and accessories, hot and cold therapy products, and skin care lotions and gels. The imaging unit, Mallinckodt, provides contrast media and delivery systems, radiopharmaceuticals and urology imaging systems. The respiratory unit is divided into Nellcor, a maker of pulse oximetry modules circuit boards; Puritan Bennett, a developer of mechanical ventilation and respiratory care devices; and Sandman, a manufacturer of sleep diagnostic systems. The pharmaceutical unit includes Mallinckrodt Pharmaceuticals, a developer of proprietary and generic drugs including addiction treatment products, and its subsidiaries: J.T. Baker and Mallinckrodt Laboratory Chemicals, producers of laboratory, biotechnology, pharmaceutical, industrial and microelectronic chemicals, and Mallinckrodt Bulk Pharmaceuticals, a bulk supplier for other pharmaceutical manufacturers. Almost every tablet made in the U.S. contains at least one of the firms product's. The firm's other subsidiaries include Ludlow Tape, as well as dental, veterinary and laboratory companies. In recent news, Tyco joined the Industry Liaison Program of the Center for the Integration of Medicine and Innovative Technology (CIMIT).

FINANCIALS: Sales and profits are in thousands of dollars—add 000 to get the full amount. Year 2004 note: Complete fiscal 2004 results were not available for all companies at press time. For this company, year 2004 is for months.

2004 Sales: $ (months)   2004 Profits: $ (months)
2003 Sales: $ 2003 Profits: $
2002 Sales: $7,899,100   2002 Profits: $
2001 Sales: $ 2001 Profits: $
2000 Sales: $ 2000 Profits: $

Stock Ticker: Subsidiary
Employees: 40,000
Fiscal Year Ends: 9/30

SALARIES/BENEFITS:
| Pension Plan: | ESOP Stock Plan: | Profit Sharing: | Top Exec. Salary: $ | Bonus: $ |
| Savings Plan: | Stock Purch. Plan: | | Second Exec. Salary: $ | Bonus: $ |

OTHER THOUGHTS:
Apparent Top Female Officers:
Hot Spot for Advancement for Women/Minorities:

LOCATIONS: ("Y" = Yes)
West:	Southwest:	Midwest:	Southeast:	Northeast:	International:
				Y	Y

Note: Financial information, benefits and other data can change quickly and may vary from those stated here.

UNIPRISE INCORPORATED

www.uniprise.com

Industry Group Code: 524114 Ranks within this company's industry group: Sales: 27 Profits:

Insurance/HMO/PPO:	Drugs:	Equipment/Supplies:	Hospitals/Clinics:	Services:	Health Care:
Insurance:	Manufacturer:	Manufacturer:	Acute Care:	Diagnostics:	Home Health:
Managed Care: Y	Distributor:	Distributor:	Sub-Acute Care:	Labs/Testing:	Long-Term Care:
Utilization Mgmt.: Y	Specialty Pharm.:	Leasing/Finance:	Outpatient Surgery:	Staffing:	Physical Therapy:
Payment Proc.: Y	Vitamins/Nutri.:	Information Sys.:	Phys. Rehab. Center:	Waste Disposal:	Phys. Practice Mgmt.:
	Clinical Trials:		Psychiatric Clinics:	Specialty Services:	

TYPES OF BUSINESS:
Employee Benefits Management
Electronic Billing & Payment Systems

BRANDS/DIVISIONS/AFFILIATES:
UnitedHealth Group
Electronic Benefit Administration Solutions
Customer Reporting System
myuhc.com
iPlan

CONTACTS: Note: Officers with more than one job title may be intentionally listed here more than once.
Tracy L. Bahl, CEO
David Astar, COO
Craig Anderson, CFO
Stephen Gage, VP-Mktg.
Al McMahon, VP/General Counsel
Stephen Gage, VP-Comm.
Vincent E. Kerr, Exec. VP-Network & Clinical Solutions
Dawn Owens, Pres.-Strategic Solutions
Nicholas Santoro, CEO-Exante Financial Services
Andy Slavitt, CEO-Consumer Solutions

Phone: 860-702-5000 Fax: 860-702-5835
Toll-Free:
Address: 450 Columbus Blvd., Hartford, CT 06115 US

GROWTH PLANS/SPECIAL FEATURES:
Uniprise Incorporated, a subsidiary of UnitedHealth Group, manages the benefit programs of the nation's leading businesses. It is the only company in the health benefits industry to focus solely on large employers, counting over half of the country's largest 100 companies as customers. The firm offers UnitedHealth products such as PPOs, POS plans, HMOs, open access plans, indemnity plans and pharmacy and prescription plans, as well as services like Electronic Benefit Administration Solutions, the Customer Reporting System, electronic billing and payment systems and myuhc.com. Through myuhc.com, customers can identify, select and locate physicians; check the status of claims; request new ID cards; and verify eligibility. The firm's iPlan controls benefit costs, encourages good health and provides employees with choices and control. Uniprise's single, unified delivery platform allows it to process over 180 million claims each year and serve over 72 million telephone callers annually.

Uniprise employees receive medical and dental coverage and commuter and education expense reimbursement.

FINANCIALS: Sales and profits are in thousands of dollars—add 000 to get the full amount. Year 2004 note: Complete fiscal 2004 results were not available for all companies at press time. For this company, year 2004 is for months.

2004 Sales: $ (months)   2004 Profits: $ (months)
2003 Sales: $3,107,000   2003 Profits: $
2002 Sales: $ 2002 Profits: $
2001 Sales: $ 2001 Profits: $
2000 Sales: $ 2000 Profits: $

Stock Ticker: Subsidiary
Employees:
Fiscal Year Ends: 12/31

SALARIES/BENEFITS:
Pension Plan: ESOP Stock Plan: Y   Profit Sharing: Top Exec. Salary: $ Bonus: $
Savings Plan: Y   Stock Purch. Plan: Y   Second Exec. Salary: $ Bonus: $

OTHER THOUGHTS:
Apparent Top Female Officers: 1
Hot Spot for Advancement for Women/Minorities:

LOCATIONS: ("Y" = Yes)
| West: | Southwest: | Midwest: | Southeast: | Northeast: Y | International: |

UNITED SURGICAL PARTNERS

www.unitedsurgical.com

Industry Group Code: 621111 Ranks within this company's industry group: Sales: 5 Profits: 4

Insurance/HMO/PPO:	Drugs:	Equipment/Supplies:	Hospitals/Clinics:	Services:	Health Care:
Insurance: Managed Care: Utilization Mgmt.: Payment Proc.:	Manufacturer: Distributor: Specialty Pharm.: Vitamins/Nutri.: Clinical Trials:	Manufacturer: Distributor: Leasing/Finance: Information Sys.:	Acute Care: Sub-Acute Care: Outpatient Surgery: Y Phys. Rehab. Center: Psychiatric Clinics:	Diagnostics: Labs/Testing: Staffing: Waste Disposal: Specialty Services:	Home Health: Long-Term Care: Physical Therapy: Phys. Practice Mgmt.:

TYPES OF BUSINESS:
Outpatient Surgical Facility Management

BRANDS/DIVISIONS/AFFILIATES:

CONTACTS:
Note: Officers with more than one job title may be intentionally listed here more than once.

William H. Wilcox, CEO
William H. Wilcox, Pres.
Mark Garvin, Sr. VP/COO
Mark A. Kopser, Sr. VP/CFO
Philip J. Parker, CIO
Dale L. Stegall, General Counsel
Jonathan R. Bond, Sr. VP-Oper.
Brett Brodnax, Sr. VP-Dev.
John J. Wellik, Chief Acc. & Compliance Officer
Pat McCann, Managing Dir.-U.K. Oper.
Dave A. Alexander, Jr., Chmn.-OrthoLink Physicians Corp.
Mark Tulloch, Pres./COO-OrthoLink Physicians Corp.
John J. Wellik, Corp. Sec.
Donald E. Steen, Chmn.

Phone: 972-713-3500 **Fax:** 972-713-3550
Toll-Free:
Address: 15305 Dallas Pkwy., Ste. 1600, Addison, TX 75001 US

GROWTH PLANS/SPECIAL FEATURES:
United Surgical Partners International, Inc. (USPI) operates more than 70 short-stay surgical facilities, including surgery centers and surgical hospitals in the U.S., Spain and the U.K. The firm acquires and develops its facilities by forming strategic relationships with physicians and health care systems. USPI hopes to attract more physician affiliations by focusing on physician satisfaction through staffing, scheduling and clinical systems and protocols that increase productivity. In the U.S., the firm generally offers physicians the opportunity to purchase equity interests in its facilities. Ownership increases the physician's involvement in facility operations, enhancing quality of patient care and reducing costs. Additionally, USPI believes this focus on physicians, combined with providing high-quality health care in a friendly and convenient environment for patients, will continue to increase case volumes. The company intends to grow through a highly selective series of acquisitions, focusing on multi-specialty centers that perform high-volume, non-emergency, lower-risk procedures and that require lower capital and operating costs than hospitals. USPI also pursues strategic relationships with not-for-profit hospitals and health care systems by allowing them to outsource their non-emergency surgical procedures to the company's facilities. The firm is well-positioned in western Europe to take advantage of the demand for privately provided surgery and cancer treatment.

FINANCIALS:
Sales and profits are in thousands of dollars—add 000 to get the full amount. Year 2004 note: Complete fiscal 2004 results were not available for all companies at press time. For this company, year 2004 is for 9 months.

2004 Sales: $294,976 (9 months)   2004 Profits: $77,498 (9 months)
2003 Sales: $446,269   2003 Profits: $29,876
2002 Sales: $329,900   2002 Profits: $19,600
2001 Sales: $244,400   2001 Profits: $2,800
2000 Sales: $138,400   2000 Profits: $-8,200

Stock Ticker: USPI
Employees: 4,350
Fiscal Year Ends: 12/31

SALARIES/BENEFITS:
Pension Plan: ESOP Stock Plan: Profit Sharing: Top Exec. Salary: $483,333   Bonus: $435,000
Savings Plan: Y   Stock Purch. Plan: Y   Second Exec. Salary: $421,667 Bonus: $379,500

OTHER THOUGHTS:
Apparent Top Female Officers:
Hot Spot for Advancement for Women/Minorities:

LOCATIONS: ("Y" = Yes)

West:	Southwest:	Midwest:	Southeast:	Northeast:	International:
Y	Y	Y	Y	Y	Y

Note: Financial information, benefits and other data can change quickly and may vary from those stated here.

UNITEDHEALTH GROUP INC
www.unitedhealthgroup.com

Industry Group Code: 524114 Ranks within this company's industry group: Sales: 2 Profits: 1

Insurance/HMO/PPO:	Drugs:	Equipment/Supplies:	Hospitals/Clinics:	Services:	Health Care:
Insurance:	Manufacturer:	Manufacturer:	Acute Care:	Diagnostics:	Home Health:
Managed Care: Y	Distributor:	Distributor:	Sub-Acute Care:	Labs/Testing:	Long-Term Care:
Utilization Mgmt.: Y	Specialty Pharm.:	Leasing/Finance:	Outpatient Surgery:	Staffing:	Physical Therapy:
Payment Proc.:	Vitamins/Nutri.:	Information Sys.:	Phys. Rehab. Center:	Waste Disposal:	Phys. Practice Mgmt.:
	Clinical Trials:		Psychiatric Clinics:	Specialty Services: Y	

TYPES OF BUSINESS:
HMO/PPO
Wellness Plans
Health Care Data Services
Benefit Administration Solutions
Chiropractic Services
International Health Care Solutions
Vision Benefit Management Services
Venture Capital Investments

BRANDS/DIVISIONS/AFFILIATES:
UnitedHealthCare
Uniprise
Specialized Care Services
Ingenix
Ovations
United Resource Networks

CONTACTS: Note: Officers with more than one job title may be intentionally listed here more than once.
William W. McGuire, CEO
Stephen J. Hemsley, Pres.
Stephen J. Hemsley, COO
Patrick J. Erlandson, CFO
Tracy L. Bahl, Sr. VP/Chief Mktg. Officer
L. Robert Dapper, Sr. VP-Human Capital
David J. Lubben, General Counsel
John S. Penshorn, Dir.-Strategy
John S. Penshorn, Dir.-Comm.
Lee deStefano, Investor Rel.
Jeannine M. Rivet, Exec. VP/CEO-Ingenix
R. Channing Wheeler, CEO-Uniprise
James B. Hudak, CEO-UnitedHealth Technologies
Robert J. Sheehy, CEO-UnitedHealthCare
William W. McGuire, Chmn.

Phone: 952-936-1300 Fax: 952-936-7430
Toll-Free: 800-328-5979
Address: 9900 Bren Rd. E., Minnetonka, MN 55343 US

GROWTH PLANS/SPECIAL FEATURES:
UnitedHealth Group specializes in health care network creation and coordination and serves approximately 52 million managed care members through more than 400,000 physicians and 3,600 hospitals. The firm is composed of five distinct, strategically aligned businesses. UnitedHealthCare organizes health markets serving the needs of individuals and employers in local geographic regions. Ovations offers health and well-being services for Americans in the second half of life, partnering with AARP to serve its customers. The Uniprise subsidiary provides leading-edge support services and health and benefit solutions to large corporations and employers, other payors and health plans. Specialized Care Services organizes specialized markets for services to meet the needs of individuals and businesses of all sizes. Subsidiary Ingenix provides health information and research to virtually all participants in the health care system. The company's subsidiaries are separated so as to be market-focused, independently branded and managed. Cairnstone Re, a managing general underwriter and medical management company, recently contracted with the firm's United Resource Networks subsidiary for access to its transplant benefit management products and services. United Resource Networks operates the nation's leading transplant network and manages over 5,000 transplant referrals each year.

The firm offers its employees flexible hours, job sharing, teleworking and compressed workweeks. Additionally, UnitedHealth Group provides tuition reimbursement, commuter expense reimbursement, domestic partner coverage, child care and elder care programs. Employees also receive medical, dental and vision coverage.

FINANCIALS: Sales and profits are in thousands of dollars—add 000 to get the full amount. Year 2004 note: Complete fiscal 2004 results were not available for all companies at press time. For this company, year 2004 is for 9 months.

2004 Sales: $26,707,000 (9 months)	2004 Profits: $1,848,000 (9 months)	**Stock Ticker: UNH**
2003 Sales: $28,823,000	2003 Profits: $1,825,000	Employees: 33,000
2002 Sales: $25,020,000	2002 Profits: $1,352,000	Fiscal Year Ends: 12/31
2001 Sales: $23,173,000	2001 Profits: $913,000	
2000 Sales: $21,122,000	2000 Profits: $736,000	

SALARIES/BENEFITS:
Pension Plan: ESOP Stock Plan: Profit Sharing: Top Exec. Salary: $1,996,154 Bonus: $5,550,000
Savings Plan: Y Stock Purch. Plan: Y Second Exec. Salary: $1,000,000 Bonus: $2,325,000

OTHER THOUGHTS:
Apparent Top Female Officers: 2
Hot Spot for Advancement for Women/Minorities:

LOCATIONS: ("Y" = Yes)
West:	Southwest:	Midwest:	Southeast:	Northeast:	International:
Y	Y	Y	Y	Y	

UNIVERSAL HEALTH SERVICES INC

www.uhsinc.com

Industry Group Code: 622110   Ranks within this company's industry group: Sales: 16   Profits: 8

Insurance/HMO/PPO:	Drugs:	Equipment/Supplies:	Hospitals/Clinics:		Services:		Health Care:	
Insurance:	Manufacturer:	Manufacturer:	Acute Care:	Y	Diagnostics:	Y	Home Health:	
Managed Care:	Distributor:	Distributor:	Sub-Acute Care:	Y	Labs/Testing:		Long-Term Care:	
Utilization Mgmt.:	Specialty Pharm.:	Leasing/Finance:	Outpatient Surgery:	Y	Staffing:		Physical Therapy:	
Payment Proc.:	Vitamins/Nutri.:	Information Sys.:	Phys. Rehab. Center:		Waste Disposal:		Phys. Practice Mgmt.:	
	Clinical Trials:		Psychiatric Clinics:		Specialty Services:			

TYPES OF BUSINESS:
Hospitals-General
Radiation Oncology Centers
Behavioral Health Hospitals
Ambulatory Surgery Centers
Women's Health Centers

BRANDS/DIVISIONS/AFFILIATES:

GROWTH PLANS/SPECIAL FEATURES:
Universal Health Services, Inc. (UHS) owns and operates acute care hospitals, behavioral health centers, ambulatory surgery centers, radiation oncology centers and women's centers. One of the nation's largest operators of hospitals, the company operates over 100 facilities across the U.S. UHS provides its facilities with capital resources as well as a variety of management services, including central purchasing, information services, finance and control systems, facilities planning, physician recruitment services, administrative personnel management, marketing and public relations. The company has spent recent years making new hospital and health care center acquisitions in the U.S.

UHS offers employment opportunities across the U.S. and in France. The company provides its employees with a comprehensive medical, dental and vision plan, as well as educational leave.

CONTACTS: Note: Officers with more than one job title may be intentionally listed here more than once.
Alan B. Miller, CEO
Alan B. Miller, Pres.
Steve G. Filton, CFO
Coleen Johns, Corp. Recruiter
Steve G. Filton, VP-Admin.
Bruce R. Gilbert, General Counsel
Richard C. Wright, VP-Dev.
Kirk E. Gorman, Treas.
O. Edwin French, Sr. VP
Michael Marquez, VP-Acute Care
Debra K. Osteen, VP
Steve G. Filton, Corp. Sec.
Alan B. Miller, Chmn.

Phone: 610-768-3300   **Fax:** 610-768-3336
Toll-Free:
Address: 367 S. Gulph Rd., King of Prussia, PA 19406-0958 US

FINANCIALS:
Sales and profits are in thousands of dollars—add 000 to get the full amount. Year 2004 note: Complete fiscal 2004 results were not available for all companies at press time. For this company, year 2004 is for 9 months.

2004 Sales: $3,049,032 (9 months)	2004 Profits: $132,318 (9 months)	**Stock Ticker:** UHS
2003 Sales: $3,643,566	2003 Profits: $199,269	Employees: 35,000
2002 Sales: $3,258,900	2002 Profits: $175,400	Fiscal Year Ends: 12/31
2001 Sales: $2,840,500	2001 Profits: $99,800	
2000 Sales: $2,242,444	2000 Profits: $93,362	

SALARIES/BENEFITS:
Pension Plan: ESOP Stock Plan: Profit Sharing: Top Exec. Salary: $1,091,800   Bonus: $737,000
Savings Plan: Y   Stock Purch. Plan: Y   Second Exec. Salary: $425,000   Bonus: $100,000

OTHER THOUGHTS:
Apparent Top Female Officers: 2
Hot Spot for Advancement for Women/Minorities:

LOCATIONS: ("Y" = Yes)
West:	Southwest:	Midwest:	Southeast:	Northeast:	International:
Y	Y			Y	Y

UNIVERSAL HOSPITAL SERVICES INC

www.uhs.com

Industry Group Code: 532400 Ranks within this company's industry group: Sales: 1 Profits: 1

Insurance/HMO/PPO:	Drugs:	Equipment/Supplies:	Hospitals/Clinics:	Services:	Health Care:
Insurance:	Manufacturer:	Manufacturer:	Acute Care:	Diagnostics:	Home Health:
Managed Care:	Distributor:	Distributor: Y	Sub-Acute Care:	Labs/Testing:	Long-Term Care:
Utilization Mgmt.:	Specialty Pharm.:	Leasing/Finance: Y	Outpatient Surgery:	Staffing:	Physical Therapy:
Payment Proc.:	Vitamins/Nutri.:	Information Sys.:	Phys. Rehab. Center:	Waste Disposal:	Phys. Practice Mgmt.:
	Clinical Trials:		Psychiatric Clinics:	Specialty Services: Y	

TYPES OF BUSINESS:
Leasing-Medical Equipment
Support Services
Outsourcing Services
Disposable Medical Supplies

BRANDS/DIVISIONS/AFFILIATES:
Asset Management Partnership Program

CONTACTS:
Note: Officers with more than one job title may be intentionally listed here more than once.
Gary D. Blackford, CEO
Gary D. Blackford, Pres.
Rex Clevenger, Sr. VP/CFO
David G. Lawson, VP-Mktg.
Walter T. Chesley, VP-Human Resources
David G. Lawson, VP-Tech.
Michael R. Johnson, VP-Admin.
Timothy W. Kuck, VP-Sales, Central
Daren Kneeland, VP-Sales, West
Darren J. Thieding, VP-Sales, East
David E. Dovenberg, Chmn.
Jeffrey L. Singer, Sr. VP-Purchasing, Logistics & Pricing

Phone: 952-893-3200 Fax: 952-893-0704
Toll-Free: 800-847-7368
Address: 3800 W. 80th St., Northland Plz., Ste. 1250, Bloomington, MN 55431-4442 US

GROWTH PLANS/SPECIAL FEATURES:
Universal Hospital Services, Inc. is the leading medical equipment lifecycle services company in the U.S., providing movable medical equipment to more than 2,600 acute care hospitals and 2,900 alternate care providers through business locations around the world. The firm has multiple rental programs, the largest of which is a pay-per-use program, which charges a per-use rental fee based on daily use of equipment per patient. This program is used most often by hospitals that need special equipment on hand but do not know when or how often it will be used. Other rental programs are based on time rentals and charge customers on a daily, weekly or monthly basis. These programs are useful for long-term care facilities that require constant equipment use. All rental programs include equipment delivery, training, technical and educational support, inspection, maintenance and comprehensive documentation. Ongoing inservice education is also available. Through Universal Hospital Services' Asset Management Partnership Program, the firm allows customers to outsource substantially all, or a significant portion of, their movable medical equipment needs by providing, maintaining, managing and tracking that equipment for them. The firm also sells disposable medical supplies to hospitals in conjunction with the equipment it rents and to alternate care providers both in connection with rental equipment and on a stand-alone basis.

FINANCIALS:
Sales and profits are in thousands of dollars—add 000 to get the full amount. Year 2004 note: Complete fiscal 2004 results were not available for all companies at press time. For this company, year 2004 is for months.

2004 Sales: $ (months)   2004 Profits: $ (months)
2003 Sales: $171,000   2003 Profits: $-19,500
2002 Sales: $153,800   2002 Profits: $- 200
2001 Sales: $125,600   2001 Profits: $-3,600
2000 Sales: $106,005   2000 Profits: $-5,078

Stock Ticker: Private
Employees: 971
Fiscal Year Ends: 12/31

SALARIES/BENEFITS:
Pension Plan: ESOP Stock Plan: Profit Sharing: Top Exec. Salary: $234,862   Bonus: $151,600
Savings Plan: Stock Purch. Plan: Second Exec. Salary: $175,784 Bonus: $118,000

OTHER THOUGHTS:
Apparent Top Female Officers:
Hot Spot for Advancement for Women/Minorities:

LOCATIONS: ("Y" = Yes)
West:	Southwest:	Midwest:	Southeast:	Northeast:	International:
Y	Y	Y	Y	Y	

UROCOR INC

www.urocor.com

Industry Group Code: 339113   **Ranks within this company's industry group:** Sales: Profits:

Insurance/HMO/PPO:	Drugs:	Equipment/Supplies:	Hospitals/Clinics:	Services:		Health Care:	
Insurance:	Manufacturer:	Manufacturer:	Acute Care:	Diagnostics:	Y	Home Health:	
Managed Care:	Distributor:	Distributor:	Sub-Acute Care:	Labs/Testing:		Long-Term Care:	
Utilization Mgmt.:	Specialty Pharm.:	Leasing/Finance:	Outpatient Surgery:	Staffing:		Physical Therapy:	
Payment Proc.:	Vitamins/Nutri.:	Information Sys.:	Phys. Rehab. Center:	Waste Disposal:		Phys. Practice Mgmt.:	
	Clinical Trials:		Psychiatric Clinics:	Specialty Services:	Y		

TYPES OF BUSINESS:
Services-Urology Diagnostics
Urological Disease Management
Urological Disease Databases
Practice Support Services

BRANDS/DIVISIONS/AFFILIATES:
Dianon Systems, Inc.
Sextant Plus
UroStone
UroSavant
UroServices
UroScore

CONTACTS:
Note: Officers with more than one job title may be intentionally listed here more than once.

Bruce Hayden, CFO
Lisa Moroski, Nat'l Account Mgr.-Mid-Atlantic Region
Dede Goehler, Nat'l Account Mgr.-Midwest Region
Bill Bauwens, Nat'l Account Mgr.-Northeast Region
Mike Roberts, Nat'l Account Mgr.-Western Region

Phone: 405-290-4000	Fax: 405-290-4002
Toll-Free:	
Address: 840 Research Pkwy., Ste. 546, Oklahoma City, OK 73104 US	

GROWTH PLANS/SPECIAL FEATURES:
UroCor, Inc. provides a broad range of diagnostic services for the clinical management of certain urological cancers and diseases. These services are used to detect major urological diseases, predict prognosis of the patient's condition, monitor the patient's therapy and identify recurrence of the disease. UroCor offers diagnostic services for prostate, bladder and kidney diseases, as well as patient support services. The company's products and services include prostate diagnostics, PSA testing, biopsies, DNA ploidy, bladder diagnostics and prognostics and kidney stone management. The company's UroServices group is designed to provide urologists and managed care organizations with access to the company's proprietary urological disease databases, disease management models and practice support services in order to improve the diagnosis and treatment of patients. UroCor is a wholly-owned subsidiary of Dianon Systems, Inc.

FINANCIALS:
Sales and profits are in thousands of dollars—add 000 to get the full amount. Year 2004 note: Complete fiscal 2004 results were not available for all companies at press time. For this company, year 2004 is for months.

2004 Sales: $ (months)	2004 Profits: $ (months)	
2003 Sales: $	2003 Profits: $	Stock Ticker: Subsidiary
2002 Sales: $	2002 Profits: $	Employees: 368
2001 Sales: $	2001 Profits: $	Fiscal Year Ends: 12/31
2000 Sales: $52,600	2000 Profits: $	

SALARIES/BENEFITS:
Pension Plan:	ESOP Stock Plan:	Profit Sharing:	Top Exec. Salary: $236,269	Bonus: $33,000
Savings Plan: Y	Stock Purch. Plan:		Second Exec. Salary: $171,385	Bonus: $

OTHER THOUGHTS:
Apparent Top Female Officers: 2
Hot Spot for Advancement for Women/Minorities:

LOCATIONS: ("Y" = Yes)
West:	Southwest:	Midwest:	Southeast:	Northeast:	International:
Y	Y	Y	Y	Y	

US ONCOLOGY INC

www.usoncology.com

Industry Group Code: 621111   Ranks within this company's industry group: Sales: 1   Profits: 2

Insurance/HMO/PPO:	Drugs:	Equipment/Supplies:	Hospitals/Clinics:	Services:	Health Care:
Insurance:	Manufacturer:	Manufacturer:	Acute Care:	Diagnostics:	Home Health:
Managed Care:	Distributor:	Distributor:	Sub-Acute Care:	Labs/Testing:	Long-Term Care:
Utilization Mgmt.:	Specialty Pharm.: Y	Leasing/Finance:	Outpatient Surgery: Y	Staffing:	Physical Therapy:
Payment Proc.:	Vitamins/Nutri.:	Information Sys.:	Phys. Rehab. Center:	Waste Disposal:	Phys. Practice Mgmt.: Y
	Clinical Trials:		Psychiatric Clinics:	Specialty Services: Y	

TYPES OF BUSINESS:
Cancer Treatment
Oncology Pharmaceutical Management
Outpatient Cancer Center Operations
Research & Development Services

BRANDS/DIVISIONS/AFFILIATES:
Welsh, Carson, Anderson and Stowe

CONTACTS:
Note: Officers with more than one job title may be intentionally listed here more than once.
R. Dale Ross, CEO
George D. Morgan, COO
Bruce Broussard, CFO
Leo E. Sands, Exec. VP/Corp. Sec.
R. Dale Ross, Chmn.

Phone: 832-601-8766   Fax: 832-601-6282
Toll-Free:
Address: 16825 Northchase Dr., Ste. 1300, Houston, TX 77060 US

GROWTH PLANS/SPECIAL FEATURES:
US Oncology, Inc. is a cancer management company that provides comprehensive management services under long-term agreements to oncology practices and serves more cancer patients than any other single health-care organization in America. The firm has affiliated physicians in all aspects of diagnosis and outpatient treatment of cancer, including medical oncology, radiation, gynecologic oncology, stem cell transplantation, diagnostic radiology and clinical research. The company's pharmacy segment concentrates on providing low-cost cancer drugs and pharmacy-related support services to affiliates. The firm's outpatient care centers provides a full suite of amenities and support services for cancer patients and doctors, with a total of 470 sites of outpatient service in 32 states, including 80 cancer centers. The clinical research group focuses on improving cancer survival rates, enhancing the patient's quality of life, reducing the cost of care and developing new approaches for diagnosis, treatment and post-treatment monitoring. The company assists in a number of aspects in the conduct of clinical trials, including protocol development, data coordination, institutional review board coordination and contract review and negotiation. In recent news, the company has agreed to be acquired by Welsh, Carson, Anderson and Stowe for $1.3 billion in cash plus $400 million in assumed debt but two class action lawsuits against the company from the stockholders of US Oncology alleging, among other things, unfair company dealings and that the company breached their fiduciary duties to the stockholders by entering into the merger agreement, may prevent the merger.

The company offers its employees dental and prescription plans, as well as service awards and employee recognition programs.

FINANCIALS:
Sales and profits are in thousands of dollars—add 000 to get the full amount. Year 2004 note: Complete fiscal 2004 results were not available for all companies at press time. For this company, year 2004 is for 6 months.

2004 Sales: $1,090,200 (6 months)   2004 Profits: $44,600 (6 months)
2003 Sales: $1,965,725   2003 Profits: $70,656
2002 Sales: $1,651,300   2002 Profits: $46,000
2001 Sales: $1,505,000   2001 Profits: $-46,300
2000 Sales: $1,324,200   2000 Profits: $-72,600

Stock Ticker: USON
Employees: 8,096
Fiscal Year Ends: 12/31

SALARIES/BENEFITS:
Pension Plan: ESOP Stock Plan: Profit Sharing: Top Exec. Salary: $701,217   Bonus: $400,680
Savings Plan: Y   Stock Purch. Plan: Second Exec. Salary: $390,247   Bonus: $140,700

OTHER THOUGHTS:
Apparent Top Female Officers:
Hot Spot for Advancement for Women/Minorities:

LOCATIONS: ("Y" = Yes)
West:	Southwest:	Midwest:	Southeast:	Northeast:	International:
Y	Y	Y	Y	Y	

US PHYSICAL THERAPY INC

www.usphysicaltherapy.com

Industry Group Code: 621490 Ranks within this company's industry group: Sales: 13 Profits: 11

Insurance/HMO/PPO:	Drugs:	Equipment/Supplies:	Hospitals/Clinics:		Services:		Health Care:	
Insurance: Managed Care: Utilization Mgmt.: Payment Proc.:	Manufacturer: Distributor: Specialty Pharm.: Vitamins/Nutri.: Clinical Trials:	Manufacturer: Distributor: Leasing/Finance: Information Sys.:	Acute Care: Sub-Acute Care: Outpatient Surgery: Phys. Rehab. Center: Psychiatric Clinics:	Y	Diagnostics: Labs/Testing: Staffing: Waste Disposal: Specialty Services:		Home Health: Long-Term Care: Physical Therapy: Phys. Practice Mgmt.:	Y

TYPES OF BUSINESS:
Clinics-Occupational & Physical Therapy

BRANDS/DIVISIONS/AFFILIATES:

CONTACTS:
Note: Officers with more than one job title may be intentionally listed here more than once.
Roy W. Spradlin, CEO
Roy W. Spradlin, Pres.
Chris Reading, COO
Larry McAfee, CFO
Stephen Rosenbloom, Sr. VP
Roy W. Spradlin, Chmn.

Phone: 713-297-7000 **Fax:** 713-297-7090
Toll-Free: 800-580-6285
Address: 1300 W. Sam Houston Pkwy., Ste. 300, Houston, TX 77043 US

GROWTH PLANS/SPECIAL FEATURES:
U.S. Physical Therapy, Inc. operates outpatient physical therapy and occupational therapy clinics. The company operates 260 clinics in 35 states, providing post-operative care and treatment for a variety of orthopedic-related disorders and sports-related injuries, treatment for neurologically related injuries, rehabilitation of injured workers and preventative care. Each clinic's staff typically includes one or more licensed physical or occupational therapist along with assistants, aides, exercise physiologists and athletic trainers. The clinics perform a tailored and comprehensive evaluation of each patient, followed by a treatment plan specific to the injury. The treatment plan may include the use of ultrasound, electrical stimulation, hot packs, iontophoresis, therapeutic exercise, manual therapy techniques, education on management of daily life skills and home exercise programs. Rather than acquire existing clinics, the firm expands its business by developing new clinics. The company attracts physical and occupational therapists by offering them a partnership interest in its new clinics. In September 2004, the company announced its intent to close eight clinics.

FINANCIALS:
Sales and profits are in thousands of dollars—add 000 to get the full amount. Year 2004 note: Complete fiscal 2004 results were not available for all companies at press time. For this company, year 2004 is for 9 months.

2004 Sales: $88,592 (9 months)   2004 Profits: $4,865 (9 months)
2003 Sales: $105,568   2003 Profits: $7,331
2002 Sales: $94,700   2002 Profits: $8,500
2001 Sales: $80,900   2001 Profits: $7,100
2000 Sales: $63,200   2000 Profits: $3,700

Stock Ticker: USPH
Employees: 1,276
Fiscal Year Ends: 12/31

SALARIES/BENEFITS:
Pension Plan: ESOP Stock Plan: Profit Sharing: Top Exec. Salary: $325,000   Bonus: $125,000
Savings Plan: Y   Stock Purch. Plan: Second Exec. Salary: $170,000   Bonus: $40,000

OTHER THOUGHTS:
Apparent Top Female Officers:
Hot Spot for Advancement for Women/Minorities:

LOCATIONS: ("Y" = Yes)
West:	Southwest:	Midwest:	Southeast:	Northeast:	International:
Y	Y	Y	Y	Y	

Note: Financial information, benefits and other data can change quickly and may vary from those stated here.

US VISION INC

www.usvision.com

Industry Group Code: 446130   **Ranks within this company's industry group:** Sales: 2   Profits:

Insurance/HMO/PPO:	Drugs:	Equipment/Supplies:		Hospitals/Clinics:		Services:		Health Care:	
Insurance:	Manufacturer:	Manufacturer:	Y	Acute Care:		Diagnostics:		Home Health:	
Managed Care:	Distributor:	Distributor:	Y	Sub-Acute Care:		Labs/Testing:		Long-Term Care:	
Utilization Mgmt.:	Specialty Pharm.:	Leasing/Finance:		Outpatient Surgery:		Staffing:		Physical Therapy:	
Payment Proc.:	Vitamins/Nutri.:	Information Sys.:		Phys. Rehab. Center:		Waste Disposal:		Phys. Practice Mgmt.:	
	Clinical Trials:			Psychiatric Clinics:		Specialty Services:	Y		

TYPES OF BUSINESS:
Eyeglasses and Related Products, Retail
Optical Products Production
Eyeglass Frames, Importing & Sales

BRANDS/DIVISIONS/AFFILIATES:
Styl-Rite

CONTACTS:
Note: Officers with more than one job title may be intentionally listed here more than once.

William A. Schwartz, Jr., CEO
William A. Schwartz, Jr., Pres.
Gayle E. Schmidt, COO
Carmen J. Nepa, III, Exec. VP/CFO
Gayle G. Schmidt, Exec. VP-Mfg.
George E. McHenry, Jr., Chief Admin. Officer
George T. Gorman, Pres.-Retail Div.

Phone: 856-228-1000   **Fax:** 856-228-3339
Toll-Free:
Address: One Harmon Dr., Glen Oaks Industrial Park, Glendora, NJ 08029 US

GROWTH PLANS/SPECIAL FEATURES:

U.S. Vision, Inc. operates 591 retail optical product locations in 47 states and Canada. The firm's retail locations are generally full-service eyewear and vision care stores, offering a broad variety of designer and private-label branded frames, prescription lenses, contact lenses and sunglasses. The majority of locations (569) are independently licensed departments within larger stores such as JC Penney and Sears. The remaining locations are freestanding stores located in malls and shopping centers. In all of the stores, an on-site independent optometrist writes prescriptions and completes optical examinations. The company's Styl-Rite subsidiary manufactures, imports and distributes optical products both for sale at its optical stores and for sale to third-party buyers. The firm operates an optical laboratory, distribution and lens grinding facility that fills customer orders for prescription eyewear and maintains a central inventory of frames for U.S. Vision. Additionally, U.S. Vision offers a selection of value-priced eyewear, as well as technologically advanced lenses such as featherweight lenses and virtually unbreakable polycarbonate lenses. Scratch-resistant and anti-reflective coatings can be added to eyewear at any U.S. Vision location. In late 2002 the company rescinded an acquisition agreement with the Norcross Investment Group in 2001 and instead went private, financed by the firm's CEO and several private investors.

FINANCIALS:
Sales and profits are in thousands of dollars—add 000 to get the full amount. Year 2004 note: Complete fiscal 2004 results were not available for all companies at press time. For this company, year 2004 is for months.

2004 Sales: $ (months)	2004 Profits: $ (months)	**Stock Ticker:** Private
2003 Sales: $172,100	2003 Profits: $	Employees: 3,000
2002 Sales: $134,800	2002 Profits: $- 300	Fiscal Year Ends: 1/31
2001 Sales: $147,617	2001 Profits: $4,795	
2000 Sales: $143,419	2000 Profits: $-1,819	

SALARIES/BENEFITS:
Pension Plan:	ESOP Stock Plan:	Profit Sharing:	Top Exec. Salary: $297,000	Bonus: $
Savings Plan: Y	Stock Purch. Plan:		Second Exec. Salary: $185,000	Bonus: $

OTHER THOUGHTS:
Apparent Top Female Officers: 2
Hot Spot for Advancement for Women/Minorities:

LOCATIONS: ("Y" = Yes)
West:	Southwest:	Midwest:	Southeast:	Northeast:	International:
Y	Y	Y	Y	Y	Y

UTAH MEDICAL PRODUCTS INC

www.utahmed.com

Industry Group Code: 339113   Ranks within this company's industry group: Sales: 129   Profits: 56

Insurance/HMO/PPO:	Drugs:	Equipment/Supplies:		Hospitals/Clinics:	Services:	Health Care:
Insurance:	Manufacturer:	Manufacturer:	Y	Acute Care:	Diagnostics:	Home Health:
Managed Care:	Distributor:	Distributor:	Y	Sub-Acute Care:	Labs/Testing:	Long-Term Care:
Utilization Mgmt.:	Specialty Pharm.:	Leasing/Finance:		Outpatient Surgery:	Staffing:	Physical Therapy:
Payment Proc.:	Vitamins/Nutri.:	Information Sys.:		Phys. Rehab. Center:	Waste Disposal:	Phys. Practice Mgmt.:
	Clinical Trials:			Psychiatric Clinics:	Specialty Services:	

TYPES OF BUSINESS:
Equipment-Obstetrics & Gynecology
Disposable Products
Electrosurgical Systems

BRANDS/DIVISIONS/AFFILIATES:
Columbia Medical, Inc.
Gesco
Intran Plus
Cordguard
Deltran-Plus
Disposa-Hood
Thora-Cath
Lumin

CONTACTS:
Note: Officers with more than one job title may be intentionally listed here more than once.
Kevin L. Cornwell, CEO
Kevin L. Cornwell, Pres.
Greg A. LeClaire, CFO
Charles F. Arthur, VP-Sales
Kevin L. Cornwell, Corp. Sec.

Phone: 801-566-1200   **Fax:** 801-566-2062
Toll-Free: 800-533-4984
Address: 7043 S. 300 West, Midvale, UT 84047 US

GROWTH PLANS/SPECIAL FEATURES:
Utah Medical Products, Inc. produces cost-effective disposable health care equipment for women and babies. The company markets a broad range of medical devices used in critical care, especially in the neonatal intensive care unit (NICU) and the labor and delivery department in hospitals, as well as outpatient clinics and physicians' offices. Mostly, the firm's own direct sales representatives and independent manufacturers' representatives sell directly to end users in the U.S. domestic market. Internationally, the products are sold through other medical device companies and through independent distributors. Utah Medical's products include obstetrics products, such as fetal monitoring accessories and vacuum-assisted delivery systems; NICU products; and gynecology, urology and electrosurgery products.

Utah Medical Products offers its employees a number of benefits, including medical, dental and vision coverage, bereavement leave, credit union membership, educational financial assistance, stock options and bonus plans for all employee classifications. The company also provides training opportunities, company-sponsored parties and picnics, free flu shots and discounted tickets for sporting and entertainment events.

FINANCIALS:
Sales and profits are in thousands of dollars—add 000 to get the full amount. Year 2004 note: Complete fiscal 2004 results were not available for all companies at press time. For this company, year 2004 is for 9 months.

2004 Sales: $20,113 (9 months)	2004 Profits: $8,823 (9 months)	**Stock Ticker:** UTMD
2003 Sales: $27,137	2003 Profits: $20,761	**Employees:** 211
2002 Sales: $27,400	2002 Profits: $7,200	**Fiscal Year Ends:** 12/31
2001 Sales: $27,000	2001 Profits: $5,900	
2000 Sales: $27,200	2000 Profits: $5,400	

SALARIES/BENEFITS:
Pension Plan:	ESOP Stock Plan:	Profit Sharing:	Top Exec. Salary: $243,207	Bonus: $228,000
Savings Plan: Y	Stock Purch. Plan:		Second Exec. Salary: $	Bonus: $

OTHER THOUGHTS:
Apparent Top Female Officers:
Hot Spot for Advancement for Women/Minorities:

LOCATIONS: ("Y" = Yes)
West:	Southwest:	Midwest:	Southeast:	Northeast:	International:
Y					Y

UTI CORPORATION

www.uticorporation.com

Industry Group Code: 339113 **Ranks within this company's industry group:** Sales: Profits:

Insurance/HMO/PPO:	Drugs:	Equipment/Supplies:	Hospitals/Clinics:	Services:	Health Care:
Insurance:	Manufacturer:	Manufacturer: Y	Acute Care:	Diagnostics:	Home Health:
Managed Care:	Distributor:	Distributor:	Sub-Acute Care:	Labs/Testing:	Long-Term Care:
Utilization Mgmt.:	Specialty Pharm.:	Leasing/Finance:	Outpatient Surgery:	Staffing:	Physical Therapy:
Payment Proc.:	Vitamins/Nutri.:	Information Sys.:	Phys. Rehab. Center:	Waste Disposal:	Phys. Practice Mgmt.:
	Clinical Trials:		Psychiatric Clinics:	Specialty Services: Y	

TYPES OF BUSINESS:
Medical Equipment Components
Product Development Services

BRANDS/DIVISIONS/AFFILIATES:
American Technical Molding
Noble-Met, Ltd.
Spectrum
Star Guide Corporation
Micro-Guide
Star Guide-Europe
Stent Technologies
Uniform Tubes

CONTACTS:
Note: Officers with more than one job title may be intentionally listed here more than once.
Ron Sparks, CEO
Ron Sparks, Pres.
Stewart Fisher, CFO

Phone: 610-489-0300 **Fax:** 610-489-1150
Toll-Free: 800-321-6285
Address: P.O. Box 26992, Collegeville, PA 19426-0992 US

GROWTH PLANS/SPECIAL FEATURES:
UTI Corporation, through its subsidiaries, provides metal and plastic components, assemblies and finished devices to original equipment manufacturers (OEMs) of medical devices internationally. The firm offers product development and manufacturing services. Product development includes design assistance, solid modeling, plastic and metallurgical analysis and testing. UTI manufactures precision metal tube and wire drawing and fabrication, machining and grinding, injection and insert molding through several subsidiaries. American Technical Molding designs and produces molds and plastic injection molded components for drug delivery systems, diagnostics, surgical instruments, blood therapy and IV disposables. Noble-Met, Ltd. in Salem, Virginia manufactures metal tube and wire components, including precious metal alloys, refractory metals and other biomedical alloys that are used in medical devices. Spectrum makes critical components for coated heart valves, implantable bone screws and soft-tissue anchors, pacemakers, bone drills, reamers, biopsy instruments, arthroscopic shavers and laparoscopic surgical devices. Star Guide Corporation, located in Arvada, Colorado, aids in precision wire component fabrication and sub-assembly through contracts with OEMs, including grinding, coil winding, straightening and welding. Star Guide has two additional divisions: Micro-Guide, based in Tehachapi, California, which offers superior micro-precision grinding for wire and tubing, and Star Guide-Europe, which provides precision wire fabrication to medical device manufacturers in Europe. Stent Technologies manufactures stents with more than 100 metals and alloys in Collegeville, Pennsylvania. Uniform Tubes and Uniform Tubes-Europe make small-diameter metal tubing and tubular components in the U.S. and Europe. Venusa is a manufacturer of disposable medical devices such as OEM specialty products and fluid disposables. UTI recently acquired MedSource Technologies, Inc. for $230 million. The acquisition makes the firm the largest design, engineering and contract manufacturing company serving the medical device market.

FINANCIALS:
Sales and profits are in thousands of dollars—add 000 to get the full amount. Year 2004 note: Complete fiscal 2004 results were not available for all companies at press time. For this company, year 2004 is for months.

2004 Sales: $ (months)   2004 Profits: $ (months)
2003 Sales: $ 2003 Profits: $
2002 Sales: $ 2002 Profits: $
2001 Sales: $ 2001 Profits: $
2000 Sales: $ 2000 Profits: $

Stock Ticker: Private
Employees:
Fiscal Year Ends:

SALARIES/BENEFITS:
Pension Plan: ESOP Stock Plan: Profit Sharing: Top Exec. Salary: $ Bonus: $
Savings Plan: Stock Purch. Plan: Second Exec. Salary: $ Bonus: $

OTHER THOUGHTS:
Apparent Top Female Officers:
Hot Spot for Advancement for Women/Minorities:

LOCATIONS: ("Y" = Yes)

West:	Southwest:	Midwest:	Southeast:	Northeast:	International:
Y	Y	Y	Y	Y	Y

VALEANT PHARMACEUTICALS INTERNATIONAL www.valeant.com

Industry Group Code: 325412 Ranks within this company's industry group: Sales: 32 Profits: 35

Insurance/HMO/PPO:	Drugs:		Equipment/Supplies:	Hospitals/Clinics:	Services:		Health Care:
Insurance:	Manufacturer:	Y	Manufacturer:	Acute Care:	Diagnostics:		Home Health:
Managed Care:	Distributor:		Distributor:	Sub-Acute Care:	Labs/Testing:		Long-Term Care:
Utilization Mgmt.:	Specialty Pharm.:		Leasing/Finance:	Outpatient Surgery:	Staffing:		Physical Therapy:
Payment Proc.:	Vitamins/Nutri.:	Y	Information Sys.:	Phys. Rehab. Center:	Waste Disposal:		Phys. Practice Mgmt.:
	Clinical Trials:			Psychiatric Clinics:	Specialty Services:	Y	

TYPES OF BUSINESS:
Drugs-Viral Disease
Oncology Drugs
Dermatology Drugs
Central Nervous System Compounds
Pain Management Drugs
Over-the-Counter Drugs
Nutritional Products
HIV Treatments

BRANDS/DIVISIONS/AFFILIATES:
Ribapharm, Inc.
Phrenilin
Efudex/Efudix
Oxsoralen-Ultra
Kinerase
Dermatix
Ancobon/Ancotil
Anapenil

CONTACTS: Note: Officers with more than one job title may be intentionally listed here more than once.
Robert W. O'Leary, CEO
Timothy C. Tyson, Pres.
Timothy C. Tyson, COO
Bary G. Bailey, Exec. VP/CFO
Wesley P. Wheeler, VP-Mktg.
Kim D. Lamon, Chief Scientific Officer
John I. Cooper, Exec. VP-Mfg.
Eileen C. Pruette, General Counsel
Wesley P. Wheeler, VP-Bus. Dev.
Robert W. O'Leary, Chmn.
John I. Cooper, Exec. VP-Supply

Phone: 714-545-0100 Fax: 714-556-0131
Toll-Free: 800-548-5100
Address: 3300 Hyland Ave., Costa Mesa, CA 92626 US

GROWTH PLANS/SPECIAL FEATURES:
Valeant Pharmaceuticals International is a global, research-based pharmaceutical company that develops, manufactures and markets a broad spectrum of pharmaceutical, over-the-counter and nutritional products under the Valeant brand name, with almost 50 marketed products. The firm operates primarily in North and Latin America, Europe and the Pacific Rim. The company's pharmaceutical products treat viral and bacterial infections, diseases of the skin, neuromuscular disorders, cancer, cardiovascular disease, diabetes and psychiatric disorders. Valeant's research and new product development, conducted primarily through its majority-owned subsidiary Ribapharm, Inc., focuses on innovative treatments for dermatology, infectious diseases and cancer. Dermatological products include Efudex/Efudix, Oxsoralen-Ultra, Kinerase and Dermatix, which are principally used for actinic keratosis, psoriasis, reducing wrinkles and other signs of aging and pigmentation disorders. Major products in the antibacterial group include Ancobon/Ancotil and Anapenil. Ancobon/Ancotil is a systemic anti-fungal product that is used in the treatment of serious infections. Anapenil is an antibiotic product that is used in the treatment of susceptible infections. Neurological drugs include Mestinon, Permax, Phrenilin and Phrenilin Forte. The company's antiviral drug, Ribavirin, is sold under the trade name Virazole in North America and most European countries, as Vilona and Virazide in Latin America and as Virazide in Spain. Ribavirin is used for the treatment of several different human viral diseases, including hepatitis, herpes, influenza, measles and chicken pox. In recent news, in an attempt to develop a more efficient delivery platform, Valeant has selected Kenco Logistic Services to operate its North American distribution network.

FINANCIALS: Sales and profits are in thousands of dollars—add 000 to get the full amount. Year 2004 note: Complete fiscal 2004 results were not available for all companies at press time. For this company, year 2004 is for 9 months.

2004 Sales: $494,502 (9 months)   2004 Profits: $-70,765 (9 months)
2003 Sales: $685,953   2003 Profits: $-55,640   Stock Ticker: VRX
2002 Sales: $737,100   2002 Profits: $-134,900   Employees: 4,437
2001 Sales: $858,100   2001 Profits: $64,100   Fiscal Year Ends: 12/31
2000 Sales: $800,300   2000 Profits: $90,200

SALARIES/BENEFITS:
| Pension Plan: | ESOP Stock Plan: | Profit Sharing: | Top Exec. Salary: $835,000 | Bonus: $500,000 |
| Savings Plan: | Stock Purch. Plan: | | Second Exec. Salary: $600,000 | Bonus: $212,500 |

OTHER THOUGHTS:
Apparent Top Female Officers: 2
Hot Spot for Advancement for Women/Minorities:

LOCATIONS: ("Y" = Yes)
West:	Southwest:	Midwest:	Southeast:	Northeast:	International:
Y		Y			Y

VARIAN MEDICAL SYSTEMS INC

www.varian.com/vms

Industry Group Code: 339113   Ranks within this company's industry group: Sales: 25   Profits: 17

Insurance/HMO/PPO:	Drugs:	Equipment/Supplies:		Hospitals/Clinics:	Services:	Health Care:
Insurance: Managed Care: Utilization Mgmt.: Payment Proc.:	Manufacturer: Distributor: Specialty Pharm.: Vitamins/Nutri.: Clinical Trials:	Manufacturer: Distributor: Leasing/Finance: Information Sys.:	Y Y	Acute Care: Sub-Acute Care: Outpatient Surgery: Phys. Rehab. Center: Psychiatric Clinics:	Diagnostics: Labs/Testing: Staffing: Waste Disposal: Specialty Services:	Home Health: Long-Term Care: Physical Therapy: Phys. Practice Mgmt.:

TYPES OF BUSINESS:
Equipment-Integrated Radiotherapy Systems
X-Ray Equipment
Oncology Systems
Software Systems
Radiation Therapy Software

BRANDS/DIVISIONS/AFFILIATES:
Clinac
Ginzton Technology Center
PortalVision
Millennium

CONTACTS: Note: Officers with more than one job title may be intentionally listed here more than once.
Richard M. Levy, CEO
Richard M. Levy, Pres.
Garry W. Rogerson, COO
Elisha M. Finney, Corp. VP/CFO
Michael S. Klein, VP-Sales & Mktg.
Jack McCarthy, VP-Human Resources
George A. Zdasiuk, VP-Ginzton Technology Center
Joseph B. Phair, Corp. VP-Admin.
Joseph B. Phair, General Counsel/Corp. Sec.
John A. Thorson, II, VP-Bus. Dev.
Kate M. Smith, Treas.
Timothy E. Guertin, Corp. VP
John C. Ford, Corp. VP
Robert H. Kluge, Corp. VP
Richard M. Levy, Chmn.

Phone: 650-493-4000   Fax: 650-842-5196
Toll-Free:
Address: 3100 Hansen Way, Palo Alto, CA 94304-1038 US

GROWTH PLANS/SPECIAL FEATURES:
Varian Medical Systems, Inc. is one of the world's leading manufacturers of integrated radiotherapy systems for treating cancer. In addition to medical equipment, the company develops software products and devices designed to enhance the productivity and quality of its equipment, devices manufactured by other companies and the general delivery of health care services. Products can be broadly classified into three principal categories: oncology systems; x-ray products, including x-ray tubes and imaging subsystems; and brachytherapy and other technologies developed by the firm's Ginzton Technology Center (GTC). The oncology systems business designs, manufactures, sells and services hardware and software products for radiation treatment of cancer. Products include linear accelerators and accessories, treatment simulators and treatment verification products, as well as software systems for planning cancer treatments and managing information and images for radiation oncology. Its Clinac series of medical linear accelerators treats cancer by producing electrons and x-rays in shaped beams that target tumors and other abnormalities in a patient. The Millennium series of multi-leaf collimators are used with a linear accelerator to define the size, shape and intensity of the radiation beams generated by the linear accelerator. Varian also manufactures and sells an electronic portal imaging product, PortalVision, which verifies a patient's treatment position, a critical component for accurate delivery of radiotherapy treatment. In October 2004, Varian entered a licensing agreement with MED-TEC whereby MED-TEC will produce patient positioning systems under a Varian patent. The agreement covers the full range of indexing systems produced by MED-TEC.
Employees enjoy a promote-from-within policy, in-house college-level courses and a work-study program for college students.

FINANCIALS:
Sales and profits are in thousands of dollars—add 000 to get the full amount. Year 2004 note: Complete fiscal 2004 results were not available for all companies at press time. For this company, year 2004 is for 9 months.

2004 Sales: $890,719 (9 months)   2004 Profits: $115,414 (9 months)
2003 Sales: $1,041,600   2003 Profits: $130,900
2002 Sales: $873,100   2002 Profits: $93,600
2001 Sales: $773,600   2001 Profits: $54,300
2000 Sales: $689,700   2000 Profits: $53,000

Stock Ticker: VAR
Employees: 2,927
Fiscal Year Ends: 9/30

SALARIES/BENEFITS:
Pension Plan: Y   ESOP Stock Plan: Profit Sharing: Y   Top Exec. Salary: $793,862   Bonus: $1,614,391
Savings Plan: Stock Purch. Plan: Second Exec. Salary: $415,228   Bonus: $665,794

OTHER THOUGHTS:
Apparent Top Female Officers: 2
Hot Spot for Advancement for Women/Minorities:

LOCATIONS: ("Y" = Yes)
West: Y   Southwest: Midwest: Southeast: Northeast: International:

VCA ANTECH INC

www.vcaantech.com

Industry Group Code: 541940   **Ranks within this company's industry group:** Sales: 1   Profits: 1

Insurance/HMO/PPO:	Drugs:	Equipment/Supplies:	Hospitals/Clinics:	Services:	Health Care:
Insurance:	Manufacturer:	Manufacturer: Y	Acute Care:	Diagnostics: Y	Home Health:
Managed Care:	Distributor:	Distributor:	Sub-Acute Care:	Labs/Testing:	Long-Term Care:
Utilization Mgmt.:	Specialty Pharm.:	Leasing/Finance:	Outpatient Surgery:	Staffing:	Physical Therapy:
Payment Proc.:	Vitamins/Nutri.:	Information Sys.:	Phys. Rehab. Center:	Waste Disposal:	Phys. Practice Mgmt.:
	Clinical Trials:		Psychiatric Clinics:	Specialty Services: Y	

TYPES OF BUSINESS:
Animal Health Care Services
Animal Diagnostic Services
Full-Service Animal Hospitals
Veterinary Equipment

BRANDS/DIVISIONS/AFFILIATES:
Antech Diagnostics
VCA Animal Hospitals
Antech News
zoasis.com
Sound Technologies, Inc.

CONTACTS:
Note: Officers with more than one job title may be intentionally listed here more than once.

Robert L. Antin, CEO
Robert L. Antin, Pres.
Arthur J. Antin, Sr. VP/COO
Tomas W. Fuller, CFO
Neil Tauber, Sr. VP-Dev.
Arthur J. Antin, Corp. Sec.
Robert L. Antin, Chmn.

Phone: 310-571-6500   **Fax:** 310-571-6700
Toll-Free: 800-966-1822
Address: 12401 W. Olympic Blvd., Los Angeles, CA 90064-1022 US

GROWTH PLANS/SPECIAL FEATURES:
VCA Antech, Inc. (VCA) provides animal health care services and operates the largest network of veterinary diagnostic laboratories and freestanding, full-service animal hospitals in the U.S. The firm's network of veterinary diagnostic laboratories, Antech Diagnostics, provides sophisticated testing and consulting services to veterinarians, who use these services in the detection, diagnosis, evaluation, monitoring, treatment and prevention of diseases and other conditions affecting animals. It offers clients access to resources such as online results through zoasis.com, a service directory, consultant guide and current and past issues of its newsletter, Antech News. VCA provides diagnostic testing daily to over 12,000 animal hospitals and zoos in all 50 states as well as government agencies worldwide. Its customer base is over twice the size of its largest competitor. VCA believes that the outsourced laboratory testing market is one of the fastest-growing segments of the animal health care services industry. VCA Animal Hospitals, the company's network of over 230 animal hospitals in 34 states, offers a full range of general medical and surgical services for animals, as well as specialized treatments including advanced diagnostic services, internal medicine, oncology, ophthalmology, dermatology and cardiology. The firm's hospital acquisition program seeks established practices in excess of $1 million with three or more full-time veterinarians on staff. The company's hospital partnership program offers more than 25 joint venture possibilities to veterinary groups that meet the same criteria as acquisitions. VCA's hospital merger program offers merger possibilities to veterinary practices of any size near a VCA hospital. In October 2004, VCA acquired Sound Technologies, Inc., the nation's largest supplier of ultrasound and digital radiology equipment to the veterinary market.

FINANCIALS:
Sales and profits are in thousands of dollars—add 000 to get the full amount. Year 2004 note: Complete fiscal 2004 results were not available for all companies at press time. For this company, year 2004 is for 9 months.

2004 Sales: $497,649 (9 months)	2004 Profits: $50,255 (9 months)	**Stock Ticker:** WOOF
2003 Sales: $544,665	2003 Profits: $43,423	Employees: 4,800
2002 Sales: $443,500	2002 Profits: $20,800	Fiscal Year Ends: 12/31
2001 Sales: $401,400	2001 Profits: $-27,400	
2000 Sales: $354,700	2000 Profits: $-8,400	

SALARIES/BENEFITS:
Pension Plan:	ESOP Stock Plan:	Profit Sharing:	Top Exec. Salary: $540,800	Bonus: $540,800
Savings Plan: Y	Stock Purch. Plan:		Second Exec. Salary: $432,640	Bonus: $389,376

OTHER THOUGHTS:
Apparent Top Female Officers:
Hot Spot for Advancement for Women/Minorities:

LOCATIONS: ("Y" = Yes)
West:	Southwest:	Midwest:	Southeast:	Northeast:	International:
Y	Y	Y	Y	Y	

VENTANA MEDICAL SYSTEMS

www.ventanamed.com

Industry Group Code: 339113 Ranks within this company's industry group: Sales: 78 Profits: 82

Insurance/HMO/PPO:	Drugs:	Equipment/Supplies:	Hospitals/Clinics:	Services:	Health Care:
Insurance:	Manufacturer:	Manufacturer: Y	Acute Care:	Diagnostics:	Home Health:
Managed Care:	Distributor:	Distributor:	Sub-Acute Care:	Labs/Testing:	Long-Term Care:
Utilization Mgmt.:	Specialty Pharm.:	Leasing/Finance:	Outpatient Surgery:	Staffing:	Physical Therapy:
Payment Proc.:	Vitamins/Nutri.:	Information Sys.:	Phys. Rehab. Center:	Waste Disposal:	Phys. Practice Mgmt.:
	Clinical Trials:		Psychiatric Clinics:	Specialty Services:	

TYPES OF BUSINESS:
Automated Tissue Preparation Systems
Instrument Reagent Systems
Consumable Products

BRANDS/DIVISIONS/AFFILIATES:
Qdot

CONTACTS:
Note: Officers with more than one job title may be intentionally listed here more than once.

Christopher M. Gleeson, CEO
Christopher M. Gleeson, Pres.
Nicholas Malden, CFO
Timothy B. Johnson, General Mgr.-Mfg. Oper.
Hany Massarany, VP-North American Oper.
Kendall B. Hendrick, General Mgr.-Diagnostic Assays & Systems
Carole Marcot, VP-Quality Systems & Regulatory
Nicholas Malden, Corp. Sec.
Jack W. Schuler, Chmn.

Phone: 520-887-2155 **Fax:** 520-887-2558
Toll-Free: 800-227-2155
Address: 1910 Innovation Park Dr., Tucson, AZ 85737 US

GROWTH PLANS/SPECIAL FEATURES:
Ventana Medical Systems, Inc. develops, manufactures and markets instruments and consumable products used to automate diagnostic and drug discovery procedures in clinical histology laboratories and drug discovery laboratories worldwide. The company's instrument reagent systems are designed to prepare and stain patient tissue or cells mounted on a microscope slide for examination by a pathologist. Ventana's consumable products include reagents and other accessories. The firm's systems provide users with automated high-quality and consistent results with high throughput and significant labor savings. Clinical products are used by anatomical pathology labs, which focus on the analysis of human tissue, to assist anatomical pathologists in the diagnosis of cancer and infectious diseases. Drug discovery products are used by research labs at large pharmaceutical and biotechnology companies and medical research centers to assist in the discovery of new drug targets. Ventana instruments are used in the majority of the top 50 U.S. cancer centers, including Johns Hopkins Hospital, the Mayo Clinic, Memorial Sloan-Kettering Cancer Center and M.D. Anderson Medical Center. In September 2004, Ventana began using, under license, Quantum Dot Corporation's (QDC) Qdot nanocrystal technology for in vitro diagnostic applications. QDC will supply Qdot nanocrystals for Ventana to incorporate into its research and pharmaceutical discovery platforms.

Ventana offers its employees education reimbursement amounting to 80% of tuition and fees up to $5,250 per year; Met Life group discounts on auto, home, property and casualty insurance; dependent care and health care spending accounts; and health, dental and vision care.

FINANCIALS:
Sales and profits are in thousands of dollars—add 000 to get the full amount. Year 2004 note: Complete fiscal 2004 results were not available for all companies at press time. For this company, year 2004 is for 9 months.

2004 Sales: $118,128 (9 months)   2004 Profits: $12,660 (9 months)
2003 Sales: $132,380   2003 Profits: $5,972
2002 Sales: $105,400   2002 Profits: $4,100
2001 Sales: $87,800   2001 Profits: $1,400
2000 Sales: $71,100   2000 Profits: $-27,300

Stock Ticker: VMSI
Employees: 618
Fiscal Year Ends: 12/31

SALARIES/BENEFITS:
Pension Plan: ESOP Stock Plan: Profit Sharing: Top Exec. Salary: $278,795   Bonus: $
Savings Plan: Y   Stock Purch. Plan: Y   Second Exec. Salary: $225,712   Bonus: $

OTHER THOUGHTS:
Apparent Top Female Officers: 1
Hot Spot for Advancement for Women/Minorities:

LOCATIONS: ("Y" = Yes)
West:	Southwest:	Midwest:	Southeast:	Northeast:	International:
	Y	Y			Y

VENTIV HEALTH INC

www.ventiv.com

Industry Group Code: 541613 Ranks within this company's industry group: Sales: 2 Profits: 2

Insurance/HMO/PPO:	Drugs:	Equipment/Supplies:	Hospitals/Clinics:	Services:	Health Care:
Insurance:	Manufacturer:	Manufacturer:	Acute Care:	Diagnostics:	Home Health:
Managed Care:	Distributor:	Distributor:	Sub-Acute Care:	Labs/Testing:	Long-Term Care:
Utilization Mgmt.:	Specialty Pharm.:	Leasing/Finance:	Outpatient Surgery:	Staffing:	Physical Therapy:
Payment Proc.:	Vitamins/Nutri.:	Information Sys.: Y	Phys. Rehab. Center:	Waste Disposal:	Phys. Practice Mgmt.:
	Clinical Trials:		Psychiatric Clinics:	Specialty Services: Y	

TYPES OF BUSINESS:
Marketing for Life Sciences and Pharmaceuticals Companies
Outsourced and Contract Sales
Telemarketing
Health Care Communications
Call Planning Systems
Data Services
Sales Force Deployment

BRANDS/DIVISIONS/AFFILIATES:
Health Products Research, Inc.
Metropolitan Area Promotional Audit
Experient Technologies, Inc.
Ventiv Health Communications
Ventiv Health Sales
Ventiv Integrated Solutions
Ventiv Valley Communications
Snyder Communications

CONTACTS:
Note: Officers with more than one job title may be intentionally listed here more than once.

Eran Broshy, CEO
John Emery, CFO
Doug Langeland, Pres.-Ventiv Integrated Solutions
Leonard Vicciardo, Pres./COO-Health Products Research
Terry Herring, Pres.-Ventiv Health Sales
Jean Francois Delaigue, Mgr.-Ventiv Health France
Daniel M. Snyder, Chmn.

Phone: 732-748-4666 Fax: 732-537-4912
Toll-Free: 800-416-0555
Address: 200 Cottontail Ln., 8th Fl., Somerset, NJ 08873 US

GROWTH PLANS/SPECIAL FEATURES:
Ventiv Health, Inc. is a comprehensive sales and marketing partner providing outsourced solutions for the pharmaceutical and life sciences industry. The firm offers a broad range of sales and marketing capabilities, including strategic and tactical sales and marketing planning, related market research and intelligence, product and brand management, operational analytics and forecasting, as well as salesforce recruitment, training, automation, professional development and campaign execution. In conjunction with these outsourced sales campaigns, the company also develops educational programs targeted to physicians and manages related public relations efforts. Clients include Aventis, Bausch and Lomb, Bristol-Myers Squibb, Eli Lilly, Novartis, Pfizer and other leading pharmaceutical and life sciences companies. Lead division Ventiv Health Sales (VHS) comprises Ventiv Health U.S. and European Contract Sales. VHS operates one of the largest contract sales organizations in the U.S., working primarily with prescription pharmaceutical and other life sciences products. VHS can recruit, train and deploy a customized, full-service and highly targeted sales force within six to 12 weeks. Ventiv's subsidiary Health Products Research uses proprietary software to analyze internal data and help a customer develop strategies for resource allocation. Ventiv Health Communications provides marketing support services including telemarketing, direct mail, symposia and congresses. Ventiv Integrated Solutions (VIS) focuses on developing fully integrated revenue-share partnerships with new and existing clients, taking on broad responsibility for analytics, sales, marketing and product management, while allowing partners to retain control of their assets. Ventiv Health, Inc. was spun off from Snyder Communications, Inc. in 1999. Daniel M. Snyder, the high profile owner of the Washington Redskins football team, retains a significant interest in Ventiv Health, Inc. and serves as the company's chairman.

FINANCIALS:
Sales and profits are in thousands of dollars—add 000 to get the full amount. Year 2004 note: Complete fiscal 2004 results were not available for all companies at press time. For this company, year 2004 is for 9 months.

2004 Sales: $234,735 (9 months)	2004 Profits: $17,022 (9 months)	
2003 Sales: $224,453	2003 Profits: $5,776	Stock Ticker: VTIV
2002 Sales: $215,400	2002 Profits: $7,900	Employees: 2,400
2001 Sales: $398,600	2001 Profits: $-58,500	Fiscal Year Ends: 12/31
2000 Sales: $416,700	2000 Profits: $16,800	

SALARIES/BENEFITS:
| Pension Plan: | ESOP Stock Plan: Y | Profit Sharing: | Top Exec. Salary: $504,587 | Bonus: $600,000 |
| Savings Plan: | Stock Purch. Plan: | | Second Exec. Salary: $291,187 | Bonus: $410,098 |

OTHER THOUGHTS:
Apparent Top Female Officers:
Hot Spot for Advancement for Women/Minorities:

LOCATIONS: ("Y" = Yes)
West:	Southwest:	Midwest:	Southeast:	Northeast:	International:
Y	Y	Y	Y	Y	Y

VIASYS HEALTHCARE INC

www.viasyshealthcare.com

Industry Group Code: 339113   Ranks within this company's industry group: Sales: 45   Profits: 55

Insurance/HMO/PPO:	Drugs:	Equipment/Supplies:		Hospitals/Clinics:	Services:	Health Care:
Insurance:	Manufacturer:	Manufacturer:	Y	Acute Care:	Diagnostics:	Home Health:
Managed Care:	Distributor:	Distributor:	Y	Sub-Acute Care:	Labs/Testing:	Long-Term Care:
Utilization Mgmt.:	Specialty Pharm.:	Leasing/Finance:		Outpatient Surgery:	Staffing:	Physical Therapy:
Payment Proc.:	Vitamins/Nutri.:	Information Sys.:		Phys. Rehab. Center:	Waste Disposal:	Phys. Practice Mgmt.:
	Clinical Trials:			Psychiatric Clinics:	Specialty Services:	

TYPES OF BUSINESS:
Health Care Devices, Instruments and Products
Respiratory Care Products
Neurocare Products
Surgical Products

BRANDS/DIVISIONS/AFFILIATES:
Bear Medical Systems, Inc.
Bird Products Corp.
Corpak MedSystems
Erich Jaeger, GmbH
Grason-Stadler, Inc.
Electro Medical Equipment, Ltd.
Nicolet Vascular
SensorMedics Corp.

CONTACTS:
Note: Officers with more than one job title may be intentionally listed here more than once.
Randy H. Thurman, CEO
Stephen Connelly, Pres.
Stephen Connelly, COO
Martin Galvan, CFO
Rebecca Mabry, VP-Global Mktg.
Gary Mathern, VP-Human Resources
Frank J. McCaney, Sr. VP-Bus. Dev.
Edward Pulwer, Group Pres.-Critical Care
Bill Murray, Group Pres.-Respiratory Tech.
Giulio Perillo, Group Pres.-Orthopedics
Randy H. Thurman, Chmn.
Mahboob Raja, Group Pres.-Int'l

Phone: 610-862-0800   Fax: 610-862-0836
Toll-Free:
Address: 277 Washington St., Ste. 200, Conshohocken, PA 19428 US

GROWTH PLANS/SPECIAL FEATURES:
Viasys Healthcare, Inc. develops, manufactures, markets and services a variety of medical devices, instruments and surgical products for use in the respiratory, neurocare and medical product markets. Viasys was spun off from Thermo Electron Corp. in 2001. The company's respiratory care group develops, manufactures and markets products for the diagnosis and treatment of respiratory, circulatory and sleep-related disorders, offered under brand names including Bird, Bear, Erich Jaeger and SensorMedics. The neurocare group offers a comprehensive line of neurodiagnostic systems under the brand names Grason-Stadler, Nicolet, Nicolet Vascular, IMEX and EME. Viasys's medical and surgical products group offers critical care disposable devices, specialty medical products and materials and a line of wireless patient monitoring systems under brand names such as Stackhouse and Corpak. The firm sells products in over 100 countries. Customers include hospitals, alternate-care sites, clinical laboratories, private physicians and original equipment manufacturers. Viasys divested itself of its Thermedics Polymer business in 2003, selling the assets to Noveon, Inc.

FINANCIALS:
Sales and profits are in thousands of dollars—add 000 to get the full amount. Year 2004 note: Complete fiscal 2004 results were not available for all companies at press time. For this company, year 2004 is for 9 months.

2004 Sales: $282,521 (9 months)   2004 Profits: $8,059 (9 months)
2003 Sales: $394,947   2003 Profits: $21,586
2002 Sales: $353,900   2002 Profits: $5,400
2001 Sales: $358,400   2001 Profits: $16,300
2000 Sales: $345,400   2000 Profits: $18,900

Stock Ticker: VAS
Employees: 1,859
Fiscal Year Ends: 12/31

SALARIES/BENEFITS:
Pension Plan: ESOP Stock Plan: Profit Sharing: Top Exec. Salary: $540,386   Bonus: $546,400
Savings Plan: Y   Stock Purch. Plan: Second Exec. Salary: $304,616 Bonus: $218,595

OTHER THOUGHTS:
Apparent Top Female Officers: 1
Hot Spot for Advancement for Women/Minorities:

LOCATIONS: ("Y" = Yes)
West:	Southwest:	Midwest:	Southeast:	Northeast:	International:
Y		Y		Y	Y

VISION SERVICE PLAN

www.vsp.com

Industry Group Code: 524114A Ranks within this company's industry group: Sales: 2 Profits:

Insurance/HMO/PPO:	Drugs:		Equipment/Supplies:	Hospitals/Clinics:	Services:	Health Care:
Insurance: Managed Care: Utilization Mgmt.: Payment Proc.:	Manufacturer: Distributor: Specialty Pharm.: Vitamins/Nutri.: Clinical Trials:	Y	Manufacturer: Distributor: Leasing/Finance: Information Sys.:	Acute Care: Sub-Acute Care: Outpatient Surgery: Phys. Rehab. Center: Psychiatric Clinics:	Diagnostics: Labs/Testing: Staffing: Waste Disposal: Specialty Services:	Home Health: Long-Term Care: Physical Therapy: Phys. Practice Mgmt.:

TYPES OF BUSINESS:
Vision Insurance

BRANDS/DIVISIONS/AFFILIATES:
Sight for Students

GROWTH PLANS/SPECIAL FEATURES:
Vision Service Plan (VSP) is one of the leading eye care benefit providers in the United States. The firm has more than 38 million members through more than 20,800 vision professionals and doctors, located in rural and metropolitan areas throughout the nation. VSP offers benefit plans that vary from general eye care and eye glasses to laser vision correction. The firm has assisted 250,000 children through its Sight for Students program, which provides vision exams and glasses to low-income and uninsured children. The program began in 1997. VSP also offers loans to assist eye doctors to buy existing practices, buy into partnerships or make down payments on private practices in California, Ohio, Texas and Colorado.

CONTACTS: Note: Officers with more than one job title may be intentionally listed here more than once.
Roger Valine, CEO
Roger Valine, Pres.
Patricia Cochran, CFO
Ric Steere, VP-Sales
Walter Grubbs, VP-Human Resources
Steve Scott, VP-IT
Barclay Westerfeld, General Counsel
Gary Brooks, Sr. VP-Oper.
Don Tee, Sr. VP-Corp. Dev. & Mktg.
Mary Ann Cavanagh, VP-Client Services
Don Price, VP-Provider Rel.
Cheryl Johnson, VP-Health Care Services
Kate Renwick-Espinosa, VP-Mktg.

Phone: 916-851-5000 Fax: 916-851-4858
Toll-Free: 800-852-7600
Address: 3333 Quality Dr., Rancho Cordova, CA 95670 US

FINANCIALS: Sales and profits are in thousands of dollars—add 000 to get the full amount. Year 2004 note: Complete fiscal 2004 results were not available for all companies at press time. For this company, year 2004 is for months.

2004 Sales: $ (months)
2003 Sales: $1,970,000
2002 Sales: $1,860,000
2001 Sales: $
2000 Sales: $

2004 Profits: $ (months)
2003 Profits: $
2002 Profits: $
2001 Profits: $
2000 Profits: $

Stock Ticker: Private
Employees: 2,000
Fiscal Year Ends: 12/31

SALARIES/BENEFITS:
Pension Plan: ESOP Stock Plan: Profit Sharing: Top Exec. Salary: $ Bonus: $
Savings Plan: Stock Purch. Plan: Second Exec. Salary: $ Bonus: $

OTHER THOUGHTS:
Apparent Top Female Officers: 4
Hot Spot for Advancement for Women/Minorities: Y

LOCATIONS: ("Y" = Yes)

West:	Southwest:	Midwest:	Southeast:	Northeast:	International:
Y	Y	Y	Y	Y	

VISX INC

www.visx.com

Industry Group Code: 339113 **Ranks within this company's industry group:** Sales: 74 Profits: 53

Insurance/HMO/PPO:	Drugs:	Equipment/Supplies:		Hospitals/Clinics:	Services:		Health Care:	
Insurance:	Manufacturer:	Manufacturer:	Y	Acute Care:	Diagnostics:		Home Health:	
Managed Care:	Distributor:	Distributor:		Sub-Acute Care:	Labs/Testing:		Long-Term Care:	
Utilization Mgmt.:	Specialty Pharm.:	Leasing/Finance:		Outpatient Surgery:	Staffing:		Physical Therapy:	
Payment Proc.:	Vitamins/Nutri.:	Information Sys.:		Phys. Rehab. Center:	Waste Disposal:		Phys. Practice Mgmt.:	
	Clinical Trials:			Psychiatric Clinics:	Specialty Services:	Y		

TYPES OF BUSINESS:
Equipment-Laser Vision Correction Systems
Marketing Education

BRANDS/DIVISIONS/AFFILIATES:
VISX STAR
VisionKey
VISX STAR S3
VISXPRESS
VISX University

CONTACTS:
Note: Officers with more than one job title may be intentionally listed here more than once.
Elizabeth H. Davila, CEO
Elizabeth H. Davila, Pres.
Timothy R. Maier, Exec. VP/CFO
Joaquin V. Wolff, VP-Mktg.
Catherine E. Murphy, VP-Human Resources
Carol F.H. Harner, VP-Research & Dev.
John F. Runkel, Jr., VP/General Counsel
Douglas H. Post, VP-Oper.
Timothy R. Maier, Treas.
Alan F. Russell, VP-Regulatory & Clinical Affairs
Donald L. Fagen, VP-Sales
John F. Runkel, Jr., Corp. Sec.

Phone: 408-733-2020 **Fax:** 408-773-7300
Toll-Free: 800-246-8479
Address: 3400 Central Expy., Santa Clara, CA 95051 US

GROWTH PLANS/SPECIAL FEATURES:

VISX, Inc. is a worldwide leader in the design, manufacture and marketing of proprietary technologies for laser vision correction. The company's main product is the VISX STAR excimer laser system, which uses a multi-variable-sized scanning beam, allows for refractive corrections in a shorter time and with less tissue removal than with other excimer lasers. An optical memory card, sold separately, controls use of the VISX system. The encoded VisionKey card is required to operate the VISX system, allowing the company to charge a licensing fee for every procedure preformed using that card. Over 2 million laser vision correction procedures have been performed in the United States using VISX laser systems. Internationally, the VISX STAR S3 system is used for the treatment of all refractive errors and, thus far, is the only U.S. system to gain approval from Japan's Ministry of Health and Welfare. VISX's marketing objective is to maximize consumer acceptance of laser vision correction by offering proven laser technology to the eye care medical community, developing improvements to that technology and providing its customers with various services and programs designed to increase operating efficiency and effectiveness. The company also operates VISX University, an educational program designed to teach laser center decision-makers how to effectively promote and market their excimer laser practices. Inrecent news, VISX agreed to be bought by Advanced Medical Optics Inc. for approximately $1.27 billion.

VISX offers its employees a comprehensive medical and insurance package plus a laser vision care program and a 24-hour fitness center.

FINANCIALS:
Sales and profits are in thousands of dollars—add 000 to get the full amount. Year 2004 note: Complete fiscal 2004 results were not available for all companies at press time. For this company, year 2004 is for 9 months.

2004 Sales: $125,452 (9 months)	2004 Profits: $32,592 (9 months)	**Stock Ticker:** EYE
2003 Sales: $143,905	2003 Profits: $23,251	**Employees:** 390
2002 Sales: $139,900	2002 Profits: $15,300	**Fiscal Year Ends:** 12/31
2001 Sales: $169,600	2001 Profits: $10,900	
2000 Sales: $200,200	2000 Profits: $35,200	

SALARIES/BENEFITS:
Pension Plan:	ESOP Stock Plan:	Profit Sharing:	Top Exec. Salary: $453,000	Bonus: $364,000
Savings Plan: Y	Stock Purch. Plan:		Second Exec. Salary: $287,000	Bonus: $215,000

OTHER THOUGHTS:
Apparent Top Female Officers: 3
Hot Spot for Advancement for Women/Minorities: Y

LOCATIONS: ("Y" = Yes)
West:	Southwest:	Midwest:	Southeast:	Northeast:	International:
Y					Y

VITAL SIGNS INC

www.vital-signs.com

Industry Group Code: 339113 **Ranks within this company's industry group:** Sales: 67 Profits: 63

Insurance/HMO/PPO:	Drugs:	Equipment/Supplies:		Hospitals/Clinics:	Services:	Health Care:
Insurance:	Manufacturer:	Manufacturer:	Y	Acute Care:	Diagnostics:	Home Health:
Managed Care:	Distributor:	Distributor:	Y	Sub-Acute Care:	Labs/Testing:	Long-Term Care:
Utilization Mgmt.:	Specialty Pharm.:	Leasing/Finance:		Outpatient Surgery:	Staffing:	Physical Therapy:
Payment Proc.:	Vitamins/Nutri.:	Information Sys.:		Phys. Rehab. Center:	Waste Disposal:	Phys. Practice Mgmt.:
	Clinical Trials:			Psychiatric Clinics:	Specialty Services:	

TYPES OF BUSINESS:
Supplies-Respiratory and Critical Care
Single-Patient-Use Medical Products
Anesthesia Products
Home Care Products

GROWTH PLANS/SPECIAL FEATURES:
Vital Signs, Inc. and its subsidiaries design, manufacture and market disposable medical products for the anesthesia, respiratory, sleep therapy, critical care and emergency care markets. Its anesthesia products include facemasks, breathing circuits, general anesthesia systems, disposable pressure infusers and single-use fiber-optic laryngoscope systems. Respiratory and critical care products include manual resuscitators, blood pressure cuffs, disposable arterial blood gas syringes and collection systems, heated humidification systems, continuous positive airway pressure systems, humidifiers and nebulizers and pediatric emergency systems. Home care products include a variety of home-use ventilators. The firm sells its products to hospitals in the United States and U.K. through its own sales force and through national distributors. Internationally, distributors sell the company's products in 55 countries.

BRANDS/DIVISIONS/AFFILIATES:

CONTACTS:
Note: Officers with more than one job title may be intentionally listed here more than once.
Terence D. Wall, CEO
Terence D. Wall, Pres.
Frederick S. Schiff, CFO
C. Barry Wicker, Exec. VP-Sales
Michael Khavinson, Exec. VP-Strategy
Joseph J. Thomas, Pres., Thompson Medical Products
Michael Khavinson, Exec. VP-Global Mktg.
Mark Felix, Exec. VP-Global Planning
Terrence D. Wall, Chmn.

Phone: 973-790-1330 **Fax:** 973-790-3307
Toll-Free: 800-932-0760
Address: 20 Campus Rd., Totowa, NJ 07152 US

FINANCIALS:
Sales and profits are in thousands of dollars—add 000 to get the full amount. Year 2004 note: Complete fiscal 2004 results were not available for all companies at press time. For this company, year 2004 is for 9 months.

2004 Sales: $136,156 (9 months)	2004 Profits: $16,565 (9 months)	**Stock Ticker:** VITL
2003 Sales: $182,163	2003 Profits: $14,222	**Employees:** 1,339
2002 Sales: $174,000	2002 Profits: $25,000	**Fiscal Year Ends:** 9/30
2001 Sales: $166,200	2001 Profits: $10,100	
2000 Sales: $150,300	2000 Profits: $13,900	

SALARIES/BENEFITS:
Pension Plan:	ESOP Stock Plan: Y	Profit Sharing:	Top Exec. Salary: $225,000	Bonus: $46,735
Savings Plan: Y	Stock Purch. Plan:		Second Exec. Salary: $175,000	Bonus: $16,011

OTHER THOUGHTS:
Apparent Top Female Officers:
Hot Spot for Advancement for Women/Minorities:

LOCATIONS: ("Y" = Yes)
West:	Southwest:	Midwest:	Southeast:	Northeast:	International:
Y		Y	Y	Y	Y

VITALWORKS INC

www.vitalworks.com

Industry Group Code: 511200   **Ranks within this company's industry group:** Sales: 6   Profits: 6

Insurance/HMO/PPO:	Drugs:	Equipment/Supplies:	Hospitals/Clinics:	Services:	Health Care:
Insurance:	Manufacturer:	Manufacturer:	Acute Care:	Diagnostics:	Home Health:
Managed Care:	Distributor:	Distributor:	Sub-Acute Care:	Labs/Testing:	Long-Term Care:
Utilization Mgmt.:	Specialty Pharm.:	Leasing/Finance:	Outpatient Surgery:	Staffing:	Physical Therapy:
Payment Proc.: Y	Vitamins/Nutri.:	Information Sys.: Y	Phys. Rehab. Center:	Waste Disposal:	Phys. Practice Mgmt.:
	Clinical Trials:		Psychiatric Clinics:	Specialty Services: Y	

TYPES OF BUSINESS:
Software-Medical Practice Management
IT Services

BRANDS/DIVISIONS/AFFILIATES:
RapidBill
Ingenuity EMR
RapidClaim
RadConnect RIS
RapidReminder

CONTACTS:
Note: Officers with more than one job title may be intentionally listed here more than once.

Stephen Kahane, CEO
Stephen Kahane, Pres.
C. Daren McCormick, COO
Joseph D. Hill, CFO
Eric Montgomery, VP-Sales
Stephen Hicks, VP/General Counsel
Kevin M. Silk, VP-Bus. Dev.
Kevin M. Silk, VP-Finance
C. Daren McCormick, VP/General Mgr.
Stephen Hicks, Corp. Sec.
Pamela Hannah, VP/General Mgr.
Joseph M. Walsh, Chmn.

Phone: 203-894-1300   **Fax:** 203-438-8416
Toll-Free: 800-278-0037
Address: 239 Ethan Allen Hwy., Ridgefield, CT 06877 US

GROWTH PLANS/SPECIAL FEATURES:
VitalWorks, Inc. is a leading nationwide provider of information management technology and services targeted toward health care practices and organizations. The company provides IT-based solutions for general medical practices and has specialty-specific products and services for practices such as radiology, anesthesiology, ophthalmology, emergency medicine, plastic surgery, internal medicine and dermatology. VitalWorks also offers enterprise-level systems designed for large physician groups and networks. Its software solutions automate image management, workflow, administrative, financial and clinical information management functions for physicians and other health care providers. VitalWorks also provides its clients with ongoing software support, training, electronic data interchange services for patient billing and claims processing and a variety of web-based services. Its software products include RapidBill, an automated patient statement processing program; RapidClaim, an electronic insurance claim program; RapidReminder, an appointment reminder program; and RadConnect RIS, an advanced radiology information system, which has shown record sales. Another product is the Ingenuity EMR web-based platform, an electronic medical records system that combines a simple browser interface with scalability, high-speed design, data security and low cost of ownership.

The company offers employees health, dental and life insurance, as well as employee and educational assistance programs.

FINANCIALS:
Sales and profits are in thousands of dollars—add 000 to get the full amount. Year 2004 note: Complete fiscal 2004 results were not available for all companies at press time. For this company, year 2004 is for 9 months.

2004 Sales: $83,088 (9 months)	2004 Profits: $-2,546 (9 months)	
2003 Sales: $111,519	2003 Profits: $7,963	**Stock Ticker:** VWKS
2002 Sales: $114,800	2002 Profits: $24,200	**Employees:** 687
2001 Sales: $106,400	2001 Profits: $-27,800	**Fiscal Year Ends:** 12/31
2000 Sales: $101,100	2000 Profits: $-78,100	

SALARIES/BENEFITS:
Pension Plan:	ESOP Stock Plan:	Profit Sharing:	Top Exec. Salary: $310,000	Bonus: $295,000
Savings Plan: Y	Stock Purch. Plan: Y		Second Exec. Salary: $230,000	Bonus: $220,000

OTHER THOUGHTS:
Apparent Top Female Officers: 1
Hot Spot for Advancement for Women/Minorities:

LOCATIONS: ("Y" = Yes)
West:	Southwest:	Midwest:	Southeast:	Northeast:	International:
Y		Y	Y	Y	

WALGREEN CO

www.walgreens.com

Industry Group Code: 446110   Ranks within this company's industry group: Sales: 1   Profits: 1

Insurance/HMO/PPO:	Drugs:	Equipment/Supplies:	Hospitals/Clinics:	Services:	Health Care:
Insurance:	Manufacturer:	Manufacturer:	Acute Care:	Diagnostics:	Home Health:
Managed Care:	Distributor:	Distributor:	Sub-Acute Care:	Labs/Testing:	Long-Term Care:
Utilization Mgmt.:	Specialty Pharm.: Y	Leasing/Finance:	Outpatient Surgery:	Staffing:	Physical Therapy:
Payment Proc.:	Vitamins/Nutri.:	Information Sys.:	Phys. Rehab. Center:	Waste Disposal:	Phys. Practice Mgmt.:
	Clinical Trials:		Psychiatric Clinics:	Specialty Services: Y	

TYPES OF BUSINESS:
Drug Stores
Mail-Order Pharmacy Services
Pharmacy Benefit Management
Health Care Maintenance Services
Online Pharmacy Services
Photo Restoration Services

BRANDS/DIVISIONS/AFFILIATES:
Walgreen's Healthcare Plus, Inc.
WHP Health Initiatives, Inc.
Walgreen Advance Care, Inc.
Intercom Plus

CONTACTS:
Note: Officers with more than one job title may be intentionally listed here more than once.

David W. Bernauer, CEO
Jeffrey A. Rein, Pres.
Jeffrey A. Rein, COO
William M. Rudolphsen, Sr. VP/CFO
Trent E. Taylor, Sr. VP/CIO
Julian A. Oettinger, General Counsel
Jerome B. Karlin, Exec. VP-Store Oper.
John W. Gleeson, VP/Treas.
George D. Wasson, VP/Pres., WHP Health Initiatives
William A. Shiel, Sr. VP-Facilities Dev.
R. Bruce Bryant, Sr. VP
George C. Eilers, Sr. VP
David W. Bernauer, Chmn.
J. Randolph Lewis, Sr. VP-Distribution & Logistics

Phone: 847-940-2500   Fax: 847-940-2804
Toll-Free:
Address: 200 Wilmot Rd., Deerfield, IL 60015 US

GROWTH PLANS/SPECIAL FEATURES:
Walgreen Co. is the leader in the U.S. chain drug store industry in sales, profits, store growth and use of technology. The company has 4,224 drugstores in 44 U.S. states and Puerto Rico and three mail service facilities. Walgreen currently averages 500 new store openings per year and expects to increase its total store count to 7,000 stores by 2010. The company's pharmacy business fills 323 million prescriptions annually. Its newest addition, Intercom Plus, a computer system for filling prescriptions, links all stores into a single network. Walgreen operates several health care-related businesses, such as Walgreen's Healthcare Plus, Inc., a mail-order drug company; WHP Health Initiatives, Inc. (WHI), a pharmacy benefits management company; and Walgreen Advance Care, Inc., a retailer of health care maintenance services. A large percentage of its stores have drive-thru pharmaciess, and most stores offer one-hour photo processing, as well as cosmetics, toiletries, liquor, beverages and tobacco. The firm also accepts prescription refill orders online through its web site, www.walgreens.com, and recently launched a web site specifically for the Latin community. Prescription sales account for approximately 62% of total sales and continue to increase each year. Its focus is on the rapid creation of a truly national drug store chain, with state-of-the-art information systems and exceptional merchandising and customer service. The company has been expanding the number of advanced services provided in its stores. For example, it recently rolled out its Photo Restoration Service nationwide, a state-of-the-art procedure that digitally restores old and damaged photographs. Walgreen also acquired 16 Oregon pharmacies from Hi-School Pharmacy. Prime Therapeutics, a pharmacy benefit solutions company, chose the firm's specialty pharmacy, a unit of WHI and a provider of injectable and biopharmaceutical medications, as its preferred provider.
The company offers its employees medical, prescription and dental plans and store discounts.

FINANCIALS:
Sales and profits are in thousands of dollars—add 000 to get the full amount. Year 2004 note: Complete fiscal 2004 results were not available for all companies at press time. For this company, year 2004 is for 12 months.

2004 Sales: $37,508,200 (12 months)   2004 Profits: $1,360,200 (12 months)
2003 Sales: $32,505,400   2003 Profits: $1,175,700
2002 Sales: $28,681,000   2002 Profits: $1,019,000
2001 Sales: $24,623,000   2001 Profits: $885,600
2000 Sales: $21,206,900   2000 Profits: $776,900

Stock Ticker: WAG
Employees: 154,000
Fiscal Year Ends: 8/31

SALARIES/BENEFITS:
Pension Plan: ESOP Stock Plan: Profit Sharing: Top Exec. Salary: $1,158,333   Bonus: $752,310
Savings Plan: Y   Stock Purch. Plan: Second Exec. Salary: $763,000   Bonus: $490,323

OTHER THOUGHTS:
Apparent Top Female Officers:
Hot Spot for Advancement for Women/Minorities:

LOCATIONS: ("Y" = Yes)
West:	Southwest:	Midwest:	Southeast:	Northeast:	International:
Y	Y	Y	Y	Y	Y

Note: Financial information, benefits and other data can change quickly and may vary from those stated here.

WARNER CHILCOTT PLC

www.wclabs.com

Industry Group Code: 325412 **Ranks within this company's industry group:** Sales: 38 Profits: 26

Insurance/HMO/PPO:	Drugs:	Equipment/Supplies:	Hospitals/Clinics:	Services:	Health Care:
Insurance:	Manufacturer: Y	Manufacturer:	Acute Care:	Diagnostics:	Home Health:
Managed Care:	Distributor:	Distributor:	Sub-Acute Care:	Labs/Testing:	Long-Term Care:
Utilization Mgmt.:	Specialty Pharm.:	Leasing/Finance:	Outpatient Surgery:	Staffing:	Physical Therapy:
Payment Proc.:	Vitamins/Nutri.:	Information Sys.:	Phys. Rehab. Center:	Waste Disposal:	Phys. Practice Mgmt.:
	Clinical Trials:		Psychiatric Clinics:	Specialty Services:	

TYPES OF BUSINESS:
Drugs-Women's Health, Dermatology & Urology

BRANDS/DIVISIONS/AFFILIATES:
Galen Holdings
Estrostep
Loestrin
Ovcon
Estrace
Femhrt
Femring
Sarafem

CONTACTS:
Note: Officers with more than one job title may be intentionally listed here more than once.

Roger Boissonneault, CEO
W. Carlton Reichel, Pres.
Geoffrey Elliot, Exec. VP/CFO
Kathleen A. Wickman, VP-Mktg.
Elizabeth Greenberg, VP-Human Resources
Herman Ellman, Sr. VP-Clinical Dev.
Leland H. Cross, Sr. VP-Tech.
Anthony D. Bruno, General Counsel
Anthony D. Bruno, Sr. VP-Corp. Dev.
Diane M. Cady, Sr. VP-Corp. Comm.
Diane M. Cady, Sr. VP-Investor Rel.
David G. Keppy, Sr. VP-Finance
John A. King, Chmn.

Phone: 353-1-709-4278 **Fax:** 353-1-662-4950
Toll-Free: 800-521-8813
Address: Lincoln House, Lincoln Pl., Dublin, Ireland

GROWTH PLANS/SPECIAL FEATURES:
Warner Chilcott plc, formerly Galen Holdings, develops and markets branded prescription pharmaceutical products in the United States directly to physician specialists, including obstetricians, gynecologists, urologists, cardiologists, dermatologists and general or family practitioners. The company is focused on women's health, dermatological and urological therapies. Warner Chilcott currently markets women's health care products in three categories: oral contraceptives, hormone replacement therapy and other products. The firm has three oral contraceptives on the market: Estrostep, Loestrin and Ovcon, the first chewable contraceptive to be given FDA approval. Ovcon is a spearmint-flavored contraceptive tablet that can be swallowed whole or chewed and swallowed. Women's hormone replacement therapy includes Estrace tablets, Estrace cream, Femhrt, and the newest product, Femring, a vaginal drug delivery ring for menopause relief, recently given FDA approval. Femring periodically delivers estradiol, a naturally occurring hormone, lasting for three months without removal. Other female products include Sarafem, a premenstrual dysphoric disorder (PMDD) reliever, and Natachew and Natafort prenatal vitamins. Warner Chilcott also offers two dermatological treatments, Doryx for acne and Dovonex for psoriasis, and two urological treatments, Estrace cream for vaginal atrophy and Pyridium Plus, a urinary tract analgesic.

FINANCIALS:
Sales and profits are in thousands of dollars—add 000 to get the full amount. Year 2004 note: Complete fiscal 2004 results were not available for all companies at press time. For this company, year 2004 is for months.

2004 Sales: $ (months)   2004 Profits: $ (months)
2003 Sales: $432,300   2003 Profits: $96,200
2002 Sales: $235,200   2002 Profits: $145,100
2001 Sales: $263,600   2001 Profits: $16,400
2000 Sales: $ 2000 Profits: $

Stock Ticker: Foreign
Employees: 960
Fiscal Year Ends: 12/31

SALARIES/BENEFITS:
Pension Plan: Y   ESOP Stock Plan: Profit Sharing: Top Exec. Salary: $ Bonus: $
Savings Plan: Y   Stock Purch. Plan: Second Exec. Salary: $ Bonus: $

OTHER THOUGHTS:
Apparent Top Female Officers: 3
Hot Spot for Advancement for Women/Minorities: Y

LOCATIONS: ("Y" = Yes)
West:	Southwest:	Midwest:	Southeast:	Northeast:	International:
					Y

WATSON PHARMACEUTICALS INC
www.watsonpharm.com

Industry Group Code: 325412 Ranks within this company's industry group: Sales: 25 Profits: 23

Insurance/HMO/PPO:	Drugs:	Equipment/Supplies:	Hospitals/Clinics:	Services:	Health Care:
Insurance: Managed Care: Utilization Mgmt.: Payment Proc.:	Manufacturer: Y Distributor: Specialty Pharm.: Vitamins/Nutri.: Clinical Trials:	Manufacturer: Distributor: Leasing/Finance: Information Sys.:	Acute Care: Sub-Acute Care: Outpatient Surgery: Phys. Rehab. Center: Psychiatric Clinics:	Diagnostics: Labs/Testing: Staffing: Waste Disposal: Specialty Services:	Home Health: Long-Term Care: Physical Therapy: Phys. Practice Mgmt.:

TYPES OF BUSINESS:
Drugs-Diversified
Generic Pharmaceuticals
Women's Health Products
Urology Products
Nephrology Products

BRANDS/DIVISIONS/AFFILIATES:
Watson Laboratories, Inc.
Watson Pharma
Oclassen Dermatologics
INFeD
Ferrlecit
Fioricet
Fiorinal
Steris Laboratories

CONTACTS:
Note: Officers with more than one job title may be intentionally listed here more than once.

Allen Y. Chao, CEO
Charles P. Slacik, Exec. VP/CFO
Susan Skara, VP-Human Resources
David C. Hsia, Sr. VP-Scientific Affairs
Maria Chow, Sr. VP-Mfg. Oper.
David Buchen, Sr. VP/General Counsel/Corp. Sec.
Charles Ebert, Sr. VP-Research & Dev.
Allen Y. Chao, Chmn.

Phone: 909-493-5300 Fax: 909-493-5836
Toll-Free:
Address: 311 Bonnie Cir., Corona, CA 92880-2882 US

GROWTH PLANS/SPECIAL FEATURES:
Watson Pharmaceuticals, Inc. develops, manufactures and markets over 30 branded and over 130 generic pharmaceutical products. With an emphasis on niche pharmaceuticals, the company offers generic versions of popular brand-name pharmaceuticals such as the asthma drugs Proventil and Ventolin. Watson continues to invest in product development and, consequently, can compete more effectively in the current health care environment. The company markets its proprietary products through its women's health, nephrology, urology and general products and divisions in order to foster close professional relationships with physicians in differing fields of medicine. Its women's health division products include oral contraceptives, a venereal disease treatment, a hormone replacement therapy and a visual cervical screening device. The urology and general products division includes urological, anti-hypertensive, neurological, psychiatric, pain management and dermatological treatment products. The nephrology division makes products for the treatment of iron-deficiency anemia. Key products within its nephrology branded product line currently include INFeD and Ferrlecit. The firm generally sells its branded products under the Watson Pharma and the Oclassen Dermatologics labels. The company also has the U.S. rights to the Fioricet and Fiorinal product lines for the treatment of tension headaches from Novartis. The company has decided to refocus its product development, sales and marketing resources on urology, nephrology and generics. The company thus intends to terminate its contract sales force agreement with Ventiv Health, Inc., to retain Steris Laboratories, its injectable manufacturing facility located in Phoenix, Arizona and to close its Miami manufacturing facility by the end of 2004. Watson Pharmaceuticals offers its employees a comprehensive benefits package including pet insurance, tuition reimbursement and prepaid legal advice.

FINANCIALS:
Sales and profits are in thousands of dollars—add 000 to get the full amount. Year 2004 note: Complete fiscal 2004 results were not available for all companies at press time. For this company, year 2004 is for 9 months.

2004 Sales: $1,217,044 (9 months) 2004 Profits: $96,227 (9 months)
2003 Sales: $1,457,722 2003 Profits: $202,864
2002 Sales: $1,223,200 2002 Profits: $175,800
2001 Sales: $1,160,700 2001 Profits: $116,400
2000 Sales: $811,500 2000 Profits: $157,500

Stock Ticker: WPI
Employees: 3,983
Fiscal Year Ends: 12/31

SALARIES/BENEFITS:
Pension Plan: ESOP Stock Plan: Y Profit Sharing: Top Exec. Salary: $890,000 Bonus: $970,000
Savings Plan: Y Stock Purch. Plan: Second Exec. Salary: $365,817 Bonus: $130,734

OTHER THOUGHTS:
Apparent Top Female Officers: 2
Hot Spot for Advancement for Women/Minorities:

LOCATIONS: ("Y" = Yes)
West	Southwest	Midwest	Southeast	Northeast	International
Y		Y	Y	Y	Y

WEBMD CORPORATION

www.webmd.com

Industry Group Code: 514199A   **Ranks within this company's industry group:** Sales: 1   Profits: 1

Insurance/HMO/PPO:	Drugs:	Equipment/Supplies:	Hospitals/Clinics:	Services:	Health Care:
Insurance: Managed Care: Utilization Mgmt.: Payment Proc.: Y	Manufacturer: Distributor: Specialty Pharm.: Vitamins/Nutri.: Clinical Trials:	Manufacturer: Y Distributor: Leasing/Finance: Information Sys.: Y	Acute Care: Sub-Acute Care: Outpatient Surgery: Phys. Rehab. Center: Psychiatric Clinics:	Diagnostics: Labs/Testing: Staffing: Waste Disposal: Specialty Services:	Home Health: Long-Term Care: Physical Therapy: Phys. Practice Mgmt.:

TYPES OF BUSINESS:
Business-to-Business Health Care Applications
Web-Based Health Care Information
Transaction Processing
Plastic Products

BRANDS/DIVISIONS/AFFILIATES:
WebMD Practice Services
Porex Corp.
WebMD Envoy
Medical Manager
ULTIA
Intergy
WebMD Health
Medscape

CONTACTS:
Note: Officers with more than one job title may be intentionally listed here more than once.
Kevin M. Cameron, CEO
Tony G. Holcombe, Pres.
Andrew C. Corbin, Exec. VP/CFO
Kirk G. Layman, Exec. VP-Admin.
Charles A. Mele, Exec. VP/General Counsel
K. Robert Draughon, Exec. VP-Bus. Dev.
Anthony Vuolo, Exec. VP-Bus. Dev.
Michael A. Singer, Exec. VP-Physician Software Strategies
Martin J. Wygod, Chmn.

Phone: 201-703-3400   **Fax:** 201-703-3401
Toll-Free:
Address: 669 River Dr., Ctr. 2, Elmwood Park, NJ 07407 US

GROWTH PLANS/SPECIAL FEATURES:
WebMD Corporation provides web-based health care information and services to facilitate connectivity and transactions among physicians, patients, payers, suppliers and consumers. The company's WebMD Envoy Internet-based information and transaction platform allows for the secure exchange of information, including patient enrollment, eligibility determination, referrals and authorizations, laboratory and diagnostic test orders and results, clinical data retrieval and claims processing. This segment processes over 2 billion transactions per year, supporting health care payers and physicians, pharmacies, dentists, hospitals, laboratory companies and other health care providers. WebMD Practice Services develops and markets information technology systems for health care providers under the Medical Manager, Intergy, ULTIA and Medical Manager Network Services brands. The WebMD Health division is a provider of general health care information, educational services and resources to online consumers. Offerings include news articles, expert presentations, interactive health management tools and a physician directory, as well as subscription services such as the Health Manager, weight loss clinic and fertility center. In addition, Medscape from WebMD is geared toward medical professionals. Through its Porex subsidiary, WebMD also manufactures porous plastic products for use in filtering, venting, wicking, diffusing and muffling. In 2004, the company announced that it would acquire Dakota Imaging and ViPS, Inc., an information technology provider.

WebMD offers employees a choice of medical insurance, bonus programs and educational assistance programs. It also provides spousal or child life insurance plans, adoption assistance, a sabbatical program and credit union benefits.

FINANCIALS:
Sales and profits are in thousands of dollars—add 000 to get the full amount. Year 2004 note: Complete fiscal 2004 results were not available for all companies at press time. For this company, year 2004 is for 9 months.

2004 Sales: $852,710 (9 months)	2004 Profits: $19,645 (9 months)	
2003 Sales: $963,980	2003 Profits: $-17,006	**Stock Ticker:** HLTH
2002 Sales: $925,900	2002 Profits: $-49,700	**Employees:** 5,635
2001 Sales: $706,600	2001 Profits: $-6,684,300	**Fiscal Year Ends:** 12/31
2000 Sales: $517,153	2000 Profits: $-3,085,608	

SALARIES/BENEFITS:
Pension Plan: ESOP Stock Plan: Profit Sharing: Top Exec. Salary: $1,308,900   Bonus: $125,000
Savings Plan: Y   Stock Purch. Plan: Y   Second Exec. Salary: $861,538   Bonus: $90,000

OTHER THOUGHTS:
Apparent Top Female Officers:
Hot Spot for Advancement for Women/Minorities:

LOCATIONS: ("Y" = Yes)
West:	Southwest:	Midwest:	Southeast:	Northeast:	International:
				Y	

WEIGHT WATCHERS INTERNATIONAL INC
www.weightwatchers.com

Industry Group Code: 446190   Ranks within this company's industry group: Sales: 1   Profits: 1

Insurance/HMO/PPO:	Drugs:	Equipment/Supplies:	Hospitals/Clinics:	Services:	Health Care:
Insurance:	Manufacturer:	Manufacturer:	Acute Care:	Diagnostics:	Home Health:
Managed Care:	Distributor:	Distributor:	Sub-Acute Care:	Labs/Testing:	Long-Term Care:
Utilization Mgmt.:	Specialty Pharm.:	Leasing/Finance:	Outpatient Surgery:	Staffing:	Physical Therapy:
Payment Proc.:	Vitamins/Nutri.:	Information Sys.:	Phys. Rehab. Center:	Waste Disposal:	Phys. Practice Mgmt.:
	Clinical Trials:		Psychiatric Clinics:	Specialty Services: Y	

TYPES OF BUSINESS:
Weight Management Programs
Franchising
Branded Diet Products

BRANDS/DIVISIONS/AFFILIATES:
Weight Watchers Corporate Solutions
Weighco Enterprises, Inc.
Weighco of Northwest, Inc.
Weighco of Southwest, Inc.
Weight Watchers eTools
WeightWatchers.com, Inc.
Weight Watchers Online

CONTACTS: Note: Officers with more than one job title may be intentionally listed here more than once.
Linda Huett, CEO
Linda Huett, Pres.
Richard McSorley, COO
Ann Sardini, VP/CFO
Robert W. Hollweg, VP/General Counsel
Maurice Kelly, VP-Oper.
Maurice Kelly, VP-Strategy
Linda W. Carilli, General Mgr.-Public Affairs
Scott R. Penn, VP-Australasia
Richard McSorley, COO-North America
Clive Brothers, COO-Europe
Robert W. Hollweg, Corp. Sec.
Raymond Debbane, Chmn.

Phone: 516-390-1400   Fax: 516-390-1334
Toll-Free:
Address: 175 Crossways Park W., Woodbury, NY 11797-2055 US

GROWTH PLANS/SPECIAL FEATURES:
Weight Watchers International, Inc. is a leading provider of weight-loss services, operating in 30 countries around the world. The company's programs help people lose weight and maintain their weight loss. At the core of its business are weekly meetings, which promote weight loss through education and group support in conjunction with a flexible, healthy diet. Each week, over 1.5 million people attend approximately 46,000 Weight Watchers meetings around the world, which are run by approximately 15,800 classroom leaders. Weight Watchers International conducts its business through a combination of company-owned and franchise operations with company-owned operations accounting for approximately 74% of total worldwide attendance. The firm has acquired the franchised territories and assets of Weighco Enterprises, Inc., Weighco of Northwest, Inc. and Weighco of Southwest, Inc., in addition to owning its San Diego, New Jersey and North Carolina franchised operations. The firm also offers Weight Watchers Corporate Solutions, a line of weight loss products that can be customized to suit the employees in any company. This at-work program addresses the weight-loss needs of working people by holding classes at their place of employment. The company's WeightWatchers.com, Inc. subsidiary offers weight loss help for meetings, members and self-help dieters. Customers can subscribe to Weight Watchers Online, designed for those who cannot join meetings but still wish to participate with other customers, and Weight Watchers eTools, which can enhance the meeting and program experience. The subsidiary also offers information on FlexPoints, the company's proprietary system for tracking and maintaining food amounts. For self-help dieters, Weight Watchers also offers an at-home kit, which is a complete mail-order system including the full set of program materials used in meetings.

As part of the Weight Watchers team, receptionists and leaders receive benefits such as flexible work schedules, free access to meetings and product discounts.

FINANCIALS:
Sales and profits are in thousands of dollars—add 000 to get the full amount. Year 2004 note: Complete fiscal 2004 results were not available for all companies at press time. For this company, year 2004 is for 9 months.

2004 Sales: $792,174 (9 months)	2004 Profits: $139,875 (9 months)
2003 Sales: $943,932	2003 Profits: $143,941
2002 Sales: $809,600	2002 Profits: $143,700
2001 Sales: $623,900	2001 Profits: $147,200
2000 Sales: $273,200	2000 Profits: $15,000

Stock Ticker: WTW
Employees: 46,000
Fiscal Year Ends: 12/31

SALARIES/BENEFITS:
Pension Plan: ESOP Stock Plan: Profit Sharing: Top Exec. Salary: $301,868   Bonus: $197,000
Savings Plan: Y   Stock Purch. Plan: Y   Second Exec. Salary: $245,698   Bonus: $151,014

OTHER THOUGHTS:
Apparent Top Female Officers: 3
Hot Spot for Advancement for Women/Minorities: Y

LOCATIONS: ("Y" = Yes)
West:	Southwest:	Midwest:	Southeast:	Northeast:	International:
Y	Y	Y	Y	Y	Y

WELCH ALLYN INC

www.welchallyn.com

Industry Group Code: 339113 **Ranks within this company's industry group:** Sales: Profits:

Insurance/HMO/PPO:	Drugs:	Equipment/Supplies:		Hospitals/Clinics:	Services:		Health Care:
Insurance:	Manufacturer:	Manufacturer:	Y	Acute Care:	Diagnostics:		Home Health:
Managed Care:	Distributor:	Distributor:		Sub-Acute Care:	Labs/Testing:		Long-Term Care:
Utilization Mgmt.:	Specialty Pharm.:	Leasing/Finance:		Outpatient Surgery:	Staffing:		Physical Therapy:
Payment Proc.:	Vitamins/Nutri.:	Information Sys.:	Y	Phys. Rehab. Center:	Waste Disposal:		Phys. Practice Mgmt.:
	Clinical Trials:			Psychiatric Clinics:	Specialty Services:	Y	

TYPES OF BUSINESS:
Equipment-Mobile Patient Monitoring Systems
Cardiac Defibrillators
Diagnostic and Therapeutic Devices
Precision Lamps
Image-Based Data Collection Systems
Training Services
Equipment Sales and Rentals

BRANDS/DIVISIONS/AFFILIATES:
Wm. Noah Allyn International Center
Everest VIT
HHP

CONTACTS:
Note: Officers with more than one job title may be intentionally listed here more than once.
Peter Soderberg, CEO
Peter Soderberg, Pres.
Kevin Cahill, CFO

Phone: 315-685-4100   **Fax:** 315-685-2546
Toll-Free: 800-535-6663
Address: 4341 State St. Rd., Skaneateles Falls, NY 13153-0220 US

GROWTH PLANS/SPECIAL FEATURES:
Welch Allyn, Inc., founded in 1915, is a leading manufacturer of medical equipment including diagnostic and therapeutic devices, cardiac defibrillators, patient monitoring systems and miniature precision lamps. Products include eye and ear care; medical index and referencing; laryngoscopes; lighting; and monitoring devices. These are used for dental health, inpatient care, pediatrics, general and family medicine, women's health, ambulatory surgery, emergency care, extended care, internal medicine and veterinary care. The firm operates numerous manufacturing, sales and distribution facilities throughout the world and operates multiple alternative businesses through subsidiaries. The Wm. Noah Allyn International Center for Training and Sales Development, known as the Lodge, is a faculty training and retreat center in Skaneateles Falls, New York. Another subsidiary, HHP, formerly Hand Held Products, designs and manufactures image-based data collection systems for transportation, postal services, warehousing, manufacturing and retail customers. Everest VIT, a full-service remote imaging company, offers technology-based training and inspection by experienced, certified technicians as well as equipment sales and rentals. Welch Allyn's lighting products division uses several proprietary manufacturing techniques.

Welch Allyn's employee benefits include medical, dental and travel insurance, child and elderly care, legal assistance, counseling, 10 to 30 vacation days annually, free health screenings, on-site fitness facilities and wellness incentives.

FINANCIALS:
Sales and profits are in thousands of dollars—add 000 to get the full amount. Year 2004 note: Complete fiscal 2004 results were not available for all companies at press time. For this company, year 2004 is for months.

2004 Sales: $ (months)	2004 Profits: $ (months)	
2003 Sales: $	2003 Profits: $	**Stock Ticker:** Private
2002 Sales: $	2002 Profits: $	Employees:
2001 Sales: $	2001 Profits: $	Fiscal Year Ends: 12/31
2000 Sales: $	2000 Profits: $	

SALARIES/BENEFITS:
Pension Plan:	ESOP Stock Plan:	Profit Sharing:	Top Exec. Salary: $	Bonus: $
Savings Plan:	Stock Purch. Plan:		Second Exec. Salary: $	Bonus: $

OTHER THOUGHTS:
Apparent Top Female Officers:
Hot Spot for Advancement for Women/Minorities:

LOCATIONS: ("Y" = Yes)
West:	Southwest:	Midwest:	Southeast:	Northeast:	International:
Y	Y	Y	Y	Y	Y

WELLCARE GROUP OF COMPANIES

www.wellcare.com

Industry Group Code: 524114   Ranks within this company's industry group: Sales: 46   Profits: 39

Insurance/HMO/PPO:	Drugs:	Equipment/Supplies:	Hospitals/Clinics:	Services:	Health Care:
Insurance: Managed Care: Y Utilization Mgmt.: Payment Proc.:	Manufacturer: Distributor: Specialty Pharm.: Vitamins/Nutri.: Clinical Trials:	Manufacturer: Distributor: Leasing/Finance: Information Sys.:	Acute Care: Sub-Acute Care: Outpatient Surgery: Phys. Rehab. Center: Psychiatric Clinics:	Diagnostics: Labs/Testing: Staffing: Waste Disposal: Specialty Services:	Home Health: Long-Term Care: Physical Therapy: Phys. Practice Mgmt.:

TYPES OF BUSINESS:
HMO Management

BRANDS/DIVISIONS/AFFILIATES:
WellCare
Staywell
HealthEase of Florida, Inc.
PreferredOne
WellCare Management Group, Inc.
WellCare HMO, Inc.
WellCare of New York, Inc.
Comprehensive Health Management of Florida

CONTACTS:
Note: Officers with more than one job title may be intentionally listed here more than once.

Todd Farha, CEO
Todd Farha, Pres.
Paul Behrens, CFO
Heath Schiesser, Sr. VP-Mktg.
Gretchen Demartini, VP-Human Resources
Robert Slepin, CIO
Thaddeus Bereday, General Counsel
Bill Keena, VP-Oper.
Donna Burtanger, Dir.-Corp. Comm.
Doug Hayward, VP-Connecticut
Dan Parietti, VP-New York
Rupesh Shah, Sr. VP-Sales
Diane Wilkosz, VP-Provider Rel.

Phone: 813-290-6200   Fax:
Toll-Free:
Address: 6800 N. Dale Mabry Hwy., Ste. 170, Tampa, FL 33614 US

GROWTH PLANS/SPECIAL FEATURES:
The WellCare Group of Companies includes WellCare Management Group, Inc.; WellCare HMO, Inc.; HealthEase of Florida, Inc.; WellCare of New York, Inc.; and Comprehensive Health Management of Florida. The company provides health care coverage for 500,000 customers in New York, Connecticut and Florida with 1,200 associates and over 20,000 physician partners. WellCare operates under the WellCare, Staywell, HealthEase and PreferredOne brand names. The company markets its products primarily to individuals who receive health care benefits through the government, such as Medicare and Medicaid. The WellCare brand caters to Medicare patients in New York and Florida. HealthEase and Staywell serve individuals that are eligible to participate in Florida's Medicaid and HealthyKids programs. PreferredOne serves Connecticut residents that are eligible for the Husky Healthcare A and B plans. In recent news, WellCare acquired Harmony Health Systems, Inc., a Medicaid managed care organization operating health plans in Illinois and Indiana, which nearly doubled the firm's number of customers.

FINANCIALS:
Sales and profits are in thousands of dollars—add 000 to get the full amount. Year 2004 note: Complete fiscal 2004 results were not available for all companies at press time. For this company, year 2004 is for months.

2004 Sales: $ (months)
2003 Sales: $1,046,000
2002 Sales: $921,800
2001 Sales: $97,300
2000 Sales: $78,600

2004 Profits: $ (months)
2003 Profits: $23,500
2002 Profits: $32,600
2001 Profits: $-1,900
2000 Profits: $-4,900

Stock Ticker: Private
Employees: 1,148
Fiscal Year Ends: 12/31

SALARIES/BENEFITS:
Pension Plan: ESOP Stock Plan: Profit Sharing: Top Exec. Salary: $ Bonus: $
Savings Plan: Stock Purch. Plan: Second Exec. Salary: $ Bonus: $

OTHER THOUGHTS:
Apparent Top Female Officers: 3
Hot Spot for Advancement for Women/Minorities: Y

LOCATIONS: ("Y" = Yes)

West:	Southwest:	Midwest:	Southeast:	Northeast:	International:
		Y	Y	Y	

Note: Financial information, benefits and other data can change quickly and may vary from those stated here.

WELLCHOICE INC

www.wellchoice.com

Industry Group Code: 524114 **Ranks within this company's industry group:** Sales: 21 Profits: 17

Insurance/HMO/PPO:	Drugs:	Equipment/Supplies:	Hospitals/Clinics:	Services:	Health Care:
Insurance: Y	Manufacturer:	Manufacturer:	Acute Care:	Diagnostics:	Home Health:
Managed Care: Y	Distributor:	Distributor:	Sub-Acute Care:	Labs/Testing:	Long-Term Care:
Utilization Mgmt.:	Specialty Pharm.:	Leasing/Finance:	Outpatient Surgery:	Staffing:	Physical Therapy:
Payment Proc.:	Vitamins/Nutri.:	Information Sys.:	Phys. Rehab. Center:	Waste Disposal:	Phys. Practice Mgmt.:
	Clinical Trials:		Psychiatric Clinics:	Specialty Services:	

TYPES OF BUSINESS:
Health Insurance

BRANDS/DIVISIONS/AFFILIATES:
Blue Cross and Blue Shield
Empire HealthChoice Assurance, Inc.
Empire HealthChoice HMO, Inc.
WellChoice Insurance of New Jersey, Inc.

GROWTH PLANS/SPECIAL FEATURES:
WellChoice, Inc. is the largest health insurance company in the State of New York based on preferred provider organization (PPO) and health maintenance organization (HMO) membership. The firm serves approximately 4.8 million members in 10 downstate New York counties and 16 counties in New Jersey, where it holds a leading market position covering over 21% of the population. WellChoice offers a broad portfolio of managed care and insurance products primarily to private and public employers including HMOs, PPOs, exclusive provider organizations, point-of-service products and dental-only coverage. The firm has the exclusive right to use the Blue Cross and Blue Shield names and marks in its New York and New Jersey areas. WellChoice subsidiaries include Empire HealthChoice Assurance, Inc.; Empire HealthChoice HMO, Inc.; and WellChoice Insurance of New Jersey, Inc.

CONTACTS:
Note: Officers with more than one job title may be intentionally listed here more than once.

Michael A. Stocker, CEO
Michael A. Stocker, Pres.
Gloria McCarthy, COO
John Remshard, CFO
Jason Gorevic, Sr. VP-Mktg. & Sales
Robert Lawrence, Sr. VP-Human Resources
Linda Tiano, General Counsel
Deborah L. Bohren, Sr. VP-Corp. Comm.
Seth I. Truwit, Corp. Sec.
John F. McGillicuddy, Chmn.

Phone: 212-476-7800 **Fax:** 212-476-1281
Toll-Free:
Address: 11 W. 42nd St., New York, NY 10036 US

FINANCIALS:
Sales and profits are in thousands of dollars—add 000 to get the full amount. Year 2004 note: Complete fiscal 2004 results were not available for all companies at press time. For this company, year 2004 is for 9 months.

2004 Sales: $4,339,612 (9 months)	2004 Profits: $186,512 (9 months)	**Stock Ticker:** WC
2003 Sales: $5,382,555	2003 Profits: $201,126	Employees: 5,400
2002 Sales: $5,105,660	2002 Profits: $376,559	Fiscal Year Ends: 12/31
2001 Sales: $	2001 Profits: $	
2000 Sales: $	2000 Profits: $	

SALARIES/BENEFITS:
Pension Plan: Y ESOP Stock Plan: Profit Sharing: Top Exec. Salary: $886,538 Bonus: $1,472,000
Savings Plan: Y Stock Purch. Plan: Second Exec. Salary: $499,615 Bonus: $521,632

OTHER THOUGHTS:
Apparent Top Female Officers: 3
Hot Spot for Advancement for Women/Minorities: Y

LOCATIONS: ("Y" = Yes)
West:	Southwest:	Midwest:	Southeast:	Northeast:	International:
				Y	

WELLPOINT HEALTH NETWORKS INC

www.wellpoint.com

Industry Group Code: 524114   Ranks within this company's industry group: Sales: 3 Profits: 2

Insurance/HMO/PPO:	Drugs:	Equipment/Supplies:	Hospitals/Clinics:	Services:	Health Care:
Insurance: Y	Manufacturer:	Manufacturer:	Acute Care:	Diagnostics:	Home Health:
Managed Care: Y	Distributor:	Distributor:	Sub-Acute Care:	Labs/Testing:	Long-Term Care:
Utilization Mgmt.:	Specialty Pharm.:	Leasing/Finance:	Outpatient Surgery:	Staffing:	Physical Therapy:
Payment Proc.: Y	Vitamins/Nutri.:	Information Sys.:	Phys. Rehab. Center:	Waste Disposal:	Phys. Practice Mgmt.:
	Clinical Trials:		Psychiatric Clinics:	Specialty Services: Y	

TYPES OF BUSINESS:
HMO/PPO
Workers' Compensation Plans
Point-of-Service Plans
Dental Plans
Pharmaceutical Plans
Managed Care Services
Actuarial Services
Claims Processing

BRANDS/DIVISIONS/AFFILIATES:
Blue Cross of California
Cobalt Corp.
Blue Cross and Blue Shield of Georgia
Blue Cross and Blue Shield of Missouri
WellPoint Pharmacy Management
HealthLink, Inc.
Golden West Vision and Dental
Anthem

CONTACTS:
Note: Officers with more than one job title may be intentionally listed here more than once.

Leonard D. Schaeffer, CEO
David C. Colby, Exec. VP/CFO
Ron J. Ponder, Exec. VP/CIO
Thomas C. Geiser, Exec. VP/General Counsel
D. Mark Weinberg, Exec. VP/Chief Dev. Officer
John Cygul, VP-Corp. Comm.
John Cygul, VP-Investor Rel.
Alice F. Rosenblatt, Exec. VP/Chief Actuary
Joan E. Herman, Pres.-Senior & Specialty Bus.
Rebecca A. Kapustay, Exec. VP-Central Services
Sandra Van Trease, Pres., UNICARE Life and Health Insurance
Leonard D. Schaeffer, Chmn.

Phone: 805-557-6655   **Fax:** 808-557-6872
Toll-Free:
Address: One WellPoint Way, Thousand Oaks, CA 91362 US

GROWTH PLANS/SPECIAL FEATURES:

WellPoint Health Networks, Inc. is one of the nation's largest suppliers of health care plans and services and the nation's second-largest health insurer. The company provides managed and indemnity health care plans to more than 13 million medical and over 49 million specialty members. The firm's managed care services include underwriting, actuarial services, network access, medical cost management and claims processing. Moreover, WellPoint offers a number of specialty products, such as mental health and life insurance, long-term care insurance and flexible spending accounts. The firm markets its products through its subsidiaries, Blue Cross of California, Blue Cross and Blue Shield of Georgia, Blue Cross and Blue Shield of Missouri and UNICARE Life and Health Insurance Company. The company's WellPoint Pharmacy Management subsidiary markets clinical management programs, drug formulary management, benefit design consultation, pharmacy network management, local network contract development, manufacturer discount programs and prescription drug databases. Other subsidiaries include HealthLink, Inc., Golden West Vision and Dental, PrecisionRx, WellPoint Behavioral Health, WellPoint Dental Services and WellPoint Workers' Compensation Managed Care Services. Recently, WellPoint signed a definitive merger agreement with Cobalt Corporation, the publicly traded holding company of Blue Cross and Blue Shield United of Wisconsin. Cobalt will be merged with one of WellPoint's subsidiaries. The company announced in late 2003 that it intends to be acquired by Anthem for about $16 billion, but multiple difficulties have indefinitely delayed the merger, although both companies remain committed to completion. This merger would combine the nation's two largest Blue Cross providers, creating a firm that will cover 26 million people in 13 states.

WellPoint offers its employees comprehensive health benefits, an employee assistance program, tuition assistance, a business-casual dress policy and commuter programs.

FINANCIALS:
Sales and profits are in thousands of dollars—add 000 to get the full amount. Year 2004 note: Complete fiscal 2004 results were not available for all companies at press time. For this company, year 2004 is for 9 months.

2004 Sales: $17,274,629 (9 months)   2004 Profits: $910,214 (9 months)
2003 Sales: $20,101,500   2003 Profits: $935,200
2002 Sales: $17,024,000   2002 Profits: $703,000
2001 Sales: $12,187,000   2001 Profits: $415,000
2000 Sales: $9,228,958   2000 Profits: $342,287

Stock Ticker: WLP
Employees: 19,100
Fiscal Year Ends: 12/31

SALARIES/BENEFITS:
| Pension Plan: | ESOP Stock Plan: | Profit Sharing: | Top Exec. Salary: $1,246,155 | Bonus: $5,690,916 |
| Savings Plan: Y | Stock Purch. Plan: Y | | Second Exec. Salary: $614,231 | Bonus: $1,025,706 |

OTHER THOUGHTS:
Apparent Top Female Officers: 4
Hot Spot for Advancement for Women/Minorities: Y

LOCATIONS: ("Y" = Yes)
West:	Southwest:	Midwest:	Southeast:	Northeast:	International:
Y	Y	Y	Y	Y	

WEST PHARMACEUTICAL SERVICES INC   www.westpharma.com

Industry Group Code: 339113   **Ranks within this company's industry group:** Sales: 40   Profits: 43

Insurance/HMO/PPO:	Drugs:	Equipment/Supplies:	Hospitals/Clinics:	Services:	Health Care:
Insurance:	Manufacturer:	Manufacturer: Y	Acute Care:	Diagnostics:	Home Health:
Managed Care:	Distributor:	Distributor:	Sub-Acute Care:	Labs/Testing: Y	Long-Term Care:
Utilization Mgmt.:	Specialty Pharm.:	Leasing/Finance:	Outpatient Surgery:	Staffing:	Physical Therapy:
Payment Proc.:	Vitamins/Nutri.:	Information Sys.:	Phys. Rehab. Center:	Waste Disposal:	Phys. Practice Mgmt.:
	Clinical Trials: Y		Psychiatric Clinics:	Specialty Services: Y	

TYPES OF BUSINESS:
Health Care Packaging
Drug Delivery Systems
Medical Device Components
Contract Packaging and Manufacturing
Contract Laboratory Services
Clinical Trials and Research

BRANDS/DIVISIONS/AFFILIATES:
Westar RS

CONTACTS:
Note: Officers with more than one job title may be intentionally listed here more than once.
Donald E. Morel, Jr., CEO
Donald E. Morel, Jr., Pres.
William J. Federici, VP/CFO
Richard D. Luzzi, Sr. VP-Human Resources
Anthony A. Sinkula, VP/Chief Scientific Officer
John R. Gailey, III, General Counsel
Michael A. Anderson, VP/Treas.
Herbert L. Hugill, Pres.-Pharmaceutical Systems Div.
John R. Gailey, III, Corp. Sec.
Linda R. Altemus, VP/Chief Compliance Officer
Donald E. Morel, Jr., Chmn.

Phone: 601-594-2900   **Fax:** 601-594-3000
Toll-Free: 800-345-9800
Address: 101 Gordon Dr., Lionville, PA 19341-0645 US

GROWTH PLANS/SPECIAL FEATURES:
West Pharmaceutical Services, Inc. brings new drug therapies and health care products to global markets. The company researches drug formulation and development, clinical research and offers laboratory services. It also designs, develops and manufactures components and systems for dispensing and delivering pharmaceutical and consumer products. West operates in two segments. The pharmaceutical systems segment designs, manufactures and sells stoppers, closures, medical device components and assemblies made from elastomers, metal and plastics and provides contract laboratory services for testing injectable drug packaging. The drug delivery systems segment identifies and develops drug delivery systems for biopharmaceutical and other drugs to improve their therapeutic performance and/or their method of administration. This segment also provides clinical research for Phase I, II and III studies and clinical and marketing research services, mostly for consumer products organizations. Westar RS is the company's line of serum stoppers, lyophilization stoppers, IV stoppers and syringe components, which are used by pharmaceutical companies to streamline the manufacturing process through the elimination of the wash, rinse and siliconizing portion of production lines. In June 2004, Westar announced that it will explore strategic alternatives for its drug delivery segment, possibly leading to discontinuing its research operations.

West offers its employees comprehensive medical, life, disability and dental plans. Furthermore, the company provides employee and educational assistance plans, as well as service recognition scholarships.

FINANCIALS:
Sales and profits are in thousands of dollars—add 000 to get the full amount. Year 2004 note: Complete fiscal 2004 results were not available for all companies at press time. For this company, year 2004 is for 9 months.

2004 Sales: $407,000 (9 months)	2004 Profits: $19,000 (9 months)	**Stock Ticker:** WST
2003 Sales: $490,700	2003 Profits: $31,900	**Employees:** 4,365
2002 Sales: $419,700	2002 Profits: $18,400	**Fiscal Year Ends:** 12/31
2001 Sales: $396,900	2001 Profits: $-5,200	
2000 Sales: $430,100	2000 Profits: $1,600	

SALARIES/BENEFITS:
Pension Plan: Y   ESOP Stock Plan: Profit Sharing: Top Exec. Salary: $482,902   Bonus: $545,510
Savings Plan: Y   Stock Purch. Plan: Y   Second Exec. Salary: $296,394   Bonus: $229,524

OTHER THOUGHTS:
Apparent Top Female Officers: 1
Hot Spot for Advancement for Women/Minorities:

LOCATIONS: ("Y" = Yes)
West:	Southwest:	Midwest: Y	Southeast: Y	Northeast: Y	International: Y

Note: Financial information, benefits and other data can change quickly and may vary from those stated here.

WRIGHT MEDICAL GROUP INC

www.wmt.com

Industry Group Code: 339113 Ranks within this company's industry group: Sales: 59 Profits: 59

Insurance/HMO/PPO:	Drugs:	Equipment/Supplies:	Hospitals/Clinics:	Services:	Health Care:
Insurance:	Manufacturer:	Manufacturer: Y	Acute Care:	Diagnostics:	Home Health:
Managed Care:	Distributor:	Distributor:	Sub-Acute Care:	Labs/Testing:	Long-Term Care:
Utilization Mgmt.:	Specialty Pharm.:	Leasing/Finance:	Outpatient Surgery:	Staffing:	Physical Therapy:
Payment Proc.:	Vitamins/Nutri.:	Information Sys.:	Phys. Rehab. Center:	Waste Disposal:	Phys. Practice Mgmt.:
	Clinical Trials:		Psychiatric Clinics:	Specialty Services:	

TYPES OF BUSINESS:
Orthopedic Implants
Reconstructive Joint Devices
Bio-Orthopedic Materials

BRANDS/DIVISIONS/AFFILIATES:
Wright Medical Technology
Allomatrix
Advance Medial Pivot Knee
Conserve Hip System
Micronail

CONTACTS: Note: Officers with more than one job title may be intentionally listed here more than once.
Laurence Y. Fairey, CEO
Laurence Y. Fairey, Pres.
John K. Bakewell, Exec. VP/CFO
R. Glen Coleman, Sr. VP-Mktg.
Jeffrey G. Roberts, VP-Research & Dev.
Jason P. Hood, General Counsel
Carl M. Stamp, VP-Bus. Dev.
Joyce B. Jones, Treas.
John R. Treace, VP-Biologics & Extremity Mktg.
Robert W. Churinetz, Sr. VP-Global Oper.
Karen L. Harris, VP-Int'l Sales & Distribution
F. Barry Bays, Chmn.
Brian T. Ennis, Pres.-Int'l

Phone: 901-867-9971 Fax: 901-867-9534
Toll-Free: 800-238-7117
Address: 5677 Airline Rd., Arlington, TN 38002 US

GROWTH PLANS/SPECIAL FEATURES:
Wright Medical Group, Inc. is a global orthopedic device company that designs, manufactures and markets reconstructive joint devices and bio-orthopedic materials. Reconstructive joint devices replace knees, hips and other joints that have failed because of disease or injury. Bio-orthopedic materials replace damaged or diseased bone and stimulate natural bone growth. Within these markets, the company focuses on the higher-growth sectors of advanced knee implants, bone-conserving hip implants, revision replacement implants and extremity implants, as well as on the integration of bio-orthopedic products into reconstructive joint procedures and other orthopedic applications. As a mid-sized orthopedic company, Wright believes its niche lies in its focus on smaller, higher-growth sectors of the market. Larger companies tend to concentrate marketing and research and development efforts on products that will have a high minimum threshold level of sales. The firm's products include the Advance Medial Pivot Knee, designed to approximate the motion of a healthy knee by using a unique spherical medial feature. The Conserve Hip System provides a bone-conserving alternative to conventional total hip reconstruction among patients diagnosed with avascular necrosis (AVN). Patients with AVN are typically younger, and Conserve replaces only the surface of the femoral, leaving the rest of the hip intact. Recently, Wright earned marketing approval from the FDA for all of its Allomatirx bone graft putties. In August 2004, the company introduced the Micronail system for wrist fracture repair.

FINANCIALS:
Sales and profits are in thousands of dollars—add 000 to get the full amount. Year 2004 note: Complete fiscal 2004 results were not available for all companies at press time. For this company, year 2004 is for 9 months.

2004 Sales: $219,832 (9 months)   2004 Profits: $17,732 (9 months)
2003 Sales: $248,932   2003 Profits: $17,397
2002 Sales: $200,900   2002 Profits: $25,100
2001 Sales: $172,900   2001 Profits: $-1,500
2000 Sales: $157,600   2000 Profits: $-39,500

Stock Ticker: WMGI
Employees: 845
Fiscal Year Ends: 12/31

SALARIES/BENEFITS:
Pension Plan: ESOP Stock Plan: Profit Sharing: Top Exec. Salary: $270,000   Bonus: $202,500
Savings Plan: Y   Stock Purch. Plan: Y   Second Exec. Salary: $212,925   Bonus: $143,724

OTHER THOUGHTS:
Apparent Top Female Officers: 2
Hot Spot for Advancement for Women/Minorities:

LOCATIONS: ("Y" = Yes)
West:	Southwest:	Midwest:	Southeast:	Northeast:	International:
		Y	Y		Y

Note: Financial information, benefits and other data can change quickly and may vary from those stated here.

WYETH

www.wyeth.com

Industry Group Code: 325412 **Ranks within this company's industry group:** Sales: 10 Profits: 12

Insurance/HMO/PPO:	Drugs:	Equipment/Supplies:	Hospitals/Clinics:	Services:	Health Care:
Insurance:	Manufacturer: Y	Manufacturer: Y	Acute Care:	Diagnostics:	Home Health:
Managed Care:	Distributor: Y	Distributor: Y	Sub-Acute Care:	Labs/Testing:	Long-Term Care:
Utilization Mgmt.:	Specialty Pharm.:	Leasing/Finance:	Outpatient Surgery:	Staffing:	Physical Therapy:
Payment Proc.:	Vitamins/Nutri.:	Information Sys.:	Phys. Rehab. Center:	Waste Disposal:	Phys. Practice Mgmt.:
	Clinical Trials:		Psychiatric Clinics:	Specialty Services:	

TYPES OF BUSINESS:
Drugs-Diversified
Wholesale Pharmaceuticals
Animal Health Care Products
Biologicals
Vaccines
Over-the-Counter Drugs

BRANDS/DIVISIONS/AFFILIATES:
American Home Products
Premarin
Dimetapp
Advil
Robitussin
Protonix
Centrum
Effexor

CONTACTS:
Note: Officers with more than one job title may be intentionally listed here more than once.

Robert A. Essner, CEO
Robert A. Essner, Pres.
Kenneth J. Martin, CFO/Exec. VP
Renè R. Lewin, VP-Human Resources
Bruce Fadem, CIO/VP-Corp. Info. Services
Lawrence V. Stein, General Counsel/Sr. VP
Thomas Hofstaetter, Sr. VP-Bus. Dev.
Marilyn H. Rhudy, VP-Public Affairs
Justin R. Victoria, VP-Investor Rel.
John C. Kelly, VP-Finance Oper.
Bernard J. Poussot, Exec. VP
Joseph M. Mahady, Sr. VP
Robert R. Ruffolo, Sr. VP
John C. Kelly, VP-Finance Oper.
Robert A. Essner, Chmn.

Phone: 973-660-5000 **Fax:** 973-660-7026
Toll-Free:
Address: 5 Giralda Farms, Madison, NJ 07940-0874 US

GROWTH PLANS/SPECIAL FEATURES:

Wyeth, formerly known as American Home products, is a global leader in pharmaceuticals, consumer health care products and animal health care products. The firm discovers, develops, manufactures, distributes and sells a diversified line of products arising from two divisions: pharmaceuticals and consumer health care. The pharmaceuticals segment sells branded and generic pharmaceuticals, biologicals and nutritionals as well as animal biologicals and pharmaceuticals. Principal products include women's health care products, neuroscience therapies, cardiovascular products, nutritionals, gastroenterology drugs, anti-infectives, vaccines, oncology therapies, musculoskeletal therapies, hemophilia treatments and immunological products. Its branded products include Premarin, Prempro, Premphase, Triphasil, Ativan, Effexor, Altace, Inderal, Zoton, Protonix and Enbrel. Principal animal health products include vaccines, pharmaceuticals, endectocides and growth implants. The consumer health care segment's products include analgesics, cough/cold/allergy remedies, nutritional supplements, lip balm and hemorrhoidal, antacid, asthma and other relief items sold over-the-counter. The segment's well-known over-the-counter products include Advil, cold medicines Robitussin and Dimetapp and nutritional supplement Centrum. In recent news, Wyeth Pharmaceuticals received FDA approval for a new formulation of the stomach acid suppressant Protonix for injection. The reformulation eliminates the need for an in-line filter, a previously required extra step in an already time-sensitive procedure to administer the medication to patients requiring immediate acid suppression.

Wyeth offers its employees child care subsidies, flextime, educational assistance and professional development programs. The company has a performance incentive award program as well as incentive programs specific to its divisions and departments.

FINANCIALS:
Sales and profits are in thousands of dollars—add 000 to get the full amount. Year 2004 note: Complete fiscal 2004 results were not available for all companies at press time. For this company, year 2004 is for 9 months.

2004 Sales: $12,709,830 (9 months)   2004 Profits: $2,998,340 (9 months)
2003 Sales: $15,850,600   2003 Profits: $2,051,600
2002 Sales: $14,584,000   2002 Profits: $4,447,200
2001 Sales: $14,128,000   2001 Profits: $2,285,000
2000 Sales: $13,262,754   2000 Profits: $-2,370,687

Stock Ticker: WYE
Employees: 52,385
Fiscal Year Ends: 12/31

SALARIES/BENEFITS:
| Pension Plan: Y | ESOP Stock Plan: | Profit Sharing: | Top Exec. Salary: $1,428,000 | Bonus: $2,000,000 |
| Savings Plan: Y | Stock Purch. Plan: Y | | Second Exec. Salary: $734,400 | Bonus: $918,000 |

OTHER THOUGHTS:
Apparent Top Female Officers: 2
Hot Spot for Advancement for Women/Minorities:

LOCATIONS: ("Y" = Yes)
West:	Southwest:	Midwest:	Southeast:	Northeast:	International:
Y	Y	Y	Y	Y	Y

YOUNG INNOVATIONS INC

www.yiinc.com

Industry Group Code: 339113 **Ranks within this company's industry group:** Sales: 102 Profits: 65

Insurance/HMO/PPO:	Drugs:	Equipment/Supplies:	Hospitals/Clinics:	Services:	Health Care:
Insurance:	Manufacturer:	Manufacturer: Y	Acute Care:	Diagnostics:	Home Health:
Managed Care:	Distributor:	Distributor:	Sub-Acute Care:	Labs/Testing:	Long-Term Care:
Utilization Mgmt.:	Specialty Pharm.:	Leasing/Finance:	Outpatient Surgery:	Staffing:	Physical Therapy:
Payment Proc.:	Vitamins/Nutri.:	Information Sys.:	Phys. Rehab. Center:	Waste Disposal:	Phys. Practice Mgmt.:
	Clinical Trials:		Psychiatric Clinics:	Specialty Services:	

TYPES OF BUSINESS:
Supplies-Dental Instruments
X-Ray Equipment

BRANDS/DIVISIONS/AFFILIATES:
D-Lish
Festival
ProCare
Plak Smacker

CONTACTS:
Note: Officers with more than one job title may be intentionally listed here more than once.
Alfred E. Brennan, Jr., CEO
Arthur L. Herbst, Jr., Pres.
Christine R. Boehning, CFO
Daniel Tarullo, VP-Bus. Dev.
Stephen Yaggy, Controller
Daniel E. Garrick, VP
Eric J. Stetzel, VP
George E. Richmond, Chmn.

Phone: 314-344-0010   **Fax:** 314-344-0021
Toll-Free: 800-325-1881
Address: 13705 Shoreline Ct. E., Earth City, MO 63045 US

GROWTH PLANS/SPECIAL FEATURES:
Young Innovations, Inc. develops, manufactures and markets supplies and equipment used by dentists and dental hygienists. The company's products include disposable and metal brush attachments, cups and brushes, panoramic x-ray machines, dental drills and related components, orthodontic toothbrushes, flavored examination gloves, children's toothbrushes, children's toothpastes, moisture control products, infection control products and ultrasonic systems and obturation products used in root canals. It operates through two business segments, professional dental and retail, selling products in North and South America, Europe and the Pacific Rim. The professional dental segment offers dental tools such as prophy angles and handpieces; D-Lish, Festival and ProCare prophy pastes; fluorides; disinfectants; gloves and masks; various x-ray systems; Plak Smacker home care kits, toothbrushes and fluorides; and root canal tools. The company has recently expanded through a series of rapid acquisitions and believes incorporating new lines of products will increase its existing sales.

FINANCIALS:
Sales and profits are in thousands of dollars—add 000 to get the full amount. Year 2004 note: Complete fiscal 2004 results were not available for all companies at press time. For this company, year 2004 is for 9 months.

2004 Sales: $59,488 (9 months)   2004 Profits: $9,123 (9 months)
2003 Sales: $76,156   2003 Profits: $13,201
2002 Sales: $72,200   2002 Profits: $11,400
2001 Sales: $63,700   2001 Profits: $9,500
2000 Sales: $51,387   2000 Profits: $8,305

Stock Ticker: YDNT
Employees: 294
Fiscal Year Ends: 12/31

SALARIES/BENEFITS:
Pension Plan: ESOP Stock Plan: Profit Sharing: Top Exec. Salary: $356,692   Bonus: $375,000
Savings Plan: Stock Purch. Plan: Second Exec. Salary: $281,692   Bonus: $300,000

OTHER THOUGHTS:
Apparent Top Female Officers: 1
Hot Spot for Advancement for Women/Minorities:

LOCATIONS: ("Y" = Yes)
West:	Southwest:	Midwest:	Southeast:	Northeast:	International:
Y	Y	Y			Y

ns
ZIMMER HOLDINGS INC

www.zimmer.com

Industry Group Code: 339113   Ranks within this company's industry group: Sales: 15   Profits: 7

Insurance/HMO/PPO:	Drugs:	Equipment/Supplies:		Hospitals/Clinics:	Services:	Health Care:
Insurance:	Manufacturer:	Manufacturer:	Y	Acute Care:	Diagnostics:	Home Health:
Managed Care:	Distributor:	Distributor:		Sub-Acute Care:	Labs/Testing:	Long-Term Care:
Utilization Mgmt.:	Specialty Pharm.:	Leasing/Finance:		Outpatient Surgery:	Staffing:	Physical Therapy:
Payment Proc.:	Vitamins/Nutri.:	Information Sys.:		Phys. Rehab. Center:	Waste Disposal:	Phys. Practice Mgmt.:
	Clinical Trials:			Psychiatric Clinics:	Specialty Services:	

TYPES OF BUSINESS:
Orthopedic Supplies
Surgical Supplies & Systems
Joint Implants
Knee & Hip Replacement Systems
Fracture Management Products

BRANDS/DIVISIONS/AFFILIATES:
NexGen
VerSys
M/DN
Orthopat
Pulsavac Plus Wound Debridemant System
ATS Tourniquet System
Implex Corp.
Trabecular Metal

CONTACTS: Note: Officers with more than one job title may be intentionally listed here more than once.
J. Raymond Elliott, CEO
J. Raymond Elliott, Pres.
Sam R. Leno, CFO
David C. Dvorak, General Counsel/Exec. VP-Corp. Services
Sam R. Leno, Exec. VP-Oper.
Sam R. Leno, Exec. VP-Corp. Finance
Bruce E. Peterson, Chmn.-Americas
J. Raymond Elliott, Chmn.
Bruno A. Melzi, Chmn.-Int'l

Phone: 219-267-6131   Fax:
Toll-Free:
Address: 345 E. Main St., Warsaw, IN 46580 US

GROWTH PLANS/SPECIAL FEATURES:

Zimmer Holdings, Inc. is a global leader in the design, development, manufacture and marketing of orthopedic reconstructive implants, trauma products and orthopedic and surgical products. Through its many subsidiaries, the company has operations in 24 countries and markets its products in over 80 countries. It sells primarily to musculoskeletal surgeons, neurosurgeons, oral surgeons, dentists, hospitals, distributors, health care dealers and health care purchasing organizations or buying groups. The company's main products are hip and knee replacements, fracture management products and various surgical products. Its NexGen knee product line is a comprehensive system for knee replacement surgery, with a leading position in posterior stabilized and revision procedures. The VerSys hip system, a Zimmer flagship brand, is an innovative, integrated family of hip products that offers surgeons design-specific options to meet varying surgical philosophies and patient needs. The firm plans to introduce approximately 340 new products to the VerSys system. Fracture management products are devices used primarily to reattach or stabilize damaged bone or tissue to support the body's natural healing process. The M/DN nail, an intramedullary nailing system for the internal fixation of long bone fractures, incorporates implants and instruments to align and fix fractures of the tibia, femur and humerus. The system has multiple screw options to provide increased surgical flexibility. Zimmer's surgical products include the OrthoPAT Autotransfusion System, the Pulsavac Plus Wound Debridement System and the ATS Tourniquet System. The company also manufactures and markets orthopedic surgical products, which include surgical supplies and instruments designed to aid in orthopedic surgical procedures. In April 2004, the company acquired Implex Corp., developer of Trabecular Metal technology, a substance that is very similar to bone.

Zimmer offers its employees a comprehensive medical plan and life insurance and disability protection plans.

FINANCIALS:
Sales and profits are in thousands of dollars—add 000 to get the full amount. Year 2004 note: Complete fiscal 2004 results were not available for all companies at press time. For this company, year 2004 is for 9 months.

2004 Sales: $2,179,800 (9 months)   2004 Profits: $341,800   (9 months)
2003 Sales: $1,901,000   2003 Profits: $346,300
2002 Sales: $1,372,400   2002 Profits: $257,800
2001 Sales: $1,178,600   2001 Profits: $149,800
2000 Sales: $1,041,000   2000 Profits: $176,000

Stock Ticker: ZMH
Employees: 6,500
Fiscal Year Ends: 12/31

SALARIES/BENEFITS:
Pension Plan: Y   ESOP Stock Plan: Profit Sharing: Top Exec. Salary: $668,269   Bonus: $1,040,656
Savings Plan: Y   Stock Purch. Plan: Second Exec. Salary: $461,365   Bonus: $433,659

OTHER THOUGHTS:
Apparent Top Female Officers:
Hot Spot for Advancement for Women/Minorities:

LOCATIONS: ("Y" = Yes)
West:	Southwest:	Midwest:	Southeast:	Northeast:	International:
Y	Y	Y		Y	Y

Note: Financial information, benefits and other data can change quickly and may vary from those stated here.

ZLB BEHRING LLC

www.zlbbehring.com

Industry Group Code: 339113 **Ranks within this company's industry group:** Sales: Profits:

Insurance/HMO/PPO:	Drugs:	Equipment/Supplies:	Hospitals/Clinics:	Services:	Health Care:
Insurance:	Manufacturer: Y	Manufacturer:	Acute Care:	Diagnostics:	Home Health:
Managed Care:	Distributor:	Distributor:	Sub-Acute Care:	Labs/Testing:	Long-Term Care:
Utilization Mgmt.:	Specialty Pharm.:	Leasing/Finance:	Outpatient Surgery:	Staffing:	Physical Therapy:
Payment Proc.:	Vitamins/Nutri.:	Information Sys.:	Phys. Rehab. Center:	Waste Disposal:	Phys. Practice Mgmt.:
	Clinical Trials:		Psychiatric Clinics:	Specialty Services:	

TYPES OF BUSINESS:
Pharmaceuticals-Coagulators

BRANDS/DIVISIONS/AFFILIATES:
CSL Limited
Humate-P
Monoclate-P
Mononine
Stimate
Helixate FS
Albuminar-5
Zemaira

CONTACTS:
Note: Officers with more than one job title may be intentionally listed here more than once.
Peter Turner, Pres.

Phone: 610-878-4155   **Fax:** 610-878-4913
Toll-Free:
Address: 1020 First Ave., King of Prussia, PA 19406 US

GROWTH PLANS/SPECIAL FEATURES:
ZLB Behring is one of the world's leading pharmaceutical companies that specializes in the manufacture of plasma products. The company is a subsidiary of CSL Limited, a worldwide pharmaceutical company based in Melbourne, Australia. The firm's product line includes drugs that treat hemophilia and other coagulation disorders, immunoglobulins that prevent and treat immune disorders, anticoagulants, surgical wound healers and plasma expanders for shock, burns and circulatory disorders. ZLB Behring also operates one of the world's largest, fully owned plasma collection networks. Patented products include coagulators; critical care and immune mediated products; and Alpha-1 inhibitors. Coagulator products include Humate-P, Monoclate-P, Mononine, Stimate and Helixate FS, for the treatment of classical hemophilia. Critical care products include Albuminar-5, Albuminar-25 and Albumin (Human) U.S.P., 5% and 25%. Immune mediated disorders are treated with Carimune NF Nanofiltered and Gammar-P I.V. The firm's Alpha-1 inhibitor, Zemaira, treats chronic augmentation and provides maintenance therapy in individuals with alpha1-proteinase inhibitor deficiency and clinical evidence of emphysema. In recent news, ZLB Behring announced that the U.S. FDA approved additional labeling information for its human plasma-derived intravenous immunoglobulin preparation, including data that show manufacturing steps used in the production of Carimune NF have the capacity to substantially decrease infectivity of transmissible spongiform encephalopathy including variant Creutzfeldt-Jakob Disease, the human form of mad cow disease.

FINANCIALS:
Sales and profits are in thousands of dollars—add 000 to get the full amount. Year 2004 note: Complete fiscal 2004 results were not available for all companies at press time. For this company, year 2004 is for   months.

2004 Sales: $ (months)	2004 Profits: $ (months)	**Stock Ticker:** Subsidiary
2003 Sales: $	2003 Profits: $	Employees:
2002 Sales: $1,119,400	2002 Profits: $	Fiscal Year Ends: 12/31
2001 Sales: $	2001 Profits: $	
2000 Sales: $	2000 Profits: $	

SALARIES/BENEFITS:
Pension Plan:	ESOP Stock Plan:	Profit Sharing:	Top Exec. Salary: $	Bonus: $
Savings Plan:	Stock Purch. Plan:		Second Exec. Salary: $	Bonus: $

OTHER THOUGHTS:
Apparent Top Female Officers:
Hot Spot for Advancement for Women/Minorities:

LOCATIONS: ("Y" = Yes)
West:	Southwest:	Midwest:	Southeast:	Northeast: Y	International: Y

Note: Financial information, benefits and other data can change quickly and may vary from those stated here.

ZOLL MEDICAL CORP

www.zoll.com

Industry Group Code: 339113 Ranks within this company's industry group: Sales: 66 Profits: 66

Insurance/HMO/PPO:	Drugs:	Equipment/Supplies:		Hospitals/Clinics:	Services:	Health Care:
Insurance:	Manufacturer:	Manufacturer:	Y	Acute Care:	Diagnostics:	Home Health:
Managed Care:	Distributor:	Distributor:		Sub-Acute Care:	Labs/Testing:	Long-Term Care:
Utilization Mgmt.:	Specialty Pharm.:	Leasing/Finance:		Outpatient Surgery:	Staffing:	Physical Therapy:
Payment Proc.:	Vitamins/Nutri.:	Information Sys.:	Y	Phys. Rehab. Center:	Waste Disposal:	Phys. Practice Mgmt.:
	Clinical Trials:			Psychiatric Clinics:	Specialty Services:	

TYPES OF BUSINESS:
Equipment-Emergency Use Noninvasive Cardiac Defibrillators and Pacemakers
Cardiac Resuscitation Devices
Mobile ECG Systems
EMS Data Management Software and Hardware

BRANDS/DIVISIONS/AFFILIATES:
ZOLL Data Control Software
ZOLL M Series
AED Defibrillator
CCT

GROWTH PLANS/SPECIAL FEATURES:
ZOLL Medical Corporation designs, manufactures and markets an integrated line of proprietary, noninvasive cardiac resuscitation devices, external pacemakers and defibrillators, disposable electrodes and mobile ECG systems. The firm also develops and sells software and associated hardware for data collection and management in the emergency medical systems market. The company's M Series defibrillators are smaller and lighter than competitive products. The M Series is designed for both hospital and pre-hospital markets. The defibrillators are equipped with the firm's proprietary biphasic waveform, which is clinically proven to be more effective than the conventional monophasic waveform. ZOLL also produces the AED defibrillator, which is intended for use by non-medical personnel. In addition, the company produces a wide variety of batteries, electrodes and emergency medical equipment.

CONTACTS:
Note: Officers with more than one job title may be intentionally listed here more than once.
Richard A. Packer, CEO
Richard A. Packer, Pres.
A. Ernest Whiton, CFO
Ward M. Hamilton, VP-Mktg.
Donald R. Boucher, VP-Research & Dev.
A. Ernest Whiton, VP-Admin.
Edward T. Dunn, VP-Oper.
John P. Bergeron, Treas.
Steven K. Flora, VP-North American Sales
E. J. Jones, VP-Int'l

Phone: 978-421-9655 Fax: 978-421-9655
Toll-Free: 800-348-9011
Address: 269 Mill Rd., Chelmsford, MA 01824-4420 US

FINANCIALS:
Sales and profits are in thousands of dollars—add 000 to get the full amount. Year 2004 note: Complete fiscal 2004 results were not available for all companies at press time. For this company, year 2004 is for 9 months.

2004 Sales: $156,057 (9 months)   2004 Profits: $6,811 (9 months)
2003 Sales: $184,603   2003 Profits: $12,850
2002 Sales: $150,200   2002 Profits: $10,200
2001 Sales: $119,200   2001 Profits: $7,600
2000 Sales: $106,336   2000 Profits: $8,802

Stock Ticker: ZOLL
Employees: 844
Fiscal Year Ends: 9/30

SALARIES/BENEFITS:
Pension Plan: Y   ESOP Stock Plan: Profit Sharing: Top Exec. Salary: $255,000   Bonus: $160,000
Savings Plan: Y   Stock Purch. Plan: Second Exec. Salary: $185,250   Bonus: $67,500

OTHER THOUGHTS:
Apparent Top Female Officers:
Hot Spot for Advancement for Women/Minorities:

LOCATIONS: ("Y" = Yes)
West:	Southwest:	Midwest:	Southeast:	Northeast:	International:
Y				Y	Y

Note: Financial information, benefits and other data can change quickly and may vary from those stated here.

ADDITIONAL INDEXES

CONTENTS:	
Index of Firms Noted as "Hot Spots for Advancement" for Women/Minorities	**p. 696**
Index by Subsidiaries, Brand Names and Selected Affiliations	**p. 697**

INDEX OF FIRMS NOTED AS HOT SPOTS FOR ADVANCEMENT FOR WOMEN & MINORITIES

ABBOTT LABORATORIES
ABIOMED INC
ADVANCED MEDICAL OPTICS INC
ADVANCEPCS INC
AFLAC INC
ALLINA HOSPITALS AND CLINICS
AMEDISYS INC
AMERICAN PHARMACEUTICAL PARTNERS INC
AMERIGROUP CORPORATION
APPLERA CORPORATION
APPLIED BIOSYSTEMS GROUP
ARQULE INC
ASCENSION HEALTH
ASSURANT INC
BARR LABORATORIES INC
BAUSCH & LOMB INC
BEVERLY ENTERPRISES INC
BLUE CARE NETWORK OF MICHIGAN
BLUE CROSS AND BLUE SHIELD OF LOUISIANA
BLUE CROSS AND BLUE SHIELD OF MICHIGAN
BLUE CROSS AND BLUE SHIELD OF MONTANA
BLUE SHIELD OF CALIFORNIA
CATHOLIC HEALTHCARE PARTNERS
CATHOLIC HEALTHCARE WEST
CENTENE CORPORATION
CIGNA CORP
COLE NATIONAL CORPORATION
COMMUNITY HEALTH SYSTEMS INC
CONTINUCARE CORP
CR BARD INC
CURATIVE HEALTH SERVICES INC
DAVITA INC
DELTA DENTAL PLANS ASSOCIATION
DIGENE CORPORATION
ELI LILLY & CO
EMERITUS CORP
ENDO PHARMACEUTICALS HOLDINGS INC
EXTENDICARE INC
FIRST HEALTH GROUP CORP
FISCHER IMAGING CORP
GAMBRO AB
GENERAL NUTRITION COMPANIES INC
GROUP HEALTH COOPERATIVE OF PUGET SOUND
GROUP HEALTH INCORPORATED
GUIDANT CORP
HARVARD PILGRIM HEALTH CARE INC
HEALTH CARE SERVICE CORPORATION
HEALTH FITNESS CORP
HEALTHNOW NEW YORK
HEARUSA INC
HEMACARE CORPORATION
HILLENBRAND INDUSTRIES
HORIZON BLUE CROSS BLUE SHIELD OF NEW JERSEY
INCYTE CORP
INTEGRA LIFESCIENCES HOLDINGS CORP
JENNY CRAIG INC
JOHNS HOPKINS MEDICINE
JOHNSON & JOHNSON
KYPHON INC
LIFE CARE CENTERS OF AMERICA
LUXOTTICA GROUP SPA
MAGELLAN HEALTH SERVICES INC
MATRIA HEALTHCARE INC
MCKESSON CORPORATION
MDS INC
MEDTRONIC VASCULAR
MERCK & CO INC
MERIDIAN BIOSCIENCE INC
MERIT MEDICAL SYSTEMS INC
MID ATLANTIC MEDICAL SERVICES INC
MILLENNIUM PHARMACEUTICALS INC
NEW YORK-PRESBYTERIAN HEALTHCARE SYSTEM
NOVATION LLC
OCCUPATIONAL HEALTH + REHABILITATION INC
ODYSSEY HEALTHCARE INC
OHIOHEALTH CORPORATION
PACIFICARE HEALTH SYSTEMS INC
PATIENT CARE INC
PDI INC
PRIORITY HEALTHCARE CORP
PROVIDENCE HEALTH SYSTEM
RENAL CARE GROUP INC
RES CARE INC
RESMED INC
SIEMENS MEDICAL SOLUTIONS
SIGNATURE EYEWEAR INC
SISTERS OF MERCY HEALTH SYSTEMS
SOLUCIENT LLC
SPECIALTY LABORATORIES INC
SSM HEALTH CARE SYSTEM INC
SUN HEALTHCARE GROUP
SYNOVIS LIFE TECHNOLOGIES INC
TECHNE CORP
THERASENSE INC
VISION SERVICE PLAN
VISX INC
WARNER CHILCOTT PLC
WEIGHT WATCHERS INTERNATIONAL INC
WELLCARE GROUP OF COMPANIES
WELLCHOICE INC
WELLPOINT HEALTH NETWORKS INC

INDEX OF SUBSIDIARIES, BRAND NAMES AND AFFILIATIONS

Brand or subsidiary, followed by the name of the related corporation

1-800-PetMeds; **PETMED EXPRESS INC**
1o2 Valve; **ICU MEDICAL INC**
300 PV; **EMPI INC**
3i; **BIOMET INC**
3TC; **SHIRE PHARMACEUTICALS PLC**
50 Gram Slam; **GENERAL NUTRITION COMPANIES INC**
800 Series; **LASERSCOPE**
AAI Development Services; **AAIPHARMA INC**
AAI International; **AAIPHARMA INC**
Aanalyst; **PERKINELMER INC**
AB500 Circulatory Support System; **ABIOMED INC**
Abbot Northwestern Hospital; **ALLINA HOSPITALS AND CLINICS**
Abbott Laboratories; **HOSPIRA INC**
Abbott Laboratories; **THERASENSE INC**
Abbott Laboratories; **I-STAT CORP**
ABI PRISM Genetic Analyzer; **APPLIED BIOSYSTEMS GROUP**
AbilityOne Products Corp.; **PATTERSON COMPANIES INC**
AbioCor; **ABIOMED INC**
ABS2000; **IMMUCOR INC**
Accelrys; **PHARMACOPEIA INC**
Access BR Monitor; **BECKMAN COULTER INC**
AccessBlue; **BLUE CROSS OF IDAHO**
Accredited Health Services, Inc.; **NATIONAL HOME HEALTH CARE CORP**
Accu-Clear; **INVERNESS MEDICAL INNOVATIONS INC**
accuDEXA; **SCHICK TECHNOLOGIES INC**
ACI Capital Co., Inc.; **JENNY CRAIG INC**
ACP; **HAEMONETICS CORPORATION**
AcrySof; **ALCON INC**
Actiq; **CEPHALON INC**
Activase; **GENENTECH INC**
Activated Checkpoint Therapy; **ARQULE INC**
Activation Control Technology (ACT); **CRYOLIFE INC**
ActiveLife; **CONVATEC**
Activelle; **NOVO-NORDISK AS**
AcuDriver Automated Osteotome System; **EXACTECH INC**

AcuMatch; **EXACTECH INC**
Acuson; **SIEMENS MEDICAL SOLUTIONS**
ADAC Laboratories; **PHILIPS MEDICAL SYSTEMS**
Adaptive Applications; **QUOVADX INC**
ADCO Surgical Supply, Inc.; **NYER MEDICAL GROUP INC**
Adderall XR; **SHIRE PHARMACEUTICALS PLC**
Adesso; **SONIC INNOVATIONS INC**
ADME/Tox; **ARQULE INC**
Administrative Services of Kansas, Inc.; **BLUE CROSS AND BLUE SHIELD OF KANSAS**
adultBasic; **CAPITAL BLUECROSS**
Advance; **QUIDEL CORP**
Advance Dynamic ROM; **EMPI INC**
Advance Insurance Company of Kansas; **BLUE CROSS AND BLUE SHIELD OF KANSAS**
Advance Medial Pivot Knee; **WRIGHT MEDICAL GROUP INC**
Advance Paradigm, Inc.; **ADVANCEPCS INC**
Advanced Bionics Corp.; **BOSTON SCIENTIFIC CORP**
Advanced Digital Imaging Research, LLC; **IRIS INTERNATIONAL INC**
Advanced Venous Access; **EDWARDS LIFESCIENCES CORP**
AdvancePCS; **CAREMARK RX INC**
Advanta; **HILL-ROM COMPANY INC**
Advantage Medical Products, LLC; **PSS WORLD MEDICAL INC**
Adventist Care Centers; **ADVENTIST HEALTH SYSTEM**
Advil; **WYETH**
Advocacy; **CORVEL CORP**
Advocate Bethany Hospital; **ADVOCATE HEALTH CARE**
Advocate Good Samaritan Hospital; **ADVOCATE HEALTH CARE**
Advocate Health Centers; **ADVOCATE HEALTH CARE**
Advocate Home Health Services; **ADVOCATE HEALTH CARE**
Advocate Hope Children's Hospital; **ADVOCATE HEALTH CARE**
Advocate Lutheran General Children's Hospital; **ADVOCATE HEALTH CARE**
Advocate Medical Group; **ADVOCATE HEALTH CARE**
AED Defibrillator; **ZOLL MEDICAL CORP**
Aegis Therapies, Inc.; **BEVERLY ENTERPRISES INC**
Aerobid; **FOREST LABORATORIES INC**
AeroChamber Plus; **FOREST LABORATORIES INC**

AERx Insulin Diabetes Management System; **ARADIGM CORPORATION**
AERx Pain Management System; **ARADIGM CORPORATION**
AERx Pulmonary Drug Delivery System; **ARADIGM CORPORATION**
AESOP; **INTUITIVE SURGICAL INC**
AEterna Laboratories; **AETERNA ZENTARIS INC**
Aetna Life Insurance Company (ALIC); **AETNA INC**
Affinity Health System; **MARIAN HEALTH SYSTEMS**
Affirm; **OSTEOTECH INC**
AFLAC Japan; **AFLAC INC**
AFLAC U.S.; **AFLAC INC**
Afrin; **SCHERING-PLOUGH CORP**
Agrylin; **SHIRE PHARMACEUTICALS PLC**
AHI Pharmacies, Inc.; **ACCREDO HEALTH INC**
AIMS/PCMS; **ARQULE INC**
AK Specialty Vehicles; **HEALTHTRONICS INC**
ALARIS Medical Systems, Inc.; **CARDINAL HEALTH INC**
Albert Einstein Healthcare Network; **JEFFERSON HEALTH SYSTEM INC**
Albuferon; **HUMAN GENOME SCIENCES INC**
Albuminar-5; **ZLB BEHRING LLC**
Alcon Surgical; **ALCON INC**
Aldurazyme; **GENZYME CORP**
Alegant Health; **CATHOLIC HEALTH INITIATIVES**
Aleve; **ROCHE GROUP**
Aleve; **BAYER CORP**
ALEXLAZR; **CANDELA CORP**
Alfigen, Inc.; **GENZYME CORP**
A-Life, Ltd.; **MENTOR CORP**
Aligners; **ALIGN TECHNOLOGY**
ALLEGRA; **SEPRACOR INC**
Allegra; **AVENTIS SA**
Allen Health Care; **NATIONAL HOME HEALTH CARE CORP**
Alliance PPO, LLC; **MID ATLANTIC MEDICAL SERVICES INC**
Allied Healthcare, Ltd.; **ALLIED HEALTHCARE INTERNATIONAL INC**
Allied Oxycare; **ALLIED HEALTHCARE INTERNATIONAL INC**
Allina Home Oxygen & Medical Equipment; **ALLINA HOSPITALS AND CLINICS**
Allina Medical Clinic; **ALLINA HOSPITALS AND CLINICS**
Allina Medical Transportation; **ALLINA HOSPITALS AND CLINICS**
Alloderm; **LIFECELL CORPORATION**

INDEX OF SUBSIDIARIES, BRAND NAMES AND AFFILIATIONS, CONT.

Allomatrix; **WRIGHT MEDICAL GROUP INC**
AllStaff, Inc.; **REHABCARE GROUP INC**
Aloe Vesta; **CONVATEC**
Alphagan; **ALLERGAN INC**
Alpha-ject; **ALPHARMA INC**
Alrex; **BAUSCH & LOMB INC**
ALSAC; **ST JUDE CHILDRENS RESEARCH HOSPITAL**
AltaGen Biosciences; **SEROLOGICALS CORP**
Altair; **SONIC INNOVATIONS INC**
Alternative Youth Services; **RES CARE INC**
Alterra Villas; **ALTERRA HEALTHCARE CORP**
Altoprev; **ANDRX CORP**
Amadeu Microkeratome; **ADVANCED MEDICAL OPTICS INC**
AMAP Chemistry Operating System; **ARQULE INC**
Ambulatory Surgery Center Program; **STRYKER CORP**
AMERICAID; **AMERIGROUP CORPORATION**
American Bankers Insurance Group, Inc.; **ASSURANT EMPLOYEE BENEFITS**
American Diversified Pharmacies, Inc.; **LONGS DRUG STORES CORPORATION**
American Family Life Assurance Company; **AFLAC INC**
American Health Packaging; **AMERISOURCEBERGEN CORP**
American Home Products; **WYETH**
American Lifestyles; **LIFE CARE CENTERS OF AMERICA**
American Medical Security Group; **PACIFICARE HEALTH SYSTEMS INC**
American Osteomedix Corp.; **INTERPORE CROSS INTERNATIONAL**
American Technical Molding; **UTI CORPORATION**
AmeriChoice Personal Care Model; **AMERICHOICE CORPORATION**
AMERIFAM; **AMERIGROUP CORPORATION**
AMERIKIDS; **AMERIGROUP CORPORATION**
AmeriPath Institute of Gastrointestinal Pathology; **AMERIPATH INC**
AMERIPLUS; **AMERIGROUP CORPORATION**
AmerisourceBergen Drug Corporation; **AMERISOURCEBERGEN CORP**
AmerisourceBergen Specialty Group; **AMERISOURCEBERGEN CORP**
AMEVIVE; **BIOGEN IDEC INC**

AMO Diplomax; **ADVANCED MEDICAL OPTICS INC**
AMO Gemini; **ADVANCED MEDICAL OPTICS INC**
Amsco; **STERIS CORP**
AMSMedOne; **AMERICAN MEDICAL SECURITY GROUP INC**
Anapenil; **VALEANT PHARMACEUTICALS INTERNATIONAL**
ANCIRC Pharmaceuticals; **ANDRX CORP**
Ancobon/Ancotil; **VALEANT PHARMACEUTICALS INTERNATIONAL**
Anda, Inc.; **ANDRX CORP**
Androcur; **SCHERING AG**
Andrx Laboratories; **ANDRX CORP**
Andrx Pharmaceuticals; **ANDRX CORP**
AneuRx; **MEDTRONIC VASCULAR**
Anexa; **ANALOGIC CORP**
Angeliq; **SCHERING AG**
AngioDynamics, Inc.; **E-Z-EM INC**
Anrad; **ANALOGIC CORP**
Ansell; **ANSELL LIMITED COMPANY**
Ansell Perry; **ANSELL LIMITED COMPANY**
AnsellCares; **ANSELL LIMITED COMPANY**
Antech Diagnostics; **VCA ANTECH INC**
Antech News; **VCA ANTECH INC**
Antegren; **ELAN CORP PLC**
ANTEGREN; **BIOGEN IDEC INC**
Antegren; **GTC BIOTHERAPEUTICS INC**
Anthem; **WELLPOINT HEALTH NETWORKS INC**
Anthrotek, Inc.; **BIOMET INC**
AO Compact; **SOLA INTERNATIONAL INC**
AO ProEasy; **SOLA INTERNATIONAL INC**
AOC Vertriebs GmbH; **PATTERSON COMPANIES INC**
Aon Market Exhange; **AON CORPORATION**
Aon Re Worldwide; **AON CORPORATION**
Aon Risk Monitor; **AON CORPORATION**
AonLine; **AON CORPORATION**
Apex; **CURATIVE HEALTH SERVICES INC**
Apex 800; **IRIDEX CORP**
Apligraph; **ORGANOGENESIS INC**
Apogent Technologies, Inc.; **FISHER SCIENTIFIC INTERNATIONAL INC**

Applera Corp.; **APPLIED BIOSYSTEMS GROUP**
Applera Corp.; **CELERA GENOMICS GROUP**
Applied Analytical Industries, Inc.; **AAIPHARMA INC**
Applied Biosystems; **APPLERA CORPORATION**
Applied Biosystems; **CELERA GENOMICS GROUP**
Aprovel; **SANOFI-SYNTHELABO**
AQUACEL; **CONVATEC**
AquaFlow; **STAAR SURGICAL CO**
Aranesp; **AMGEN INC**
Arden Courts; **MANOR CARE INC**
Arixtra; **SANOFI-SYNTHELABO**
Arkansas FirstSource PPO; **ARKANSAS BLUE CROSS AND BLUE SHIELD**
Arkansas National Life Insurance Company; **HILLENBRAND INDUSTRIES**
Arlington Memorial Hospital; **TEXAS HEALTH RESOURCES**
Arrow LionHeart; **ARROW INTERNATIONAL INC**
ARROWguard; **ARROW INTERNATIONAL INC**
Arrow-Howes; **ARROW INTERNATIONAL INC**
ARTWorks Clinical Information System; **INTEGRAMED AMERICA INC**
ARTWorks Practice Management Information System; **INTEGRAMED AMERICA INC**
Ascend Specialty Pharmacy Services, Inc.; **NATIONAL MEDICAL HEALTH CARD SYSTEMS INC**
Ascension Health Ventures; **ASCENSION HEALTH**
askyoursurgeon.com; **I FLOW CORPORATION**
Aspartate Aminotransferase Test; **CHOLESTECH CORP**
Asset Management Partnership Program; **UNIVERSAL HOSPITAL SERVICES INC**
Assisted Living Concepts, Inc.; **EXTENDICARE INC**
Associated Healthcare; **HARBORSIDE HEALTHCARE CORP**
Associated Hospital Service Corp. of Massachusetts; **BLUE CROSS AND BLUE SHIELD OF MASSACHUSETTS**
Assurant Employee Benefits; **ASSURANT INC**
Assurant Group; **ASSURANT EMPLOYEE BENEFITS**
Assurant Health; **ASSURANT INC**
Assurant PreNeed; **ASSURANT INC**

INDEX OF SUBSIDIARIES, BRAND NAMES AND AFFILIATIONS, CONT.

Assurant Solutions; **ASSURANT INC**
Assurant, Inc.; **ASSURANT EMPLOYEE BENEFITS**
ASTA Medica Oncology; **BAXTER INTERNATIONAL INC**
Astellas Pharma, Inc.; **FUJISAWA PHARMACEUTICALS COMPANY LTD**
AstroSachs; **SOLUCIENT LLC**
ATL Ultrasound; **PHILIPS MEDICAL SYSTEMS**
Atlanta Neonatal Physician Group; **PEDIATRIX MEDICAL GROUP INC**
AtmosAir; **KINETIC CONCEPTS INC**
Atrion Medical Products; **ATRION CORPORATION**
Atrium Biotechnologies, Inc.; **AETERNA ZENTARIS INC**
AtroPen; **MERIDIAN MEDICAL TECHNOLOGIES INC**
ATS Open Pivot; **ATS MEDICAL INC**
ATS Tourniquet System; **ZIMMER HOLDINGS INC**
Augmentin; **GLAXOSMITHKLINE PLC**
Aura; **MISONIX INC**
AuraZyme Pharmaceuticals, Inc.; **CRYOLIFE INC**
Aureomycin; **ALPHARMA INC**
AutoCAT; **ARROW INTERNATIONAL INC**
AutoCyte; **TRIPATH IMAGING INC**
Automated Intelligent Microscopy; **IRIS INTERNATIONAL INC**
AutoMed Technologies; **AMERISOURCEBERGEN CORP**
AVA 3Xi; **EDWARDS LIFESCIENCES CORP**
Availity, Inc.; **BLUE CROSS AND BLUE SHIELD OF FLORIDA**
AvantGuard; **HILL-ROM COMPANY INC**
Avastin; **GENENTECH INC**
Avastin; **ROCHE GROUP**
Avatec; **ALPHARMA INC**
Aventis; **SANOFI-SYNTHELABO**
Aventis Pasteur; **AVENTIS SA**
Aventis Pharma; **AVENTIS SA**
Avera Health Foundation; **AVERA HEALTH**
Avera Health Plans; **AVERA HEALTH**
Avera Marshall; **AVERA HEALTH**
Avera McKennan; **AVERA HEALTH**
Avera Queen of Peace; **AVERA HEALTH**
Avera Sacred Heart; **AVERA HEALTH**
Avera Select; **AVERA HEALTH**
Avera St. Luke's; **AVERA HEALTH**
Aviane; **BARR LABORATORIES INC**
aVidaRx; **ADVANCEPCS INC**
AVONEX; **BIOGEN IDEC INC**

Aware Cross and Blue Shield Associati; **BLUE CROSS AND BLUE SHIELD OF MINNESOTA**
AXA Group; **AXA PPP HEALTHCARE**
Axcis; **CARDIOGENESIS CORP**
Axon Instruments, Inc.; **MOLECULAR DEVICES CORP**
AxSYM; **ABBOTT LABORATORIES**
Azasan; **AAIPHARMA INC**
Azelex; **ALLERGAN INC**
AZO; **POLYMEDICA CORPORATION**
Balanced Gold; **OUTLOOK POINTE CORP**
Balfor Medical, Ltd.; **ALLIED HEALTHCARE INTERNATIONAL INC**
Band-Aid; **JOHNSON & JOHNSON**
Baptist Care Centers; **OCCUPATIONAL HEALTH + REHABILITATION INC**
Barbara Ann Karmanos Cancer Institute; **DETROIT MEDICAL CENTER**
Bard Access Systems; **CR BARD INC**
Bard Devices, Inc.; **CR BARD INC**
Bard Medical Systems; **CR BARD INC**
BarnesCare; **BJC HEALTHCARE**
Barnes-Jewish Hospital; **BJC HEALTHCARE**
Barnstead International; **APOGENT TECHNOLOGIES INC**
Barr Research, Inc.; **BARR LABORATORIES INC**
Basic Care; **HILLENBRAND INDUSTRIES**
BasicBlue; **ARKANSAS BLUE CROSS AND BLUE SHIELD**
Basil; **STERIS CORP**
Batesville Casket Company; **HILLENBRAND INDUSTRIES**
Baublys; **EXCEL TECHNOLOGY INC**
Bayer Chemicals; **BAYER AG**
Bayer Chemicals Corp.; **BAYER CORP**
Bayer Corporation; **BAYER AG**
Bayer CropScience; **BAYER AG**
Bayer CropScience, LP; **BAYER CORP**
Bayer Group; **BAYER CORP**
Bayer HealthCare; **BAYER CORP**
Bayer HealthCare; **BAYER AG**
Bayer Industry Services; **BAYER AG**
Bayer MaterialScience; **BAYER AG**
Bayer MaterialSciences, LLC; **BAYER CORP**
Bayer Polymers; **BAYER CORP**
Bayer Technology Services; **BAYER AG**
Bear Medical Systems, Inc.; **VIASYS HEALTHCARE INC**
bebe eyes; **SIGNATURE EYEWEAR INC**
Beckman Instruments, Inc.; **BECKMAN COULTER INC**

Becton Dickinson Biosciences; **BECTON DICKINSON & CO**
Becton Dickinson Diagnostics; **BECTON DICKINSON & CO**
Becton Dickinson Medical; **BECTON DICKINSON & CO**
Behavioral Health Resources, Inc.; **BLUE CROSS AND BLUE SHIELD OF NORTH CAROLINA**
behavioralhealthonline.com; **PHC INC**
Beijing United Family Hospital and Clinics; **CHINDEX INTERNATIONAL INC**
Belfab; **PERKINELMER INC**
Belle; **SYBRON DENTAL SPECIALTIES INC**
Benadryl; **PFIZER INC**
Beni Stabili; **LUXOTTICA GROUP SPA**
Benicar; **FOREST LABORATORIES INC**
Berman; **ARROW INTERNATIONAL INC**
Beta-Cath; **NOVOSTE CORPORATION**
Betapace; **SCHERING AG**
Betaseron; **CHIRON CORP**
Betaseron; **SCHERING AG**
Betoptic; **ALCON INC**
BioBalance Corp.; **NEW YORK HEALTH CARE INC**
Bio-d; **OSTEOTECH INC**
BIODESIGN; **MERIDIAN BIOSCIENCE INC**
BioFoam; **CRYOLIFE INC**
BioGlue; **CRYOLIFE INC**
Bio-Intact PTH; **QUEST DIAGNOSTICS INC**
BioKnowledge Library; **INCYTE CORP**
Biolab Group (The); **CANTEL MEDICAL CORP**
BioLink; **COVANCE INC**
Biomec 3000; **BECKMAN COULTER INC**
Biomedics; **OCULAR SCIENCES INC**
Biomek NX; **BECKMAN COULTER INC**
Biomet; **INTERPORE CROSS INTERNATIONAL**
Biomet Merck Group; **BIOMET INC**
BioPartners In Care; **ACCREDO HEALTH INC**
Bio-Plexus, Inc.; **ICU MEDICAL INC**
Biora AB; **INSTITUT STRAUMANN AG**
BioSafety; **MEDICAL ACTION INDUSTRIES INC**
BioScrip; **MIM CORP**
BIOSTER; **PHARMACOPEIA INC**
BioTek; **IMMUCOR INC**
Biovail Pharmaceuticals Canada; **BIOVAIL CORPORATION**

INDEX OF SUBSIDIARIES, BRAND NAMES AND AFFILIATIONS, CONT.

Biovail Pharmaceuticals, Inc.; **BIOVAIL CORPORATION**
Biovail Ventures; **BIOVAIL CORPORATION**
Bird Products Corp.; **VIASYS HEALTHCARE INC**
BIS Module Kit; **ASPECT MEDICAL SYSTEMS INC**
BIS Pediatric Sensor; **ASPECT MEDICAL SYSTEMS INC**
BIS Sensor Plus; **ASPECT MEDICAL SYSTEMS INC**
BIS Sensors; **ASPECT MEDICAL SYSTEMS INC**
BIS System; **ASPECT MEDICAL SYSTEMS INC**
Bispectral Index; **ASPECT MEDICAL SYSTEMS INC**
Bi-Ventricular Support System; **ABIOMED INC**
BJC Corporate Health Services; **BJC HEALTHCARE**
BJC Home Care Services; **BJC HEALTHCARE**
BJC Medical Group; **BJC HEALTHCARE**
BJ's Wholesale Club; **COLE NATIONAL CORPORATION**
B-K Medical A/S; **ANALOGIC CORP**
Block Medical de Mexico, S.A. de C.V.; **I FLOW CORPORATION**
Bloodless Surgery Station; **HAEMONETICS CORPORATION**
Blue Care Network HMO; **BLUE CROSS AND BLUE SHIELD OF MICHIGAN**
Blue Care Network of Michigan; **BLUE CROSS AND BLUE SHIELD OF MICHIGAN**
Blue Choice New England; **BLUE CROSS AND BLUE SHIELD OF MASSACHUSETTS**
Blue Choice POS; **BLUE CROSS AND BLUE SHIELD OF MICHIGAN**
Blue Cross and Blue Shield; **WELLCHOICE INC**
Blue Cross and Blue Shield of Georgia; **WELLPOINT HEALTH NETWORKS INC**
Blue Cross and Blue Shield of Illinois; **HEALTH CARE SERVICE CORPORATION**
Blue Cross and Blue Shield of Missouri; **WELLPOINT HEALTH NETWORKS INC**
Blue Cross and Blue Shield of New Mexico; **HEALTH CARE SERVICE CORPORATION**
Blue Cross and Blue Shield of Texas; **HEALTH CARE SERVICE CORPORATION**

Blue Cross and Blue Shield System; **BLUE CROSS AND BLUE SHIELD ASSOCIATION**
Blue Cross Association; **BLUE CROSS AND BLUE SHIELD ASSOCIATION**
Blue Cross Blue Shield; **HORIZON BLUE CROSS BLUE SHIELD OF NEW JERSEY**
Blue Cross Blue Shield; **MEDCO HEALTH SOLUTIONS**
Blue Cross Blue Shield Association; **BLUE SHIELD OF CALIFORNIA**
Blue Cross Blue Shield Association; **BLUE CROSS AND BLUE SHIELD OF MINNESOTA**
Blue Cross Blue Shield Association; **BLUE CROSS AND BLUE SHIELD OF WYOMING**
Blue Cross Blue Shield of Michigan; **BLUE CARE NETWORK OF MICHIGAN**
Blue Cross Blue Shield of Ohio; **MEDICAL MUTUAL OF OHIO**
Blue Cross of California; **WELLPOINT HEALTH NETWORKS INC**
Blue HealthSolutions; **BLUE CROSS AND BLUE SHIELD OF VERMONT**
Blue MedSave; **BLUE CROSS AND BLUE SHIELD OF MICHIGAN**
Blue Network P; **BLUE CROSS AND BLUE SHIELD OF TENNESSEE INC**
Blue Perks; **BLUE CROSS AND BLUE SHIELD OF TENNESSEE INC**
Blue Plus; **BLUE CROSS AND BLUE SHIELD OF MINNESOTA**
Blue Prefferred PPO; **BLUE CROSS AND BLUE SHIELD OF MICHIGAN**
Blue Shield of California Foundation; **BLUE SHIELD OF CALIFORNIA**
Blue Shield of California Life & Health Insurance; **BLUE SHIELD OF CALIFORNIA**
Blue Traditional; **BLUE CROSS AND BLUE SHIELD OF MICHIGAN**
Blue Value; **BLUE CROSS AND BLUE SHIELD OF GEORGIA INC**
Blue Vision PPO; **BLUE CROSS AND BLUE SHIELD OF MICHIGAN**
BlueAdvantage; **BLUE CROSS AND BLUE SHIELD OF NORTH CAROLINA**
BlueCard; **BLUE CROSS AND BLUE SHIELD ASSOCIATION**
BlueCard Program; **ARKANSAS BLUE CROSS AND BLUE SHIELD**
BlueCare; **BLUE CROSS OF IDAHO**
BlueCare; **BLUE CROSS AND BLUE SHIELD OF NORTH CAROLINA**
BlueChoice; **BLUE CROSS AND BLUE SHIELD OF NEBRASKA**
BlueChoice Vision; **BLUE CROSS AND BLUE SHIELD OF GEORGIA INC**

BlueClassic; **BLUE CROSS AND BLUE SHIELD OF NEBRASKA**
BlueCross BlueShield of Delaware; **CAREFIRST INC**
BlueCross BlueShield of Western New York; **HEALTHNOW NEW YORK**
bluecrossmontana.com; **BLUE CROSS AND BLUE SHIELD OF MONTANA**
BlueEdge PPO; **BLUE CROSS AND BLUE SHIELD OF TEXAS**
BlueHealthConnection; **BLUE CARE NETWORK OF MICHIGAN**
BlueLincs HMO; **BLUE CROSS AND BLUE SHIELD OF OKLAHOMA**
BlueOptions; **BLUE CROSS AND BLUE SHIELD OF NORTH CAROLINA**
BluePreferred; **BLUE CROSS AND BLUE SHIELD OF NEBRASKA**
BluePrime; **BLUE CROSS AND BLUE SHIELD OF NEBRASKA**
BlueSelect; **BLUE CROSS AND BLUE SHIELD OF LOUISIANA**
BlueShield of Northeastern New York; **HEALTHNOW NEW YORK**
BlueTest; **QUIDEL CORP**
BMD; **ALPHARMA INC**
BN II; **DADE BEHRING HOLDINGS INC**
BN Prospec; **DADE BEHRING HOLDINGS INC**
BN100; **DADE BEHRING HOLDINGS INC**
BNA; **DADE BEHRING HOLDINGS INC**
BonePlast Bone Void Filler; **INTERPORE CROSS INTERNATIONAL**
Boost; **BRISTOL MYERS SQUIBB CO**
Boston; **BAUSCH & LOMB INC**
Botox; **ALLERGAN INC**
Bovatec; **ALPHARMA INC**
Brace Shop Prosthetic Orthotic Centers, Inc. (The); **HANGER ORTHOPEDIC GROUP INC**
Bradford Particle Design; **NEKTAR THERAPEUTICS**
Brain Tumor Center of Minnesota; **FAIRVIEW HEALTH SERVICES**
Brandywine Hospital; **COMMUNITY HEALTH SYSTEMS INC**
BRAVO; **NOVOSTE CORPORATION**
Breathe Right Nasal Strips; **CNS INC**
Breathe Right Vapor Shot!; **CNS INC**
Breg; **ORTHOFIX INTERNATIONAL NV**
Brethine; **AAIPHARMA INC**
Bridge; **MEDTRONIC VASCULAR**
Brigham and Women's Hospital; **PARTNERS HEALTHCARE SYSTEM**

INDEX OF SUBSIDIARIES, BRAND NAMES AND AFFILIATIONS, CONT.

Bright Now! Dental, Inc.; **CASTLE DENTAL CENTERS INC**
Bright Now! Dental, Inc.; **MONARCH DENTAL CORP**
Brimonidine; **ALCON INC**
Bristol-Myers Squibb; **CONVATEC**
BUDDE Halo Retractor System; **INTEGRA LIFESCIENCES HOLDINGS CORP**
Buffalo Hospital; **ALLINA HOSPITALS AND CLINICS**
BUPA; **BRITISH UNION PROVIDENT ASSOCIATION (BUPA)**
BUPA Care Homes; **BRITISH UNION PROVIDENT ASSOCIATION (BUPA)**
BUPA Childcare; **BRITISH UNION PROVIDENT ASSOCIATION (BUPA)**
BUPA Health Insurance; **BRITISH UNION PROVIDENT ASSOCIATION (BUPA)**
BUPA Heartbeat; **BRITISH UNION PROVIDENT ASSOCIATION (BUPA)**
BUPA International; **BRITISH UNION PROVIDENT ASSOCIATION (BUPA)**
BUPA TravelCover; **BRITISH UNION PROVIDENT ASSOCIATION (BUPA)**
Bupropion; **EON LABS INC**
Bupropion; **TEVA PHARMACEUTICAL INDUSTRIES**
BVS-5000; **ABIOMED INC**
Bx SONIC Stent; **CORDIS CORP**
California Dental Health Plan; **PACIFICARE HEALTH SYSTEMS INC**
Callisto; **PERKINELMER INC**
Calumet Coach Company; **HEALTHTRONICS INC**
Cambridge Technology; **EXCEL TECHNOLOGY INC**
Camitro Corporation; **ARQULE INC**
Camp Riley; **CLARIAN HEALTH PARTNERS INC**
Camtronics Medical Systems; **ANALOGIC CORP**
Cantel Medical Corp.; **MINNTECH CORP**
Capital Administrative Services; **CAPITAL BLUECROSS**
Capital Advantage Insurance Company; **CAPITAL BLUECROSS**
Capitol Vial, Inc.; **APOGENT TECHNOLOGIES INC**
Capture; **IMMUCOR INC**
CAPVRF44; **GISH BIOMEDICAL INC**
Carbatrol; **SHIRE PHARMACEUTICALS PLC**
Cardiac Healthways; **AMERICAN HEALTHWAYS INC**
Cardinal Health; **CARDINAL MEDICAL PRODUCTS AND SERVICES**

cardinal.com; **CARDINAL HEALTH INC**
Cardio CRP; **QUEST DIAGNOSTICS INC**
CardioBeeper; **SHL TELEMEDICINE**
CardioBeeper; **MERIDIAN MEDICAL TECHNOLOGIES INC**
CardioPocket; **MERIDIAN MEDICAL TECHNOLOGIES INC**
CardioPocket; **SHL TELEMEDICINE**
CardioTech International, Inc.; **GISH BIOMEDICAL INC**
CARDIOVATIONS; **ETHICON INC**
Cardizem LA; **BIOVAIL CORPORATION**
Care Choice; **TRINITY HEALTH COMPANY**
CareAssist; **HILL-ROM COMPANY INC**
Carecast; **IDX SYSTEMS CORP**
CareCentrix; **GENTIVA HEALTH SERVICES INC**
careevolve.com; **BIO REFERENCE LABORATORIES INC**
CareFirst BlueChoice; **CAREFIRST INC**
CareFirst BlueCross BlueShield; **CAREFIRST INC**
CareFirst of Maryland, Inc.; **CAREFIRST INC**
Carelink Health Plans; **COVENTRY HEALTH CARE INC**
Caremark Rx, Inc.; **ADVANCEPCS INC**
CareMC; **CORVEL CORP**
caremc.com; **CORVEL CORP**
CarePlus Health Plan; **AMERIGROUP CORPORATION**
Caring Foundation; **BLUE CROSS AND BLUE SHIELD OF WYOMING**
Caring Foundation of Montana, Inc.; **BLUE CROSS AND BLUE SHIELD OF MONTANA**
CARITAS Health Services; **CATHOLIC HEALTH INITIATIVES**
Carmeda End-Point Attached Heparin; **CORDIS CORP**
Carpentier-Edwards; **EDWARDS LIFESCIENCES CORP**
Carsen Group, Inc.; **CANTEL MEDICAL CORP**
CashBack; **AXA PPP HEALTHCARE**
Catholic Health Ministries; **TRINITY HEALTH COMPANY**
C-beam; **CANDELA CORP**
CCT; **ZOLL MEDICAL CORP**
CD Horizon Eclipse Spinal System; **MEDTRONIC SOFAMOR DANEK**
CD Horizon Sextant; **MEDTRONIC INC**
CD Horizon Sextant System; **MEDTRONIC SOFAMOR DANEK**
CDR; **SCHICK TECHNOLOGIES INC**

CDR Wireless; **SCHICK TECHNOLOGIES INC**
CDRPan; **SCHICK TECHNOLOGIES INC**
Cedara Imaging Application Platform; **CEDARA SOFTWARE CORP**
Cedara OpenEyes; **CEDARA SOFTWARE CORP**
Cedara OrthoWorks; **CEDARA SOFTWARE CORP**
Cedara Vivace; **CEDARA SOFTWARE CORP**
Celera Diagnostics; **APPLIED BIOSYSTEMS GROUP**
Celera Diagnostics; **CELERA GENOMICS GROUP**
Celera Diagnostics; **APPLERA CORPORATION**
Celera Discovery System; **CELERA GENOMICS GROUP**
Celera Genomics; **APPLERA CORPORATION**
Celexa; **FOREST LABORATORIES INC**
Cell Saver; **HAEMONETICS CORPORATION**
Celltech Pharmaceuticals; **CELLTECH GROUP PLC**
Celltech R&D; **CELLTECH GROUP PLC**
Cemex; **EXACTECH INC**
CenCorp Health Solutions; **CENTENE CORPORATION**
Cenestine; **BARR LABORATORIES INC**
Cenpatico Behavior Health; **CENTENE CORPORATION**
Center for Advanced Diagnostics; **AMERIPATH INC**
Centerpulse Orthopedics, Inc.; **CENTERPULSE AG**
Centerpulse Orthopedics, Ltd.; **CENTERPULSE AG**
Centerpulse Spine-Tech, Inc.; **CENTERPULSE AG**
CentreVu Customer Care Solution; **AMERICAN HEALTHWAYS INC**
Centricity; **GE HEALTHCARE**
Centrum; **WYETH**
Centura Health; **CATHOLIC HEALTH INITIATIVES**
Ceprotin; **BAXTER INTERNATIONAL INC**
Ceres Purchasing Solutions; **BEVERLY ENTERPRISES INC**
Cerezyme; **GENZYME CORP**
Cermax Xenon; **PERKINELMER INC**
Cerner Millennium; **CERNER CORP**
Cerulean Companies, Inc.; **BLUE CROSS AND BLUE SHIELD OF GEORGIA INC**

INDEX OF SUBSIDIARIES, BRAND NAMES AND AFFILIATIONS, CONT.

Cerveillance Scope; **COOPER COMPANIES INC**
Cetrorelix; **AETERNA ZENTARIS INC**
Cetrotide; **AETERNA ZENTARIS INC**
Cetrotide; **SERONO SA**
CGI Management, Inc.; **CAPITAL SENIOR LIVING CORP**
CGMS System Gold; **MEDTRONIC MINIMED INC**
Charlie Hospital; **HEALTH MANAGEMENT ASSOCIATES INC**
Charlotte Regional Medical Center; **HEALTH MANAGEMENT ASSOCIATES INC**
Chattanooga Group; **ENCORE MEDICAL CORPORATION**
Chemicon International, Inc.; **SEROLOGICALS CORP**
Children's Infection Defense Center; **ST JUDE CHILDRENS RESEARCH HOSPITAL**
Children's Medical Ventures; **NOVAMETRIX MEDICAL SYSTEMS INC**
ChillTip; **LUMENIS LTD**
CHIP; **CAPITAL BLUECROSS**
Chiron Biopharmaceuticals; **CHIRON CORP**
Chiron Blood Testing; **CHIRON CORP**
Chiron Vaccines; **CHIRON CORP**
Chromacol, Ltd.; **APOGENT TECHNOLOGIES INC**
Chronimed; **MIM CORP**
Chugai Pharmaceuticals; **ROCHE GROUP**
CIBA Vision; **NOVARTIS AG**
CIGNA Behavioral Health; **CIGNA CORP**
CIGNA Dental & Vision Care; **CIGNA CORP**
CIGNA Group Insurance; **CIGNA CORP**
CIGNA HealthCare; **CIGNA CORP**
CIGNA International; **CIGNA CORP**
CIGNA Pharmacy Management; **CIGNA CORP**
CIMA Labs, Inc.; **CEPHALON INC**
Ciprofloxacin; **EON LABS INC**
Cisplatin; **AMERICAN PHARMACEUTICAL PARTNERS INC**
Citadel Group (The); **RES CARE INC**
Citrucel; **GLAXOSMITHKLINE PLC**
City Optical; **ESSILOR INTERNATIONAL SA**
ClaimPassXL; **PLANVISTA CORP**
Clairol, Inc.; **BRISTOL MYERS SQUIBB CO**
Claravis; **BARR LABORATORIES INC**
Clare Bridge; **ALTERRA HEALTHCARE CORP**

Clare Bridge Cottage; **ALTERRA HEALTHCARE CORP**
Clarian West Medical Center; **CLARIAN HEALTH PARTNERS INC**
ClariFlex; **ADVANCED MEDICAL OPTICS INC**
CLARINEX; **SEPRACOR INC**
CLARION CII Bionic Ear System; **ADVANCED BIONICS CORPORATION**
ClassicBlue; **BLUE CROSS AND BLUE SHIELD OF NORTH CAROLINA**
ClassicBlue; **BLUE CROSS OF IDAHO**
CLAVE; **ICU MEDICAL INC**
CLC2000; **ICU MEDICAL INC**
CleanOp; **MICROTEK MEDICAL HOLDINGS INC**
Clearblue; **INVERNESS MEDICAL INNOVATIONS INC**
Clearview; **INVERNESS MEDICAL INNOVATIONS INC**
Clinac; **VARIAN MEDICAL SYSTEMS INC**
ClinCheck; **ALIGN TECHNOLOGY**
Clinical Product Suite; **QUALITY SYSTEMS INC**
Cobalt Corp.; **WELLPOINT HEALTH NETWORKS INC**
Coblation; **ARTHROCARE CORP**
Codexis, Inc.; **MAXYGEN INC**
Codman and Shurtleff, Inc.; **DEPUY INC**
ColdBlue; **PERKINELMER INC**
Cole Managed Vision; **COLE NATIONAL CORPORATION**
Cole National Corp.; **LUXOTTICA GROUP SPA**
Cole Vision Corp.; **COLE NATIONAL CORPORATION**
Colilert-18; **IDEXX LABORATORIES INC**
Colisure; **IDEXX LABORATORIES INC**
Collamer; **STAAR SURGICAL CO**
Collezione Rathschuler; **LUXOTTICA GROUP SPA**
Col-Sur P.A.D.; **MEDTRONIC VASCULAR**
Columbia Medical, Inc.; **UTAH MEDICAL PRODUCTS INC**
Combi-12; **MOLECULAR DEVICES CORP**
Combined Benefits Management, Inc.; **BLUE CROSS AND BLUE SHIELD OF MONTANA**
Comfort; **RESMED INC**
Community Blue; **HEALTHNOW NEW YORK**
Community Health Partners; **CATHOLIC HEALTHCARE PARTNERS**

Community Mercy Health Partners; **CATHOLIC HEALTHCARE PARTNERS**
Compass Group; **MORRISON MANAGEMENT SPECIALISTS INC**
Compex Sport; **COMPEX TECHNOLOGIES INC**
Composix; **CR BARD INC**
Comprehensive Benefits Administrators; **BLUE CROSS AND BLUE SHIELD OF VERMONT**
Comprehensive Health Management of Florida; **WELLCARE GROUP OF COMPANIES**
CompScript, Inc.; **OMNICARE INC**
Computer Motion, Inc.; **INTUITIVE SURGICAL INC**
CONCENTRA Managed Care; **CONCENTRA INC**
Concentra Operating Corporation; **CONCENTRA INC**
Concorde Microsystem, Inc.; **CTI MOLECULAR IMAGING**
Conforma; **SONIC INNOVATIONS INC**
ConnectiCare Holding Company; **HEALTH INSURANCE PLAN OF GREATER NEW YORK**
Connecticut Staffing Works Corp.; **NATIONAL HOME HEALTH CARE CORP**
Connecticut Vision Correction; **OPTICARE HEALTH SYSTEMS**
Conserve Hip System; **WRIGHT MEDICAL GROUP INC**
Consolidated Benefits, Inc.; **CAPITAL BLUECROSS**
Continuum; **EXCEL TECHNOLOGY INC**
Contour Profile Moderate Plus Gel; **MENTOR CORP**
Control Laser; **EXCEL TECHNOLOGY INC**
Control Systemation, Inc.; **EXCEL TECHNOLOGY INC**
ConvaTec; **BRISTOL MYERS SQUIBB CO**
Conway Associates, Inc.; **NYER MEDICAL GROUP INC**
CooperSurgical, Inc.; **COOPER COMPANIES INC**
CooperVision, Inc.; **COOPER COMPANIES INC**
Coppertone; **SCHERING-PLOUGH CORP**
COR Therapeutics, Inc.; **MILLENNIUM PHARMACEUTICALS INC**
Coral Blood Services, Inc.; **HEMACARE CORPORATION**
Cordguard; **UTAH MEDICAL PRODUCTS INC**

INDEX OF SUBSIDIARIES, BRAND NAMES AND AFFILIATIONS, CONT.

Cordis Neurovascular, Inc.; **CORDIS CORP**
CoreCare; **CORVEL CORP**
Cornerstone Equity Investors; **TEAM HEALTH**
CORONA; **NOVOSTE CORPORATION**
Corpak MedSystems; **VIASYS HEALTHCARE INC**
Cosgrove-Edwards; **EDWARDS LIFESCIENCES CORP**
CostTrack; **OWENS & MINOR INC**
Coulter Corporation; **BECKMAN COULTER INC**
Covance Clinical Research Unit, Inc.; **COVANCE INC**
Covance Pharmaceutical Packaging Services, Inc.; **COVANCE INC**
Coventry Health and Life; **COVENTRY HEALTH CARE INC**
Coventry Health Care, Inc.; **FIRST HEALTH GROUP CORP**
Cozaar; **MERCK & CO INC**
CQI+TM Outcomes Measurement Systems; **HORIZON HEALTH CORPORATION**
Cre Lox Technology; **BRISTOL MYERS SQUIBB CO**
Crinone; **SERONO SA**
Critical Care Systems; **CURATIVE HEALTH SERVICES INC**
Crizal Alize; **ESSILOR INTERNATIONAL SA**
CROSSAIL; **GUIDANT CORP**
Crothall Services; **MORRISON MANAGEMENT SPECIALISTS INC**
Crown of Texas Hospice; **ODYSSEY HEALTHCARE INC**
Cruise Control; **STAAR SURGICAL CO**
CryoLife Europa, Ltd.; **CRYOLIFE INC**
CryoLife International, Inc.; **CRYOLIFE INC**
Crystal Health, LLC; **ALTERRA HEALTHCARE CORP**
CSL Limited; **ZLB BEHRING LLC**
CSS Informatics; **PHARMACEUTICAL PRODUCT DEVELOPMENT INC**
CT Smoothies; **E-Z-EM INC**
C-TEK Anterior Cervical Plate; **INTERPORE CROSS INTERNATIONAL**
CTI Molecular Technologies, Inc.; **CTI MOLECULAR IMAGING**
CuffPatch; **ORGANOGENESIS INC**
CuraScript; **EXPRESS SCRIPTS INC**
Customer Reporting System; **UNIPRISE INCORPORATED**
CustomLASIK; **TLC VISION CORPORATION**
CVS ProCare; **CVS CORPORATION**
CVS Realty Co.; **CVS CORPORATION**

cvs.com; **CVS CORPORATION**
CVX-300; **SPECTRANETICS CORP**
Cymetra; **LIFECELL CORPORATION**
CYPHER; **CORDIS CORP**
Cystosar-U; **AMERICAN PHARMACEUTICAL PARTNERS INC**
D.A.W., Inc.; **NYER MEDICAL GROUP INC**
D.H. Baker Dental Laboratory; **NATIONAL DENTEX CORP**
da Vinci Surgical System; **INTUITIVE SURGICAL INC**
Daig; **ST JUDE MEDICAL INC**
Dakota Smith; **SIGNATURE EYEWEAR INC**
Dana-Farber/Partners CancerCare; **PARTNERS HEALTHCARE SYSTEM**
Darvocet; **AAIPHARMA INC**
Darvon; **AAIPHARMA INC**
DataLink Data Management System; **LIFESCAN INC**
Datex-Ohmeda; **INSTRUMENTARIUM CORPORATION**
Daughters of Charity National Health System; **ASCENSION HEALTH**
Davis Medical Center; **HEALTH MANAGEMENT ASSOCIATES INC**
Davis Vision; **HIGHMARK INC**
DaVita Clinical Research, Inc.; **DAVITA INC**
DB Capital Partners, Inc.; **JENNY CRAIG INC**
DBS Holdings, Inc.; **MIV THERAPEUTICS INC**
DCA Medical Services, Inc.; **MEDICORE INC**
de'MEDICI Systems; **HEALTHSTREAM INC**
Deccox; **ALPHARMA INC**
Decision Power; **HEALTH NET INC**
Deio; **INSTRUMENTARIUM CORPORATION**
DELFIA Xpress; **PERKINELMER INC**
DeltaCare USA; **DELTA DENTAL PLANS ASSOCIATION**
DeltaPreferred Option USA; **DELTA DENTAL PLANS ASSOCIATION**
DeltaPremier USA; **DELTA DENTAL PLANS ASSOCIATION**
DeltaSelect USA/TRICARE; **DELTA DENTAL PLANS ASSOCIATION**
DeltaUSA; **DELTA DENTAL PLANS ASSOCIATION**
Deltran-Plus; **UTAH MEDICAL PRODUCTS INC**
Demand Generics; **BLUE CROSS AND BLUE SHIELD OF TENNESSEE INC**
Demetron; **SYBRON DENTAL SPECIALTIES INC**

Dental Indemnity USA; **BLUE CROSS AND BLUE SHIELD OF TEXAS**
Dental Network of America, Inc.; **HEALTH CARE SERVICE CORPORATION**
DentalBlue; **ARKANSAS BLUE CROSS AND BLUE SHIELD**
DentalBlue; **BLUE CROSS AND BLUE SHIELD OF NORTH CAROLINA**
DentalBlue; **BLUE CROSS OF IDAHO**
Dentrix Dental Systems, Inc.; **HENRY SCHEIN INC**
Depakine; **SANOFI-SYNTHELABO**
Depakote; **ABBOTT LABORATORIES**
Depend; **KIMBERLY CLARK CORP**
DePuy International; **DEPUY INC**
DePuy Orthopaedics; **DEPUY INC**
DePuy Spine, Inc.; **DEPUY INC**
DePuy Trauma & Extremities; **DEPUY INC**
Dermatix; **VALEANT PHARMACEUTICALS INTERNATIONAL**
Dermpath Diagnostics; **AMERIPATH INC**
Detach; **STERIS CORP**
DeVilbiss; **SUNRISE MEDICAL INC**
DeVos Children's Hospital; **SPECTRUM HEALTH**
Dharmacon, Inc.; **FISHER SCIENTIFIC INTERNATIONAL INC**
Diabetes Healthways; **AMERICAN HEALTHWAYS INC**
Dialysis Corporation of America; **MEDICORE INC**
DIANON Systems, Inc.; **LABORATORY CORP OF AMERICA HOLDINGS**
Dianon Systems, Inc.; **UROCOR INC**
DIAS Plus; **IMMUCOR INC**
Dictation Tracking System; **MEDQUIST INC**
Diflucan; **PFIZER INC**
DigitalDiagnost; **PHILIPS MEDICAL SYSTEMS**
Digitek; **MYLAN LABORATORIES INC**
Dimension; **PREMERA BLUE CROSS**
Dimetapp; **WYETH**
DioLite 532; **IRIDEX CORP**
Direct Dental Supply Co.; **PATTERSON COMPANIES INC**
Disetronic Injection Systems; **THERASENSE INC**
Diskus; **BESPAK PLC**
Disposa-Hood; **UTAH MEDICAL PRODUCTS INC**
Diversicare Canada Management Services Co., Inc.; **ADVOCAT INC**
DiversiCare Rehab Services; **REHABCARE GROUP INC**
D-Lish; **YOUNG INNOVATIONS INC**

INDEX OF SUBSIDIARIES, BRAND NAMES AND AFFILIATIONS, CONT.

DNAShuffling; **MAXYGEN INC**
DNAwithPap; **DIGENE CORPORATION**
DocQment Enterprise Platform; **MEDQUIST INC**
Doctor's Express; **OPTICARE HEALTH SYSTEMS**
Doctors Hospital Nelsonville; **OHIOHEALTH CORPORATION**
DonJoy; **DJ ORTHOPEDICS INC**
DoubleCheck; **INVERNESS MEDICAL INNOVATIONS INC**
Doxycycline; **AMERICAN PHARMACEUTICAL PARTNERS INC**
Dr. Scholl's; **SCHERING-PLOUGH CORP**
Dreyer Medical Clinic; **ADVOCATE HEALTH CARE**
Driver; **MEDTRONIC INC**
drugmax.com; **DRUGMAX INC**
drugmaxtrading.com; **DRUGMAX INC**
Duling Optical; **EMERGING VISION INC**
DuoDerm; **CONVATEC**
Dupel Iontophoresis System; **EMPI INC**
Duracon Total Knee System; **STRYKER CORP**
Dura-Flow Chronic Dialysis catheter; **E-Z-EM INC**
DuraGen Dural Graft Matrix; **INTEGRA LIFESCIENCES HOLDINGS CORP**
Durex; **SSL INTERNATIONAL**
Dyersburg Regional Medical Center; **COMMUNITY HEALTH SYSTEMS INC**
Dynacare, Inc.; **LABORATORY CORP OF AMERICA HOLDINGS**
Dynacord; **TELEX COMMUNICATIONS INC**
Dynacq International, Inc.; **DYNACQ HEALTHCARE INC**
DynaVox; **SUNRISE MEDICAL INC**
East Pointe Hospital; **HEALTH MANAGEMENT ASSOCIATES INC**
Easton Hospital; **COMMUNITY HEALTH SYSTEMS INC**
Eaton Apothecary; **NYER MEDICAL GROUP INC**
Ebenezer; **FAIRVIEW HEALTH SERVICES**
EBI Medical, Inc.; **INTERPORE CROSS INTERNATIONAL**
EBI, LP; **BIOMET INC**
eBioCare; **CURATIVE HEALTH SERVICES INC**
Ecabet; **AAIPHARMA INC**
Eckerd; **CVS CORPORATION**
ECLiPS; **PHARMACOPEIA INC**
eData Entry; **ERESEARCH TECHNOLOGY INC**

Eddie Bauer Eyewear; **SIGNATURE EYEWEAR INC**
Edge; **OCULAR SCIENCES INC**
EDI Midwest; **BLUE CROSS AND BLUE SHIELD OF KANSAS**
EDiX Corp.; **IDX SYSTEMS CORP**
Education Design, Inc.; **HEALTHSTREAM INC**
Effexor; **WYETH**
Efudex/Efudix; **VALEANT PHARMACEUTICALS INTERNATIONAL**
eKendleCollege; **KENDLE INTERNATIONAL INC**
EKG Enabler; **EPIC SYSTEMS CORPORATION**
Electro Medical Equipment, Ltd.; **VIASYS HEALTHCARE INC**
Electronic Benefit Administration Solutions; **UNIPRISE INCORPORATED**
Electronic Medical Records; **QUALITY SYSTEMS INC**
Electro-Optics; **COHERENT INC**
Electro-Voice; **TELEX COMMUNICATIONS INC**
eLoader 3.5; **PHARMACEUTICAL PRODUCT DEVELOPMENT INC**
Eloxatin; **SANOFI-SYNTHELABO**
eMaxx; **QUEST DIAGNOSTICS INC**
Embla 96/384; **MOLECULAR DEVICES CORP**
Emdogain; **INSTITUT STRAUMANN AG**
eMed Technologies Corporation; **CEDARA SOFTWARE CORP**
Emergency Medical Internetwork; **HEALTHSTREAM INC**
Empi, Inc.; **ENCORE MEDICAL CORPORATION**
Empire HealthChoice Assurance, Inc.; **WELLCHOICE INC**
Empire HealthChoice HMO, Inc.; **WELLCHOICE INC**
Employee Assistance Programs International, Inc.; **HORIZON HEALTH CORPORATION**
Employer Plan Services; **BLUE CROSS AND BLUE SHIELD OF WYOMING**
EMSA Military Services, Inc.; **AMERICA SERVICE GROUP INC**
EMTrack; **LOGISTICARE INC**
Enbrel; **AMGEN INC**
Encore Medical Corporation; **EMPI INC**
Endo Pharmaceuticals, Inc.; **ENDO PHARMACEUTICALS HOLDINGS INC**
Endocardial Solutions; **ST JUDE MEDICAL INC**
Endoscope Reprocessing System; **CANTEL MEDICAL CORP**

Endovascular Laser Venous System; **E-Z-EM INC**
EndoWrist; **INTUITIVE SURGICAL INC**
Enterprise Appointment Scheduling; **QUALITY SYSTEMS INC**
Enterprise EDC; **ERESEARCH TECHNOLOGY INC**
Enterprise Master Patient Index; **QUALITY SYSTEMS INC**
Enterprise Practice Management; **QUALITY SYSTEMS INC**
Enterra; **MEDTRONIC INC**
Entex LA; **ANDRX CORP**
EnVision; **PERKINELMER INC**
EpicCare; **EPIC SYSTEMS CORPORATION**
Epicor Medical, Inc.; **ST JUDE MEDICAL INC**
EpiLaser; **PALOMAR MEDICAL TECHNOLOGIES INC**
EpiPen; **MERIDIAN MEDICAL TECHNOLOGIES INC**
Epix VT; **EMPI INC**
Epogen; **AMGEN INC**
eResearch Community; **ERESEARCH TECHNOLOGY INC**
eResearch Network; **ERESEARCH TECHNOLOGY INC**
Erich Jaeger, GmbH; **VIASYS HEALTHCARE INC**
ESPrit 3G; **COCHLEAR LTD**
Essilor of America, Inc.; **ESSILOR INTERNATIONAL SA**
EsteLux; **PALOMAR MEDICAL TECHNOLOGIES INC**
Esthetica Partners, Inc.; **PALOMAR MEDICAL TECHNOLOGIES INC**
ESTORRA; **SEPRACOR INC**
Estrace; **WARNER CHILCOTT PLC**
Estrofem; **NOVO-NORDISK AS**
Estrostep; **WARNER CHILCOTT PLC**
ETHICON Products; **ETHICON INC**
Ever; **AFLAC INC**
Everest VIT; **WELCH ALLYN INC**
EVI; **TELEX COMMUNICATIONS INC**
Evidence Based Medicine; **HEALTH NET INC**
Evolis; **BIO RAD LABORATORIES INC**
eWebIT; **ECLIPSYS CORPORATION**
EXACT; **ANALOGIC CORP**
ExamOne; **LABONE INC**
Excedrin; **BRISTOL MYERS SQUIBB CO**
EX-CYTE; **SEROLOGICALS CORP**
Experient Technologies, Inc.; **VENTIV HEALTH INC**
EXPeRT; **ERESEARCH TECHNOLOGY INC**

INDEX OF SUBSIDIARIES, BRAND NAMES AND AFFILIATIONS, CONT.

eXplore Optix; **ART ADVANCED RESEARCH TECHNOLOGIES**
Extended FAMILI; **SPECTRANETICS CORP**
Extendicare Health Services, Inc.; **EXTENDICARE INC**
Eye Care for a Lifetime; **OPTICARE HEALTH SYSTEMS**
EyeMed Vision Care, LLC; **LUXOTTICA GROUP SPA**
EZBrace; **ORTHOFIX INTERNATIONAL NV**
F. Hoffmann-La Roche, Ltd.; **ROCHE GROUP**
Fabrazyme; **GENZYME CORP**
Facet Technologies, Inc.; **MATRIA HEALTHCARE INC**
Fact Plus; **INVERNESS MEDICAL INNOVATIONS INC**
Failed Reactions Database; **PHARMACOPEIA INC**
Fairview Foundation; **FAIRVIEW HEALTH SERVICES**
Fairview Hand Center; **FAIRVIEW HEALTH SERVICES**
Fairview Press; **FAIRVIEW HEALTH SERVICES**
Fairview-University Medical Center; **FAIRVIEW HEALTH SERVICES**
Familymeds Group, Inc.; **DRUGMAX INC**
Faulkner Hospital; **PARTNERS HEALTHCARE SYSTEM**
Fax And Scan Today (FAST); **HOOPER HOLMES INC**
FCG Management Services, LLC; **FIRST CONSULTING GROUP INC**
FeatherTouch; **MEDTRONIC XOMED SURGICAL PRODUCTS INC**
Femhrt; **WARNER CHILCOTT PLC**
Femring; **WARNER CHILCOTT PLC**
femScript; **ADVANCEPCS INC**
Ferrlecit; **WATSON PHARMACEUTICALS INC**
FertilityMarKit; **INTEGRAMED AMERICA INC**
FertilityPartners; **INTEGRAMED AMERICA INC**
FertilityWeb; **INTEGRAMED AMERICA INC**
Festival; **YOUNG INNOVATIONS INC**
FFI Health Services; **ADVANCEPCS INC**
FiberChoice; **CNS INC**
Filtek; **3M COMPANY**
FineTech; **PAR PHARMACEUTICAL COMPANIES INC**
Finn Knee Replacement System; **BIOMET INC**
Finn-Aqua; **STERIS CORP**
Fioricet; **WATSON PHARMACEUTICALS INC**
Fiorinal; **WATSON PHARMACEUTICALS INC**
First Coast Service Options, Inc.; **BLUE CROSS AND BLUE SHIELD OF FLORIDA**
First Health Group; **COVENTRY HEALTH CARE INC**
First Health Network; **FIRST HEALTH GROUP CORP**
First Seniority; **HARVARD PILGRIM HEALTH CARE INC**
FirstStep; **KINETIC CONCEPTS INC**
Fisher Clinical Services, Inc.; **FISHER SCIENTIFIC INTERNATIONAL INC**
Fisher Hamilton; **FISHER SCIENTIFIC INTERNATIONAL INC**
Fisher HealthCare; **FISHER SCIENTIFIC INTERNATIONAL INC**
Fisher Research; **FISHER SCIENTIFIC INTERNATIONAL INC**
Fisher Science Education; **FISHER SCIENTIFIC INTERNATIONAL INC**
Fisher Scientific International, Inc.; **APOGENT TECHNOLOGIES INC**
FlashDose; **BIOVAIL CORPORATION**
FLAVORx; **RITE AID CORPORATION**
Flexicair Eclipse; **HILL-ROM COMPANY INC**
FlexPlus; **BLUE CROSS AND BLUE SHIELD OF GEORGIA INC**
FlexTip Plus; **ARROW INTERNATIONAL INC**
FLIPR; **MOLECULAR DEVICES CORP**
Flomax; **ABBOTT LABORATORIES**
Florida Combined Life Insurance Company, Inc.; **BLUE CROSS AND BLUE SHIELD OF FLORIDA**
Florida Hospital; **ADVENTIST HEALTH SYSTEM**
Flouroscan; **HOLOGIC INC**
Flovent; **GLAXOSMITHKLINE PLC**
Flowcast; **IDX SYSTEMS CORP**
Fluad; **CHIRON CORP**
Fludara; **SCHERING AG**
Fluoxetine; **EON LABS INC**
FocalPoint SlideProfiler; **TRIPATH IMAGING INC**
FOCUS; **OWENS & MINOR INC**
Fogarty; **EDWARDS LIFESCIENCES CORP**
Forethought Federal Savings Bank; **HILLENBRAND INDUSTRIES**
Forethought Financial Services; **HILLENBRAND INDUSTRIES**
Forethought Group, Inc. (The); **HILLENBRAND INDUSTRIES**
Forethought Life Insurance Company; **HILLENBRAND INDUSTRIES**
Fort Bend Hospital; **MEMORIAL HERMANN HEALTHCARE SYSTEM**
Fort Dearborn Life Insurance Company; **HEALTH CARE SERVICE CORPORATION**
FortaFlex; **ORGANOGENESIS INC**
FortaGen; **ORGANOGENESIS INC**
Fortamet; **ANDRX CORP**
FortaPerm; **ORGANOGENESIS INC**
Fortis Benefits Insurance Co.; **ASSURANT HEALTH**
Fortis Benefits Insurance Company; **ASSURANT EMPLOYEE BENEFITS**
Fortis Health; **ASSURANT HEALTH**
Fortis Insurance Co.; **ASSURANT HEALTH**
Fortis, Inc.; **ASSURANT INC**
Fosamax; **MERCK & CO INC**
Franciscan Health System; **CATHOLIC HEALTH INITIATIVES**
Franciscan Sisters of Mary; **SSM HEALTH CARE SYSTEM INC**
Frankford Hospitals; **JEFFERSON HEALTH SYSTEM INC**
Franklin Square Hospital Center; **MEDSTAR HEALTH**
Freedom; **OXFORD HEALTH PLANS INC**
Freedom Home Health; **AMEDISYS INC**
FreeStyle; **THERASENSE INC**
FreeStyle Flash; **THERASENSE INC**
FreeStyle Tracker; **THERASENSE INC**
Fresenius Biotech; **FRESENIUS AG**
Fresenius Biotech; **FRESENIUS AG**
Fresenius Health Care Group; **FRESENIUS AG**
Fresenius Kabi; **FRESENIUS AG**
Fresenius Medical Care AG; **FRESENIUS AG**
Fresenius Netcare; **FRESENIUS AG**
Fresenius ProServe; **FRESENIUS AG**
Fujisawa GmbH; **FUJISAWA PHARMACEUTICALS COMPANY LTD**
Fujisawa Healthcare, Inc.; **FUJISAWA PHARMACEUTICALS COMPANY LTD**
GABRITRIL; **CEPHALON INC**
Galen Holdings; **WARNER CHILCOTT PLC**
Galesburg Cottage Hospital; **COMMUNITY HEALTH SYSTEMS INC**
Galileo; **IMMUCOR INC**
Gambro BCT; **GAMBRO AB**
Gambro Healthcare Laboratory Services, Inc.; **GAMBRO AB**
Gambro Healthcare, Inc.; **GAMBRO AB**
Gambro Renal Products; **GAMBRO AB**
Gambro, Inc.; **GAMBRO AB**
Gamma Locking Nail System; **STRYKER CORP**
Gammex; **ANSELL LIMITED COMPANY**

INDEX OF SUBSIDIARIES, BRAND NAMES AND AFFILIATIONS, CONT.

Gatekeeper Reflux Repair System; **MEDTRONIC INC**
Gateway Regional Medical Center; **COMMUNITY HEALTH SYSTEMS INC**
GCG Wisconsin Package; **PHARMACOPEIA INC**
GDX System; **CHOLESTECH CORP**
GE Aviation Services; **GE COMMERCIAL FINANCE**
GE Commercial Equipment Financing; **GE COMMERCIAL FINANCE**
GE Corporate Financial Services; **GE COMMERCIAL FINANCE**
GE Electric Co.; **GE HEALTHCARE**
GE European Equipment Finance; **GE COMMERCIAL FINANCE**
GE Healthcare Bio-Sciences; **GE HEALTHCARE**
GE Healthcare Financial Services; **GE COMMERCIAL FINANCE**
GE Healthcare Information Technologies; **GE HEALTHCARE**
GE Healthcare Technologies; **GE HEALTHCARE**
GE Medical Systems; **INSTRUMENTARIUM CORPORATION**
GE Real Estate; **GE COMMERCIAL FINANCE**
GE Vendor Financial Services; **GE COMMERCIAL FINANCE**
Gemini; **MOLECULAR DEVICES CORP**
Genentech; **ROCHE GROUP**
General Electric Co.; **GE COMMERCIAL FINANCE**
Genesis; **MATRIA HEALTHCARE INC**
Genesis Health Ventures, Inc.; **NEIGHBORCARE INC**
GENESIS II; **SMITH & NEPHEW PLC**
Genevac, Ltd.; **APOGENT TECHNOLOGIES INC**
GenomeLab SNPstream Genotyping System; **BECKMAN COULTER INC**
Gentamicin; **AMERICAN PHARMACEUTICAL PARTNERS INC**
Gentiva Business Services; **GENTIVA HEALTH SERVICES INC**
Gentiva Orthopedic Services; **GENTIVA HEALTH SERVICES INC**
GentleLASE; **CANDELA CORP**
GentleYAG; **CANDELA CORP**
Genyx Medical, Inc.; **CR BARD INC**
Genzyme Biosurgery; **GENZYME CORP**
Genzyme Genetics; **IMPATH INC**
Genzyme Molecular Oncology; **GENZYME CORP**

Genzyme Transgenics Corp.; **GTC BIOTHERAPEUTICS INC**
GEO Structure; **INTERPORE CROSS INTERNATIONAL**
Geo-Matt; **SPAN AMERICA MEDICAL SYSTEMS INC**
Georgetown University Hospital; **MEDSTAR HEALTH**
Gesco; **UTAH MEDICAL PRODUCTS INC**
GHI HMO; **GROUP HEALTH INCORPORATED**
GHS General Insurance Agency; **BLUE CROSS AND BLUE SHIELD OF OKLAHOMA**
GHS Holding Company, Inc.; **BLUE CROSS AND BLUE SHIELD OF OKLAHOMA**
GHS Property and Casualty Insurance Company; **BLUE CROSS AND BLUE SHIELD OF OKLAHOMA**
GI Monitor; **BECKMAN COULTER INC**
Ginzton Technology Center; **VARIAN MEDICAL SYSTEMS INC**
Giraffe OmniBed; **GE HEALTHCARE**
Gish Biocompatible Surfaces Coating; **GISH BIOMEDICAL INC**
GK Financing, LLC; **AMERICAN SHARED HOSPITAL SERVICES**
GNC Corporation; **GENERAL NUTRITION COMPANIES INC**
GNC Live Well; **GENERAL NUTRITION COMPANIES INC**
Golden West Vision and Dental; **WELLPOINT HEALTH NETWORKS INC**
GONAL-f; **SERONO SA**
Good Samaritan Health Systems; **CATHOLIC HEALTH INITIATIVES**
Good Samaritan Hospital; **MEDSTAR HEALTH**
Graft Jacket; **LIFECELL CORPORATION**
Grafton Demineralized Bone Matrix; **OSTEOTECH INC**
Grand Laboratories, Inc.; **NOVARTIS AG**
Grant Medical Center; **OHIOHEALTH CORPORATION**
Grason-Stadler, Inc.; **VIASYS HEALTHCARE INC**
Great Escapes Travel Program; **APRIA HEALTHCARE GROUP INC**
Greater Georgia Life Insurance Company, Inc.; **BLUE CROSS AND BLUE SHIELD OF GEORGIA INC**
GreenLight; **LASERSCOPE**
Group Benefits of Georgia, Inc.; **BLUE CROSS AND BLUE SHIELD OF GEORGIA INC**

Group Health Community Foundation; **GROUP HEALTH COOPERATIVE OF PUGET SOUND**
Group Health Options, Inc.; **GROUP HEALTH COOPERATIVE OF PUGET SOUND**
Group Health Permanente; **GROUP HEALTH COOPERATIVE OF PUGET SOUND**
Group Heatlh Center for Health Studies; **GROUP HEALTH COOPERATIVE OF PUGET SOUND**
Group Hospitalization and Medical Services, Inc.; **CAREFIRST INC**
Group Insurance Services, Inc.; **BLUE CROSS AND BLUE SHIELD OF NORTH CAROLINA**
Group Practice Affiliates, LLC; **CENTENE CORPORATION**
Groupcast; **IDX SYSTEMS CORP**
GroupMedChoice; **AMERICAN MEDICAL SECURITY GROUP INC**
Guardian Continuous Glucose Monitor System; **MEDTRONIC MINIMED INC**
GuardiaNet Systems, Inc.; **3M COMPANY**
GuardWire Plus; **MEDTRONIC VASCULAR**
Gulf South Medical Supply, Inc.; **PSS WORLD MEDICAL INC**
GYNECARE; **ETHICON INC**
Gyrus International, Ltd.; **GYRUS GROUP**
Gyrus North America Sales, Inc.; **GYRUS GROUP**
Hager Dental GmbH; **HENRY SCHEIN INC**
Halkey-Roberts Corp.; **ATRION CORPORATION**
Hall Surgical; **CONMED CORP**
Hanger Prosthetics & Orthotics, Inc.; **HANGER ORTHOPEDIC GROUP INC**
Hardin Memorial Hospital; **OHIOHEALTH CORPORATION**
Harlem Hospital Center; **NEW YORK CITY HEALTH AND HOSPITALS CORPORATION**
HARMONIC SCALPEL; **ETHICON INC**
Harper University Hospital; **DETROIT MEDICAL CENTER**
Harris Methodist Health System; **TEXAS HEALTH RESOURCES**
Hart Schaffner & Marx Eyewear; **SIGNATURE EYEWEAR INC**
Harvard Medical School; **PARTNERS HEALTHCARE SYSTEM**
Harvard Pilgrim Health Care of New England; **HARVARD PILGRIM HEALTH CARE INC**

INDEX OF SUBSIDIARIES, BRAND NAMES AND AFFILIATIONS, CONT.

Hawe; **SYBRON DENTAL SPECIALTIES INC**
HCR Manor Care; **MANOR CARE INC**
HCR Manor Care Foundation; **MANOR CARE INC**
Health Acquisition Corp.; **NATIONAL HOME HEALTH CARE CORP**
Health Advantage; **ARKANSAS BLUE CROSS AND BLUE SHIELD**
Health Alliance Plan of Michigan; **HENRY FORD HEALTH SYSTEMS**
Health Care Service Corporation; **BLUE CROSS AND BLUE SHIELD OF TEXAS**
Health e-Blue; **BLUE CARE NETWORK OF MICHIGAN**
Health Enhancement; **MATRIA HEALTHCARE INC**
Health Information Network, Inc. (The); **HEALTH CARE SERVICE CORPORATION**
Health Net Dental, Inc.; **SAFEGUARD HEALTH ENTERPRISES INC**
Health Net Vision, Inc.; **SAFEGUARD HEALTH ENTERPRISES INC**
Health Options, Inc.; **BLUE CROSS AND BLUE SHIELD OF FLORIDA**
Health Plan of Nevada, Inc.; **SIERRA HEALTH SERVICES INC**
Health Products Research, Inc.; **VENTIV HEALTH INC**
HealthAmerica; **COVENTRY HEALTH CARE INC**
HealthAssurance; **COVENTRY HEALTH CARE INC**
Healthcare Learning Center; **HEALTHSTREAM INC**
Healthcare Staffing Solutions, Inc.; **REHABCARE GROUP INC**
HealthCare USA; **COVENTRY HEALTH CARE INC**
Healthdyne Technologies; **MATRIA HEALTHCARE INC**
HealthEase of Florida, Inc.; **WELLCARE GROUP OF COMPANIES**
HealthLink, Inc.; **WELLPOINT HEALTH NETWORKS INC**
HealthNow; **HEALTHNOW NEW YORK**
HealthPlan Services; **PLANVISTA CORP**
HealthReach PPO; **OHIOHEALTH CORPORATION**
HealthViewPlus; **SOLUCIENT LLC**
Healthy Extensions; **BLUE CROSS AND BLUE SHIELD OF GEORGIA INC**
Healthy Families Program; **BLUE CROSS OF CALIFORNIA**
Healthy First Steps; **AMERICHOICE CORPORATION**
Heartland; **MANOR CARE INC**

Heartpoint, Inc.; **ETHICON INC**
HEARx; **HEARUSA INC**
Heathwise Knowledgebase; **BLUE CROSS AND BLUE SHIELD OF VERMONT**
Helixate FS; **ZLB BEHRING LLC**
Hematronix, Inc.; **BIO RAD LABORATORIES INC**
Hemed; **GISH BIOMEDICAL INC**
Hemophilia Health Services, Inc.; **ACCREDO HEALTH INC**
Hemophilia Resources of America, Inc.; **ACCREDO HEALTH INC**
Henry Ford Heart and Vascular Institute; **HENRY FORD HEALTH SYSTEMS**
Henry Ford Hospital; **HENRY FORD HEALTH SYSTEMS**
Henry Ford Wyandotte Hospital; **HENRY FORD HEALTH SYSTEMS**
HEPTIMAX; **QUEST DIAGNOSTICS INC**
Herceptin; **GENENTECH INC**
Herceptin; **ROCHE GROUP**
HerdCheck; **IDEXX LABORATORIES INC**
Heritage Labs; **HOOPER HOLMES INC**
Heritage Labs; **HOOPER HOLMES INC**
HERMES; **INTUITIVE SURGICAL INC**
Heska Corp.; **I-STAT CORP**
HFC Assessment Services; **HEALTH FITNESS CORP**
HFC Fitness Programs; **HEALTH FITNESS CORP**
HFC Treatment Services; **HEALTH FITNESS CORP**
HFC Wellness Programs; **HEALTH FITNESS CORP**
HGSAdministrators; **HIGHMARK INC**
HHC Health and Home Care; **NEW YORK CITY HEALTH AND HOSPITALS CORPORATION**
HHP; **WELCH ALLYN INC**
Highly Maneuverable Vehicle; **INVACARE CORP**
Highmark Life and Casualty Group (The); **HIGHMARK INC**
Highpoint Healthcare Distribution; **PSS WORLD MEDICAL INC**
Hillenbrand Industries; **HILL-ROM COMPANY INC**
Hill-Rom, Inc.; **HILLENBRAND INDUSTRIES**
HIP Integrative Wellness; **HEALTH INSURANCE PLAN OF GREATER NEW YORK**
HiResolution Bionic Ear System; **ADVANCED BIONICS CORPORATION**

HMO Blue; **BLUE CROSS AND BLUE SHIELD OF MASSACHUSETTS**
HMO Blue New England; **BLUE CROSS AND BLUE SHIELD OF MASSACHUSETTS**
HMO Blue Texas; **BLUE CROSS AND BLUE SHIELD OF TEXAS**
HMO Louisiana, Inc.; **BLUE CROSS AND BLUE SHIELD OF LOUISIANA**
HMOBlue; **BLUE CROSS OF IDAHO**
HMS Holdings Corp.; **HEALTH MANAGEMENT SYSTEMS INC**
Home Care Bed; **INVACARE CORP**
HomeCall, Inc.; **MID ATLANTIC MEDICAL SERVICES INC**
HomeReach; **OHIOHEALTH CORPORATION**
Horizon Behavioral Services, Inc.; **HORIZON HEALTH CORPORATION**
Horizon Casualty Services, Inc.; **HORIZON BLUE CROSS BLUE SHIELD OF NEW JERSEY**
Horizon Healthcare Dental, Inc.; **HORIZON BLUE CROSS BLUE SHIELD OF NEW JERSEY**
Horizon Healthcare Insurance Agency, Inc.; **HORIZON BLUE CROSS BLUE SHIELD OF NEW JERSEY**
Horizon Healthcare Insurance Company of New York; **HORIZON BLUE CROSS BLUE SHIELD OF NEW JERSEY**
Horizon HMO; **HORIZON BLUE CROSS BLUE SHIELD OF NEW JERSEY**
Horizon Medical Products, Inc.; **RITA MEDICAL SYSTEMS INC**
Horizon Mental Health Management, Inc.; **HORIZON HEALTH CORPORATION**
Horizon NJ Health; **HORIZON BLUE CROSS BLUE SHIELD OF NEW JERSEY**
Hornell International; **3M COMPANY**
Hospal; **GAMBRO AB**
Hospira; **ABBOTT LABORATORIES**
Hospital Comparison Report; **HEALTH NET INC**
Houston Health Hour Radio Show; **MEMORIAL HERMANN HEALTHCARE SYSTEM**
HPHC Insurance Company; **HARVARD PILGRIM HEALTH CARE INC**
HPHConnect; **HARVARD PILGRIM HEALTH CARE INC**
HRA Holding Corporation; **ACCREDO HEALTH INC**
Huggies; **KIMBERLY CLARK CORP**
HumanaOne; **HUMANA INC**
Humate-P; **ZLB BEHRING LLC**

INDEX OF SUBSIDIARIES, BRAND NAMES AND AFFILIATIONS, CONT.

Humility of Mary Health Partners; **CATHOLIC HEALTHCARE PARTNERS**
Huron Valley-Sinai Hospital; **DETROIT MEDICAL CENTER**
Hutzel Hospital; **DETROIT MEDICAL CENTER**
Hybrid Capture 2; **DIGENE CORPORATION**
Hybrid Capture Gene Analysis System; **DIGENE CORPORATION**
HydroBrader; **MEDTRONIC XOMED SURGICAL PRODUCTS INC**
HydroFlex; **CR BARD INC**
Hydrogenics; **OCULAR SCIENCES INC**
Hydron; **OCULAR SCIENCES INC**
Hylaform Plus; **INAMED CORP**
Hypak; **BECTON DICKINSON & CO**
IDXtend for the Web; **IDX SYSTEMS CORP**
iE33 Intelligent Echocardiography System; **PHILIPS MEDICAL SYSTEMS**
iECHO; **AMERISOURCEBERGEN CORP**
Ifosfamide; **AMERICAN PHARMACEUTICAL PARTNERS INC**
IGC-Medical Advances, Inc.; **INTERMAGNETICS GENERAL CORP**
IGC-Polycold Systems, Inc.; **INTERMAGNETICS GENERAL CORP**
IHC Health Plans; **INTERMOUNTAIN HEALTH CARE**
IHC HomeCare; **INTERMOUNTAIN HEALTH CARE**
IHC Physician Group; **INTERMOUNTAIN HEALTH CARE**
IHC/AmeriNet; **INTERMOUNTAIN HEALTH CARE**
ILEX Oncology, Inc.; **GENZYME CORP**
Illomedin; **SCHERING AG**
Image Control System; **QUALITY SYSTEMS INC**
Imagecast; **IDX SYSTEMS CORP**
Imaging Choice Consortium; **CTI MOLECULAR IMAGING**
ImmTech Biologics, Inc.; **NOVARTIS AG**
IMMULITE; **DIAGNOSTIC PRODUCTS CORPORATION**
IMMULITE 1000; **DIAGNOSTIC PRODUCTS CORPORATION**
IMMULITE 2000; **DIAGNOSTIC PRODUCTS CORPORATION**
IMMULITE Turbo; **DIAGNOSTIC PRODUCTS CORPORATION**
Immunex Corp.; **AMGEN INC**

ImmunoCAP; **QUEST DIAGNOSTICS INC**
Impavido; **AETERNA ZENTARIS INC**
Implex Corp.; **ZIMMER HOLDINGS INC**
Impressive Staffing Corp.; **NATIONAL HOME HEALTH CARE CORP**
IMS Inpatient Therapy Profiler; **IMS HEALTH INC**
IMS Knowledge Link 2; **IMS HEALTH INC**
INAMED Aesthetics; **INAMED CORP**
INAMED Health; **INAMED CORP**
INAMED International; **INAMED CORP**
Incepture, Inc.; **BLUE CROSS AND BLUE SHIELD OF FLORIDA**
Incyte Genomics; **INCYTE CORP**
Indiana University Hospital; **CLARIAN HEALTH PARTNERS INC**
InDuo; **LIFESCAN INC**
Infasurf; **FOREST LABORATORIES INC**
INFeD; **WATSON PHARMACEUTICALS INC**
Infolink; **HOOPER HOLMES INC**
INFUSE Bone Graft; **MEDTRONIC SOFAMOR DANEK**
InfuSystem, Inc.; **I FLOW CORPORATION**
ING Groep N.V.; **AETNA INC**
Ingenix; **UNITEDHEALTH GROUP INC**
Ingenuity EMR; **VITALWORKS INC**
Inhale Therapeutic Systems, Inc.; **NEKTAR THERAPEUTICS**
InnoCentive, LLC; **ELI LILLY & CO**
Innosense Minnova; **EMPI INC**
Innova; **GE HEALTHCARE**
Innova LifeSciences Corporation; **SYBRON DENTAL SPECIALTIES INC**
Innovative Neurotronics, Inc.; **HANGER ORTHOPEDIC GROUP INC**
Innovex; **QUINTILES TRANSNATIONAL CORP**
InpatientView; **SOLUCIENT LLC**
Insight Managed Vision Care; **EMERGING VISION INC**
Insignia; **HANGER ORTHOPEDIC GROUP INC**
InSite; **INTUITIVE SURGICAL INC**
InstaTrak; **GE HEALTHCARE**
Institute for Athletic Medicine; **FAIRVIEW HEALTH SERVICES**
Insurer Physicians Services Organization, Inc.; **HIGHMARK INC**
INTEGRA Bilayer Matrix Wound Dressing; **INTEGRA LIFESCIENCES HOLDINGS CORP**

INTEGRA Dermal Regeneration Template; **INTEGRA LIFESCIENCES HOLDINGS CORP**
Integra NeuroSciences; **INTEGRA LIFESCIENCES HOLDINGS CORP**
Integra Plastic and Reconstructive Surgery; **INTEGRA LIFESCIENCES HOLDINGS CORP**
Integrail, Inc.; **NATIONAL MEDICAL HEALTH CARD SYSTEMS INC**
IntegraMed Financial Services; **INTEGRAMED AMERICA INC**
IntegraMed Pharmaceutical Services, Inc.; **INTEGRAMED AMERICA INC**
Integrated Medical Systems, Inc.; **ELI LILLY & CO**
Integrilin; **MILLENNIUM PHARMACEUTICALS INC**
Integris Allura; **PHILIPS MEDICAL SYSTEMS**
Integrity Healthcare Services; **PRIORITY HEALTHCARE CORP**
intelihealth.com; **AETNA INC**
Intense Pulsed Light; **LUMENIS LTD**
Intercom Plus; **WALGREEN CO**
Intergen Company; **SEROLOGICALS CORP**
Intergy; **WEBMD CORPORATION**
International Outreach Program; **ST JUDE CHILDRENS RESEARCH HOSPITAL**
International Remote Imaging Systems, Inc.; **IRIS INTERNATIONAL INC**
International Technidyne Corp.; **THORATEC CORPORATION**
Interpore International; **BIOMET INC**
InterVascular, Inc.; **DATASCOPE CORP**
Intraject; **ARADIGM CORPORATION**
Intran Plus; **UTAH MEDICAL PRODUCTS INC**
Intuition; **SIGNATURE EYEWEAR INC**
Investors Guaranty Life Insurance Company; **OXFORD HEALTH PLANS INC**
Invisalign; **ALIGN TECHNOLOGY**
Iosorb; **MICROTEK MEDICAL HOLDINGS INC**
iPlan; **UNIPRISE INCORPORATED**
IQ Guide Wire; **BOSTON SCIENTIFIC CORP**
iQ200 Automated Urine Microscopy Analyzer; **IRIS INTERNATIONAL INC**
IRIS Medical IQ 810; **IRIDEX CORP**
Irvine Biomedical, Inc.; **ST JUDE MEDICAL INC**
IsoSeed; **THERAGENICS CORP**
i-STAT Canada, Ltd.; **I-STAT CORP**
i-STAT System; **I-STAT CORP**
I-TRAC Plus; **IMMUCOR INC**

INDEX OF SUBSIDIARIES, BRAND NAMES AND AFFILIATIONS, CONT.

Ivpcare, Inc.; **INTEGRAMED AMERICA INC**
James Whitcomb Riley Museum Home; **CLARIAN HEALTH PARTNERS INC**
JARIT Surgical Instruments, Inc.; **INTEGRA LIFESCIENCES HOLDINGS CORP**
Jefferson HealthCARE; **JEFFERSON HEALTH SYSTEM INC**
Jefferson Radiation Oncology; **JEFFERSON HEALTH SYSTEM INC**
John Alden Life Insurance Co.; **ASSURANT HEALTH**
Johns Hopkins Bayview Medical Center; **JOHNS HOPKINS MEDICINE**
Johns Hopkins Health System; **JOHNS HOPKINS MEDICINE**
Johns Hopkins HealthCare; **JOHNS HOPKINS MEDICINE**
Johns Hopkins Hospital and Outpatient Center; **JOHNS HOPKINS MEDICINE**
Johns Hopkins University School of Medicine; **JOHNS HOPKINS MEDICINE**
Johnson & Johnson; **CORDIS CORP**
Johnson & Johnson; **DEPUY INC**
Johnson & Johnson; **ETHICON INC**
Johnson & Johnson; **LIFESCAN INC**
Johnson & Johnson Wound Management; **ETHICON INC**
Kadian; **ALPHARMA INC**
Kaiser Foundation Health Plans; **KAISER PERMANENTE**
Kaiser Foundation Hospitals; **KAISER PERMANENTE**
Kali Laboratories, Inc.; **PAR PHARMACEUTICAL COMPANIES INC**
Katy Hospital; **MEMORIAL HERMANN HEALTHCARE SYSTEM**
KD Innovation; **DJ ORTHOPEDICS INC**
Kendall; **TYCO HEALTHCARE GROUP**
Kent Community Campus; **SPECTRUM HEALTH**
Kerr; **SYBRON DENTAL SPECIALTIES INC**
Ketek; **AVENTIS SA**
Keystone Health Plan Central; **CAPITAL BLUECROSS**
Killer Loop; **LUXOTTICA GROUP SPA**
KinAir; **KINETIC CONCEPTS INC**
Kinerase; **VALEANT PHARMACEUTICALS INTERNATIONAL**
Kineret; **AMGEN INC**
King Pharmaceuticals; **MERIDIAN MEDICAL TECHNOLOGIES INC**
King Pharmaceuticals; **MYLAN LABORATORIES INC**
Kingsworth Hospital; **HENRY FORD HEALTH SYSTEMS**
Klark-Teknik; **TELEX COMMUNICATIONS INC**
Kleenex; **KIMBERLY CLARK CORP**
Kliogest; **NOVO-NORDISK AS**
Kotex; **KIMBERLY CLARK CORP**
Kresge Eye Institute; **DETROIT MEDICAL CENTER**
KRG Capital Partners; **CIVCO MEDICAL INSTRUMENTS**
KTP/532; **LASERSCOPE**
KyphOs; **KYPHON INC**
KyphX; **KYPHON INC**
KyphX HV-R; **KYPHON INC**
Lab-Line Instruments, Inc.; **APOGENT TECHNOLOGIES INC**
LabLink; **COVANCE INC**
LACI; **SPECTRANETICS CORP**
Lady Lite; **MEDICORE INC**
Lakeland Protective Wear, Inc.; **LAKELAND INDUSTRIES INC**
Lambda Physik; **COHERENT INC**
Lanoxin; **GLAXOSMITHKLINE PLC**
LANXESS; **BAYER AG**
LANXESS Corp.; **BAYER CORP**
Laser Vision Centers, Inc.; **TLC VISION CORPORATION**
LasikPlus; **LCA VISION INC**
Laura Ashley Eyewear; **SIGNATURE EYEWEAR INC**
Laurel Lake Retirement Community; **CATHOLIC HEALTHCARE PARTNERS**
LDX Analyzer; **CHOLESTECH CORP**
LDX System; **CHOLESTECH CORP**
LeadQuest; **TRIPOS INC**
Lee County Community Hospital; **HEALTH MANAGEMENT ASSOCIATES INC**
LensCrafters; **LUXOTTICA GROUP SPA**
LENSender Direct Lens Delivery; **BAUSCH & LOMB INC**
Lexapro; **FOREST LABORATORIES INC**
Liberty; **OXFORD HEALTH PLANS INC**
Liberty Diabetes; **POLYMEDICA CORPORATION**
Liberty Respiratory; **POLYMEDICA CORPORATION**
Lidoderm; **ENDO PHARMACEUTICALS HOLDINGS INC**
Life Care; **SENTARA HEALTHCARE**
Life Care at Home; **LIFE CARE CENTERS OF AMERICA**
LIFELINE; **LIFELINE SYSTEMS INC**
LifeManagement; **MAGELLAN HEALTH SERVICES INC**
Lifepath AAA; **EDWARDS LIFESCIENCES CORP**
Lifepoint Hospitals, Inc.; **PROVINCE HEALTHCARE CO**
Lifescape; **SIGNATURE EYEWEAR INC**
LifeStyles; **ANSELL LIMITED COMPANY**
LightSheer; **LUMENIS LTD**
LightSheer; **PALOMAR MEDICAL TECHNOLOGIES INC**
Lindig Men's Health Center and Resource Library; **MEMORIAL HERMANN HEALTHCARE SYSTEM**
Link S.T.A.R.; **EXACTECH INC**
Linkia; **HANGER ORTHOPEDIC GROUP INC**
Linux Global Partners, Inc.; **MEDICORE INC**
Linvatec Corporation; **CONMED CORP**
Lippincott & Marguiles; **MARSH & MCLENNAN COMPANIES INC**
Lite Touch; **MEDICORE INC**
LITHIUM; **TRIPOS INC**
Little Company of Mary; **PROVIDENCE HEALTH SYSTEM**
Little Company of Mary Hospital; **PROVIDENCE HEALTH SYSTEM**
Little Ones; **CONVATEC**
Lobaplatin; **AETERNA ZENTARIS INC**
Loestrin; **WARNER CHILCOTT PLC**
LORAD; **HOLOGIC INC**
Louisville Bedding Products, Inc.; **SPAN AMERICA MEDICAL SYSTEMS INC**
Lovenox; **AVENTIS SA**
LSO; **CTI MOLECULAR IMAGING**
LSO HI-REZ Reveal PET/CT; **CTI MOLECULAR IMAGING**
LTL; **ESSILOR INTERNATIONAL SA**
LTS-Plus; **MICROTEK MEDICAL HOLDINGS INC**
Ludlow Tape; **TYCO HEALTHCARE GROUP**
Lumigan; **ALLERGAN INC**
Lumin; **UTAH MEDICAL PRODUCTS INC**
Luveris; **SERONO SA**
Luxottica Group SpA; **COLE NATIONAL CORPORATION**
LymphoStat-B; **HUMAN GENOME SCIENCES INC**
Lyovac; **STERIS CORP**
Lyra; **LASERSCOPE**
Lyra XP; **LASERSCOPE**
M.D. IPA Surgicenter, Inc.; **MID ATLANTIC MEDICAL SERVICES INC**
M/DN; **ZIMMER HOLDINGS INC**
Madison Dearborn Capital Partners; **TEAM HEALTH**

INDEX OF SUBSIDIARIES, BRAND NAMES AND AFFILIATIONS, CONT.

Magee Rehabilitation; **JEFFERSON HEALTH SYSTEM INC**
Magellan Behavioral Health; **MAGELLAN HEALTH SERVICES INC**
Magellan Behavioral Health; **BLUE CROSS AND BLUE SHIELD OF TEXAS**
Magellan Behavioral Health; **HORIZON BLUE CROSS BLUE SHIELD OF NEW JERSEY**
magellanassist.com; **MAGELLAN HEALTH SERVICES INC**
magellanprovider.com; **MAGELLAN HEALTH SERVICES INC**
Magnaflow; **ARROW INTERNATIONAL INC**
Main Line Health; **JEFFERSON HEALTH SYSTEM INC**
Mallinckodt; **TYCO HEALTHCARE GROUP**
Mallinckordt Imaging; **MALLINCKRODT INC**
Mallinckordt Respiratory; **MALLINCKRODT INC**
Mallinckrodt Pharmaceuticals; **MALLINCKRODT INC**
MammoTest; **FISCHER IMAGING CORP**
MAMSI Life and Health Insurance Company; **MID ATLANTIC MEDICAL SERVICES INC**
Managed Care Server; **QUALITY SYSTEMS INC**
Management by Information, Inc.; **OPTION CARE INC**
ManorCare; **MANOR CARE INC**
Mar Cor Services; **CANTEL MEDICAL CORP**
Marconi Medical Systems; **PHILIPS MEDICAL SYSTEMS**
Mark I Nerve Agent Antidote Kit; **MERIDIAN MEDICAL TECHNOLOGIES INC**
Market Planner Plus (The); **SOLUCIENT LLC**
Marketplace@Novation; **NOVATION LLC**
Marquis DR ICD; **MEDTRONIC INC**
Marriott Senior Living Services; **SUNRISE SENIOR LIVING**
Marsh, Inc.; **MARSH & MCLENNAN COMPANIES INC**
Massachusetts General Hospital; **PARTNERS HEALTHCARE SYSTEM**
MaternaLink; **MATRIA HEALTHCARE INC**
Matrix Fault Current Limiter; **INTERMAGNETICS GENERAL CORP**
MatureRx; **ADVANCEPCS INC**

MatureRx-Plus; **ADVANCEPCS INC**
Maxim Total Knee System; **BIOMET INC**
Maximo; **MEDTRONIC INC**
Maxxim Meadical; **MEDICAL ACTION INDUSTRIES INC**
MaxyScan; **MAXYGEN INC**
Maxzide; **MYLAN LABORATORIES INC**
Mayo Clinic; **MAYO FOUNDATION FOR MEDICAL EDUCATION AND RESEARCH**
Mayo Clinic College of Medicine; **MAYO FOUNDATION FOR MEDICAL EDUCATION AND RESEARCH**
Mayo Clinic Hospital; **MAYO FOUNDATION FOR MEDICAL EDUCATION AND RESEARCH**
Mayo Health System; **MAYO FOUNDATION FOR MEDICAL EDUCATION AND RESEARCH**
Mayo School of Health Sciences; **MAYO FOUNDATION FOR MEDICAL EDUCATION AND RESEARCH**
McKesson Automation; **MCKESSON CORPORATION**
McKesson Corporation; **MOORE MEDICAL CORP**
McKesson HBOC, Inc.; **MCKESSON CORPORATION**
McKesson Medical-Surgical; **MCKESSON CORPORATION**
McKesson Medication Management; **MCKESSON CORPORATION**
McKesson Pharmaceutical; **MCKESSON CORPORATION**
McKesson Pharmacy Systems; **MCKESSON CORPORATION**
MD-Individual Practice Association, Inc.; **MID ATLANTIC MEDICAL SERVICES INC**
MDS Capital Corp.; **MDS INC**
MDS Diagnostic Services; **MDS INC**
MDS Nordion; **MDS INC**
MDS Pharma Services; **MDS INC**
MDS Proteomics; **MDS INC**
MDS Sciex; **MDS INC**
Mead Johnson Nutritionals; **BRISTOL MYERS SQUIBB CO**
MEDai; **ADVENTIST HEALTH SYSTEM**
Medex; **BLUE CROSS AND BLUE SHIELD OF MASSACHUSETTS**
Medex, Inc.; **MEDEX HOLDINGS CORPORATION**
medformation.com; **ALLINA HOSPITALS AND CLINICS**
Medfusion 3500 Syringe Pump; **MEDEX HOLDINGS CORPORATION**
Medicaid NEMT; **LOGISTICARE INC**

Medi-Cal; **BLUE CROSS OF CALIFORNIA**
Medical Analysis Systems, Inc.; **FISHER SCIENTIFIC INTERNATIONAL INC**
Medical Center of Southeastern Oklahoma; **HEALTH MANAGEMENT ASSOCIATES INC**
Medical Device Alliance, Inc.; **ARTHROCARE CORP**
Medical Dictation Center, Inc.; **MEDQUIST INC**
Medical Life Insurance Company; **HEALTH CARE SERVICE CORPORATION**
Medical Manager; **WEBMD CORPORATION**
Medical Resources Home Health Corp.; **NATIONAL HOME HEALTH CARE CORP**
Medical Transcription System; **MEDQUIST INC**
Medicare Enhance; **HARVARD PILGRIM HEALTH CARE INC**
Medicine Centre, LLC; **NEIGHBORCARE INC**
Medicine Shoppe International, Inc.; **CARDINAL HEALTH INC**
Medic-One Group; **ALLIED HEALTHCARE INTERNATIONAL INC**
Medigas; **ALLIED HEALTHCARE INTERNATIONAL INC**
MediLux; **PALOMAR MEDICAL TECHNOLOGIES INC**
Mediquest Dictation Tracking System; **MEDQUIST INC**
Medko; **INSTRUMENTARIUM CORPORATION**
MedOne; **AMERICAN MEDICAL SECURITY GROUP INC**
MedPlus; **QUEST DIAGNOSTICS INC**
Medscape; **WEBMD CORPORATION**
MedsInfo-ED; **BLUE CROSS AND BLUE SHIELD OF MASSACHUSETTS**
MedSpan Health Options, Inc.; **OXFORD HEALTH PLANS INC**
MedStar Diabetes Institute; **MEDSTAR HEALTH**
MedStar Health Visiting Nurse Association; **MEDSTAR HEALTH**
MedStar Physician Partners; **MEDSTAR HEALTH**
MedStar Research Institute; **MEDSTAR HEALTH**
Medtronic; **MEDTRONIC VASCULAR**
Medtronic CareLink Therapy Management System; **MEDTRONIC MINIMED INC**
Medtronic, Inc.; **MEDTRONIC MINIMED INC**

INDEX OF SUBSIDIARIES, BRAND NAMES AND AFFILIATIONS, CONT.

Medtronic, Inc.; **MEDTRONIC XOMED SURGICAL PRODUCTS INC**
Medtronic, Inc.; **MEDTRONIC SOFAMOR DANEK**
Mega Men; **GENERAL NUTRITION COMPANIES INC**
Meltus; **SSL INTERNATIONAL**
Member Service Life Insurance Company; **BLUE CROSS AND BLUE SHIELD OF OKLAHOMA**
Memorial Hermann Children's Hospital; **MEMORIAL HERMANN HEALTHCARE SYSTEM**
Memorial Hermann Garden Spa; **MEMORIAL HERMANN HEALTHCARE SYSTEM**
Memorial Hermann Heart and Vascular Institute; **MEMORIAL HERMANN HEALTHCARE SYSTEM**
Memorial Hospital for Cancer and Allied Diseases; **MEMORIAL SLOAN KETTERING CANCER CENTER**
Meniett; **MEDTRONIC XOMED SURGICAL PRODUCTS INC**
Menjugate; **CHIRON CORP**
Mental Health Outcomes, Inc.; **HORIZON HEALTH CORPORATION**
Mentor Medical, Ltd.; **MENTOR CORP**
Mercer Consulting Group, Inc.; **MARSH & MCLENNAN COMPANIES INC**
Mercer Delta Consulting; **MARSH & MCLENNAN COMPANIES INC**
Merck, Corp.; **MEDCO HEALTH SOLUTIONS**
Merck Institute for Science Education; **MERCK & CO INC**
Mercy Health Partners; **CATHOLIC HEALTHCARE PARTNERS**
Mercy Healthcare Sacramento; **CATHOLIC HEALTHCARE WEST**
Merial; **AVENTIS SA**
Merit Sensor Systems; **MERIT MEDICAL SYSTEMS INC**
Mesna; **AMERICAN PHARMACEUTICAL PARTNERS INC**
Metcare; **METROPOLITAN HEALTH NETWORKS**
Metcare RX, Inc.; **METROPOLITAN HEALTH NETWORKS**
Metformin; **EON LABS INC**
MetHealth; **METROPOLITAN HEALTH NETWORKS**
Methodist Health Foundation; **CLARIAN HEALTH PARTNERS INC**
Methodist Hospital; **CLARIAN HEALTH PARTNERS INC**
Metra; **QUIDEL CORP**
Metrex; **SYBRON DENTAL SPECIALTIES INC**

MetroPlus; **NEW YORK CITY HEALTH AND HOSPITALS CORPORATION**
Metropolitan Area Promotional Audit; **VENTIV HEALTH INC**
METRx MicroDiscectomy System; **MEDTRONIC SOFAMOR DANEK**
METRx MicroDiscectomy System; **MEDTRONIC INC**
MGH Institute of Health Professions; **PARTNERS HEALTHCARE SYSTEM**
M-I Vascular, Inc.; **MIV THERAPEUTICS INC**
Michigan Evaluation Group; **HOOPER HOLMES INC**
Micro Bio-Medics, Inc.; **HENRY SCHEIN INC**
Microgenics Corp.; **APOGENT TECHNOLOGIES INC**
Micro-Guide; **UTI CORPORATION**
Micronail; **WRIGHT MEDICAL GROUP INC**
MicroPlaner; **MEDTRONIC XOMED SURGICAL PRODUCTS INC**
MicroScan; **DADE BEHRING HOLDINGS INC**
Microtek Medical, Inc.; **MICROTEK MEDICAL HOLDINGS INC**
Microvascular Anastomotis Coupler; **SYNOVIS LIFE TECHNOLOGIES INC**
Midas Consoles; **TELEX COMMUNICATIONS INC**
Midland Medical Technologies; **SMITH & NEPHEW PLC**
Midodrine; **EON LABS INC**
Midtown Dental; **NATIONAL DENTEX CORP**
Milburn Distributions, Inc.; **PATTERSON COMPANIES INC**
Millennium; **VARIAN MEDICAL SYSTEMS INC**
Mind/Body Institute for Clinical Wellness; **MEMORIAL HERMANN HEALTHCARE SYSTEM**
Ministry Health Care; **MARIAN HEALTH SYSTEMS**
Minnesota Heart and Vascular Center; **FAIRVIEW HEALTH SERVICES**
Minnesota Mining and Manufacturing Company; **3M COMPANY**
Minntech Corp.; **CANTEL MEDICAL CORP**
Minntech Fibercor; **MINNTECH CORP**
Minntech International; **MINNTECH CORP**
Minntech Renal Systems; **MINNTECH CORP**
Mirada Solutions, Ltd.; **CTI MOLECULAR IMAGING**
Mirage; **RESMED INC**

Mister Baby; **SSL INTERNATIONAL**
MIVI Technologies, Inc.; **MIV THERAPEUTICS INC**
MMC Capital; **MARSH & MCLENNAN COMPANIES INC**
Mobile Meals; **SENTARA HEALTHCARE**
MolecularBreeding; **MAXYGEN INC**
Monistat; **JOHNSON & JOHNSON**
Monoclate-P; **ZLB BEHRING LLC**
Mononine; **ZLB BEHRING LLC**
Morphine Auto-Injector; **MERIDIAN MEDICAL TECHNOLOGIES INC**
Morrison Healthcare Food Services; **MORRISON MANAGEMENT SPECIALISTS INC**
Morrison Human Resource Services; **MORRISON MANAGEMENT SPECIALISTS INC**
Morrison Senior Dining; **MORRISON MANAGEMENT SPECIALISTS INC**
Mountain State Blue Cross Blue Shield; **HIGHMARK INC**
MPS Myocardial Protection System; **ATRION CORPORATION**
MRI Devices Corp.; **INTERMAGNETICS GENERAL CORP**
MSA Safety Works; **MINE SAFETY APPLIANCES CO**
M-Series; **EXACTECH INC**
MULTI-LINK; **GUIDANT CORP**
Multimedia Marketing, Inc.; **HEALTHSTREAM INC**
My Health Plan; **BLUE CROSS OF IDAHO**
MyChoice Blue; **ARKANSAS BLUE CROSS AND BLUE SHIELD**
MyHealthways; **AMERICAN HEALTHWAYS INC**
Mylan Bertek Pharmaceuticals; **MYLAN LABORATORIES INC**
Mylan Pharmaceuticals; **MYLAN LABORATORIES INC**
Mylan Technologies; **MYLAN LABORATORIES INC**
Mylanta; **JOHNSON & JOHNSON**
Mystaire; **MISONIX INC**
myuhc.com; **UNIPRISE INCORPORATED**
Nafion; **SIGMA ALDRICH CORP**
Namenda; **FOREST LABORATORIES INC**
NanoCrystal; **BRISTOL MYERS SQUIBB CO**
Nanomask; **EMERGENCY FILTRATION PRODUCTS INC**
NanoStat; **NANOBIO CORPORATION**
NanoView; **BIOPHAN TECHNOLOGIES INC**

INDEX OF SUBSIDIARIES, BRAND NAMES AND AFFILIATIONS, CONT.

National Association of Blue Shield Plans; **BLUE CROSS AND BLUE SHIELD ASSOCIATION**
National Economic Research Associates; **MARSH & MCLENNAN COMPANIES INC**
National Health Investors, Inc.; **NATIONAL HEALTHCARE CORP**
National Health Realty, Inc.; **NATIONAL HEALTHCARE CORP**
National Preferred Provider Network; **PLANVISTA CORP**
National Senior Care, Inc.; **MARINER HEALTH CARE INC**
Natura; **SONIC INNOVATIONS INC**
NaturalBlue; **BLUE CROSS AND BLUE SHIELD OF NEBRASKA**
Navigant Biotechnologies, Inc.; **GAMBRO AB**
Navigy, Inc; **BLUE CROSS AND BLUE SHIELD OF FLORIDA**
Nebulizer; **MISONIX INC**
NeighborCare At Home; **NEIGHBORCARE INC**
Nellcor; **TYCO HEALTHCARE GROUP**
Neovastat; **AETERNA ZENTARIS INC**
Neupogen; **AMGEN INC**
NeuraGen Nerve Guide; **INTEGRA LIFESCIENCES HOLDINGS CORP**
Neurontin; **PFIZER INC**
NeutroSpec; **MALLINCKRODT INC**
New England Home Care, Inc.; **NATIONAL HOME HEALTH CARE CORP**
New Jersey Staffing Works Corp.; **NATIONAL HOME HEALTH CARE CORP**
New Mountain Partners; **NATIONAL MEDICAL HEALTH CARD SYSTEMS INC**
New Star PMR; **CARDIOGENESIS CORP**
New York-Presbyterian Hospital; **NEW YORK-PRESBYTERIAN HEALTHCARE SYSTEM**
NexGen; **ZIMMER HOLDINGS INC**
NextGen Healthcare Information Systems, Inc.; **QUALITY SYSTEMS INC**
Niagara; **LASERSCOPE**
Nice n' Easy; **BRISTOL MYERS SQUIBB CO**
Nichols Institute; **QUEST DIAGNOSTICS INC**
Nicolet Vascular; **VIASYS HEALTHCARE INC**
Nifedipine ER; **MYLAN LABORATORIES INC**
Nightingale; **SENTARA HEALTHCARE**

Nightingale Nursing Bureau, Ltd.; **ALLIED HEALTHCARE INTERNATIONAL INC**
Nimbus Logic 200; **HUNTLEIGH TECHNOLOGIES PLC**
Nipro Corp.; **THERASENSE INC**
NMHCRX Mail Order, Inc.; **NATIONAL MEDICAL HEALTH CARD SYSTEMS INC**
Noble-Met, Ltd.; **UTI CORPORATION**
Norditropin SimpleXx; **NOVO-NORDISK AS**
North Shore Medical Center; **PARTNERS HEALTHCARE SYSTEM**
Northwest Toxicology; **LABONE INC**
Nova Factor, Inc.; **ACCREDO HEALTH INC**
NovaMed Eyecare, Inc.; **NOVAMED INC**
NOVAPLUS; **NOVATION LLC**
Novartis Institute for Biomedical Research, Inc.; **NOVARTIS AG**
NovoPen; **NOVO-NORDISK AS**
NovoSeven; **NOVO-NORDISK AS**
NOW Flu A&B; **THERMO ELECTRON CORP**
NOW RSV; **THERMO ELECTRON CORP**
Nucleus 3; **COCHLEAR LTD**
Nurse Healthline, Inc.; **AMERICAN MEDICAL SECURITY GROUP INC**
NurseWise; **CENTENE CORPORATION**
NuTex; **ANSELL LIMITED COMPANY**
Nutravail Technologies, Inc.; **BIOVAIL CORPORATION**
Nutropin Depot; **GENENTECH INC**
NWL; **LASERSCOPE**
Nyer Internet, Inc.; **NYER MEDICAL GROUP INC**
Oak Hill Capital Partners; **DUANE READE INC**
OASIS; **ORTHOFIX INTERNATIONAL NV**
OccuLogix, LP; **TLC VISION CORPORATION**
OccuMed; **BJC HEALTHCARE**
Oclassen Dermatologics; **WATSON PHARMACEUTICALS INC**
OcuCare Systems, Inc.; **OPTICARE HEALTH SYSTEMS**
Ocu-Guard; **SYNOVIS LIFE TECHNOLOGIES INC**
Oculex Pharmaceuticals, Inc; **ALLERGAN INC**
OcuLight; **IRIDEX CORP**
Ocuvite; **BAUSCH & LOMB INC**
OhioHealth Group; **OHIOHEALTH CORPORATION**

Ohmeda Medical; **INSTRUMENTARIUM CORPORATION**
Oklahoma Caring Foundation (The); **BLUE CROSS AND BLUE SHIELD OF OKLAHOMA**
OM DIRECT; **OWENS & MINOR INC**
Omnicare Clinical Research; **OMNICARE INC**
OMNI-ReSound ApS; **SONIC INNOVATIONS INC**
On Call; **AVMED HEALTH PLAN**
One 2 One; **HOSPIRA INC**
OneTouch; **LIFESCAN INC**
OneTouch Diabetes Management Software; **LIFESCAN INC**
ON-Q Post-Operative Pain Relief System; **I FLOW CORPORATION**
OnSite; **CARDINAL MEDICAL PRODUCTS AND SERVICES**
Opal-Lite; **ESSILOR INTERNATIONAL SA**
OPENSAIL; **GUIDANT CORP**
Operating Room for the 21st Century (The); **AMERICAN SHARED HOSPITAL SERVICES**
OPSM Group, Ltd.; **LUXOTTICA GROUP SPA**
Optefil; **EXACTECH INC**
Opteform; **EXACTECH INC**
Optetrak; **EXACTECH INC**
OptiEdge; **ADVANCED MEDICAL OPTICS INC**
Opti-Free; **ALCON INC**
Optimal Chemical Entities; **ARQULE INC**
OptiMARK; **MALLINCKRODT INC**
Optimum Choice of the Carolinas, Inc.; **MID ATLANTIC MEDICAL SERVICES INC**
Optimum Choice, Inc.; **MID ATLANTIC MEDICAL SERVICES INC**
Opus Medical; **ARTHROCARE CORP**
OpusDent; **LUMENIS LTD**
ORALCDx; **HENRY SCHEIN INC**
Oraqix; **DENTSPLY INTERNATIONAL INC**
OREX Processor; **MICROTEK MEDICAL HOLDINGS INC**
OREX Technologies International; **MICROTEK MEDICAL HOLDINGS INC**
Ormco; **SYBRON DENTAL SPECIALTIES INC**
Ortho DX; **COMPEX TECHNOLOGIES INC**
Orthodontic Centers of America; **OCA INC**
Orthofix; **ORTHOFIX INTERNATIONAL NV**
Orthofuser; **GISH BIOMEDICAL INC**

INDEX OF SUBSIDIARIES, BRAND NAMES AND AFFILIATIONS, CONT.

OrthoPAT; **HAEMONETICS CORPORATION**
Orthopat; **ZIMMER HOLDINGS INC**
Orthotrac; **ORTHOFIX INTERNATIONAL NV**
Osiris; **BIO RAD LABORATORIES INC**
OsteoPure; **OSTEOTECH INC**
Othy; **SYMMETRY MEDICAL INC**
Ovation; **OSTEOTECH INC**
Ovations; **UNITEDHEALTH GROUP INC**
Ovcon; **WARNER CHILCOTT PLC**
Ovidrel/Ovitrelle; **SERONO SA**
Oxford Health Insurance, Inc.; **OXFORD HEALTH PLANS INC**
Oxford Health Plans, Inc.; **OXFORD HEALTH PLANS INC**
oxfordhealth.com; **OXFORD HEALTH PLANS INC**
OxiFirst; **MALLINCKRODT INC**
Oxsoralen-Ultra; **VALEANT PHARMACEUTICALS INTERNATIONAL**
Pacific Dunlop Limited; **ANSELL LIMITED COMPANY**
PacifiCare Behavioral Health of California, Inc.; **PACIFICARE HEALTH SYSTEMS INC**
PacifiCare Health Systems; **AMERICAN MEDICAL SECURITY GROUP INC**
PacifiCare Life and Health Insurance Company; **PACIFICARE HEALTH SYSTEMS INC**
PacifiCare Life Assurance Company; **PACIFICARE HEALTH SYSTEMS INC**
Pamidronate; **AMERICAN PHARMACEUTICAL PARTNERS INC**
Pandac; **OWENS & MINOR INC**
Panorama Patient Monitoring Network; **DATASCOPE CORP**
Par Pharmaceutical, Inc.; **PAR PHARMACEUTICAL COMPANIES INC**
Paradigm; **MEDTRONIC MINIMED INC**
Parallux; **IDEXX LABORATORIES INC**
Partners Community HealthCare; **PARTNERS HEALTHCARE SYSTEM**
Partners in Wound Care Program; **AMEDISYS INC**
Partners National Health Plans of North Carolina; **BLUE CROSS AND BLUE SHIELD OF NORTH CAROLINA**
Patanol; **ALCON INC**
Patterson Dental Company; **PATTERSON COMPANIES INC**

Patterson Dental Supply, Inc.; **PATTERSON COMPANIES INC**
Paxil; **GLAXOSMITHKLINE PLC**
PayerServ; **PLANVISTA CORP**
PCS Health Systems; **ELI LILLY & CO**
PCS Health Systems; **ADVANCEPCS INC**
PDC Funding Company, LLC; **PATTERSON COMPANIES INC**
Pearle Vision; **COLE NATIONAL CORPORATION**
Pediatrix Screening, Inc.; **PEDIATRIX MEDICAL GROUP INC**
PediDyne; **KINETIC CONCEPTS INC**
Peer-A-Med; **SOLUCIENT LLC**
Pentasa; **SHIRE PHARMACEUTICALS PLC**
Peoplefirst Rehabilitation; **KINDRED HEALTHCARE INC**
Percepta; **SOLA INTERNATIONAL INC**
Percocet; **ENDO PHARMACEUTICALS HOLDINGS INC**
Percodan; **ENDO PHARMACEUTICALS HOLDINGS INC**
PerFix; **CR BARD INC**
Peri-Strips; **SYNOVIS LIFE TECHNOLOGIES INC**
Permanente Medical Groups; **KAISER PERMANENTE**
Per-Se Exchange; **PER SE TECHNOLOGIES INC**
Persona; **INVERNESS MEDICAL INNOVATIONS INC**
PersonalBlue; **BLUE CROSS OF IDAHO**
PETNET Pharmaceuticals, Inc.; **CTI MOLECULAR IMAGING**
PETNET Solutions; **CTI MOLECULAR IMAGING**
Phacoflex II; **ADVANCED MEDICAL OPTICS INC**
Pharma Services Holding; **QUINTILES TRANSNATIONAL CORP**
PharmaBio Development; **QUINTILES TRANSNATIONAL CORP**
PharmaCare Management Services; **CVS CORPORATION**
Pharmacare Resources, Inc.; **ACCREDO HEALTH INC**
Pharmaceutical Buyers, Inc.; **D & K HEALTHCARE RESOURCES INC**
Pharmaceutical Resources, Inc.; **PAR PHARMACEUTICAL COMPANIES INC**
Pharmachemie BV; **TEVA PHARMACEUTICAL INDUSTRIES**
Pharmacia Corporation; **PFIZER INC**
Pharmacopeia Drug Discovery; **PHARMACOPEIA INC**

Pharmacy Healthcare Solutions; **AMERISOURCEBERGEN CORP**
pharmacymax.com; **DRUGMAX INC**
Pharmakon LLC; **PDI INC**
PharmAssure; **GENERAL NUTRITION COMPANIES INC**
PharMerica, Inc.; **AMERISOURCEBERGEN CORP**
PharmGuard Medication Safety Software; **MEDEX HOLDINGS CORPORATION**
PhD Workstation; **BIO RAD LABORATORIES INC**
Philips Medcare; **PHILIPS MEDICAL SYSTEMS**
Philips Telemedicine Services; **SHL TELEMEDICINE**
Phillips Eye Institute; **ALLINA HOSPITALS AND CLINICS**
Phoenixville Hospital; **COMMUNITY HEALTH SYSTEMS INC**
Photo Research; **EXCEL TECHNOLOGY INC**
Phrenilin; **VALEANT PHARMACEUTICALS INTERNATIONAL**
Physicians Dialysis, Inc.; **DAVITA INC**
Physiotherapy Associates; **STRYKER CORP**
Pinnacle; **SYBRON DENTAL SPECIALTIES INC**
Pioneer Behavioral Health; **PHC INC**
Pioneer Pharmaceutical Research; **PHC INC**
Pipracil; **AMERICAN PHARMACEUTICAL PARTNERS INC**
Plak Smacker; **YOUNG INNOVATIONS INC**
PlanServ; **PLANVISTA CORP**
PlanVista Solutions, Inc.; **PLANVISTA CORP**
Plasco, Inc.; **MICROTEK MEDICAL HOLDINGS INC**
PlasmaKinetic; **GYRUS GROUP**
Plavix; **SANOFI-SYNTHELABO**
Polamar Medical Products, Inc.; **PALOMAR MEDICAL TECHNOLOGIES INC**
Porex Corp.; **WEBMD CORPORATION**
PortalVision; **VARIAN MEDICAL SYSTEMS INC**
Portamedic; **HOOPER HOLMES INC**
Portamedic Select; **HOOPER HOLMES INC**
Post-it; **3M COMPANY**
Posurdex; **ALLERGAN INC**
Pottstown Memorial Medical Center; **COMMUNITY HEALTH SYSTEMS INC**

INDEX OF SUBSIDIARIES, BRAND NAMES AND AFFILIATIONS, CONT.

Power Programs for Managing Diseases; **RESPIRONICS INC**
PowerInsight; **CERNER CORP**
PowerPac HC; **BIO RAD LABORATORIES INC**
PowerSculpt Cosmetic System; **MEDTRONIC XOMED SURGICAL PRODUCTS INC**
PPD Development; **PHARMACEUTICAL PRODUCT DEVELOPMENT INC**
PPD Discovery; **PHARMACEUTICAL PRODUCT DEVELOPMENT INC**
PPD Medical Communications; **PHARMACEUTICAL PRODUCT DEVELOPMENT INC**
PPD Medical Device; **PHARMACEUTICAL PRODUCT DEVELOPMENT INC**
PPD Virtual; **PHARMACEUTICAL PRODUCT DEVELOPMENT INC**
Preferred Financial Group; **HEALTH CARE SERVICE CORPORATION**
Preferred Provider Organization of Michigan; **BLUE CROSS AND BLUE SHIELD OF MICHIGAN**
PreferredOne; **WELLCARE GROUP OF COMPANIES**
Premarin; **WYETH**
Premier Blue; **BLUE CROSS AND BLUE SHIELD OF KANSAS**
Premier Health Partners; **CATHOLIC HEALTH INITIATIVES**
Premier Health, Inc.; **BLUE CROSS AND BLUE SHIELD OF KANSAS**
Premier Insurance Management; **PREMIER INC**
Premier Medical Insurance Group, Inc.; **SSM HEALTH CARE SYSTEM INC**
Premier Sourcing Partners; **PREMIER INC**
PrepStain; **TRIPATH IMAGING INC**
Presbyterian Healthcare Resources; **TEXAS HEALTH RESOURCES**
Prescription Solutions; **PACIFICARE HEALTH SYSTEMS INC**
PreserVision; **BAUSCH & LOMB INC**
PressureGuard; **SPAN AMERICA MEDICAL SYSTEMS INC**
PressureGuard Easy Air; **SPAN AMERICA MEDICAL SYSTEMS INC**
PREVACARE; **ETHICON INC**
Prevacid; **ABBOTT LABORATORIES**
Preventive Nutrition; **GENERAL NUTRITION COMPANIES INC**
Prialt; **ELAN CORP PLC**
PRIME ECG; **MERIDIAN MEDICAL TECHNOLOGIES INC**
Prime Medical Services, Inc.; **HEALTHTRONICS INC**
Priority Health; **SPECTRUM HEALTH**

Priority Healthcare Pharmacy; **PRIORITY HEALTHCARE CORP**
Pro Osteon Implant 500; **INTERPORE CROSS INTERNATIONAL**
ProActive; **OCULAR SCIENCES INC**
Proamatine; **SHIRE PHARMACEUTICALS PLC**
PROBACTRIX; **NEW YORK HEALTH CARE INC**
ProCallus; **ORTHOFIX INTERNATIONAL NV**
ProCare; **YOUNG INNOVATIONS INC**
ProCare One Nurses, LLC; **HORIZON HEALTH CORPORATION**
Producers of Quality Medical Disposables; **MEDICORE INC**
Profile Therapeutics plc; **RESPIRONICS INC**
PROFIX; **SMITH & NEPHEW PLC**
Prograf; **FUJISAWA PHARMACEUTICALS COMPANY LTD**
Proleukin; **CHIRON CORP**
Prometheus Assisted Living, LLC; **ATRIA SENIOR LIVING GROUP**
Pronto Heavy Duty Power Wheelchair; **INVACARE CORP**
PROTECT Emergency Response Systems, Inc.; **LIFELINE SYSTEMS INC**
Protonix; **WYETH**
Protopic; **FUJISAWA PHARMACEUTICALS COMPANY LTD**
Providence Holy Cross; **PROVIDENCE HEALTH SYSTEM**
Providence Milwaukie Hospital; **PROVIDENCE HEALTH SYSTEM**
Providence St. Peter Hospital; **PROVIDENCE HEALTH SYSTEM**
Providence Valdez Medical Center; **PROVIDENCE HEALTH SYSTEM**
PROVIGIL; **CEPHALON INC**
ProxyMed; **PLANVISTA CORP**
Prozac; **ELI LILLY & CO**
PSIMedica; **BIO REFERENCE LABORATORIES INC**
PsychScope; **HORIZON HEALTH CORPORATION**
Pull-Ups; **KIMBERLY CLARK CORP**
Pulmozyme; **GENENTECH INC**
Pulsavac Plus Wound Debridemant System; **ZIMMER HOLDINGS INC**
Punctur-Guard; **ICU MEDICAL INC**
PuraPly; **ORGANOGENESIS INC**
Puritan-Bennett; **MALLINCKRODT INC**
Putnam Investments, LLC; **MARSH & MCLENNAN COMPANIES INC**
Q TRAP; **APPLIED BIOSYSTEMS GROUP**

Qdot; **VENTANA MEDICAL SYSTEMS**
QDR; **HOLOGIC INC**
QDX Care Management System; **QUOVADX INC**
QDX Cash Accelerator; **QUOVADX INC**
QDX Enterprise Data Exchange; **QUOVADX INC**
QDX Phoenix Solution Sourcing; **QUOVADX INC**
QDX Platform V; **QUOVADX INC**
QDX Quick Trials; **QUOVADX INC**
QS-10 Guidewire; **MEDTRONIC VASCULAR**
QSTAR; **APPLIED BIOSYSTEMS GROUP**
Quality Medical Transcription, Inc.; **MEDQUIST INC**
Quality Oncology, Inc.; **MATRIA HEALTHCARE INC**
Quantronix; **EXCEL TECHNOLOGY INC**
Quartet; **SONIC INNOVATIONS INC**
Quest Medical, Inc.; **ATRION CORPORATION**
Quest Total Care Pharmacy; **NEIGHBORCARE INC**
Quick Study, Inc.; **HEALTHSTREAM INC**
Quickie; **SUNRISE MEDICAL INC**
Quickie Chameleon; **SUNRISE MEDICAL INC**
QuickVue; **QUIDEL CORP**
Quorum Health Group; **TRIAD HOSPITALS INC**
QUS-2; **QUIDEL CORP**
Q-Yag 5; **PALOMAR MEDICAL TECHNOLOGIES INC**
R&D Systems Europe, Ltd.; **TECHNE CORP**
R&D Systems GmbH; **TECHNE CORP**
RadConnect RIS; **VITALWORKS INC**
Radianse, Inc.; **ASCENSION HEALTH**
RadNet Management, Inc.; **PRIMEDEX HEALTH SYSTEMS INC**
Rapid Capture System; **DIGENE CORPORATION**
Rapid D-10; **BIO RAD LABORATORIES INC**
RapidBill; **VITALWORKS INC**
RapidClaim; **VITALWORKS INC**
RapidReminder; **VITALWORKS INC**
RapidVue; **QUIDEL CORP**
Raytel Medical Corp.; **SHL TELEMEDICINE**
ReACT; **IMMUCOR INC**
Readi-CAT; **E-Z-EM INC**
ReadyNurse; **HARBORSIDE HEALTHCARE CORP**
Rebif; **SERONO SA**

Plunkett's Health Care Industry Almanac 2005

INDEX OF SUBSIDIARIES, BRAND NAMES AND AFFILIATIONS, CONT.

REFLECTION; **SMITH & NEPHEW PLC**
Reflex; **CONMED CORP**
Regence BlueCross BlueShield of Oregon; **REGENCE GROUP (THE)**
Regence BlueCross BlueShield of Utah; **REGENCE GROUP (THE)**
Regence BlueShield of Idaho; **REGENCE GROUP (THE)**
Regence BlueShield of Washington; **REGENCE GROUP (THE)**
Regence Life & Health Insurance; **REGENCE GROUP (THE)**
Regentek; **DJ ORTHOPEDICS INC**
Regional Spinal Cord Injury Centers; **JEFFERSON HEALTH SYSTEM INC**
Rehab Designs of America Corporation; **HANGER ORTHOPEDIC GROUP INC**
Rehab Without Walls; **GENTIVA HEALTH SERVICES INC**
Rehabilicare; **COMPEX TECHNOLOGIES INC**
Rehabilitation Institute of Michigan; **DETROIT MEDICAL CENTER**
Rehabilitation Institute of St. Louis (The); **BJC HEALTHCARE**
Rehabilitative Care Systems of America; **REHABCARE GROUP INC**
Relafen; **GLAXOSMITHKLINE PLC**
RelayHealth; **BLUE CROSS AND BLUE SHIELD OF FLORIDA**
Reliance; **STERIS CORP**
Remicade; **GTC BIOTHERAPEUTICS INC**
Reminyl; **SHIRE PHARMACEUTICALS PLC**
RenaClear; **MINNTECH CORP**
Renagel; **GENZYME CORP**
Renalin 100 Cold Sterilant; **MINNTECH CORP**
Renatron II; **MINNTECH CORP**
Rennie; **ROCHE GROUP**
RENOVA Internal Hex; **LIFECORE BIOMEDICAL INC**
ReNu; **BAUSCH & LOMB INC**
Renucci Hospitality House; **SPECTRUM HEALTH**
Repliform; **LIFECELL CORPORATION**
ResCare Premier; **RES CARE INC**
ResCare Training Technologies; **RES CARE INC**
ResControl; **RESMED INC**
Research and Diagnostic Systems, Inc.; **TECHNE CORP**
RespAide; **EMERGENCY FILTRATION PRODUCTS INC**
Respiratory Healthways; **AMERICAN HEALTHWAYS INC**
Respironics, Inc.; **NOVAMETRIX MEDICAL SYSTEMS INC**

Restasis; **ALLERGAN INC**
RESTORE; **LIFECORE BIOMEDICAL INC**
RETAANE; **ALCON INC**
RetroX; **GYRUS GROUP**
Reverset; **INCYTE CORP**
Rheopheresis; **TLC VISION CORPORATION**
Ribapharm, Inc.; **VALEANT PHARMACEUTICALS INTERNATIONAL**
Riley Children's Foundaton; **CLARIAN HEALTH PARTNERS INC**
Riley Hospital for Children; **CLARIAN HEALTH PARTNERS INC**
Risperdal; **JOHNSON & JOHNSON**
Rita Ann; **AMERISOURCEBERGEN CORP**
RITA System; **RITA MEDICAL SYSTEMS INC**
Rituxan; **GENENTECH INC**
River Region Home Health; **AMEDISYS INC**
Robitussin; **WYETH**
Roche Holding, Ltd.; **ROCHE GROUP**
Rochester Medical Hospital; **MAYO FOUNDATION FOR MEDICAL EDUCATION AND RESEARCH**
Rock Bottom; **DUANE READE INC**
Rogue Wave C++; **QUOVADX INC**
Rolaids; **PFIZER INC**
Rosetta Stone; **HEALTH NET INC**
ROSYS Plato; **IMMUCOR INC**
Rotech Medical Corporation; **ROTECH HEALTHCARE INC**
Roto Rest Delta; **KINETIC CONCEPTS INC**
Royal Philips Electronics; **MEDQUIST INC**
Royal Philips Electronics; **PHILIPS MEDICAL SYSTEMS**
RTS; **TELEX COMMUNICATIONS INC**
Rush Home Care Network; **PATIENT CARE INC**
Rx Nebraska; **BLUE CROSS AND BLUE SHIELD OF NEBRASKA**
RxAmerica; **LONGS DRUG STORES CORPORATION**
SAF-Clens; **CONVATEC**
SafeGuard Health Plans, Inc.; **SAFEGUARD HEALTH ENTERPRISES INC**
Safeskin; **KIMBERLY CLARK CORP**
Sahara; **HOLOGIC INC**
Saint Clair's Health System; **MARIAN HEALTH SYSTEMS**
Saint John Health System; **MARIAN HEALTH SYSTEMS**
Saizen; **SERONO SA**
Salem Dental; **NATIONAL DENTEX CORP**

Sample Management System; **DIAGNOSTIC PRODUCTS CORPORATION**
Samuel Merritt College; **SUTTER HEALTH**
San Pedro Peninsula Hospital; **PROVIDENCE HEALTH SYSTEM**
Sanatis GmbH; **KYPHON INC**
Sanitas; **BRITISH UNION PROVIDENT ASSOCIATION (BUPA)**
Sanofi-Synthelabo; **AVENTIS SA**
Sarafem; **WARNER CHILCOTT PLC**
SARNavigator; **TRIPOS INC**
Sauber; **SSL INTERNATIONAL**
Saunders/Pronex Traction Devices; **EMPI INC**
Scan One; **CORVEL CORP**
SCBA, Inc.; **NYER MEDICAL GROUP INC**
Schein Empire Dental Chair; **HENRY SCHEIN INC**
Schering-Plough Animal Health; **SCHERING-PLOUGH CORP**
Schering-Plough Healthcare Products; **SCHERING-PLOUGH CORP**
Schering-Plough Pharmaceuticals; **SCHERING-PLOUGH CORP**
Schering-Plough Research Institute; **SCHERING-PLOUGH CORP**
Scholl; **SSL INTERNATIONAL**
Scotch Tape; **3M COMPANY**
Scotch-Brite; **3M COMPANY**
Scotchgard; **3M COMPANY**
Scott; **KIMBERLY CLARK CORP**
ScriptAssist; **CENTENE CORPORATION**
SE Biliary Stent Ststem; **MEDTRONIC VASCULAR**
Seabury & Smith, Inc.; **MARSH & MCLENNAN COMPANIES INC**
SealChip; **MOLECULAR DEVICES CORP**
Sears Optical; **COLE NATIONAL CORPORATION**
SEASONALE; **BARR LABORATORIES INC**
Secure Horizons; **TUFTS ASSOCIATED HEALTH PLANS**
Secure Horizons Medicare Supplement Plan; **PACIFICARE HEALTH SYSTEMS INC**
Secure IV; **SPAN AMERICA MEDICAL SYSTEMS INC**
SELAN+ Zinc Oxide; **SPAN AMERICA MEDICAL SYSTEMS INC**
Select Blue Advantage PPO; **BLUE CROSS AND BLUE SHIELD OF TEXAS**
Select Optical; **ESSILOR INTERNATIONAL SA**
Select Saver; **BLUE CROSS AND BLUE SHIELD OF TEXAS**

INDEX OF SUBSIDIARIES, BRAND NAMES AND AFFILIATIONS, CONT.

SelecTEMP; **BLUE CROSS AND BLUE SHIELD OF TEXAS**
Selenia; **HOLOGIC INC**
Semi-Q; **QUIDEL CORP**
SenoScan; **FISCHER IMAGING CORP**
Sensar; **ADVANCED MEDICAL OPTICS INC**
Sensipar; **AMGEN INC**
SensorMedics Corp.; **VIASYS HEALTHCARE INC**
Sentara Bayside; **SENTARA HEALTHCARE**
Sentara CarePlex; **SENTARA HEALTHCARE**
Sentara Leigh; **SENTARA HEALTHCARE**
Sentara Norfolk General; **SENTARA HEALTHCARE**
Sentara Virginia Beach; **SENTARA HEALTHCARE**
Sentinel; **OSTEOTECH INC**
Separation Technology, Inc.; **APOGENT TECHNOLOGIES INC**
Septi-Soft; **CONVATEC**
Serax; **ALPHARMA INC**
Serologicals Proteins, Inc.; **SEROLOGICALS CORP**
Serologicals, Ltd.; **SEROLOGICALS CORP**
Serostim; **SERONO SA**
Sextant Plus; **UROCOR INC**
Shanghai United Family Hospital and Clinics; **CHINDEX INTERNATIONAL INC**
Shearwater Corp.; **NEKTAR THERAPEUTICS**
Shire Laboratories; **SHIRE PHARMACEUTICALS PLC**
SHUSA; **PACIFICARE HEALTH SYSTEMS INC**
Sicor, Inc.; **TEVA PHARMACEUTICAL INDUSTRIES**
Siemens AG; **SIEMENS MEDICAL SOLUTIONS**
Sierra BioSource; **SEROLOGICALS CORP**
Sierra Health-Care Options; **SIERRA HEALTH SERVICES INC**
Sight for Students; **VISION SERVICE PLAN**
Signature Eyewear Collection; **SIGNATURE EYEWEAR INC**
Silkair; **HILL-ROM COMPANY INC**
Similac; **ABBOTT LABORATORIES**
Sinai-Grace Hospital; **DETROIT MEDICAL CENTER**
Singer Specs; **EMERGING VISION INC**
Singulair; **MERCK & CO INC**
Sister Kenny Rehabilitation Insitute; **ALLINA HOSPITALS AND CLINICS**

Sisters of Bon Secours; **BON SECOURS HEALTH SYSTEM INC**
Sisters of Charity of the Incarnate Word; **CHRISTUS HEALTH**
Sisters of Providence; **PROVIDENCE HEALTH SYSTEM**
Sisters of St. Joseph Health System; **ASCENSION HEALTH**
Sisters of St. Joseph of Carondelet; **ASCENSION HEALTH**
Sisters of the Sorrowful Mother; **MARIAN HEALTH SYSTEMS**
Site For Sore Eyes; **EMERGING VISION INC**
Skintonic; **CANDELA CORP**
SKY Computers; **ANALOGIC CORP**
Sloan-Kettering Institute; **MEMORIAL SLOAN KETTERING CANCER CENTER**
SLP 1000; **PALOMAR MEDICAL TECHNOLOGIES INC**
SmartCare; **INVERNESS MEDICAL INNOVATIONS INC**
SmartCell; **HAEMONETICS CORPORATION**
SmartChoice; **OCULAR SCIENCES INC**
SmartPReP; **LIFECELL CORPORATION**
SmartSpec Plus; **BIO RAD LABORATORIES INC**
SmartSuction; **HAEMONETICS CORPORATION**
Smit Mobile Equipment Company; **HEALTHTRONICS INC**
Smith & Nephew Group; **SMITH & NEPHEW PLC**
Smith Holden, Inc.; **HENRY SCHEIN INC**
Smoothbeam; **CANDELA CORP**
SNAP; **IDEXX LABORATORIES INC**
Snyder Communications; **VENTIV HEALTH INC**
Soarian; **SIEMENS MEDICAL SOLUTIONS**
SOCRATES; **INTUITIVE SURGICAL INC**
SofLens; **BAUSCH & LOMB INC**
SofPort; **BAUSCH & LOMB INC**
SoftScan; **ART ADVANCED RESEARCH TECHNOLOGIES**
SOLAMax; **SOLA INTERNATIONAL INC**
SOLAOne; **SOLA INTERNATIONAL INC**
Sologrip III; **CARDIOGENESIS CORP**
Solstice; **MEDTRONIC VASCULAR**
Somatom Sensation 16; **SIEMENS MEDICAL SOLUTIONS**
Sonicator; **MISONIX INC**
SonicWAVE; **STAAR SURGICAL CO**

Sonoline; **SIEMENS MEDICAL SOLUTIONS**
Sonomist; **MISONIX INC**
Sonora Medical Systems, Inc.; **MISONIX INC**
Sordin AB; **MINE SAFETY APPLIANCES CO**
Soredex; **INSTRUMENTARIUM CORPORATION**
Sound Technologies, Inc.; **VCA ANTECH INC**
Sound Technology; **ANALOGIC CORP**
Source Medical; **MDS INC**
South Bay Medical; **MENTOR CORP**
South Pacific Tyres; **ANSELL LIMITED COMPANY**
Southern Health; **COVENTRY HEALTH CARE INC**
Southern National Life Insurance Company, Inc.; **BLUE CROSS AND BLUE SHIELD OF LOUISIANA**
Southern Ohio Medical Center; **OHIOHEALTH CORPORATION**
Southern Prosthetic Supply, Inc.; **HANGER ORTHOPEDIC GROUP INC**
Southwest Medical Associates; **SIERRA HEALTH SERVICES INC**
Sowerby Health Centers; **HARBORSIDE HEALTHCARE CORP**
Space Traveler; **ENVIRONMENTAL TECTONICS CORP**
Spacelabs Medical, Inc.; **INSTRUMENTARIUM CORPORATION**
Span+Aids; **SPAN AMERICA MEDICAL SYSTEMS INC**
Specialized Care Services; **UNITEDHEALTH GROUP INC**
Specialty Rehab Management, Inc.; **HORIZON HEALTH CORPORATION**
SpectraMax; **MOLECULAR DEVICES CORP**
SPECTRON; **SMITH & NEPHEW PLC**
Spectrum; **UTI CORPORATION**
Spectrum Healthcare Resources; **TEAM HEALTH**
Spherecom Dental Supply, Inc.; **HENRY SCHEIN INC**
Spinal-Stim; **ORTHOFIX INTERNATIONAL NV**
Spirometer Enabler; **EPIC SYSTEMS CORPORATION**
SportSafe; **BIOVAIL CORPORATION**
Springfusor Mechanical Infusion System; **MEDEX HOLDINGS CORPORATION**
Springhouse; **MANOR CARE INC**
Springs Memorial Hospital; **COMMUNITY HEALTH SYSTEMS INC**

INDEX OF SUBSIDIARIES, BRAND NAMES AND AFFILIATIONS, CONT.

SPrint; **COCHLEAR LTD**
St. Elizabeth Health Partners; **CATHOLIC HEALTHCARE PARTNERS**
St. Louis Children's Hospital; **BJC HEALTHCARE**
St. Luke's Hospital; **MAYO FOUNDATION FOR MEDICAL EDUCATION AND RESEARCH**
St. Mary's Health Partners; **CATHOLIC HEALTHCARE PARTNERS**
St. Marys Hospital; **MAYO FOUNDATION FOR MEDICAL EDUCATION AND RESEARCH**
STAARVISC II; **STAAR SURGICAL CO**
Staffing Enterprise, Ltd.; **ALLIED HEALTHCARE INTERNATIONAL INC**
STAGE-1; **LIFECORE BIOMEDICAL INC**
Star Guide Corporation; **UTI CORPORATION**
Star Guide-Europe; **UTI CORPORATION**
STARFlex; **NMT MEDICAL INC**
StarMed Staffing, Inc.; **REHABCARE GROUP INC**
StatSat; **GISH BIOMEDICAL INC**
StatSpin, Inc.; **IRIS INTERNATIONAL INC**
Staywell; **WELLCARE GROUP OF COMPANIES**
Stent Technologies; **UTI CORPORATION**
Stentgenix; **MIV THERAPEUTICS INC**
STERIS Isomedix Services; **STERIS CORP**
Steris Laboratories; **WATSON PHARMACEUTICALS INC**
STERIS SYSTEM 1; **STERIS CORP**
Sterling House; **ALTERRA HEALTHCARE CORP**
Sterling Optical; **EMERGING VISION INC**
Sterling Vision; **EMERGING VISION INC**
Stilnox; **SANOFI-SYNTHELABO**
Stimate; **ZLB BEHRING LLC**
Straumann Dental Implant System; **INSTITUT STRAUMANN AG**
Stryker Biotech; **STRYKER CORP**
Stryker Howmedica Osteonics; **STRYKER CORP**
Stryker Leibinger; **STRYKER CORP**
Stryker MedSurg; **STRYKER CORP**
Study Tracker; **COVANCE INC**
Styl-Rite; **US VISION INC**
SuccessWorks; **EPIC SYSTEMS CORPORATION**
Sucralfate; **EON LABS INC**

Sullivan Dental Products; **HENRY SCHEIN INC**
Sulzer Medical; **CENTERPULSE AG**
Sunbelt Home Health Care; **ADVENTIST HEALTH SYSTEM**
Sunbelt Systems Concepts; **ADVENTIST HEALTH SYSTEM**
SunBridge Healthcare Corp.; **SUN HEALTHCARE GROUP**
SunDance Rehabilitation Corp.; **SUN HEALTHCARE GROUP**
Sunrise Access Manager; **ECLIPSYS CORPORATION**
Sunrise Assisted Living; **SUNRISE SENIOR LIVING**
Sunrise Clinical Manager; **ECLIPSYS CORPORATION**
Sunrise Decision Support Manager; **ECLIPSYS CORPORATION**
Sunrise Health Management; **ACCREDO HEALTH INC**
Sunrise Medical Education; **SUNRISE MEDICAL INC**
Sunrise Patient Financial Manager; **ECLIPSYS CORPORATION**
Sunrise Record Manager; **ECLIPSYS CORPORATION**
SunriseXA; **ECLIPSYS CORPORATION**
Sunsoft; **OCULAR SCIENCES INC**
SunStone; **PSYCHIATRIC SOLUTIONS INC**
Super Arrow-Flex; **ARROW INTERNATIONAL INC**
Superior Consulting Company, Inc.; **SUPERIOR CONSULTANT HOLDINGS CORP**
SuperPower, Inc.; **INTERMAGNETICS GENERAL CORP**
Superstat; **EMERGENCY FILTRATION PRODUCTS INC**
SurePath; **TRIPATH IMAGING INC**
SureStep; **LIFESCAN INC**
SurgiTrack; **OWENS & MINOR INC**
SURPASS; **IDEXX LABORATORIES INC**
Sutter GammaKnife; **SUTTER HEALTH**
Swan-Ganz; **EDWARDS LIFESCIENCES CORP**
SYBYL; **TRIPOS INC**
Symmetry Jet; **SYMMETRY MEDICAL INC**
Symmetry Othy; **SYMMETRY MEDICAL INC**
Symmetry PolyVac; **SYMMETRY MEDICAL INC**
Symmetry Thornton; **SYMMETRY MEDICAL INC**
Symmetry UltreXX; **SYMMETRY MEDICAL INC**
Syndol; **SSL INTERNATIONAL**

SynerGraft; **CRYOLIFE INC**
Synergy; **MEDTRONIC INC**
SYNERGY Spinal System; **INTERPORE CROSS INTERNATIONAL**
SynOcta; **INSTITUT STRAUMANN AG**
Synovis Interventional Solutions; **SYNOVIS LIFE TECHNOLOGIES INC**
Synovis Micro Companies Alliance; **SYNOVIS LIFE TECHNOLOGIES INC**
Synovis Precision Engineering; **SYNOVIS LIFE TECHNOLOGIES INC**
Synovis Surgical Innovations; **SYNOVIS LIFE TECHNOLOGIES INC**
SynQuest Technologies; **HEALTHSTREAM INC**
Synrad; **EXCEL TECHNOLOGY INC**
System 37; **MATRIA HEALTHCARE INC**
Systemed, LLC; **MEDCO HEALTH SOLUTIONS**
Syva; **DADE BEHRING HOLDINGS INC**
TAB Tumescent Absorbent Bandage; **MEDTRONIC XOMED SURGICAL PRODUCTS INC**
Tamoxifen; **BARR LABORATORIES INC**
TAP Pharmaceutical Products; **ABBOTT LABORATORIES**
TaqMan; **APPLIED BIOSYSTEMS GROUP**
Target Optical; **COLE NATIONAL CORPORATION**
Taxotere; **AVENTIS SA**
Taxus; **BOSTON SCIENTIFIC CORP**
Taylor Medical, Inc.; **PSS WORLD MEDICAL INC**
Tazorac; **ALLERGAN INC**
TE; **INSTITUT STRAUMANN AG**
Teflon EasyCare; **SOLA INTERNATIONAL INC**
TeleBreather; **SHL TELEMEDICINE**
Telemedicine; **AMERICHOICE CORPORATION**
TelePress; **SHL TELEMEDICINE**
TeleWeight; **SHL TELEMEDICINE**
Telex; **TELEX COMMUNICATIONS INC**
Teraklin AG; **GAMBRO AB**
Term Guard; **MATRIA HEALTHCARE INC**
TerryFoam; **SPAN AMERICA MEDICAL SYSTEMS INC**
Testoviron; **SCHERING AG**
TESTSKIN II; **ORGANOGENESIS INC**

INDEX OF SUBSIDIARIES, BRAND NAMES AND AFFILIATIONS, CONT.

Teva North America; **TEVA PHARMACEUTICAL INDUSTRIES**
Teva Pharmaceuticals USA; **TEVA PHARMACEUTICAL INDUSTRIES**
Texas Health Research Institute; **TEXAS HEALTH RESOURCES**
Theracor; **HARBORSIDE HEALTHCARE CORP**
Therapeutic Systems, Ltd.; **REHABCARE GROUP INC**
TheraPulse; **KINETIC CONCEPTS INC**
TheraSeed; **THERAGENICS CORP**
TheraSense, Inc.; **ABBOTT LABORATORIES**
TheraSource; **THERAGENICS CORP**
TherMatrx, Inc.; **AMERICAN MEDICAL SYSTEMS HOLDINGS INC**
Thermo Cardiosystems; **THORATEC CORPORATION**
Things Remembered; **COLE NATIONAL CORPORATION**
ThinPrep Pap; **QUEST DIAGNOSTICS INC**
Thoele Dental; **NATIONAL DENTEX CORP**
Thomas Jefferson University Hospitals; **JEFFERSON HEALTH SYSTEM INC**
Thora-Cath; **UTAH MEDICAL PRODUCTS INC**
Thoratec IVAD; **THORATEC CORPORATION**
Thoratec VAD; **THORATEC CORPORATION**
Threshold ImmunoLigand; **MOLECULAR DEVICES CORP**
ThromboSol; **LIFECELL CORPORATION**
Tiazac; **FOREST LABORATORIES INC**
Tidewater Healthcare Shared Services Group, Inc.; **NEIGHBORCARE INC**
Tinactin; **SCHERING-PLOUGH CORP**
TLC; **OPTICARE HEALTH SYSTEMS**
TLC Laser Eye Centers, Inc.; **TLC VISION CORPORATION**
TMR 2000; **CARDIOGENESIS CORP**
TNKase; **GENENTECH INC**
TOBI; **CHIRON CORP**
Top Quality Partials; **NATIONAL DENTEX CORP**
Total Lean; **GENERAL NUTRITION COMPANIES INC**
Total Renal Care Holdings, Inc.; **DAVITA INC**
Total Renal Research, Inc.; **DAVITA INC**
Total Solutions; **SYMMETRY MEDICAL INC**

TotalCare; **HILL-ROM COMPANY INC**
Trabecular Metal; **ZIMMER HOLDINGS INC**
Traditional Blue; **HEALTHNOW NEW YORK**
Transitions; **SOLA INTERNATIONAL INC**
TranStar; **HILL-ROM COMPANY INC**
Trexell; **BARR LABORATORIES INC**
Tri Supreme; **ESSILOR INTERNATIONAL SA**
TriaDyne; **KINETIC CONCEPTS INC**
Trial Tracker; **COVANCE INC**
TrialBase; **KENDLE INTERNATIONAL INC**
TriAlert; **KENDLE INTERNATIONAL INC**
TriaLine; **KENDLE INTERNATIONAL INC**
TrialView; **KENDLE INTERNATIONAL INC**
TrialWare; **KENDLE INTERNATIONAL INC**
TrialWeb; **KENDLE INTERNATIONAL INC**
TRIANO; **SIEMENS MEDICAL SOLUTIONS**
Tribute; **SONIC INNOVATIONS INC**
TriCare; **BLUE CROSS AND BLUE SHIELD OF WYOMING**
TriCenturion, Inc.; **BLUE CROSS AND BLUE SHIELD OF FLORIDA**
Tri-Hospital Home Health and Hospice; **PATIENT CARE INC**
Trinity Design; **TRINITY HEALTH COMPANY**
Trinity Health International; **TRINITY HEALTH COMPANY**
Trinity Health Plans; **TRINITY HEALTH COMPANY**
TriPath Oncology; **TRIPATH IMAGING INC**
Trisequens; **NOVO-NORDISK AS**
Tristar Optical Co., Ltd.; **LUXOTTICA GROUP SPA**
TriWest; **BLUE SHIELD OF CALIFORNIA**
Trogard Finesse; **CONMED CORP**
True Blue; **BLUE CROSS OF IDAHO**
Trypsin; **SEROLOGICALS CORP**
Tufts Associated Health Maintenance Organization; **TUFTS ASSOCIATED HEALTH PLANS**
Tufts Benefit Administrators, Inc.; **TUFTS ASSOCIATED HEALTH PLANS**
Tufts Insurance Company; **TUFTS ASSOCIATED HEALTH PLANS**
Tufts Preferred Provider Option; **TUFTS ASSOCIATED HEALTH PLANS**

Tufts Total Health Plan; **TUFTS ASSOCIATED HEALTH PLANS**
Tularik, Inc.; **AMGEN INC**
Tums; **GLAXOSMITHKLINE PLC**
TurbiTime System; **DADE BEHRING HOLDINGS INC**
Tyco Healthcare Group; **MALLINCKRODT INC**
Tyco International, Ltd.; **TYCO HEALTHCARE GROUP**
Tykon, Inc.; **D & K HEALTHCARE RESOURCES INC**
Tylenol; **JOHNSON & JOHNSON**
U.S. Surgical; **TYCO HEALTHCARE GROUP**
U.S.-China Industrial Exchange, Inc.; **CHINDEX INTERNATIONAL INC**
UCB SA; **CELLTECH GROUP PLC**
UDL Laboratories; **MYLAN LABORATORIES INC**
ULTIA; **WEBMD CORPORATION**
Ultraflex; **OCULAR SCIENCES INC**
Ultra-Pro II Needle Guide; **CIVCO MEDICAL INSTRUMENTS**
UltraPulse; **LUMENIS LTD**
UltraVIEW; **PERKINELMER INC**
Ultraview; **INSTRUMENTARIUM CORPORATION**
Ultrazyme; **ADVANCED MEDICAL OPTICS INC**
UltreXX; **SYMMETRY MEDICAL INC**
Uniform Tubes; **UTI CORPORATION**
Union Memorial Hospital; **MEDSTAR HEALTH**
UniPatch; **TYCO HEALTHCARE GROUP**
Uniprise; **UNITEDHEALTH GROUP INC**
Unistik; **LIFESCAN INC**
United Concordia; **HIGHMARK INC**
United Research China Shanghai; **IMS HEALTH INC**
United Resource Networks; **UNITEDHEALTH GROUP INC**
UnitedHealth Group; **DENTAL BENEFITS PROVIDERS**
UnitedHealth Group; **OXFORD HEALTH PLANS INC**
UnitedHealth Group; **UNIPRISE INCORPORATED**
UnitedHealth Group; **AMERICHOICE CORPORATION**
UnitedHealth Group; **MID ATLANTIC MEDICAL SERVICES INC**
UnitedHealthCare; **UNITEDHEALTH GROUP INC**
Universal; **CONMED CORP**
UrinQuick; **QUIDEL CORP**
UroSavant; **UROCOR INC**
UroScore; **UROCOR INC**
UroServices; **UROCOR INC**

INDEX OF SUBSIDIARIES, BRAND NAMES AND AFFILIATIONS, CONT.

UroStone; **UROCOR INC**
Uryxr; **CR BARD INC**
USAble MCO; **ARKANSAS BLUE CROSS AND BLUE SHIELD**
V.A.C. System; **KINETIC CONCEPTS INC**
Vacutainer; **BECTON DICKINSON & CO**
Vagifem; **NOVO-NORDISK AS**
Vagus Nerve Stimulation Therapy System; **CYBERONICS INC**
Valley Drug Company; **DRUGMAX INC**
Valleylab; **TYCO HEALTHCARE GROUP**
Value Drug; **DUANE READE INC**
Varibar dysphagia line; **E-Z-EM INC**
VariLite; **IRIDEX CORP**
Varilux Ipseo; **ESSILOR INTERNATIONAL SA**
Vascu-Guard; **SYNOVIS LIFE TECHNOLOGIES INC**
VasoSeal; **DATASCOPE CORP**
Vasotec; **MERCK & CO INC**
VASOVIEW; **GUIDANT CORP**
Vbeam; **CANDELA CORP**
VBR; **OSTEOTECH INC**
VCA Animal Hospitals; **VCA ANTECH INC**
VELCADE; **MILLENNIUM PHARMACEUTICALS INC**
Venodyne; **MICROTEK MEDICAL HOLDINGS INC**
Ventiv Health Communications; **VENTIV HEALTH INC**
Ventiv Health Sales; **VENTIV HEALTH INC**
Ventiv Integrated Solutions; **VENTIV HEALTH INC**
Ventiv Valley Communications; **VENTIV HEALTH INC**
Veritus Medicare Services; **HIGHMARK INC**
Vermont Freedom Plan; **BLUE CROSS AND BLUE SHIELD OF VERMONT**
Vermont Health Partnership Plan; **BLUE CROSS AND BLUE SHIELD OF VERMONT**
Vermont Health Plan; **BLUE CROSS AND BLUE SHIELD OF VERMONT**
Veronis Suhler Stevenson Partners; **SOLUCIENT LLC**
VersArray; **BIO RAD LABORATORIES INC**
VersiTor; **ARTHROCARE CORP**
VerSys; **ZIMMER HOLDINGS INC**
VHA, Inc.; **SOLUCIENT LLC**
Via Christi Health System; **MARIAN HEALTH SYSTEMS**
ViaSpan; **BARR LABORATORIES INC**
Viral Antigens, Inc.; **MERIDIAN BIOSCIENCE INC**

ViroSeq; **APPLERA CORPORATION**
Visine; **PFIZER INC**
Vision; **GISH BIOMEDICAL INC**
VisionCare of California, Inc.; **EMERGING VISION INC**
VisionKey; **VISX INC**
VISTA BRITE TIP Guiding Catheter; **CORDIS CORP**
Vista Fertility Institute; **DYNACQ HEALTHCARE INC**
Vista Medical Center Hospital; **DYNACQ HEALTHCARE INC**
VISX STAR; **VISX INC**
VISX STAR S3; **VISX INC**
VISX University; **VISX INC**
VISXPRESS; **VISX INC**
VITALITY; **GUIDANT CORP**
VitalView; **CRITICARE SYSTEMS INC**
VNU N.V.; **SOLUCIENT LLC**
Voyager Biospectrometry Workstation; **APPLIED BIOSYSTEMS GROUP**
Vytra Health Plans; **HEALTH INSURANCE PLAN OF GREATER NEW YORK**
Walgreen Advance Care, Inc.; **WALGREEN CO**
Walgreen's Healthcare Plus, Inc.; **WALGREEN CO**
Walter Lorenz Surgical, Inc.; **BIOMET INC**
Walton Medical Center; **HEALTH MANAGEMENT ASSOCIATES INC**
Wampole; **INVERNESS MEDICAL INNOVATIONS INC**
Watchman; **SHL TELEMEDICINE**
Watson Laboratories, Inc.; **WATSON PHARMACEUTICALS INC**
Watson Pharma; **WATSON PHARMACEUTICALS INC**
Wavelight; **LASERSCOPE**
Wayne State University School of Medicine; **DETROIT MEDICAL CENTER**
WebMD Envoy; **WEBMD CORPORATION**
WebMD Health; **WEBMD CORPORATION**
WebMD Practice Services; **WEBMD CORPORATION**
Webster Veterinary Supply, Inc.; **PATTERSON COMPANIES INC**
Weighco Enterprises, Inc.; **WEIGHT WATCHERS INTERNATIONAL INC**
Weighco of Northwest, Inc.; **WEIGHT WATCHERS INTERNATIONAL INC**
Weighco of Southwest, Inc.; **WEIGHT WATCHERS INTERNATIONAL INC**
Weight Watchers Corporate Solutions; **WEIGHT WATCHERS INTERNATIONAL INC**

Weight Watchers eTools; **WEIGHT WATCHERS INTERNATIONAL INC**
Weight Watchers Online; **WEIGHT WATCHERS INTERNATIONAL INC**
WeightWatchers.com, Inc.; **WEIGHT WATCHERS INTERNATIONAL INC**
Wellbutrin XL; **BIOVAIL CORPORATION**
WellCare; **WELLCARE GROUP OF COMPANIES**
WellCare HMO, Inc.; **WELLCARE GROUP OF COMPANIES**
WellCare Management Group, Inc.; **WELLCARE GROUP OF COMPANIES**
WellCare of New York, Inc.; **WELLCARE GROUP OF COMPANIES**
WellChoice Insurance of New Jersey, Inc.; **WELLCHOICE INC**
WellPath; **COVENTRY HEALTH CARE INC**
WellPoint Health Networks; **BLUE CROSS OF CALIFORNIA**
WellPoint Health Networks, Inc.; **ANTHEM INC**
WellPoint Health Networks, Inc.; **BLUE CROSS AND BLUE SHIELD OF GEORGIA INC**
WellPoint Pharmacy Management; **WELLPOINT HEALTH NETWORKS INC**
Welsh, Carson, Anderson & Rowe; **AMERIPATH INC**
Welsh, Carson, Anderson and Stowe; **US ONCOLOGY INC**
West Central Ohio Health Partners; **CATHOLIC HEALTHCARE PARTNERS**
Westar RS; **WEST PHARMACEUTICAL SERVICES INC**
Western Biomedical Technologies; **RESPIRONICS INC**
Western Pennsylvania Caring Foundation; **HIGHMARK INC**
Whole Blood Flow Cytometry Control; **TECHNE CORP**
Whole Blood Glucose/Hemoglobin Control; **TECHNE CORP**
WHP Health Initiatives, Inc.; **WALGREEN CO**
William C. Conner Research Center; **ALCON INC**
WISDOM; **OWENS & MINOR INC**
Wittgensteiner Kliniken-WKA; **FRESENIUS AG**
Wm. Noah Allyn International Center; **WELCH ALLYN INC**
WorkHealth; **OHIOHEALTH CORPORATION**

INDEX OF SUBSIDIARIES, BRAND NAMES AND AFFILIATIONS, CONT.

WorldMed International, Inc.; **PSS WORLD MEDICAL INC**
WP Domus GmbH; **INVACARE CORP**
Wright Medical Technology; **WRIGHT MEDICAL GROUP INC**
www.gncgear.com; **GENERAL NUTRITION COMPANIES INC**
www.medicalmailorder.com; **NYER MEDICAL GROUP INC**
www.natalu.com; **PEDIATRIX MEDICAL GROUP INC**
www.physicianequipment.com; **NYER MEDICAL GROUP INC**
Wynwood; **ALTERRA HEALTHCARE CORP**
Wypall; **KIMBERLY CLARK CORP**
Xatral; **SANOFI-SYNTHELABO**
XCaliber; **ORTHOFIX INTERNATIONAL NV**
XenoLogiX; **EDWARDS LIFESCIENCES CORP**

Xolair; **GENENTECH INC**
XOPENEX; **SEPRACOR INC**
XUSA/XYZAL; **SEPRACOR INC**
YAGLAZR; **CANDELA CORP**
Yakima Medical Center; **HEALTH MANAGEMENT ASSOCIATES INC**
Yamanouchi Pharmaceutical Company; **FUJISAWA PHARMACEUTICALS COMPANY LTD**
Yasmin; **SCHERING AG**
Youthtrack; **RES CARE INC**
Zantac; **GLAXOSMITHKLINE PLC**
Zavesca; **CELLTECH GROUP PLC**
Zemaira; **ZLB BEHRING LLC**
Zentaris GmbH; **AETERNA ZENTARIS INC**
Zepharma, Inc.; **FUJISAWA PHARMACEUTICALS COMPANY LTD**
ZEUS; **INTUITIVE SURGICAL INC**

Zimmer Dental, Inc.; **CENTERPULSE AG**
Zimmer Holdings, Inc.; **CENTERPULSE AG**
Zippie; **SUNRISE MEDICAL INC**
Zithromax; **PFIZER INC**
zoasis.com; **VCA ANTECH INC**
Zocor; **MERCK & CO INC**
ZOLL Data Control Software; **ZOLL MEDICAL CORP**
ZOLL M Series; **ZOLL MEDICAL CORP**
Zoloft; **PFIZER INC**
Zonegran; **ELAN CORP PLC**
Zydis; **CARDINAL HEALTH INC**
Zydone; **ENDO PHARMACEUTICALS HOLDINGS INC**
ZYRTEC; **SEPRACOR INC**

Ref.
RA
410.53
.P137

0060146 6